Psychiatric Nursing

Contemporary Practice

SEVENTH EDITION

Mary Ann Boyd, PhD, DNS,
RN, PMHCNS-BC

Professor Emerita
Southern Illinois University Edwardsville
Edwardsville, Illinois

Rebecca Luebbert, PhD,
RN, PMHCNS-BC

Associate Professor
Department Chair, Primary Care & Health
 Systems Nursing
Southern Illinois University Edwardsville
Edwardsville, Illinois

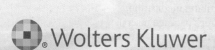 Wolters Kluwer

Philadelphia • Baltimore • New York • London
Buenos Aires • Hong Kong • Sydney • Tokyo

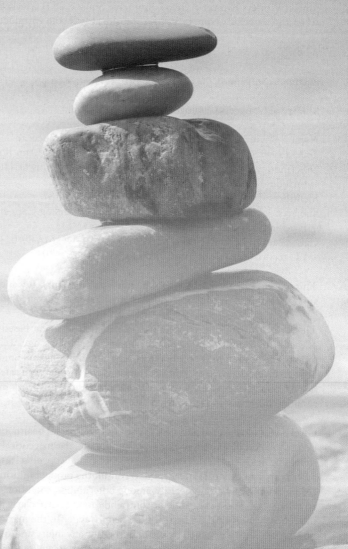

Vice President, Nursing Segment: Julie K. Stegman
Director, Nursing Education and Practice Content: Jamie Blum
Senior Development Editor: Julie M. Vitale
Editorial Coordinator: Vinodhini Varadharajalu
Editorial Assistant: Molly Kennedy
Marketing Manager: Brittany K. Riney
Production Project Manager: Barton Dudlick
Design Coordinator: Stephen Druding
Art Director: Jennifer Clements
Manufacturing Coordinator: Margie Orzech-Zeranko
Prepress Vendor: Lumina Datamatics

Seventh Edition

Copyright © 2022 Wolters Kluwer

9 8 7 6 5 4 3 2 1

Printed in Singapore

Library of Congress Cataloging-in-Publication Data

Names: Boyd, M. (Mary Ann), author. Luebbert, R. (Rebecca)
Title: Psychiatric Nursing: Contemporary Practice/Mary Ann Boyd & Rebecca Luebbert
Description: Seventh edition. | Philadelphia: Wolters Kluwer, [2022] |
   Includes bibliographical references.
Identifiers: LCCN 2017024303 | ISBN 9781975161187
Subjects: | MESH: Mental Disorders–nursing | Nursing Care–methods |
   Psychiatric Nursing–methods
Classification: LCC RC440 | NLM WY 160 | DDC 616.89/0231–dc23
   LC record available at https://lccn.loc.gov/2017024303

shop.LWW.com

MKO721

*To Jim with love and gratitude for your constant support and
sacrifice throughout this journey.*

MAB

*In loving memory of my mom, Linda. And to my dad, Joseph,
for his never-ending support and encouragement.*

RL

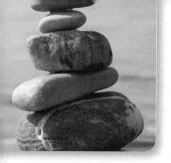

Contributors

Beverly Baliko, PhD, RN, PMHNP-BC
Associate Professor
College of Nursing
University of South Carolina
Columbia, South Carolina
Chapter 23: Mental Health Care for Survivors
of Violence

Andrea C. Bostrom, PhD, PMHCNS-BC
Professor, retired
Kirkhof College of Nursing at Grand Valley State University
Allendale, Michigan
Chapter 24: Schizophrenia and Related Disorders

Mary Ann Boyd, PhD, DNS, RN, PMHCNS-BC
Professor Emerita
Southern Illinois University Edwardsville
Edwardsville, Illinois

Jeanne Clement-Alvarez, EdD, MSN, RN, FAAN
Retired
The Ohio State University
Columbus, Ohio
Chapter 13: Cognitive Interventions in Psychiatric
Nursing

Sheri Compton-McBride, DNP, RN
Assistant Professor
Director of RN/BS Nursing Program and Contract
Management
Southern Illinois University Edwardsville – School of
Nursing
Edwardsville, Illinois
Chapter 34: Sleep–Wake Disorders

Dorothy M. Corrigan, D.Min., DNP(c), APRN,
BC-GNP, CARN-AP, C-GCS
CEO-The Knock Institute LLC
La Crosse Wisconsin
Chapter 43: Care of Persons Who Are Medically
Compromised

Susan Dawson, EdD, PMHNP-BC
Adult Psychiatric Nurse Practitioner
Adjunct Professor
Compassionate Healthcare
Maryville University
St. Louis, Missouri
Chapter 31: Addiction and Substance-Related Disorders

Catherine Gray Deering, PhD, RN
Professor
Clayton State University
Morrow, Georgia
Chapter 16: Mental Health Promotion for Children and
Adolescents

Cheryl Forchuk PhD, RN, O Ont, FCAHS
Beryl and Richard Ivey Research Chair in Aging, Mental
Health, Rehabilitation and Recovery
Lawson Health Research Institute
Parkwood Institute Research
Distinguished University Professor
Nursing and Psychiatry
Western University
London, Ontario, Canada
Chapter 10: Communication and the Therapeutic
Relationship

Patricia E. Freed, MSN, EdD
Associate Professor
Trudy Bush Valentine School of Nursing
Saint Louis University
St. Louis, Missouri
Chapter 1: Psychiatric-Mental Health Nursing and
Evidence-Based Practice
Chapter 28: Obsessive-Compulsive and Related
Disorders
Chapter 31: Addiction and Substance-Related Disorders

Kimberlee Hansen, MS, RN, CNS, NP
Nurse Practitioner
Jefferson Barracks Division
VA St. Louis Health Care System
St. Louis, Missouri
Chapter 30: Personality and Impulse-Control Disorders

Rebecca Luebbert, PhD, RN, PMHCNS-BC
Associate Professor
Department Chair, Primary Care & Health Systems
Nursing
Southern Illinois University Edwardsville
Edwardsville, Illinois

Kelley McGuire, PhD, CNE, RN
Assistant Professor
School of Nursing
Southern Illinois University Edwardsville
Edwardsville, Illinois
Chapter 19: Stress and Mental Health

Victoria Soltis-Jarrett, PhD, PMHCNS/NP-BC, FAANP, FAAN
Carol Morde Ross Distinguished Professor of
  Psychiatric-Mental Health Nursing
Family Psychiatric Nurse Practitioner
University of North Carolina at Chapel Hill
Chapel Hill, North Carolina
Chapter 33: Somatic Symptom and Dissociative
  Disorders

Sandra P. Thomas, PhD, RN, FAAN
Editor, "Issues in Mental Health Nursing"
Sara and Ross Croley Endowed Professor in Nursing
University of Tennessee, Knoxville
College of Nursing
Knoxville, Tennessee
Chapter 20: Management of Anger, Aggression, and
  Violence

Barbara Jones Warren, PhD, RN, PMHCNS-BC, FNAP, FAAN
Professor of Clinical Nursing
Director
Psychiatric Mental Health Nursing Across the Lifespan
  Specialty Track
NIH ANA Racial/Ethnic Minority Fellow
College of Nursing
The Ohio State University
Columbus, Ohio
Chapter 25: Depression

Valerie Yancey, PhD, RN
Associate Professor
School of Nursing
Southern Illinois University Edwardsville
Edwardsville, Illinois
Chapter 6: Ethics, Standards, and Nursing Frameworks

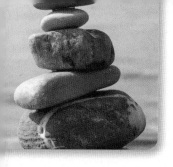

Reviewers

(Essentials of Psychiatric Nursing, Second Edition)

Pamela Adamshick, PhD, RN, PMHCNS-BC
Associate Professor
Nursing and Public Health Department
Moravian College
Bethlehem, Pennsylvania

Abbey Devers, RN, BSN
Psychiatric/Mental Health Nursing Instructor
Nursing Program
Iowa Central Community College
Fort Dodge, Iowa

Nancy Elkins, EdD, MSN, RN
Associate Professor
School of Nursing
Marshall University
Huntington, West Virginia

Mary Beth Hutches, DNP, RN
Chair, BSN Programs
Assistant Professor
School of Nursing
Aurora University
Aurora, Illinois

Sheila G. Jacobs, RN, MSN
Professor, BSN Program
School of Nursing
George Mason University
Fairfax, Virginia

Deborah Johnson, MSN, RN
Assistant Professor
Department of Nursing
Ivy Tech Community College
Columbus, Indiana

Karen Lillie, RN, BS, MS, FNPC, PMHNP
Lecturer, Undergraduate Program Director
Department of Nursing
California State University, Bakersfield
Bakersfield, California

Kathy T. Morris, EdD, MSN, RN
Assistant Professor
School of Nursing
Georgia Southern University—Armstrong Campus
Savannah, Georgia

Colleen M. Quinn, EdD, MSN, RN
Professor
Department of Nursing
Broward College
Fort Lauderdale, Florida

Robi Thomas, PhD, RN, PMHNP-BC
Associate Professor
McAuley School of Nursing
University of Detroit Mercy
Grand Rapids, Michigan

Maureen Vidrine, DNP, APRN-PMH, BC
Associate Professor
Mary Inez Grindle School of Nursing
Brenau University
Gainesville, Georgia

Pamela Worrell-Carlisle, RN, MA, CHPN, PhD
Assistant Professor
School of Nursing
Georgia Southern University
Statesboro, Georgia

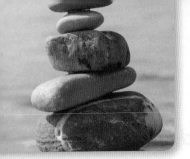

Preface

The impact of the coronavirus pandemic on mental health and well-being is felt worldwide. As most of the world focused on survival of the coronavirus, mental health needs were unattended. Now, we are faced with untreated mental disorders complicated by the mental health consequences of the pandemic. While the negative economic and social consequences of the pandemic are well-known, research is just emerging detailing the significant aftereffects to children, adults, families, and communities. Anxiety and contamination fears plague children as they return to schools. Depression, intimate partner violence, and anxiety are on the rise in the adult population. The pandemic accelerated economic inequality affecting underserved and low-income communities.

Virtual health care access was available to people in communities with internet access. Many rural communities did not have internet access. In-person health care was available for only emergency treatment with little access to prevention and treatment of chronic disorders. Since the pandemic is having such a world wide impact on mental health, COVID-19 discussions are woven throughout the chapters.

The primary purpose of this text is to prepare nurses to care for persons with mental health issues and problems. Mental disorders are recognized as one of the major burdens to society. These disorders contribute to high morbidity and mortality rates, as well as lost economic productivity. One in five persons will suffer a mental disorder in a lifetime. The duty of every nurse in all settings is to have the knowledge and skills to implement evidence-based practice for persons with mental disorders. As a result of the pandemic, it is more critical than ever that nurses are prepared to care for persons suffering from stress, depression, anxiety, and trauma.

The seventh edition of *Psychiatric Nursing: Contemporary Practice* evolved during the pandemic as virtual mental health care became the norm and mental health care providers were challenged to deliver innovative quality care in an electronic environment. As electronic access to mental health applications increased, it became obvious that nurses would be key players in the expansion of the delivery of mental health care. This text includes discussions and recommendations on the use of electronic platforms in nursing practice and their ethical implications.

The special needs and mental health issues of the lesbian, gay, bisexual, transgender, queer or questioning (LGBTQ) communities have long been ignored. Stigma-

tization and discrimination can prevent persons who identify as LGBTQ from accessing quality mental health care and, in turn, contribute to mental health problems. This text discusses the mental health needs and care of persons who identify as LGBTQ. Gender-neutral, bias-free language is used throughout the text.

Based on the request of several reviewers, a new chapter is included on the care of military veterans. This chapter discusses the relationship between the military experience and the health care needs of veterans. The mental health issues and disorders of veterans are explained within the context of their military experiences. There is also a discussion of the role of the Veterans Health Administration in providing mental health care to veterans.

TEXT ORGANIZATION

The first three units of *Psychiatric Nursing: Contemporary Practice, Seventh Edition* present the conceptual underpinnings and principles of psychiatric–mental health nursing. In Unit I, students are introduced to mental health nursing care in contemporary society as an evidenced-based practice. Students are introduced to stigma and recovery in Chapter 2, which sets the stage for a more detailed discussion of recovery in Chapter 9.

Unit II provides the theoretical foundations of psychiatric nursing including several nursing and recovery frameworks as well as biological and psychosocial theoretical underpinnings. Unit III is the essence of psychiatric–mental health nursing with a detailed discussion of the psychiatric–mental health nursing process including explanations of evidence-based interventions. Therapeutic communication skills, psychopharmacology, cognitive interventions, group interventions, and family assessment and interventions are presented in a clear and understandable language. This unit prepares the student for making clinical judgments and sound decisions in caring for patients.

Units IV and V present mental health promotion and prevention content, including comprehensive chapters on stress and mental health, crises, violence, and suicide prevention. Unit VI discusses the care of persons with mental disorders within a recovery-oriented, evidence-based practice.

Units VII and VIII focus on the assessment and care of children and older adults with mental disorders characteristic of each age group. Unit IX introduces the student to a new chapter, Care of Veterans with Mental Health Needs as well as caring for persons who are experiencing homelessness and co-occurring mental disorders. Chapter 43 addresses the care of persons with selected medical disorders that are typical of persons with mental disorders.

The text presents complex concepts in easy-to-understand language with multiple examples and explanations. Students find the text easy to comprehend, filled with meaningful information, and applicable to all areas of nursing practice.

PEDAGOGICAL FEATURES

The seventh edition of *Psychiatric Nursing: Contemporary Practice* incorporates a multitude of pedagogical features to focus and direct student learning, including the following:

By including evidence-based content from which students can draw valid inferences, students can develop clinical judgment and decision-making skills.

- **Expanded Table of Contents** allows readers to find and refer to concepts from one location.
- **Learning Objectives, Key Terms,** and **Key Concepts** in the chapter openers cue readers on what will be encountered and what is important to understand in each chapter.
- **Summary of Key Points** listed at the end of each chapter provides quick access to important chapter content to facilitate study and review.
- **Critical Thinking Challenges** ask questions that require students to think critically about chapter content and apply psychiatric nursing concepts to nursing practice.
- **Movie Viewing Guides** list current examples of movies that depict various mental health disorders and that are widely available. Viewing points are provided to serve as a basis for discussion in class and among students.

SPECIAL FEATURES

Case Studies threaded in the disorder chapters are related to the Nursing Care Plan and Therapeutic Dialogue features, giving students the opportunity to apply content. Cases will come from the Patient Experience Videos, to help tie content from the book to the videos. For chapters without a corresponding video, a new case study has been created. Exposure to patients builds student confidence and provides a seamless transition to the practice world.

- **Wellness Challenges** threaded in disorder chapters focus on keeping patients healthy and utilize case study "patient" information to apply the content.

- **Integration with Primary Care,** also threaded in disorder chapters and utilizing case study content, addresses integration of psychiatric disorders with basic health needs blended.
- **NCLEX Notes** help students focus on important application areas to prepare for the NCLEX.
- **Emergency Care Alerts** highlight important situations in psychiatric nursing care that the nurse should recognize as emergencies.
- **Research for Best Practice** boxes highlight today's focus on evidence-based practice for best practice, presenting findings and implications of studies that are applicable to psychiatric nursing practice.
- **Therapeutic Dialogue** boxes compare and contrast therapeutic and nontherapeutic conversations to encourage students by example to develop effective communication skills.
- **Psychoeducation Checklists** identify content areas for patient and family education related to specific disorders and their treatment. These checklists support critical thinking by encouraging students to develop patient-specific teaching plans based on chapter content.
- **Clinical Vignette** boxes present reality-based clinical portraits of patients who exhibit the symptoms described in the text. Questions are posed to help students express their thoughts and identify solutions to issues presented in the vignettes.
- **Medication Profile** boxes present a thorough picture of commonly prescribed medications for patients with mental health problems. The profiles complement the text discussions of biologic processes known to be associated with various mental health disorders.
- **Key Diagnostic Characteristics** summaries describe diagnostic criteria, target symptoms, and target associated findings for select disorders, adapted from the *DSM-5* by the American Psychiatric Associations.
- **Concept Mastery Alerts** clarify common misconceptions as identified by Lippincott's Adaptive Learning Powered by prepU.
- **Evidence-Based Nursing Practice of Persons with Selected Mental Health Disorders** sections provide an in-depth study of the more commonly occurring major psychiatric disorders.
- **Patient Education** 📖, **family** 🏠, **and emergency** 🚑 **icons** highlight content related to these topics to help link concepts to practice.

TEACHING/LEARNING PACKAGE

To facilitate mastery of this text's content, a comprehensive teaching and learning package has been developed to assist faculty and students.

Instructor Resources

Tools to assist you with teaching your course are available upon adoption of this text at http://thePoint.lww.com/Boyd7e

- **A Test Generator** lets you put together exclusive new tests from a bank containing hundreds of questions to help you in assessing your students' understanding of the material. Test questions link to chapter learning objectives.
- **PowerPoint Presentations** provide an easy way for you to integrate the textbook with your students' classroom experience, either via slide shows or handouts. Multiple-choice and true/false questions are integrated into the presentations to promote class participation and allow you to use i-clicker technology.
- **An Image Bank** lets you use the photographs and illustrations from this textbook in your PowerPoint slides or as you see fit in your course.
- **Case Studies** with related questions (and suggested answers) give students an opportunity to apply their knowledge to a client case similar to one they might encounter in practice.
- **Pre-Lecture Quizzes** (and answers) are quick, knowledge-based assessments that allow you to check students' reading.
- **Guided Lecture Notes** walk you through the chapters, objective by objective.
- **Discussion Topics** (and suggested answers) can be used as conversation starters or in online discussion boards.
- **Plus Assignments, Lesson Plans, QSEN Competency Maps, Strategies for Effective Teaching,** and **Syllabi.**

Student Resources

An exciting set of free resources is available to help students review material and become even more familiar with vital concepts. Students can access all these resources at http://thePoint.lww.com/Boyd6e using the codes printed in the front of their textbooks.

- **NCLEX-Style Review Questions** for each chapter help students review important concepts and practice for the NCLEX.
- **Watch & Learn Videos,** *Lippincott Theory to Practice Video Series: Psychiatric–Mental Health Nursing,* includes videos of true-to-life patients displaying mental health disorders, allowing students to gain experience and a deeper understanding of mental health patients.

- **Journal Articles** provided for each chapter offer access to current research available in Wolters Kluwer journals.
- **Movie Viewing Guides** list current examples of movies that depict various mental health disorders and that are widely available. Viewing points are provided to serve as a basis for discussion in class and among students.

A FULLY INTEGRATED COURSE EXPERIENCE

We are pleased to offer an expanded suite of digital solutions and ancillaries to support instructors and students using *Psychiatric Nursing: Contemporary Practice,* Seventh Edition. To learn more about any solution, please contact your local Wolters Kluwer representative.

Lippincott CoursePoint+

The same trusted solution, innovation and unmatched support that you have come to expect from *Lippincott CoursePoint+* is now enhanced with more engaging learning tools and deeper analytics to help prepare students for practice. This powerfully integrated, digital learning solution combines learning tools, case studies, virtual simulation, real-time data, and the most trusted nursing education content on the market to make curriculum-wide learning more efficient and to meet students where they're at in their learning. And now, it's easier than ever for instructors and students to use, giving them everything they need for course and curriculum success!

Lippincott CoursePoint+ includes the following:

- Engaging course content provides a variety of learning tools to engage students of all learning styles.
- A more personalized learning approach, including adaptive learning powered by PrepU, gives students the content and tools they need at the moment they need it, giving them data for more focused remediation and helping to boost their confidence.
- Varying levels of case studies, virtual simulation, and access to Lippincott Advisor help students learn the critical thinking and clinical judgment skills to help them become practice-ready nurses.
- Unparalleled reporting provides in-depth dashboards with several data points to track student progress and help identify strengths and weaknesses.
- Unmatched support includes training coaches, product trainers, and nursing education consultants to help educators and students implement CoursePoint with ease.

vSim for Nursing

vSim for Nursing, jointly developed by Laerdal Medical and Wolters Kluwer Health, offers innovative scenario-based learning modules consisting of web-based virtual simulations, course learning materials, and curriculum tools designed to develop critical thinking skills and promote clinical confidence and competence. vSim for Nursing | Mental Health includes 10 mental health scenarios authored by the National League for Nursing. Students can progress through suggested readings, pre- and post-simulation assessments, documentation assignments, and guided reflection questions, and will receive an individualized feedback log immediately upon completion of the simulation. Throughout the student learning experience, the product offers remediation back to trusted Lippincott resources, including Lippincott Nursing Advisor and Lippincott Nursing Procedures—two online, evidence-based, clinical information solutions used in healthcare facilities throughout the United States. This innovative product provides a comprehensive patient-focused solution for learning and integrating simulation into the classroom.

Contact your Wolters Kluwer sales representative or visit http://thepoint.lww.com/vsim for options to enhance your mental health nursing course with vSim for Nursing.

Lippincott DocuCare

Lippincott DocuCare combines web-based academic electronic health record (EHR) simulation software with clinical case scenarios, allowing students to learn how to use an EHR in a safe, true-to-life setting, while enabling instructors to measure their progress. Lippincott DocuCare's nonlinear solution works well in the classroom, simulation lab, and clinical practice.

Contact your Wolters Kluwer sales representative or visit http://thepoint.lww.com/DocuCare for options to enhance your mental health nursing course with DocuCare.

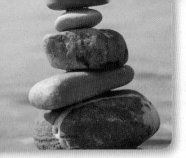

Acknowledgments

This text is a result of many long hours of diligent work by the contributors, editors, and assistants. Psychiatric nurses are constantly writing about and discussing new strategies for caring for persons with mental disorders. Consumers of mental health services provided directions for nursing care and validated the importance of nursing interventions. I wish to acknowledge and thank these individuals.

Jamie Blum and Julie Vitale of Wolters Kluwer were extraordinary partners in this project. I want to especially acknowledge their attention to detail and their commitment to excellence. They provided direction, support, and valuable input throughout this project. They were extraordinary partners during revision of this update. They brought a broad knowledge base and extreme patience during the whole update process. I want to thank Ann Francis for the organizational skills that kept the project on target. This text would not be possible without Indu Jawwad and the highly committed team of Lumina Datamatics.

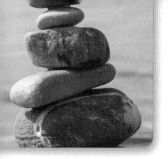

Contents

UNIT VII   CARE OF CHILDREN AND ADOLESCENTS 695

UNIT VIII   CARE OF OLDER ADULTS 745

UNIT IX   CARE OF SPECIAL POPULATIONS 785

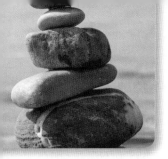

Case Studies in This Book

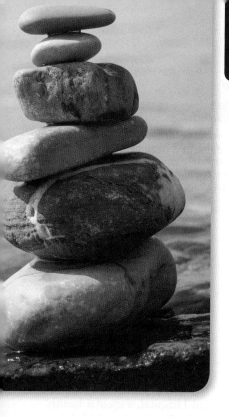

UNIT I

Mental Health Care in Contemporary Society

1

Psychiatric–Mental Health Nursing and Evidence-Based Practice

Patricia E. Freed and Mary Ann Boyd

KEYCONCEPTS

- evidence-based practice
- psychiatric–mental health nursing

LEARNING OBJECTIVES

After studying this chapter, you will be able to:

1. Identify the dynamic scope of psychiatric–mental health nursing practice.

2. Relate the history of psychiatric–mental health nursing to contemporary nursing practice.

3. Discuss the importance of evidence-based psychiatric–mental health nursing practice in all health care settings.

4. Outline the evolution of recovery in mental health care.

5. Discuss the impact of recent legislative and policy changes in the delivery of mental health evidence.

KEY TERMS

- Asylum • Deinstitutionalization • Institutionalization • Moral treatment • Neurosis • Psychoanalysis • Psychosis

INTRODUCTION

Everyone experiences emotional and mental health issues at some time in their lives. During periods of illness and stress, mental health issues often become overwhelming to individuals and their families. Every nurse provides mental health interventions, no matter the practice site. Nurses in acute care settings are likely to care for persons in mental health crises because medical problems are treated before any mental health issues (e.g., physical injuries from a suicide attempt are treated before the underlying depression). Like anyone else,

people with psychiatric disorders seek health care for their medical illnesses. The stress of the medical illness can also exacerbate psychiatric symptoms.

Psychiatric nurses care for patients with a wide range of emotional problems and mental disorders (Box 1.1). These nurses, specializing in mental health nursing, are experts in caring not only for persons with a primary diagnosis of a mental disorder but also for those with self-concept and body image issues, developmental crises, co-occurring disorders, end-of-life changes, and emotional stress related to illness, disability, or loss. It is a psychiatric nurse who is called when violence, suicide, or a disaster erupts. In this

---

BOX 1.1

Psychiatric–Mental Health Nursing Phenomena of Concern

Phenomena of concern for psychiatric–mental health nurses are dynamic, exist in all populations across the life span, and include but are not limited to the following:
- Promotion of optimal mental and physical health and well-being
- Prevention of mental and behavioral distress and illness
- Promotion of social inclusion of mentally and behaviorally fragile individuals
- Co-occurring mental health and substance use disorders
- Co-occurring mental health and physical disorders
- Alterations in thinking, perceiving, communicating, and functioning related to psychological and physiologic distress
- Psychological and physiologic distress resulting from physical, interpersonal, and/or environmental trauma or neglect

- Psychogenesis and individual vulnerability
- Complex clinical presentations confounded by poverty and poor, inconsistent, or toxic environmental factors
- Alterations in self-concept related to loss of physical organs and/or limbs, psychic trauma, developmental conflicts, or injury
- Individual, family, or group isolation and difficulty with interpersonal relations
- Self-harm and self-destructive behaviors including mutilation and suicide
- Violent behavior including physical abuse, sexual abuse, and bullying
- Low health literacy rates contributing to treatment nonadherence

---

text, the terms *psychiatric nursing* and *psychiatric–mental health nursing* are used interchangeably. The standards of practice are discussed in Chapter 6.

> **KEYCONCEPT** Grounded in nursing theories, **psychiatric–mental health nursing** is defined as the "nursing practice specialty committed to promoting mental health through the assessment, diagnosis, and treatment of behavioral problems, mental disorders, and comorbid conditions across the life span. Psychiatric–mental health nursing intervention is an art and a science, employing purposeful use of self and a wide range of nursing, psychosocial, and neurobiological evidence to produce effective outcomes" (American Nurses Association, American Psychiatric Nurses Association, & International Society of Psychiatric–Mental Health Nurses, 2014, p. 1).

THE PAST AND PRESENT

Psychiatric nursing has a history that can be traced back to the early days of nursing practice. Today, the specialty has developed into one of the core mental health professions with an emphasis on evidence-based practice.

Early Founders

The roots of contemporary psychiatric–mental health nursing can be traced to Florence Nightingale's holistic view of a patient who lives within a family and community. She was especially sensitive to human emotions and recommended interactions that today would be classified as therapeutic communication (see Chapter 10). For example, this early nursing leader's intervention for reducing anxiety about an illness was to encourage independence and self-care (Nightingale, 1859).

Linda Richards, the first trained nurse in the United States, opened the Boston City Hospital Training School for Nurses in 1882 at McLean Hospital, a mental health facility (Box 1.2) (Cowles, 1887). Employees of McLean were recruited into the nursing program to learn to provide physical care for patients with mental disorders who developed medical illnesses. In 1913, Effie Taylor integrated psychiatric nursing content into the curriculum at Johns Hopkins' Phipps Clinic. Taylor, like Nightingale before her, encouraged nurses to avoid the dichotomy of mind and body (Church, 1987). The first psychiatric nursing textbook, *Nursing Mental Disease*, was written by Harriet Bailey in 1920 (Bailey, 1920). Gradually, nursing education programs in psychiatric hospitals were phased into mainstream nursing education programs.

Emergence of Modern Nursing Perspectives

As psychiatric–mental health nursing developed as a profession in the 20th century, modern perspectives of mental illness emerged, and these new theories profoundly shaped mental health care (see Units II and III). In 1952, Hildegard E. Peplau published the landmark work *Interpersonal Relations in Nursing* (Peplau, 1952). This publication introduced psychiatric–mental health nursing practice to the concepts of interpersonal relations and the therapeutic relationship. Peplau conceptualized nursing practice as independent of physicians. The use of self as a nursing tool was outside the dominance of both hospital administrators and physicians.

Peplau also contributed to educational programs for psychiatric nursing, developing a specialty training program in psychiatric nursing—the first graduate nursing program—in 1954 at Rutgers University. Subspecialties began to emerge, focusing on children, adolescents, and older adults.

In 1967, the Division of Psychiatric and Mental Health Nursing Practice of the ANA published the first

BOX 1.2

History of Psychiatric–Mental Health Nursing

1882 First training school for psychiatric nursing at McLean Asylum by E. Cowles; first nursing program to admit men

1913 First nurse-organized program of study for psychiatric training by Euphemia (Effie) Jane Taylor at Johns Hopkins Phipps Clinic

1914 Mary Adelaide Nutting emphasized nursing role development

1920 First psychiatric nursing text published, *Nursing Mental Disease,* by Harriet Bailey

1950 Accredited schools required to offer a psychiatric nursing experience

1952 Publication of Hildegard E. Peplau's *Interpersonal Relations in Nursing*

1954 First graduate program in psychiatric nursing established at Rutgers University by Hildegard E. Peplau

1963 *Perspectives in Psychiatric Care and Journal of Psychiatric Nursing* published

1967 *Standards of Psychiatric–Mental Health Nursing Practice* published; American Nurses Association (ANA) initiated the certification of generalists in psychiatric–mental health nursing

1979 *Issues in Mental Health Nursing* published; ANA initiated the certification of specialists in psychiatric–mental health nursing

1980 *Nursing: A Social Policy Statement* published by the ANA

1982 *Revised Standards of Psychiatric and Mental Health Nursing Practice* issued by the ANA

1985 *Standards of Child and Adolescent Psychiatric and Mental Health Nursing Practice* published by the ANA

1987 *Archives of Psychiatric Nursing and Journal of Child and Adolescent Psychiatric and Mental Health Nursing* published

1994 *Statement on Psychiatric–Mental Health Clinical Nursing Practice and Standards of Psychiatric–Mental Health Clinical Nursing Practice* published

1996 Guidelines specifying course content and competencies published by the Society for Education and Research in Psychiatric–Mental Health Nursing

2000 *Scope and Standards of Psychiatric–Mental Health Nursing Practice* published

2003 A second advanced practice role, Psychiatric–Mental Health Nurse Practitioner, was delineated

2014 *Psychiatric–Mental Health Nursing: Scope and Standards of Practice* was revised to reflect the expanding role of psychiatric–mental health nurses practicing in a recovery-oriented environment.

Statement on Psychiatric Nursing Practice. This publication was the first official sanction of a holistic approach of psychiatric–mental health nurses practicing in a variety of settings with a diverse clientele, emphasizing health promotion as well as health restoration. Since 1967, there have been several updates of the official practice statement that reflect the expansion of the role of psychiatric nurses with a delineation of functions.

Over the past century, psychiatric nursing practice expanded from the hospital to the community. Today in the United States, many nursing graduate degree programs offer specializations in psychiatric–mental health. Psychiatric nurses sit on corporate boards; serve in the armed forces; lead major health care initiatives; teach in major universities; and care for young and old people, families, and disadvantaged and homeless individuals. Psychiatric nursing is truly a versatile and rewarding field of nursing practice (Fig. 1.1).

Evidence-Based Practice and Current Psychiatric Nursing

Evidence-based practice is the standard of care in psychiatric nursing and mental health care. Clinical decisions that lead to high-quality patient outcomes are based on

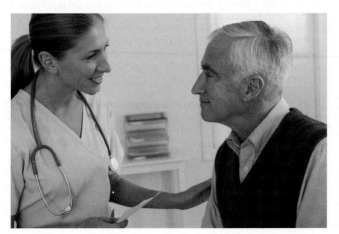
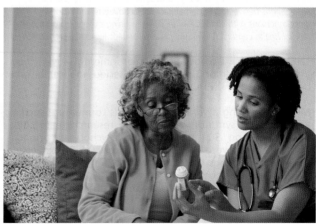

FIGURE 1.1 Contemporary psychiatric–mental health nursing is a versatile and rewarding field of practice.

research and evidence-based theories, clinical expertise, and patient preferences and values. By combining data from various sources such as expert opinion, patient data, and clinical experiences, the nurse is able to be objective, yet open to new ideas. For example, using epidemiologic data alerts nurses to the increase in suicide rates among young men, that experts were predicting it, but that whether the trend continues or the factors behind it remains unknown.

> **KEYCONCEPT Evidence-based practice** is a lifelong problem-solving approach to clinical practice that integrates
> • a systematic search for and critical appraisal of the most relevant and best research (i.e., external evidence) to answer a burning clinical question;
> • one's own clinical expertise, including use of internal evidence generated from outcomes management or evidence-based quality improvement projects, a thorough patient assessment, and evaluation and use of available resources necessary to achieve desired patient outcomes (Melnyk & Fineout-Overholt, 2021, p. 8).

In an evidence-based approach, clinical questions are defined; evidence is discovered and analyzed; the research findings are applied in a practical manner and in collaboration with the patient; and outcomes are evaluated. One of the first steps is seeking out a mentor who can help through the evidence-based process because this approach requires using literature search skills, followed by careful reading and critiquing of the current studies and seeking the advice of experts in the field. A nurse might start with a clinical question, such as "Do social and environmental adversities effect recovery among persons with serious mental illness being treated in community mental health centers?"

The nurse and mentor will narrow the question and begin a critique of the literature. Even though the process results in directions for practice, the nurse will face many challenges. See Box 1.3.

EVOLUTION OF MENTAL HEALTH RECOVERY

Throughout history, popular beliefs of the time served as the basis for understanding and treating people with mental illnesses. Prehistoric healers practiced an ancient surgical technique of removing a disk of bone from the skull to let out the evil spirits. In the early Christian period (1–100 CE), when sin or demonic possession was thought to cause mental disorders, clergymen treated patients, often through prescribed exorcisms. If such measures did not succeed, patients were excluded from the community and sometimes even put to death. Later in the medieval era (1000–1300 CE), contaminated environments were believed to cause *mental illness*. Consequently, individuals were removed from their "sick" environments and placed in protected **asylums**. Table 1.1 provides a summary of historical events and correlating perspectives on mental health during the premoral treatment era (800 CE to the colonial period).

Moral Treatment and Asylums

As evidence mounted that insanity was an illness and recovery was a possibility, existing primitive physical treatments, such as venesections (bloodletting) and gyrations (strapping patients to a rotating board), began to be

---

BOX 1.3

Research for Best Practice: Associations between Two Domains of Social Adversity and Recovery among Persons with Serious Mental Illnesses Being Treated in Community Mental Health Centers.

Compton, M. T., Bakeman, R., Capulong, L., Pauselli, L., Alolayan, Y., Drisafio, A., King, K., Reed, T., Broussard, B., & Shim, R. (2020). Associations between two domains of social adversity and recovery among persons with serious mental illnesses being treated in community mental health centers. Community Mental Health Journal, 56(1), 22–31.

THE QUESTION: Do social and environmental adversities affect recovery among persons with serious mental illness being treated in CMHCs?

METHODS: Using a variety of methods to measure social adversity and symptom severity, the research team collected data on 300 persons with psychosis or mood disorders who were receiving treatment at five diverse community settings. After controlling for the effects of gender and diagnostic categories, statistical exploratory methods were applied to explain the relationships among a large number of variables.

FINDINGS: Social and economic adversities and home environment adversities jointly accounted for 3.4% of the variance in recovery. Symptom severity had a partial influence on social and economic adversities and a substantial influence on home environment adversities. The researchers concluded that recovery in persons with serious mental illness is influenced by their social and environmental circumstances as well as their symptoms.

IMPLICATIONS FOR NURSING: These findings validate the relationship between recovery and the determinants of mental health, highlighting the need for referrals to community services, and helping nurses realize that their advocacy obligations need to address social policies and programs directed at adversities that negatively impact recovery. The challenge will be in securing change as resources for helping vulnerable populations are targeted for reduction or elimination.

TABLE 1.1	PREMORAL TREATMENT ERA	
Period	Beliefs About *Mental Illness*	Mental Health Care
Ancient times to 800 BCE	Sickness was an indication of the displeasure of deities for sins; viewed as supernatural.	Persons with psychiatric symptoms were driven from homes and ostracized by relatives. When behavioral manifestations were viewed as supernatural powers, the persons who exhibited them were revered.
Periods of inquiry: 800 BCE to 1 CE	Egypt and Greek periods of inquiry. Physical and mental health were viewed as interrelated. Hippocrates argued abnormal behaviors were due to brain disturbances. Aristotle related mental disorders to physical disorders.	Counseling, work, and music were provided in temples by priests to relieve the distress of those with mental disorders. Observation and documentation were a part of the care. The mental disorders were treated as diseases. The aim of treatment was to correct imbalances.
Early Christian and early medieval: 1–1000 CE	Power of Christian church grew. St. Augustine pronounced all diseases were ascribed to demons.	Persons with psychiatric symptoms were incarcerated in dungeons, beaten, and starved.
Later medieval: 1000–1300	In Western Europe, spirit of inquiry was dead. Healing was taken over by theologians and witch doctors. Persons with psychiatric symptoms were incarcerated in dungeons, beaten, and starved. In the Middle East, Avicenna said mental disorders are illnesses.	First asylums were built by Muslims. Persons with psychiatric symptoms were treated as being sick.
Renaissance: 1300–1600	In England, insane were differentiated from criminal. In colonies, mental illnesses were believed to be caused by demonic possession. Witch hunts were common.	Persons with psychiatric symptoms who presented a threat to society were apprehended and locked up. There were no public provisions for persons with mental disorders except jail. Private hospitalization for the wealthy who could pay. Bethlehem Asylum was used as a private institution.
Colonial: 1700–1790	1751: Benjamin Franklin established Pennsylvania Hospital (in Philadelphia)—the first institution in United States to receive those with mental disorders for treatment and cure. 1773: First public, freestanding asylum at Williamsburg, Virginia. 1783: Benjamin Rush categorized mental illnesses and began to treat mental disorders with medical interventions, such as bloodletting, mechanical devices.	The beginnings of mental diseases were viewed as illness to be treated.

From U.S. National Library of Medicine. Images from the history of medicine. National Institutes of Health, Department of Health and Human Services. http://resource.nlm.gov/10139406; http://resource.nlm.nih.gov/101436673

viewed as either painful or barbaric (Fig. 1.2). With science not advanced enough to offer reasonable treatment approaches, a safe haven, or **asylum**, was considered the best option for treatment. In the moral treatment period (1790–1900), **moral treatment**, that is, the use of kindness, compassion, and a pleasant environment, was adopted. Individuals with mental disorders were routinely removed from their communities and placed in asylums, which were thought to be best for their safety and comfort (Fig. 1.3).

Despite the good intentions that may have been at the root of the moral treatment movement, within the asylums, patients were often treated inhumanely. A turning point occurred at Bicêtre, a men's hospital in France that had the distinction of being the worst asylum in the world, when physician Philippe Pinel (1745–1826) ordered the removal of the chains, stopped the abuses of drugging and bloodletting, and placed the patients under the care of physicians. Three years later, the same standards were extended to Salpêtrière, the asylum for female patients.

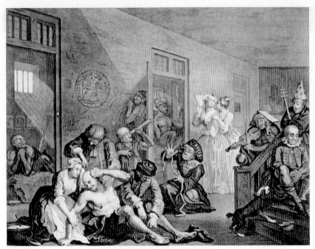

FIGURE 1.2 Interior of Bethlehem Asylum, London. (William Hogarth, 1697–1765. The Rake's Progress: Scene in Bedlam.) (From U.S. National Library of Medicine. Images from the history of medicine. Washington, DC: National Institutes of Health, Department of Health and Human Services. http://resource.nlm.nih.gov/101394076)

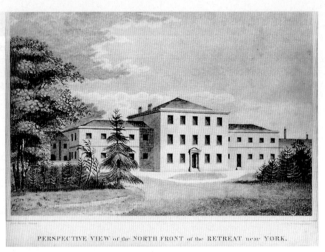

FIGURE 1.4 The perspective view of the north front of the retreat near York Samuel Tuke, 1784–1857 (1813). (From U.S. National Library of Medicine. Images from the history of medicine. National Institutes of Health, Department of Health and Human Services. http://resource.nlm.nih.gov/101436033)

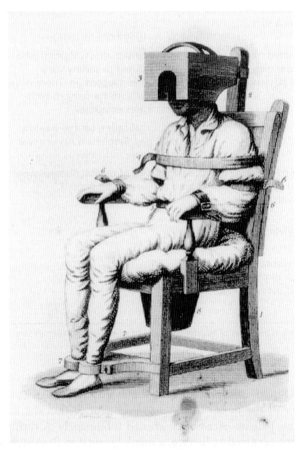

FIGURE 1.3 The Tranquilizer Chair of Benjamin Rush. A patient is sitting in a chair, his body immobilized, a bucket attached beneath the seat. (Benjamin Rush, 1746–1813. [1811]). (From U.S. National Library of Medicine. Images from the history of medicine. Washington, DC: National Institutes of Health, Department of Health and Human Services. http://resource.nlm.nih.gov/101436673)

At about the same time in England, William Tuke (1732–1822), a member of the Society of Friends, raised funds for a retreat for members who had mental disorders. The York Retreat was opened in 1796; restraints were abandoned, and sympathetic care in quiet, pleasant surroundings with some form of industrial occupation, such as weaving or farming, was provided (Fig. 1.4).

In the United States, the Quakers were instrumental in stopping the practice of bloodletting; they also placed great emphasis on providing a proper religious atmosphere (Deutsch, 1949). The Quaker Friends Asylum was proposed in 1811 and opened 6 years later in Frankford, Pennsylvania (now Philadelphia), to become the second asylum in the United States. The humane and supportive rehabilitative attitude of the Quakers was seen as an extremely important influence in changing techniques of caring for those with mental disorders. As states were founded, new hospitals were opened that were dedicated to the care of patients with mental disorders.

Even with these hospitals, only a fraction of people with mental disorders received treatment. Those who were judged dangerous were hospitalized; those deemed harmless or mildly insane were treated the same as other indigents and given no public support. In farm communities, as was the custom during the first half of the 19th century, poor and indigent individuals were often auctioned and bought by landowners to provide cheap labor. Landowners eagerly sought them for their strong backs and weak minds. The arrangement had its own economic usefulness because it provided the community with a low-cost way to care for people with mental illness. Some states used almshouses (poorhouses) for housing mentally ill individuals.

Public Funding, Dorothea Dix, and State Hospitals

Hospitals for individuals with mental illness were few because of financing; there were no funding mechanisms to support these large institutions. The first step in resolving the funding problem was defining responsibility—that is, which agency would be responsible for paying for care. In 1828, Horace Mann, a representative in the Massachusetts state legislature, saw his plea that the "insane are wards of the state" become a reality. State governments were mandated to assume financial responsibility for the care of people with mental illnesses (Beers, 1908).

After states were designated as being financially responsible for the treatment of their residents with mental illnesses, the next step was ensuring that each state appropriated funds. Dorothea Lynde Dix (1802–1887), a vigorous crusader for the humane treatment of patients with mental illness, was responsible for much of the reform of the mental health care system in the 19th century. Her solution was state hospitals. She first influenced the Massachusetts legislature to expand the Massachusetts State Hospital. Then, through public awareness campaigns and lobbying efforts, she managed to convince state after state to build hospitals. At the end of Dix's long career, 20 states had responded directly to her appeals by establishing or enlarging state hospitals (Box 1.4).

Institutionalization and Its Outcomes

In state hospitals, **institutionalization**, the forced confinement of individuals for long periods of time in large facilities, became the primary treatment for more than 50 years (1900–1955). Institutions had little more to offer than food, clothing, pleasant surroundings, and perhaps some means of employment and exercise. Outcomes of institutionalization were consistently negative. Thousands of people were warehoused within the walls of institutions for months and years with little hope of reentering society. Patients were socially isolated from their families and normal community life. The medical superintendent's major concern was the day-to-day operation of the large, aging physical structures. Untrained attendants who had little understanding of mental illnesses were responsible for the care, which was often cruel and inhumane. There were few educated nurses. Patients suffered adverse physical and psychological effects. There were few trained mental health providers. Early institutions eventually evolved into self-contained communities that produced their own food and made their own clothing. Institutionalization was a dismal failure.

BOX 1.4
Dorothea Lynde Dix

At nearly 40 years of age, Dorothea Dix, a retired school teacher living in Massachusetts, was solicited by a young theology student to help in preparing a Sunday school class for women inmates at the East Cambridge Jail. Dix led the class herself and was shocked by the filth and dirt in the jail. She was particularly struck by the treatment of inmates with mental disorders. It was the dead of winter, and no heat was provided. When she questioned the jailer about the lack of heat, his answer was that "the insane need no heat." The prevailing myth was that people with mental illnesses were insensible to extremes of temperature. Dix's outrage initiated a long struggle in the reform of care.

An early feminist, Dix disregarded the New England role of a Puritan woman and diligently investigated the conditions of jails and the plight of the mentally ill. During the Civil War, she was appointed to the post of Superintendent of Women Nurses, the highest position held by a woman during the war.

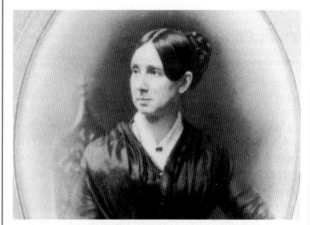

Dorothea Lynde Dix.

From U.S. National Library of Medicine. Images from the history of medicine. National Institutes of Health, Department of Health and Human Services. http://resource.nlm.nih.gov/101413738.

Women had a particularly difficult time and often were institutionalized at the convenience of their fathers or husbands. Because a woman's role in the late 1800s was to function as a domestic extension of her husband, any behaviors or beliefs that did not conform to male expectations could be used to justify the claim of insanity. Women were literally held prisoner for years. In the asylums, women were psychologically degraded, used as servants, and physically tortured by male physicians and female attendants (Bly, 1887).

The relatively primitive and often misguided biologic treatments were unsuccessful. For example, the use of hydrotherapy, or baths, was an established procedure in mental institutions. Warm baths and, in some instances, ice cold baths produced calming effects for patients with mental disorders. However, this treatment's success was attributed to the restraint of patients during the bath rather than the physiologic responses that hydrotherapy produced. Baths were then applied indiscriminately and used as a form of restraint rather than a therapeutic practice.

Clifford Beers (1876–1943) recovered from a mental disorder, became an advocate of humane treatment, and published an autobiography, *A Mind That Found Itself* (1908), depicting his 3-year hospitalization experience in the 18th century. He was beaten; choked; imprisoned for long periods in dark, dank, padded cells; and confined for many days in a straightjacket. By 1909, Beers formed a National Committee for Mental Hygiene. Through the committee's advocacy efforts, other mental health services were initiated, such as child guidance clinics, prison clinics, and industrial mental health care.

Freud's Contribution

At the same time that the institutionalization movement was gaining strength, Sigmund Freud (1856–1939) and the psychoanalytic movement of the early 1900s exerted influence on the mental health community. Freud, trained as a neuropathologist, developed a personality theory based on unconscious motivations for behavior or drives. According to the Freudian model, normal development occurred in stages, with the first three—oral, anal, and genital—being the most important. Infants progressed through the oral stage, experiencing the world through symbolic oral ingestion; through the anal stage, in which toddlers develop a sense of autonomy through withholding; and on to the genital stage, in which a beginning sense of sexuality emerges within the framework of the oedipal relationship. If there was any interference in normal development, such as psychological trauma, psychosis or neurosis would develop (Freud, 1905).

Freud and his followers believed the primary causes of mental illnesses were psychological and a result of disturbed personality development and faulty parenting (Freud, 1927). Mental illnesses were categorized either as a **psychosis** (severe) or as a **neurosis** (less severe). A psychosis impaired daily functioning because of breaks in contact with reality. A neurosis was less severe, but individuals were often distressed about their problems. Soon, Freud's ideas represented the forefront of psychiatric thought and began to shape society's view of mental health care. Freudian ideology dominated psychiatric thought well into the 1970s.

Intensive **psychoanalysis**, therapy that focused on repairing the trauma of the original psychological injury, was the Freudian treatment of choice. However, psychoanalysis was costly and time-consuming and required lengthy training. Few could perform it. Thousands of patients in state institutions with severe mental illnesses were essentially ignored.

Freud's view of mental illness as a psychological disorder gained credibility. He was a prolific writer who reported that his patients improved through psychoanalysis and interpretation of dreams (Freud, 1900). His outcomes were not judged by contemporary standards or subjected to meta-analysis processes. Today, psychoanalysis remains as a treatment option for a select group of patients who have the cognitive abilities to discuss and understand complex psychological concepts.

National Action

During World War II (1939–1945), mental illness was beginning to be seen as a problem that could happen to anyone. Many "normal" people who volunteered for the armed services were disqualified on the grounds that they were psychologically unfit to serve. Others who had already served tours of duty developed psychiatric and emotional problems related to their wartime experiences. Today, these problems are recognized as a distinct disorder: posttraumatic stress disorder (see Chapter 29).

In 1946, the National Mental Health Act created a six-member National Mental Health Advisory Council that established the National Institute of Mental Health, which was responsible for overseeing and coordinating research and training. Under the Act's provisions, the federal government also provided grants to states to support existing outpatient facilities and programs to establish new ones. Before 1948, more than half of all states had no clinics; by 1949, all but five had one or more. Six years later, there were 1,234 outpatient clinics. During the same time period, the Hill–Burton Act provided substantial federal support for hospital construction, which expanded the number of psychiatric units in general hospitals.

Impact of Psychopharmacology

Psychopharmacology revolutionized the treatment of people with mental illness. Initially, barbiturates, particularly amobarbital sodium (Amytal sodium), were tried for treating mental diseases in the 1930s (Malamud, 1944). When chlorpromazine was introduced in the 1950s, the mental health community was rather hopeful that a medication had been discovered to cure severe mental illness. In reality, the phenothiazines were the first of many antipsychotics to be developed (see Chapter 12). The medications calmed the patients and reduced some of the symptoms. With calmer patients and fewer symptoms, the negative effects of living in a restrictive and coercive institutional environment became evident.

A New National Objective: Community Treatment

In 1961, *Action for Mental Health*, a report of the Joint Commission on Mental Illness and Health Commission, called for larger investments in basic research; national personnel recruitment and training programs; one full-time clinic for every 50,000 individuals supplemented by general hospital units and state-run regional intensive psychiatric treatment centers; and access to emergency care and treatment in general, both in mental hospitals and in community clinics. The funding for the construction and operation of the community mental health system would be shared by federal, state, and local governments. The ideas expressed in the report clearly shifted authority for mental health programming to the federal government and were the basis of the federal legislation, the Mental Retardation Facilities and Community Mental Health Centers Construction Act, signed into law by John F. Kennedy in 1963. Unfortunately, this Act funded only some of the approaches proposed by the Commission and did not support the operation of state-run regional intensive psychiatric centers.

The supporters of this 1963 legislation believed the exact opposite of what Dorothea Dix believed during the previous century. That is, instead of viewing an institution as a peaceful asylum, institutionalization was viewed as contributing to the illness. If patients were moved into a "normal" community-living setting, it was believed that the symptoms of mental disorders could easily be treated and eventually would disappear. Thus, **deinstitutionalization**, the release of those confined to mental institutions for long periods of time into the community for treatment, support, and rehabilitation, became a national movement.

The inpatient state hospital population fell by about 15% between 1955 and 1965 and by about 59% during the succeeding decade. The 2,000 projected community mental health centers (CMHCs) that should have been in place by 1980 never materialized. By 1990, only about 1,300 programs provided various types of psychosocial rehabilitation services, such as vocational, educational, or social-recreational services (International Association of Psychosocial Rehabilitation, 1990).

Deinstitutionalization: A Failed Approach

There is no evidence that the majority of persons discharged from state hospitals benefited from CMHC services. The CMHCs, by and large, ignored the legions of people with serious mental illnesses and instead focused on the treatment of alcoholism and drug addiction. Individual psychotherapy, the primary treatment offered in most centers, was insufficient for those who needed other types of treatment, housing, and vocational opportunities. By the 1990s, deinstitutionalization was considered a failure.

CONTEMPORARY MENTAL HEALTH CARE

Millions of adults and children are disabled by mental illness every year. Compared with all other diseases, major depressive disorder, anxiety disorder, and opioid use disorders rank in the top eight conditions responsible for chronic disability in the United States from 1990 to 2016 (U.S. Burden of Disease Collaborators, 2018). Government initiatives are attempting to increase the public's understanding of mental disorders and related issues.

In 1999, *Mental Health: A Report of the Surgeon General* summarized evidence for the treatment of mental illness. As the first report addressing mental health by the Office of the Surgeon General, two main findings were presented (U.S. Department of Health and Human Services [U.S. DHHS], 1999):

* The efficacy of mental health treatments is well documented.

* A range of treatments exist for most mental disorders.

The following year, another landmark report, *Report of the Surgeon General's Conference on Children's Mental Health: A National Action Agenda*, was published. This report highlights consensus recommendations for identifying, recognizing, and referring children to services; increasing access to services for families; and using evidence for evaluating treatment services, systems of care, and financing (U.S. Public Health Service, 2000).

In 2003, the *President's New Freedom Commission on Mental Health* recommended that the mental health system be transformed. The report identified six goals as the foundation for transforming mental health care in the United States into a consumer-centered, family-centered, and recovery-oriented system (Box 1.5) (New Freedom Commission on Mental Health, 2003).

BOX 1.5

U.S. Goals in a Transformed Mental Health System

Goal 1 Americans understand that mental health is essential to overall health.
Goal 2 Mental health care is consumer and family driven.
Goal 3 Disparities in mental health services are eliminated.
Goal 4 Early mental health screening, assessment, and referral to services are common practices.
Goal 5 Excellent mental health care is delivered, and research is accelerated.
Goal 6 Technology is used to access mental health care and information.

New Freedom Commission on Mental Health. (2003). Achieving the promise: Transforming mental healthcare in America (p. 8). DHHS Publication No. SMA-03–3831. U.S. Department of Health and Human Services.

The Mental Health Parity and Addiction Equity Act was enacted in 2008 to ensure fairness between mental health and/or substance use disorder benefits and medical/surgical benefits covered by a health plan. The final rules were not effective until July 1, 2014, and implemented in 2015. Under this rule, a plan may not allow a patient to have unlimited visits with a medical provider and only a few visits to a mental health provider. In 2010, the Patient Protection and Affordable Care Act was passed that provided more people with access to affordable, effective treatments for their mental health needs. This law also prevents insurance companies from excluding people because of preexisting conditions. The intent of this legislation was to put the consumers of mental health care back in charge of their care. A study by the Commonwealth Fund in 2017 reported that access through Medicaid coverage and establishing state marketplaces improved access to care for millions of Americans, who, unlike those who remained uninsured, were less likely to experience delays or be unable to get care due to costs (Glied et al., 2017). A variety of provisions under the Affordable Care Act brought the biggest expansion of substance abuse services in a generation. It seemed the future of mental health care looked good, as legislation was propelling mental health care forward.

But today, the future does not look so promising. Advocacy groups are warning that despite growing demand for behavioral health services, rollbacks are coming. According to the National Alliance on Mental Illness, multiple bills proposed by the executive branch will weaken market placement protections (Palanker et al., 2020). The Cohen Veterans Network, a national not-for-profit philanthropic organization for veterans and their families, and the National Council for Behavioral Health (2018) concluded that lack of access to care is fueling a mental health crisis, which is hitting rural and lower-income communities especially hard. The future of America's mental health services may hang in the balance of what advocates, consumers, and voters are able to accomplish in an unfriendly environment. This is a time in history to be ever vigilant of the gains previously made and to speak loudly on behalf of our mental health clients if we expect to keep them.

Recovery and the Consumer Movement

Recovery from mental illness is realistic and now a worldwide goal. Consumers are demanding that mental health services receive the same support and attention as other health services. The traditional medical model, which is viewed as autocratic and paternalistic, is being replaced by a collaborative model whereby mental health professionals work in partnership with consumers to help rebuild their lives. Consumer advocacy efforts have led to the implementation of recovery philosophy and practices (see Chapter 2). In this text, the terms *consumers* and *patients* are used interchangeably.

National Mental Health Objectives

The vision of (*Healthy People 2030*) is building a healthier future for all. The overarching goal of *Healthy People 2030* is to improve mental health based on the following objectives:

- General Mental Health and Mental Disorders
  - Increase the proportion of people with substance use and mental health disorders who get treatment for both.
  - Increase the proportion of primary care visits where adolescents and adults are screened for depression.
- Adolescents
  - Increase the proportion of adolescents with depression who get treatment.
  - Increase the proportion of children and adolescents with symptoms of trauma who get treatment.
  - Increase the number of children and adolescents with serious emotional disturbance who get treatment.
- Cancer
  - Increase quality of life for cancer survivors.
- Children
  - Increase the proportion of children and adolescents with attention deficit/hyperactivity disorder who get appropriate treatment.
  - Increase the proportion of children with mental health problems who get treatment.
  - Increase the proportion of children with autism spectrum disorder who receive special services by age 4 years.
  - Increase the proportion of children and adolescents who get appropriate treatment for anxiety or depression.
  - Increase the proportion of children and adolescents who get appropriate treatment for behavior problems.
  - Increase the proportion of children and adolescents who get preventive mental health care in school.
- Hospital and Emergency Services
  - Reduce emergency department visits related to nonmedical use of prescription opioids.
- Injury Prevention
  - Reduce the suicide rate.
  - Reduce the suicide attempts by adolescents.
- LGBT
  - Reduce suicidal thoughts in lesbian, gay, or bisexual high school students.
  - Reduce suicidal thoughts in transgender students.
- Parents or Caregivers
  - Reduce anxiety and depression in family caregivers of people with disabilities.

- People with Disabilities
  - Reduce the proportion of adults with disabilities who delay preventive care because of cost.
  - Reduce the proportion of adults with disabilities who experience serious psychological distress.
- Pregnancy and Childbirth
  - Increase the proportion of women who get screened for postpartum depression.
- Schools
  - Increase the proportion of public schools with a counselor, social worker, and psychologist.
- Violence Prevention
  - Reduce emergency department visits for nonfatal intentional self-harm injuries.

The mental health goal is to improve mental health through prevention and by ensuring access to appropriate, quality mental health services. Three new mental health issues have emerged in the past decade: physical and mental trauma experienced by military members and veterans, large-scale psychological trauma in communities caused by violence and natural disasters, and the understanding and treatment of older adults with dementia and mood disorders. Objectives focusing on mental health and mental disorders provide guidance for all health care professionals (Box 1.6).

The challenge for psychiatric nursing is to work toward these goals through direct practice, advocating for persons with emotional and mental disorders, and improving the social and physical environments of care.

SUMMARY OF KEY POINTS

- Every practicing nurse cares for persons with an emotional or mental disorder. Every nurse needs basic psychiatric nursing knowledge and skills.
- Psychiatric–mental health nursing is a specialized area of nursing that promotes mental health through applying the nursing process. Psychiatric nurses care for people with a wide range of emotional problems and mental disorders.
- The need for psychiatric–mental health nursing was recognized near the end of the 19th century when Linda Richards opened the Boston City Hospital Training School for Nurses in 1882. Today, psychiatric nursing is recognized as one of the core mental health professions.
- Evidence-based practice is the standard of care in psychiatric nursing and in the mental health field. Historically, popular beliefs about the source of mental illnesses and treatment served as evidence.
- Over time, most treatment approaches, including institutionalization and deinstitutionalization, did not result in positive outcomes.
- Freud contributed to the psychoanalytic understanding of personality development and showed the strength of psychoanalysis. However, the psychoanalytic model was not effective in the treatment of people with severe mental illnesses.
- The U.S. Surgeon General's reports, the President's New Freedom Commission on Mental Health, and the goals of *Healthy People 2030* continue to highlight the need for resources for the care of persons with mental illness.
- The Patient Protection and Affordable Care Act prevents third-party payers from excluding people from insurance coverage for preexisting disorders.
- Today, consumers of mental health services insist on building partnerships with providers in order to recover from mental illness. The traditional medical model is being replaced by a collaborative approach in which consumers and mental health care providers develop a partnership in recovery-oriented care.

CRITICAL THINKING CHALLENGES

1. Discuss whether these patients will have mental health needs:

   a. A 32-year-old recently divorced woman with obesity and diabetes, who recently lost her job and can no longer pay for her medications.

   b. A 25-year-old veteran whose war injuries have left him paralyzed from the waist down.

   c. An 86-year-old woman whose husband recently died and now must move to a nursing home.

2. Give three examples of changes in nursing practice based on new evidence.

3. Present an argument for the moral treatment of people with mental disorders.

4. Identify common themes in the 1999 *Mental Health: A Report of the Surgeon General*, the President's New Freedom Commission of Mental Health Report, and *Healthy People 2030: National Health Promotion and Disease Prevention Objectives*.

Movie Viewing Guides

One Flew over the Cuckoo's Nest: 1975. This classic film stars Jack Nicholson as Randle P. McMurphy, who takes on the state hospital establishment. This movie won all five of the top Academy Awards: Best Picture, Best Actor, Best Actress, Best Director, and Best Adapted Screenplay. The film depicts life in an inpatient psychiatric ward of the late 1960s and increased public awareness of the potential human rights violations inherent in a large, public mental system. However, the portrayal of electroconvulsive therapy is stereotyped and inaccurate, and the suicide of Billy appears to be simplistically linked to his domineering mother. This film depicts the loss of patients' rights and the use of coercion and punishment in mental institutions before the deinstitutionalization movement.

VIEWING POINTS: This film should be viewed from several different perspectives: What is the basis of McMurphy's admission? How does Nurse Ratchet interact with the patients? How are patient rights violated?

I Never Promised You a Rose Garden: 1977. This movie, now available on streaming services and DVD (Digital Video Disc), stars Kathleen Quinlan as Deborah Blake, a 16-year-old young woman who is institutionalized for her mental illness. Her treatment in the institution was typical of the 1960s. In this film, the therapeutic relationship between Deborah and her physician was considered ideal.

VIEWING POINTS: How were patients, especially adolescent girls with emotional problems, treated in the 1960s? How would Deborah's treatment be judged today?

REFERENCES

American Nurses Association, American Psychiatric Nurses Association, & International Society of Psychiatric-Mental Health Nurses. (2014). *Psychiatric-mental health nursing: Scope and standards of practice* (2nd ed.). Nursebooks.org.

Bailey, H. (1920). *Nursing mental diseases*. Macmillan.

Beers, C. W. (1908). *A mind that found itself*. Longmans, Green, & Co.

Bly, N. (1887). *Ten days in a mad-house*. Ian L. Munro.

Church, O. M. (1987). From custody to community in psychiatric nursing. *Nursing Research, 36*(10), 48–55.

Cohen Veterans Network, & The National Council for Behavioral Health. (2018). New Study Reveals Lack of Access a root Cause for Mental Health Crisis in America. https://www.thentionalcouncil.org/press-releases

Compton, M. T., Bakeman, R., Capulong, L., Pauselli, L., Alolayan, Y., Drisafio, A., King, K., Reed, T., Broussard, B., & Shim, R. (2020). Associations between two domains of social adversity and recovery among persons with serious mental illnesses being treated in community mental health centers. *Community Mental Health Journal, 56*(1), 22–31.

Cowles, E. (1887). Nursing reform for the insane. *American Journal of Insanity, 44*(176), 191.

Deutsch, S. (1949). *The mentally ill in America*. Oxford University Press.

Freud, S. (1900). Interpretation of dreams. In J. Strachey, A. Freud, A. Strachey, & A. Tyson (Eds.), (1953). *The standard edition of the complete psychological works of Sigmund Freud* (Vol. 4). Hogarth Press.

Freud, S. (1905). Three essays on the theory of sexuality. In J. Strachey, A. Freud, A. Strachey, & A. Tyson (Eds.), (1953). *The standard edition of the complete psychological works of Sigmund Freud* (pp. 135–248). Hogarth Press.

Freud, S. (1927). The ego and the id. In E. Jones (Ed.), (1957). *The international psycho-analytical library, N. 12*. Hogarth Press.

Glied, S. A., Ma, S., & Borja, A. (2017). Effect of the Affordable Care Act on Health Care Access. The Commonwealth Fund. https://www.commonwealthfund.org/publications/issue-briefs/2017/may/effect-affordable-care-act-health-care-accessInternational

International Association of Psychosocial Rehabilitation. (1990). A national directory: Organizations providing psychosocial rehabilitation and related community support services in the United States. Center for Psychiatric Rehabilitation, Boston University.

Malamud, W. (1944). The history of psychiatric therapies. In J. K. Hall, G. Zilboorg, & H. Bunker (Eds.), *One hundred years of American psychiatry* (pp. 273–323). Columbia University Press.

Melnyk, B. M., & Fineout-Overholt, E. (2019). *Evidence-based practice in nursing & healthcare: A guide to best practice* (4th ed.). Wolters Kluwer.

New Freedom Commission on Mental Health. (2003). Achieving the promise: Transforming mental health care in America (Publication No. SMA-03-3831). Department of Health and Human Services.

Nightingale, F. (1859). *Notes on nursing: What it is and what it is not*. Harrison & Son.

Office of Disease Prevention and Health Promotion. 2021. *Healthy People 2030*. U.S. Department of Health and Human Services. Mental Health and Mental Disorders; Healthy People 2030. health.gov

Palanker, D., Volk, K., Thomas, L., & Thomas, K. (2020). Mental health parity at risk. National Alliance for Mental Illness. https://www.nami.org/About-NAMI/Publications-Reports/Public-Policy-Reports/Parity-at-Risk/ParityatRisk.pdf

Peplau, H. (1952). *Interpersonal relations in nursing*. Putnam.

U.S. Burden of Disease Collaborators, Mokdad, A. H., Ballestros, K., Echko, M., Glenn, S., et al. (2018). The State of US Health, 1990–2016: Burden of diseases, injuries, and risk factors among US states. *JAMA, 319*(14), 1444–1472. https://doi.org/10.1001/jama.2018.0158

U.S. Department of Health and Human Services. (1999). Mental health: A report of the surgeon general. U.S. Department of Health and Human Services, Substance Abuse and Mental Health Services Administration, Center for Mental Health Services, National Institutes of Health, National Institute of Mental Health.

U.S. Public Health Service. (2000). *Report of the Surgeon General's Conference on Children's Mental Health: A national action agenda*. Department of Health and Human Services.

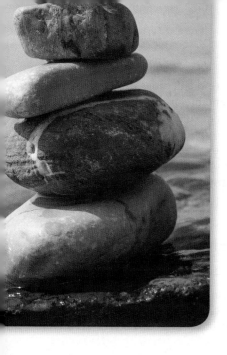

2
Mental Health and Mental Disorders
Fighting Stigma and Promoting Recovery

Mary Ann Boyd and Rebecca Luebbert

KEYCONCEPTS

- mental disorders
- mental health
- recovery
- stigma
- trauma
- wellness

LEARNING OBJECTIVES

After studying this chapter, you will be able to:

1. Relate the concept of mental health to wellness.

2. Identify the rationale for promoting wellness for people with mental health challenges.

3. Differentiate the concepts of mental health and mental illness.

4. Discuss the significance of epidemiologic evidence in studying the occurrence of mental disorders.

5. Describe the consequences of the stigma of mental illness on individuals and families.

6. Identify recovery components and their role in the treatment of mental illness.

7. Discuss the role of trauma-informed care in recovery-oriented nursing practice.

KEY TERMS

- Cultural explanation • Cultural idiom of distress • Cultural syndrome • Culture-bound syndromes • *DSM-5* • Epidemiology
- Incidence • Label avoidance • Point prevalence • Prevalence • Public stigma • Rate • Recovery-oriented care • Self-stigma
- Syndrome • Trauma-informed care

INTRODUCTION

To understand health and illness in any practice area, nurses need a basic understanding of mental health and its relationship with wellness. This chapter discusses concepts of mental health and wellness, the diagnosis of mental disorders, how the stigma of mental illness can be a barrier to treatment, and the importance of focusing on recovery from mental illness.

MENTAL HEALTH AND WELLNESS

Mental health is defined as a state of well-being in which the individual realizes their own abilities, can cope with life's normal stresses, can work productively and fruitfully, and can make a contribution to society. A person cannot be healthy without being *mentally* healthy, but it is possible to be mentally healthy and have a mental or physical disorder (World Health Organization [WHO], 2018).

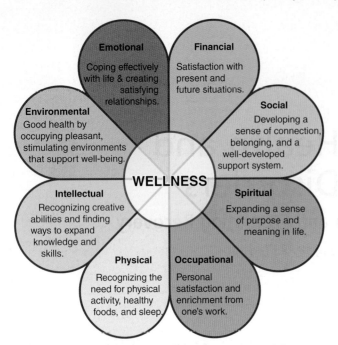

FIGURE 2.1 Eight dimensions of wellness. (Adapted from U.S. DHHS, SAMHSA. [2020b]. *The eight dimensions of wellness.* https://www.samhsa.gov/wellness-initiative/eight-dimensions-wellness)

Mental health is essential to personal well-being, interpersonal relationships, and contributing to the community.

KEYCONCEPT **Mental health** is the emotional and psychological well-being of an individual who has the capacity to interact with others, deal with ordinary stress, and perceive one's surroundings realistically (adapted from American Nurses Association, American Psychiatric Nurses Association, & International Society of Psychiatric–Mental Health Nurses, 2014).

Mental health is an essential piece of total wellness. The concept of wellness encompasses both physical and mental health. Problems in one area impact the other area. Wellness is not the absence of disease or stress; it involves having a purpose in life, being actively involved in satisfying work and play, having joyful relationships, having a healthy body and living environment, and being happy. It includes the mental, emotional, physical, occupational, intellectual, and spiritual aspects of a person's life (U.S. Department of Health and Human Services, Substance Abuse & Mental Health Services Administration [U.S. DHHS, SAMHSA], 2020b) (see Fig. 2.1).

KEYCONCEPT **Wellness** is being in good physical and mental health. Improving physical health can benefit mental health, and vice versa. Wellness is not the absence of disease. There are eight dimensions of wellness: emotional, financial, social, spiritual, occupational, physical, intellectual, environmental (U.S. DHHS, SAMHSA, 2020b). See Figure 2.1.

Mental health problems significantly impact the process of wellness. Individuals with mental health problems are more likely to die decades earlier than the general public from preventable diseases (Heiberg et al., 2018). People with serious mental health problems often face social, economic, and/or environmental disadvantages that result in lack of access to health care, lack of information, and lack of culturally and linguistically competent care and programs (U.S. DHHS, SAMHSA, 2020c).

OVERVIEW OF MENTAL HEALTH DISORDERS

Mental disorders can disrupt mental health and result in one of the most common causes of disability. In this text, the terms *mental disorder* and *mental illness* will be used interchangeably.

KEYCONCEPT **Mental disorders** are clinically significant disturbances in cognition, emotion regulation, or behavior that reflect a dysfunction in the psychological, biologic, or developmental processes underlying mental dysfunction. They are usually associated with distress or impaired functioning (American Psychiatric Association [APA], 2013).

A mental illness or mental disorder is a **syndrome**, a set of symptoms that cluster together that may have multiple causes and may represent several different disease states that have not yet been defined. Unlike many medical diseases, mental disorders are defined by clusters of behaviors, thoughts, and feelings, not by underlying biologic pathology. Laboratory tests are not generally used in diagnosing mental disorders.

The landmark study *Global Burden of Disease 2010* found an alarming impact of mental and behavioral disorders on health and productivity in the world. Depression is one of the leading disease burdens in middle- and high-income countries such as the United States. In 2019, in the United States, 1 in 5 adults, or 47.6 million people, had a mental illness (National Institute of Mental Health [NIMH], 2019).

Evidence for this very high occurrence of mental disorders is established through epidemiologic research. **Epidemiology**, the study of patterns of disease distribution and determinants of health within populations, contributes to the overall understanding of the mental health status of population groups, or aggregates, and associated factors. Epidemiologic studies examine associations among possible factors related to an area of investigation, but they do not determine causes of illnesses. The Centers for Disease Control and Prevention (CDC) tracks and reports mental health epidemiologic data. Throughout this book, epidemiologic data are included in discussions of mental health problems and mental disorders. See Box 2.1 for an explanation of terms.

Adapted from Durá-Vilá, G., & Hodes, M. (2012). Cross-cultural study of idioms of distress among Spanish nationals and Hispanic American migrants: *susto, nervios* and *ataque de nervios*. *Social Psychiatry and Psychiatric Epidemiology, 47*(10), 1627–1637.

BOX 2.1
Epidemiologic Terms

In epidemiology, certain terms have specific meanings relative to what they measure. When expressing the number of cases of a disorder, population rates, rather than raw numbers, are used.

Rate is the proportion of the cases in the population when compared with the total population. It is expressed as a fraction, in which the numerator is the number of cases and the denominator is the total number in the population, including the cases and non-cases. The term *average rate* is used for measures that involve rates over specified time periods:

$$Rate = \frac{Case\ in\ population}{Total\ population\ (cases\ and\ non\text{-}cases)}$$

Prevalence refers to the total number of people who have the disorder within a given population at a specified time regardless of how long ago the disorder started.

Point prevalence is a basic measure that refers to the proportion of individuals in the population who have the disorder at a specified point in time (t). This point can be a day on the calendar, such as April 1, 2020, or a point defined in relation to the study assessment, such as the day of the interview. This is also expressed as a fraction:

$$Point\ prevalence\ rate = \frac{Cases\ at\ t}{Population\ at\ t}$$

Incidence refers to a rate that includes only *new* cases that have occurred within a clearly defined time period. The most common time period evaluated is 1 year. A study of incidence cases is more difficult than a study of prevalent cases because a study of incidence cases requires at least two measurements to be taken: one at the start of the prescribed time period and another at the end of it.

BOX 2.2
Frequently Reported Cultural Syndromes and Idioms

Ataque de nervios: frequent episodes of loss of control, uncontrollable crying, tremors, and severe anxiety and sadness with somatization symptoms including muscle ache and headache, nausea, loss of appetite, insomnia, fatigue, and psychomotor agitation. Reported among women over 45 years old, with little education and who have experienced a loss (such as a divorce) or acute distress.

Susto: fright characterized by symptoms of psychomotor agitation, anorexia, insomnia, fever, diarrhea, confusion, apathy, depression, and introversion following an emotional trauma or witnessing a traumatic experience.

Diagnosis of Mental Health Conditions

Mental disorders are organized and diagnosed according to the criteria published in the *Diagnostic and Statistical Manual of Mental Disorders, Fifth Edition* (*DSM-5*; APA, 2013). The current **DSM-5** system contains subtypes and other specifiers that further classify disorders. Although the *DSM-5* specifies criteria for diagnosing mental disorders, there are no absolute boundaries separating one disorder from another, and disorders often have different manifestations at different points in time.

In a mental disorder, alterations in behaviors, thoughts, and feelings are unexpected and are outside normal, culturally defined limits. If a behavior is considered normal within a specific culture, it is not viewed as a psychiatric symptom. For example, members of some religious groups "speak in tongues." To an observer, it appears that the individuals are hallucinating (see Chapter 24), but this behavior is normal for this group within a particular setting.

The amount of disability or impairment in functioning is an important consideration when assessing a person with a mental disorder. A person's ability to understand, communicate, and get along with others is important in the recovery process. If symptoms impair an individual's ability to independently perform self-care and daily activities, recovery will be more difficult. The World Health Organization's Disability Assessment Schedule 2.0 is an instrument that can be used for measuring the amount of impairment that the individual experiences.

Culture-bound syndromes, which are illnesses that occur only within a specific culture, have been studied for years. The *DSM-5* replaced the term with three concepts: **Cultural syndrome** is a group of co-occurring symptoms that occurs in one culture, for example, *ataque de nervios*. **Cultural idiom of distress** is a phrase or way of talking about distress within a culture, for example, *susto*. **Cultural explanation** or cause is an etiology that is culturally conceived (APA, 2013). There is little research that reliably describes cultural syndromes or idioms of distress, but there are two conditions—*ataque de nervios* and *susto*—that are frequently reported in a small number of persons (Durá-Vilá & Hodes, 2012) (Box 2.2).

Stigma

Stigma is one of the major barriers to treatment, recovery, and social integration. A major reason individuals with mental health problems do not seek or continue with treatment is the stigma they encounter. Stigma, myths, and misconceptions surrounding mental illness contribute to the discrimination and human rights violations experienced by people living with mental illness.

KEYCONCEPT Stigma is a dynamic social/interactional process in which the stigmatized person is labeled as different and linked to negative stereotypes. Persons with stigmatizing beliefs socially distance themselves from the stigmatized person. Public stigma, self-stigma, and label avoidance are three types of stigma people with mental illnesses experience.

Public Stigma

Public stigma occurs after individuals are publicly "marked" as having a mental illness. When they act or say things that are odd or unusual or tell others that they have a mental illness, these individuals are at risk of being subjected to prejudice and discrimination. Common stereotypes include being dangerous, unpredictable, and incapable of functioning independently. People with mental illness are sometimes treated as if they are responsible for their disabilities and are inaccurately accused of being weak or immoral (Corrigan & Al-Khouja, 2018). Stigmatization robs individuals of work, independent living, and meaningful relationships.

When people with mental illnesses or emotional problems are stigmatized by society, they are often ostracized by the society in which they live. The stigma associated with all forms of mental illness is strong but generally increases the more an individual's behavior differs from the cultural norm. Reducing stigma has been identified as a public health priority (National Academy of Sciences, 2016).

Media perpetuates the stigma of mental disorders and treatment. News coverage often associates violence with mental illness (McGinty et al., 2018). Few describe successful treatment or recovery. Additionally, mental health treatment and providers are often stigmatized (Henderson, 2018). In films, psychiatric hospitals are often portrayed as dangerous and unwelcoming places, as in *The Snake Pit* (1948), *One Flew Over the Cuckoo's Nest* (1975), *Instinct* (1999), *Twelve Monkeys* (1995), *Sling Blade* (1996), *Girl, Interrupted* (1999), *Don Juan Demarco* (1994), *A Beautiful Mind* (2001), and *Analyze That* (2002). Nurses are dressed in white in contrast to the dark, gloomy surroundings, and patients have little to do other than to walk the halls of the institution, acting odd.

One of the best ways to counteract the negative effects of stigma is to have contact with the stigmatized group (Corrigan & Al-Khouja, 2018). Another way is to use non-stigmatizing language. Just as a person with diabetes mellitus should not be referred to as a "diabetic" but rather as a "person with diabetes," a person with a mental disorder should never be referred to as a "schizophrenic" or "bipolar" but rather as a "person with schizophrenia" or a "person with bipolar disorder." Using words such as *psycho*, *nuts*, *funny farm*, and *maniac* reinforces negative images of mental illness. Jokes that depict people with mental illness as stupid, dangerous, or incompetent perpetuate negative myths.

Self-Stigma

Self-stigma occurs when negative stereotypes are internalized by people with mental illness. Patients are aware of the public's negative view of mental illness and agree with the public's perceptions. As they become aware of the negative stereotypes, they begin agreeing with the stereotype. Then they may begin applying the stigma to themselves: "I have a mental illness, so I must be incompetent." As a result of the application of the negative stereotype to self, they develop low self-esteem (Corrigan & Nieweglowski, 2019).

Label Avoidance

Label avoidance, avoiding treatment or care in order not to be labeled as being mentally ill, is another type of stigma and one of the reasons that so few people with mental health problems actually receive help. By avoiding treatment, they avoid the stigma of mental illness. For example, negative views of mental illness by several of the Asian cultures influence the willingness of their members to seek treatment. They may ignore their symptoms or refuse to seek treatment because of the stigma associated with being mentally ill (Corrigan & Nieweglowski, 2019).

RECOVERY FROM MENTAL ILLNESS

Recovery is the single most important goal for individuals with mental disorders. The following definition of recovery was released following a lengthy consensus-seeking process that began in 2010 and involved government agency officials, experts, consumers, family members, advocates, researchers, managed care representatives, and others.

> **KEYCONCEPT Recovery** from mental disorders and/or substance use disorders is a process of change through which individuals improve their health and wellness, live a self-directed life, and strive to reach their full potential (U.S. DHHS, SAMHSA, 2020a).

Recovery-oriented treatment is based on the belief that mental illnesses and emotional disturbances are treatable and that recovery is an expectation. There are four dimensions that support recovery: *health* (managing disease and living in a physically and emotionally healthy way), *home* (a safe and stable place to live), *purpose* (meaningful daily activities and independence, resources, and income), and *community* (relationships and social networks) (U.S. DHHS, SAMHSA, 2020a). Consumers and families have real and meaningful choices about treatment options and providers. In **recovery-oriented care**, the person with a mental health problem develops a partnership with a clinician to manage the illness, strengthen coping abilities, and build resilience for life's challenges (Box 2.3).

Mental health recovery benefits not only the individual and family but also society by ultimately reducing the global burden of mental health problems. Recovery is guided by 10 fundamental principles. (Box 2.4). See Chapter 9 for further discussion of recovery.

BOX 2.3

Cultural Change: Implementation of a Recovery Program

McDonagh, J. G., Haren, W. B., Valvano, M., Grubaugh, A. L., Wainwright, F. C., Rhue, C. H., Pelic, C. M., Pelic, C. G., Koval, R., & York, J. A. (2019). Cultural change: Implementation of a recovery program in a Veterans Health Administration Medical Center inpatient unit. Journal of the American Psychiatric Nurses Association, 25(3), 208–217.

THE QUESTION: How does an inpatient mental health unit implement recovery-oriented services?

METHODS: A recovery-oriented inpatient program on a 24-bed locked unit consisted of several critical components, including the development of an interprofessional committee, creation of vision and mission statement, education of staff, integration of the peer support specialist role, development and delivery of recovery-oriented curriculum, development of the interprofessional program partnership, and adoption of the *Veteran's Recovery Self-Help Resource*

Book and the Veterans Recovery Worksheet. An interprofessional Partnership for Wellness conducted evidence-based recovery and holistic health programs for 4 to 6 hours per day. The measurement indicators included veteran feedback, program requirements, and system measures.

FINDINGS: Preliminary indicators over a 2-year period suggest that the veterans rated group content and relevance high, per-post psychiatric rehospitalization rates decreased by 46%, and fidelity to the recommended strategies was high.

IMPLICATIONS FOR NURSING: Recovery-oriented practice is realistic in an inpatient mental health unit if there are committed interprofessional staff, effective training, and an organizational culture exemplifying recovery-oriented principles.

Recovery-Oriented Care and Trauma-Informed Care

Mental health professionals increasingly focus on the harmful effects of trauma on health and mental health status. Individuals who experience trauma, particularly in childhood, have a higher incidence of chronic disease and behavior health issues. Trauma is a universal experience for people with mental and substance abuse disorders, and addressing it is a critical component of mental health care (U.S. DHHS, SAMHSA, 2014).

> **KEYCONCEPT** Individual **trauma** results from an event, a series of events, or a set of circumstances that is experienced by an individual as physically or emotionally harmful or life threatening and that has lasting adverse effects on the individual's functioning and mental, physical, social, emotional, or spiritual well-being (U.S. DHHS, SAMHSA, 2014).

BOX 2.4

Guiding Principles of Recovery

Recovery emerges from hope: The belief that recovery is real provides the essential and motivating message of a better future—that people can and do overcome the internal and external challenges, barriers, and obstacles that confront them.

Recovery is person driven: Self-determination and self-direction are the foundations for recovery, as individuals define their own life goals and design their unique path(s).

Recovery occurs via many pathways: Individuals are unique with distinct needs, strengths, preferences, goals, culture, and backgrounds, including trauma experiences that affect and determine their pathway(s) to recovery. Abstinence is the safest approach for those with substance use disorders.

Recovery is holistic: Recovery encompasses an individual's whole life, including mind, body, spirit, and community. The array of services and supports available should be integrated and coordinated.

Recovery is supported by peers and allies: Mutual support and mutual aid groups, including the sharing of experiential knowledge and skills, as well as social learning, play an invaluable role in recovery.

Recovery is supported through relationship and social networks: An important factor in the recovery process is the presence and involvement of people who believe in the person's ability to recover; who offer hope, support, and encouragement; and who also suggest strategies and resources for change.

Recovery is culturally based and influenced: Culture and cultural background in all of its diverse representations including values, traditions, and beliefs are key in determining a person's journey and unique pathway to recovery.

Recovery is supported by addressing trauma: Services and supports should be trauma informed to foster safety (physical and emotional) and trust as well as to promote choice, empowerment, and collaboration.

Recovery involves individual, family, and community strengths and responsibility: Individuals, families, and communities have strengths and resources that serve as a foundation for recovery.

Recovery is based on respect: Community, systems, and societal acceptance and appreciation for people affected by mental health and substance use problems—including protecting their rights and eliminating discrimination—are crucial in achieving recovery.

From U.S. DHHS, SAMHSA. (2020a). Recovery and recovery support. https://www.samhsa.gov/find-help/recovery.

An important aspect of recovery-oriented care is preventing re-traumatization by exposing individuals to triggers—such as confinement to a mental health unit or applying restraints—only when accompanied by the proper support and sensitivity (National Council for Behavioral Health, 2020). **Trauma-informed care** is integral to recovery-oriented nursing care for people with emotional problems and mental disorders. Trauma-informed care incorporates a basic realization and understanding of the impact of trauma on individuals, families, groups, organizations, and communities. In trauma-informed care, nurses recognize the signs of trauma and respond by fully integrating knowledge about the trauma into policies, procedures, and practice.

Individuals with mental illnesses can regain mental health with the support of families, mental health providers, and society. The contributions of these individuals strengthen communities and support the overall health of a nation.

SUMMARY OF KEY POINTS

- Mental health is the emotional and psychological well-being of an individual. To be mentally healthy means that one can interact with others, deal with daily stress, and perceive the world realistically. Mental disorders are health conditions characterized by alterations in thinking, mood, or behavior and are associated with distress or impaired functioning.

- Good physical and mental health characterize wellness. Individuals can have a mental disorder and experience wellness.

- Epidemiology is important to understanding the distribution of mental illness and determinants of health within a given population. The rate of occurrence refers to the proportion of the population that has the disorder. Incidence is the rate of new cases within a specified time. Prevalence is the rate of occurrence of all cases at a particular point in time.

- Stigma toward mental illness can be viewed in three ways. Public stigma marks a person as having a mental illness. When a person with a mental illness shares the public's negative view of mental illness, self-stigma occurs. If a person with a mental illness does not seek treatment because of fear of being labeled "mentally ill," label avoidance occurs.

- The *DSM-5* organizes psychiatric diagnoses according to behaviors and symptom patterns.

- Cultural syndromes are specific disorders found within a particular culture. There is little research on the syndromes, but *ataque de nervios* and *susto* are well documented.

- Mental health recovery is the single most important goal for the mental health delivery system. Recovery is viewed a process of changes through which individuals improve their health and wellness, live a self-directed life, and strive to reach their full potential.

- Trauma is experienced by many individuals as physically or emotionally harmful or life threatening and has lasting adverse effects on the individual. Trauma-informed care is integral to recovery-oriented care.

CRITICAL THINKING CHALLENGES

1. A person who is seeking help for a mental disorder asks why the individual's physical health is important to the nurse.

2. Compare the meaning of the epidemiologic terms *prevalence*, *incidence*, and *rate*. Access the CDC's website (www.cdc.gov) and identify major mental health problems in the United States.

3. Examine the description of people with mental illness in the media, including television programs, news, and newspapers. Are negative connotations evident?

4. Examine how family and friends describe people with mental illness. Do you think their description of mental illness is based on fact or myth? Explain.

5. Explain the three forms of stigma and give examples.

6. Discuss the negative impact of labeling someone with a psychiatric diagnosis.

7. Using the components of mental health recovery as a framework, compare the goals for a person with schizophrenia with the goals for a person with a medical disease such as diabetes.

8. Discuss the application of trauma-informed care with a person who has experienced a trauma such as rape or a life-threatening event.

To Write Love On Her Arms (2015). This 2015 Substance Abuse and Mental Health Services Administration Voice Award winner is a true story that presents a vision of hope, healing, and redemption. Renee, played by Kat Dennings, is a Florida girl living with addiction and mental illness. She has also experienced abuse and is trying to come to grips with that trauma. Renee discovers the value of friendships and courageously embarks on a daunting journey toward recovery.

VIEWING POINTS: Observe the stigma that is associated with having a mental illness. Identify the trauma Renee experienced and how it influences her ability to engage in treatment.

Unfolding Patient Stories: Sandra Littlefield

Part 1

Sandra Littlefield is a 36-year-old female with borderline personality disorder. Her history includes several divorces, drug and alcohol abuse, poor impulse control, anxiety, cutting, suicide attempts, prostitution, and jail time. Why could she be subject to stereotypes and bias? Describe the stigma of mental illness and how it can affect her as an inmate, in the community, and with recovery? What actions by Sandra may be influenced by internalizing the perceived stigma people have of her?

REFERENCES

American Nurses Association, American Psychiatric Nurses Association, & International Society of Psychiatric–Mental Health Nurses. (2014). *Psychiatric–mental health nursing: Scope and standards of practice* (2nd ed.). American Nurses Association.

American Psychiatric Association. (2013). *Diagnostic and statistical manual of mental disorders* (5th ed.). Author.

Corrigan, P. W., & Al-Khouja, A. (2018). Three agendas for changing the public stigma of mental illness. *Psychiatric Rehabilitation Journal, 41*(1), 1–7.

Corrigan, P. W., & Nieweglowski, K. (2019). How does familiarity impact the stigma of mental illness? *Clinical Psychology Review, 70*, 40–50.

Durá-Vilá, G., & Hodes, M. (2012). Cross-cultural study of idioms of distress among Spanish nationals and Hispanic American migrants: *susto*, *nervios* and *ataque de nervios*. *Social Psychiatry and Psychiatric Epidemiology, 47*(10), 1627–1637.

Heiberg, I. H., Jacobsen, B. K., Nesvåg, R., Bramness, J. G., Reichborn-Kjennerud, T., Næss, Ø., Ystrom, E., Hultman, C. M., & Høye, A. (2018). Total and cause-specific standardized mortality ratios in patients with schizophrenia and/ or substance use disorder. *PLoS ONE, 13*(8), e0202028.

Henderson, L. (2018). Popular television and public mental health: Creating media entertainment from mental distress. *Critical Public Health, 28*(1), 106–117.

McGinty, E. E., Goldman, H. H., Pescosolido, B. A., & Barry, C. L. (2018). Communicating about mental illness and violence: Balancing stigma and increased support for services. *Journal of Health Politics, Policy and Law, 43*(2), 185–228. https://doi.org/10.1215/03616878-4303507

National Academy of Sciences. (2016). *Ending discrimination against people with mental substance use disorders: The evidence for stigma change.* National Academies Press.

National Council for Behavioral Health. (2020). Fostering resilience and recovery: A change package for advancing trauma-informed primary care. https://www.thenationalcouncil.org/wp-content/uploads/2019/12/FosteringResilienceChangePackage_Final.pdf?daf=375ateTbd56

National Institute of Mental Health. (2019). Mental health by the numbers. https://nami.org/mhstats

U.S. DHHS, SAMHSA. (2014). SAMHSA's concept of trauma and guidance for trauma-informed approach. https://store.samhsa.gov/product/SAMHSA-s-Concept-of-Trauma-and-Guidance-for-a-Trauma-Informed-Approach/SMA14-4884

U.S. DHHS, SAMHSA. (2020a). Recovery and recovery support. https://www.samhsa.gov/find-help/recovery

U.S. DHHS, SAMHSA. (2020b). The eight dimensions of wellness. https://store.samhsa.gov/sites/default/files/d7/priv/sma16-4953.pdf

U.S. DHHS, SAMHSA. (2020c). Behavioral health equity. https://www.samhsa.gov/behavioral-health-equity

WHO. (2018). Mental health: Strengthening our response. Author. https://www.who.int/news-room/fact-sheets/detail/mental-health-strengthening-our-response

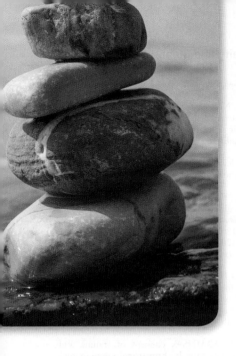

3
Cultural and Spiritual Issues Related to Mental Health Care

Mary Ann Boyd

KEYCONCEPTS

- cultural competence
- culture
- spirituality

LEARNING OBJECTIVES

After studying this chapter, you will be able to:

1. Discuss the ways that cultural competence is demonstrated in psychiatric–mental health nursing.

2. Describe the beliefs about mental health and illness in different cultural and social groups.

3. Differentiate concepts of religiousness and spirituality.

4. Discuss the role of spirituality and religiousness in persons with mental illness.

5. Discuss the beliefs of major religions and their role in shaping views on mental illnesses.

KEY TERMS

- Acculturation • Cultural explanations • Cultural identity • Cultural idiom of distress • Health literacy • Linguistic competence • Religiousness

INTRODUCTION

All cultural groups have sets of values, beliefs, and patterns of accepted behavior, and it is often difficult for those of one culture to understand those of another. This is especially true regarding mental illness—whereas some cultures view it as a condition for which the ill person must be punished and ostracized from society; other cultures are more tolerant and believe that family and community members are key to the care and treatment of mentally ill people. Nurses' and patients' religious backgrounds and cultural heritages may be different, so it is important for nurses to clearly understand the thinking and perspectives of other cultures and groups.

This chapter examines cultural and social mores of various cultural and religious groups. Understanding cultural and religious beliefs and the significance of spirituality is especially important when caring for people with mental health problems. These beliefs and practices can define and shape the experience of being mentally ill and influence the willingness to seek care. Treating mental disorders is intertwined with people's attitudes about themselves, their beliefs, values, and ways.

KEYCONCEPT Culture is not only a way of life for people who identify or associate with one another on the basis of some common purpose, need, or similarity of background but also the totality of learned, socially transmitted beliefs, values, and behaviors that emerge from its members' interpersonal transactions that can be used to define them as a collective. Culture is a term that goes beyond just race or ethnicity. It can also refer to such characteristics as age, gender, sexual orientation, disability, religion, income level, education, geographical location, or profession.

Cultures are dynamic and continually changing. When immigrants arrive in the United States with their own cultures, they begin to adapt to their new environment. **Acculturation** is the term used to describe the socialization process by which underrepresented groups learn and adopt selective aspects of the dominant culture. Their culture changes because of the influences of the new environment. Eventually, a new minority culture evolves that is different than the native culture and different from the dominant culture, which in turn is transformed by the new residents.

Everyone has a **cultural identity** or a set of cultural beliefs with which one looks for standards of behavior. Because culture is broadly defined, many people consider themselves to have multiple cultural identities. Often, the nurse is challenged to provide culturally appropriate care for persons from cultures other than the nurse's culture. Uncertainty about cultural beliefs and practices can result in feelings of anxiety and vulnerability when interacting with patients from other cultures. Patients may interpret the nurse's anxiety as a lack of caring or competence. It is important to learn and understand each patient's cultural background and identity to provide culturally competent care and avoid miscommunication and knowledge barriers (Markey & Okantey, 2019).

CULTURAL AND LINGUISTIC COMPETENCE

Cultural and linguistic competence is especially important for psychiatric–mental health nurses because of the significance of therapeutic communication. There are several definitions of cultural and linguistic competence, but there is a consensus that cultural and linguistic competence involves an adjustment or recognition of one's own culture to understand the culture of another person.

Linguistic competence, the capacity to communicate effectively and convey information that is easily understood by diverse audiences, is an important part of cultural competence (Harris-Haywood et al., 2014). Linguistic competence not only refers to the appropriate use of words, grammar, and syntax, but also to the practical aspects such as choice of discussion topics, taking turns, use of metaphors, and the "hidden rules" of interactions. The following is an example of a hidden rule: For one patient, it is a cultural expectation for a nurse to sit down and "chit chat" before providing care; for another patient, limited eye contact is best. A nurse who is culturally competent understands and appreciates cultural differences in health care practices and similarities within, among, and between groups.

KEYCONCEPT Cultural competence, the ability to interact effectively with people of different cultures, involves a set of academic and interpersonal skills that are respectful of and responsive to the health beliefs, health care practices, and

cultural and linguistic needs of diverse patients to bring about positive health care outcomes (U.S. Department of Health and Human Services [U.S. DHHS], 2020; Substance Abuse and Mental Health Services Administration, 2014).

Cultural competence can reinforce a person's engagement in treatment, therapeutic relations, and treatment outcomes. It is essential in decreasing disparities in mental health services. There are linguistic variations within cultural groups as well as cultural variations within a language group. Speaking the same language does not guarantee shared meaning and understanding. Communication may be adversely affected when patients are unable to fully express themselves in English. Understanding the impact of literacy levels is integral to providing culturally competent care. Demonstrating an understanding that literacy levels contribute to the interpretation of personal, psychological experiences is critical.

The ability to obtain, process, and understand basic health information and services in order to make health decisions is dependent upon a person's **health literacy**, that is, the ability to use reading, writing, verbal, and numerical skills in the context of health (Agency for Healthcare Research & Quality [AHRQ], 2018). If a person has limited health literacy and cannot process and understand basic health information and services, it is unlikely the individual will be able to follow discharge instruction, take prescribed medication, and adhere to a treatment plan (Glick et al., 2019; Polster, 2018). (See Box 3.1.)

BOX 3.1

Health Literacy Universal Precautions

- Health professionals should assume that all patients and caregivers may have difficulty comprehending health information.
- Health professionals should communicate in ways that anyone can understand.
- Health literacy universal precautions are aimed at the following:
  - Simplifying communication with and confirming comprehension for all patients, so that the risk of miscommunication is minimized.
  - Making the office environment and health care system easier to navigate.
  - Supporting patient's efforts to improve their health.
- Four domains are important for promoting health literacy.
  - Spoken communication
  - Written communication
  - Self-management and empowerment
  - Supportive systems

Agency for Healthcare Research & Quality. (2018). *Health literacy universal precautions toolkit* (2nd ed.). Agency for Healthcare Research and Quality. https://www.ahrq.gov/health-literacy/quality-resources/tools/literacy-toolkit/health-littoolkit2-intro.html

CULTURAL AND SOCIAL FACTORS AND BELIEFS ABOUT MENTAL ILLNESS

Cultural beliefs and practices influence how patients communicate and manifest their symptoms, cope with their illnesses, and receive family and community support. The *DSM-5* differentiates **cultural idiom of distress**, a commonly used term or phrase that describes the suffering within a cultural group from **cultural explanations**, perceived causes for symptoms (American Psychiatric Association [APA], 2013). For example, the term *nervios* is an idiom used by Hispanics in the Western Hemisphere that explains a wide range of somatic and emotional symptoms such as headache, irritability, nervousness, insomnia, and difficulty concentrating. The term *susto* (extreme fright causing the soul to leave the body) is believed to be the cause of a group of varied symptoms including appetite disturbance, sleep problems, and low self-worth among people in Central and South America. See Chapter 2.

Social factors contribute to the development of mental disorders. Ethnic and racial minorities in the United States live in a social environment of inequality that increases their exposure to racism, discrimination, violence, and poverty, which contribute to the experience of their illnesses (Hauenstein et al., 2019). Racially and ethnically diverse groups are less likely to receive mental health services and more likely to receive poorer quality care. Poverty is found in all cultural groups and is present in other groups, such as older adults, people with physical disabilities, individuals with psychiatric impairments, and single-parent families. In the United States in 2019, 22.2% of people living below the poverty line are single mothers and their children; 26.4% of Blacks live below the poverty level, as do 20.9% of Hispanic Americans and 12.3% of Whites. Currently in the United States, the poverty guidelines for a family of four is a yearly income of $26,200 or less in the 48 mainland states; $32,750 or less in Alaska; and $30,130 or less in Hawaii (U.S. DHHS, 2020). These figures do not include the financial impact of the coronavirus pandemic.

Families living in poverty are under tremendous financial and emotional stress, which may trigger or exacerbate mental problems. Along with the daily stressors of trying to provide food and shelter for themselves and their families, their lack of time, energy, and money prevents them from attending to their psychological needs. Often, these families become trapped in a downward economic spiral as tension and stress mount. The inability to gain employment and the lack of financial independence only add to the feelings of powerlessness and low self-esteem. Being self-supporting gives one a feeling of control over life and bolsters self-esteem. Dependence on others or the government causes frustration, anger, apathy, and feelings of depression and meaninglessness. Alcoholism, depression, and child and partner abuse may become a means of coping with such hopelessness and despair. The homeless population is the group most at risk for being unable to escape this spiral of poverty.

Hispanic Americans

The number of Hispanic or Latinx Americans living in the United States has been gradually increasing, and this group is now the largest underrepresented in the United States, constituting 59 million (18.3% of the total population). Countries of origin include Mexico (62%), Central and South American (15%), Puerto Rico (10%), and Cuba (4%). Hispanic populations are largest in urban areas, such as New York, Chicago, Los Angeles, San Francisco, and Miami–Fort Lauderdale (U.S. Census Bureau, 2018).

Studies indicate that Hispanic Americans tend to use all other resources before seeking help from mental health professionals. They are more likely to seek help at nonprofit hospitals or community health centers that also offer mental health services. Reasons for this are unclear, but barriers for treatment include beliefs that mental health facilities do not accommodate their cultural needs (e.g., language, beliefs, values), cost of care, availability of services, accessibility of services, and concerns regarding immigration status (Rosales & Calvo, 2019; Stafford & Draucker, 2020).

Black and African Americans

In 2018, the estimated population of Black or African Americans was 47.8 million or 13.4% of the U.S. population (U.S. Census Bureau, 2020). Although Black Americans share many beliefs, attitudes, values, and behaviors, there are also many subcultural and individual differences based on social class, country of origin, occupation, religion, educational level, and geographic location. African Americans have extensive family networks in which members can be relied on for moral support, help with child rearing, financial aid, and help in crises. Older family members are treated with great respect. But Blacks with mental illness suffer from the stresses of double stigma—not only from their own cultural group but also from longtime racial discrimination. To make matters worse, racial discrimination may come from within the health community itself (Box 3.2).

Several studies show that diagnoses and treatment for African Americans often are racially biased. African Americans are disproportionately diagnosed as having schizophrenia when compared to other groups. This disparity in diagnosis in schizophrenia has been stable over the past 3 decades. There is some indication that using a structured interview (rather than a subjective clinical interview) may reduce this disparity (Schwartz et al., 2019).

BOX 3.2

Barriers and Facilitators to Mental Health Help-Seeking among African American Youth and Their Families: A Systematic Review Study.

Planey, A. M., Smith, S. M., Moore, S., & Walker, T. D. (2019). Barriers and facilitators to mental health help-seeking among African American youth and their families: A systematic review study. Children & Youth Services Review, 101, 190–200.

THE QUESTIONS: 1. What are the barriers to African American youth mental health help-seeking outpatient mental health service use? 2. What are the facilitators of African American youth mental health help-seeking outpatient mental health service use?

METHODS: A systematic approach was used to retrieve relevant research studies related to barriers to and facilitators of mental health service use among Black/African American youth. Articles published between 2000 and 2017 were selected from electronic databases (CINAHL, PsychINFO, and SocINDEX) using keywords that covered the following domains: race, child, mental health, use, and barrier/facilitator. Only empirical qualitative, quantitative, and mixed methods studies were included.

Fifteen articles met study criteria. Six used quantitative methods, eight used qualitative methods, and one used a mixed methods approach. Six studies were reported by the youth, six were reported by parents/caregivers, and two were from gatekeepers (teachers, clinicians). One provided data from youth and caregiver.

FINDINGS: Seven themes identified barriers of mental health help-seeking and service use. (1) Child-related factors included beliefs that the child does not have a mental health problem or the problem is not serious; beliefs that youth should be self-reliant and handle their own problems, and child or youth refused to attend mental health treatment. (2) Clinician-therapeutic barriers included negative prior experiences with mental health care, perceptions that treatments were not effective, lack of trust of the provider, and fear of negative consequences of seeking and using mental health care services. (3) Stigma and shame included fears that friends would laugh, joke, or tease them or that family members might feel offended because they were not able to help and the fear of the caregivers that would find out or what would others think about them. (4) The ideals and values of faith communities were a barrier as well as the lack of information about mental illness shared by religious leaders. (5) Mental health care was not affordable, available, and accessible to many youths. (6) School systems were identified as a barrier by both parents and teachers. Teachers found it difficult to communicate with the parents; parents perceived the school and teachers as part of the problem.

Seven themes identified facilitators of mental health help-seeking and service use. They include severity of child mental health, the caregiver experiences and commitment, a supportive social network, therapeutic factors (positive therapeutic relations), religion and spirituality, referrals and mandates by parents and gatekeepers, and geographic region. (Residence in urban area had more access.)

IMPLICATIONS FOR NURSING: The nurse should recognize that the use of mental health services by African American children and youth involves many barriers and facilitators. In one situation, the school system is a barrier and in another, a facilitator. The children and youth face difficult challenges in accessing quality mental health care. Nurses can identify facilitators and support the caregiver's access to services.

Asian Americans, Polynesians, and Pacific Islanders

In 2018 more than 22.2 million (5.9% of the U.S. population) Asian Americans, Polynesians, and Pacific Islanders lived in the United States, and this group represents one of the fastest growing underrepresented populations in the United States. This large multicultural group includes Chinese, Filipino, Japanese, Asian Indian, Korean, Vietnamese, Laotian, Cambodian, Hawaiian, Samoan, and Guamanian people. Most Chinese, Japanese, Korean, Asian Indian, and Filipino immigrants have migrated to urban areas; the Vietnamese have settled throughout the United States (U.S. Census Bureau, 2020).

Generally, Asian cultures have a tradition of denying or disguising the existence of mental illnesses. In many of these cultures, it is an embarrassment to have a family member treated for mental illness, which may explain the extremely low utilization of mental health services (Chu et al., 2021).

Asian Americans may experience a culture-bound syndrome, such as neurasthenia, which is characterized by fatigue, weakness, poor concentration, memory loss, irritability, aches and pains, and sleep disturbances. Associated with the Korean culture, *hwa-byung*, "suppressed anger syndrome," is characterized by subjective and expressed anger, sensations of heat, and feelings of hate (Im et al., 2017). Research regarding specific mental health problems in Asian cultures is sparse, but various data suggest that rates of suicide within American Indian/Alaska Native adolescents are higher than those of other adolescents in the United States (American Foundation for Suicide Prevention, 2020).

Native Americans

In 2016, the estimated population of Native Americans was more than 6.9 million people, 1.3% of the U.S. population (U.S. Census Bureau, 2018). Native American cultures emphasize respect and reverence for the earth and nature, from which come survival and comprehension of life and one's relationships with a separate, higher spiritual being and with other human beings. Shamans, or medicine men, are central to most cultures. They are healers believed to possess psychic abilities. Healing treatments rely on herbal medicines and healing ceremonies and feasts. Self-understanding derives from observing nature; relationships with others emphasize interdependence and sharing.

Traditional views about mental illnesses vary among the tribes. In some, mental illness is viewed as a supernatural possession, as being out of balance with nature. In certain Native American groups, people with mental illnesses are stigmatized. However, the degree of stigmatization is not the same for all disorders. In tribal groups that make little distinction between physical and mental illnesses, there is little stigma. In other groups, an event, such as suicide, is stigmatized. Different illnesses may be encountered in different Native American cultures and gene pools.

Arab Americans

The Arab American community includes immigrants and their descendants from several Arab world countries including Syria, Lebanon, Egypt, Palestine, Iraq, Jordan, and Yemen. There are an estimated 3.7 million Arab Americans in the United States with two-third living in ten states (California, Michigan, New York, Florida, Texas, New Jersey, Illinois, Ohio, Pennsylvania, and Virginia.) More than one-third live in Los Angeles, Detroit, and New York. More than 82% are U.S. citizens. Arab Americans have a strong commitment to family, economic and educational achievements, and making contributions to all aspects of American life. The first wave of Arab immigrants that came to the United States during the 19th and 20th centuries were primarily Christian. Since the 1960s, Muslim Arabs began immigrating in greater numbers to the United States. Most Arab Americans in the United States practice Christianity (Arab American Institute Foundation, 2020).

Mental illness and seeking mental health care are highly stigmatized in all Arab countries. Although there is little research about the views of Arab Americans, there is emerging evidence that stigma toward mental health treatment is preventing individuals from accessing treatment. They are more likely to visit a primary care provider with somatic problems that represent a mental health problem (Dallo et al., 2018; Dardas & Simmons, 2015; Jaber et al., 2015). An additional stressor is discrimination against the Muslim Arab American community, particularly for men (Lowe et al., 2019).

Women of Underrepresented Groups

Women within underrepresented groups may experience more conflicting feelings and psychological stressors than do men in trying to adjust to both their defined role in the underrepresented culture and a different role in the larger predominant society. Stress from acculturation, stigma toward mental illness, and lack of social support contribute to depression among immigrant women (Ganann et al., 2020). Negative stereotypic attitudes of health care providers may also contribute to reluctance to access mental health care (Kapadia et al., 2018).

Rural Cultures

Most mental health services are in urban areas because most people live near cities. Those living in rural areas have limited access to health care, which leads to fewer people being diagnosed with a mental health problem. Even though rural residents are less likely than urban residents to have mental health diagnoses or receive mental health care, the suicide rate is higher in the rural areas with firearms most commonly used (Marino et al., 2018; Stein et al., 2017). Rural areas are also diverse in both geography and culture. For example, access to mental health for those in the deep South is different from access for those with the same problems in the Northwest. Treatment approaches may be accepted in one part of the country but not in another. Suicide rates are higher in rural areas when compared to urban areas.

SPIRITUALITY, RELIGION, AND MENTAL ILLNESS

Both spirituality and religion are factors that may influence beliefs about mental illness and impact treatment and recovery.

KEYCONCEPT Spirituality develops over time and is a dynamic, conscious process. Although it is not easily defined, there is general agreement that five attributes best describe the essence of spirituality: meaning, belief, connecting, self-transcendence, and value .*Meaning* involves making sense of life and having a purpose to exist. *Belief* provides a coping mechanism and facilitates hope by having something to have faith in. *Connecting* with a higher power and relationships with family and friends serve as an important support for persons in crisis. *Self-transcendence*, the experience and appreciation of a dimension beyond oneself, facilitates spiritual growth. *Value* identifies objects that have value to the person (Stephenson et al., 2017).

Related but different than spirituality, **religiousness** is the participation in a community of people who gather around common ways of worshiping. Spirituality can be expressed through adhering to a set of religious beliefs. Religious beliefs often define an individual's relationship within a family and community. Many different religions are practiced throughout the world. Judeo-Christian thinking tends to dominate Western societies. Other religions, such as Islam, Hinduism, and Buddhism, dominate Eastern and Middle Eastern cultures (Table 3.1). Because religious beliefs often influence approaches to mental health, it is important to understand the basis of various religions that appear to be growing in the United States.

Both religion and spirituality can provide support and strength in dealing with mental illnesses and emotional problems.

People with mental illness benefit from spiritual assessment and interventions (see Chapter 11). Perception of well-being and health in persons with severe mental illness has been positively associated with spirituality and

TABLE 3.1   MAJOR WORLD RELIGIONS AND BELIEF FORMS

Source of Power or Force (Deity)	Historical Sacred Texts or Beliefs	Key Beliefs or Ethical Life Philosophy
Buddhism		
Buddha individual responsibility and logical or intuitive thinking Buddhist subjects include • *Lamaism* (Tibet), in which Buddhism is blended with spirit worship; • *Mantrayana* (Himalayan area, Mongolia, Japan), in which intimate relationship with a guru and recitations of secret mantras are emphasized; belief in sexual symbolism and demons; • *Ch'an* (China) *Zen* (Japan), in which self-reliance and awareness through intuitive understanding are stressed; • *Satori* (enlightenment) may come from "sudden insight" or through self-discipline, meditation, and instruction.	Tripitaka (scripture) Middle Path (way of life) The Four Noble Truths Eightfold Path (guides for life) The Texts of Taoism (include the Tao Te Ching of Lao Tzu and The Writings of Chuang Tzu) Sutras (Buddhist commentaries) Sangha (Buddhist Community)	Buddhism attempts to deal with problems of human existence such as suffering and death. Life is misery, unhappiness, and suffering with no ultimate reality in the world or behind it. The cause of all human suffering and misery is desire. The "middle path" of life avoids the personal extremes of self-denial and self-indulgence. Visions can be gained through personal meditation and contemplation; good deeds and compassion also facilitate the process toward nirvana, the ultimate mode of existence. The end of suffering is the extinction of desire and emotion and ultimately the unreal self. Present behavior is a result of past deed.
Christianity		
God, a unity in tripersonality; Father, Son, and Holy Ghost.	Bible Teachings of Jesus through the apostles and the church fathers	God's love for all creatures is a basic belief. Salvation is gained by those who have faith and show humility toward God. Brotherly love is emphasized in acts of charity, kindness, and forgiveness.
Confucianism		
No doctrine of a God or Gods or life after death. Individual responsibility and logical and intuitive thinking.	Five Classics (Confucian thought) Analects (conversations and sayings of Confucius)	A philosophy or a system of ethics for living rather than a religion that teaches how people should act toward one another. People are born "good." Moral character is stressed through sincerity in personal and public behavior. Respect is shown for parents and figures of authority. Improvement is gained through self-responsibility, introspection, and compassion for others.
Hinduism		
Brahma (the Infinite Being and Creator that pervades all reality) Other Gods: Vishnu (preserver), Shiva (destroyer), Krishna (love)	Vedas (doctrine and commentaries)	All people are assigned to castes (permanent hereditary orders, each having different privileges in society; each was created from different parts of Brahma): 1. *Brahmans:* includes priests and intellectuals. 2. *Kshatriyas:* includes rulers and soldiers. 3. *Vaisya:* includes farmers, skilled workers, and merchants. 4. *Sudras:* includes those who serve the other three castes (servants, laborers, peasants). 5. *Untouchables:* the outcasts; those not included in the other castes.

TABLE 3.1	MAJOR WORLD RELIGIONS AND BELIEF FORMS (Continued)	
Source of Power or Force (Deity)	Historical Sacred Texts or Beliefs	Key Beliefs or Ethical Life Philosophy
Islam		
Allah (the only God) Has two major sects: • *Sunni* (orthodox): traditional and simple practices are followed; human will is determined by outside forces. • *Shiite*: practices are rapturous and trancelike; human beings have free will.	Koran (the words of God delivered to Mohammed by the angel Gabriel) Hadith (commentaries by Mohammed) Five Pillars of Islam (religious conduct) Islam was built on Christianity and Judaism	God is just and merciful; humans are limited and sinful. God rewards the good and punishes the sinful. Mohammed, through the Koran, guides people and teaches them truth. Peace is gained through submission to Allah. The sinless go to Paradise, and the evil go to Hell. A "good" Muslim obeys the Five Pillars of Islam.
Judaism		
God	Hebrew Bible (Old Testament) Torah (first five books of Hebrew Bible) Talmud (commentaries on the Torah)	Jews have a special relationship with God: obeying God's law through ethical behavior and ritual obedience earns the mercy and justice of God. God is worshiped through love, not out of fear.
Shintoism		
Gods of nature, ancestor worship, national heroes.	Tradition and custom (the way of the Gods) Beliefs were influenced by Confucianism and Buddhism	Reverence for ancestors and a traditional Japanese way of life are emphasized. Loyalty to places and locations where one lives or works and purity and balance in physical and mental life are major motivators of personal conduct.
Taoism		
All the forces in nature.	Tao-te-Ching ("The Way and the Power")	Quiet and happy harmony with nature is the key belief. Peace and contentment are found in the personal behaviors of optimism, passivity, humility, and internal calmness. Humility is an especially valued virtue. Conformity to the rhythm of nature and the universe leads to a simple, natural, and ideal life.
Tribal Beliefs		
Animism: Souls or spirits embodied in all beings and everything in nature (trees, rivers, mountains). *Polytheism:* Many Gods, in the basic powers of nature (sun, moon, earth, water).	Passed on through ceremonies, rituals, myths, and legends Oral history, rather than written literature, is the common medium	All living things are related. Respect for powers of nature and pleasing the spirits are fundamental beliefs to meet the basic and practical needs for food, fertility, health, and interpersonal relationships and individual development. Harmonious living is comprehension and respect of natural forces.
Summary of Other Belief Forms		

• *Agnosticism:* the belief that whether there is a God and a spiritual world, or any ultimate reality is unknown and probably unknowable.
• *Atheism:* the belief that no God or Deity exists.
• *Maoism:* the faith that is centered in the leadership of the Communist Party and all the people; the major belief goal is to move away from individual personal desires and ambitions toward viewing and serving all people as a whole.
• *Scientism:* the belief that values and guidance for living come from scientific knowledge, principles, and practices; systematic study and analysis of life, rather than superstition, lead to true understanding and practice of life.

BOX 3.3
The Effects of Religiosity and Spirituality on Mental Health

Peres, M. F. P., Kamei, H. H., Tobo, P. R., & Lucchetti, G. (2018). Mechanisms behind religiosity and spirituality's effect on mental health, quality of life and well-being. Journal of Religion & Health, 57(5), 1843–1855.

THE QUESTION: What spirituality and religiosity aspects are related to quality of life, well-being, and mental health in a general population?

METHODS: A cross-sectional sample of 967 Brazilians were asked to complete questionnaires related to religiousness, faith-peace-meaning, optimism, life satisfaction, happiness, and quality of life.

FINDINGS: From the sample, 80% completed the survey. Participants had a mean age of 34 years, and 51% were female. All participants were married and had a university-level education. Participants identified as Catholics (43.5%), Protestants (7.4%), Spiritists (5.9%), and no religious affiliation or were atheists/agnostics (15.7%).

Meaning and peace were associated with less depressive symptoms and more physical, psychological, social, and environmental quality of life. Peace was also associated with less perceived stress. Faith was associated with more psychological and social quality of life. Meaning and peace were more strongly associated than religiousness with quality of life, mental health, and less stress. Religious participants found greater meaning and peace than nonreligious participants.

IMPLICATIONS FOR NURSING: Helping a person develops meaning, and peace supports positive mental health and quality of life.

religiousness (Box 3.3). To carry out spiritual interventions, the nurse enters a therapeutic relationship with the patient and uses the self as a therapeutic tool. Examples of spiritual interventions include meditation; guided imagery; and, when appropriate, prayer to connect with inner sources of solace and hope.

SUMMARY OF KEY POINTS

- The term *culture* is defined as a way of life that manifests the learned beliefs, values, and accepted behaviors that are transmitted socially within a specific group. Culture also refers to age, gender, sexual orientation, disability, religion, income level, education, geographical location, or profession.

- Everyone has a cultural identity, which helps define expected behavior.

- Cultural and linguistic competence is based on a set of skills that allows individuals to increase their understanding and appreciation of cultural differences and similarities within, among, and between groups. Cultural competence is demonstrated by valuing the culture beliefs, bridging any language gap, and considering the patient's literacy level when planning and implementing care.

- Mental illnesses are stigmatized in many cultural groups. A variety of cultural and religious beliefs underlie the stigmatization.

- Access to mental health treatment is particularly limited for those living in rural areas or those who live in poverty.

- Spirituality can be a source of strength and support for both the patient with mental illness and the nurse providing the care.

- Religious beliefs are closely intertwined with beliefs about health and mental illness.

CRITICAL THINKING CHALLENGES

1. Assess your cultural competence with groups that have the following heritage: African, Asian, Hispanic, Arabic, and Native American.

2. Compare beliefs about mental illnesses within African and Asian American groups.

3. Compare the access to mental health services in your state or county in rural areas versus urban areas.

4. Discuss the differences between spirituality and religiousness. Is it possible that someone can be spiritual and not religious?

5. Identify the religious groups that are associated with the following sacred texts: *Bible, Koran, Vedas,* Texts of Taoism, and *Talmud.*

Unfolding Patient Stories: Li Na Chen

Part 1 (Chinese Family)

Li Na Chen is a 40-year-old Chinese female diagnosed with major depressive disorder who attempted suicide by drug overdose. She is married with two children, ages 12 and 14. Why is it important for the nurse to conduct a cultural assessment of the client and her family? Describe methods the nurse can use to demonstrate cultural competence and avoid inaccurate assumptions about the Chinese culture? What questions can the nurse ask to assess cultural beliefs, practices, and influences on Li Na's mental illness and family functioning?

Movie Viewing Guides
The Big Sick (2017), a comedy, is based on a true story of Kumail Nanjiani (comedian) and Emily Gardner (writer). Kumail Nanjiani, who stars as himself, immigrated to the United States from Pakistan with his family. Kumail and Emily (Zoe Kazan) fall in love

but struggle when their cultures clash. Kumail is expected to live by the traditions of his Muslim parents. Kumail's family is very close and always have dinner together; Emily lives far from her family. Kumail's mother is constantly trying to set up an arranged marriage for him. Emily develops a mysterious illness that forces her to be placed in a medically induced coma, which forces Kumail to negotiate Emily's medical crisis and her parents with his family's expectations.

VIEWING POINTS: Identify the cultural differences between Kumail's and Emily's families. Are any cultural stereotypes depicted in the film? Discuss the role of prejudice and discrimination in the outcome of the movie.

REFERENCES

Agency for Healthcare Research & Quality. (2018). *Health literacy universal precautions toolkit* (2nd ed.). Agency for Healthcare Research and Quality. https://www.ahrq.gov/health-literacy/quality-resources/tools/literacy-toolkit/healthlittoolkit2-intro.html

American Foundation for Suicide Prevention. (2018). Suicide statistics. https://afsp.org/suicide-statistics/.

American Psychiatric Association. (2013). *Diagnostic and statistical manual of mental disorders, DSM-5.* (5th ed.). American Psychiatric Association.

Arab American Institute Foundation. (2020). *Who are Arab Americans?* https://www.aaiusa.org/demographics.

Chu, K. M., Garcia, S., Koka, H., Wynn, G. H., & Kao, T. C. (2021). Mental health care utilization and stigma in the military: Comparison of Asian Americans to other racial groups. *Ethnicity and Health, 26*(2), 235–250. https://doi.org/10.1080/13557858.2018.1494823

Dallo, F. J., Prabhakar, D., Ruterbusch, J., Schwartz, K., Peterson, E. L., Liu, B., & Ahmedani, B. K. (2018). Screening and follow-up for depression among Arab Americans. *Depression and Anxiety, 35*(12), 1198–1206. https://doi.org/10.1002/da.22817

Dardas, L. A., & Simmons, L. A. (2015). The stigma of mental illness in Arab families: A concept analysis. *Journal of Psychiatric and Mental Health Nursing, 22*(9), 668–679.

Fontenot, K., Jessica, S., & Kollar, M. (2018). *Income and Poverty in the United States: 2017.* U.S. Census Bureau, Current Population Reports, P60-263, U.S. Government Printing Office.

Ganann, R., Sword, W., Newbold, K. B., Thabane, L., Armour, L., & Kint, B. (2020). Influences on mental health and health services accessibility in immigrant women with post-partum depression: An interpretive descriptive study. *Journal of Psychiatric and Mental Health Nursing, 27*(1), 87–96.

Glick, A. F., Farkas, J. S., Mendelsohn, A. L., Fierman, A. H., Tomopoulos, S., Rosenberg, R. E., Dreyer, B. P., Melgar, J., Varriano, J., & Yin, H. S. (2019). Discharge instruction comprehension and adherence errors: Interrelationship between plan complexity and parent health literacy. *The Journal of Pediatrics, 214*, 193–200.e3. https://doi.org/10.1016/j.jpeds.2019.04.052

Harris-Haywood, S., Goode, T., Gao, Y., Smith, K., Bronheim, S., Flocke, S. A., & Zyzanski, S. (2014). Psychometric evaluation of a cultural competency assessment instrument for health professionals. *Medical Care, 52*(2), e7–e15. www.lww-medicalcare.com.

Hauenstein, E. J., Clark, R. S., & Merwin, E. I. (2019). Modeling health disparities and outcomes in disenfranchised populations. *Community Mental Health Journal, 55*(1), 9–23.

Im, C. S., Baeg, S., Choi, J. H., Lee, M., Kim, H. J., Chee, I. S., Ahn, S. H., & Kim, J. L. (2017). Comparative analysis of emotional symptoms in elderly Koreans with hwa-byung and depression. *Psychiatry Investigation, 14*(6), 864–870. https://doi.org/10.4306/pi.2017.14.6.864

Jaber, R. M., Farroukh, M., Ismail, M., Najda, J., Sobh, H., Hammad, A., & Dalack, G. W. (2015). Measuring depression and stigma towards depression and mental health treatment among adolescents in an Arab-American community. *International Journal of Culture and Mental Health, 8*(3), 247–254.

Kapadia, D., Nazroo, J., & Tranmer, T. (2018). Ethnic differences in women's use of mental health services: Do social networks plan a role? Findings from a national survey. *Ethnicity & Health, 23*(3), 293–306.

Lowe, S. R., Tineo, P., & Young, M. N. (2019). Perceived discrimination and major depression and generalized anxiety symptoms: In Muslim American College Students. *Journal of Religion & Health, 58*(4), 1136–1145. https://doi.org/10.1007/s10943-018-0684-1

Marino, E., et al. (2018). Addressing the cultural challenges of firearm restriction in suicide prevention: A test of public health messaging to protect those at risk. *Archives of Suicide Research, 22*(3), 394–404.

Markey, K., & Okantey, C. (2019). Nurturing cultural competence in nurse education through a values-based learning approach. *Nurse Education in Practice, 38*, 153–156.

Planey, A. M., Smith, S. M., Moore, S., & Walker, T. D. (2019). Barriers and facilitators to mental health help-seeking among African American youth and their families: A systematic review study. *Children and Youth Services Review, 101*(C), 190–200.

Polster, D. S. (2018). Confronting barriers to improve healthcare literacy and cultural competency in disparate populations. *Nursing2018, 48*(12), 28–33.

Rosales, R., & Calvo, R. (2019). Characteristics of Hispanic-serving mental health organizations in the U.S. *Journal of Health Care for the Poor and Underserved, 30*(2), 547–559. https://doi.org/10.1353/hpu.2019.0032

Schwartz, E. K., Docherty, N. M., Najolia, G. M., & Cohen, A. S. (2019). Exploring the racial diagnostic bias of schizophrenia using behavioral and clinical-based measures. *Journal of Abnormal Psychology, 128*(3), 263–271.

Stafford, A. M., & Draucker, C. B. (2020). Barriers to and facilitators of mental health treatment engagement among Latina adolescents. *Community Mental Health Journal, 56*(4), 662–669. https://doi.org/10.1007/s10597-019-00527-0

Stein, E. M., Gennuso, K. P., Ugboaja, D. C., & Remington, P. L. (2017). The epidemic of despair among white Americans: Trends in the leading causes of premature death, 1999–2015. *American Journal of Public Health, 107*(10), 1541–1547. https://doi.org/10.2105/AJPH.2017.303941

Stephenson, P. S., Sheehan, D., & Shahrour, G. (2017). Support for using five attributes to describe spirituality among families with a parent in hospice. *Palliative & Supportive Care, 15*(3), 320–327. https://doi.org/10.1017/S1478951516000778

Substance Abuse and Mental Health Services Administration. (2014). Improving cultural competence. Treatment improvement protocol (TIP) Series, No. 59. HHS Publication No. (SMA) 14-4849. Substance Abuse and Mental Health Services Administration.

U.S. Census Bureau. (2018). Hispanic or Latino origin by specific origin. Survey/Program: American Community Survey TableID: B03001 https://data.census.gov/cedsci/table?q=Hispanic%20&hidePreview=false&tid=ACSDT1Y2018.B03001&t=Hispanic%20or%20Latino&vintage=2018

U.S. Census Bureau. (2020). Quick facts United States. https://www.census.gov/quickfacts/fact/table/US/PST045219#PST045219

U.S. Department of Health and Human Services. (2020). The annual update of the HHS poverty guidelines. *Federal Register, 12*(85), 3060. https://www.govinfo.gov/content/pkg/FR-2020-01-17/pdf/2020-00858.pdf

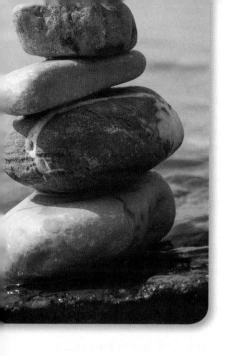

4

Patient Rights and Legal Issues

Rebecca Luebbert

KEYCONCEPT

- self-determinism

LEARNING OBJECTIVES

After studying this chapter, you will be able to:

1. Define self-determinism and its implications in mental health care.

2. Discuss the legal protection of the rights of people with mental illness.

3. Discuss the legal determination of competency.

4. Delineate the differences between voluntary and involuntary treatment.

5. Discuss the difference between privacy and confidentiality.

6. Discuss Health Insurance Portability and Accountability Act and mandates to inform and their implications in psychiatric–mental health care.

7. Describe the persons with mental illness in forensic settings.

8. Discuss the stigma of mental illness and criminality.

9. Describe legal outcomes for persons with mental illness in forensic settings.

10. Identify the importance of accurate, quality documentation in electronic and nonelectronic patient records.

KEY TERMS

- Accreditation • Advance care directives • Assault • Breach of confidentiality • Chemical restraint • Competence • Confidentiality • External advocacy system • Incompetent • Informed consent • Internal rights protection system • Involuntary commitment • Least restrictive environment • Living will • Medical battery • Negligence • Power of attorney • Privacy • Restraint • Seclusion • Voluntary admission • Voluntary commitment

INTRODUCTION

Because individuals with mental disorders are often vulnerable to mistreatment and abuse, their legal rights and the ethical health care practices of mental health providers are ongoing concerns for psychiatric–mental health nurses. For example, can a person be forced into a hospital if their behavior is bizarre but harmless? What human rights can be denied to a person who has a mental disorder and under what circumstances? These questions are not easily answered. This chapter summarizes some of the key patient rights and legal issues that underlie psychiatric–mental health nursing practice across the continuum of care.

SELF-DETERMINISM: A FUNDAMENTAL RIGHT AND NEED

At the foundation of many questions related to the rights of mental health patients is the issue of self-determinism and preservation of this right.

A self-determined individual is internally motivated to make choices based on personal goals, not to please others or to be rewarded. That is, a person engages in activities that are interesting, challenging, pleasing, exciting, or fun, requiring no rewards other than the positive feelings that accompany them because of inner goals, needs, drives, or preferences. Personal autonomy and avoidance of dependence on others are key values of self-determinism, which is integral to the recovery process (see Chapter 2).

In mental health care, self-determinism is the right to choose one's own health-related behaviors, which at times differ from those recommended by health professionals. A patient's right to refuse treatment, to choose an alternate treatment, and to seek a second opinion are all self-deterministic acts. In mental health care, adhering to treatment regimens may be at odds with the self-deterministic views of an individual. Patients may decline taking medication for many reasons, including denial or lack of insight of their illness, concerns about potential side effects or cost of medications, and perceived stigma associated with taking a psychotropic medication (Barloon & Hilliard, 2016). Supporting a person's ability to choose treatment becomes complex because of related issues of competency, informed consent, voluntary and involuntary commitment, and public safety; these issues are discussed later in this chapter.

> **KEYCONCEPT Self-determinism** is based on a person's fundamental right to autonomy. Exercising this right, patients may choose to "accept, refuse, or terminate treatment without deceit, undue influence, duress, coercion, or prejudice" (American Nurses Association, 2015, p. 2).

PROTECTION OF PATIENT RIGHTS

Because people with psychiatric problems are vulnerable to mistreatment and abuse, laws exist that guarantee them legal protection. These laws offer protection of self-determinism, protection against discrimination in employment, and protection against mistreatment in health care settings.

Self-Determination Act

The Patient Self-Determination Act was implemented on December 1, 1991, as a part of the Omnibus Budget Reconciliation Act of 1990 and requires hospitals, health maintenance organizations, skilled nursing facilities, home health agencies, and hospices receiving Medicare and Medicaid reimbursement to inform patients at the time of admission of their right to be a central part of any and all health care decisions made about them or for them. Patients have the following rights:

- Be provided with information regarding advance care documents.
- Be asked at admission or enrollment whether they have an advance care document and that this fact be recorded in the medical record.
- Be provided with information on their rights to complete advance care documents and refuse medical care (*Omnibus Budget Reconciliation Act*, 1990).

The Act also requires health care institutions receiving Medicare and Medicaid reimbursement to educate health care personnel and the local community about advance care planning.

Advance Care Directives in Mental Health

At different times during the course of an illness, people with mental disorders may be unable to make sound decisions regarding their treatment and care. Fortunately, advance care directives legally protect them from their periodic poor decision-making abilities. A competent individual can make a decision about a treatment—a decision that can be honored even if the person is no longer able to make decisions. (See later discussion for how competency is determined.)

Advance care directives are written instructions for health care when individuals are incapacitated. Living wills and appointment directives, often referred to as **power of attorney** or health proxies, are recognized under state laws and their courts. A **living will** specifies what treatment should be omitted or refused in the event that a person is unable to make those decisions. A **durable power of attorney** for health care appoints a proxy, usually a relative or trusted friend, to make health care decisions on an individual's behalf if that person is incapacitated.

An advance directive does not need to be written, reviewed, or signed by an attorney. It must be witnessed by two people and notarized and applies only if the individual is unable to make their own decisions as a result of being incapacitated or if, in the opinion of two physicians, the person is otherwise unable to make decisions for themselves.

Psychiatric advance directives (PADs) allow patients, while competent, to document their choices of treatment and care. This declaration must be made in advance and signed by the patient and two witnesses. Through the use of a PAD, individuals are empowered to direct their treatment such as choice of medication and hospitalization. Although a physician can override this declaration during times when the patient's decision-making capacity is clearly distorted because of mental illness, the patient must be informed first and the order made by the court. During periods of competency, the PAD can be revoked.

Bill of Rights for Mental Health Patients

Rights of people with mental disorders receive additional protection beyond that afforded to patients in other health care areas (Box 4.1). The Mental Health Systems Act [42 U.S.C. 9501 et seq.] of 1980 requires that each state review and revise, if necessary, its laws to ensure that mental health patients receive these human rights protections and services that they require.

Americans with Disabilities Act and Job Discrimination

The Americans with Disabilities Act of 1990 ensures that people with disabilities, including those with mental illnesses and addictions, have legal protection against discrimination in the workplace, housing, public programs, transportation, and telecommunications. An employer is free to select the most qualified applicant available, but if the most qualified person has a mental disorder, this law mandates that reasonable accommodations need to be made for that individual. Accommodations include any adjustments to a job or work environment, such as restructuring a job, modifying work schedules, and acquiring or modifying equipment (U.S. Equal Employment Opportunity Commission, Office of the Americans with Disabilities Act, 2020).

Access to Mental Health Services

Mental health services are one of the 10 designated Essential Health Benefits requiring coverage through plans established by the Patient Protection and Affordable Care Act. Services required include behavioral health treatment, counseling, and psychotherapy. The Mental Health Parity and Addiction Equity Act requires insurance plans to offer comparable benefits and coverage for mental and substance disorders that are offered for medical and surgical coverage. Treatment fees and limitations for mental health services cannot be any more restrictive than those designated for medical care (Substance Abuse and Mental Health Services Administration [SAMHSA], 2020).

BOX 4.1

Bill of Rights for Persons Receiving Mental Health Services

- The right to appropriate treatment and related services under conditions that support the person's personal liberty and restrict such liberty only as necessary to comply with treatment needs, laws, and judicial orders.
- The right to an individualized, written treatment or service plan (to be developed promptly after admission), treatment based on the plan, periodic review and reassessment of needs, and appropriate revisions of the plan, including a description of services that may be needed after discharge.
- The right to ongoing participation in the planning of services to be provided and in the development and periodic revision of the treatment plan, and the right to be provided with a reasonable explanation of all aspects of one's own condition and treatment.
- The right to refuse treatment, except during an emergency situation or as permitted under law in the case of a person committed by a court for treatment.
- The right not to participate in experimentation in the absence of the patient's informed, voluntary, written consent; the right to appropriate protections associated with such participation; and the right to an opportunity to revoke such consent.
- The right to freedom from restraints or seclusion, other than during an emergency situation.

- The right to a humane treatment environment that affords reasonable protection from harm and appropriate privacy.
- The right to confidentiality of records.
- The right to access, upon request, one's own mental health care records.
- The right (in residential or inpatient care) to converse with others privately and to have access to the telephone and mails unless denial of access is documented as necessary for treatment.
- The right to be informed promptly, in appropriate language and terms, of the rights described in this section.
- The right to assert grievances with respect to infringement of the Bill of Rights, including the right to have such grievances considered in a fair, timely, and impartial procedure.
- The right of access to protection, service, and a qualified advocate in order to understand, exercise, and protect one's rights.
- The right to exercise the rights described in this section without reprisal, including reprisal in the form of denial of any appropriate, available treatment.
- The right to referral as appropriate to other providers of mental health services upon discharge.

From 42 (U.S. Code § 10841)—Restatement of bill of rights. Title V of the Mental Health Systems Act [42.U.S.C. 9501 et seq].

Internal Rights Protection Systems

Mental health care systems have **internal rights protection systems** or mechanisms to combat any violation of their patients' rights. Public Law 99–319, the Protection and Advocacy for Mentally Ill Individuals Act of 1986, requires each state mental health provider to establish and operate a system that protects and advocates for the rights of individuals with mental illnesses and investigates any incidents of abuse and neglect.

External Advocacy Systems

Health organizations such as the American Hospital Association, American Healthcare Association, and the American Public Health Association serve as advocates for the rights and treatment of mental health patients and are a part of an **external advocacy system**. They are financially and administratively independent from the mental health agencies. These groups advocate through negotiation and recommendations but have no legal authority. They can resort to litigation that leads to lawsuits and consent decrees (legal mandates that are monitored by the U.S. Department of Justice) or, in some instances, a denial of accreditation to the health care institution by their certifying body.

Accreditation of Mental Health Care Delivery Systems

Patient rights are also assured of protection by an agency's **accreditation**, the recognition or approval of an institution according to the accrediting body's criteria. Accrediting bodies such as The Joint Commission require patient rights standards. The Centers for Medicare and Medicaid Services (CMS) sets patient rights standards for institutions seeking Medicare and Medicaid funding. Community mental health centers are not accredited by either the Joint Commission or CMS but by another agency, the Commission on Accreditation of Rehabilitation Facilities.

TREATMENT AND PATIENT RIGHTS

In caring for patients receiving mental health services or treatment, it is important for nurses to understand several issues related to the patient's rights to determine choices about their own treatment. These issues are related to competency, informed consent, least restrictive environment, and voluntary and involuntary treatment.

Competency

One of the most important concepts underlying the legal rights of individuals is competency to consent to or to refuse treatment. Although competency is a legal determination, it is not clearly defined across the states. It is generally agreed that **competence**, or the degree to which the patient can understand and appreciate the information given during the consent process, refers to a patient's cognitive ability to process information at a specific time. A patient may be competent to make a treatment decision at one time and not be competent at another time. Similarly, competence is also decision specific, so that a patient may be competent to decide on a simple treatment with a relatively clear consequence but may not be competent to decide about a treatment with a complex set of outcomes. A competent patient can refuse any aspect of the treatment plan.

Competency is different from rationality, which is a characteristic of a patient's decision, not of the patient's ability to make a decision. An irrational decision is one that involves hurting oneself pointlessly, such as stopping recommended treatment even though symptoms return. A person who is competent may make what appears to be an irrational decision, and it cannot be overruled by health care providers; however, if a person is judged **incompetent** (i.e., unable to understand and appreciate the information given during the consent process), it is possible to force treatment on the individual. Strong arguments are, however, made against forced treatment under these circumstances. Forced treatment denigrates individuals, and according to self-determinism theory and recovery concepts, individuals are not as likely to experience treatment success if it is externally imposed.

How is it determined that a patient is competent? Mental health legal experts generally agree that four areas should be directly assessed (Appelbaum, 2007). Table 4.1 outlines these assessment areas. A patient who is competent to give informed consent should be able to achieve the following:

- Communicate choices.
- Understand relevant information.
- Appreciate the situation and its consequences.
- Use a logical thought process to compare the risks and benefits of treatment options.

Informed Consent

Individuals seeking mental health care must provide **informed consent**, a legal procedure to ensure that the patient knows the benefits and costs of treatment. Merely signing a consent document does not imply an informed consent. To provide informed consent for care, the patient must be given adequate information upon which to base decisions and actively participate in the decision-making process. Informed consent is not an option but is mandated by state laws. In most states, the

TABLE 4.1	DETERMINATION OF COMPETENCY	
Assessment Area	**Definition**	**Patient Attributes**
Communicate choices	Ability to express choices	Patient should be able to clearly indicate their treatment choice.
Understand relevant information	Capacity to comprehend the meaning of the information given about treatment	Patient should be able to paraphrase understanding of treatment.
Appreciate the situation and its consequence	Capacity to grasp what the information means specifically to the patient	Patient should be able to discuss the disorder, the need for treatment, the likely outcomes, and the reason the treatment is being suggested.
Use a logical thought process to compare the risks and benefits of treatment options	Capacity to reach a logical conclusion consistent with the starting premise	Patient should be able to discuss logical reasons for the choice of treatment.

Adapted from Appelbaum, P. (2007). Assessment of patients' competence to consent to treatment. *New England Journal of Medicine, 357*(18), 1834–1840.

law mandates that a mental health provider must inform a patient in such a way that an average reasonable person would be able to make an educated decision about the interventions.

Informed consent is complicated in mental health treatment. A patient must be competent to give consent, but the individual's decision-making ability often is compromised by the mental illness. This dilemma might be illustrated by a situation in which a person who is informed of medication side effects refuses treatment, not because of the potential negative impact of the medication but because they deny the illness outright. The health care provider knows that when the person begins taking the medication, the symptoms of the illness may subside, and the decision-making ability will return.

Most institutions have policies that outline the nursing responsibilities within the informed consent process. The nurse has a key role in the process of informed consent, from structuring the written informed consent document to educating the patient about a particular procedure. The nurse makes sure that consent has been obtained before any treatment is given. Informed consent is especially important in research projects involving experimental drugs or therapies.

Least Restrictive Environment

The right to refuse treatment is related to a larger concept—the right to be treated in the **least restrictive environment**, which means that an individual cannot be restricted to an institution when they can be successfully treated in the community. In 1975, the courts ruled that a person committed to psychiatric treatment had a right to be treated in the least restrictive environment (*Dixon v. Weinberger*, 1975). Medication cannot be given

unnecessarily. An individual cannot be restrained or locked in a room unless all other *less restrictive* interventions are tried first.

Seclusion and Restraint

Seclusion is the involuntary confinement of a person in a room or an area where the person is physically prevented from leaving (CMS, 2015). A patient is placed in seclusion for purposes of safety or behavioral management. The seclusion room has no furniture except a mattress and a blanket. The walls are usually padded. The room is environmentally safe, with no hanging devices, electrical outlets, or windows from which the patient could jump. When a patient is placed in seclusion, they are observed at all times.

There are several types of seclusion arrangements. Some facilities place seclusion rooms next to the nurses' stations. These seclusion rooms have an observation window. Other facilities use a modified patient room and assign a staff member to view the patient at all times. Seclusion is an extremely negative patient experience; consequently, its use is seriously questioned, and many facilities have completely abandoned its practice (Box 4.2). Patient outcomes may actually be worse if seclusion is used.

The most restrictive safety intervention is the use of **restraint**, any manual method, physical or mechanical, that immobilizes or reduces the ability of the patient to move. The nurse must choose the least restrictive type of restraint to keep a patient safe. Wrist restraints restrict arm movement. Walking restraints or ankle restraints are used if a patient cannot risk the impulse to run from a facility but is safe to go outside and to activities. Three- and four-point restraints are applied to the wrist and ankles in bed. When five-point restraints are used, all extremities are secured, and another restraint is placed

---

BOX 4.2

Evidence for Seclusion and Restraint Use

Sailas, E., & Fenton, M. (2012). Seclusion and restraint for people with serious mental illnesses. The Cochrane Database of Systematic Reviews, (2), CD001163.

THE QUESTION: How effective are seclusion, restraint, or alternative controls for people with serious mental illness?

METHODS: A meta-analysis of the effectiveness of seclusion and restraint compared with the alternatives for persons with serious mental illnesses was conducted. Randomized controlled trials were included if they focused on the use of restraint or seclusion or strategies designed to reduce the need for restraint or seclusion in the treatment of serious mental illness. The search yielded 2155 citations. Of these, 35 studies were obtained.

FINDINGS: No controlled studies exist that evaluate the value of seclusion or restraint in those with serious mental illness. There are reports of serious adverse effects for these techniques in qualitative reviews.

IMPLICATIONS FOR NURSING: Alternative ways of dealing with unwanted or harmful behaviors need to be developed. Continuing use of seclusion or restraint must, therefore, be questioned.

---

across the chest. **Chemical restraint** is the use of medications for restricting patients' behavior or their freedom of movement. These chemical restraints include medications that are not a part of their standard psychiatric treatment or that are at a higher dosage of their standard medication.

Restraints should be applied only after every other intervention is used and the patient continues to be a danger to self or others. Documentation must reflect a careful assessment of the patient that indicates the need for an intervention to protect the patient from harm (CMS, 2015). In addition, nurses should document all of the previously tried de-escalation interventions before the application of restraints (see Chapter 10). Restraints should be removed when the patient regains control over their behavior. The nurse should closely observe the patient and protect them from self-injury continuously while the patient is in seclusion and/or restraints.

Definite risks are associated with the use of seclusion and restraint; consequently, its use is seriously questioned (see Box 4.2). The use of seclusion and restraint can result in psychological harm and physical injury to both the patient and staff members involved in its use. Injury rates to staff in settings involving the use of seclusion and restraint are found to be higher than in other high-risk industries. Additionally, studies have shown that patients who have been secluded or restrained prolong their treatment time and are more likely to be readmitted for further treatment (SAMHSA, 2019).

In recovery-oriented practice, the nurse is particularly sensitive to recognizing the relationship between earlier trauma and retraumatizing a person by using restraint. Trauma-informed care, being aware of, and sensitive to doing no further harm to survivors of trauma, is important in recovery-oriented practice. There is general agreement that in order to use a trauma-informed approach, the patient needs to feel connected, valued, informed, and hopeful of recovery (SAMHSA, 2014); the staff recognize the connection between earlier trauma and adult mental health problems; and staff work in mindful and empowering ways with individuals and families (Muskett, 2014).

The use of both seclusion and restraints must follow the Medicare regulations contained in the Patients' Rights Condition of Participation (CMS, 2015). Agencies that do not follow the regulations may lose their Medicare and Medicaid certification and, consequently, their funding. The application of physical restraints should also follow hospital policies. Fundamental principles for the nurse to follow when considering the use of seclusion and restraints include the following:

- Seclusion or restraint must never be used out of convenience, as a punishment, or as a means of coercion.
- Seclusion or restraint must only be used as a last resort, when all other least restrictive means are shown to be ineffective.
- Seclusion or restraint must be used for the minimal amount of time necessary to ensure the safety of the patient or others.
- When mechanical restraint is necessary, only the least number of the restraint points must be used and the individual must be under continuous observation (APNA Position Statement on the Use of Seclusion and Restraint, 2018).

Voluntary and Involuntary Treatment

Accessing the mental health delivery system is similar to seeking any other type of health care. Whether in a public or private system, the treatment setting is usually for outpatient. Treatment strategies (e.g., medication, psychotherapy) are recommended and agreed on by both the provider and the individual. Arrangements for treatment and follow-up are then made. The patient leaves the outpatient setting and is responsible for following the plan.

Inpatient treatment is generally reserved for patients who are acutely ill or have a forensic commitment. If hospitalization is required, the person enters the treatment facility, participates in the treatment planning process, and follows through with the treatment. The individual maintains all civil rights and is free to leave at any time even if it is against medical advice. In most settings, this type of admission is called a **voluntary admission**. If an individual is admitted to a public facility, the state statute may refer to the process as **voluntary commitment** rather than admission; however, in both instances, full legal rights are retained.

Involuntary commitment is the mandated treatment without the person's consent but with a court order. There are also legal provisions for people to be involuntarily committed to outpatient mental health facilities through state civil laws. Because involuntary commitment is a prerogative of the state agency, each state and the District of Columbia have separate commitment statutes; however, three common elements are found in most of these statutes. There should be evidence that the individual is (1) mentally disordered, (2) dangerous to self or others, or (3) unable to provide for basic needs (i.e., *gravely disabled*).

Patients who are involuntarily committed have the right to receive treatment, but they also may have the right to refuse it. Arguments over the rights of civilly committed patients to refuse treatment first surfaced in 1975 when a federal district court judge issued a temporary restraining order prohibiting the use of psychotropic medication against the patient's will at a state hospital in Boston. Laws about commitment and refusal of medication vary from state to state. A separate judicial process may be necessary if an individual is determined to be incompetent to refuse medication. Forcing a patient to take medication against their will without a legal provision to do so may expose the nurse to liability (Barloon & Hilliard, 2016).

Commitment procedures vary considerably among the states. Most have provisions for an emergency short-term hospitalization of 48 to 92 hours authorized by a certified mental health provider without court approval. These emergency hospitalizations are often initiated by a concerned family member or friend. At the end of this time-limited period, either the individual agrees to voluntary treatment or extended commitment procedures are begun. The judge must order the commitment, and the individual is afforded several legal rights, including notice of the proceedings, a full hearing (jury trial if requested) in which the government must prove the grounds for commitment, and the right to legal counsel at state expense.

PRIVACY AND CONFIDENTIALITY

In addition to issues related to self-determinism, privacy and confidentiality are rights requiring protection for mental health patients. **Privacy** refers to the part of an individual's personal life that is not governed by society's laws and government intrusion. Protecting an individual from intrusion is a responsibility of health care providers. **Confidentiality** pertains to an ethical duty of nondisclosure. Patients often share intimate details of their lives during the course of treatment, including personal thoughts, experiences, and behaviors. Providers who receive confidential information within their nurse–patient relationship must protect that information from being accessed by others and resist disclosing it. Confidentiality involves two people: the individual who discloses and the person with whom the information is shared. If confidentiality is broken, a person's privacy is also violated; however, a person's privacy can be violated but confidentiality maintained. For example, if a nurse observes an adult patient reading pornography alone in their room, the patient's privacy has been violated. If the patient asks the nurse not to tell anyone and the request is honored, confidentiality is maintained.

A **breach of confidentiality** occurs when a nurse divulges a patient's personal information without the patient's consent. Examples of a breach in confidentiality include discussing a patient's problem with one of their relatives without the patient's consent and sharing patient information with another professional who is not involved in the patient's care when the individual has not given permission for the information to be shared. Maintaining confidentiality is not as easy as it first appears. For example, family members are legally excluded from receiving any information about an adult member without consent even if that member is receiving care from the family. Ideally, a patient gives consent for information to be shared with the family or has psychiatric advance care directive. Ultimately, it is the nurse's duty to safeguard both personal and clinical information in the work setting as well as off duty in all venues, including social media (American Nurses Association, 2015).

NCLEXNOTE Which patient is most likely a candidate for involuntary commitment? A patient who refuses to take medication or one who is singing in the street in the middle of the night disturbing the neighbors?

Answer: The patient who is singing in the night disturbing the neighbors. Rationale: Patients have a right to refuse medication in many states and provinces. Refusing medication does not pose an immediate danger to self or others. The patient who is singing in the street is more likely to be judged as a danger to self or others.

 Concept Mastery Alert

Privacy is the part of the person's life that is not governed by laws. *Confidentiality* is the responsibility of the health care worker to limit sharing of patient information with only those mandated to know. Confidentiality affords the patient privacy.

Health Insurance Portability and Accountability Act and Protection of Health Information

The Health Insurance Portability and Accountability Act of 1996 (HIPAA) provides legal protection in several areas of health care, including privacy and confidentiality. This act protects working Americans from losing existing health care coverage when changing jobs and increases opportunities for purchasing health care. It regulates the use and release of patient information, especially electronic transfer of health information. Effective April 2003, HIPAA regulations require patient authorization for the release of information with the exception of that required for treatment, payment, and health care administrative operations. The release of information related to psychotherapy requires patient permission. The underlying intent is to prevent the release of information to agencies not related to health care, such as employers, without the patient's consent. When information is released, the patient must agree to the exact information that is being disclosed, the purpose of disclosure, the recipient of the information, and an expiration date for the disclosure of information (U.S. Department of Health and Human Services, 2002).

The American Recovery and Reinvestment Act of 2009 includes several provisions affecting the management of health information. For the most part, this law focuses on maintaining privacy of electronic transfer and storage of health information and communication. In the clinical area, one way of maintaining privacy is by restricting access to records by staff members unless there is a specific reason such as caring for a patient.

Mandates to Inform

At certain times, health care professionals are legally obligated to breach confidentiality. When there is a judgment that the patient has harmed any person or is about to injure someone, professionals are mandated by law to report it to authorities. The legal *duty to warn* was a result of the 1976 decision of *Tarasoff v. Regents of the University of California* (1976). In this case, a 26-year-old graduate student told university psychologists about his obsession with another student, Tatiana Tarasoff, whom he subsequently killed. Tatiana Tarasoff's parents initiated a separate civil action and brought a lawsuit against the therapist, the university, and the campus police, claiming that Tatiana's death was a result of negligence on the part of the defendants.

The plaintiffs claimed that the therapists should have warned Ms. Tarasoff that the graduate student presented a danger to her and that he should have been confined to a hospital. Both claims were originally dismissed in the lower courts, but in 1974, the California Supreme Court reversed the lower courts' decisions and said that Ms.

Tarasoff should have been warned. The high court said that psychotherapists have a duty to warn the foreseeable victims of their patients' violent actions. Because of the outcry from professional mental health organizations, the court agreed to review the case, and in 1976, the original decision was revised by the ruling that psychotherapists have a duty to exercise reasonable care in protecting the foreseeable victims of their patients' violent actions. The results of this case have had far-reaching consequences and have influenced many decisions in the United States. Although many lawsuits have been based on the *Tarasoff* case, most have failed. Usually, if there are clear threats of violence toward others, the therapist is mandated to warn potential victims.

> **NCLEXNOTE** What guides the intervention for a patient who tells the nurse that they want to hurt a family member: mandate to inform or HIPAA?
> Answer: Mandate to inform. Rationale: Because others are at risk for injury, the *Tarasoff* decision will prevail.

CRIMINAL JUDICIAL PROCESSES

In mental health, the term *forensic* pertains to legal proceedings and mandated treatment of persons with a mental illness. Individuals with mental illnesses are at higher risk for arrest than the general population and are more likely to have encounters with the criminal justice system and be convicted of a crime than those without a mental illness (Gottfried & Christopher, 2017). Despite the large number of people with mental illnesses that commit crimes, the majority of the encounters with the justice system occur when individuals with mental illness are victims of crime (National Alliance on Mental Illness, 2020).

As the number of state hospitals was dramatically reduced beginning in the 1960s, the number of persons with mental illness incarcerated in jails and prisons increased. Individuals in crisis are more likely to encounter the police versus the mental health care system. Approximately 2 million individuals with mental illness are incarcerated in prisons and jails in the United States per year, including 15% of incarcerated men and 30% of incarcerated women (National Alliance on Mental Illness, 2020). High rates of substance use and substance use disorders are found in incarcerated adults and youth, and among both men and women. The prevalence of post-traumatic stress disorder and mood and anxiety disorders are also higher in incarcerated individuals than in the general population (Gottfried & Christopher, 2017). Individuals with schizophrenia or bipolar disorder are 10 times more likely to be in a prison or jail than in a psychiatric treatment facility (Treatment Advocacy Center, 2020).

Individuals with mental illnesses are treated in a variety of forensic settings, including county jails, correctional facilities, psychiatric hospitals, and the community. The number of admissions to state psychiatric hospitals is increasing for the first time since the 1970s because of an increase of forensic patients (Torrey et al, 2014). Forensic patients often do not receive sufficient treatment for their illness while they are incarcerated, however, and are at risk for further deterioration and revictimization (Gottfried & Christopher, 2017; National Alliance on Mental Illness, 2020).

Stigma of Criminality

Incarcerated patients suffer the combined effects of the stigma of mental illness and criminality. Although stigma is an issue for all persons with a mental illness, it is magnified for those who have committed a crime. There is often reluctance on the part of mental health professionals to treat these patients, especially if murder and childhood sexual abuse are involved. Even if the worry is unfounded, clinicians express safety concerns for themselves and other patients and may refuse to care for these patients.

When nonforensic patients receive the maximum benefit from hospitalization, they are normally discharged back into the community. For forensic patients, the community often wants a more stringent discharge threshold and unrealistically expects the hospital to guarantee compliance with community rules and structure. Treatment and the criminal justice systems are often in conflict with each other.

Fitness to Stand Trial

Once a mental illness is diagnosed in a person who has committed a crime, the individual's **fitness to stand trial** is determined. Fitness means that a person is able to consult with a lawyer with a reasonable degree of rational understanding of the facts of the alleged crime and of the legal proceedings as spelled out in the court case of *Dusky v. United States* of 1960 (Beran & Tommey, 1979, p. 12). A person is found **unfit to stand trial** if, because of mental or physical condition, they are unable to understand the nature and purpose of the proceedings or to assist in the defense (West, 2017).

In most states, when an individual with a mental illness is found unfit to stand trial, hospitalization in a forensic mental health facility follows. The goal of this hospitalization is to help the person become *fit* to stand trial, not to treat the mental illness. Sometimes, the patient's mental illness has to be treated to attain fitness. Simply stated, to be fit to stand trial, the person must be able to communicate with counsel and assist in the defense;

be able to appreciate their presence in relation to time, place, and things; be able to understand that they are in a court of justice charged with a criminal offense; show an understanding of the charges and their consequences, as well as court procedures and the roles of the judge, jury, prosecutor, and defense attorney; and have sufficient memory to relate the circumstances surrounding the alleged criminal offense.

An individual cannot be *unfit* forever. If fitness cannot be attained usually within 1 year, a hearing is held, during which the facts of the alleged crime are presented to a judge who rules on the case. If the charges are dismissed, the judge could order a civil commitment. If there is sufficient evidence to convict, the individual could be sent back to the hospital for further treatment to attain fitness. The maximum length of this additional treatment is based on the severity of the charge. For those accused of sexual-related offenses (because of mental disorder), states usually have special statutes for hospitalization and discharge (e.g., registration and community notification).

Not Guilty by Reason of Insanity

Once fitness to stand trial is established, the trial or hearing can proceed. One possible outcome is **not guilty by reason of insanity (NGRI)**. The accused is judged unable to distinguish right from wrong or to be unable to control their actions at the time of the crime. The rationale underlying this ruling is one of fairness. It is unfair to hold a person responsible if that individual does not know that the action is wrong or does not have control over their behavior.

Nearly all individuals found NGRI are also subject to involuntary commitment in a *secure* setting. The patient cannot leave hospital grounds without court approval. A person sentenced NGRI is given a date that is equal to the time or sentence to be served if they had been guilty of the crime.

Guilty but Mentally Ill

Different from NGRI, in which *not guilty* individuals are committed to the mental health system, **guilty but mentally ill (GBMI)** is a criminal conviction, and the person is sent to the correctional system. Mental illness is considered a factor in the crime but not to the extent that the individual is incapable of knowing right from wrong or controlling their actions. The sentence for the GBMI is the same type of determinate sentence any inmate receives. Before release, every effort is made to ensure that patients will receive proper follow-up care in the community and close monitoring by parole staff. Both NGRI and GBMI persons are treated for their mental disorders, but one is treated in jail and the other in a hospital. The conditions of release are different. Whereas individuals with a GBMI are subject to the correctional system's parole decisions, those with an NGRI are discharged from the hospital through the courts upon recommendations of the forensic mental health professionals.

Probation

Probation is a sentence of conditional or revocable release under the supervision of a probation officer for a specified time. For individuals with a mental illness who have committed minor offenses, probation is sometimes used instead of jail as long as care in a treatment facility can be arranged. If treatment and rehabilitation are successful, criminal charges may be dropped and a prison record avoided. Probation is also used when a criminal has served time and continued monitoring is needed after being released from the correctional facility.

Misconceptions Regarding Insanity Pleas

There are many misconceptions about the insanity plea. One is that the insanity defense provides a loophole through which criminals can escape punishment for illegal acts. In reality, the insanity defense is extremely difficult to use even in the cases of severely ill individuals. As a result, despite popular belief, the insanity defense is used in fewer than 1% of criminal cases (Box 4.3).

Countless newspaper articles, talk shows, and news commentaries concerning the insanity defense have bombarded the public. Some of the cases have been highly

---

BOX 4.3

The Case of Andrea Yates

In March 2002, Andrea Yates, age 37 years, was convicted of murder for drowning her five children. She was sentenced to life in prison despite past treatment for postpartum depression and psychosis, four hospitalizations, and two suicide attempts. Andrea Yates was found guilty because in her testimony to the police, she stated that she knew the criminal justice system would punish her for her actions, implying that she knew the acts were wrong in the eyes of the law. Texas law does not recognize that for someone as ill as Andrea Yates, mental illnesses can create more powerful hierarchies of right and wrong than societal law. In July 2006, Andrea was granted a retrial because the previous verdict was overturned on appeal because of erroneous testimony. At the second trial, Andrea was found not guilty by reason of insanity. She was committed to a state mental hospital with periodic hearings before a judge to determine whether she should be released (Biography.com, 2020).

---

publicized. One such case was that of John Hinckley, who attempted to assassinate President Ronald Reagan in 1981 and who was found NGRI. On psychiatric examination, Hinckley was found to be living in a "fantasy world with magical and grandiose expectations of impressing and winning over" his love, actress Jodie Foster (Goldstein, 1995, p. 309). Hinckley attempted to commit a historic deed that would make him famous and unite him with the love object of his delusions. His acquittal stimulated public cries for reform of the insanity defense. Within 2.5 years of John Hinckley's acquittal, 34 states changed their insanity defense statutes to limit its use or to prevent the premature release of dangerous people.

Gun Laws and Mental Illness

The Brady Handgun Violence Prevention Act of 1993, commonly referred to as the Brady Act or Brady Bill, was originally proposed in response to Hinckley's assassination attempt on President Reagan. The Brady Act requires a background check on individuals seeking ownership of a firearm. Under this Act, individuals considered mentally incompetent, having severe mental illness, or those having been committed to a mental institution are prohibited from gun ownership. There is much controversy surrounding gun control for persons with mental illness. While the laws are intended to restrict firearms in those determined to be of significant danger to others, the reality is that only a very small percentage of all violent crimes are perpetrated by individuals diagnosed with mental illness. Therefore, insisting that gun violence is strictly a mental health problem unfairly stigmatizes those with mental illness (Philpott-Jones, 2018).

ACCOUNTABILITY FOR NURSES AND OTHER MENTAL HEALTH CARE PROFESSIONALS

Nurses and other health care professionals are accountable for the care they provide in mental health as well as any other practice area.

Legal Liability in Psychiatric Nursing Practice

Malpractice is based on a set of torts (a civil wrong not based on contract committed by one person that causes injury to another). An **assault** is the threat of unlawful force to inflict bodily injury upon another. An assault must be imminent and cause reasonable apprehension in the individual. Battery is the intentional and unpermitted contact with another. **Medical battery**, intentional and unauthorized harmful or offensive contact, occurs when a patient is treated without informed consent. For example, a clinician who fails to obtain consent before performing a procedure is subject to being accused of medical battery. Also, failure to respect a patient's advance directives is considered medical battery. False imprisonment is the detention or imprisonment contrary to provision of the law. Facilities that do not discharge voluntarily committed patients upon request can be subject to this type of litigation.

Negligence is a breach of duty of reasonable care for a patient for whom a nurse is responsible that results in personal injuries. A clinician who does get consent but does not disclose the nature of the procedure and the risks involved is subject to a negligence claim. Five elements are required to prove negligence: duty (accepting assignment to care for patient), breach of duty (failure to practice according to acceptable standards of care), cause in fact (the injury would not have happened if the standards had been followed), cause in proximity (harm actually occurred within the scope of foreseeable consequence), and damages (physical or emotional injury caused by breach of standard of care). Simple mistakes are not negligent acts.

Lawsuits in Psychiatric Mental Health Care

Few lawsuits are filed against mental health clinicians and facilities compared with other health care areas. If psychiatric nurses are included in lawsuits, they are usually included in the lawsuit filed against agency. Common areas of litigation surround the nursing care of patients who are suicidal or violent. Maintaining and documenting an appropriate standard of care can protect nurses from complicated legal proceedings. The following can help prevent negative outcomes of malpractice litigations:

- Evaluate risks, especially when privileges broaden or care is transferred.
- Document decisional processes and reasons for choices among alternatives.
- Involve family in important decisions.
- Make decisions within team model and document this shared responsibility.
- Adhere to agency's policy and procedures.
- Seek consultation and record input.

Nursing Documentation

Careful documentation is important both to help ensure protection of patient rights and for nurse accountability.

Documentation can be handwritten or electronic. It is very common in psychiatric facilities that all disciplines record one progress note. Nursing documentation is based on nursing standards (see Chapter 6) and the policies of the particular facility. Many documentation styles are problem focused. That is, documentation is structured to address specific problems that are identified on the nursing care plan or interdisciplinary treatment plan. No matter the setting or structure of the documentation, nurses are responsible for documenting the following:

- Observations of the patient's subjective and objective physical, psychological, and social responses to mental disorders and emotional problems
- Interventions implemented and the patient's response
- Observations of therapeutic and side effects of medications
- Evaluation of outcomes of interventions

Particular attention should be paid to the reason the patient is admitted for care. If the person's initial problem was suicide or homicidal ideation, the patient should routinely be assessed for suicidal and homicidal thoughts even if the treatment plan does not specifically identify suicide and homicide as potential problems. Careful documentation is always needed for patients who are suicidal, homicidal, aggressive, or restrained in any way. Medications prescribed as needed (pro re nata) also require a separate entry, including reason for administration, dosage, route, and response to the medication.

A patient record is the primary documentation of a patient's problems, verifies the behavior of the patient at the point of care, and describes the care provided. The patient record is considered a legal document. Courts consider acts not recorded as acts not done. Patients also have legal access to their records. For handwritten documentation, the entries should always be written in pen with no erasures. If an entry is corrected, it should be initialed by the person making the correction. All entries should be clear, well written, and void of jargon. Judgmental statements, such as *patient is manipulating staff*, have no place in patients' records. Only meaningful, accurate, objective descriptions of behavior should be used. General, stereotypic statements, such as *had a good night* or *no complaints*, are meaningless and should be avoided.

With the universal use of electronic records, meaningful documentation is sometimes more difficult. Many institutions require health care workers to enter observations, assessment data, and interventions into a template that requires a *click* in a box on the monitor screen. Additional narrative entries are usually required to provide quality, individualized care. Nurses should adhere to the same standards of practice and documentation when entering electronic data as when entering data in a non-electronic record.

SUMMARY OF KEY POINTS

- The right of self-determination entitles all patients to refuse treatment, to obtain other opinions, and to choose other forms of treatment. It is one of the basic patients' rights established by Title II, Public Law 99–139, outlining the Universal Bill of Rights for Mental Health Patients.

- Laws and systems are established to protect the rights of people with mental health issues. Some of these include the Self-Determination Act, advance directives, a patient Bill of Rights, the Americans with Disabilities Act, internal rights protection systems, external advocacy systems, and accreditation of mental health care delivery systems.

- The internal rights protection system and the external advocates combat violations of human rights.

- Informed consent is another protective right that helps patients decide what can be done to their bodies and minds. It must be obtained from a competent individual before any treatment is begun to ensure that the information is not only received but also understood.

- A competent person can refuse any treatment. Incompetence is determined by the court when the patient cannot understand the information.

- The right to the least restrictive environment entitles patients to be treated in the least restrictive setting and by the least restrictive interventions and protects patients from unnecessary confinement and medication.

- Seclusion or restraint should be used as a last resort and only when there is risk of harm to the patient or someone else. Patients secluded or restrained should be under continuous observation by staff.

- Involuntary commitment procedures are specified at the state level. Patients who are involuntarily committed have the right to refuse treatment and medication.

- Patient privacy is protected through HIPAA regulations related to the transfer and storage of information. A breach in confidentiality is legally mandated when there is a threat of violence toward others.

- Nursing documentation is guided by practice standards and policies of the agency. Nurses are responsible for individualized documentation in both electronic and nonelectronic health records.

CRITICAL THINKING CHALLENGES

1. Consider the relationship of self-determinism to competence by differentiating patients who are competent to give consent and those who are incompetent. Discuss the steps in determining whether a patient is competent to provide informed consent for a treatment.

2. Define competency to consent to or refuse treatment and relate the definition to the Self-Determination Act.

3. A patient is involuntarily admitted to a psychiatric unit and refuses all medication. After being unable to persuade the patient to take prescribed medication, the nurse documents the patient's refusal and notifies the prescriber. Should the nurse attempt to give the medication without patient consent? Support your answer.

4. A person who is homeless with a mental illness refuses any treatment. Although he is clearly psychotic and would benefit from treatment, he is not a danger to himself or others and seems to be able to provide for his basic needs. His family is desperate for him to be treated. What are the ethical issues underlying this situation?

5. Discuss the purposes of living wills and health proxies. Discuss their use in psychiatric–mental health care.

6. Identify the legal and ethical issues underlying the *Tarasoff* case and mandates to inform.

7. Compare the authority and responsibilities of the internal rights protection system with those of the external advocacy system.

Movie Viewing Guides

Lady in the Van: (2015). This movie is based on a true story about Miss Mary Shepherd (Maggie Smith), an eccentric, homeless woman, who temporarily parked her old van in the driveway of Allen Bennett's (Alex Jennings) upper-middle-class home in Camden, England. She stayed for 15 years. The story depicts the strained relationship as he tried to humanely move her to more suitable housing. As the story develops, Bennett learns that Miss Shepherd is really Margaret Fairchild (died in 1989), a former gifted pupil of the pianist Alfred Cortot. She had played Chopin in a promenade concert, had tried to become a nun, was committed to an institution by her brother, had escaped, had had an accident when her van was hit by a motorcyclist for which she believed herself to blame, and thereafter lived in fear of arrest.

VIEWING POINTS: How does the relationship between Mary Shepard and Allen Bennett change during the 15-year period. Are Miss Shepard's rights being violated? Does she have the right to remain parked in Mr. Bennett's driveway. What legal measures were used in the movie?

REFERENCES

American Nurses Association. (2015). *Code of ethics for nurses with interpretive statements*. American Nurses Association.

American Psychiatric Nurses Association. (2018). *APNA position statement on the use of seclusion and restraint*. https://www.apna.org/i4a/pages/index.cfm?pageid=3728

Appelbaum, P. (2007). Assessment of patients' competence to consent to treatment. *New England Journal of Medicine, 357*(18), 1834–1840.

Barloon, L. F., & Hilliard, W. (2016). Legal considerations of psychiatric nursing practice. *Nursing Clinics of North America, 51*(2), 161–171.

Beran, N. J., & Tommey, B. G. (1979). Mentally ill offenders and the criminal justice system. In *Issues in forensic services* (pp. 1–23). Proeger Special Studios.

Biography.com (Editors). (2020). Andrea Yates biography. https://www.biography.com/crime-figure/andrea-yates

Brady Handgun Violence Prevention Act of 1993. 18 U.S. Code §921-922 (Public Law 103–159, 107 Stat. 1536, November 30, 1993).

Centers for Medicare and Medicaid Services. (2015). *Interpretive guidelines for hospital CoP for patient rights: Quality of care information, quality standards 418.54*. https://www.cms.gov/Regulations-and-Guidance/Guidance/manuals/downloads/som107ap_m_hospice.pdf

Dixon v. Weinberger, 405 F. Supp. 974 (D. D. C. 1975).

Goldstein, R. (1995). Paranoids in the legal system: The litigious paranoid and the paranoid criminal. *Psychiatric Clinics of North America, 18*(2), 303–315.

Gottfried, E. D., & Christopher, S. C. (2017). Mental disorders among criminal offenders: A review of the literature. *Journal of Correctional Health Care, 23*(3), 336–346.

Muskett, C. (2014). Trauma-informed care in inpatient mental health settings: A review of the literature. *International Journal of Mental Health Nursing, 23*(1), 51–59.

National Alliance on Mental Illness. (2020). Jailing people with mental illness. https://www.nami.org/Advocacy/Policy-Priorities/Divert-from-Justice-Involvement/Jailing-People-with-Mental-Illness

Omnibus Budget Reconciliation Act of 1990. Public Law No. 101–158, Paragraph 4206, 4751.

Philpott-Jones, S. (2018). Mass shootings, mental illness, and gun control. *Hastings Center Report, 48*(2), 7–9.

Sailas, E., & Fenton, M. (2012). Seclusion and restraint for people with serious mental illness. *The Cochrane Database of Systematic Reviews*, https://doi.org/10.1002/14651858.CD001163.

Substance Abuse and Mental Health Services Administration. (2014). SAMHSA's concept of trauma and guidance for a trauma-informed approach. HHS Publication No. (SMA) 14-4884. Substance Abuse and Mental Health Services Administration.

Substance Abuse and Mental Health Services Administration. (2019). Alternatives to seclusion and restraint. https://www.samhsa.gov/trauma-violence

Substance Abuse and Mental Health Services Administration. (2020). Laws, regulations, and guidelines. https://www.samhsa.gov/about-us/who-we-are/laws-regulations

Tarasoff v. Regents of the University of California, 551P. 2d 334 (Cal. 1976).

Torrey, E. F., Zdanowicz, M. T., Kennard, A. D., Lamb, H. R., Eslinger, D. F., Biasotti, M. C., & Fuller, D. A. (2014). *The treatment of persons with mental illness in prisons and jails: A state survey*. Arlington, VA: Treatment Advocacy Center. http://www.treatmentadvocacycenter.org/storage/documents/treatment-behind-bars/treatment-behind-bars.pdf

Treatment Advocacy Center. (2020). Serious mental illness: By the numbers. https://www.treatmentadvocacycenter.org/storage/documents/smi_infographic.pdf

U.S. Code § 10841-Restatement of bill of rights. Title V of the Mental Health Systems Act [42.U.S.C. 9501 et seq]. https://www.law.cornell.edu/uscode/text/42/10841

U.S. Department of Health and Human Services. (2002). Standards for privacy of individually identifiable health information; final rule. *Federal Register, 65*, 53182–53273.

U.S. Equal Employment Opportunity Commission, Office of the Americans with Disabilities Act. (2020). Your employment rights as an individual with a disability. https://www.eeoc.gov/laws/guidance/your-employment-rights-individual-disability

West, T. (Ed.). (2017). *West Illinois criminal law and procedure* (2017 ed.). Thompson Reuters.

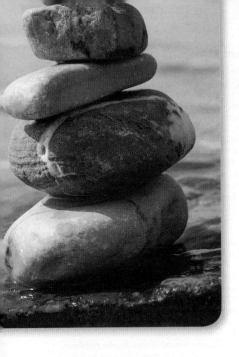

5
Mental Health Care in the Community

Mary Ann Boyd

KEYCONCEPTS

- case management
- continuum of care

LEARNING OBJECTIVES

After studying this chapter, you will be able to:

1. Define and explain continuum of care for mental health services.

2. Explain how the concept of the least restrictive environment influences the choice of treatment settings.

3. Identify various mental health treatment settings and associated programs along the continuum of care.

4. Discuss the role of the psychiatric nurse at different points along the continuum of care.

5. Describe the integration of psychiatric and medical care in community settings.

KEY TERMS

- 23-hour observation • Assertive community treatment • Board-and-care homes • Case management
- Coordination of care • Crisis intervention • Crisis intervention teams • Digital applications
- In-home mental health care • Integrated care • Intensive case management • Intensive outpatient program
- Intensive residential services • Medical home • Outpatient detoxification • Partial hospitalization
- Peer support services • Psychiatric rehabilitation programs • Recovery centers • Reintegration • Relapse
- Residential services • Telehealth • Therapeutic foster care • Transfer • Transitional care

INTRODUCTION

The evolution of a behavioral health care system is affected by scientific advances and social factors. Recovery from mental illness is a goal at all stages of treatment. The long-term nature of mental illnesses requires varying levels of care at different stages of the disorders as well as family and community support. Treatment costs are shared among public and private sectors. A demand exists for a comprehensive, holistic approach to care that encompasses all levels of need. Consumers, families, providers, advocacy groups, and third-party payers of mental health care no longer accept long-term institutionalization, once the

hallmark of psychiatric care. Instead, they advocate for short-term treatment in an environment that promotes dignity and well-being while meeting the patient's biologic, psychological, and social needs.

Reimbursement issues influence health care delivery. In the United States, health maintenance organizations, preferred provider organizations, Medicaid, and Medicare have set limits on the types and lengths of treatment for which they provide reimbursement coverage, which in turn influences the kind of care the patient receives. In other countries, other regulatory bodies influence access and treatment options. Fragmentation of services is a constant threat. Today, psychiatric–mental health nurses face the challenge of providing mental health care within a complex system that is affected by financial constraints and narrowed treatment requirements.

DEFINING THE CONTINUUM OF CARE

A continuum of care that supports recovery can be viewed from various perspectives and ranges from intensive treatment (hospitalization) to supportive interventions (outpatient therapy). An individual's needs for ongoing clinical treatment and care are matched with the intensity of professional health services.

In a continuum, continuity of care is provided over an extended time. The appropriate medical, nursing, psychological, or social services may be delivered within one organization or across multiple organizations. The continuum facilitates the stability, continuity, and comprehensiveness of service to an individual and maximizes the coordination of care and services.

> KEYCONCEPT A **continuum of care** consists of an integrated system of settings, services, health care clinicians, and care levels, spanning illness-to-wellness states.

Least Restrictive Environment

The primary goal of the continuum of care is to provide treatment that supports recovery in the **least restrictive environment** (see Chapter 4). In 1999, the U.S. Supreme Court reinforced the principle of least restrictive environment with the Olmstead decision, which states that it is a violation of the Americans with Disabilities Act to institutionalize people with severe mental illnesses when services in the community are equally effective (*Olmstead v. L.C.*, 1999). Therefore, treatment is usually delivered in the community (as opposed to a hospital or institution) and, ideally, in an outpatient setting.

Coordination of Care

Coordination of care is the integration of appropriate services so that individualized care is provided. Appropriate services are those that are tailored to address a client's strengths and weaknesses, cultural context, service preferences, and recovery goals, including referral to community resources and liaisons with others (e.g., physician, health care organizations, and community services). Several agencies could be involved, but when care is coordinated, a person's needs are met without duplication of services. Coordination of care requires collaborative and cooperative relationships among many services, including primary care, public health, mental health, social services, housing, education, and criminal justice, to name a few.

In some instances, a whole array of integrated services is needed. For example, children can benefit from treatment and specialized support at home and school. These wraparound services represent a unique set of community services and natural supports individualized for the child or adult and family to achieve a positive set of outcomes.

Case Management

Coordinated care is often accomplished through a **case management** service model in which a case manager locates services, links the patient with these services, and then monitors the patient's receipt of these services. This type of case management is referred to as the *broker* model. Case management can be provided by an individual or a team; it may include both face-to-face and telephone contact with the patient as well as contact with other service providers. **Intensive case management** is targeted for adults with serious mental illnesses and children with serious emotional disturbances. Managers of such cases have fewer caseloads and higher levels of professional training than do traditional case managers.

> KEYCONCEPT **Case management** is a professional and collaborative process that assesses, plans, implements, coordinates, monitors, and evaluates the options and services required to meet an individual's health needs. It uses communication and available resources to promote health, quality, and cost-effective outcomes in support of the 'Triple Aim,' of improving the experience of care, improving the health of populations, and reducing per capita costs of healthcare (Commission for Case Manger Certification [CCMC], 2015, p. 4).

Case management services are built on a strong working alliance between the patient and the case manager. Quality is assessed by measuring patient outcomes that result from the services, such as symptom reduction, improved functioning and community integration, and patient satisfaction with the services provided. In addition, case managers can optimize a patient's use of resources by developing a treatment plan that closely matches the individual needs of the patient and by matching the most appropriate treatment to the patient's phase of illness.

The Nurse as Case Manager

Case managers work in a variety of settings, including insurance companies, hospitals, workmen compensation, and independent organizations (Armold, 2019). Psychiatric nurse case managers serve in various pivotal functions across the continuum of care. These functions can involve both direct care and coordination of the care delivered by others. The repertoire of required skills includes collaboration with members of a multidisciplinary team, teaching, management, leadership, group, and research skills. The nurse case manager must have firm knowledge of psychiatric nursing and be able to function independently. This role is probably the most diverse role within the psychiatric continuum.

Virtual Health Care

Telehealth, the delivery of health-related services and information via digital communication technologies, is rapidly appearing as a primary strategy in the delivery of health care, particularly mental health throughout the continuum of care. The coronavirus disease (COVID-19) pandemic drove dramatic acceleration in the use and acceptance of digital health care as a credible option to in-person visits. Now, telehealth is preferred by many clinicians and patients in certain situations (Peek et al., 2020).

Telehealth had its beginning in the early 1900s, and as technology advanced, the impact of digital communication has assumed increasing importance (see Table 5.1). The technology was initially used as a method of storing and forwarding medical information, but its use quickly expanded to remote medical monitoring. Today, it is widely used for real-time interactive services. **Digital applications** or apps are used for all three—storing and forwarding, remote medical monitoring, and interactive services (Cassatly & Cassatly, 2017).

In mental health care, telehealth was initially viewed as a way of providing access to mental health services in rural communities because of clinician shortages, lack of public transportation, and poverty. Telehealth contact with patients after discharge from the hospital allowed nurses to assess psychiatric symptoms, check on medication adherence, discuss approaches to solving problems associated with community living, and provide emotional support. As technology advanced, more telehealth applications became available to those in rural areas.

Even though the technology supported virtual interaction, there were several barriers that prevented utilization of the service. Internet connectivity was not always available in rural areas. Clinicians were often reluctant to use technology for fear of missing indications of suicide or other safety issues. Third-party insurers were unwilling to pay for telehealth visits. An in-person visit was required before controlled substances could be prescribed, and Health Insurance Portability and Accountability Act and Privacy Standards required strict secure two-way communication preventing the use of Zoom, Skype, or FaceTime.

These barriers were relaxed or removed during the COVID-19 pandemic. Medicare began paying for office, hospital, and other visits furnished via telehealth across the country in 2020. Health Insurance Portability and Accountability Act and Privacy Standards were relaxed; visits were no longer limited to rural settings. Prescribers were able to issue prescriptions for controlled substances to patients using telemedicine without a prior in-person patient medical evaluation.

Telehealth interventions for the treatment, prevention, diagnosis, and management of depression, serious mental illness, and substance use are now used in most urban and rural settings (Box 5.1). Videoconferencing, e-mail, mobile apps, and texting are being used (Naslund et al., 2017).

TABLE 5.1	HISTORY OF TELEHEALTH IN U.S. HEALTH CARE
Date	**Events**
Early 1900s	Patient interview over telephone.
1950s	Psychiatrist–patient interaction over closed-circuit television.
1960s	U.S. space program introduced remote medical monitoring.
1990s	Internet is introduced. Health professionals began sharing information electronically.
1996	Institute of Medicine report—Telemedicine: A Guide to Assessing Telecommunication for Healthcare.
2010	Affordable Care Act resulted in improvement in broadband support, medical networks, electronic health records.
2020	Coronavirus pandemic caused a need for remote health care delivery leading to reduction in barriers and widespread use of telehealth.

BOX 5.1

Use of a Mobile App to Improve Distress

Stallman, H. M. (2019). Efficacy of the My Coping Plan mobile application in reducing distress: A randomised controlled trial. Clinical Psychologist, 23(3), 206–212.

THE QUESTION: Is the strengths-focused My Coping Plan app effective in improving mental health and coping?

METHODS: Fifty-six university students with self-reported elevated levels of distress (K10 total ≥ 16) were randomly assigned to the intervention (My Coping Plan) or waitlist control condition.

RESULTS: At 1-month follow-up, participants in the intervention condition reported significantly lower psychological distress ($d = 0.31$), improved well-being ($d = -0.42$), and improved healthy coping strategies ($d = 0.39$) compared with those in the control condition. There was no significant difference between groups in reported unhealthy coping strategies. The majority of participants downloaded the app and made a coping plan. Just over half used their plan when they were distressed.

IMPLICATIONS FOR NURSING: Mobile apps have potential to improve mental health and well-being in the short term, likely through increased self-efficacy.

MENTAL HEALTH SERVICES IN A CONTINUUM OF CARE

Crisis Care

An organized approach is required to treat individuals in crisis, including a mechanism for rapid access to care (within 24 hours), a referral for hospitalization, or access to outpatient services.

Crisis Intervention

Crisis intervention—a specialized short-term, goal-directed therapy for those in acute distress—is brief, usually lasting fewer than 6 hours (see Chapter 21). This type of short-term care focuses on stabilization, symptom reduction, and prevention of relapse requiring inpatient services.

Crisis intervention units can be found in the emergency departments of general and psychiatric hospitals and in crisis centers within community mental health centers. Patients in crisis demonstrate severe symptoms of acute mental illness, including labile mood swings, suicidal ideation, or self-injurious behaviors. Therefore, this treatment option commands a high degree of nursing expertise. Patients in crisis usually require medications such as anxiolytics or benzodiazepines for symptom management. Key nursing roles include assessment of short-term therapeutic interventions and medication administration. Nurses also facilitate referrals for admission to the hospital or for outpatient services.

Crisis intervention teams (CTI)—interdisciplinary mental health specialists and first responders—provide protection to individuals with mental illness symptoms who are a threat to self or others. Law enforcement personnel, such as police officers, are often the first responders when crises occur in the community. Police officers need to accurately assess and intervene in crisis situations and determine whether the people involved in the crisis are experiencing behavioral problems due to symptoms of mental illness. CIT have been developed to train police officers to recognize and intervene in crisis situations in the community and determine whether emergency psychiatric services are needed. Crisis intervention by CIT-trained police officers can avoid inappropriate involvement of the patient in the criminal justice system and ensure that patients with behavioral problems due to mental illnesses receive appropriate psychiatric treatment (Crisanti et al., 2019).

23-Hour Observation

The use of **23-hour observation** is a short-term treatment that serves the patient in immediate but short-term crisis. This type of care admits individuals to an inpatient setting for as long as 23 hours, during which time services are provided at a less-than-acute care level. The clinical problem usually is a transient disruption of baseline function, which will resolve quickly. Usually, the individual is experiencing suicidal or homicidal ideation, which presents a threat to themselves or others. The nurse's role in this treatment modality is assessment and monitoring. Medications also are usually administered. This treatment is used for acute trauma, such as rape and alcohol and narcotic detoxification, and for individuals with personality disorders who present with self-injurious behaviors.

Crisis Stabilization

When the immediate crisis does not resolve quickly, crisis stabilization is the next step. This type of care usually lasts fewer than 7 days and has a symptom-based indication for hospital admission. The primary purpose of stabilization is control of precipitating symptoms through medications, behavioral interventions, and coordination with other agencies for appropriate aftercare. The major focus of nursing care in a short-term inpatient setting is symptom management. Ongoing assessment; short-term, focused interventions; and medication administration and monitoring of efficacy and side effects are major components of nursing care during stabilization. Nurses may also provide focused group psychotherapy designed to develop and strengthen the personal management strategies of patients. When treating aggressive or violent patients, the nurse implements the appropriate use of seclusion and restraints according to facility policy.

Acute Inpatient Care

Acute inpatient hospitalization is the most intensive treatment and occurs in the most restrictive setting in the continuum. Inpatient treatment is reserved for acutely ill patients who, because of a mental illness, meet one or more of three criteria: high risk for harming themselves, high risk for harming others, or unable to care for their basic needs. Delivery of inpatient care can occur in a psychiatric hospital, psychiatric unit within a general hospital, or public-operated facility. Nursing care is critical in the acute care setting and is provided around the clock.

Admission to inpatient environments can be voluntary or involuntary (see Chapter 4). The average length of stay for an involuntary admission ranges between 24 hours and several days, depending on the state or province laws; the length of stay for a voluntary admission depends on the acuity of symptoms and the patient's ability to pay the costs of treatment. It is unconstitutional in the United States to confine a nondangerous person with a mental illness with an involuntary hospitalization when the patient can survive independently with the help of willing and responsible family or friends. Nevertheless, the interdisciplinary treatment team determines that the patient is no longer at risk to themselves or others before discharge can occur.

Both the number of available beds in psychiatric hospitals in the United States and length of inpatient stay have continually decreased since the 1980s, a trend attributed to managed care and expansion of multidisciplinary, intensive community-based services, such as **assertive community treatment (ACT)**. Additional contributors to decreased length of stay include strict admission criteria and regulations that determine the need for continued hospitalization. Currently, admission to a hospital is determined based on medical necessity, such as dangerousness or the need for crisis stabilization. Discharge is a complex process that varies from setting to setting often depending on the resources of individual, hospital, and community systems (Xiao et al., 2019).

Partial Hospitalization

Partial hospitalization programs (PHPs), also referred to as day treatment programs, were developed to complement inpatient mental health care and outpatient services and provide treatment to patients with acute psychiatric symptoms who are experiencing a decline in social or occupational functioning, who cannot function autonomously on a daily basis, or who do not pose imminent danger to themselves or others. It is a time-limited, ambulatory, active treatment program that offers therapeutically intensive, coordinated, and structured clinical services within a stable milieu. The aim of PHPs is patient stabilization without hospitalization or reduced length of inpatient care. An alternative to inpatient treatment, PHP usually provides the resources to support therapeutic activities both for full-day and half-day programs. This level of care does not include overnight hospital care; however, the patient can be admitted for inpatient care within 24 hours.

In **partial hospitalization**, the interdisciplinary treatment team partners with the patient and devises and executes a comprehensive plan of care encompassing behavioral therapy, social skills training, basic living skills training, education regarding illness and symptom identification and relapse prevention, community survival skills training, relaxation training, nutrition and exercise counseling, and other forms of expressive therapy. Group-based services such as wellness education and counseling for comorbid serious mental illnesses and substance abuse are also provided (Taube-Schiff et al., 2019). Compared with other outpatient programs, PHPs offer more intensive nursing care.

Residential Services

Residential services provide a place for people to reside during a 24-hour period or any portion of the day on an ongoing basis. A residential facility can be publicly or privately owned. **Intensive residential services** are intensively staffed for patient treatment. These services may include medical, nursing, psychosocial, vocational, recreational, or other support services. Combining residential care and mental health services, this treatment form offers rehabilitation and therapy to people with serious and persistent mental illnesses, including chronic schizophrenia, bipolar disorder, and unrelenting depression. These services may provide short-term treatment for stays from 24 hours to 3 or 6 months or long-term treatment for several months to years.

As a result of deinstitutionalization, many patients who were unable to live independently were discharged from state hospitals to intermediate- or skilled-care nursing facilities. The use of nursing homes for residential care is controversial because many of these facilities lack mental health services. Residential care in nursing homes varies from state to state. If a facility serves a primarily geriatric population, placement of younger persons there can be problematic. If a facility with more than 16 beds is engaged primarily in providing diagnosis, treatment, or care of persons with mental disorders (including medical attention, nursing care, and related services), it is designated by the federal government as an institution for mental disease (IMD). A Medicare-certified facility having more than 16 beds and at least 50% of residents with a mental disorder is also considered an IMD. An IMD may not qualify for matching federal Medicaid dollars, which means that the state has principal responsibility for funding inpatient psychiatric services (Congressional Research Service, July 30, 2019).

Nursing plays an important role in the care of people who have severe and persistent mental illnesses and who require partial hospitalization or long-term stays at residential treatment facilities. Nurses provide recovery-oriented psychiatric nursing care with a focus on psychoeducation, basic social skills training, aggression management, activities of daily living training, and group living. Education on symptom management, understanding mental illnesses, and medication is essential for recovery. The *Psychiatric–Mental Health Nursing: Scope and Standards of Practice* guides the nurse in delivering patient care (American Nurses Association, American Psychiatric Nurses Association, & International Society of Psychiatric-Mental Health Nurses, 2014) (see Chapter 11).

Respite Residential Care

Sometimes, the family of a person with mental illness who lives at home may be unable to provide care continuously.

In such cases, respite residential care can provide short-term necessary housing for the patient and periodic relief for the caregivers.

Transitional Care

Health service systems have established a goal of reducing readmission following discharge from the hospital. Risk for 30-day readmission following discharge is high among people diagnosed with mental illnesses (Lewis et al., 2019). People with serious mental illnesses need support and access to community resources when they are discharged from inpatient hospitalization but are often unable to access resources due to cognitive impairments, poor problem-solving skills, social isolation, unstable housing, and poverty. Access to these resources is critically important to promote medication adherence and attendance at the first follow-up appointment following discharge from the hospital.

Transitional care interventions have been used in the community to ensure that people with mental illnesses stay engaged in treatment between discharge from the hospital and the first follow-up appointment. Some programs provide intensive interventions immediately after discharge with reducing the intensity when the person returns for a follow-up appointment; some use peer support specialists over a long length of time (Tyler et al., 2019).

In-Home Mental Health Care

If at all possible, people with mental illnesses live at home, not in a residential treatment setting. The goals are choices, not placement; physical and social integration, not segregated and congregate grouping by disability; and individualized flexible services and support, not standardized levels of service. When a person can live at home but outpatient care does not meet the treatment needs, **in-home mental health care** may be provided. Home care emphasizes the personal autonomy of the patient and the need for a trusting, collaborative relationship between the nurse and the patient (Roldán-Merino et al., 2013). In this setting, direct patient care and case management skills are used to decrease hospital stays and increase the functionality of the patient within the home. Individuals who most benefit from in-home mental health care include patients with chronic, persistent mental illness or patients with mental illness and comorbid medical conditions that require ongoing monitoring.

In-home mental health care services rely on the skills of the mental health nurse in providing ongoing assessment and implementing a comprehensive, individualized treatment plan of care. Components of the care plan and the ongoing assessment include data on mental health status, the environment, medication compliance, family dynamics and home safety, supportive psychotherapy, psychoeducation, coordination of services delivered by other home care staff, and communication of clinical issues to the patient's psychiatrist. In addition, the plan should address care related to collecting laboratory specimens (blood tests) and crisis intervention to reduce rehospitalization.

Outpatient Care

Outpatient care is a level of care that occurs outside of a hospital or institution. Outpatient services usually are less intensive and are provided to patients who do not require inpatient, residential, or home care environments. Many patients enroll in outpatient services immediately upon discharge from an inpatient setting. Outpatient treatment can include ongoing medication management, skills training, supportive group therapy, substance abuse counseling, social support services, and case management. People with severe mental illnesses have high rates of comorbid medical illnesses, and many outpatient mental health clinics have developed integrated mental health–primary care treatment models to address the physical health needs of those with mental illnesses. These varying services promote community **reintegration** (return and acceptance of a person as a fully participating member of a community), symptom management, and healthy lifestyle (Murphy et al., 2019).

Intensive Outpatient Programs

The primary focus of **intensive outpatient programs** is on stabilization and relapse prevention for highly vulnerable individuals who function autonomously on a daily basis. People who meet these criteria have returned to their previous lifestyles (e.g., interacting with family, resuming work, and returning to school). Attendance in this type of program benefits individuals who still require frequent monitoring and support within a therapeutic milieu that enables them to remain connected to the community. The duration of treatment and level of services rendered are based on the patient's immediate needs. The treatment duration usually is time limited, with sessions offered 3 to 4 hours per day and 2 to 3 days per week. The treatment activities of the intensive outpatient program are similar to those offered in PHPs; whereas PHPs emphasize social skills training, intensive outpatient programs teach patients about stress management, illness, medication, and relapse prevention.

Other Services Integrated into a Continuum of Care

Within the continuum of care, other outpatient services may be received separately or simultaneously within various settings. They involve discrete services and patient variables.

Peer Support Services

Peer support services are provided by mental health consumers who have experienced symptom remission and are actively involved in their own recovery from mental illness. Peer support specialists typically work in outpatient settings, such as community mental health centers, therapeutic rehabilitation centers, and **recovery centers**. The peer support specialist works with other mental health consumers who are in the process of moving toward recovery goals. The relationship between peer specialists and mental health consumers offers an opportunity for offering mutual support for coping with mental illness and reciprocal sharing of personal experiences in the process of recovery. Peer support specialists assist consumers with self-determination and personal responsibility for recovery. They can also teach mental health consumers effective self-management skills and self-advocacy and encourage participation in wellness and recovery activities (Lapidos et al., 2018).

Outpatient Detoxification

There is an increasing shift toward providing alcohol and drug detoxification in an outpatient setting. The decision to use outpatient detoxification depends on symptom severity and types of drugs the patient uses. Patients with alcohol dependence who show signs of tolerance and withdrawal can undergo detoxification in an outpatient setting. However, patients who undergo ambulatory detoxification must have reliable family members who are available to provide monitoring. Outpatient detoxification is not suitable for situations involving severe or complicated withdrawal, especially with delirium. In addition, patients who are pregnant or have a history of a seizure disorder are hospitalized for detoxification.

Outpatient detoxification is a specialized form of partial hospitalization for patients requiring medical supervision. During the initial withdrawal phase, use of a 23-hour bed may be a treatment option, depending on the stage of withdrawal and the type of addictive substance used. Or the patient may be required to attend a detoxification program 4 to 5 days per week until symptoms resolve. The length of participation depends on the severity of addiction.

Outpatient detoxification includes a 12-step recovery model, such as Alcoholics Anonymous (AA) and Narcotics Anonymous (NA), which provides outpatient involvement with professionals experienced in addiction counseling. It encourages abstinence and provides training in stress management and relapse prevention. Al-Anon and Alateen rely on 12-step support for families, who are usually included in the treatment program.

In-Home Detoxification

Detoxification from alcohol may be done in the home. For home detoxification to be safe and effective, symptoms of withdrawal must be mild, and a family member must be present at all times. The nurse is required to visit the patient daily for medication monitoring during the patient's first week of sobriety. Daily visits are necessary until the patient is in a medically stable condition. Referrals may come from primary care physicians, court mandates, or employee assistance programs.

Assertive Community Treatment

The ACT model is a multidisciplinary clinical team approach providing 24-hour, intensive community-based services. ACT typically includes low staff-to-patient ratios, but this may not be possible in rural areas with shortages of qualified mental health professionals and few services (Spivak et al., 2019). The ACT model helps individuals with serious mental illness live in the community by providing a comprehensive range of treatments, rehabilitation, and supportive services to help patients meet the requirements of community living. Concentration of services for high-risk patients within a single multiservice team enhances continuity and coordination of care, which improves the quality of care. ACT can reduce length of hospitalization and emergency department services, which reduces the cost of mental health treatment for patients with serious mental illnesses (Thoegersen et al., 2019).

RECOVERY-ORIENTED REHABILITATION SETTINGS

Psychiatric rehabilitation programs, also termed *psychosocial rehabilitation*, focus on the reintegration of people with psychiatric disabilities into the community through work, education, and social avenues while addressing their medical and residential needs. The goal is to empower patients to achieve the highest level of functioning possible. Therapeutic activities or interventions are provided individually or in groups. They may include development and maintenance of daily and community living skills, such as communication (basic language), vocational, self-care (grooming, bodily care, feeding), and social skills that help patients function in the community. These programs promote increased functioning with the least necessary ongoing professional intervention. Psychiatric rehabilitation provides a highly structured environment, similar to a PHP, in a variety of settings, such as office buildings, hospital outpatient units, and freestanding structures.

The mental health nurse's role continues to focus on the consumer's recovery goals in all treatment settings. As behavioral health care delivery occurs more in outpatient settings, so does the work of nurses. Most rehabilitation programs have a full-time nurse who functions as part of the multidisciplinary team.

Psychiatric rehabilitation nurses are concerned with the recovery-oriented, holistic evaluation of the person and with assessing and educating the patient on compliance issues, necessary laboratory work, and environmental and lifestyle issues. This evaluation assesses the five dimensions of a person—physical, emotional, intellectual, social, and spiritual—and emphasizes recovery. Issues of psychotropic medication—evaluation of response, monitoring of side effects, and connection with pharmacy services—also fall to the nurse.

Self-Help Groups

Self-help groups are available in the community. These include AA, NA, and related 12-step programs. AA and NA use peer support as a strategy for helping people who are attempting to abstain from alcohol or drug use. Counseling, mentoring, and support are provided by individuals with alcohol or drug dependence who successfully abstain from substance use. In many cases, people with comorbid substance abuse and psychiatric diagnoses, such as schizophrenia and bipolar disorder, are unable to benefit from traditional AA self-help groups because of their psychiatric symptoms. For this reason, AA groups are available to meet the needs of individuals with comorbid psychiatric and substance abuse issues. Nurses may be asked to serve as consultants to these groups.

Relapse Prevention Aftercare Programs

Relapse of mental illness symptoms and substance abuse is the major reason for rehospitalization in the United States. **Relapse** is the recurrence or marked increase in severity of the symptoms of a disease, especially after a period of apparent improvement or stability. Many issues affect a person's well-being. First and foremost, patients must believe that their lives are meaningful and worthwhile. Homelessness and unemployment create tremendous threats to a person's identity and feelings of wellness.

Much work has gone into relapse prevention programs for the major mental illnesses and addiction disorders. Relapse prevention programs involve both patients and families and seek to (1) educate them about the illness, (2) enable them to cope with the chronic nature of the illness, (3) teach them to recognize early warning signs of relapse, (4) educate them about prescribed medications and the need for compliance, and (5) inform them about other disease management strategies (i.e., stress management, exercise) in preventing relapse.

Nurses become involved in relapse prevention programs in several different ways. They can act as referral sources for the programs, trainers or leaders of the programs, or aftercare sources for patients when the programs are completed. In addition, mental health nurses can help patients and family members by promoting optimism, sticking to goals and aspirations, and focusing on individual strengths.

Supported Employment

The ability to work in a competitive job is important in recovery from severe mental illness. Supported employment services assist individuals to find work; assess individuals' skills, attitudes, behaviors, and interest relevant to work; offer vocational rehabilitation or other training; and provide work opportunities. Consumers receive onsite support and job-coaching services on a one-to-one basis. They occur in real work settings and are used for patients with severe mental illnesses. The primary focus is to maintain attachment between the mentally ill person and the work force.

ALTERNATIVE HOUSING ARRANGEMENTS

Housing is an important factor in successful community transition. Patients with psychiatric disabilities who are homeless are a vulnerable population. One of the largest hurdles to overcome in treating the persons with a mental illness is finding appropriate housing that will meet the individual's immediate social, financial, and safety needs. Caring for people with severe mental illnesses in the home can be very stressful for family members because of the person's symptom severity and unpredictable behaviors. Many individuals with a mental illness live in some form of supervised or supported community living situation, which ranges from highly supervised congregate settings to independent apartments. The following discussion focuses on four models of alternative housing and the role of the nurse. These are personal care homes, board-and-care homes, therapeutic foster care, and supervised apartments.

Personal Care Homes

Personal care homes operate within houses in the community. Usually, 6 to 10 people live in one house with a health care attendant providing 24-hour supervision to assist with medication monitoring or other minor activities, including transportation to appointments, meals, and self-care skills. The clientele generally is heterogeneous and includes older adults, people with mild mental retardation, and patients with chronic and subacute mental illness. Most states require these homes to be licensed.

Board-and-Care Homes

Board-and-care homes provide 24-hour supervision and assistance with medications, meals, and some self-care skills. Individualized attention to self-care skills and other activities of daily living generally is not available. These homes are licensed to house 50 to 150 people in one location. Rooms are shared, with two to four occupants per bedroom.

Therapeutic Foster Care

Therapeutic foster care is indicated for patients in need of a family-like environment and a high level of support. Therapeutic foster care is available for child, adolescent, and adult populations. This level of care actually places patients in residences of families specially trained to handle individuals with mental illnesses. The training usually consists of crisis management, medication education, and illness education. The family provides supervision, structure, and support for the individual living with them. The person who receives these services shares the responsibility of completing household chores and may be required to attend an outpatient program during the day.

Supervised Apartments

In a supervised apartment setting, individuals live in their own apartments, usually alone or with one roommate, and are responsible for all household chores and self-care. A staff member or *supervisor* stops by each apartment routinely to evaluate how well the patients are doing, make sure they are taking their medications, and ensure that the household is being maintained. The supervisor may also be required to mediate disagreements between roommates.

Role of Nurses in Alternative Housing

Professional registered nurses typically are not employed in alternative housing settings. However, nurses play a pivotal role in the successful reintegration of patients from more restrictive inpatient settings into society. Nurses are employed in PHPs and inpatient units and as case managers. Therefore, nurses act as liaisons for the residential placement of patients. Nurses are employed directly as consultants or provide consultation to treatment teams during discharge planning in determining appropriate outpatient settings, evaluating medication follow-up needs, and making recommendations for necessary medical care for existing physical conditions. Feedback from the residential care providers and follow-up by the treatment team regarding the patient's response to treatment interventions are essential. Rehospitalization can be curtailed if the residential care operators identify and forward specific problems to the treatment teams. Patient interventions can be modified in an outpatient setting.

INTEGRATED CARE

People diagnosed with psychiatric disorders frequently have complex comorbid medical illnesses, such as hypertension, cardiac disease, metabolic syndrome, and diabetes, that require regular and ongoing treatment and engagement in self-management. However, access to care for complex health problems is often very limited in this population. Collaboration between medical and psychiatric providers is important to ensure that patients receive holistic care that addresses all illnesses. **Integrated care** is a health systems delivery model that ensures people receive a continuum of health promotion, disease management, rehabilitation, and palliative care services at different levels and settings according to their needs throughout life (World health Organization [WHO], 2015).

Medical Home

Integrated care can also be delivered in a **medical home**, a treatment setting that uses a team approach to deliver comprehensive patient-centered care that addresses all aspects of patients' health-related needs. There are five key functions of the medical home:

- comprehensive care that meets the majority of the person's physical and mental health care needs through a team-based approach
- patient-centered care that delivers primary care that is oriented toward the whole person
- coordinated care across all elements of the health care system
- accessible services through minimizing wait times, enhanced office hours, and after-hours access to providers through alternative methods such as telephone or mail

- quality and safety through providing safe, high-quality care through clinical judgment, decision support tools, evidence-based care, shared decision-making, performance measurement, improvement activities (Agency for Healthcare Quality and Research, 2020)

Health and Illness Management in the Community

High rates of medical illnesses among people with serious mental illnesses are often attributed to side effects of medication and lifestyle factors. Rates of smoking and obesity are very high among people diagnosed with posttraumatic stress disorder. They often do not engage in wellness and health promotion activities because of psychiatric symptoms, of lack of understanding of what they need to do to promote health, and their residing in unsafe communities (van der Berk-Clark et al., 2018).

Community mental health centers and therapeutic rehabilitation centers are convenient and safe settings to provide services that promote wellness in this population. These community centers can provide health education, self-management programs, healthy eating and cooking classes, group exercise or walking programs, weight loss groups, smoking cessation counseling, and screening for medical comorbidities.

MANAGED CARE

The concept of managed care emerged in efforts to coordinate patient care efficiently and cost effectively. **Managed care organizations** provide services through health maintenance organizations or preferred provider organizations. Purchasers of health care, such as employers and government health agencies, contract with managed care organizations to provide mental health services. Traditionally, these services were separated from general medical care packages and reimbursed differently than other health care services. With the passage of the Affordable Care Act (see Chapter 1), the mental health services are supposed to be reimbursed at the same level as other health care problems. The recent trend is integration of many mental health services within a primary care setting. The goals of this approach to care are to increase access to care and to provide the most appropriate level of services in the least restrictive setting. Efforts focus on providing more outpatient and alternative treatment programs and avoiding costly inpatient hospitalizations. When properly conducted and administered, an integrated primary care allows patients better access to quality services while using health care dollars wisely.

Today, managed behavioral health care has succeeded in standardizing admissions criteria, reducing length of patient stay, and directing patients to the proper level of care—inpatient and outpatient—all while attempting to control the costs. Across the continuum of care nurses encounter integrated or collaborative organizations, and they must be familiar with the policies, procedures, and clinical judgment criteria established by managed care organizations. As the delivery of mental health care services becomes more integrated into primary care and growing numbers of patients with mental illnesses reach older age, increasing demands are placed on the health and mental health care systems to accommodate the needs of this population. Rates of comorbid medical illnesses are high in older adults with severe mental illnesses, and the need is great for services that provide adequate psychiatric and medical care for this population, ideally in the same treatment setting (Bartels et al., 2018).

The Nurse's Role in Negotiating the Mental Health Delivery Systems

Because of shorter inpatient stays, inpatient psychiatric–mental health nurses maximize the short time they have by educating patients about their illness, available community resources, and medications to minimize the potential for relapse. These nurses focus on teaching social skills and self-reliance and creating empowering environments that in turn build self-confidence and help the patient move toward recovery.

The interface of psychiatric–mental health nurses with other nurses in managed care organizations and integrated primary care systems is primarily in the form of communicating the progress of individual patients to the nurses (mental health and nonmental health) and other health care workers who maintain a long-term relationship with the patient and family.

Public and Private Collaboration

Today, there are many public–private sector collaborations. The need for public–private collaboration prompted the National Association of State Mental Health Program Directors, an organization representing the 55 state and territorial public mental health systems, and the American Managed Behavioral Healthcare Association, an organization representing private managed behavioral health care firms, to work together. Nurses can expect to see more strategic alliances and joint ventures between the public and private sectors.

NURSING PRACTICE IN THE CONTINUUM OF CARE

Throughout this chapter, nurses' roles in different settings have been explained. Regardless of the situation or setting, nurses conduct assessments at the point of first patient contact. The individual's needs are then matched with the most appropriate setting, service, or program that will meet those needs. If a patient is admitted for services, the nurse also begins discharge planning upon first admission.

Assessment and Identification of Services

Choosing the level of care begins with an initial assessment to determine the need for care, the type of care to be provided, and the need for additional assessment. The nurse must discuss with the patient with suicidal and homicidal thoughts. Nurses also need to consider financial issues because funding considerations may play a part in placement options. Other factors affecting the selection of care include the type of treatment the individual seeks, their current physical condition and ability to consent to treatment, and the organization's ability to provide direct care or to deflect care to another service provider.

Based on the results of the initial assessment, the nurse may admit the patient into services provided at that agency or initiate a referral or transfer to provide the intensity and scope of treatment required by the individual at that point in time (Fig. 5.1). Referral involves sending an individual from one clinician to another or from one service setting to another for care or consultation. **Transfer** involves formally shifting responsibility for the care of an individual from one clinician to another or from one care unit to another. The processes of referral and transfer to other levels of care are integral for effective use of services along the continuum. These processes are based on the individual's assessed needs and the organization's capability to provide the care. Figure 5.1 depicts the process of assessment, treatment, transfer, and referral when considering appropriate levels of care.

Discharge Planning

Discharge planning begins upon admission of the individual to any level of health care. Most facilities have a written procedure for discharge planning. This procedure often provides for a transfer of clinical care information when a person is referred, transferred, or discharged to another facility or level of care. All discharge planning activities should be documented in the clinical record, including the patient's response to proposed aftercare treatment, follow-up for psychiatric and physical health problems, and discharge instructions. Medication education, food–drug interactions, drug–drug interactions, and special diet instructions (if applicable) are extremely important in ensuring patient safety. Discharge planning is an integral part of psychiatric nursing care and should be considered a part of the psychiatric rehabilitation process. In addressing an individual's needs, one can

coordinate aftercare and discharge interventions for optimal outcomes. The overall goal of discharge planning is to provide the patient with all of the resources they need to function as independently as possible in the least restrictive environment and to avoid rehospitalization.

The nurse can optimize discharge plan compliance by partnering with the patient from the first encounter. Because patients with mental illnesses may have limited cognitive abilities and residual motivational and anxiety problems, the nurse should explain in detail all aftercare plans and instructions to the patient. It is helpful also to schedule all aftercare appointments before the patient leaves the facility. The nurse should then give the patient written instructions about where and when to go for the appointment and a contact person's name and telephone number at the aftercare placement. Finally, the nurse should review emergency telephone numbers and contacts and medication instructions with the patient.

SUMMARY OF KEY POINTS

- The continuum of care is a comprehensive system of services and programs designed to match the needs of the individual with the appropriate treatment in settings that vary according to levels of service, structure, and intensity of care.

- Psychiatric–mental health nurses' specific responsibilities vary according to the setting. In most settings, nurses function as members of a multidisciplinary team and assume responsibility for assessment and selection of level of care, education, evaluation of response to treatment, referral or transfer to a more appropriate level of care, and discharge planning. Discharge planning provides patients with all the resources they need to function effectively in the community and avoid rehospitalization.

- Mental health care can be given within an integrated primary care setting or a separate system. The nurse's role will vary depending upon the setting and the needs of the patient.

CRITICAL THINKING CHALLENGES

1. Define the continuum of care in mental health care and discuss the importance of the least restrictive environment.

2. Differentiate the role of the nurse in each of the following continuum settings:

   a. Crisis stabilization

   b. In-home detoxification

   c. Partial hospitalization

   d. Assertive community treatment

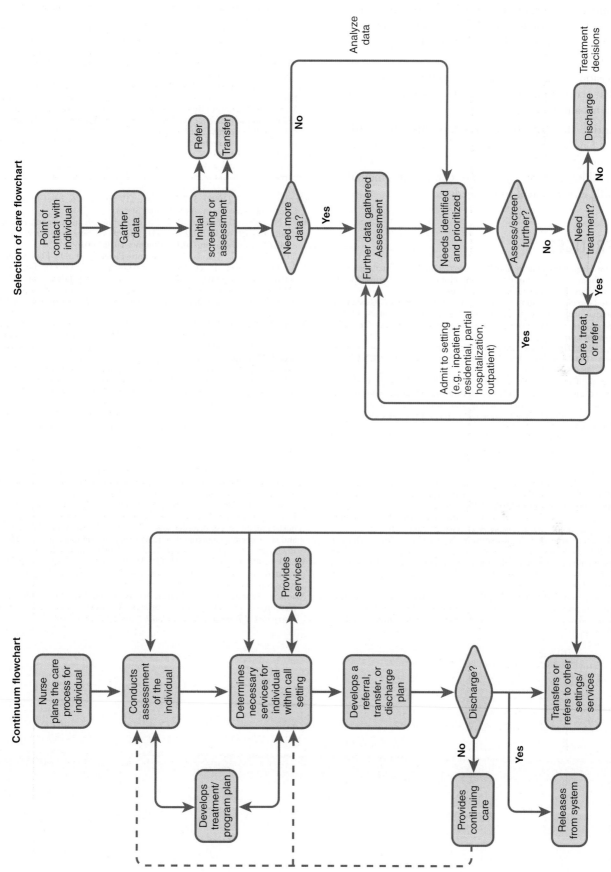

FIGURE 5.1 Flowcharts illustrating nursing care in the mental health care continuum and selection of care.

3. Compare alternative housing arrangements, including personal care homes, board-and-care homes, therapeutic foster care, and supervised apartments.

4. Envision using more than one service at a time. What combinations of services could benefit patients and families?

5. Identify the specific community mental health service needs of patients across the lifespan. Include the unique needs of children, adolescents, adults, and older patients. How do community mental health services meet these needs?

REFERENCES

Agency for Healthcare Quality and Research. (2020). 5 key functions of the Medical home. Department of Health and Human Services. https://pcmh.ahrq.gov/page/5-key-functions-medical-home

American Nurses Association, American Psychiatric Nurses Association, & International Society of Psychiatric Mental Health Nurses. (2014). *Psychiatric-mental health nursing: Scope and standards of practice* (2nd ed.). Nursesbooks.org.

Armold, S. (2019). Case management: An overview for nurses. *Nursing 2019, 49*(9), 43–45. https://doi.org/10.1097/01.NURSE.0000577708.49429.83

Bartels, S. J., DiMilia, P. R., Fortuna, K. L., & Naslund, J. A. (2018). Integrated care for older adults with serious mental illness and medical comorbidity: Evidence-based models and future research directions. *Psychiatric Clinics of North America, 41*(1), 153–164. https://doi.org/10.1016/j.psc.2017.10.012

Commission for Case Manger Certification (2015). Definition of case management. Case management body of knowledge. https://cmbodyofknowledge.com/content/introduction-case-management-body-knowledge

Congressional Research Service. (July 30, 2019). Medicaid's Institutions for Mental Disease (IMD) exclusion. www.crs.gov IF 10222 Version 10 Updated. https://fas.org/sgp/crs/misc/IF10222.pdf

Cassatly, S., & Cassatly, M. (2017). The Affordable Care Act and digital health applications. *Practice Management*, www.greenbranch.com.

Crisanti, A. S., Earheart, J. A., Rosenbaum, N. A., Tinney, M., & Duhigg, D. J. (2019). Beyond crisis intervention team (CIT) classroom training: Videoconference continuing education for law enforcement. *International Journal of Law and Psychiatry, 62*, 104–110. https://doi.org/10.1016/j.ijlp.2018.12.003

Lapidos, A., Jester, J., Ortquist, M., Werner, P., Ruffolo, M. C., & Smith, M. (2018). Survey of peer support specialists: Professional activities, self-rated skills, job satisfaction, and financial well-being. *Psychiatric Services (Washington, D.C.), 69*(12), 1264–1267. https://doi.org/10.1176/appi.ps.201800251

Lewis, K. L., Fanaian, M., Kotze, B., & Grenyer, F. S. (2019). Mental health presentations to acute psychiatric services: 3-year study of prevalence and readmission risk for personality disorders compared with psychotic, affective, substance or other disorders. *BJPsych Open, 5*(1), e1. https://doi.org/10.1192/bjo.2018.72

Murphy, J. A., Oliver, G., Ng, C. H., Wain, C., Magennis, J., Opie, R. S., Bannatyne, A., & Sarris, J. (2019). Pilot-testing of "Healthy Body Healthy Mind": An integrative lifestyle program for patients with a mental illness and co-morbid metabolic syndrome. *Frontiers in Psychiatry, 10*, 91. https://doi.org/10.3389/fpsyt.2019.00091

Naslund, J. A., Aschbrenner, K. A., Araya, R., Marsch, L. A., Unützer, J., Patel, V., & Bartels, S. J. (2017). Digital technology for treating and preventing mental orders in low-income and middle-income countries: A narrative review of the literature. *Lancet Psychiatry, 4*(6), 486–500. https://doi.org/10.1016/S2215-0366(17)30096-2

Olmstead v. L.C. (1999). 527 U.S. 581; 119 S.Ct. 2176. Brief Filed: 3/99 Court: Supreme Court of the United States.

Peek, N., Sujan, M., & Scott, P. (2020). Digital health and care in pandemic times: Impact of COVID-19. *BMJ Health & Care Informatics, 27*(1), e100166. https://doi.org/10.1136/bmjhci-2020-100166

Roldán-Merino, J., García, I. C., Ramos-Pichardo, J. D., Foix-Sanjuan, A., Quilez-Jover, J., & Montserrat-Martinez, M. (2013). Impact of personalized in-home nursing care plans on dependence in ADLs/IADLs and on family burden among adults diagnosed with schizophrenia: A randomized controlled study. *Perspectives in Psychiatric Care, 49*(3), 171–178.

Spivak, S., Cullen, B. A., Green, C., Firth, T., Sater, H., & Mojtabai, R. (2019). Availability of assertive community treatment in the United States: 2010 to 2016. *Psychiatric Services, 70*(10), 948–951. https://doi.org/10.1176/appi.ps.201900032

Taube-Schiff, M., Mehak, A., Marangos, S., Kalim, A., & Ungar, T. (2019). Advancing care within an adult mental health day hospital: Program re-design and evaluation. *Journal of Behavioral Health Service & Research, 46*(1), 15–28. https://doi.org/10.1007/s11414-017-9568-5

Thoegersen, M. H., Morthorst, B. R., & Nordentoft, M. (2019). Assertive community treatment versus standard treatment for severely mentally ill patients in Denmark: A quasi-experimental trial. *Nordic Journal of Psychiatry, 73*(2), 149–158. https://doi.org/10.1080/08039488.2019.1576765

Tyler, N., Wright, N., & Waring, J. (2019). Interventions to improve discharge from acute adult mental health inpatient care. *BMC Health Service and Research, 19*(1), 883. https://doi.org/10.1186/s12913-019-4658-0

van der Berk-Clark, C., Secrest, S., Walls, J., Hallberg, E., Lustman, P. J., Schneider, F. D., & Scherrer, J. F. (2018). Association between posttraumatic stress disorder and a lack of exercise, poor diet, obesity and co-occurring smoking: A systematic review and meta-analysis. *Health Psychology, 37*(5), 407–416. https://doi.org/10.1037/hea0000593

World health Organization. (2015). WHO global strategy on people-centred and integrated health services: Interim report, *4*(6), 486–500. https://apps.who.int/iris/handle/10665/155002

Xiao, S., Tourangeau, A., Widger, K., & Berta, W. (2019). Discharge planning in mental healthcare settings: A review and concept analysis. *International Journal of Mental Health Nursing, 28*, 816–832.

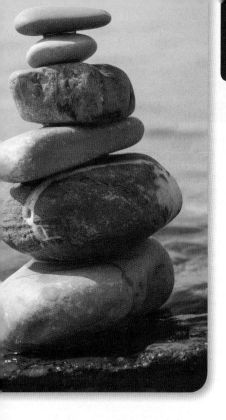

UNIT II

Foundations of Psychiatric Nursing

6

Ethics, Standards, and Nursing Frameworks

Valerie Yancey and Mary Ann Boyd

KEYCONCEPTS

- biopsychosocial framework
- ethical principles
- standards of practice

LEARNING OBJECTIVES

After studying this chapter, you will be able to:

1. Describe the importance of the ethical principles of beneficence, fidelity, justice, nonmaleficence, respect for autonomy, and veracity for considering ethical situations in psychiatric–mental health (PMH) nursing practice.

2. Delineate the scope and standards of PMH nursing practice.

3. Describe how professional nursing organizations influence and strengthen PMH nursing practice.

4. Discuss the relationship between the biopsychosocial model and wellness and recovery models used as frameworks for PMH nursing practice.

5. Identify the basic tools used in PMH nursing practice.

6. Discuss emerging challenges for PMH nursing.

7. Discuss the benefits of using standardized nursing languages.

KEY TERMS

- Beneficence • Clinical judgment • Fidelity • Justice • Nonmaleficence • Nursing process • Paternalism
- Psychiatric–mental health advanced practice registered nurse • Psychiatric–mental health registered nurse
- Reflection • Respect for autonomy • Scope and standards of practice • Standardized nursing language • Veracity

INTRODUCTION

This chapter opens with a discussion of the ethical principles used by psychiatric nurses daily. The scope and standards of practice are then highlighted. This chapter explains how the biopsychosocial model provides a framework for psychiatric–mental health (PMH) nursing and relates to recovery and wellness models. A discussion of the challenges facing PMH nursing helps create a vision for the changing nature of this dynamic nursing specialty.

ETHICS OF PSYCHIATRIC NURSING

PMH nursing practice is guided by the *Code of Ethics for Nurses with Interpretive Statements* (Box 6.1). The *Code* communicates nursing's ethical values, obligations, duties, and professional ideals; establishes ethical standards; and confirms the profession's commitment to society (American Nurses Association [ANA], 2015). When faced with ethical concerns, the nurse can reflect on a series of questions, outlined in Box 6.2.

BOX 6.1

Code of Ethics for Nurses

1. The nurse practices with compassion and respect for the inherent dignity, worth, and unique attributes of every person.
2. The nurse's primary commitment is to the patient, whether an individual, family, group, or community.
3. The nurse promotes, advocates for, and protects the rights, health, and safety of the patient.
4. The nurse has authority, accountability, and responsibility for nursing practice; makes decisions; and takes action consistent with the obligation to promote health and to provide optimal care.
5. The nurse owes the same duties to self as to others, including the responsibility to promote health and safety, preserve wholeness of character and integrity, maintain competence, and continue personal and professional growth.
6. The nurse, through individual and collective effort, establishes, maintains, and improves the ethical environment of the work setting and conditions of employment that are conducive to safe, quality health care.
7. The nurse, in all roles and settings, advances the profession through research and scholarly inquiry, professional standards development, and the generation of both nursing and health policy.
8. The nurse collaborates with other health professionals and the public to protect human rights, promote health diplomacy, and reduce health disparities.
9. The profession of nursing, collectively through its professional organizations, must articulate nursing values, maintain the integrity of the profession, and integrate principles of social justice into nursing and health policy.

Reprinted with permission from American Nurses Association. (2015). *Code of ethics for nurses with interpretive statements.* Nursesbooks.org. All rights reserved.

BOX 6.2

Basic Questions for Ethical Decision-Making

- What do I know about this patient situation?
- What do I know about the patient's values and moral preferences?
- What assumptions am I making that need more data to clarify?
- What are my own feelings (and values) about the situation, and how might they be influencing how I view and respond to this situation?
- Are my own values in conflict with those of the patient?
- What else do I need to know about this case, and where can I obtain this information?
- What can I never know about this case?
- Given my primary obligation to the patient, what should I do to be ethical?

Reprinted with permission from Davis, A. (2008). Provision two. In M. Fowler (Ed.), *Guide to the code of ethics for nursing: Interpretation and application* (p. 18). Nursebooks.org.

Four primary health care **ethical principles**—respect for autonomy, beneficence, nonmaleficence, and justice—guide nurses' consideration of ethical concerns. In health care decisions and conduct, these principles highlight the ethical aspects of the patient situations, decision dilemmas, and relationships.

The principle of **respect for autonomy** is based on the understanding that each person has the fundamental right to make voluntary decisions about their health care and life decisions. Persons are to be regarded as self-determining. The principle of respect for autonomy gives rise to expectations for ethical conduct, namely, the use of informed consent in health care practices. To give consent to a treatment or procedure, a person must have the needed relevant information, be able to rationally deliberate, and not be forced into a decision. The PMH nurse protects autonomy by assessing a person's decisional capacity to act in their own best interests as they see it. Nurses are also obligated by the principle of respect for autonomy to protect individuals' privacy. A person loses the ability to be self-determining if information about their health conditions is shared with others without permission. Privacy can be important especially in mental health practice because of the potential for stigmatization and the patient's potential vulnerability. The meaning of the principle of **beneficence** (goodness) rests on the assumption that professionals have a duty to act in ways that benefit a patient or community, and that they take steps necessary to minimize harm. The scope and standards of nursing practice (discussed later in this chapter) delineate the ways that nurses are to act in a beneficent way toward those in their care. Nurses use their knowledge and skills to create environments in which people can thrive. **Nonmaleficence** is the duty one has to never intentionally harm another. Often in health care decisions, negative outcomes may occur as a result of any choice that is made. The professional is obligated to minimize the harm and risks as much as possible for both the individual and others who may be involved. The principle of **justice** encourages providers to consider how the goods of a society, including health care, are distributed. As noted in the first provision of the *Code of Ethics for Nurses*, providers have an ethical duty to treat all people with dignity, respect, and fairness. Those "goods" are to be distributed equally. All people should have access to health care. Justice also requires that we consider instances when basic goods should be distributed so that those who need more get what they need for health and survival, even if they use more resources than others get. Mental health services are often not readily available to those most in need, a violation of the principle of justice.

Each of the four primary principles prompts nurses to focus on different aspects of an ethical decision or relationship. Sometimes, one principle may be in tension with one or more of the other principles. For example, a patient may decide to stop taking a medication (autonomy), but the nurse wants to avoid the harm that could likely come to the patient or others when the patient discontinues medication use. In ethical dilemmas, all of the principles are important and relevant. The PMH nurse must be able to weigh the relative merits of the principles when there is a conflict and help others to see the competing ethical claims. The nurse strives to promote a decision that achieves the most good and avoids harm as much as possible.

> **NCLEXNOTE** Be prepared to think of patient situations that illustrate the principles of respect for autonomy and beneficence and identify how patients' and nurses' views may differ.

Two secondary ethical principles, veracity and fidelity, provide additional guidance for mental health care practice. **Veracity** highlights one's duty to tell the truth. Nurses guided by the principle of veracity understand that honesty provides a foundation for the development of trust in a helping, healing relationship. There are times, however, when "telling the truth" requires judgment and sensitivity to the patient's situation. For example, giving others more information than is necessary, even if that information is true, could cause an excess of fear, anxiety, and harm. Or, there may be times when the nurse cannot truthfully respond to a patient's question. A nurse cannot guarantee or truthfully assure a patient that a medication will eliminate all mental health symptoms. Nurses use good moral reasoning and judgment when they consider how to be truthful, using the principle of beneficence (doing the good) in their responses to others. **Fidelity** implies that nurses should be faithful to their obligations and duties toward others, society, and the nursing profession. Fidelity is also essential for the maintenance of trusting relationships because it is centered on doing what one says will be done (keeping promises). At times, health care professionals use the principle of **paternalism** to guide their actions and decisions. The paternalism is based on the belief that professionals have the knowledge and education needed to make decisions for others and should do so. Often professionals' expert knowledge of the technical and medical aspects of a situation makes their judgment most valuable. Professionals may not know, however, the details of a person's life and values. Nurses protect against unwarranted use of a paternalistic approach by encouraging patient, family, and community involvement in decisions. Paternalism may be justified in some mental health conditions in which a person is temporarily unable to deliberate in the best interests of self or others. Socially, some health care decisions, such as the mandated use of seat belts or motorcycle helmets, are made paternalistically to protect others. Paternalism can be in direct conflict with the mental health recovery belief of self-determination (see Chapters 1 and 7).

> **NCLEXNOTE** Be able to identify ethical situations encountered by psychiatric–mental health nurses in inpatient and outpatient settings.

SCOPE AND STANDARDS OF PRACTICE

The legal authority to practice nursing is regulated by law and granted by each state or province. The **scope and standards of practice** are defined by the nursing profession and describe the responsibilities to which nurses are legally, professionally, and ethically held accountable.

The American Nurses Association (ANA) and psychiatric nursing organizations (discussed later in this chapter) further clarify the boundaries of PMH nursing and establish the scope of practice for nurses at different educational levels and in various nursing roles. Nurses are ethically obligated to abide by the scope and standards of practice to honor their commitments made to patients, communities, and society.

Scope of Psychiatric–Mental Health Nursing

PMH nurses address a wide range of actual and potential mental health problems or psychiatric disorders, including emotional stress or crisis, self-concept changes, addictive patterns, developmental issues, physical symptoms that occur with psychological changes, and mental health and treatment symptom management. To understand an individual's mental health condition and select appropriate interventions, nurses integrate knowledge from the biologic, psychological, and social domains.

> **KEYCONCEPT** Six **standards of practice** define the parameters of PMH nursing and are organized according to the nursing process steps: assessment, diagnosis, outcome identification, planning, implementation, and evaluation (Box 6.3).

Standards of Practice

The **nursing process** serves as a framework for clinical judgment decision-making and nursing practice.

BOX 6.3

Standards of Practice

STANDARD 1: ASSESSMENT

The PMH-RN collects and synthesizes comprehensive health data that are pertinent to the health care consumer's health and/or situation.

STANDARD 2: DIAGNOSIS

The PMH-RN analyzes the assessment data to determine diagnoses, problems, and areas of focus for care and treatment, including level of risk.

STANDARD 3: OUTCOMES IDENTIFICATION

The PMH-RN identifies expected outcomes and the health care consumer's goals for a plan individualized to the health care consumer or to the situation.

STANDARD 4: PLANNING

The PMH-RN develops a plan that prescribes strategies and alternatives to assist the health care consumer in attainment of expected outcomes.

STANDARD 5: IMPLEMENTATION

The PMH-RN implements the specified plan.

Standard 5A: Coordination of Care

The PMH-RN coordinates care delivery.

Standard 5B: Health Teaching and Health Promotion

The PMH-RN employs strategies to promote health and a safe environment.

Standard 5C: Consultation

The PMH-APRN provides consultation to influence the identified plan, enhance the abilities of other clinicians to provide services for health care consumers, and effect change.

Standard 5D: Prescriptive Authority and Treatment

The PMH-APRN uses prescriptive authority, procedures, referrals, treatments, and therapies in accordance with state and federal laws and regulations.

Standard 5E: Pharmacologic, Biologic, and Integrative Therapies

The PMH-APRN incorporates knowledge of pharmacologic, biologic, and complementary interventions with applied clinical skills to restore the health care consumer's health and prevent further disability.

Standard 5F: Milieu Therapy

The PMH-APRN provides, structures, and maintains a safe, therapeutic, recovery-oriented environment in collaboration with health care consumers, families, and other health care clinicians.

Standard 5G: Therapeutic Relationship and Counseling

The PMH-RN uses the therapeutic relationship and counseling interventions to assist health care consumers in their individual recovery journeys by improving and regaining their previous coping abilities, fostering mental health, and preventing mental disorder and disability.

Standard 5H: Psychotherapy

The PMH-APRN conducts individual, couples, group, and family psychotherapy using evidence-based psychotherapeutic frameworks and the nurse–client therapeutic relationship.

STANDARD 6: EVALUATION

The PMH-RN evaluates progress toward attainment of expected outcomes.

Reprinted with permission from American Nurses Association, American Psychiatric Nurses Association, & International Society of Psychiatric–Mental Health Nurses. (2014). *Psychiatric–mental health nursing: Scope and standards of practice* (2nd ed.). Nursesbooks.org.

Each of the six standards includes competencies for a **Psychiatric–Mental Health Registered Nurse** (PMH-RN) and **Psychiatric–Mental Health Advanced Practice Registered Nurses** (PMH-APRN) practice. The fifth standard, implementation, has several subcategories that define the standards for specific interventions.

Standards of Professional Performance

Ten standards of professional performance for PMH nurses flow from the six standards of practice. The 10 standards for professional performance include ethics, education, evidence-based practice and research, quality of practice, communication, leadership, collaboration, professional practice evaluation, resource utilization, and environmental health. Each standard of performance includes expected competencies (Table 6.1) (American Nurses Association, American Psychiatric Nurses Association, & International Society of Psychiatric–Mental Health Nurses, 2014).

Levels of Practice

There are two levels of PMH nursing practice. The first level is the PMH-RN whose educational preparation is at the bachelor's or associate's degree level. The PMH-APRN receives educational preparation at the master's or doctoral level. A PMH-APRN can practice as a psychiatric–mental health clinical nurse specialist or as a psychiatric–mental health nurse practitioner (Box 6.4).

Psychiatric–Mental Health Nursing Practice

According to the *Psychiatric–Mental Health Nursing: Scope and Standards of Practice*, the PMH nurse is a registered nurse who demonstrates specialized competence and knowledge, skills, and abilities in caring for persons with mental health issues and problems and psychiatric disorders. Competency is obtained through education and experience. The preferred educational preparation for a PMH-RN is at the baccalaureate level, with credentialing

TABLE 6.1	STANDARDS OF PROFESSIONAL PERFORMANCE	
Standard	**Area of Performance**	**Description**
Standard 7	Ethics	Integrates ethical provisions in all areas of practice.
Standard 8	Education	Attains knowledge and competency that reflect current nursing practice.
Standard 9	Evidence-based practice and research	Integrates evidence and research findings into practice.
Standard 10	Quality of practice	Systematically enhances the quality and effectiveness of nursing practice.
Standard 11	Communication	Communicates effectively in a variety of formats in all areas of practice.
Standard 12	Leadership	Provides leadership in the professional practice setting and the profession.
Standard 13	Collaboration	Collaborates with the health care consumer, family, interprofessional health team, and others in the conduct of nursing practice.
Standard 14	Professional practice evaluation	Evaluates one's own practice in relation to the professional practice standards and guidelines, relevant statutes, rules, and regulations.
Standard 15	Resource utilization	Considers factors related to safety, effectiveness, cost, and impact on practice in the planning and delivery of nursing services.
Standard 16	Environmental health	Practices in an environmentally safe and healthy manner.

Reprinted with permission from American Nurses Association, American Psychiatric Nurses Association, & International Society of Psychiatric–Mental Health Nurses. (2014). *Psychiatric–mental health nursing: Scope and standards of practice* (2nd ed.). Nursesbooks.org.

BOX 6.4

Clinical Activities of Psychiatric–Mental Health Nurses

PSYCHIATRIC–MENTAL HEALTH REGISTERED NURSE

Health promotion and health maintenance
Intake screening, evaluation, and triage
Case management
Provision of therapeutic and safe environments
Milieu therapy
Promotion of self-care activities
Administration of psychobiologic treatment and monitoring responses
Complementary interventions
Crisis intervention and stabilization
Psychiatric rehabilitation

ADVANCED PRACTICE REGISTERED NURSE

Psychopharmacologic interventions
Psychotherapy
Community interventions
Case management
Program development and management
Clinical supervision
Consultation and liaison

---

by the American Nurses Credentialing Center or a recognized certification organization (ANA et al., 2014).

PMH-RNs are "characterized by the use of the nursing process to treat people with actual or potential mental health problems, psychiatric disorders and co-occurring psychiatric and substance use disorders" (ANA et al., 2014, p. 25). By using the nursing process, the PMH-RN promotes and fosters health and safety, assesses dysfunction and areas of strength, and assists individuals in achieving personal recovery goals. The nurse performs a wide range of interventions, including health promotion and health maintenance strategies, intake screening and evaluation and triage, case management, milieu therapy, promotion of self-care activities, psychobiologic interventions, complementary interventions, health teaching, counseling, crisis care, and psychiatric rehabilitation. An overview of psychiatric nursing interventions is provided in Unit 3.

Psychiatric–Mental Health Advanced Practice Registered Nurse

The PMH-APRN, a licensed registered nurse educationally prepared at the master's or doctoral level, is nationally certified as a clinical nurse specialist or a psychiatric nurse practitioner by the American Nurses Credentialing Center. A PMH-APRN educated in a Doctor of Nursing program focuses on nursing practice knowledge development, quality improvement, action research, health systems leadership, and health policy. Nurses with doctoral preparation at the Doctor of Philosophy level focus on the development of nursing science and acquire skills in designing, conducting, and analyzing research. Doctor of Nursing Science degrees, offered at some universities, have a research focus. Nurse administrators and educators, depending on setting and role requirements, can be PMH-RNs, or APRNs.

Psychiatric–Mental Health Nursing Organizations

Nursing professional organizations provide leadership and give legitimacy and definition to PMH nursing. They advocate for nurses to function within the fullest extent of their professional scope of practice and provide health policy advocacy at local, state, and national levels.

The ANA, nursing's largest organization, fosters high standards of practice, promotes safe and ethical work environments for nurses, and advocates for needed health care policy and legislation. The ANA supports and advocates for PMH nursing practice at national and state levels and works closely with PMH nursing organizations.

Two organizations for psychiatric nurses, the American Psychiatric Nurses Association (APNA) and the International Society of Psychiatric Nursing (ISPN), focus on the specific interests of PMH care and nursing practice. The APNA, the largest PMH nursing organization, advances PMH nursing practice and helps shape mental health policy thereby improving mental health care for culturally diverse individuals, families, groups, and communities. The ISPN consists of four specialist divisions: the Association of Child and Adolescent Psychiatric Nurses, International Society of Psychiatric Consultation Liaison Nurses, Society for Education and Research in Psychiatric–Mental Health Nursing, and Adult and Geropsychiatric–Mental Health Nurses. The ISPN unites and strengthens PMH nurses and promotes quality care for individuals and families experiencing mental health problems. The International Nurses Society on Addictions is committed to the prevention, intervention, treatment, and management of addictive disorders. These organizations have annual meetings at which new research is presented. Student memberships are available.

THE BIOPSYCHOSOCIAL FRAMEWORK

The biopsychosocial framework (Fig. 6.1) is a well-recognized, holistic model for organizing nursing practice. Each of the model's three domains—biologic, psychological, and social—has an independent knowledge and treatment focus but interacts and is mutually interdependent with the other domains. Each domain (described in the following section) influences an individual's mental health and provides a framework for implementing the nursing process.

A nurse using a biopsychosocial framework assesses a patient's physical, psychological, and social strengths and needs and considers the interaction of those three domains in making a nursing diagnosis. The biopsychosocial framework is congruent with the recovery and wellness models and guides recovery-oriented care (see Chapter 1). Standardized nursing languages, such as the International Classification for Nursing Practice, Clinical Care Classification, and the Omaha System, can be used with this framework (da Cruz Sequeira & Sampaio, 2018; Kerr et al., 2016; Saba, 2018).

> **KEYCONCEPT** The **biopsychosocial framework** consists of three separate but interdependent domains: biologic, psychological, and social. Each domain has an independent knowledge and treatment focus but interacts and is mutually interdependent with the other domains.

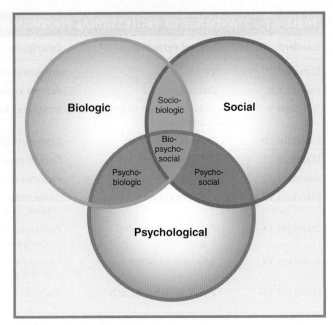

FIGURE 6.1 The biopsychosocial model.

Biologic Domain

The *biologic* domain is concerned with the physiological aspects of all health conditions, including the biologic aspects of mental health conditions or disorders. Biologic theories and concepts consider vital functional health patterns, essential when assessing a person's mental health: exercise, elimination patterns, sleep, and nutrition. Neurobiologic theories serve as a basis for understanding and administering pharmacologic agents (see Chapters 8 and 12).

Psychological Domain

The *psychological* domain involves the theoretical basis of the psychological processes—thoughts, feelings, and behavior (intrapersonal dynamics) that influence one's emotion, cognition, and behavior. Psychological and nursing sciences generate theories and research critical to a nurse's understanding and assessment of patients' mental health symptoms and responses to treatment. Although some mental disorders have a neurobiological basis, symptoms are experienced and observed as psychological. For example, even though manic behavior is caused by dysfunction in the brain, there are no laboratory tests to confirm a diagnosis, only a pattern of behavior.

PMH nurses use many behavioral interventions, including cognitive approaches, behavior therapy, and patient education. In using therapeutic communication and in developing therapeutic relationships, a nurse should have self-awareness and the capacity to be aware of and interpret a patient's feelings, psychological states, and behaviors (see Chapter 10).

Social Domain

The *social* domain includes theories that describe the influence of social forces on the patient, family, and community within cultural settings. Social and nursing sciences illustrate how social connections within families and communities influence mental health, treatment, and recovery. Psychiatric disorders are not caused solely by social factors, but their mental health manifestations and treatment can be significantly affected by the society in which a patient lives. For example, the presence of social and family support often improves treatment outcomes. Moreover, families of origin, extended families, or other significant relationships can positively influence or complicate a patient's mental health condition and treatment outcomes. Community forces, including cultural and ethnic groups within larger communities, shape the patient's manifestation of disorders, response to treatment, and overall view of mental illness.

TOOLS OF PSYCHIATRIC NURSING PRACTICE

Self

The most important tool of psychiatric nursing is the self. Through relationship building, patients learn to trust the nurse who then guides, teaches, and advocates for quality care and treatment. This text emphasizes the primary importance of the patient–nurse relationship.

Clinical Judgment and Reflection

Sound **clinical judgment** depends on critical thinking skills and reflection. Using the critical thinking skills of problem-solving and decision-making, nurses analyze, evaluate, explain, infer, and interpret biopsychosocial data. Some critical thinking activities such as nursing assessments occur in an orderly fashion, over a predictable period of time. Some decisions based on critical thinking must occur in response to an emergency or are made moment to moment, such as deciding whether a patient can leave a unit or whether a patient should receive a medication. Critical thinking is an ongoing process that undergirds safe, ethical, and effective PMH nursing care (Box 6.5).

Reflection involves ongoing self-evaluation through observing, monitoring, and judging of one's own and others' behaviors with the goal of providing effective and meaningful nursing care. Reflective skills are used to enhance all aspects of PMH nursing practice, including self-awareness, nurse–patient interactions, and evaluating systems of care.

Interdisciplinary Care

The PMH nurse collaborates with other professionals, patients, and family members in all settings. In the hospital, a patient may see a psychiatrist or psychiatric nurse practitioner who treats the symptoms and prescribes the medication; a case manager who coordinates care; a psychiatric social worker for individual psychotherapy; a

---

BOX 6.5

Research for Best Practices: Practice Development Strategies

Cheng, S., Backonja, U., Buck, B., Monroe-DeVita, M., & Walsh, E. (2020). Facilitating pathways to care: A qualitative study of the self-reported needs and coping skills of caregiver of young adults diagnosed with early psychosis. Journal of Psychiatric and Mental Health Nursing, 27(4), 368–379. https://doi.org/10.1111/jpm.12591

THE QUESTION: What is the lived experience of family members of a young adult newly diagnosed with psychosis? What do family members with no prior experience with a serious mental health issue want to know to be better prepared to offer support and help to a family member?

METHODS: This qualitative study used focus groups to gather information about family members' lived experiences, fears, knowledge deficits, and uncertainties in providing in-home care to a young adult with new onset of psychosis. The researchers used what they learned from the focus groups to propose strategies for the use of mobile and online technologies to enhance family coping.

FINDINGS: Family members needed more information about early psychotic symptoms, symptom monitoring, resources, access to care and hospitalization, and how to maintain safety for the patient and themselves. Focus group participants expressed a desire to educate others in the public with whom young adults interact about the symptoms of early psychotic episodes and agreed that mobile and online technologies were helpful coping devises.

IMPLICATIONS FOR NURSING: PMH nurses provide care for patients and family caregivers, knowing that positive patient outcomes depend significantly on caregiver coping and strengths. Especially early in the process of learning how to support a person with mental illness, family members need innovative approaches that address their specific needs for support and information.

psychiatric nurse for management of responses related to the mental disorder, administration of medication, and monitoring side effects; and an occupational therapist for transition into the workplace. In the community clinic, a patient may meet weekly with a therapist, monthly with a mental health provider who prescribes medication, and twice a week with a group leader in a day treatment program. An interdisciplinary group of professionals bring specialized skills to the patient's care.

Plan of Care

As with patients receiving treatment for a physical condition, patients receiving PMH services also have written plans of care. The patient and family (if appropriate) should participate in the development of the plan. In situations where nurses are the primary caregivers, as in-home care, a nursing care plan is used. When professionals from other disciplines provide services to the same patient, as in a hospital or outpatient treatment facility, an interdisciplinary treatment plan may be used with or instead of a traditional nursing care plan. When an interdisciplinary plan is used, nurses should make sure the nursing components of the plan are easily identified and take responsibility for implementation and team input. The nurse provides care within the PMH nurse's scope of practice, so a traditional nursing care plan may or may not be used, depending on institutional policies.

Both nursing care plans and interdisciplinary treatment plans are individualized, based on the patient's needs and strengths. At times, third-party payers, who reimburse the costs of the service, review and approve the plan. This text places an emphasis on developing nursing care plans because they serve as a basis of nursing practice and can also be used in a multidisciplinary or interdisciplinary individual treatment plan.

CHALLENGES OF PSYCHIATRIC NURSING

The challenges of PMH nursing are increasing. New knowledge is being generated, technology has radically transformed health care, and nursing practice is becoming more specialized, evidence based, and autonomous. This section discusses some of these challenges.

Knowledge Development, Dissemination, and Application

Knowledge is rapidly expanding in the PMH field. Genetic research has opened new areas of investigation into the etiology of several disorders such as schizophrenia, bipolar disorders, dementia, and autism and in drug dosing and metabolism. The science of psychoneuroimmunology investigates the inseparable connections among a person's psychological state, immune system, and the nervous system. Consistent with the biopsychosocial model, psychoneuroimmunology encourages PMH nurses to think holistically about mental health conditions and treatment. Understanding the influence on mental health of comorbid medical conditions—for example, hypertension, hypothyroidism, hyperthyroidism, and diabetes mellitus—contributes to the expansion of the nurses' necessary knowledge base. Psychiatric nurses must stay abreast of the advances in genetic science, psychoneuroimmunology, and comorbid disease states and incorporate into practice the most recent evidence-based findings and research to provide safe, competent care to individuals with mental disorders. Accessing new information through journals, electronic databases, and continuing education takes time and vigilance but provides a sound basis for application of new knowledge.

Overcoming Stigma

All nurses, based on their knowledge and adherence to the professional code of ethics, play an important role in dispelling myths and stigma often associated with mental illness. Stigma often prevents individuals from seeking help for mental health problems and is a form of injustice (see Chapter 2). PMH nurses have a unique insight into the harms caused by stigmatization. The principle of beneficence underlies the nurse's responsibility to reduce the burden of mental illness by addressing stigma, improving access to care, and educating patients, family members, communities, and society about the etiology, symptoms, and treatment of mental illnesses.

Holistic Nursing Care

PMH nursing has long been viewed as different and set apart from the practice of nurses in medical and surgical settings. PMH nurses' practice is now shaped by a holistic, comprehensive understanding of the people and communities in their care, as nurses consider the physical, psychological, spiritual, and social dynamics that influence mental health. PMH nurses accept the challenge of including mental health promotion and wellness approaches as part of their professional obligation.

Health Care Delivery System Challenges

PMH nurses face challenges posed by the systems in which mental health care is provided. Mental health care now features integrated community-based services where culturally competent, high-quality nursing care is needed

TABLE 6.2	EXAMPLES OF THE RELATIONSHIP OF THE BIOPSYCHOSOCIAL MODEL TO STRUCTURED NURSING LANGUAGES		
	Interventions		
Nursing Language	**Biologic**	**Psychological**	**Social**
Clinical Care Classification *Diagnosis:* Sleep pattern disturbance	Care related to improving pattern of sleep.	Teach sleep pattern control.	Manage sleep pattern control.
Omaha System *Diagnosis:* Insomnia	Take medication therapy as prescribed.	Establish routine. Use guided imagery.	Use community resources.

Adapted from Saba, V. K. (2018). *Clinical care classification (CCC) system. A guide to nursing documentation.* Springer Publishing Company; Martin, K. S. (2005). *The Omaha System: A key to practice, documentation, and information management* (2nd ed.). Elsevier Saunders.

to meet the mental health care needs of patients and communities. In caring for patients who require social welfare support—housing, job opportunities, welfare, or transportation—nurses need to know how to navigate those systems to help the patient get needed assistance. Addressing the social problem can help alleviate mental health stressors and chronic illness exacerbations. Sometimes, the nurse is the only person with an understanding of medical conditions such as human immunodeficiency virus, acquired immunodeficiency syndrome, and other somatic health problems, drawing on the nurse's teaching and mentoring skills. Despite some of the increased challenges to PMH practice in outpatient settings, assertive community treatment reduces inpatient service use, promotes continuity of outpatient care, and increases the stability of people with serious mental illnesses (see Chapter 10). Nurses are challenged to expand their knowledge and help move the currently fragmented health care system toward one focusing on patients and community-centered care.

The Challenges of Technology in Health Care

Technologic advances have had an unprecedented impact on health care, posing challenges to PMH nurses. The electronic storing and sharing of health records, increased use of video conferences and telehealth appointments for patient psychological assessments and therapy sessions, and the advent of technologies to track patients' medications compliance pose potential threats to patient privacy and self-determination. Nurses accept the challenge of protecting patients' medical information and have a duty to minimize any mismanagement of technology that can cause harm.

Electronic documentation has been helpful in making readily available the use of standardized nursing terminologies. Nurses improve patient care by using **standardized nursing language** when communicating with nurses and other disciplines, giving visibility to nursing activities, enhancing data collection, communicating outcome

evaluations, and documenting adherence to standards of care.

There are several terminology sets being evaluated for use in electronic records (MBL Technologies, & Clinovations, 2017). Table 6.2 provides an example of how some of these standardized languages relate to the biopsychosocial framework. These terminologies vary in their scope of practice and their applicability to psychiatric nursing practice. For example, the International Classification for Nursing Practice® is more inclusive of mental health phenomena than the Perioperative Nursing Data Set. To be useful in psychiatric nursing, standardized languages must specifically address responses to mental disorders and emotional problems.

> **KEYCONCEPT A standardized nursing language** is readily understood by all nurses to describe care. It provides a common means of communication.

Professionals use telemedicine in many ways from communicating with remote sites to completing educational programs. Patients and family members often use internet access to learn about their disorders and treatment and locate resources. Persons with cognitive dysfunction benefit from software programs designed to accommodate cognitive deficits.

SUMMARY OF KEY POINTS

- The ANA's code of ethics establishes the ethical standards used by nurses in all areas of practice and communicates those standards to others.

- Several primary and secondary ethical principles provide guidance to PMH nurses for making ethical decisions and forming trusting, healing relationships with patients.

- *Psychiatric–Mental Health Nursing: Scope and Standards of Practice* (2014) establishes the areas of concern, standards of practice (using the nursing process), and standards of professional performance for basic and advanced practice nurses.

- Professional nursing organizations, such as the ANA, APNA, ISPN, and International Nurses Society on Addictions, provide leadership in shaping mental health care and advocate for patients and nurses.

- The biopsychosocial framework focuses on three separate but interdependent dimensions—biologic, psychological, and social—used in the assessment and treatment of mental disorders. This comprehensive and holistic framework provides the foundation for effective PMH nursing practice and is consistent with the principles of recovery and wellness models.

- Nursing care plans and interdisciplinary treatment plans are developed for each patient. Nurses use clinical reasoning skills to develop and revise plans of care.

- The PMH nurse collaborates with other disciplines to develop plans of care and often coordinates care delivery.

- Emerging challenges face PMH nurses as they incorporate advances in genetics, integrated models, evidence-based practice, and research findings into the care of persons with psychiatric disorders.

- As PMH nurses become more established as leaders in community-based health care, their roles will expand and evolve.

Unfolding Patient Stories: Linda Waterfall

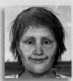 Linda Waterfall, a 48-year-old Native American with an aggressive form of breast cancer, is scheduled for a mastectomy. She is extremely nervous, refusing the preoperative medication, lorazepam, and reconsidering her family's request to meet with tribal healers. How can the code of ethics for nurses be applied to ethical issues identified in this situation? What values and beliefs of a nurse might conflict with Linda's? How does understanding the differences in values influence the nurse's response to Linda's beliefs and inform ethical decision-making?

CRITICAL THINKING CHALLENGES

1. A nurse is asked to witness a wedding for two patients (one with schizophrenia and the other with bipolar disorder) who recently met while being hospitalized. They are grateful to the nurse for their care. Discuss which ethical principles apply and may be in conflict.

2. Describe how the values represented in each of the primary ethical principles help in ethical deliberations and consider how they might be in tension or conflict in some situations.

3. Describe how social conditions—environment, safety, access to resources, job opportunities, and housing—may influence a person's mental health and recovery.

4. Visit the ANA's website for a description of the certification credential requirements for PMH nursing. Compare the functions of a PMH-RN with those of an advanced practice psychiatric nurse.

5. Explain the biopsychosocial framework and apply it to the following three clinical examples:

    a. A loud noise triggers a rapid heart rate and anxiety in a person who has recently experienced an acute traumatic event.

    b. A teenager, depressed by social isolation, begins to eat unhealthy food.

    c. A person with bipolar disease develops insomnia, worried that they will lose their job if someone informs the boss about their mental health diagnosis.

6. Describe how each of the following nursing organizations promotes quality mental health care and supports nursing practice. Visit the organizations' websites to find the information you need to make comparisons.

    a. American Nurses Association

    b. American Psychiatric Nurses Association

    c. International Society of Psychiatric–Mental Health Nurses

    d. International Nurses Society on Addictions

REFERENCES

American Nurses Association. (2015). *Code of ethics for nurses with interpretive statements.* Nursesbooks.org.

American Nurses Association, American Psychiatric Nurses Association, & International Society of Psychiatric–Mental Health Nurses. (2014). *Psychiatric–mental health nursing: Scope and standards of practice* (2nd ed.). Nursesbooks.org.

da Cruz Sequeira, C. A., & Sampaio, F. M. C. (2018). Taxonomies: Towards a shared nomenclature and language. In J. Santos & J. Cutcliffe (Eds.), *European Psychiatric/Mental Health Nursing in the 21st Century.* Principles of Specialty Nursing (Under the auspices of the European Specialist Nurses Organisations (ESNO) (pp. 37–47). https://doi.org/10.1007/978-3-319-31772-4_4

Davis, A. (2008). Provision two. In M. Fowler (Ed.), *Guide to the code of ethics for nurses: Interpretation and application* (p. 18). Nursebooks.org.

Kerr, M. J., Flaten, C., Honey, M. L., Gargantua-Aguila, S., Nahcivan, N. O., Martin, K. S., & Monsen, K. A. (2016). Feasibility of using the Omaha System for community-level observations. *Public Health Nursing, 33*(3), 256–263.

Martin, K. S. (2005). *The Omaha System: A key to practice, documentation, and information management* (2nd ed.). Elsevier Saunders.

MBL Technologies, & Clinovations. (2017). *Standard nursing terminologies: A landscape analysis.* The Office of the National coordinator for Health Information Technology. https://www.healthit.gov/sites/default/files/snt_final_05302017.pdf

Moorhead, S., Johnson, M., Maas, M. L., & Swanson, E. (2018). *Nursing outcomes classification (NOC)* (6th ed.). St. Louis.

Saba, V. K. (2018). *Clinical care classification system.* Sabacare. https://www.sabacare.com/framework/

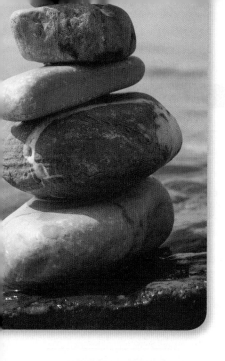

7
Psychosocial Theoretic Basis of Psychiatric Nursing

Mary Ann Boyd

KEYCONCEPTS

- anxiety
- empathic linkage

LEARNING OBJECTIVES

After studying this chapter, you will be able to:

1. Discuss psychosocial theories that support psychiatric nursing practice.

2. Identify the underlying theories that contribute to the understanding of human beings and behavior.

3. Compare the key elements of each theory that provides a basis for psychiatric–mental health nursing practice.

4. Identify common nursing theoretic models used in psychiatric–mental health nursing.

KEY TERMS

- Behaviorism • Classical conditioning • Cognitions • Cognitive theory • Connections • Countertransference • Defense mechanisms • Disconnections • Empathy • Family dynamics • Formal support systems • Informal support systems • Interpersonal relations • Libido • Modeling • Object relations • Operant behavior • Psychoanalysis • Self-efficacy • Self-system • Social distance • Transaction • Transference • Unconditional positive regard

INTRODUCTION

This chapter presents an overview of selected psychodynamic, cognitive behavioral, developmental, social, and nursing theories that serve as the knowledge base for psychiatric–mental health nursing practice. Many of these theories are covered in more depth in other chapters. Biologic theories are discussed in Chapters 8 and 12.

PSYCHODYNAMIC THEORIES

Psychodynamic theories explain the development of mental or emotional processes and their effects on behavior and relationships. Many of the psychodynamic concepts and models that are important in psychiatric

nursing began with the Austrian physician Sigmund Freud (1856–1939). Since his time, Freud theories have been enhanced by interpersonal and humanist models. These theories proved to be especially important in the development of therapeutic relationships, techniques, and interventions (Table 7.1).

Psychoanalytic Theory

In Freud psychoanalytic model, the human mind is conceptualized in terms of conscious mental processes (an awareness of events, thoughts, and feelings with the ability to recall them) and unconscious mental processes (thoughts and feelings that are outside awareness and are not remembered).

TABLE 7.1	PSYCHODYNAMIC MODELS		
Theorist	Overview	Major Concepts	Applicability
Psychoanalytic Models			
Sigmund Freud (1856–1939)	Founder of psychoanalysis Believed that the unconscious could be accessed through dreams and free association Developed a personality theory and theory of infantile sexuality	Id, ego, superego Consciousness Unconscious mental processes Libido Object relations Anxiety and defense mechanisms Free associations, transference, and countertransference	Individual therapy approach used for enhancement of personal maturity and personal growth
Anna Freud (1895–1982)	Application of ego psychology to psychoanalytic treatment and child analysis with emphasis on the adaptive function of defense mechanisms	Refinement of concepts of anxiety, defense mechanisms	Individual therapy, childhood psychoanalysis
Neo-Freudian Models			
Alfred Adler (1870–1937)	First defected from Freud Founded the school of individual psychology	Inferiority	Added to the understanding of human motivation
Carl Gustav Jung (1875–1961)	After separating from Freud, founded the school of psychoanalytic psychology Developed new therapeutic approaches	Redefined libido Introversion Extroversion Persona	Personalities are often assessed on the introversion and extroversion dimensions
Otto Rank (1884–1939)	Introduced idea of primary trauma of birth Active technique of therapy, including more nurturing than Freud Emphasized feeling aspect of analytic process	Birth trauma Will	Recognized the importance of feelings within psychoanalysis
Erich Fromm (1900–1980)	Emphasized the relationship of the individual to society	Society and individual are not separate	Individual desires are formed by society
Melanie Klein (1882–1960)	Devised play therapy techniques Believed that complex unconscious fantasies existed in children younger than 6 months of age Principal source of anxiety arose from the threat to existence posed by the death instinct	Pioneer in object relations Identification	Developed different ways of applying psychoanalysis to children; influenced present-day English and American schools of child psychiatry
Karen Horney (1885–1952)	Opposed Freud theory of castration complex in women and his emphasis on the oedipal complex Argued that neurosis was influenced by the society in which one lived	Situational neurosis Character	Beginning of feminist analysis of psychoanalytic thought
Interpersonal Relations			
Harry Stack Sullivan (1892–1949)	Impulses and striving need to be understood in terms of interpersonal situations	Participant observer Parataxic distortion Consensual validation	Provided the framework for the introduction of the interpersonal theories in nursing
Humanist Theories			
Abraham Maslow (1908–1970)	Concerned himself with healthy rather than sick people Approached individuals from a holistic-dynamic viewpoint	Needs Motivation	Used as a model to understand how people are motivated and needs that should be met
Frederick S. Perls (1893–1970)	Awareness of emotion, physical state, and repressed needs would enhance the ability to deal with emotional problems	Reality Here and now	Used as a therapeutic approach to resolve current life problems that are influenced by old, unresolved emotional problems
Carl Rogers (1902–1987)	Based theory on the view of human potential for goodness Used the term *client* rather than *patient* Stressed the relationship between therapist and client	Empathy Positive regard	Individual therapy approach that involves never giving advice and always clarifying client's feelings

Study of the Unconscious

Freud believed that the unconscious part of the human mind is only rarely recognized by the conscious, as in remembered dreams (see Movies at the end of this chapter). The term *preconscious* is used to describe unconscious material that is capable of entering consciousness.

Personality and Its Development

Freud personality structure consists of three parts: the id, ego, and superego (Freud, 1927). The *id* is formed by unconscious desires, primitive instincts, and unstructured drives, including sexual and aggressive tendencies that arise from the body. The *ego* consists of the sum of certain mental mechanisms, such as perception, memory, and motor control, as well as specific defense mechanisms (discussed in the following). The ego controls movement, perception, and contact with reality. The capacity to form mutually satisfying relationships is a fundamental function of the ego, which is not present at birth but is formed throughout the child's development. The *superego* is that part of the personality structure associated with ethics, standards, and self-criticism. A child's identification with important and esteemed people in early life, particularly parents, helps form the superego.

Object Relations and Identification

Freud introduced the concept of **object relations**, the psychological attachment to another person or object. He believed that the choice of a sexual partner in adulthood and the nature of that relationship depended on the quality of the child's object relationships during the early formative years.

The child's first love object is the mother, who is the source of nourishment and the provider of pleasure. Gradually, as the child separates from the mother, the nature of this initial attachment influences future relationships. The development of the child's capacity for relationships with others progresses from a state of narcissism to social relationships, first within the family and then within the larger community. Although the concept of object relations is fairly abstract, it can be understood in terms of a child who imitates their mother and then becomes like their mother in adulthood. This child incorporates their mother as a love object, identifies with her, and grows up to become like her. This process is especially important in understanding an abused child who, under certain circumstances, becomes an adult abuser.

Anxiety and Defense Mechanisms

For Freud, anxiety is the reaction to danger and is experienced as a specific state of physical unpleasantness. **Defense mechanisms** are coping styles that protect a person from unwanted anxiety. Although they are defined differently than in Freud day, defense mechanisms still play an explanatory role in contemporary psychiatric–mental health practice. Defense mechanisms are discussed in the chapter on Communication and the Therapeutic Relationship (Chapter 10).

Sexuality

The energy or psychic drive associated with the sexual instinct, or **libido**, literally translated from Latin to mean "pleasure" or "lust," resides in the id. When sexual desire is controlled and not expressed, tension results and is transformed into anxiety (Freud, 1905). Freud believed that adult sexuality is an end product of a complex process of development that begins in early childhood and involves a variety of body functions or areas (oral, anal, and genital zones) that correspond to stages of relationships, especially with parents.

Psychoanalysis

Freud developed **psychoanalysis**, a therapeutic process of accessing the unconscious conflicts that originate in childhood and then resolving the issues with a mature adult mind. As a system of psychotherapy, psychoanalysis attempts to reconstruct the personality by examining free associations (spontaneous, uncensored verbalizations of whatever comes to mind) and the interpretation of dreams. Therapeutic relationships had their beginnings within the psychoanalytic framework.

Transference and Countertransference

Transference is the displacement of thoughts, feelings, and behaviors originally associated with significant others from childhood onto a person in a current therapeutic relationship (Moore & Fine, 1990). For example, a woman's feelings toward her parents as a child may be directed toward the therapist. If a woman were unconsciously angry with her parents, she may feel unexplainable anger and hostility toward her therapist. In psychoanalysis, the therapist uses transference as a therapeutic tool to help the patient understand emotional problems and their origin.

Countertransference, on the other hand, is defined as the direction of all of the therapist's feelings and attitudes toward the patient. Countertransference becomes a problem when these feelings and perceptions are based on other interpersonal experiences. For example, a patient may remind a nurse of a beloved grandmother. Instead of therapeutically interacting with the patient from an objective perspective, the nurse feels an unexplained attachment to her and treats the patient as if she were the nurse's grandmother. The nurse misses important assessment and intervention data.

Neo-Freudian Models

Many of Freud's followers ultimately broke away, establishing their own forms of psychoanalysis. Freud did not receive criticism well. The rejection of some of his basic tenets often cost his friendship as well. Various psychoanalytic schools have adopted other names because their doctrines deviated from Freudian theory.

Adler's Foundation for Individual Psychology

Alfred Adler (1870–1937), a Viennese psychiatrist and founder of the school of individual psychology, was a student of Freud, who believed that the motivating force in human life is an intolerable sense of inferiority. Some people try to avoid these feelings by developing an unreasonable desire for power and dominance. This compensatory mechanism can get out of hand, and these individuals become self-centered and neurotic, overcompensate, and retreat from the real world and its problems.

Today, Adler's theories and principles are adapted and applied to both psychotherapy and education. Adlerian theory is based on principles of mutual respect, choice, responsibility, consequences, and belonging.

Jung Analytical Psychology

One of Freud's earliest students, Carl Gustav Jung (1875–1961), a Swiss psychoanalyst, created a model called analytical psychology. Jung believed in the existence of two basically different types of personalities: extroverted and introverted. Whereas extroverted people tend to be generally interested in other people and objects of the external world, introverted people are more interested in themselves and their internal environment. According to Jung, both extroverted and introverted tendencies exist in everyone, but the libido usually channels itself mainly in one direction or the other. He also developed the concept of *persona*—what a person appears to be to others in contrast to who they really are (Jung, 1966).

Horney Feminine Psychology

Karen Horney (1885–1952), a German American psychiatrist, challenged many of Freud's basic concepts and introduced principles of feminine psychology. Recognizing a male bias in psychoanalysis, Horney was the first to challenge the traditional psychoanalytic belief that women felt disadvantaged because of their genital organs. Freud believed that women felt inferior to men because their bodies were less completely equipped, a theory he described as "penis envy." Horney rejected this concept, as well as the oedipal complex, arguing that

there are significant cultural reasons why women may strive to obtain qualities or privileges that are defined by a society as being masculine. For example, in Horney time, most women did not have access to a university education, the right to vote, or economic independence. She argued that women truly were at a disadvantage because of the paternalistic culture in which they lived (Horney, 1939).

Other Neo-Freudian Theories

Otto Rank: Birth Trauma

Otto Rank (1884–1939), an Austrian psychologist and psychotherapist, was also one of Freud's students. He attributed all neurotic disturbances to the primary trauma of birth. For Rank, human development is a progression from complete dependence on the mother and family to physical independence coupled with intellectual dependence on society and finally to complete intellectual and psychological emancipation. A person's will guides and organizes the integration of self.

Erich Fromm: Societal Needs

Erich Fromm (1900–1980), an American psychoanalyst, focused on the relationship of society and the individual. He argued that individual and societal needs are not separate and opposing forces; their relationship is determined by the historic background of the culture. Fromm also believed that the needs and desires of individuals are largely formed by their society. For Fromm, the fundamental purpose of psychoanalysis and psychology is to bring harmony and understanding between the individual and society (Fromm-Reichmann, 1950).

Melanie Klein: Play Therapy

Melanie Klein (1882–1960), an Austrian psychoanalyst, devised play therapy techniques to demonstrate how a child's interaction with toys reveals earlier infantile fantasies and anxieties. She believed that complex, unconscious fantasies exist in children younger than 6 months of age. She is generally acknowledged as a pioneer in presenting an object relations viewpoint to the psychodynamic field, introducing the idea of early identification, a defense mechanism by which one patterns oneself after another person, such as a parent (Klein, 1963).

Harry Stack Sullivan: Interpersonal Forces

Interpersonal theories stress the importance of human relationships; instincts and drives are less important. Harry Stack Sullivan (1892–1949), an American psychiatrist, viewed **interpersonal relations** as a basis of human development and behavior. He believed that the health or sickness of one's personality is determined by the characteristic patterns in which one deals with other people. For example, one man is passive aggressive to everyone who contradicts him. This maladaptive behavior began when he was unable to express his disagreement to his parents. Health depends on managing the constantly changing physical, social, and interpersonal environment as well as past and current life experiences (Sullivan, 1953).

Humanistic Theories

Humanistic theories are based on the belief that all human beings have the potential for goodness. Humanist therapists focus on patients' ability to learn about and accept themselves. They do not investigate repressed memories. Through therapy, patients explore personal capabilities in order to develop self-worth. They learn to experience the world in a different way.

Rogers Client-Centered Therapy

Carl Rogers (1902–1987), an American psychologist, introduced client-centered therapy. **Empathy**, the capacity to assume the internal reference of the client in order to perceive the world in the same way as the client, is used in the therapeutic process (Rogers, 1980). The counselor is genuine but nondirect and also uses **unconditional positive regard**, a nonjudgmental caring for the client. In this therapy, the counselor's attitude and nonverbal communication are crucial. The therapist's emotional investment (i.e., true caring) in the client is essential in the therapeutic process (Rogers, 1980).

Gestalt Therapy

Another humanistic approach is Gestalt therapy, developed by Frederick S. (Fritz) Perls (1893–1970), a German-born former psychoanalyst who immigrated to the United States. Perls believed the root of human anxiety is frustration with inability to express natural biologic and psychological desires in modern civilization. The repression of these basic desires causes anxiety. In Gestalt therapy, these unmet needs are brought into awareness through individual and group exercises (Perls, 1969).

Abraham Maslow's Hierarchy of Needs

Abraham Maslow's (1921–1970) hierarchy of needs is fixture in social science and nursing (Maslow, 1970) (Figure 7.1). In nursing, Maslow model is used to prioritize care. Basic needs (food, shelter) should be met before higher-level needs (self-esteem) can be met.

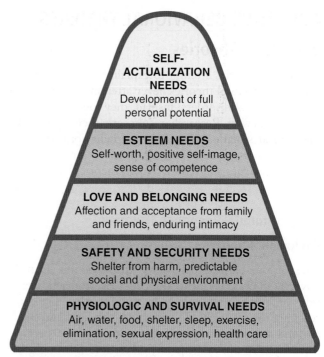

FIGURE 7.1 Maslow's hierarchy of needs.

Applicability of Psychodynamic Theories to Psychiatric–Mental Health Nursing

Several psychodynamic concepts are important in the practice of psychiatric–mental health nursing, such as interpersonal relationships, defense mechanisms, transference, countertransference, and internal objects. In particular, a therapeutic interpersonal relationship is a core of psychiatric–mental health nursing intervention (see Chapter 11 for nursing interventions). Even though there is general consensus that most of these theories are useful, the nurse should continue to critically analyze them for utility and relevance. For example, Maslow theory may be useful when a person with mental illness is homeless and wants food and shelter. But, another person in a similar situation may reject food and shelter because self-esteem is associated with being free to reject the confines of an institution. In this case, self-esteem need is more important than food or shelter.

Recently, there is renewed interest in psychodynamic treatment for depression. Psychodynamic therapists have a strong emphasis on affect and emotional expression, examination of topics that the patient avoids, recurring patterns of behaviors, feelings, experiences and relationships, the past and its influence on the present, interpersonal relationships, and exploration of wishes, dreams, and fantasies (Pitman & Knauss, 2020).

COGNITIVE-BEHAVIORAL THEORIES

Behavioral Theories

Behavioral theories attempt to explain how people learn and act. Behavioral theories never attempt to explain the cause of mental disorders; instead, they focus on normal human behavior. Research results are then applied to the clinical situation. Two areas of behavioral theories relevant to psychiatric–nursing practice are stimulus–response theories and reinforcement theories (Table 7.2).

Early Stimulus–Response Theories

Pavlovian Theory

One of the earliest behavioral theorists was Ivan P. Pavlov (1849–1936), who noticed that stomach secretions of dogs were stimulated by triggers other than food reaching the stomach. He found that the sight and smell of food triggered stomach secretions, and he became interested in this anticipatory secretion. Through his experiments, he was able to stimulate secretions with a variety of other laboratory nonphysiologic stimuli. Thus, a clear connection was made between thought processes and physiologic responses.

In Pavlov model, there is an unconditioned stimulus (not dependent on previous training) that elicits an unconditioned (i.e., specific) response. In his experiments, meat is the unconditioned stimulus, and salivation is the

unconditioned response. Pavlov taught the dog to associate a bell (conditioned stimulus) with the meat (unconditioned stimulus) by repeatedly ringing the bell before presenting the meat. Eventually, the dog salivated when he heard the bell. This phenomenon is called **classical conditioning** (or Pavlovian conditioning) (Pavlov, 1927/1960).

John B. Watson and the Behaviorist Revolution

At about the same time Pavlov was working in Russia, **behaviorism**, a learning theory that only focuses on objectively observable behaviors and discounts any independent activities of the mind, was introduced in the United States by John B. Watson (1878–1958). He rejected the distinction between body and mind and emphasized the study of objective behavior (Watson & Rayner, 1920). He developed two principles: frequency and recency. The *principle of frequency* states that the more often a response is made to a stimulus, the more likely the response to that stimulus will be repeated. The *principle of recency* states that the closer in time a response is to a particular stimulus, the more likely the response will be repeated.

Reinforcement Theories

Edward L. Thorndike

A pioneer in experimental animal psychology, Edwin L. Thorndike (1874–1949) studied the problem-solving behavior of cats to determine whether animals solved

Theorist	Overview	Major Concepts	Applicability
TABLE 7.2 BEHAVIORAL THEORISTS			
Stimulus–Response			
Edwin R. Guthrie (1886–1959)	Continued with understanding conditioning as being important in learning	Recurrence of responses tends to follow a specific stimulus	Important in analyzing habitual behavior
Ivan P. Pavlov (1849–1936)	Classical conditioning	Unconditioned stimuli Unconditioned response Conditioned stimuli	Important in understanding learning of automatic responses such as habitual behaviors
John B. Watson (1878–1958)	Introduced behaviorism Believed that learning was classical conditioning called *reflexes* Rejected distinction between mind and body	Principle of frequency Principle of recency	Focuses on the relationship between the mind and body
Reinforcement Theories			
B. F. Skinner (1904–1990)	Developed an understanding of the importance of reinforcement and differentiated types and schedules	Operant behavior Respondent behavior Continuous reinforcement Intermittent reinforcement	Important in behavior modification
Edward L. Thorndike (1874–1949)	Believed in the importance of effects that followed behavior	Reinforcement	Important in behavior modification programs

problems by reasoning or instinct. He found that neither choice was completely correct; animals gradually learn the correct response by "stamping in" the stimulus–response connection. The major difference between Thorndike and behaviorists such as Watson was that Thorndike believed that reinforcement of positive behavior was important in learning. He was the first reinforcement theorist, and his view of learning became the dominant view in American learning theory (Thorndike, 1906).

B. F. Skinner

One of the most influential behaviorists, B. F. Skinner (1904–1990) studied **operant behavior** or conditioning. In this type of learning, the focus is on the consequence of the behavioral response, not on a specific stimulus. If a behavior is reinforced or rewarded with success, praise, money, and so on, the behavior will probably be repeated. For example, if a child climbs on a chair, reaches the faucet, and is able to get a drink of water successfully, it is more likely that the child will repeat the behavior (Skinner, 1935). If a behavior does not have a positive outcome, it is less likely that the behavior will be repeated. Nurses use this knowledge to create behavior management plans to reinforce healthy, positive behaviors.

Cognitive Theories

The initial behavioral studies focused on human actions without much attention to the internal thinking process. When complex behaviors could not be accounted for by strictly behavioral explanations, thought processes became new subjects for study. **Cognitive theory**, an outgrowth of different theoretic perspectives, including the behavioral and the psychodynamic, attempted to link internal thought processes with human behavior (Table 7.3).

Albert Bandura Social Cognitive Theory

Learning by watching others is the basis of Albert Bandura (b. 1925) social cognitive theory. He developed his ideas after being concerned about television violence contributing to aggression in children. He showed learning occurs by internalizing behaviors of others through a process of **modeling** called pervasive imitation, or one person trying to be like another. The model does not have to be a real person but could be a character in history or generalized to an ideal person (Bandura, 1977, 1986).

An important concept of Bandura's is **self-efficacy**, a person's sense of ability to deal effectively with the environment (Bandura, 1993). Efficacy beliefs influence how people feel, think, motivate themselves, and behave. The stronger the self-efficacy, the higher the goals people set for themselves and the firmer their commitment to them (Maine et al., 2017).

One of Bandura's recent contributions is showing that intentions and self-motivation play roles in determining behavior, significantly expanding the reinforcement model. He believes that the human mind is not only reactive to a stimulus but is also creative, proactive, and reflective (Bandura, 2001). Recent research supports Bandura ideas in accounting for goal achievement in entrepreneurship (Gielnik et al., 2020).

Aaron Beck: Thinking and Feeling

American psychiatrist Aaron T. Beck (b. 1921) of the University of Pennsylvania devoted his career to understanding the relationship between cognition and mental health. For Beck, **cognitions** are verbal or pictorial events in the stream of consciousness. He realized the importance of cognitions when treating people with depression. He found that depression improved when patients began viewing themselves and situations in a positive light.

He believes that people with depression have faulty information-processing systems that lead to biased cognitions. These faulty beliefs cause errors in judgment that become habitual errors in thinking. These individuals incorrectly interpret life situations, judge themselves too harshly, and jump to inaccurate negative conclusions. A person may truly believe that they have no friends, and

TABLE 7.3	COGNITIVE THEORISTS		
Theorist	**Overview**	**Major Concepts**	**Applicability**
Aaron Beck (b. 1921)	Conceptualized distorted cognitions as a basis for depression	Cognitions Beliefs	Important in cognitive therapy
Kurt Lewin (1890–1947)	Developed field theory, a system for understanding learning, motivation, personality, and social behavior	Life space Positive valences	Important in understanding motivation for changing behavior
Edward Chace Tolman (1886–1959)	Introduced the concept of cognitions: believed that human beings act on beliefs and attitudes and strive toward goals	Negative valences Cognition	Important in identifying person's beliefs

BOX 7.1

Caregiver Beliefs and Depression

Crano, C., Lucidi, F., & Violani, C. (2017). The relationship between caregiving self-efficacy and depressive symptoms in family caregivers of patients with Alzheimer disease: a longitudinal study. International Psychogeriatrics, 29(7), 1095–1103.

THE QUESTION: Is there an association between caregiver's beliefs and depression?

METHODS: A three-wave design was used with initial assessment and follow-ups three months later and one year later. One hundred and seventy caregivers of patients with AD responded to measures of caregiver burden, caregiving self-efficacy (including control over upsetting beliefs about caregiving), and depressive symptoms.

FINDINGS: The caregiving burden at the time of the first assessment influenced the severity of depression one year later. The depressive symptoms were less severe when the caregivers believed that they had control over their upsetting thoughts about caregiving.

IMPLICATIONS FOR NURSING: Interventions that target caregivers' negative thoughts about the caregiving role may help them in coping with their situation.

therefore no one cares. On examination, the evidence for the beliefs is based on the fact that there has been no contact with anyone because of moving from one city to another. Thus, a distorted belief is the basis of the cognition. Beliefs are important because they are related to a person's mood. For example, negative beliefs of caregivers of family members with Alzheimer disorder are related to depression (see Box 7.1). Beck and his colleagues continue to develop cognitive therapy, a successful approach for the treatment of depression (Beck, 2021).

Applicability of Cognitive-Behavioral Theories to Psychiatric–Mental Health Nursing

Basing interventions on behavioral theories is widespread in psychiatric nursing. For example, patient education interventions are usually derived from the behavioral theories. Teaching patients new coping skills for their symptoms of mental illnesses is another example. Changing an entrenched habit involves helping patients identify what motivates them and how these new lifestyle habits can become permanent. In psychiatric units, behavioral interventions include the privilege systems and token economies. Cognitive behavioral approaches are discussed throughout this text.

DEVELOPMENTAL THEORIES

Developmental theories explain normal human growth and development over time. Many developmental theories are presented in terms of stages based on the assumption that normal development proceeds longitudinally from the beginning to the ending stage.

Erik Erikson: Psychosocial Development

Freud and Sullivan both published treatises on stages of human development, but Erik Erikson (1902–1994) outlined the psychosocial developmental model that is most often used in nursing. Erikson model is an expansion of Freud psychosexual development theory. Whereas Freud model emphasizes intrapsychic experiences, Erikson model recognizes the role of the psychosocial environment. For example, parental divorce disrupts the family interaction pattern, and the financial and housing environment impact the development of the children.

Each of Erikson's eight stages is organized by age and developmental conflicts: basic trust versus mistrust, autonomy versus shame and doubt, initiative versus guilt, industry versus inferiority, identity versus role diffusion, intimacy versus isolation, generativity versus stagnation, and ego integrity versus despair. Successful resolution of a conflict or crisis leads to essential strength and virtues (Table 7.4). For example, a positive outcome of the trust versus mistrust crisis is the development of a basic sense of trust. If the crisis is unsuccessfully resolved, the infant moves into the next stage without a sense of trust. According to this model, a child who is mistrustful will have difficulty completing the next crisis successfully and, instead of developing a sense of autonomy, will more likely be full of shame and doubt (Erikson, 1963).

Identity and Adolescence

One of Erikson's major contributions is the recognition of the turbulence of adolescence and identity formation. When adolescence begins, childhood ways are given up, and bodily changes occur. An identity is formed. Trying to reconcile a personal view of self with society's perception can be overwhelming and lead to role confusion and alienation (Erikson, 1968).

Research Evidence for Erikson Models

Evidence is mixed that every person follows the eight stages of development as outlined by Erikson. In an early study, male college students who measured low on identity also scored low on intimacy ratings (Orlofsky et al., 1973). These results lend support to the idea that identity precedes

TABLE 7.4	ERIKSON'S EIGHT AGES OF MAN	
Approximate Chronologic Age	Developmental Conflict*	Long-Term Outcome of Successful Resolution
Infant	Basic trust vs. mistrust	Drive and hope
Toddler	Autonomy vs. shame and doubt	Self-control and willpower
Preschool-aged child	Initiative vs. guilt	Direction and purpose
School-aged child	Industry vs. inferiority	Method and competence
Adolescence	Identity vs. role diffusion	Devotion and fidelity
Young adult	Intimacy vs. isolation	Affiliation and love
Adulthood	Generativity vs. stagnation	Production and care
Maturity	Ego integrity vs. despair	Renunciation and wisdom

*Successful outcome is evidenced by the development of the characteristic listed first.
Adapted from Erikson, E. (1963). *Childhood and society* (pp. 273–274). W. W. Norton & Company.

intimacy. In another study, intimacy was found to begin developing early in adolescence before the development of identity (Ochse & Plug, 1986). Studying fathers with young children, Christiansen and Palkovitz (1998) found that *generativity* (defined as the need or drive to produce, create, or effect a change) was associated with a paternal identity, psychosocial identity, and psychosocial intimacy. In addition, fathers who had a religious identification also had higher generativity scores than did others.

A longitudinal study of 86 men beginning at age 21 years with reassessment 32 years later at age 53 years supports Erikson psychosocial eight-stage model (Westermeyer, 2004). In this study, 48 men (56%) achieved generativity at follow-up. Successful young adults as predicted by Erikson model at midlife lived within a warm family environment; had an absence of troubled parental discipline; experienced a mentor relationship; and, most importantly, had favorable peer group relationships. The model is also used as a framework for psychodynamic psychotherapy (Knight, 2017).

Erikson model may apply differently to men and women. In one study, generativity is associated with well-being in both men and women, but in men, generativity is related to the urge for self-protection, self-assertion, self-expansion, and mastery. In women, the antecedents may be the desire for contact, connection, and union (Ackerman et al., 2000).

Studies show that generativity is significantly associated with successful marriage, work achievements, close friendships, altruistic behaviors, and overall mental health. Generativity is also associated with optimism and forgiveness in dealing with grandparenting problems within the family (Ehlman & Ligon, 2012; Pratt et al., 2008) and contemplating the meaning of life to older adults (Jonsén et al., 2015).

Jean Piaget: Learning in Children

One of the most influential people in child psychology is Jean Piaget (1896–1980), who contributed more than 40 books and 100 articles on child psychology alone. Piaget theory views intelligence as an adaptation to the environment. He proposes that cognitive growth is like embryologic growth: an organized structure becomes more and more differentiated over time. Piaget system explains how knowledge develops and changes (Table 7.5).

Each stage of cognitive development represents a particular structure with major characteristics. Piaget theory was developed through observation of his own children and therefore never received formal testing.

The major strength of his model is its recognition of the central role of cognition in development and the discovery of surprising features of young children's thinking. For example, children in middle childhood become capable of considering more than one aspect of an object or situation at a time. Their thinking becomes more complex. They can understand that the area of a rectangle is determined by the length *and* width. For psychiatric–mental health nurses, Piaget model provides a framework to recognize different levels of thinking in the assessment and intervention processes. For example, the assessment of concrete thinking is typical of some people with schizophrenia who are unable to perform abstract thinking.

Carol Gilligan: Gender Differentiation in Moral Development

Carol Gilligan (b. 1936) argues that most development models are male centered and therefore inappropriate

TABLE 7.5	PIAGET PERIODS OF INTELLECTUAL DEVELOPMENT		
Age (years)	Period	Cognitive Developmental Characteristics	Description
Birth to 2	Sensorimotor	Divided into six stages, characterized by (1) inborn motor and sensory reflexes, (2) primary circular reaction and first habit, (3) secondary circular reaction, (4) use of familiar means to obtain ends, (5) tertiary circular reaction and discovery through active experimentation, and (6) insight and object permanence	The infant understands the world in terms of overt, physical action on that world. The infant moves from simple reflexes through several steps to an organized set of schemes. Significant concepts are developed, including space, time, and causality. Above all, during this period, the child develops the scheme of the permanent object.
2–7	Preoperational	Deferred imitation; symbolic play, graphic imagery (drawing); mental imagery; and language egocentrism, rigidity of thought, semilogical reasoning, and limited social cognition	Child no longer only makes perceptual and motor adjustment to objects and events. Child can now use symbols (mental images, words, gestures) to represent these objects and events; uses these symbols in an increasingly organized and logical fashion.
7–11	Concrete operations	Conservation of quantity, weight, volume, length, and time based on reversibility by inversion or reciprocity; operations: class inclusion and seriation	Conservation is the understanding of what values remain the same. For example, if liquid is poured from a short, wide glass into a tall, narrow one, the preoperational child thinks that the quantity has changed. For the concrete operation child, the amount stays the same.
11 through the end of adolescence	Formal operations	Combination system whereby variables are isolated and all possible combinations are examined; hypothetical-deductive thinking	Mental operations are applied to objects and events. The child classifies, orders, and reverses them. Hypotheses can be generated from these concrete operations.

for girls and women. She challenges Erik Erikson (psychosocial development) and Kohlberg (moral) theories as being biased against women because they are based on primarily privileged, White men and boys. For Gilligan, attachment within relationships is the important factor for successful development. After comparing male and female personality development, she highlights differences (Gilligan, 2004). In developing identity, boys separate from their mothers, and girls attach. Girls probably learn to value relationships and become interdependent at an earlier age. They learn to value the ideal of care, begin to respond to human need, and want to take care of the world by sustaining attachments so no one is left alone. Her model of moral development, *Ethic of Care*, is divided into three stages beginning with *preconventional* or selfishness (what is best for me) to *conventional* or responsibility to others (self-sacrifice is goodness) to *postconventional* or do not hurt others or self (she is a person too) (Gilligan, 2011).

Gilligan conclusion that female development depends on relationships has implications for everyone who provides care to women. Traditional models that advocate separation as the primary goal of human development immediately place women at a disadvantage. By negating the value and importance of attachments within relationships, the natural development of women is impaired. If Erikson model is applied to women, their failure

to separate then becomes defined as a developmental failure (Gilligan, 1982).

Jean Baker Miller: A Sense of Connection

Jean Baker Miller (1927–2006) conceptualized female development within the context of experiences and relationships. Her landmark book, *Toward a New Psychology of Women* (1976/1986), led to the development of the relational-cultural theory, which identified a sense of connection as the central organizing feature of women's development. The goal of development is to increase a woman's ability to build and enlarge mutually enhancing relationships (Miller, 1994). **Connections** (mutually responsive and enhancing relationships) lead to mutual engagement (attention), empathy, and empowerment. In relationships in which everyone interacts beneficially, mutual psychological development can occur. **Disconnections** (lack of mutually responsive and enhancing relationships) occur when a child or adult expresses a feeling or explains an experience and does not receive any response from others. The most serious types of disconnection arise from the lack of response that occurs after abuse or attacks. The theory is currently evolving and serves as a model for psychotherapy and nursing practice on psychiatric units (Kress et al., 2018; Walker & Rosen, 2004).

Applicability of Developmental Theories to Psychiatric–Mental Health Nursing

Developmental theories are used in understanding childhood and adolescent experiences and their manifestations as adult problems. When working with children, nurses can use developmental models to help gauge development and mood. However, because most of the models are based on the assumptions of the linear progression of stages and have not been adequately tested, applicability has limitations. Most do not account for gender differences and diversity in lifestyles and cultures.

SOCIAL THEORIES

Numerous social theories underlie psychiatric–mental health nursing practice. Chapter 3 presents some of the sociocultural issues and discusses various social groups. This section represents a sampling of important social theories that a nurse uses. This discussion is not exhaustive and should be viewed by the student as including a few of the important social theoretic perspectives.

Family Dynamics

Family dynamics are the patterned interpersonal and social interactions that occur within the family structure over the life of a family. Family dynamics models are based on systems theory in which the change of one part affects the total functioning of the system. The family is viewed organizationally as an open system in which one member's actions influence the functioning of the total system. Family theories are especially useful to nurses who are assessing family dynamics and planning interventions. Family systems models are used to help nurses form collaborative relationships with patients and families dealing with health problems. Generalist psychiatric–mental health nurses will not be engaged in family therapy. However, they will be caring for individuals and families. Understanding family dynamics is important in every nurse's practice.

Formal and Informal Social Support

Assisting patients in the recovery process means helping patients identify supportive family and community systems. **Formal support systems** are large organizations, such as hospitals and nursing homes that provide care to individuals. **Informal support systems** are family, friends, and neighbors. Individuals with strong informal support networks actually live longer than those without this type of support. Adolescents who are survivors of sexual assault are more likely to seek support from informal support systems than formal supports (Fehler-Cabral & Campbell, 2013). In addition, classic studies showed that those without informal support have significantly higher mortality rates when the causes of death are accidents (e.g., smoking in bed) or suicides (Litwak, 1985).

An important concept is **social distance**, the degree to which the values of the formal organization and primary group members differ. In the United States, the most closely located, accessible, and available family member is expected to provide the care to a family member. Spouses are the first choice, then children, other family members, friends, and finally formal support. On the other, care-related stress can result in the informal caregiver changing the balance by placing a family member in an institution (Friedemann et al., 2014).

Formal and informal support systems are balanced when they are at a midpoint of social distance, that is, close enough to communicate but not so close to destroy each other—neither enmeshment nor isolation (Litwak et al., 1990; Messeri et al., 1993). Conflicts arise when the relationship becomes unbalanced. For example, if the primary group and the formal care system begin performing similar caregiving services, there may be disagreements. Balance is reestablished when the formal system increases the social distance by developing relationships and providing support to the caregiver and reducing contact with the patient. Thus, a balance is maintained between the two systems. In another instance, when a patient relies only on the health care provider for care and support (e.g., calls the nurse every day, visits the physician weekly, refuses any help from family), balance can be reestablished by linking the patient to an informal support system for help with some of the caregiving tasks.

By applying frameworks of formal and informal support systems to their patients, psychiatric nurses can understand the complex social forces that patient's with mental disorders and their caregivers experience (McPherson et al., 2013) (Box 7.2). Nurses can help adjust the social distance between the formal and informal systems by identifying communication barriers and helping the two groups work together. For example, a patient misses an appointment because of a lack of transportation. The case manager helps the patient communicate the problem to the system to obtain another appointment. Informal caregivers are valued by the case manager, who recognizes the important services performed by family and friends. Thus, linkages between mental health providers (formal support) and the consumer network (informal support) are reinforced.

Role Theories

A role is a person's social position and function within an environment. Anthropologic theories explain members' roles that relate to a specific society. For example, the

---

BOX 7.2

Formal and Informal Support to Caregivers

Verbakel, E., Metzelthin, S.F., & Kempen, G.I.J.M. (2018). Caregiving to older adults: Determinants of informal caregivers' subjective well-being and formal and informal support as alleviating conditions. The Journals of Gerontology. Series B, Psychological Sciences, 73(6), 1099–1111. https://doi.org/10.1093/geronb/gbw047

THE QUESTION: Are there relationships among informal caregivers' subjective well-being and primary stressors, hours of informal caregiving, and burden? Does formal (professional home care) and informal support (from other caregivers, family, and friends) alleviate well-being losses due to providing informal care?

METHODS: Data from 4,717 dyads of informal caregivers and their older care recipients were analyzed.

FINDINGS: Caregivers' subjective well-being was directly related to the burden, hours of informal caregiving, and problem behavior of the care recipients. Formal and informal support reduced the impact of the primary stressors and caregiving hours. Reduction of formal/professional care may increase the negative well-being of caregivers.

IMPLICATIONS FOR NURSING: Formal and informal support to caregivers can promote well-being for caregivers.

BOX 7.3

Cultural Knowledge of Mental Health Beliefs and Practices

Wolf, K.M. (2016). Somali immigrant perceptions of mental health and illness: An ethnonursing study. Journal of Transcultural Nursing, 27(4), 349–358.

QUESTION: What are the mental health meanings, beliefs, and practices from the perspective of immigrant Somalis?

METHODS: Qualitative ethnonursing research methods were used. Thirty informants (9 key and 21 general) were interviewed in community settings.

FINDINGS: Analysis of the interviews revealed 21 categories and 9 patterns. Two main themes emerged: Religion significantly influences their mental health, and religious beliefs and practices influence their health care choices.

IMPLICATIONS FOR NURSING: Culturally congruent care will improve care for Somali immigrants.

---

universal roles of healer may be assumed by a nurse in one culture and a spiritual leader in another. Societal expectations, social status, and rights are attached to these roles. Psychological theories, which are concerned about roles from a different perspective, focus on the relationship of an individual's role: the self. The responsibilities of a parent are often in conflict with the personal needs for time alone. All of the neo-Freudian and humanist models that have been discussed focus on reciprocal social relationships or interactions that determine how the mind develops.

Role theories emphasize the importance of social interaction in either the individual's choice of a particular role or society's recognition of it. Psychiatric–mental health nursing uses role concepts in understanding group interaction and the role of the patient in the family and community. In addition, milieu therapy approaches discussed in later chapters are based on the patient's assumption of a role within the psychiatric environment.

Sociocultural Perspectives

Margaret Mead: Culture and Gender

American anthropologist Margaret Mead (1901–1978) is widely known for her studies of primitive societies and her contributions to social anthropology. She conducted studies in New Guinea, Samoa, and Bali and devoted much of her studies to the patterns of child-rearing in various cultures. She was particularly interested in the cultural influences determining male and female behavior (Mead, 1970). Influenced by Carl Jung and Erik Erikson, she had a vision of unity and diversity of the psychosocial development of a single human species (Sullivan, 2004). Although her research is often criticized as not having scientific rigor and being filled with misinterpretations, it is accepted as a classic in the field of anthropology (Sullivan, 2004). She established the importance of culture in determining human behavior.

Madeleine Leininger: Transcultural Health Care

Concern about the impact of culture on the treatment of children with psychiatric and emotional problems led Madeleine Leininger (1924–2012) to develop a new field, transcultural nursing, directed toward holistic, congruent, and beneficent care. Leininger developed the *Theory of Culture Care Diversity and Universality*, which explains diverse and universal dimensions of human caring (Figure 7.2). Nursing care in one culture is different from another because definitions of health, illness, and care are culturally defined (Leininger & McFarland, 2006). The goal of Leininger theory is to discover culturally based care (Leininger, 2007). Leininger model continues to be used today as a framework for understanding mental health beliefs of various ethnic groups (Wolf et al., 2016), Alzheimer disease (Barbosa et al., 2020), and violence against women (Broch et al., 2017) (see Box 7.3).

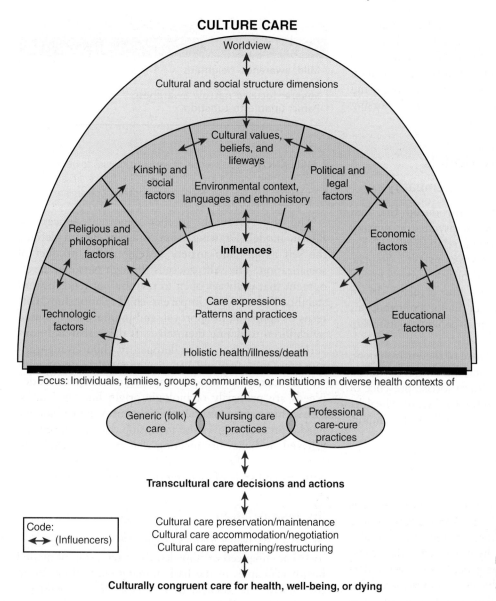

FIGURE 7.2 Leininger sunrise model to depict theory of cultural care diversity and universality.

Applicability of Social Theories to Psychiatric–Mental Health Nursing

The use of social and sociocultural theories is especially important for psychiatric–mental health nurses. In any individual or family assessment, the sociocultural aspect is integral to mental health. It would be impossible to complete an adequate assessment without considering the role of the individual within the family and society. Interventions are based on the understanding and significance of family and cultural norms. It would be impossible to interact with the family in a meaningful way without an understanding of the family's cultural values. In the inpatient setting, the nurse is responsible for designing the social environment of the unit as well

as ensuring that the patient is safe from harm. To accomplish this complex task, an understanding of the unit as a small social community helps the nurse use the environment in patient treatment (see Chapter 11). In addition, many group interventions are based on sociocultural theories (see Chapter 14).

NURSING THEORIES

Nursing theories are useful to psychiatric–mental health nursing in conceptualizing the individual, family, or community and in planning nursing interventions (see Chapter 11). The use of a specific theory depends on the patient situation. For example, in people with schizophrenia who have problems related to maintaining self-care, Dorothea Orem theory of self-care is useful. By contrast, Hildegarde Peplau theories are appropriate when a nurse is developing a relationship with a patient. Because of the wide range of possible problems requiring different approaches, familiarity with several nursing theories is essential.

Interpersonal Relations Models

Hildegarde Peplau: The Power of Empathy

Hildegarde Peplau (1909–1999) introduced the first systematic theoretic framework for psychiatric nursing and focused on the nurse–patient relationship in her book *Inter-personal Relations in Nursing* in 1952 (Peplau, 1952). She led psychiatric–mental health nursing out of the confinement of custodial care into a theory-driven professional practice. One of her major contributions was the introduction of the nurse–patient relationship (see Chapter 10).

Peplau believed in the importance of the environment, defined as external factors considered essential to human development (Peplau, 1992): cultural forces, presence of adults, secure economic status of the family, and a healthy prenatal environment. Peplau emphasized the importance of empathic linkage.

> **KEYCONCEPT Empathic linkage** is the ability to feel in oneself the feelings experienced by another person.

The interpersonal transmission of anxiety or panic is the most common empathic linkage. According to Peplau, other feelings, such as anger, disgust, and envy, can also be communicated nonverbally by way of empathic transmission to others. Although the process is not yet understood, she explains that empathic communication occurs. She believes that if nurses pay attention to what they feel during a relationship with a patient, they can gain invaluable observations of feelings a patient is experiencing and has not yet noticed or talked about.

Anxiety is a key concept for Peplau, who contends that professional practice is unsafe if this concept is not understood.

> **KEYCONCEPT Anxiety,** according to Peplau, is an energy that arises when expectations that are present are not met.

If anxiety is not recognized, it continues to rise and escalates toward panic. There are various levels of anxiety, each having its observable behavioral cues (Box 7.4). These cues are sometimes called *defensive*, but Peplau argues that they are often "relief behaviors." For example, some people may relieve their anxiety by yelling and swearing; others seek relief by withdrawing. In both instances, anxiety was generated by an unmet security need.

BOX 7.4

Levels of Anxiety

Mild: awareness heightens
Moderate: awareness narrows
Severe: focused narrow awareness
Panic: unable to function

NCLEXNOTE Peplau model of anxiety continues to be an important concept in psychiatric nursing. Severe anxiety interferes with learning. Mild anxiety is useful for learning.

The **self-system** is another important concept in Peplau model. Drawing from Sullivan, Peplau defined the self as an "anti-anxiety system" and a product of socialization. The self proceeds through personal development that is always open to revision but tends toward stability. For example, in parent–child relationships, patterns of approval, disapproval, and indifference are used by children to define themselves. If the verbal and nonverbal messages have been derogatory, children incorporate these messages and also view themselves negatively.

The concept of need is important to Peplau model. Needs are primarily of biologic origin but need to be met within a sociocultural environment. When a biologic need is present, it gives rise to tension that is reduced and relieved by behaviors meeting that need. According to Peplau, nurses should recognize and support the patients' patterns and style of meeting their health care needs.

Ida Jean Orlando

In 1954, Ida Jean Orlando (1926–2007) studied the factors that enhanced or impeded the integration of mental health principles in the basic nursing curriculum. From this study, she published *The Dynamic Nurse–Patient Relationship* to offer nursing students a theory of effective nursing practice. She studied nursing care of patients on medical–surgical units, not people with psychiatric problems in mental hospitals. Orlando identified three areas of nursing concern: the nurse–patient relationship, the nurse's professional role, and the identity and development of knowledge that is distinctly nursing (Orlando, 1961). A nursing situation involves the behavior of the patient, the reaction of the nurse, and anything that does not relieve the distress of the patient. Patient distress is related to the inability of the individual to meet or communicate their own needs (Orlando, 1961, 1972).

Orlando helped nurses focus on the whole patient rather than on the disease or institutional demands. Her ideas continue to be useful today, and current research supports her model (Olson & Hanchett, 1997). A small nursing study investigated whether Orlando nursing theory–based practice had a measurable impact on patients' immediate distress when compared with nonspecified nursing interventions. Orlando approach consisted of the nurse validating the patient's distress before taking any action to reduce it. Patients being cared for by the Orlando group experienced significantly less stress than those receiving traditional nursing care (Potter & Bockenhauer, 2000). Orlando model has been used in many settings, including fall prevention in a hospital (Abraham, 2011). Orlando theory is also proposed as a model for teaching communication in nursing programs (Gaudet & Howett, 2018).

Existential and Humanistic Theoretical Perspectives

Rosemarie Rizzo Parse

The *Humanbecoming Theory* views humans as indivisible, unpredictable, ever-changing coauthors and experts about their lives (Parse, 1998, 2007). Three major themes underlie this theory: meaning (personal meaning to the situation), rhythmicity (the paradoxical patterning of the human–universe mutual processes—the ups and downs of life), and transcendence (power and originating of transforming) (Parse, 1996, 1998, 2008). The postulates involved in living a human life are *illuminating* (unbound knowing extended to infinity), *paradox* (intricate rhythm expressed as a pattern preference), *freedom* (liberation), and *mystery* (unexplainable) (Parse, 2007).

The theory was expanded to address the ethos of humanbecoming with the core knowings of living quality. The four tenets of humanbecoming are *reverence* (solemn regard for humanuniverse presence), *awe* (beholding the unexplainable of humanuniverse existence), *betrayal* (the violation of humanuniverse trust), and *shame* (humiliation with dishonoring humanuniverse worth) (Parse, 2018).

As one of the more abstract nursing theories, *humanbecoming* can be used in understanding patients' life experiences and connecting psychologically with a patient. This theory has been widely studied in nursing and adds qualitative dimension to understanding the patient's human experience. For example, one of the studies explores freedom from a humanbecoming perspective (Bunkers, 2020). Parse theory is recommended as an alternative to the medical approach for a grieving family who has experienced a pregnancy loss, still birth, or neonatal death. The theory of humanbecoming focuses of quality of life as experienced and the meaning of the experience as perceived by the parents (Wilson et al., 2016).

Jean Watson

The theory of transpersonal caring was initiated by Jean Watson (b. 1940). Watson believes that caring is the foundation of nursing and recommends that specific theories of caring be developed in relation to specific human conditions and health and illness experiences (Watson, 2005). Her conceptualizations transcend conventional views of illness and focus on the meaning of health and quality of life (Watson, 2007). There are three foundational concepts of her theory:

- Transpersonal Caring–Healing Relations: a relational process related to philosophic, moral, and spiritual foundation.
- Ten Caritas Process: the original 10 Carative Factors have evolved into the 10 Caritas Processes (Box 7.5).
- Caritas Field: a field of consciousness created when the nurse focuses on love and caring as their way of being and consciously manifests a healing presence with others.

BOX 7.5

Nursing: Human Science and Human Care Assumptions, and Factors in Care

ASSUMPTIONS

1. Caring can be effectively demonstrated and practiced only interpersonally.
2. Caring consists of factors that result in the satisfaction of certain human needs.
3. Effective caring promotes health and individual or family growth.
4. Caring responses accept a person not only as they are now but also as what they may become.
5. A caring environment offers the development of potential while allowing the person to choose the best action for themselves at a given point in time.
6. Caring is more "healthogenic" than is curing. It integrates biophysical knowledge with knowledge of human behavior to generate or promote health and provide ministrations to those who are ill. A science of caring is complementary to the science of curing.
7. The practice of caring is central to nursing.

10 CARITAS PROCESSES™

1. Embrace altruistic values and practice loving kindness with self and others.
2. Instill faith, hope, and honor in others.
3. Be sensitive to self and others by nurturing individual beliefs and practices.
4. Develop helping–trusting–caring relationships.
5. Promote and accept positive and negative feelings as you authentically listen to another's story.
6. Use creative scientific problem-solving methods for caring decision-making.
7. Share teaching and learning that address the individual needs and comprehension styles.
8. Create a healing environment for the physical and spiritual self that respects human dignity.
9. Assist with basic physical, emotional, and spiritual human needs.
10. Be open to mystery and allow miracles to enter.

Watson theory is especially applicable to the care of those who seek help for mental illness. This model emphasizes the importance of sensitivity to self and others; the development of helping and trusting relations; the promotion of interpersonal teaching and learning; and provision for a supportive, protective, and corrective mental, physical, sociocultural, and spiritual environment. Watson caring science-based interventions have been shown to decrease patient's emotional strains, increase patients' self-management confidence and emotional well-being, increase nurses' job satisfaction and engagement, and improve nursing students' confidence in the conical performance and the awareness of caring behaviors (Holly et al., 2019).

Systems Models

Imogene M. King

The theory of goal attainment developed by Imogene King (1923–2007) is based on a systems model that includes three interacting systems: personal, interpersonal, and social. In this model, human beings interact with the environment, and the individual's perceptions influence reactions and interactions (Figure 7.3). Nursing involves caring for the human being, with the goal of health defined as adjusting to the stressors in both internal and external environments (King, 2007). She defines nursing as a "process of human interactions between nurse and patient whereby each perceives the other and the situation; and through communication, they set goals, explore means, and agree on means to achieve goals" (King, 1981, p. 144). This model focuses on the process that occurs between a nurse and a patient. The process is initiated to help the patient cope with a health problem that compromises their ability to maintain social roles, functions, and activities of daily living (King, 1992).

In this model, the person is goal oriented and purposeful, reacting to stressors, and is viewed as an open system interacting with the environment. The variables in nursing situations are as follows:

- Geographic place of the transacting system, such as the hospital
- Perceptions of the nurse and patient
- Communications of the nurse and patient
- Expectations of the nurse and patient
- Mutual goals of the nurse and patient
- The nurse and patient as a system of interdependent roles in a nursing situation (King, 1981, p. 88)

The quality of nurse–patient interactions may have positive or negative influences on the promotion of health in any nursing situation. It is within this inter personal system of nurse and patient that the healing process is performed. Interaction is depicted in which the outcome is a **transaction**, defined as the transfer of value between two or more people. This behavior is unique, based on experience, and is goal directed.

King's work reflects her understanding of the systematic process of theory development. Her model continues to be developed and applied in national and international settings, including psychiatric–mental health care (Shanta & Connolly, 2013). The model also serves as a basis for a recent nursing theory related to work team/group empowerment. The theory is applied to improve nurses' empowerment within health care organizations (Friend & Sieloff, 2018).

Betty Neuman

Betty Neuman (b. 1924) uses a systems approach as a model of nursing care. Neuman wants to extend care beyond an illness model, incorporating concepts of problem finding and prevention and the newer behavioral science concepts and environmental approaches to wellness. Neuman developed her framework in the late 1960s as chairwoman of the University of California at Los Angeles graduate nursing program. The key components of the model are a client system (physiological, psychological, sociocultural, developmental, spiritual) interacting with the environment. The wholistic model can be applied to prevention and treatment. Expansion of the model is an area of interest because of the need to define and describe her concept of social issues (Aronowitz & Fawcett, 2016).

Neuman was one of the first psychiatric nurses to include the concept of stressors in understanding nursing care. The Neuman systems model is applied to practice and educational settings, including community health,

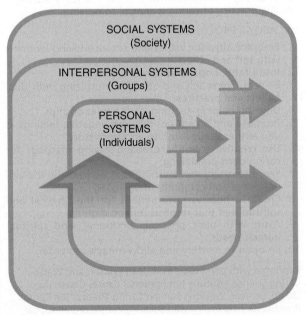

FIGURE 7.3 Imogene King's conceptual framework for nursing: dynamic interacting systems.

family therapy, renal nursing, perinatal nursing, and mental health nursing of older adults (Beckman et al., 2012; Neuman & Fawcett, 2011). This model has been applied to the practice and educational setting, including international programs (Greco et al., 2016; Olowokere & Okanlawon, 2015; Vanaki & Rafiei, 2020).

Dorothea Orem

Self-care is the focus of the general theory of nursing initiated by Dorothea Orem (1914–2007) in the early 1960s. The Self-Care Deficit Nursing Theory consists of three separate parts: a theory of self-care, theory of self-care deficit, and theory of nursing systems (Biggs, 2008; Orem, 2001; Orem & Taylor, 2011). The theory of self-care defines the term as activities performed independently by an individual to promote and maintain personal well-being throughout life. The central focus of Orem theory is the self-care deficit theory, which describes how people can be helped by nursing. Nurses can help meet self-care requisites through five approaches: acting or doing for, guiding, teaching, supporting, and providing an environment to promote the patient's ability to meet current or future demands. The nursing systems theory refers to a series of actions a nurse takes to meet the patient's self-care requisites. This system varies from the patient being totally dependent on the nurse for care to needing only some education and support.

Orem model is used in psychiatric–mental health nursing because of its emphasis on promoting independence of the individual and on self-care activities (Burdette, 2012; Seed & Torkelson, 2012; Wazni & Gifford, 2017). Although many psychiatric disorders have an underlying problem, such as motivation, these problems are generally manifested as difficulties conducting ordinary self-care activities (e.g., personal hygiene) or developing independent thinking skills.

Other Nursing Theories

Other nursing models are applied in psychiatric settings. Martha Rogers model of unitary human beings and Calista Roy adaptation model have been the basis of many psychiatric nursing approaches.

SUMMARY OF KEY POINTS

- The traditional psychodynamic framework helped form the basis of early nursing interpersonal interventions, including the development of therapeutic relationships and the use of such concepts as transference, countertransference, empathy, and object relations.

- The behavioral theories are often used in strategies that help patients change behavior and thinking.

- Sociocultural theories remain important in understanding and interacting with patients as members of families and cultures.

- Nursing theories form the conceptual basis for nursing practice and are useful in a variety of psychiatric–mental health settings.

CRITICAL THINKING CHALLENGES

1. Discuss the similarities and differences among Freud ideas and those of the neo-Freudians, including Jung, Adler, Horney, and Sullivan.

2. Compare and contrast the basic ideas of psychodynamic and behavioral theories.

3. Compare and differentiate classic conditioning from operant conditioning.

4. Define the following terms and discuss their applicability to psychiatric–mental health nursing: classical conditioning, operant conditioning, positive reinforcement, and negative reinforcement.

5. List the major developmental theorists and their main ideas.

6. Discuss the cognitive therapy approaches to mental disorders and how they can be used in psychiatric–mental health nursing practice.

7. Define formal and informal support systems. How does the concept of social distance relate to these two systems?

8. Compare and contrast the basic ideas of the nursing theorists.

Unfolding Patient Stories: Randy Adams

Part 1 (Cognitive Behavioral Social Theories)

Randy Adams, a 28-year-old veteran exposed to bomb blasts during combat in the Middle East, has symptoms of posttraumatic stress disorder and neurocognitive problems. How can cognitive-behavioral and social theories be applied to his condition? How does an understanding of psychosocial theories assist the nurse in selecting suitable interventions to promote psychological and social functioning?

Movie Viewing Guides
Freud: 1962. This film depicts Sigmund Freud as a young physician, focusing on his early psychiatric theories and treatments. His struggles for acceptance of his ideas among the Viennese medical community are depicted. This fascinating film is well done and gives an interesting overview of the impact of psychoanalysis.

VIEWING POINTS: Watch for the impact on political thinking during the gradual acceptance of Freud ideas. Discuss the "dream sequence" and its impact on the development of psychoanalysis as a therapeutic technique.

An Angel at My Table: 1990, New Zealand. This three-part television miniseries tells the story of Janet Frame, New Zealand's premiere novelist and poet. Based on her autobiography, the film portrays Frame as a shy, awkward child who experiences a family tragedy that alienates her socially. She studies in England to be a teacher, but her shyness and social ineptness cause extreme anxiety. Seeking mental health care, she receives a misdiagnosis of schizophrenia and spends 8 years in a mental institution. She barely escapes a lobotomy when she is notified of a literary award. She then begins to develop friendships and a new life.

VIEWING POINTS: Observe Janet Frame's childhood development. Does she "fit" any of the models that are discussed in this chapter? Consider her life in light of Gilligan and Miller theories that it is important for women to have a sense of connection.

REFERENCES

Abraham, S. (2011). Fall prevention conceptual framework. *Health Care Manager (Frederick), 30*(20), 179–184.

Ackerman, S., Zuroff, D. C., & Moskowitz, D. S. (2000). Generativity in midlife and young adults: Links to agency, communion, and subjective well-being. *International Journal of Aging and Human Development, 5*(1), 17–41.

Aronowitz, T., & Fawcett, J. (2016). Thoughts about social issues: A Neuman systems Model perspective. *Nursing Science Quarterly, 29*(2), 173–176.

Bandura, A. (1977). *Social learning theory.* Prentice-Hall.

Bandura, A. (1986). *Social foundations of thought and action: A social-cognitive theory.* Prentice Hall.

Bandura, A. (1993). Perceived self-efficacy in cognitive development and function. American Educational Research Association Annual Meeting. *Educational Psychologist, 28*(2), 117–148.

Bandura, A. (2001). Social cognitive theory: An agentic perspective. *Annual Review of Psychology, 52,* 1–26.

Barbosa, M., Corso, M. E., & Rabel, E. (2020). Interdisciplinarity of care to the elderly with Alzheimer's disease: Reflection to the light of the theories of Leininger and Heller. *Anna Nery School Journal of Nursing, 24*(1), 1–8.

Beck, J. S. (2021). *Cognitive behavior therapy: Basics and beyond* (3rd ed.). Guilford Press.

Beckman, S. J., Boxley-Harges, S. L., & Kaskel, B. L. (2012). Experience informs: Spanning three decades with the Neuman Systems Model. *Nursing Science Quarterly, 25*(4), 341–346.

Biggs, A. (2008). Orem's Self-Care Deficit Nursing Theory: Update on the state of the art and science. *Nursing Science Quarterly, 21*(3), 200–206.

Broch, D., Crossetti, M. G. O., & Riquinho, D. L. (2017). Reflections on violence against women in the perspective of Madeleine Leininger. *Journal of Nursing UFPE On Line, 11*(12). https://periodicos.ufpe.br/revistas/revistaenfermagem/article/view/22588

Bunkers, S. S. (2020). Freedom and humanbecoming. *Nursing Science Quarterly, 33*(1), 7–11.

Burdette, L. (2012). Relationship between self-care agency, self-care practices and obesity among rural midlife women. *Self-Care, Dependent-Care & Nursing, 19*(1), 5–14.

Christiansen, S. L., & Palkovitz, R. (1998). Exploring Erikson's psychosocial theory and development: Generativity and its relationship to paternal identity, intimacy, and involvement in childcare. *The Journal of Men's Studies, 7*(1), 133–156.

Ehlman, K., & Ligon, M. (2012). The application of a generativity model for the older adults. *International Journal of Aging and Human Development, 74*(4), 331–344.

Erikson, E. (1963). *Childhood and society* (2nd ed.). W. W. Norton & Company.

Erikson, E. (1968). *Identity: Youth and crisis.* W. W. Norton & Company.

Fehler-Cabral, F., & Campbell, R. (2013). Adolescent sexual assault disclosure: The impact of peers, families, and schools. *American Journal of Community Psychology, 52*(1–2), 73–83.

Freud, S. (1905). Three essays on the theory of sexuality. In J. Strachey, A. Freud, A. Strachey, & A. Tyson (Eds.). (1953). *The standard edition of the complete psychological works of Sigmund Freud* (pp. 135–248). Hogarth Press.

Freud, S. (1927). The ego and the id. In E. Jones (Ed.): (1957). *The international psychoanalytical library* (No. 12). Hogarth Press.

Friedemann, M., Newman, F. L., Buckwalter, K. C., & Montgomery R. J. (2014). Resource need and use of multiethnic caregivers of elders in their homes. *Journal of Advanced Nursing, 70*(3), 662–673.

Friend, M. L., & Sieloff, C. L. (2018). Empowerment in nursing literature: An update and look to the future. *Nursing Science Quarterly, 31*(4), 355–361.

Fromm-Reichmann, F. (1950). *Principles of intensive psychotherapy.* University of Chicago Press.

Gaudet, D., & Howett, M. (2018). Communication and technology: Ida Orland's theory applied. *Nursing Science Quarterly, 31*(4), 369–373.

Gielnik, M. M., Bledow, R., & Stark, M. S. (2020). A dynamic account of self-efficacy in entrepreneurship. *The Journal of Applied Psychology, 105*(5), 487–505. https://doi.org/10.1037/apl0000451

Gilligan, C. (1982). *In a different voice.* Harvard University Press.

Gilligan, C. (2004). Recovering psyche: Reflections on life-history and history. *Annual of Psychoanalysis, 32,* 131–147.

Gilligan, C. (2011). *Joining the resistance.* Polity Press.

Greco, R. M., Alves de Moura, D. C., Arreguy-Sena, C., Alvarenga Martins, N., & da Silva Alves, M. (2016). Labour conditions and theory of Betty Neuman; Third-party workers of a public university. *Journal of Nursing URPE On Line, Suppl 2*; 727–735. https://doi.org/10.5205/reuol.6884-59404-2-SM-1.1002sup201605

Holly, W., Fazzone, P. A., Sitzman, K., & Hardin, S. R. (2019). The current intervention studies based on Watson's Theory of Human Caring: A systematic review. *International Journal for Human Caring, 23*(1), 4–22.

Horney, K. (1939). *New ways in psychoanalysis.* W. W. Norton & Company.

Jonsén, E., Norberg, A., & Lundman, B. (2015). Sense of meaning in life among the oldest old people living in a rural area in northern Sweden. *International Journal of Older People Nursing, 10*(3), 221–229.

Jung, C. (1966). On the psychology of the unconscious. The personal and the collective unconscious. In C. Jung (Ed.), *Collected works of C. G. Jung* (2nd ed., Vol. 7, pp. 64–79). Princeton University Press.

King, I. (1981). *A theory for nursing: Systems, concepts, process.* Wiley.

King, I. (1992). King's theory of goal attainment. *Nursing Science Quarterly, 5*(1), 19–26.

King, I. (2007). King's conceptual system, theory of goal attainment, and transaction process in the 21st century. *Nursing Science Quarterly, 20*(2), 109–116.

Klein, M. (1963). *Our adult world and other essays.* Heinemann Medical Books.

Knight, Z. G. (2017). A proposed model of psychodynamic psychotherapy linked to Erik Erikson's eight stages of psychosocial development. *Clinical Psychology & Psychotherapy, 24*(5), 1047–1058.

Kress, V. E., Haiyasoso, M., Zoldan, C. A., Headley, J. A., & Trepal, H. (2018). The use of relational-cultural theory in counseling clients who have traumatic stress disorders. *Journal of Counseling & Development, 96*(1), 106–114.

Leininger, M. (2007). Theoretical questions and concerns: Response from the theory of culture care diversity and universality perspective. *Nursing Science Quarterly, 20,* 9–13.

Leininger, M., & McFarland, M. (2006). *Cultural care diversity and universality theory. A theory of nursing* (2nd ed.). Jones & Bartlett Publishers.

Litwak, E. (1985). Complementary roles for formal and informal support groups: A study of nursing homes and mortality rates. *Journal of Applied Behavioral Science, 21*(4), 407–425.

Litwak, E., Messeri, P., & Silverstein, M. (1990). The role of formal and informal groups in providing help to older people. *Marriage and Family Review, 15*(1–2), 171–193.

Maine, A., Dickson, A., Truesdale, M., & Brown, M. (2017). An application of Bandura's 'Four Sources of Self-Efficacy' to the self-management of type 2 diabetes in people with intellectual disability: An inductive and deductive thematic analysis. *Research in Developmental Disabilities, 70,* 75–84. https://doi.org/10.1016/j.ridd.2017.09.004

Maslow, A. (1970). *Motivation and personality* (rev. ed.). Harper & Brothers.

McPherson, K. M., Kayes, N. K., Moloczij, N., & Cummins, C. (2013). Improving the interface between informal carers and formal health and social services: A qualitative study. *International Journal of Nursing Studies, 51*(3), 418–429. https://doi.org/10.1016/j.ijnurstu.2013.07.006

Mead, M. (1970). *Culture and commitment: A study of the generation gap.* Natural History Press/Doubleday & Co.

Messeri, P., Silverstein, M., & Litwak, E. (1993). Choosing optimal support groups: A review and reformulation. *Journal of Health and Social Behavior, 34*(6), 122–137.

Miller, J. B. (1976). *Toward a new psychology of women.* Beacon Press.

Miller, J. B. (1994). Women's psychological development. Connections, disconnections, and violations. In M. Berger (Ed.), *Women beyond Freud: New concepts of feminine psychology* (pp. 79–97). Brunner Mazel.

Moore, B., & Fine, B. (Eds.). (1990). *Psychoanalytic terms and concepts.* The American Psychoanalytic Association and Yale University Press.

Neuman, B., & Fawcett, J. (Eds.). (2011). *The Neuman systems model* (5th ed.). Prentice Hall.

Ochse, R., & Plug, C. (1986). Cross-cultural investigation of the validity of Erikson's theory of personality development. *Journal of Personality and Social Psychology, 50*(6), 1240–1252.

Olowokere, A. E., & Okanlawon, F. A. (2015). Application of Neuman System model to psychosocial support of vulnerable school children. *West African Journal of Nursing, 26*(1), 14–25.

Olson, J., & Hanchett, E. (1997). Nurse-expressed empathy, patient outcomes, and the development of a middle-range theory. *Image: The Journal of Nursing Scholarship, 29*(1), 71–76.

Orem, D. (2001). *Nursing concepts of practice* (6th ed.). Mosby.

Orem, D. E., & Taylor, S. G. (2011). Reflections on nursing practice science: The nature, the structure, and the foundation of nursing sciences. *Nursing Science Quarterly, 24*(1), 35–41.

Orlando, I. J. (1961). *The dynamic nurse–patient relationship.* G. P. Putnam's Sons.

Orlando, I. J. (1972). *The discipline and teaching of nursing process.* G. P. Putnam's Sons.

Orlofsky, J., Marcia, J., & Lesser, I. (1973). Ego identity status and the intimacy versus isolation crisis of young adulthood. *Journal of Personality and Social Psychology, 27*(2), 211–219.

Parse, R. R. (1996). Reality: A seamless symphony of becoming. *Nursing Science Quarterly, 9*, 181–184.

Parse, R. R. (1998). *The humanbecoming school of thoughts: A perspective for nurses and other health professionals.* Sage.

Parse, R. R. (2007). The humanbecoming school of thought in 2050. *Nursing Science Quarterly, 20*, 308–311.

Parse, R. R. (2008). The humanbecoming leading-following model. *Nursing Science Quarterly, 21*, 369–375.

Parse, R. R. (2018). Dignity: The ethos of humanbecoming. *Nursing Science Quarterly, 31*(3), 259–262.

Pavlov, I. P. (1927/1960). *Conditioned reflexes.* Dover Publications.

Peplau, H. (1952). *Interpersonal relations in nursing.* G. Putnam & Sons.

Peplau, H. (1992). Interpersonal relations: A theoretical framework for application in nursing practice. *Nursing Science Quarterly, 5*(1), 13–18.

Perls, F. (1969). *In and out of the garbage pail.* Real People Press.

Pitman, S. R., & Knauss, D. (2020). Contemporary psychodynamic approaches to treating anxiety: Theory, research, and practice. *Advances in Experimental Medicine and Biology, 1191*, 451–464. https://doi.org/10.1007/978-981-32-9705-0_23

Potter, M. L., & Bockenhauer, B. J. (2000). Implementing Orlando's nursing theory. *Journal of Psychosocial Nursing and Mental Health Services, 38*(13), 14–21.

Pratt, M. W., Norris, J. E., Cressman, K., Lawford, H., & Hebblethwaite, S. (2008). Parents' stories of grandparenting concerns in the three-generational family: Generativity, optimism, and forgiveness. *Journal of Personality, 76*(3), 581–604.

Rogers, C. (1980). *A way of being.* Houghton Mifflin.

Seed, M. S., & Torkelson, D. J. (2012). Beginning the recovery journey in acute psychiatric care: Using concepts from Orem's self-care deficit nursing theory. *Issues in Mental Health Nursing, 33*(6), 394–398.

Shanta, L. L., & Connolly, M. (2013). Using King's interacting systems theory to link emotional intelligence and nursing practice. *Journal of Professional Nursing, 29*(3), 174–180.

Skinner, B. F. (1935). The generic nature of the concepts of stimulus and response. *Journal of General Psychology, 12*, 40–65.

Sullivan, G. (2004). A four-fold humanity: Margaret Mead and psychological types. *Journal of the History of the Behavioral Sciences, 40*(2), 183–206.

Sullivan, H. (1953). *The interpersonal theory of psychiatry.* W. W. Norton & Company.

Thorndike, E. L. (1906). *The principles of teaching, based on psychology.* A.G. Seiler.

Vanaki, Z., & Rafiei, H. (2020). Application of Betty Neuman system Theory in management of pressure injury in patients following stroke. *MEDSURG Nursing, 29*(2), 129–133.

Walker, M., & Rosen, W. B. (2004). *How connections heal: Stories from relational-cultural therapy.* Guilford Press.

Watson, J. (2005). *Caring science as sacred science.* F. A. Davis.

Watson, J. (2007). Theoretical questions and concerns: Response from a caring science framework. *Nursing Science Quarterly, 20*, 13–15.

Watson, J. B., & Rayner, R. (1920). Conditioned emotional reactions. *Journal of Experimental Psychology, 3*, 1–14.

Wazni, L., & Gifford, W. (2017). Addressing physical health needs of individuals with schizophrenia using Orem's theory. *Journal of Holistic Nursing, 35*(3), 271–279.

Westermeyer, J. F. (2004). Predictors and characteristics of Erikson's life cycle model among men: A 32-year longitudinal study. *International Journal of Aging & Human Development, 58*(1), 29–48.

Wilson, D. R. (2016). Parse's nursing theory and its application to families experiencing empty arms. *International Journal of Childbirth Education, 31*(2), 29–33.

Wolf, K. M., Zoucha, R., McFarland, M., Salman, K., Dagne, A., & Hashi, N. (2016). Somali immigrant perceptions of mental health and illness: An ethnonursing study. *Journal of Transcultural Nursing, 27*(4), 349–358.

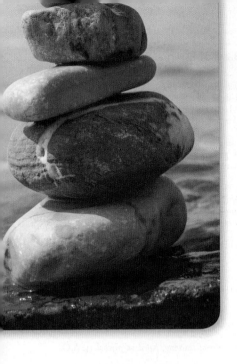

8
Biologic Foundations of Psychiatric Nursing

Mary Ann Boyd

KEYCONCEPTS

- neuroplasticity
- neurotransmitters

LEARNING OBJECTIVES

After studying this chapter, you will be able to:

1. Describe the association between biologic functioning and symptoms of psychiatric disorders.

2. Locate brain structures primarily involved in psychiatric disorders and describe the primary functions of these structures.

3. Describe basic mechanisms of neuronal transmission.

4. Identify the location and function of neurotransmitters significant to hypotheses regarding major mental disorders.

5. Discuss the role of genetics in the development of psychiatric disorders.

6. Discuss the basic utilization of new knowledge gained from fields of study, including psychoneuroimmunology and chronobiology.

KEY TERMS

- Acetylcholine • Amino acids • Autonomic nervous system • Basal ganglia • Biogenic amines • Biologic markers
- Brain stem • Cerebellum • Chronobiology • Circadian cycle • Cortex • Dopamine • Enteric nervous system
- Extrapyramidal motor system • Frontal, parietal, temporal, and occipital lobes • Functional imaging
- Gut–brain axis • Gut microbiota • GABA • Genetic susceptibility • Glutamate • Hippocampus • Histamine
- Hypothalamus–pituitary–thyroid axis • Limbic system • Locus coeruleus • Neurocircuitry • Neurohormones
- Neurons • Neuromodulators • Neuropeptides • Norepinephrine • Phenotype • Pineal body • Population genetics
- Proband • Psychoneuroimmunology • Receptor • Serotonin • Structural imaging • Synaptic cleft • Working memory
- Zeitgebers

INTRODUCTION

All behavior recognized as human results from actions that originate in the brain and its amazing interconnection of neural networks. Modern research has increased understanding of how the complex circuitry of the brain interacts with the external environment, memories, and experiences.

Through the spinal column and peripheral nerves, along with other systems, such as the endocrine and immune systems, the brain constantly receives and processes information. As the brain shifts and sorts through the amazing amount of information it processes every hour, it decides on actions and initiates behaviors, allowing each person to act in entirely unique and very human ways.

Mental disorders cannot be traced to specific physiologic problems but rather are complex syndromes consisting of symptoms that more or less cluster together. Therefore, it is important for the nurse to understand basic nervous system functioning, as well as some of the research that is exploring the biologic basis of mental disorders.

This chapter reviews the basic information necessary for understanding neuroscience as it relates to the role of the psychiatric–mental health nurse. It reviews basic central nervous system (CNS) structures and functions, the peripheral nervous system (PNS), general functions of the major neurotransmitters and **receptors**, basic principles of neurotransmission, genetic models, circadian rhythms, and biologic tests. The chapter assumes that the reader has a basic knowledge of human biology, anatomy, and pathophysiology. It is not intended as a full presentation of neuroanatomy and physiology but rather as an overview of the structures and functions most critical to understanding the role of the psychiatric–mental health nurse. Psychiatric–mental health nurses must be able to make the connection between (1) patients' psychiatric symptoms, (2) the probable alterations in brain functioning linked to those symptoms, and (3) the rationale for treatment and care practices.

NEUROANATOMY OF THE CENTRAL NERVOUS SYSTEM

Although this section discusses functioning areas of the brain separately, each area is intricately connected with the others, and each functions interactively. The CNS contains the brain, **brain stem**, and spinal cord, and the PNS consists of the **neurons** that connect the CNS to the muscles, organs, and other systems in the periphery of the body. Whatever affects the CNS may also affect the PNS and vice versa.

Cerebrum

The largest region of the human brain, the cerebrum fills the entire upper portion of the cranium. The **cortex**, or outermost surface of the cerebrum, makes up about 80% of the human brain. The cortex is four to six cellular layers thick, and each layer is composed of cell bodies mixed with capillary blood vessels. This mixture makes the cortex gray brown (thus the term *gray matter*). The cortex consists of numerous bumps and grooves in a fully developed adult brain, as shown in Figure 8.1. This "wrinkling" allows for a large amount of surface area to be confined in the limited space of the skull. The increased surface area allows for more potential connections among cells within the cortex. The grooves are called *fissures* if they extend deep into the brain and *sulci* if they are shallower. The bumps or convolutions are called *gyri*. Together they provide many of the landmarks for the subdivisions of the cortex. The longest and deepest groove, the longitudinal fissure, separates the cerebrum into left and right hemispheres. Although these two divisions are nearly symmetric, there is some variation in the location and size of the sulci and gyri in each hemisphere. Substantial variation in these convolutions is found in the cortex of different individuals.

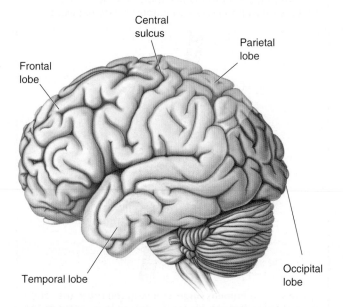
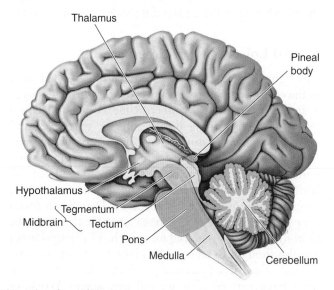

FIGURE 8.1 Lateral and medial surfaces of the brain. **Left:** The left lateral surface of the brain. **Right:** The medial surface of the right half of a sagittally hemisected brain. (Reprinted with permission from Bear, M. F., Conners, B. W., & Paradiso, M. A. [2016]. *Neuroscience: Exploring the brain* [4th ed.]. Wolters Kluwer.)

Left and Right Hemispheres

The cerebrum can be roughly divided into two halves, or hemispheres. The left hemisphere is dominant in about 95% of people, but about 5% of individuals have mixed dominance. Each hemisphere controls functioning mainly on the opposite side of the body. Aside from controlling activities on the left side of the body, the right hemisphere also provides input into receptive nonverbal communication, spatial orientation and recognition, intonation of speech and aspects of music, facial recognition and facial expression of emotion, and nonverbal learning and memory. In general, the left hemisphere is more involved with verbal language function, including areas for both receptive and expressive speech control, and provides strong contributions to temporal order and sequencing, numeric symbols, and verbal learning and memory.

The two hemispheres are connected by the corpus callosum, a bundle of neuronal tissue that allows information to be exchanged quickly between the right and left hemispheres. An intact corpus callosum is required for the hemispheres to function in a smooth and coordinated manner.

Lobes of the Brain

The lateral surface of each hemisphere is further divided into four lobes: **the frontal, parietal, temporal, and occipital lobes** (see Fig. 8.1). The lobes work in coordinated ways, but each is responsible for specific functions. An understanding of these unique functions is helpful in understanding how damage to these areas produces the symptoms of mental illness and how medications that affect the functioning of these lobes can produce certain effects.

Frontal Lobes

The right and left frontal lobes make up about one fourth of the entire cerebral cortex and are proportionately larger in humans than in any other mammal. The precentral gyrus, the gyrus immediately anterior to the central sulcus, contains the primary motor area, or homunculi. Damage to this gyrus or to the anterior neighboring gyri causes spastic paralysis in the opposite side of the body. The frontal lobe also contains Broca area, which controls the motor function of speech. Damage to Broca area produces expressive aphasia or difficulty with the motor movements required for speech. The frontal lobes are also thought to contain the highest or most complex aspects of cortical functioning, which collectively make up a large part of what we call personality. **Working memory** is an important aspect of frontal lobe function, including the ability to plan and initiate activity with future goals in mind. Insight, judgment, reasoning, concept formation, problem-solving skills, abstraction, and self-evaluation are all abilities that are modulated and affected by the actions of the frontal lobes. These skills are often referred to as *executive functions* because they modulate more primitive impulses through numerous connections to other areas of the cerebrum.

When normal frontal lobe functioning is altered, executive functioning is decreased, and modulation of impulses can be lost, leading to changes in mood and personality. The importance of the frontal lobe and its role in the development of symptoms common to psychiatric disorders are emphasized in later chapters that discuss disorders such as schizophrenia, attention-deficit hyperactivity disorder, and dementia. Box 8.1 describes how altered frontal lobe function can affect mood and personality.

BOX 8.1

Frontal Lobe Syndrome

In the 1860s, Phineas Gage became a famous example of frontal lobe dysfunction. Mr. Gage was a New England railroad worker who had a thick iron-tamping rod propelled through his frontal lobes by an explosion. He survived but suffered significant changes in his personality. Mr. Gage, who had previously been a capable and calm supervisor, began to show impatience, labile mood, disrespect for others, and frequent use of profanity after his injury (Harlow, 1868). Similar conditions are often called *frontal lobe syndrome*. Symptoms vary widely from individual to individual. In general, after damage to the dorsolateral (upper and outer) areas of the frontal lobes, the symptoms include a lack of drive and spontaneity. With damage to the most anterior aspects of the frontal lobes, the symptoms tend to involve more changes in mood and affect, such as impulsive and inappropriate behavior.

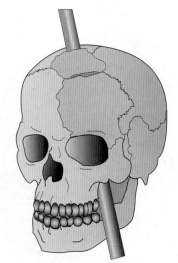

The skull of Phineas Gage, showing the route the tamping rod took through his skull. The angle of entry of the rod shot it behind the left eye and through the front part of the brain, sparing regions that are directly concerned with vital functions like breathing and heartbeat.

Parietal Lobes

The postcentral gyrus, immediately behind the central sulcus, contains the primary somatosensory area. Damage to this area and neighboring gyri results in deficits in discriminative sensory function but not in the ability to perceive sensory input. The posterior areas of the parietal lobe appear to coordinate visual and somatosensory information. Damage to this area produces complex sensory deficits, including neglect of contralateral sensory stimuli and spatial relationships. The parietal lobes contribute to the ability to recognize objects by touch, calculate, write, recognize fingers of the opposite hands, draw, and organize spatial directions (e.g., how to travel to familiar places).

Temporal Lobes

The temporal lobes contain the primary auditory and olfactory areas. Wernicke area, located at the posterior aspect of the superior temporal gyrus, is primarily responsible for receptive speech. The temporal lobes also integrate sensory and visual information involved in control of written and verbal language skills as well as visual recognition. The hippocampus, an important structure discussed later, lies in the internal aspects of each temporal lobe and contributes to memory. Other internal structures of this lobe are involved in the modulation of mood and emotion.

Occipital Lobes

The primary visual area is in the most posterior aspect of the occipital lobes. Damage to this area results in a condition called *cortical blindness*. In other words, the retina and optic nerve remain intact, but the individual cannot see. The occipital lobes are involved in many aspects of visual integration of information, including color vision, object and facial recognition, and the ability to perceive objects in motion.

Association Cortex

Although not a lobe, the association cortex is an important area that allows the lobes to work in an integrated manner. Areas of one lobe of the cortex often share functions with an area of the adjacent lobe. When these neighboring nerve fibers are related to the same sensory modality, they are often referred to as *association areas*. For example, an area in the inferior parietal, posterior temporal, and anterior occipital lobes integrates visual, somatosensory, and auditory information to provide the abilities required for basic academic skills. These areas, along with numerous connections beneath the cortex, are part of the mechanisms that allow the human brain to work as an integrated whole.

Subcortical Structures

Beneath the cortex are layers of tissue composed of the axons of cell bodies. The axonal tissue forms pathways that are surrounded by glia, a fatty or lipid substance, which has a white appearance, and give these layers of neuron axons their name—white matter. Structures inside the hemispheres, beneath the cortex, are considered subcortical. Many of these structures, essential in the regulation of emotions and behaviors, play important roles in our understanding of mental disorders. Figure 8.2 provides a coronal section view of the gray matter, white matter, and important subcortical structures.

The **basal ganglia** are subcortical gray matter areas in both the right and the left hemispheres that contain many cell bodies or nuclei. The primary subdivisions of the basal ganglia are the putamen, globus pallidus, and caudate. The basal ganglia are involved with motor functions and the learning and the programming of behavior or activities that are repetitive and, done over time, become automatic. The basal ganglia have many connections with the cerebral cortex, thalamus, midbrain structures, and spinal cord. Damage to portions of these nuclei may produce changes in posture or muscle tone. In addition, damage may produce abnormal movements, such as twitches or tremors. The basal ganglia can be adversely affected by some of the medications used to treat psychiatric disorders, leading to side effects and other motor-related problems.

Limbic System

The **limbic system** is essential to understanding the many hypotheses related to psychiatric disorders and emotional behavior in general. The limbic system is called a "system" because it comprises several small structures that work in a highly organized way. These structures include the hippocampus, thalamus, hypothalamus, amygdala, and limbic midbrain nuclei. See Figure 8.3 for identification and location of the structures within the limbic system and their relationships to other common CNS structures.

Basic emotions, needs, drives, and instinct begin and are modulated in the limbic system. Hate, love, anger, aggression, and caring are basic emotions that originate within the limbic system. Not only does the limbic system function as the seat of emotions, but because emotions are often generated based on our personal experiences, the limbic system also is involved with aspects of memory. Hypothesized changes in the limbic system play a significant role in many theories of major mental disorders, including schizophrenia, depression, and anxiety disorders (discussed in later chapters).

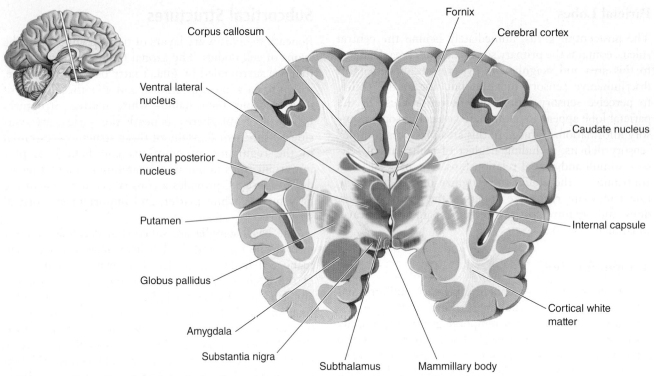

FIGURE 8.2 Coronal section of the brain, illustrating the corpus callosum, basal ganglia, and lateral ventricles. (Reprinted with permission from Bear, M. F., Conners, B. W., & Paradiso, M. A. [2016]. *Neuroscience: Exploring the brain* [4th ed.]. Wolters Kluwer.)

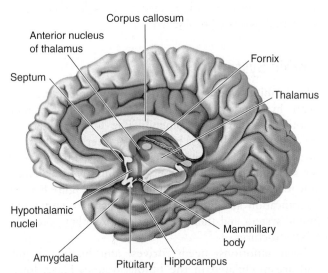

FIGURE 8.3 The structures of the limbic system are integrally involved in memory and emotional behavior. Theories link changes in the limbic system to many major mental disorders, including schizophrenia, depression, and anxiety disorders.

Hippocampus

The **hippocampus** is involved in storing information, especially the emotions attached to a memory. Our emotional responses to memories and our associations with other related memories are functions of how information is stored within the hippocampus. Although memory storage is not limited to one area of the brain, destruction of the left hippocampus impairs verbal memory, and damage to the right hippocampus results in difficulty with recognition and recall of complex visual and auditory patterns. Deterioration of the nerves of the hippocampus and other related temporal lobe structures found in Alzheimer disease produces the disorder's hallmark symptoms of memory dysfunction.

Thalamus

Sometimes called the "relay-switching center of the brain," the thalamus functions as a regulatory structure to relay all sensory information, except smell, sent to the CNS from the PNS. From the thalamus, the sensory information is relayed mostly to the cerebral cortex. The thalamus relays and regulates by filtering incoming information and determining what to pass on or not pass on to the cortex. In this fashion, the thalamus prevents the cortex from becoming overloaded with sensory stimulus. The thalamus is thought to play a part in controlling electrical activity in the cortex. Because of its primary relay function, damage to a very small area of the thalamus may produce deficits in many cortical functions, thus causing behavioral abnormalities.

Hypothalamus

Basic human activities, such as sleep–rest patterns, body temperature, and physical drives such as hunger and sex, are regulated by another part of the limbic system that rests deep within the brain and is called the hypothalamus. Dysfunction of this structure, whether from disorders or because of an adverse effect of drugs used to treat mental illness, produces common psychiatric symptoms, such as appetite and sleep problems.

Nerve cells within the hypothalamus secrete hormones, for example, antidiuretic hormone, which, when sent to the kidneys, accelerates the reabsorption of water; and oxytocin, which acts on smooth muscles to promote contractions, particularly within the walls of the uterus. Because cells within the nervous system produce these hormones, they are often referred to as **neurohormones** (hormones that are produced by cells within the nervous system) and form a communication mechanism through the bloodstream to control organs that are not directly connected to nervous system structures.

The pituitary gland, often called the *master gland*, is directly connected by thousands of neurons that attach it to the ventral aspects of the hypothalamus. Together with the pituitary gland, the hypothalamus functions as one of the primary regulators of many aspects of the endocrine system. Its functions are involved in control of visceral activities, such as body temperature, arterial blood pressure, hunger, thirst, fluid balance, gastric motility, and gastric secretions. Deregulation of the hypothalamus can be manifested in symptoms of certain psychiatric disorders. For example, in schizophrenia, patients often wear heavy coats during the hot summer months and do not appear hot. Before the role of the hypothalamus in schizophrenia was understood, psychological reasons were used to explain such symptoms. Now it is increasingly clear that such a symptom relates to deregulation of the hypothalamus's normal role in temperature regulation and is a biologically based symptom (Tan & Knight, 2018).

Amygdala

The amygdala is directly connected to more primitive centers of the brain involving the sense of smell. It has numerous connections to the hypothalamus and lies adjacent to the hippocampus. The amygdala provides an emotional component to memory and is involved in modulating aggression and sexuality. Impulsive acts of aggression and violence have been linked to dysregulation of the amygdala, and erratic firing of the nerve cells in the amygdala is a focus of investigation in bipolar mood disorders (see Chapter 26).

Limbic Midbrain Nuclei

The limbic midbrain nuclei are a collection of neurons (including the ventral tegmental area and the locus coeruleus) that appear to play a role in the biologic basis of addiction. Sometimes referred to as the pleasure center or reward center of the brain, the limbic midbrain nuclei function to chemically reinforce certain behaviors, ensuring their repetition. Emotions such as feeling satisfied with good food, the pleasure of nurturing young, and the enjoyment of sexual activity originate in the limbic midbrain nuclei. The reinforcement of activities such as nutrition, procreation, and nurturing young are all primitive aspects of ensuring the survival of a species. When functioning in abnormal ways, the limbic midbrain nuclei can begin to reinforce unhealthy or risky behaviors, such as drug abuse. Exploration of this area of the brain is in its infancy but offers potential insight into addictions and their treatment.

Other Central Nervous System Structures

The **extrapyramidal motor system** is a bundle of nerve fibers connecting the thalamus to the basal ganglia and cerebral cortex. Muscle tone, common reflexes, and automatic voluntary motor functioning (e.g., walking) are controlled by this nerve track. Dysfunction of this motor track can produce hypertonicity in muscle groups. In Parkinson disease, the cells that compose the extrapyramidal motor system are severely affected, producing many involuntary motor movements. A number of medications, which are discussed in Chapter 12, also affect this system.

The **pineal body** is located above and medial to the thalamus. Because the pineal gland easily calcifies, it can be visualized by neuroimaging and often is a medial landmark. Its functions remain somewhat of a mystery despite long knowledge of its existence. It contains secretory cells that emit the neurohormone melatonin and other substances. These hormones are thought to have several regulatory functions within the endocrine system. Information received from light–dark sources controls release of melatonin, which has been associated with sleep and emotional disorders. In addition, a modulation of immune function has been postulated for melatonin from the pineal gland.

The **locus coeruleus** is a tiny cluster of neurons that fan out and innervate almost every part of the brain, including most of the cortex, the thalamus and hypothalamus, the **cerebellum**, and the spinal cord. Just one neuron from the coeruleus can connect to more than 250,000 other neurons. Despite its small size, the wide-ranging neuronal connections allow this tiny structure to influence the regulation of attention, time perception, sleep–rest cycles, arousal, learning, pain, and mood. It also plays a role in information processing of new, unexpected, and novel experiences. Some think its function or dysfunction may explain why individuals become addicted to substances and seek out risky behaviors despite awareness of negative consequences.

The brain stem, which is located beneath the thalamus and composed of the midbrain, pons, and medulla, has important life-sustaining functions. Nuclei of numerous neural pathways to the cerebrum are in the brain stem. They are significantly involved in mediating symptoms of emotional dysfunction. These nuclei are also the primary source of several neurochemicals, such as serotonin, that are commonly associated with psychiatric disorders.

The cerebellum is in the posterior aspect of the skull beneath the cerebral hemispheres. This large structure controls movements and postural adjustments. To regulate postural balance and positioning, the cerebellum receives information from all parts of the body, including the muscles, joints, skin, and visceral organs, as well as from many parts of the CNS.

Autonomic Nervous System

Closely associated with the spinal cord but not lying entirely within its column is the **autonomic nervous system**, a subdivision of the PNS. It was originally given this name for being independent of conscious thought, that is, automatic. However, it does not necessarily function as autonomously as the name indicates. This system contains efferent (nerves moving away from the CNS), or motor system neurons, which affect target tissues such as cardiac muscle, smooth muscle, and the glands. It also contains afferent nerves, which are sensory and conduct information from these organs back to the CNS.

The autonomic nervous system is further divided into the sympathetic and parasympathetic nervous systems. These systems, although peripheral, are included here because they are involved in the emergency, or "fight-or-flight," response as well as the peripheral actions of many medications (see Chapter 12). Figure 8.4 illustrates the innervations of various target organs by the autonomic nervous system. Table 8.1 identifies the actions of the sympathetic and parasympathetic nervous systems on various target organs.

TABLE 8.1	PERIPHERAL ORGAN RESPONSE IN THE AUTONOMIC NERVOUS SYSTEM	
Effector Organ	Sympathetic Response (Mostly Norepinephrine)	Parasympathetic Response (Acetylcholine)
Eye		
• Iris sphincter muscle	Dilation	Constriction
• Ciliary muscle	Relaxation	Accommodation for near vision
Heart		
• Sinoatrial node	Increased rate	Decrease in rate
• Atria	Increased contractility	Decrease in contractility
• Atrioventricular node	Increased contractility	Decrease in conduction velocity
Blood Vessels	Constriction	Dilation
Lungs		
• Bronchial muscles	Relaxation	Bronchoconstriction
• Bronchial glands		Secretion
Gastrointestinal Tract		
• Motility and tone	Relaxation	Increased
• Sphincters	Contraction	Relaxation
• Secretion		Stimulation
Urinary Bladder		
• Detrusor muscle	Relaxation	Contraction
• Trigone and sphincter	Contraction	Relaxation
Uterus	Contraction (pregnant) Relaxation (nonpregnant)	Variable
Skin		
• Pilomotor muscles	Contraction	No effect
• Sweat glands	Increased secretion	No effect
Glands		
• Salivary, lachrymal		Increased secretion
• Sweat		Increased secretion

NEUROPHYSIOLOGY OF THE CENTRAL NERVOUS SYSTEM

At their most basic level, the human brain and connecting nervous system are composed of billions of cells. Most are connective and supportive glial cells with ancillary functions in the nervous system.

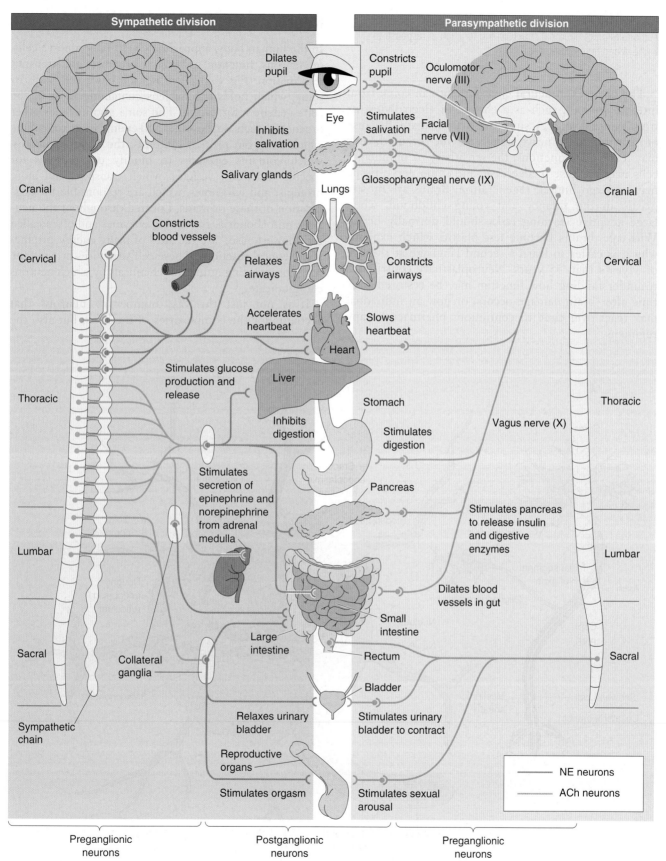

FIGURE 8.4 Diagram of the autonomic nervous system. Note that many organs are innervated by both sympathetic and parasympathetic nerves. (Reprinted with permission from Bear, M. F., Conners, B. W., & Paradiso, M. A. [2016]. *Neuroscience: Exploring the brain* [4th ed.]. Wolters Kluwer.)
Note. ACh = acetylcholine; NE = norepinephrine.

KEYCONCEPT Neuroplasticity is a continuous process of modulation of neuronal structure and function in response to the changing environment.

The changes in neural environment can come from internal sources, such as a change in electrolytes, or from external sources, such as a virus or toxin. Because of neuroplasticity, nerve signals may be rerouted, cells may learn new functions, the sensitivity or number of cells may increase or decrease, and some nerve tissue may undergo limited regeneration. Brains are mostly plastic during infancy and young childhood, when large adaptive learning tasks should normally occur. With age, brains become less plastic, which explains why it is easier to learn a second language at the age of 5 years than 55 years. Neuroplasticity contributes to understanding how function may be restored over time after brain damage occurs, or how an individual may react over time to continuous pharmacotherapy regimens.

Neurons and Nerve Impulses

In the human body, approximately 10 billion nerve cells, or neurons, function to receive, organize, and transmit information (Fig. 8.5). Each neuron has a cell body, or soma, which holds the nucleus containing most of the cell's genetic information. The soma also includes other organelles, such as ribosomes and endoplasmic reticulum, which carry out protein synthesis; the Golgi apparatus, which contains enzymes to modify the proteins for specific functions; vesicles, which transport and store proteins; and lysosomes, which are responsible for degradation of these proteins. Located throughout the neurons, mitochondria, containing enzymes and often called the "powerhouse," are the sites of many energy-producing chemical reactions. These cell structures provide the basis for secreting numerous chemicals by which neurons communicate.

It is not just the vast number of neurons that accounts for the complexities of the brain but also the

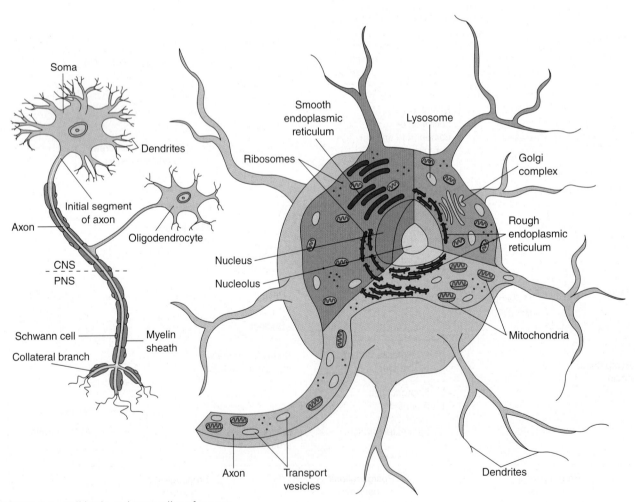

FIGURE 8.5   Cell body and organelles of neuron.
Note. CNS = central nervous system; PNS = peripheral nervous system.

enormous number of neurochemical interconnections and interactions among neurons. A single motor neuron in the spinal cord may receive signals from more than 10,000 sources of interconnections with other nerves. Although most neurons have only one axon, which varies in length and conducts impulses away from the soma, each has numerous dendrites, receiving signals from other neurons. Because axons may branch as they terminate, they also have multiple contacts with other neurons.

Nerve signals are prompted to fire by a variety of chemical or physical stimuli. This firing produces an electrical impulse. The cell's membrane is a double layer of phospholipid molecules with embedded proteins. Some of these proteins provide water-filled channels through which inorganic ions may pass (Fig. 8.6). Each of the common ions—sodium, potassium, calcium, and chloride—has its own specific molecular channel. Many of these channels are voltage gated and thus open or close in response to changes in the electrical potential across the membrane. At rest, the cell membrane is polarized with a positive charge on the outside and about a 270 mV charge on the inside, owing to the resting distribution of sodium and potassium ions. As potassium passively diffuses across the membrane, the sodium pump uses energy to move sodium from the inside of the cell against a concentration gradient to maintain this distribution. An action potential, or *nerve impulse*, is generated as the membrane is depolarized and a threshold value is reached, which triggers the opening of the voltage-gated sodium channels, allowing sodium to surge into the cell. The inside of the cell briefly becomes positively charged and the outside negatively charged. Once initiated, the action potential becomes self-propagating, opening nearby sodium channels. This electrical communication moves into the soma from the dendrites or down the axon by this mechanism.

Synaptic Transmission

For one neuron to communicate with another, the electrical process described must change to a chemical communication. The **synaptic cleft**, a junction between one nerve and another, is the space where the electrical intracellular signal becomes a chemical extracellular signal. Various substances are recognized as the chemical messengers among neurons.

As the electrical action potential reaches the ends of the axons, called *terminals*, calcium ion channels are opened, allowing an influx of Ca^{++} ions into the neuron. This increase in calcium stimulates the release of neurotransmitters into the synapse. Rapid signaling among neurons requires a ready supply of neurotransmitter. These neurotransmitters are stored in small vesicles grouped near the cell membrane at the end of the axon. When stimulated, the vesicles containing the neurotransmitter fuse with the cell membrane, and the neurotransmitter is released into the synapse (Fig. 8.7). The neurotransmitter then crosses the synaptic cleft to a receptor site on the postsynaptic neuron and stimulates adjacent neurons. This is the process of neuronal communication.

When the neurotransmitter has completed its interaction with the postsynaptic receptor and stimulated that cell, its work is done, and it needs to be removed. It can be removed by natural diffusion away from the area of high neurotransmitter concentration at the receptors by being broken down by enzymes in the synaptic cleft or through reuptake through highly specific mechanisms into the presynaptic terminal. The primary steps in synaptic transmission are summarized in Figure 8.7.

Neurotransmitters

As described in the overview earlier, neurotransmitters are key in the process of synaptic transmission.

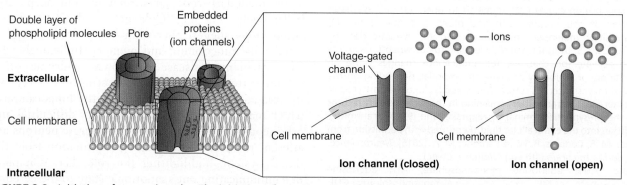

FIGURE 8.6 Initiation of a nerve impulse. The initiation of an action potential, or nerve impulse, involves the opening and closing of the voltage-gated channels on the cell membrane and the passage of ions into the cell. The resulting electrical activity sends communication impulses from the dendrites or axon into the body.

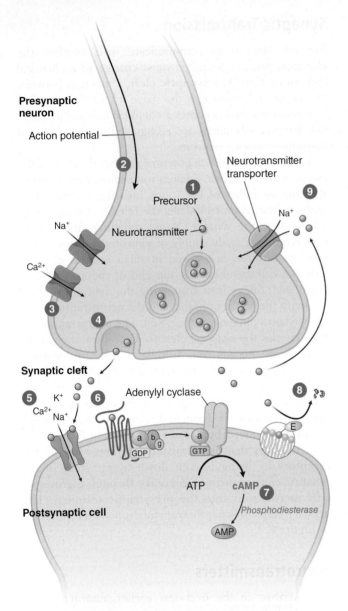

FIGURE 8.7 Synaptic transmission. The most significant events that occur during synaptic transmission are as follows: (1) the action potential reaches the presynaptic terminal; (2) membrane depolarization causes Ca⁺⁺ terminals to open; (3) Ca⁺⁺ mediates fusion of the vesicles with the presynaptic membrane; (4) transmitter molecules are released into the synaptic cleft by exocytosis; (5) transmitter molecules bind to postsynaptic receptors and activate ion channels; (6) conductance changes cause an excitatory or inhibitory postsynaptic potential, depending on the specific transmitter; (7) current flow spreads along the postsynaptic membrane; (8) transmitter remaining in the synaptic cleft returns to the presynaptic terminal by reuptake; and (9) the transmitter diffuses into the extracellular fluid. (Reprinted with permission from Bear, M. F., Conners, B. W., & Paradiso, M. A. [2016]. *Neuroscience: Exploring the brain* [4th ed.]. Wolters Kluwer.)
Note. AMP, adenosine monophosphate; ATP, adenosine triphosphate; cAMP, cyclic adenosine monophosphate; GDP, guanosine diphosphate; GTP, guanosine triphosphate.

Neurotransmitters are small molecules that directly and indirectly control the opening or closing of ion channels. **Neuromodulators** are chemical messengers that make the target cell membrane or postsynaptic membrane susceptible to the effects of the primary neurotransmitter.

> **KEYCONCEPT Neurotransmitters** are small molecules that directly and indirectly control the opening or closing of ion channels.

Excitatory neurotransmitters reduce the membrane potential and enhance the transmission of the signal between neurons. *Inhibitory neurotransmitters* have the opposite effect and slow down nerve impulses. Although some are synthesized from dietary precursors, such as tyrosine or tryptophan, most synthesis occurs in the terminals or the neuron itself. Neurotransmitters are commonly classified as the following: cholinergic, biogenic amine (monoamines or bioamines), amino acid, and neuropeptides. Table 8.2 summarizes some of the key neurotransmitters and their proposed functions.

Acetylcholine

Acetylcholine (ACh) is the primary cholinergic neurotransmitter. Found in the greatest concentration in the PNS, ACh provides the basic synaptic communication for the parasympathetic neurons and part of the sympathetic neurons, which send information to the CNS.

ACh is an excitatory neurotransmitter that is found throughout the cerebral cortex and limbic system. It arises primarily from cell bodies in the basal forebrain constellation, which provides innervations to the cerebral cortex, amygdala, hippocampus, and thalamus as well as from the dorsolateral tegmentum of the pons that projects to the basal ganglia, thalamus, hypothalamus, medullary reticular formation, and deep cerebellar nuclei (Fig. 8.8) (Colangelo et al., 2019). These connections suggest that ACh is involved in higher intellectual functioning and memory. Individuals who have Alzheimer disease or Down syndrome often exhibit patterns of cholinergic neuron loss in regions innervated by these pathways (e.g., the hippocampus), which may contribute to their memory difficulties and other cognitive deficits. Some cholinergic neurons are afferent to these areas bringing information from the limbic system, highlighting the role that ACh plays in communicating one's emotional state to the cerebral cortex.

TABLE 8.2	CLASSIC AND PUTATIVE NEUROTRANSMITTERS: THEIR DISTRIBUTION AND PROPOSED FUNCTIONS		
Neurotransmitter	Cell Bodies	Projections	Proposed Function
Acetylcholine			
Dietary precursor: choline	Basal forebrain Pons Other areas	Diffuse throughout the cortex, hippocampus PNS	Important role in learning and memory Some role in wakefulness and basic attention Peripherally activates muscles and is the major neurochemical in the autonomic system
Monoamines			
Dopamine (dietary precursor: tyrosine)	Substantia nigra Ventral tegmental area Arcuate nucleus Retina olfactory bulb	Striatum (basal ganglia) Limbic system and cerebral cortex Pituitary	Involved in involuntary motor movements Some role in mood states, pleasure components in reward systems, and complex behavior (e.g., judgment, reasoning, insight)
Norepinephrine (dietary precursor: tyrosine)	Locus coeruleus Lateral tegmental area and others throughout the pons and medulla	Very widespread throughout the cortex, thalamus, cerebellum, brain stem, and spinal cord Basal forebrain, thalamus, hypothalamus, brain stem, and spinal cord	Proposed role in learning and memory, attributing value in reward systems, fluctuates in sleep and wakefulness Major component of the sympathetic nervous system responses, including "fight or flight"
Serotonin (dietary precursor: tryptophan)	Raphe nuclei Others in the pons and medulla	Very widespread throughout the cortex, thalamus, cerebellum, brain stem, and spinal cord	Proposed role in the control of appetite, sleep, mood states, hallucinations, pain perception, and vomiting
Histamine (precursor: histidine)	Hypothalamus	Cerebral cortex Limbic system Hypothalamus Found in all mast cells	Control of gastric secretions, smooth muscle control, cardiac stimulation, stimulation of sensory nerve endings, and alertness
Amino Acids			
GABA	Derived from glutamate without localized cell bodies	Found in cells and projections throughout the CNS, especially in intrinsic feedback loops and interneurons of the cerebrum; also in the extrapyramidal motor system and cerebellum	Fast inhibitory response postsynaptically inhibits the excitability of the neurons and therefore contributes to seizure, agitation, and anxiety control
Glycine	Primarily the spinal cord and brain stem	Limited projection, but especially in the auditory system and olfactory bulb Also found in the spinal cord, medulla, midbrain, cerebellum, and cortex	Inhibitory Decreases the excitability of spinal motor neurons but not cortical
Glutamate	Diffuse	Diffuse, but especially in the sensory organs	Excitatory Responsible for the bulk of information flow
Neuropeptides			
Endogenous opioids (i.e., endorphins, enkephalins)	A large family of neuropeptides that has three distinct subgroups, all of which are manufactured widely throughout the CNS	Widely distributed within and outside of the CNS	Suppress pain, modulate mood and stress Likely involvement in reward systems and addiction Also may regulate pituitary hormone release Implicated in the pathophysiology of diseases of the basal ganglia
Melatonin (one of its precursors: serotonin)	Pineal body	Widely distributed within and outside of the CNS	Secreted in dark and suppressed in light, helps regulate the sleep–wake cycle as well as other biologic rhythms
Substance P	Widespread, significant in the raphe system and spinal cord	Spinal cord, cortex, brain stem, and especially sensory neurons associated with pain perception	Involved in pain transmission, movement, and mood regulation
Cholecystokinin	Predominates in the ventral tegmental area of the midbrain	Frontal cortex, where it is often colocalized with dopamine Widely distributed within and outside of the CNS	Primary intestinal hormone involved in satiety; also has some involvement in the control of anxiety and panic

Note. CNS = central nervous system; GABA = gamma-aminobutyric acid; PNS = peripheral nervous system.

Acetylcholine system

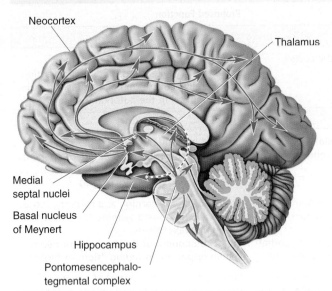

FIGURE 8.8 Cholinergic pathways. (Reprinted with permission from Bear, M. F., Conners, B. W., & Paradiso, M. A. [2016]. *Neuroscience: Exploring the brain* [4th ed.]. Wolters Kluwer.)

Biogenic Amines

The **biogenic amines** (bioamines) consist of small molecules manufactured in the neuron that contain an amine group, thus the name. The catecholamines (amine attached to a catechol group) include dopamine, norepinephrine, and epinephrine, which are all synthesized from the amino acid tyrosine. Another monoamine, serotonin, is synthesized from tryptophan. Melatonin is derived from serotonin. All of these neurotransmitters are critical in many of the mental disorders.

Dopamine

Dopamine is an excitatory neurotransmitter found in distinct regions of the CNS and is involved in cognition, motor, and neuroendocrine functions. Dopamine is the neurotransmitter that stimulates the body's natural "feel good" reward pathways, producing pleasant euphoric sensation under certain conditions. It is involved in the regulation of action, emotion, motivation, and attention. Dopamine levels are decreased in Parkinson disease, and abnormally high activity of dopamine has been associated with schizophrenia (discussed in more detail in Chapter 24). Abnormalities of dopamine activity within the reward system pathways are suspected to be a critical aspect of the development of drug and other addictions. The dopamine pathways are distinct neuronal areas within the CNS in which the neurotransmitter dopamine predominates. Three major dopaminergic pathways have been identified.

The *mesocortical* and *mesolimbic pathways* originate in the ventral tegmental area and project into the medial aspects of the cortex (mesocortical) and the limbic system inside the temporal lobes, including the hippocampus and amygdala (mesolimbic). Sometimes, they are considered to be one pathway and at other times two separate pathways. The mesocortical pathway has major effects on cognition, including functions such as judgment, reasoning, insight, social conscience, motivation, the ability to generalize learning, and reward systems in the human brain. It contributes to some of the highest seats of cortical functioning. The mesolimbic pathway also strongly influences emotions and has projections that affect memory and auditory reception. Abnormalities in these pathways have been associated with schizophrenia.

Another major dopaminergic pathway begins in the substantia nigra and projects into the basal ganglia, parts of which are known as the *striatum*. Therefore, this pathway is called the *nigrostriatal pathway*. This influences the extrapyramidal motor system, which serves the voluntary motor system and allows involuntary motor movements. Destruction of dopaminergic neurons in this pathway has been associated with Parkinson disease.

The final dopamine pathway originates from projections of the mesolimbic pathway and continues into the hypothalamus, which then projects into the pituitary gland. Therefore, this pathway, called the *tuberoinfundibular pathway*, has an impact on endocrine function and other functions, such as metabolism, hunger, thirst, sexual function, circadian rhythms, digestion, and temperature control. Figure 8.9 illustrates the dopaminergic pathways.

Norepinephrine

Norepinephrine is an excitatory neurochemical that plays a major role in generating and maintaining mood states. Because norepinephrine is so heavily concentrated in the terminal sites of sympathetic nerves, it can be released quickly to ready the individual for a fight-or-flight response to threats in the environment. For this reason, norepinephrine is thought to play a role in the physical symptoms of anxiety (Bastos et al., 2018).

Nerve tracts and pathways containing predominantly norepinephrine are called *noradrenergic* and are less clearly delineated than the dopamine pathways. In the CNS, noradrenergic neurons originate in the locus coeruleus, where more than half of the noradrenergic cell bodies are located. Because the locus coeruleus is one of the major timekeepers of the human body, norepinephrine is involved in sleep and wakefulness. From the locus coeruleus, noradrenergic pathways ascend into the neocortex, spread diffusely (Fig. 8.10), and enhance the ability of neurons to respond to whatever input they may be receiving. In addition, norepinephrine appears to be involved in the process of reinforcement,

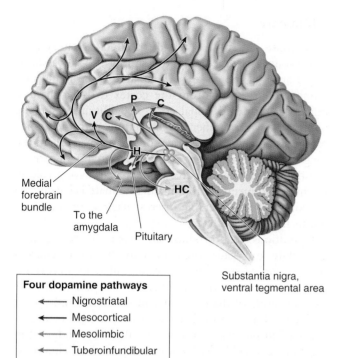

FIGURE 8.9 Dopaminergic pathways. C, caudate nucleus; H, hypothalamus; HC, hippocampal formation; P, putamen; S, striatum; V, ventral striatum. The dopaminergic diffuse modulatory systems arising from the substantia nigra and the ventral tegmental area. The substantia nigra and ventral tegmental area lie close together in the midbrain. The project to the striatum (caudate nucleus and putamen) and limbic and frontal cortical regions, respectively. (Reprinted with permission from Bear, M. F., Conners, B. W., & Paradiso, M. A. [2016]. *Neuroscience: Exploring the brain* [4th ed.]. Wolters Kluwer.)

which facilitates learning. Noradrenergic pathways innervate the hypothalamus and thus are involved to some degree in endocrine function. Anxiety disorders and depression are examples of psychiatric illnesses in which dysfunction of the noradrenergic neurons may be involved. (Refer to Table 8.1 for the effects of ACh on various organs in the parasympathetic system.)

Serotonin

Serotonin (also called 5-hydroxytryptamine or 5-HT) is primarily an excitatory neurotransmitter that is diffusely distributed within the cerebral cortex, limbic system, and basal ganglia of the CNS. Serotonergic neurons also project into the hypothalamus and cerebellum. Figure 8.11 illustrates serotonergic pathways. Serotonin plays a role in emotions, cognition, sensory perceptions, and essential biologic functions, such as sleep and appetite. During the rapid eye movement (REM) phase of sleep, or the dream state, serotonin concentrations decrease, and muscles subsequently relax. Serotonin is also involved in the control of food intake, hormone secretion, sexual behavior, thermoregulation, and cardiovascular regulation. Some serotonergic fibers reach the cranial blood vessels within the brain and the *piamater* where they have a vasoconstrictive effect. The potency of some new medications for migraine headaches is related to their ability to block serotonin transmission in the cranial blood vessels. Descending serotonergic

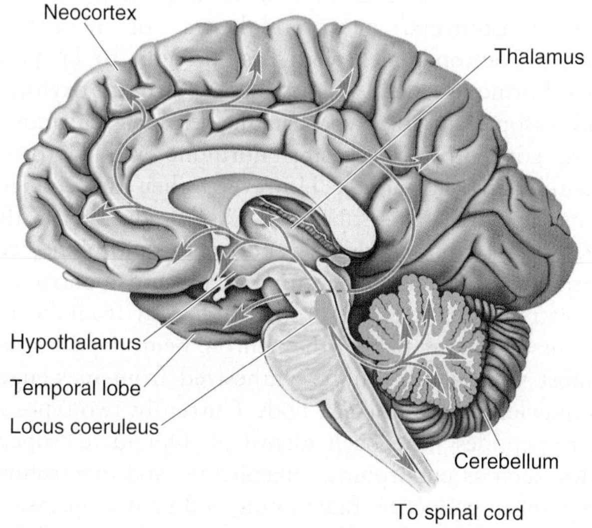

FIGURE 8.10 Noradrenergic pathways. (Reprinted with permission from Bear, M. F., Conners, B. W., & Paradiso, M. A. [2016]. *Neuroscience: Exploring the brain* [4th ed.]. Wolters Kluwer.)

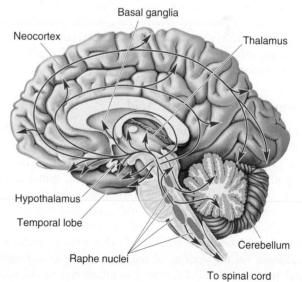

FIGURE 8.11 The serotonergic diffuse modulatory systems arising from the raphe nuclei. The raphe nuclei are clustered along the midline of the brain stem and project extensively to all levels of the central nervous system. (Reprinted with permission from Bear, M. F., Conners, B. W., & Paradiso, M. A. [2016]. *Neuroscience: Exploring the brain* [4th ed.]. Wolters Kluwer.)

pathways are important in central pain control. Whereas depression and insomnia have been associated with decreased levels of 5-HT, mania has been associated with increased 5-HT. Some of the most well-known antidepressant medications, such as Prozac and Zoloft, which are discussed in more depth in Chapter 12, function by raising serotonin levels within certain areas of the CNS. Melatonin, which is derived from serotonin, is produced by the pineal gland and plays a role in sleep, aging, and mood changes.

Amino Acids

Amino acids, the building blocks of proteins, have many roles in intraneuronal metabolism. In addition, amino acids can function as neurotransmitters in as many as 60% to 70% of the synaptic sites in the brain. Amino acids are the most prevalent neurotransmitters. Virtually all of the neurons in the CNS are activated by excitatory amino acids, such as glutamate, and inhibited by inhibitory amino acids, such as **gamma-aminobutyric acid (GABA)** and glycine. Many of these amino acids coexist with other neurotransmitters.

Histamine

Histamine, derived from the amino acid histidine, has been identified as a neurotransmitter. Its cell bodies originate predominantly in the hypothalamus and project to all major structures in the cerebrum, brain stem, and spinal cord. Its functions are not well known, but it appears to have a role in autonomic and neuroendocrine regulation. Many psychiatric medications can block the effects of histamine postsynaptically and produce side effects such as sedation, weight gain, and hypotension.

Gamma-Aminobutyric Acid

GABA is the primary inhibitory neurotransmitter for the CNS. The pathways of GABA exist almost exclusively in the CNS, with the largest GABA concentrations in the hypothalamus, hippocampus, basal ganglia, spinal cord, and cerebellum. GABA functions in an inhibitory role in control of spinal reflexes and cerebellar reflexes. It has a major role in the control of neuronal excitability through the brain. In addition, GABA has an inhibitory influence on the activity of the dopaminergic nigrostriatal projections. GABA also has interconnections with other neurotransmitters. For example, dopamine inhibits cholinergic neurons, and GABA provides feedback and balance. Dysregulation of GABA and GABA receptors has been associated with anxiety disorders, and decreased GABA activity is involved in the development of seizure disorders.

Glutamate

Glutamate, the most widely distributed excitatory neurotransmitter, is the main transmitter in the associational areas of the cortex. Glutamate can be found in a number of pathways from the cortex to the thalamus, pons, striatum, and spinal cord. In addition, glutamate pathways have a number of connections with the hippocampus. Some glutamate receptors may play a role in the long-lasting enhancement of synaptic activity. In turn, in the hippocampus, this enhancement may have a role in learning and memory. Too much glutamate is harmful to neurons, and considerable interest has emerged regarding its neurotoxic effects.

Conditions that produce an excess of endogenous glutamate can cause neurotoxicity by overexcitation of neuronal tissue. This process, called excitotoxicity, increases the sensitivity of glutamate receptors, produces overactivation of the receptors, and is increasingly being understood as a critical piece of the cascade of events involved in physical symptoms of alcohol withdrawal in dependent individuals. Excitotoxicity is also believed to be part of the pathology of conditions such as ischemia, hypoxia, hypoglycemia, and hepatic failure. Damage to the CNS from chronic malfunctioning of the glutamate system may be involved in the psychiatric symptoms seen in neurodegenerative diseases such as Huntington, Parkinson, and Alzheimer diseases; vascular dementia; amyotrophic lateral sclerosis; and AIDS-related dementia. Degeneration of glutamate neurons is implicated in the development of schizophrenia.

Neuropeptides

Neuropeptides, short chains of amino acids, exist in the CNS and have a number of important roles as neurotransmitters, neuromodulators, or neurohormones. Neuropeptides were first thought to be pituitary hormones, such as adrenocorticotropin, oxytocin, and vasopressin, or hypothalamic-releasing hormones (e.g., corticotropin-releasing hormone and thyrotropin-releasing hormone). However, when an endogenous morphine–like substance was discovered in the 1970s, the term *endorphin*, or endogenous morphine, was introduced. Although the amino acids and monoamine neurotransmitters can be produced directly from dietary precursors in any part of the neuron, neuropeptides are, almost without exception, synthesized from messenger ribonucleic acid in the cell body. Currently, two types of neuropeptides have been identified. Opioid neuropeptides, such as endorphins, enkephalins, and dynorphins, function in endocrine functioning and pain suppression. The nonopioid neuropeptides, such as substance P and somatostatin, play roles in pain transmission and endocrine functioning, respectively.

There are considerable variations in the distribution of individual neuropeptides, but some areas are especially rich in cell bodies containing neuropeptides. These areas include the amygdala, striatum, hypothalamus, raphe nuclei, brain stem, and spinal cord. Many of the interneurons of the cerebral cortex contain neuropeptides, but there are considerably fewer in the thalamus and almost none in the cerebellum.

Receptors

Embedded in the postsynaptic membrane are a number of proteins that act as receptors for the released neurotransmitters. Each neurotransmitter has a specific receptor, or protein, for which it and only it will fit.

Lock and Key

The "lock-and-key" analogy has often been used to describe the fit of a given neurotransmitter to its receptor site. The target cell, when stimulated by the neurotransmitter, will then respond by evoking its own action potential and either producing some action common to that cell or acting as a relay to keep the messages moving throughout the CNS. This pattern of the electrical signal from one neuron, converted to chemical signal at the synaptic cleft, picked up by an adjacent neuron, again converted to an electrical action potential, and then to a chemical signal, occurs billions of times a day in billions of different neurons. This electrical–chemical communication process allows the structures of the brain to function together in a coordinated and organized manner.

Receptor Sensitivity

Both presynaptic and postsynaptic **receptors** have the capacity to change, developing either a greater-than-usual response to the neurotransmitter, known as supersensitivity, or a less-than-usual response, called subsensitivity. These changes represent the concept of neuroplasticity of brain tissue discussed earlier in the chapter. The change in sensitivity of the receptor is most commonly caused by the effect of a drug on a receptor site or by disease that affects the normal functioning of a receptor site. Drugs can affect the sensitivity of the receptor by altering the strength of attraction or affinity of a receptor for the neurotransmitter, by changing the efficiency with which the receptor activity translates the message inside the receiving cell, or by decreasing over time the number of receptors.

These mechanisms may account for the long-term, sometimes severely adverse, effects of psychopharmacologic drugs, the loss of effectiveness of a given medication, or the loss of effectiveness of a medication after repeated use in treating recurring episodes of a psychiatric disorder. Disease may cause a change in the normal number or function of receptors, thereby altering their sensitivity. For example, depression is associated with a reduction in the normal number of certain receptors, leading to an abnormality in their sensitivity to neurotransmitters such as serotonin and norepinephrine (Crispino et al., 2020). A decreased response to continued stimulation of these receptors is usually referred to as *desensitization* or *refractoriness*. This suspected subsensitivity is referred to as *downregulation* of the receptors.

Receptor Subtypes

The nervous system uses many different neurochemicals for communication, and each specific chemical messenger requires a specific receptor on which the chemical can act. More than 100 different chemical messengers have been identified, with new ones being uncovered. In addition to the sheer number of receptors needed to accommodate these chemicals, the neurotransmitters may produce different effects at different synaptic sites.

Each major neurotransmitter has several different subtypes of receptors, allowing the neurotransmitter to have different effects in different areas of the brain. The receptors usually have the same name as the neurotransmitter, but the classification of the subtypes varies. For example, dopamine receptors are named D1, D2, D3, and so on. Serotonin receptors are grouped in families such as 5HT 1a and 5HT 1b. The receptors for Ach have completely different names: muscarinic and nicotinic. Two specific subtype receptors have been identified for GABA: A and B (see Table 8.3).

Brain structures such as the prefrontal cortex, striatum, hippocampus, and amygdala are linked through complex neural functional networks (Uddin et al., 2019). Recent

TABLE 8.3	SELECTED NEUROTRANSMITTERS AND RECEPTORS
Neurotransmitter	**Receptor Subtypes**
Acetylcholine (ACH)	Muscarinic receptors (M_1, M_2, M_3, M_4, M_5) Nicotinic receptor
Glutamate (Glu)	AMPA, NMDA, kainate receptors
Gamma-aminobutyric acid (GABA)	$GABA_A$, $GABA_B$
Serotonin (5-HT)	5-HT_{1A}, 5-HT_{1B}, 5-HT_{1D}, 5-HT_{1E}, 5-HT_{2A}, 5-HT_{2B}, 5-HT_C, 5-HT_4, 5-HT_{5A}
Dopamine (DA)	D1, D2, D3, D4, D5
Norepinephrine (NE)	α_1, α_2, β_1, β_2

Reprinted with permission from Bear, M. F., Connors, B. W., & Paradiso, M. A. (2016). *Neuroscience: Exploring the brain* (4th ed.). Wolters Kluwer.

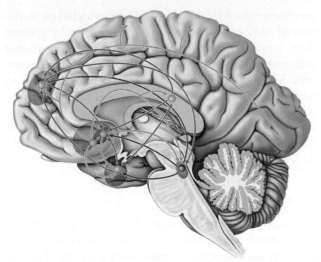

FIGURE 8.12 Complex neural functional networks involved in psychiatric disorders. *Arrows* illustrate projections. (Redrawn by permission from Nature: Haber, S. N., & Rauch, S. L. [2010]. Neurocircuitry: A window into the networks underlying neuropsychiatric disease. *Neuropsychopharmacology, 35*[1], 1–3. Copyright © 2009 Springer Nature.)

Note. ACC = anterior cingulate cortex; Amy = amygdala; Cd = caudate nucleus; DPFC = dorsal prefrontal cortex; GP = globus pallidus; Ex Amy = extended amygdala; Hipp = hippocampus; MD = medial dorsal nucleus of the thalamus; MTL = medial temporal lobe; OFC = orbital frontal cortex; Pu = Putamen; SN = substantia nigra; Thal = thalamus; vmPFC = ventral medial prefrontal cortex; VP = ventral pallidum; VS = ventral striatum; VTA = ventral tegmental area.

research indicates that a dysfunctional **neurocircuitry** underlies most psychiatric disorders (Fig. 8.12). Various neurocircuits are the focus of study of different illness. For example, the cingulo-frontal-parietal network is associated with attention-deficit disorder, and the amygdalocortical circuitry is the focus in psychosis and schizophrenia.

STUDIES OF THE BIOLOGIC BASIS OF MENTAL DISORDERS

As described earlier, mental disorders are complex syndromes consisting of clusters of biopsychosocial symptoms. These syndromes are not specific physiologic disorders, and research efforts are focused on piecing the puzzle together. One important area of study is genetics; it is well established that genetic factors play an important role in the development of mental disorders. In addition, as the complexity of the nervous system and its interrelationship with other body systems and the environment have become more fully understood, new fields of study have emerged. One field worth noting is **psychoneuroimmunology (PNI)**. Although it has long been observed that individuals under stress have compromised immune systems and are more likely to acquire common diseases, only recently have changes in

the immune system been noted as widespread in some psychiatric illnesses. Another field, **chronobiology**, has provided new information suggesting that dysfunction of biologic rhythms may not only result from a psychiatric illness but also contribute to its development.

Genetics

The sequence of the human genome is the beginning of our understanding of complex genetic connections that leads to a **phenotype** or observable characteristics or expressions of a specific trait. The genome provides researchers with a road map of the exact sequence of the three billion nucleotide bases that make up human organisms. Many thought that after the human genome was mapped, it would be easy to determine the genes responsible for mental disorders. Unfortunately, it is not that simple. Knowing the location of the gene and its sequence is just a piece of the complex puzzle. The location of the genes does not tell us which genes are responsible for a mental illness or how mutations occur.

Population Genetics

Inheritance of mental disorders is studied by using epidemiologic methods that identify risks and patterns of illness or traits from generation to generation. Beginning with a **proband**, a person who has the disorder or trait, **population genetics** relies on the following principal epidemiologic methods:

- **Family studies** analyze the occurrence of a disorder in first-degree relatives (biologic parents, siblings, and children), second-degree relatives (grandparents, uncles, aunts, nieces, nephews, and grandchildren), and so on.

- **Twin studies** analyze the presence or absence of the disorder in pairs of twins. The *concordance rate* is the measure of similarity of occurrence in individuals with a similar genetic makeup.

- **Adoption studies** compare the risk for the illness developing in offspring raised in different environments. The strongest inferences may be drawn from studies that involve children separated from their parents at birth.

Mental disorders and their symptoms are not an expression of a single gene. The transmission pattern does not follow classic Mendelian genetics in which the dominant allele (variant) on only one chromosome or recessive alleles on both chromosomes are responsible for manifestation of a disorder. Monozygotic (identical) twins do not manifest the same mental disorder with 100% concordance rate, but they have a higher rate of a disorder than dizygotic (fraternal) twins, who share roughly the same proportion of genes that ordinary siblings do (50%). Internal and external environmental events influence the development of a disorder with a genetic contribution. This interaction between the environment and a genetic predisposition underlies several mental disorders such as schizophrenia, autism, and attention-deficit hyperactivity disorder.

Molecular Genetics

A gene comprises short segments of deoxyribonucleic acid and is packed with the instructions for making proteins that have a specific function. When genes are absent or malfunction, protein production is altered, and bodily functions are disrupted. In this fashion, genes play a role in cancer, heart disease, diabetes, and many psychiatric disorders. Although no conclusive evidence exists for a complete genetic cause of most psychiatric disorders, significant evidence suggests that strong genetic contributions exist for most (McCutcheon et al., 2020).

Intracellular genes direct protein production responsible for genetic expression. Individual nerve cells outside of the cell respond to these changes, modifying proteins to adapt to the new environment. This dynamic nature of gene function highlights the manner in which the body and the environment interact and in how environmental factors influence gene expression.

The study of molecular genetics in psychiatric disorders is in its infancy. It is likely that psychiatric disorders are polygenic. This means that psychiatric disorders develop when genes interact with each other and with environmental factors such as stress, infections, poor nutrition, catastrophic loss, complications during pregnancy, and exposure to toxins. Thus, genetic makeup conveys vulnerability, or a risk for the illness, but the right set of environmental factors must be present for the disorder to develop in an at-risk individual (Renzi et al., 2018).

Genetic Susceptibility

The concept of **genetic susceptibility** suggests that an individual may be at increased risk for a psychiatric disorder. Specific risk factors for psychiatric disorders are just beginning to be understood, and environmental influences are examples of risk factors. In the absence of one specific gene for the major psychiatric disorders, risk factor assessment is a logical alternative for predicting who is more likely to experience psychiatric disorders or certain conditions, such as aggression or suicidality (Musci et al., 2019).

When considering information regarding risks for genetic transmission of psychiatric disorders, there are several key points to remember:

• Psychiatric disorders have been described and labeled quite differently across generations, and errors in diagnosis may occur.

• Similar psychiatric symptoms may have considerably different causes, just as symptoms such as chest pain may occur in relation to many different causes.

• Genes that are present may not always cause the appearance of the trait.

• Several genes work together in an individual to produce a given trait or disorder.

• A biologic cause is not necessarily solely genetic in origin. Environmental influences alter the body's functioning and often mediate or worsen genetic risk factors.

Psychoneuroimmunology

PNI examines the relationships among the immune system, nervous system, and endocrine system and our behaviors, thoughts, and feelings. The immune system is composed of the thymus, spleen, lymph nodes, lymphatic vessels, tonsils, adenoids, and bone marrow, which manufacture all the cells that eventually develop into T cells, B cells, phagocytes, macrophages, and natural killer (NK) cells (Fig. 8.13). Many contemporary stress research studies are examining the role of the NK cells in the early recognition of foreign bodies. Lower NK

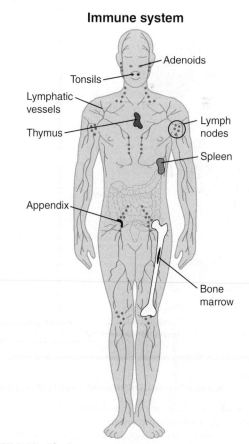

Immune system

Adenoids

Tonsils

Lymphatic vessels

Thymus

Lymph nodes

Spleen

Appendix

Bone marrow

FIGURE 8.13   The immune system.

cell function is related to increased disease susceptibility. NK cell function is affected by stress-induced physiologic arousal in humans. NK cell activity has been shown to vary in response to many emotional, cognitive, and physiologic stressors, including anxiety, depression, perceived lack of personal control, bereavement, pain, and surgery (Costello et al., 2019; Furtado & Katzman, 2015).

Overactivity of the immune system can occur in autoimmune diseases such as systemic lupus erythematosus, allergies, and anaphylaxis. Evidence suggests that the nervous system regulates many aspects of immune function.

Specific immune system dysfunctions may result from damage to the hypothalamus, hippocampus, or pituitary and may produce symptoms of psychiatric disorders. Figure 8.14 illustrates the interaction between stress and the immune system. This figure also demonstrates the true biopsychosocial nature of the complex interrelationship of the nervous system, the endocrine system, the immune system, and environmental or emotional stress.

Immune dysregulation may also be involved in the development of psychiatric disorders. This can occur by allowing neurotoxins to affect the brain, damaging

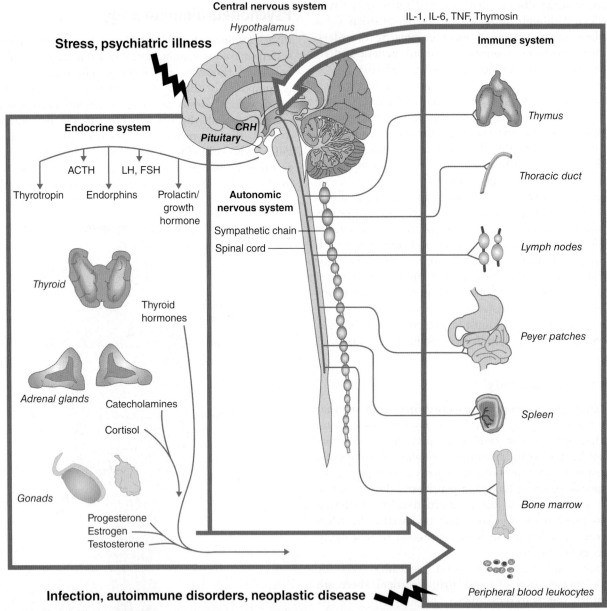

FIGURE 8.14 Examples of the interaction between stress or psychiatric illness and the immune system through the endocrine system.
Note. ACTH = adrenocorticotropic hormone; CRH = corticotropin-releasing hormone; FSH = follicle-stimulating hormone; IL = interleukin; LH = luteinizing hormone; TNF = tumor necrosis factor.

neuroendocrine tissue, or damaging tissues in the brain at locations such as the receptor sites. Some antidepressants have been thought to have antiviral effects. Symptoms of diseases such as depression may occur after an occurrence of serious infection, and prenatal exposure to infectious organisms has been associated with the development of schizophrenia. Stress and conditioning have specific effects on the suppression of immune function (Liu & Tang, 2018; Vidal & Pacheco, 2020).

Normal functioning of the endocrine system is often disturbed in people with psychiatric disorders. For example, thyroid functioning is often low in those with bipolar disorder, and people with schizophrenia have a higher incidence of diabetes (see Unit VI). The hypothalamus sends and receives information through the pituitary, which then communicates with structures in the peripheral aspects of the body. Figure 8.15 presents an example of the communication of the anterior pituitary with a number of organs and structures.

Axes, the structures within which the neurohormones are providing messages, are the most often studied aspect of the neuroendocrine system. These axes always involve a feedback mechanism. For example, the **hypothalamus–pituitary–thyroid axis (HPA)** regulates

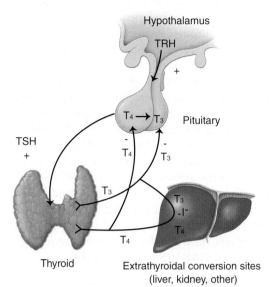

FIGURE 8.16 Hypothalamic–pituitary–thyroid axis. This figure shows the regulation of thyroid-stimulating hormone (or thyrotropin) secretion by the anterior pituitary. Also depicted are the positive effects of thyrotropin-releasing hormone from the hypothalamus and negative effects of circulating triiodothyronine (T_3) and T_3 from intrapituitary conversion of thyroxine (T_4).
Note. TRH = thyrotropin-releasing hormone; TSH = thyroid-stimulating hormone.

the release of thyroid hormone by the thyroid gland using thyrotropin-releasing hormone from the hypothalamus to the pituitary and thyroid-stimulating hormone (TSH) from the pituitary to the thyroid. Figure 8.16 illustrates the HPA. The hypothalamic–pituitary–gonadal axis regulates estrogen and testosterone secretion through luteinizing hormone and follicle-stimulating hormone. Interest in the endocrine system is heightened by various endocrine disorders that produce psychiatric symptoms. Addison disease (hypoadrenalism) produces depression, apathy, fatigue, and occasionally psychosis. Hypothyroidism produces depression and some anxiety. Administration of steroids can cause depression, hypomania, irritability, and in some cases, psychosis. Some psychiatric disorders have been associated with endocrine system dysfunction. For example, some individuals with mood disorders show evidence of dysregulation in adrenal, thyroid, and growth hormone axes (see Chapter 26).

Gut–Brain Axis

The **gut–brain axis** is the term used to define the relationship among the CNS, neuroendocrine and neuroimmune systems including the HPA, sympathetic and autonomic nervous systems, the **enteric nervous system (ENS)**, the vagus nerve, and the gut microbiota. The ENS or "second brain" is a mesh-like system of neurons

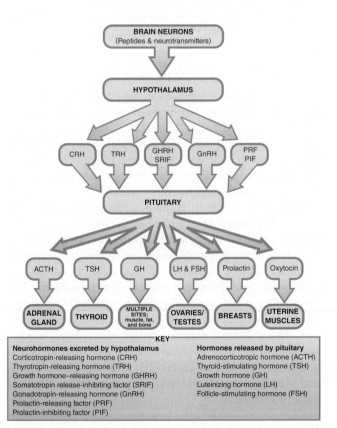

FIGURE 8.15 Hypothalamic and pituitary communication system. The neurohormonal communication system between the hypothalamus and the pituitary exerts effects on many organs and systems.

that governs the function of the gastrointestinal system. The ENS can operate independently and communicates with the CNS through the parasympathetic (vagus nerve) and sympathetic (prevertebral ganglia) nervous system (Li & Owyang, 2003).

The **gut microbiota** is the complex bacterial community located in the gastrointestinal tract (Strandwitz, 2018). Recent research shows that gut microbiota not only is essential for maintaining metabolic and immune health but also influences brain development and neurogenesis and interacts with the ENS and CNS. There is evidence that the gut microbiota has a role in depression, anxiety, Alzheimer disease, and autism spectrum disorder (Bostanciklioglu, 2019; Foster & Neufeld, 2013). It appears that bacteria can respond to and produce neurotransmitters such as the dopamine, norepinephrine, serotonin, and GABA (Strandwitz, 2018).

Chronobiology

Chronobiology involves the study and measure of time structures or biologic rhythms. Some rhythms have a **circadian cycle**, or 24-hour cycle, but others, such as the menstrual cycle, operate in different periods. Rhythms exist in the human body to control endocrine secretions, sleep–wake, body temperature, neurotransmitter synthesis, and more. These cycles may become deregulated and may begin earlier than usual, known as a phase advance, or later than usual, known as a phase delay.

Zeitgebers are specific events that function as time givers or synchronizers and that set biologic rhythms. Light is the most common example of an external zeitgeber. The suprachiasmatic nucleus of the hypothalamus is an example of an internal zeitgeber. Some theorists think that psychiatric disorders may result from one or more biologic rhythm dysfunctions. For example, depression may be, in part, a phase advance disorder, including early morning awakening and decreased time of onset of REM sleep. Seasonal affective disorder may be the result of shortened exposure to light during the winter months. Exposure to specific artificial light often relieves symptoms of fatigue, overeating, hypersomnia, and depression (see Chapters 12, 26, and 34.).

DIAGNOSTIC APPROACHES

Although no commonly used laboratory tests exist that directly confirm a mental disorder, they are still used as part of the diagnosis of these illnesses. **Biologic markers** are diagnostic test findings that occur only in the presence of the psychiatric disorder and include such findings as laboratory and other diagnostic test results and neuropathologic changes noticeable in assessment. These markers increase diagnostic certainty and reliability and may have predictive value, allowing for the possibility of preventive interventions to forestall or avoid the onset of illness. In addition, biologic markers could assist in developing evidence-based care practices. If markers are used reliably, it is much easier to identify the most effective treatments and to determine the expected prognoses for given conditions. The psychiatric–mental health nurse should be aware of the most current information on biologic markers so that information, limitations, and results can be discussed knowledgeably with the patient.

Laboratory Tests

For many years, laboratory tests have attempted to measure levels of neurotransmitters and other CNS substances in the bloodstream. Many of the metabolites of neurotransmitters can be found in the urine and cerebrospinal fluid as well. However, these measures have had only limited utility in elucidating what is happening in the brain. Levels of neurotransmitters and metabolites in the bloodstream or urine do not necessarily equate with levels in the CNS. In addition, availability of the neurotransmitter or metabolite does not predict the availability of the neurotransmitter in the synapse, where it must act, or directly relate to the receptor sensitivity. Nonetheless, numerous research studies have focused on changes in neurotransmitters and metabolites in blood, urine, and cerebrospinal fluid. These studies have provided clues but remain without conclusive predictive value and therefore are not routinely used.

Another laboratory approach to the study of some of the psychiatric disorders is the challenge test. A challenge test has been most often used in the study of panic disorders. These tests are usually conducted by intravenously administering a chemical known to produce a specific set of psychiatric symptoms. For example, lactate or caffeine may be used to induce the symptoms of panic in a person who has panic disorder. The biologic response of the individual is then monitored.

Beyond their role in helping to diagnose mental disorders, laboratory tests are also an active part of the normal care and assessment of patients with psychiatric disorders. Many physical conditions mimic the symptoms of mental illness, and many of the medications used to treat psychiatric illness can produce health problems. For these reasons, the routine care of patients with psychiatric disorders includes the use of laboratory tests such as complete blood counts, thyroid studies, electrolytes, hepatic enzymes, and other evaluative tests. Psychiatric–mental health nurses need to be familiar with these procedures and assist patients in understanding the use and implications of such tests.

Neurophysiologic Procedures

Several neurophysiologic procedures are used in mental health for diagnostic purposes.

Electroencephalography

Electroencephalography (EEG) is a tried and true method for investigating what is happening inside the living brain. Developed in the 1920s, EEG measures electrical activity in the uppermost nerve layers of the cortex. Usually, 16 electrodes are placed on the patient's scalp. The EEG machine, equipped with graph paper and recording pens, is turned on, and the pens then trace the electrical impulses generated over each electrode. Until the use of computed tomography (CT) in the 1970s, the EEG was the only method for identifying brain abnormalities. It remains the simplest and most noninvasive method for identifying some disorders. It is increasingly being used to identify individual neuronal differences.

An EEG may be used in psychiatry to differentiate possible causes of the patient's symptoms. For example, some types of seizure disorders, such as temporal lobe epilepsy, head injuries, or tumors, may present with predominantly psychiatric symptoms. In addition, metabolic dysfunction, delirium, dementia, altered levels of consciousness, hallucinations, and dissociative states may require EEG evaluation.

Spikes and wave-pattern changes are indications of brain abnormalities. Spikes may be the focal point from which a seizure occurs. However, abnormal activity often is not discovered on a routine EEG while the individual is awake. For this reason, additional methods are sometimes used. Nasopharyngeal leads may be used to get physically closer to the limbic regions. The patient may be exposed to a flashing strobe light while the examiner looks for activity that is not in phase with the flashing light or the patient may be asked to hyperventilate for 3 minutes to induce abnormal activity if it exists. Sleep deprivation may also be used. This involves keeping the patient awake throughout the night before the EEG evaluation. The patient may then be drowsy and fall asleep during the procedure. Abnormalities are more likely to occur when the patient is asleep. Sleep may also be induced using medication; however, many medications change the wave patterns on an EEG. For example, the benzodiazepine class of drugs increases the rapid and fast beta activity. Many other prescribed and illicit drugs, such as lithium, which increases theta activity, can cause EEG alterations.

In addition to reassuring, preparing, and educating the patient for the examination, the nurse should carefully assess the history of substance use and report this information to the examiner. If a sleep deprivation EEG is to be done, caffeine or other stimulants that might assist the patient in staying awake should be withheld because they may change the EEG patterns.

Polysomnography

Polysomnography is a special procedure that involves recording the EEG throughout a night of sleep. This test is usually conducted in a sleep laboratory. Other tests are usually performed at the same time, including electrocardiography and electromyography. Blood oxygenation, body movement, body temperature, and other data may be collected as well, especially in research settings. This procedure is usually conducted for evaluating sleep disorders, such as sleep apnea, enuresis, or somnambulism. However, sleep pattern changes are frequently researched in mental disorders as well.

Researchers have found that normal sleep divisions and stages are affected by many factors, including drugs, alcohol, general medical conditions, and psychiatric disorders. For example, REM latency, the length of time it takes an individual to enter the first REM episode, is shortened in depression. Reduced delta sleep is also observed. These findings have been replicated so frequently that some researchers consider them biologic markers for depression.

 Concept Mastery Alert

Polysomnography involves recording an EEG throughout a night of sleep. A sleep deprivation EEG involves keeping a client awake the night before the EEG evaluation.

Structural and Functional Imaging

Neuroimaging of the brain involves **structural imaging**, which visualizes the structure of brain and allows diagnosis of gross intracranial disease and injury, and **functional imaging**, which visualizes processing of information. One of the most well-known examples of structural imaging is magnetic resonance imaging (MRI), which produces two- or three-dimensional images of brain structures without the use of x-rays or radioactive tracers. An MRI creates a magnetic field around the patient's head through which radio waves are sent. A functional MRI (fMRI) that creates functional images relies on the properties of oxygenated and deoxygenated hemoglobin to see images of changes in blood flow. The advantage of fMRI is that it is possible to see how the brain works when different stimuli are presented and problems that exist, such as a stroke. The fMRI has replaced most use of positron emission tomography (PET), which measures blood flow and oxygen and glucose metabolism. The emissions from the injected radioactive tracers are rapidly decayed and limit the monitoring of PET to short tasks.

Neuroimaging has limited clinical use in mental health, but its use is increasing in diagnosis and treatment of some disorders such as Alzheimer disease and traumatic brain injury (Henderson et al., 2020). Neuroimaging has promising potential for unlocking the pathophysiology of several mental disorders. With the introduction of the fMRI, it is now possible to study the circuitry and pinpoint genetic-based predisposing factors. An MRI technique, diffusion tensor imaging, allows for viewing macroscopic changes that occur at the axon level (Tǿnnesen et al., 2018).

Other Neurophysiologic Methods

Evoked potentials (EPs), also called event-related potentials, use the same basic principles as an EEG. They measure changes in electrical activity of the brain in specific regions as a response to a given stimulus. Electrodes placed on the scalp measure a large waveform that stands out after the administration of repetitive stimuli, such as a click or flash of light. There are several different types of EPs to be measured, depending on the sensory area affected by the stimulus, the cognitive task required, or the region monitored, any of which can change the length of time until the wave occurrence. EPs are used extensively in psychiatric research. In clinical practice, EPs are used primarily in the assessment of demyelinating disorders, such as multiple sclerosis.

However, brain electrical activity mapping studies, which involve a 20-electrode EEG that generates computerized maps of the brain's electrical activity, have found a slowing of electrical activity in the frontal lobes of individuals who have schizophrenia.

SUMMARY OF KEY POINTS

- Neuroscientists now view behavior and cognitive function as a result of complex interactions within the CNS and its plasticity, or its ability to adapt and change in both structure and function.

- Each hemisphere of the brain is divided into four lobes: the frontal lobe, which controls motor speech function, personality, and working memory—often called the executive functions that govern one's ability to plan and initiate action; the parietal lobe, which controls the sensory functions; the temporal lobe, which contains the primary auditory and olfactory areas; and the occipital lobe, which controls visual integration of information.

- The structures of the limbic system are integrally involved in memory and emotional behavior. Dysfunction of the limbic system has been linked with major mental disorders, including schizophrenia, depression, and anxiety disorders.

- Neurons communicate with each other through synaptic transmission. Neurotransmitters excite or inhibit a response at the receptor sites and have been linked to certain mental disorders. These neurotransmitters include Ach, dopamine, norepinephrine, serotonin, GABA, and glutamate.

- Although no one gene has been found to produce any psychiatric disorder, significant evidence indicates that most psychiatric disorders have a genetic predisposition or susceptibility. For individuals who have such genetic susceptibility, the identification of risk factors is crucial in helping to plan interventions to prevent development of that disorder or to prevent certain behavior patterns, such as aggression or suicide.

- PNI examines the relationship among the immune system; the nervous system; the endocrine system; and thoughts, emotions, and behavior.

- The gut microbiota is not only essential for maintaining metabolic and immune health, but also has a role in depression, anxiety, and other mental disorders. It appears that the bacteria can respond to and produce neurotransmitters.

- Chronobiology focuses on the study and measure of time structures or biologic rhythms occurring in the body and associates dysregulation of these cycles as contributing factors to the development of psychiatric disorders.

- Biologic markers are physical indicators of disturbances within the CNS that differentiate one disease process from another, such as biochemical changes or neuropathologic changes. These biologic markers can be measured by several methods of testing, including challenge tests, EEG, polysomnography, EPs, CT scanning, MRI, PET, and single-photon emission CT; the psychiatric nurse must be familiar with all of these methods.

CRITICAL THINKING CHALLENGES

1. A woman who has experienced a "ministroke" continues to regain lost cognitive function months after the stroke. Her husband takes this as evidence that she never had a stroke. How would you approach patient teaching and counseling for this couple to help them understand this occurrence if the stroke did damage to her brain?

2. Your patient has "impaired executive functioning." Consider what would be a reasonable follow-up schedule for this patient for counseling sessions. Would it be reasonable to schedule visits at 1 p.m. weekly? Is the patient able to keep to this schedule? Why or why not? What would be the best schedule?

3. Mr. S is unable to sleep after watching an upsetting documentary. Identify the neurotransmitter activity that may be interfering with sleep. (Hint: fight or flight.)

4. Describe what behavioral symptoms or problems may be present in a patient with dysfunction of the following brain area:
   a. Basal ganglia
   b. Hippocampus
   c. Limbic system
   d. Thalamus
   e. Hypothalamus
   f. Frontal lobe

5. Compare and contrast the functions of the sympathetic and parasympathetic nervous systems.

6. Discuss the steps in synaptic transmission, beginning with the action potential and ending with how the neurotransmitter no longer communicates its message to the receiving neuron.

7. Examine how a receptor's usual response to a neurotransmitter might change.

8. Compare the roles of dopamine and Ach in the CNS.

9. Explain how dopamine, norepinephrine, and serotonin all contribute to endocrine system regulation. Suggest some other transmitters that may affect endocrine function.

10. Discuss how the fields of PNI and chronobiology overlap.

11. Compare the methods used to find biologic markers of psychiatric disorders reviewed in this chapter. Consider the potential risks and benefits to the patient.

REFERENCES

Bastos, D. B., Sarafim-Silva, B. A., Sundefeld, M. L., Ribeiro, A. A., Brandão, J. D., Biasoli, É. R., Miyahara, G. I., Casarini, D. E., & Bernabé, D. G. (2018). Circulating catecholamines are associated with biobehavioral factors and anxiety symptoms in head and neck cancer patients. *PLoS One*, *13*, e0202515. https://doi.org/10.1371/journal.pone.0202515

Bear, M. F., Conners, B. W., & Paradiso, M. A. (2016). *Neuroscience: Exploring the brain* (4th ed.). Wolters Kluwer.

Bostancikloglu, M. (2019). The role of gut microbiota in pathogenesis of Alzheimer's disease. *Journal of Applied Microbiology*, *127*, 954–967. https://doi.org/10.1111/jam.14264

Colangelo, C., Shichkova, P., Keller, D., Markram, H., & Ramaswamy, S. (2019). Cellular, synaptic and network effects of acetylcholine in the neocortex. *Frontiers in Neural Circuits*, *13*, 24. https://doi.org/10.3389/fncir.2019.00024

Costello, H., Gould, R. L., Abrol, E., & Howard, R. (2019). Systematic review and meta-analysis of the association between peripheral inflammatory cytokines and generalised anxiety disorder. *BMJ Open*, *9*, e027925. https://doi.org/10.1136/bmjopen-2018-027925

Crispino, M., Volpicelli, F., & Perrone-Capano, C. (2020). Role of the serotonin receptor 7 in brain plasticity: From development to disease. *International Journal of Molecular Sciences*, *21*(2), 505. https://doi.org/10.3390/ijms21020505

Foster, J., & Neufeld, K. A. (2013). Gut–brain axis: How the microbiome influences anxiety and depression. *Trends in Neurosciences*, *36*(5), 305–312. https://doi.org/10.1016/j.tins.2013.01.005

Furtado, M., & Katzman, M. A. (2015). Neuroinflammatory pathways in anxiety, posttraumatic stress, and obsessive compulsive disorders. *Psychiatric Research*, *229*(1–2), 37–38.

Haber, S. N., & Rauch, S. L. (2010). Neurocircuitry: A window into the networks underlying neuropsychiatric disease. *Neuropsychopharmacology Reviews*, *35*(1), 1–3.

Harlow, J. M. (1868). Recovery after severe injury to the head. *Publication of the Massachusetts Medical Society*, *2*, 327.

Henderson, T. A., van Lierop, M. J., McLean, M., Uszler, J. M., Thornton, J. F., Siow, Y. H., Pavel, D. G., Cardaci, J., & Cohen, P. (2020). Functional neuroimaging in psychiatry-aiding in diagnosis and guiding treatment. What the American Psychiatric Association does not know. *Frontiers in Psychiatry*, *11*, 276. https://doi.org/10.3389/fpsyt.2020.00276

Li, Y., & Owyang, C. (2003). Musings on the Wanderer: What's new in our understanding of vago-vagal reflexes? V. remodeling of vagus and enteric neural circuitry after vagal injury. *American Journal of Physiology. Gastrointestinal and Liver Physiology*, *285*(3), G461–G469. https://doi.org/10.1152/ajpgi.00119.2003

Liu, Y., & Tang, X. (2018). Depressive syndromes in autoimmune disorders of the nervous system: Prevalence, etiology, and influence. *Frontiers in Psychiatry*, *9*, 451. https://doi.org/10.3389/fpsyt.2018.00451

McCutcheon, R. A., Reis, M. T., & Howes, O. D. (2020). Schizophrenia: An overview. *JAMA Psychiatry*, *77*(2), 201–210. https://doi.org/10.1001/jamapsychiatry.2019.3360

Musci, R. J., Augustinavicius, J. L., & Volk, H. (2019). Gene-environment interactions in psychiatry: Recent evidence and clinical implications. *Current Psychiatry Reports*, *21*(9), 81. https://doi.org/10.1007/s11920-019-1065-5

Renzi, C., Provencal, N., Bassil, K. C., Evers, K., Kihlbom, U., Radford, E. J., Koupil, I., Mueller-Myhsok, B., Hansson, M. G., & Rutten, B. P. (2018). From epigenetic associations to biological and psychosocial explanations in mental health. *Progress in Molecular Biology and Translational Science*, *158*, 299–323.

Strandwitz, P. (2018). Neurotransmitter modulation by the gut microbiota. *Brain Research*, *1693*(Pt B), 128–133. https://doi.org/10.1016/j.brainres.2018.03.015

Tan, C. L., & Knight, Z. A. (2018). Regulation of body temperature by the nervous system. *Neuron*, *98*(1), 31–48. https://doi.org/10.1016/j.neuron.2018.02.022

Tónnesen, S., Kaufmann, T., Doan, N. T., Alnæs, D., Córdova-Palomera, A., Van Der Meer, D., Rokicki, J., Moberget, T., Gurholt, T. P., Haukvik, U. K., & Ueland, T. (2018). White matter aberrations and age-related trajectories in patients with schizophrenia and bipolar disorder revealed by diffusion tensor imaging. *Scientific Reports*, *8*(1), 14229. https://doi.org/10.1038/s41598-018-32355-9

Uddin, L. Q., Yeo, B., & Spreng, R. N. (2019). Towards a universal taxonomy of macro-scale functional human brain networks. *Brain Topography*, *32*(6), 926–942. https://doi.org/10.1007/s10548-019-00744-6

Vidal, P. M., & Pacheco, R. (2020). The cross-talk between the dopaminergic and the immune system involved in schizophrenia. *Frontiers in Pharmacology*, *11*, 394. https://doi.org/10.3389/fphar.2020.00394

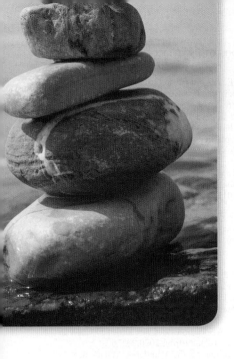

9
Recovery Framework for Mental Health Nursing

Mary Ann Boyd

KEYCONCEPTS

- advocacy
- peer support specialists
- person-centered care
- psychoeducation
- recovery-oriented nursing care
- shared decision-making

LEARNING OBJECTIVES

After studying this chapter, you will be able to:

1. Identify major concepts underlying the recovery framework.

2. Identify the barriers to recover from mental health problems.

3. Discuss the factors that contribute to a recovery-oriented environment.

KEY TERMS

- Empowerment • Engagement • Informed choice model • Paternalistic model • Positive mental health
- Shared decision-making model • Social inclusion • Stigma resilience

INTRODUCTION

The practice of psychiatric–mental health nursing incorporates the whole person, not only active symptoms and treatment.

> **KEYCONCEPT Recovery-oriented nursing care** is a holistic approach characterized by collaborating with persons with mental health problems and disorders to improve health and wellness, live a self-directed life, and strive to meet their full potential.

The overall goal of nursing care is to facilitate a person's recovery. Chapter 1 discussed the concept of recovery and delineated the principles of recovery. This chapter explores recovery concepts, identifies barriers, and covers approaches that promote recovery.

MENTAL HEALTH RECOVERY

Recovering from mental health disorders is not a new concept. In 1830, John Perceval, son of one of England prime ministers, wrote of his personal recovery from schizophrenia despite the psychiatric treatment he received (Bateson, 1974). In the United States, the recovery model was initially applied only to the care of persons with substance abuse problems. Recently, the recovery model application was expanded to all persons with mental health problems. This change grew out of the consumer/survivor/ex-patient movement following the civil rights movement in the late 1960s. Today, recovery concepts and principles are embraced worldwide in the care and treatment of persons with mental disorders.

Recovery involves achieving a balance between clinical and personal recovery. There are often differing views of mental health recovery between the person with mental health issues and the clinician. The person is often more focused on developing meaning in life and transforming an illness identity to a healthy one, whereas the clinician may want to focus on reduction of symptoms, a return to pre-illness states, and a reduction or cessation of medication (Jacob et al., 2017). It is important that clinicians understand that the therapeutic relationship is collaborative and involves much more than symptom reduction. Building upon trust, the clinician acknowledges the negative impact of mental illness on self-esteem, builds a supportive relationship, listens to personal viewpoints, conveys the belief that recovery is possible, recognizes the person's capacity for recovery, and promotes access to resources.

Positive Mental Health

An emerging concept that is useful in collaborating with a person with mental health issues is **positive mental health**, experiencing more desirable health-related quality of life events than undesirable ones (Sirgy, 2019). Positive mental health can be viewed from a biologic perspective. For example, increasing serotonin and dopamine activity is associated with positive moods. It can also be viewed from a psychosocial view such as spending more time in social activities than in social isolation.

Positive mental health includes satisfying experiences with family, friends, and work. Feelings of well-being are important. Well-being comprises overall life satisfaction, as well as cognitive, emotional, social, and moral growth and development. Self-acceptance, personal growth, purpose in life, autonomy, and positive relations with others contribute to a positive mental health (Sirgy, 2019).

Person-Centered Care

One of the key concepts in recovery-oriented care is person-centered care. The person is at the center of care—that is, the person is actively involved in determining the best options for their health care circumstances and no longer passively receives a prescription for treatment of a disease. For a person to participate in their care and make meaningful decisions, the individual must be educated about the disorder and treatment options and use collaboration skills to interact with the clinician.

> **KEYCONCEPT Person-centered care** is an approach to health care that is organized around health needs and expectations, rather than diseases. The person, family, and community participate in and benefit from a trusted health care system (World Health Organization [WHO], 2015).

In person-centered care, the person is actively engaged in planning interventions based upon individual strengths and needs. The plan, which reflects the person's preferences and values, provides the structure in which the individual, in partnership with the clinician, can identify long- and short-term life goals and skills (Hamovitch et al., 2018). The person–clinician partnership plans and manages mental health and health care issues, provides an opportunity for collaborative and creative thinking, and serves as a tool for gauging progress toward goals (Hamovitch et al., 2018). Research on this approach shows improved engagement in health care and medication adherence (Stanhope et al., 2013).

Person-centered care in nursing practice is built on a strong nurse–patient relationship. A solid therapeutic relationship can help reduce symptom severity and improve global function, community living skills, quality of life, and patient satisfaction with treatment (Kidd et al., 2017). The therapeutic relationship and the person-centered care planning process are linked to each other, each influencing the other. A sense of connection based on caring, support, and continuity enables the person to engage in behavior change needed to improve health and well-being (Hamovitch et al., 2018).

Empowerment

A related concept is **empowerment**, the process of supporting people and communities to take control of their own health needs with the goal of healthy behaviors, positive mental health, self-management of illnesses, and well-being (Grealish et al., 2017; WHO, 2015). Empowerment facilitates patient independence, self-management, and self-efficacy.

Empowerment can lead to better decision-making and foster permanent changes in health. For a person to feel empowered, the individual must have the knowledge and skill to manage a particular issue. By sharing health and mental health care information with patients, they will be able to develop self-management skills. Empowerment and hope are enhanced through patient self-management.

Engagement

Engaging a person in mental health care is the first step in supporting recovery. The interaction between a clinician and a person seeking help can set the tone and course of treatment. The first interaction can start the recovery journey, or it can leave the person feeling hopeless and unwilling to return. Many people who seek mental health care drop out after their first or second visit. Engagement in treatment begins with a trusting and respectful relationships with providers (National Alliance on Mental Illness [NAMI], 2016).

Engagement is the strengths-based process through which individuals with mental health conditions form a healing connection with people that support their recovery and wellness within the context of family, culture, and community (NAMI, 2016). Engagement is not adherence or compliance but a broader concept involving active participation from people who are seeking care and those who deliver care. Lack of effective engagement can result in serious consequences such as hospitalization, homelessness, or even death.

Stigma and discrimination can prevent individuals from seeking help or engaging in a therapeutic relationship. Hospital policies and procedures requiring removal of personal items, locked doors, and sterile environments can magnify feelings of dehumanization and self-stigma. Preventing or treating self-stigma may be important in promoting active engagement in some persons (Hack et al., 2020).

Shared Decision-Making

The **shared decision-making model** is central in the recovery model; in this approach, the individual is an active participant, and decision-making is shared (Alguera-Lara et al., 2017). In this model, clinician–patient communication and decision-making differ from the following two types of models: a **paternalistic model**, in which the decisions are made by only the clinician and given to the patient, and the **informed choice model**, in which information is given to the patient and the patient makes the decision. (See Figure 9.1 for the continuum of decision-making.) Because patients almost always view psychiatric hospitalization and treatment as unwanted, many people believe that having a mental disorder means a lifelong process of losing power and control over their lives, particularly if their treatment is not voluntary. In the paternalistic model, individuals can feel coerced into treatment and believe they have lost their ability to make decisions. However, empowering the patient to make the decision, as in the informed choice model, excludes clinician expertise and support, which may lead to poor choices.

> **KEYCONCEPT Shared decision-making** helps people make decisions about their care and treatment based on facts and recommendations provided by the clinician. It changes the power imbalance, where the clinician makes the decision, to shared decisions based on relevant information. Shared decision-making is *how* a decision is made, not *what* the final decision is.

The advantages of shared decision-making are reduced symptoms, improved self-esteem, increased service satisfaction, and improved treatment compliance. Other positive outcomes include improved patient knowledge, increased confidence in decision-making, and more active patient involvement (Alguera-Lara et al., 2017).

RECOVERY INTERVENTIONS

The ultimate aim of every intervention is recovery. Along the way, there are important interventions that focus on treating underlying illnesses that places the person in the best position to continue the recovery journey. Effective interventions are based on the person's needs, preparedness to engage, and stage of recovery. Successful outcomes of these interventions lead to engagement of other evidence-based strategies that support the journey (Sly et al., 2020; Winsper et al., 2020).

Psychoeducation

> **KEYCONCEPT Psychoeducation (PE)** is an individual, family, group, or community education intervention with systematic, structured, and didactic teaching–learning interaction that focuses on enhancing knowledge and skills related to a mental health and wellness through emotional support and motivation to enable person to recover from mental health problems and disorders and lead meaningful, productive lives.

Psychoeducation is not a new idea in mental health care with its beginnings in the early 20th century and the de-institutional movement of the 1950s and 1960s (see Chapter 1). As psychoeducation developed, it became recognized as a useful and effective approach in helping persons with mental health problems actively participate in treatment. Psychoeducation combines cognitive behavioral, educational, and motivational approaches with the goal of providing the person and family with knowledge about the disorder and treatment, and the skills to participate in treatment decisions. Essential elements of psychoeducation include briefing the person about the disorder, problem-solving training, communication techniques, and self-assertiveness (Sarkhel et al., 2020).

Paternalistic Model	Shared Decision-Making Model	Informed Choice Model
• Clinician knows best and makes choices. • Patient will do best if instructions are followed.	• Clinician shares evidence and offers options. • Patient is supported to consider options.	• Clinician shares evidence and offers options but does not offer an opinion. • The patient chooses.

FIGURE 9.1 Continuum of decision-making.

Psychoeducation is conducted by several mental health disciplines, including nurses, psychiatrists, social workers, psychologists, peer support specialists, and others. Not only does psychoeducation provide knowledge and competence about the disorder, it also promotes insight into the disorders, promotes relapse prevention, and provides skills for crisis management and suicide prevention.

Social Inclusion

Social inclusion, receiving social support and participation in a family and community, is important in successful recovery. Social inclusion is multidimensional with interrelated dimensions including employment or education, housing and neighborhood, and participation in social activities (Filia et al., 2018).

Employment and Education

Employment is one of the most important factors that impacts mental health recovery. Employment gives individuals a sense of purpose and a reason to get up in the morning. Mental health problems, including functional impairment and psychosocial disability, frequently interfere with the ability to work, resulting in absences, interpersonal conflicts, and poor work performance. Symptoms of the illness, side effects of medications, stigma, poor social support, academic underachievement, and poor workplace environment are factors that contribute to difficulty in obtaining and maintaining employment. Individuals who quit work or are fired often find that it is difficult to regain employment. Even when their symptoms are treated, they still may not be hired (Isaacs et al., 2019).

Lack of educational opportunities can lead to lack of skills or qualifications required for employment. Unrecognized learning disabilities can lead to mental health problems that culminate in dropping out of school prior to high school completion (Aro et al., 2019). Education and employment are important goals for persons with mental illness. Employment improves mental health and reduces the overall cost of mental health care (Gibbons& Salkever, 2019). Recovery-oriented care recognizes employment potential and provides social support for gaining meaningful employment. Factors that facilitate obtaining and maintaining employment include personal strengths, social support, accommodative work environment, disclosure, and support from mental health professionals and services (Thomas et al., 2019b).

Housing and Neighborhood

Housing is critical to recovery from mental and substance abuse disorders. Recovery-oriented care promotes safe, affordable, and permanent support housing in the community, with access to benefits and services for individuals, families, and communities. In some instances, housing is sought after the mental disorder is treated and is in remission. In other instances, securing housing is a necessary first step to set the stage for strengthening coping skills and addressing the mental disorder (see Chapter 41).

Housing is more than a place to live. Housing within a safe neighborhood with low crime rates, grocery stores, and access to transportation is critical for a recovery. There should be opportunities to develop social relationships within the neighborhood environment.

Social Activities

The opportunity to engage in social activities results in several positive outcomes. The person is not alone in a room or apartment and can interact and connect with others. Social activities provide opportunities for the person to grow and develop as a member of society. Within the context of social activities, social support from others can emerge (Filia et al., 2019).

Peer Support

Peer support is an integral component of the recovery model.

KEYCONCEPT Peer support specialists are people who have been successful in their recovery who help others experiencing similar situations. These specialists are trained and certified to use their experiences to help others and work with the other mental health disciplines in recovery-oriented care. They have well-defined competencies (see Box 9.1).

Peer support specialists form voluntary relationships with patients on the basis of mutual fit. Peer support

---

BOX 9.1

Core Competencies for Peer Workers in Behavior Health Services

1. Engages peers in collaborative and caring relationships
2. Provides support
3. Shares lived experiences of recovery
4. Personalizes peer support
5. Supports recovery planning
6. Links to resources, services, and supports
7. Provides information about skills related to health, wellness, and recovery
8. Helps peers to manage crises
9. Values communication
10. Supports collaboration and teamwork
11. Promotes leadership and advocacy
12. Promotes growth and development

Reprinted from Substance Abuse and Mental Health Services Administration. (2015). Core competencies for peer workers in behavioral health services. https://www.samhsa.gov/sites/default/files/programs_campaigns/brss_tacs/core-competencies_508_12_13_18.pdf specialists engage in a wide range of activities, including advocacy, linkage to resources, sharing of experiences, community and relationship building, group facilitation, skill building mentoring, and goal setting. They also may plan and develop groups, services, or activities, provide training, and administer programs. Because they are able to describe their mental health experiences and can explain their journey of recovery, they are especially well suited to educate the public and policymakers and can challenge negative stereotypes. Patients have the option to decline services of a peer support specialist (Chinman et al., 2019).

Research supports the effectiveness of peer support specialists in a variety of settings, including urban and rural areas (Castellanos et al., 2018). For example, the Veterans Administration is using certified peer support specialists in remote, community-based clinics to support trauma-affected veterans in a group setting. The veterans are able to share their experiences involving service-related trauma and interpersonal violence in a supportive environment with other veterans and a peer specialist. In this setting, skills are taught to defuse violent thoughts and to prevent further violence (Azevedo et al., 2020).

BARRIERS TO RECOVERY

Poverty

A major barrier in accessing recovery-oriented care is poverty. Individuals with schizophrenia are more likely than the general population to experience poverty and homelessness (see Chapter 41). Poverty is associated with mental disorders such as depression (Jokela et al., 2019) and schizophrenia (Thomas et al., 2019a).

The lack of monetary resources is the primary definition of what it means to be poor (Sylvestre et al., 2018). Without economic resources such as an income or savings, people are unable to fully participate in society. Individuals and families who meet a certain income threshold are eligible for government supplement, which is minimal and cannot meet basic needs. People with a disability such as a mental illness may qualify for additional support through Social Security Disability Insurance. Their ability to survive on this income will depend on the availability of other resources, such as support from family, friends, and neighbors, available social services, and cost of living (which varies depending on where people live).

Poverty can result in lack of permanent housing, no transportation, and inability to pay for services. Access to health care in the United States is highly dependent on employment; many people with mental health problem are unemployed, resulting in lack of income and health insurance. People with mental illnesses are frequently reliant on public health care, but they may not be able to access services. Public mental health care often involves long wait times for appointments at inconvenient hours. Medications may not be affordable, and even if individuals are able to obtain them, they may have no place to store them. Interpersonal aspects of health care also play a role in people seeking mental health care. Individuals may perceive that they cannot talk to their provider or that their provider does not care about them (Bellamy et al., 2016).

Homelessness

Homelessness is a lack of a fixed, regular, and adequate nighttime residence, and it can be considered as either sheltered or unsheltered. The homeless shelters provide temporary or transitional housing operated by public and private agencies for individuals and families who have no stable housing, including a hotel or motel paid for by government or charitable organization. The unsheltered homeless live in the places that are not ordinarily used for housing such as cars, parks, abandoned building, tents, and bus/train stations (National Alliance to End Homelessness, 2020).

Homelessness is stressful and coping with homelessness is challenging. Substance abuse can be an issue, and people who are homeless are often victims of crime. The incidence of posttraumatic stress disorder among individuals who are homeless may be higher than in the general population. Homeless women are especially in danger of being assaulted, abused, and raped. Individuals with mental illnesses who are homeless are trying to survive and fear being hospitalized or "locked up." See Chapter 41.

Stigma

Anti-stigma approaches have had the positive impact of reducing public stigma for persons with mental illness (Corrigan & Nieweglowski, 2019) (see Chapter 2). Self-stigma is a barrier to recovery because individuals internalize the community's negative views of persons with mental disorders. Self-stigma is associated with increased severity of symptoms of mental disorders. The challenge for nurses and other clinicians is to support **stigma resilience**, a personal trait that means the patient has the capacity to withstand or recover from significant challenges that threaten stability, viability, or development (Hofer et al., 2019).

Lack of Services

Mental health services vary from state to state. Factors that contribute to whether persons with mental health disorders can be treated include access to insurance, access to treatment, quality and cost of insurance, access to special education, and workforce availability. In the United States, 10.3% of adults with mental illness are uninsured, limiting access to services. The number of uninsured declined under the Affordable Care Act, but this law is being challenged, and the number of uninsured is expected to increase if the law is determined to be unconstitutional. The state prevalence of uninsured adults with mental illness ranges from 2.4% in Massachusetts to 22.9% in Wyoming (Mental Health America [MHA], 2020).

More than 57% of adults with a mental health disorder receive no treatment in the United States (ranging from 40.7% in Vermont to 64.8% in California [MHA, 2020]). One out of five adults with a mental illness report inability to receive needed services. There are several reasons for lack of treatment, including no insurance or limited coverage of services; shortage of psychiatrists, nurses, and other mental health professionals; and lack of treatment services such as inpatient treatment, individual therapy, and community services. Additionally, there is a disconnect between primary care systems and mental health systems (MHA, 2020).

Services for children and youth are even more sparse. Only 28.2% of youth with severe depression receive some consistent treatment (7–25 visits per year). These services vary by state, with 53.9% of youth with severe depression in Maryland receiving some outpatient treatment compared to 13.5% in South Carolina (MHA, 2020).

Access to mental health care is very limited in rural areas. Health care providers are concentrated in urban areas, leaving rural counties without an adequate number of health care professionals. It is estimated that 1,600 counties in the United States do not have an accredited mental health provider. Farmers and their families need mental health support and treatment; stress among farm families is high, and they need to know how to manage the stress effectively. The National Health Service Corps and telemedicine are providing some help to the rural communities (National Association for Rural Mental Health [NARMH], 2020).

SOCIETAL ROLE IN PROMOTING A RECOVERY-ORIENTED ENVIRONMENT

Advocacy

The World Health Organization recognized the need for mental health advocacy to promote the human rights of persons with mental disorders and to reduce stigma and discrimination in a 2003 publication, *Advocacy for Mental Health* (WHO, 2003).

KEYCONCEPT Advocacy is various actions aimed at changing the major structural and attitudinal barriers to achieving positive mental health outcomes. It is an important means of raising awareness of mental health issues.

Mental health advocacy began when families of people with mental disorders made their voices heard and raised awareness of the needs and mistreatment of their loved ones. Individuals with the disorders joined their families to develop advocacy organizations to influence legislation and policy development. Today, many mental health workers and their organizations have joined the movement to advocate for the mental health needs, rights, and recovery of the general population.

The concept of advocacy includes several elements such as awareness raising; providing information, education, training, and counseling; and mutual help, mediating, defending, and denouncing. Through the advocacy movement, society's negative perception of persons with mental disorders is being challenged and gradually replaced with more realistic, empathic perceptions.

Advocacy occurs at many levels. Individuals with mental disorders advocate for their own recovery. They are often motivated to contact advocacy groups in the hope that advocates will intervene on their behalf through effective communication with health care providers (Morrison et al., 2018). They may contact the local advocacy service in their facility or a local community advocacy group such as National Alliance on Mental Illness or Mental Health America.

Advocacy groups and organizations play important roles promoting national and international agendas. These groups develop databases with patient groups, families, and organizations. Establishing a regular flow of information with governmental decision-making groups and other organizations, they are instrumental in formulating and evaluating policy, plans, programs, legislation, and quality improvement standards. Other activities include establishing educational initiatives, conducting media activities, and organizing public events to raise awareness of mental health issues.

Removing Social, Economic, and Political Barriers

An important step in promoting a recovery-oriented environment is the reduction of stigma and stigmatizing messages. Education about mental health disorders and treatment is critical in reducing discrimination of persons with mental disorders. National media organizations should use nonstigmatizing language in their publications.

Universal access to mental health services would help reduce the disparities between those who are insured and those who are not. More national mental health programs such as the National Suicide Hotline, a 24-hour crisis intervention hotline offering counseling and referral, would also be helpful.

Health care workers can play an important role in advocating for quality mental health care through participating in activities of patient and family groups. They can educate communities and support access to services.

RECOVERY-ORIENTED PSYCHIATRIC– MENTAL HEALTH NURSING PRACTICE

Recovery-oriented care is integral to the practice of psychiatric–mental health nursing and consistent with relationship-based care (American Nurses Association [ANA], American Psychiatric Nursing Association [APNA], International society of Psychiatric-Mental Health Nurses [ISPN], 2014). Psychiatric–mental health nurses develop partnerships with patients through therapeutic relationships. Psychiatric–mental health nursing approaches are based on shared decision-making. Interventions are determined by both the nurse and the patient.

As the care paradigm has shifted from nurse-directed care to recovery-oriented care with shared decision-making, nurses have the opportunity to truly practice from a holistic perspective. Also, nurses are now able to engage peer support specialists in supporting patients through recovery.

SUMMARY OF KEY POINTS

- Mental health recovery is based on concepts of person-centered care, empowerment, shared decision-making, employment, housing, and peer support.

- Empowering the patient to engage in the care process requires that the individual is educated on health and mental health issues and approaches. The person must have the knowledge and skills to engage in a meaningful collaborative process.

- Person-centered care places the person in the center of the care process. The individual becomes a partner to the clinician and together they decide the best approach based on persons circumstances. The care approach is individualized; one person's care plan will look different from another.

- In shared decision-making, the patient is an active participant in the decision. The advantages of shared decision-making include reduced symptoms, improved self-esteem, increased service satisfaction, and improved treatment compliance.

- Employment is a goal of recovery. In some instances, supportive employment will be needed to accommodate disabilities.

- Housing is critical to recovery. There are several types of housing arrangements such as independent, transitional, and supportive.

- Peer support is an integral component of recovery. Peer support specialists are new members of the mental health team who are recovering from mental health problems. These individuals use their experiences to help others.

- Barriers to recovery include poverty, homelessness, stigma, and lack of services. Advocacy plays an important role in promoting a recovery-oriented environment and seeks to remove social, economic, and political barriers.

- Recovery-oriented psychiatric–mental health nursing practice is based on developing partnerships with patients through the use of the therapeutic relationship.

CRITICAL THINKING CHALLENGES

1. Compare a traditional medical approach to care with recovery-oriented care.

2. Using the nursing process, describe the inclusion of the person-centered approach.

3. Compare and contrast the paternalistic, informed-choice, and shared decision-making approaches for a patient who has schizophrenia and can be treated with an oral or long-acting injectable.

4. Discuss with a patient how mental health issues impact employment and housing.

5. What factors might interfere with the ability of the person who is mentally ill to participate in treatment?

6. What barriers to communication might the nurse experience when relating to the person who is homeless and mentally ill?

 Movie Viewing Guides
Home: (2013). Jack (Gbenga Akinnagbe) lives in a group home and is suffering from a mental illness. He wants to have his own home and reconnect with his son. When he moves into an apartment, he finds that living alone is more difficult than he expected.

VIEWING POINTS: How does Jack's illness affect his ability to maintain his independence? What does having his own home represent to Jack?

REFERENCES

Alguera-Lara, V., Dowsey, M. M., Ride, J., Kinder, S., & Castle, D. (2017). Shared decision making in mental health: The importance for current clinical practice. *Australasian Psychiatry, 25*(6), 578–582.

American Nurses Association, American Psychiatric Nursing Association, International society of Psychiatric-Mental Health Nurses. (2014). *Scope and standards of practice psychiatric-mental health nursing* (2nd ed.).

Aro, T., Eklund, K., Eloranta, A. K., Närhi, V., Korhonen, E., & Ahonen, T. (2019). Associations between childhood learning disabilities and adult-age mental health problems, lack of education, and unemployment. *Journal of Learning Disabilities, 52*(1), 71–83. https://doi.org/10.1177/0022219418775118

Azevedo, K. J., Ramirez, J. C., Kumar, A., LeFevre, A., Factor, A., Hailu, E., Lindley, S. E., & Jain, S. (2020). Rethinking violence prevention in rural and underserved communities: How Veteran peer support groups help participants deal with sequelae from violent traumatic experiences. *Journal of Rural Health. 36*(2), 266–273. https://doi.org/10.1111/jrh.12362

Bateson, G. (Ed.). (1974). *Perceval's narrative: A patient's account of his psychosis, 1830–1832*. William Morrow & Company.

Bellamy, C. D., Flanagan, E., Costa, M., O'Connell-Bonarrigo, M., Tana Le, T., Guy, K., Antunes, K., & Steiner, J. L. (2016). Barriers and facilitators of healthcare for people with mental illness: Why integrated patient centered healthcare is necessary. *Issues in Mental Health Nursing*, 37(6), 421–428. https://doi.org/10.3109/01612840.2016.1162882

Castellanos, D., Capo, M., Valderrama, D., Jean-Francois, M., & Luna, A. (2018). Relationship of peer specialists to mental health outcomes in South Florida. *International Journal of Mental Health Systems*, 12(59). https://doi.org/10.1186/s13033-018-0239-6

Chinman, M., McCarthy, S., Mitchell-Miland, C., Bachrach, R. L., Schutt, R. K., & Ellison, M. (2019). Predicting engagement with mental health peer specialist services. *Psychiatric Services*, 70(4), 333–336. https://doi.org/10.1176/appi.ps.201800368

Corrigan, P. W., & Nieweglowski, K. (2019). How does familiarity impact the stigma of mental illness?. *Clinical Psychology Review*, 70, 40–50. https://doi.org/10.1016/j.cpr.2019.02.001

Filia, K., Jackson, H., Cotton, S., & Killackey, E. (2019). Understanding what it means to be socially included for people with a lived experience of mental illness. *The International Journal of Social Psychiatry*, 65(5), 413–424. https://doi.org/10.1177/0020764019852657

Filia, K. M., Jackson, H. J., Cotton, S. M., Gardner, A., & Killackey, E. J. (2018). What is social inclusion? A thematic analysis of professional opinion. *Psychiatric Rehabilitation Journal*, 41(3), 183–195. https://doi.org/10.1037/prj0000304

Gibbons, B. J., & Salkever, D. S. (2019). Working with a severe mental Illness: Estimating the causal effects of employment on mental health status and total mental health costs. *Administration and Policy in Mental Health*. https://doi.org/10.1007/s10488-019-00926-1

Grealish, A., Tai, S., Hunter, A., Emsley, R., Murrells, T., & Morrison, A. P. (2017). Does empowerment mediate the effects of psychological factors on mental health, well-being, and recovery in young people? *Psychology Psychotherapy*, 90(3), 314–335. https://doi.org/10.1111/papt.12111

Hack, S. M., Muralidharan, A., Brown, C. H., Drapalski, A. L., & Lucksted, A. A. (2020). Stigma and discrimination as correlates of mental health treatment engagement among adults with serious mental illness. *Psychiatric Rehabilitation Journal*, 43(2), 106–110. https://doi.org/10.1037/prj0000385.ck

Hamovitch, E. K., Choy-Brown, M., & Stanhope, V. (2018). Person-centered care and the therapeutic alliance. *Community Mental Health Journal*, 54(7), 951–958. https://doi.org/10.1007/s10597-018-0295-z

Hofer, A., Post, F., Pardeller, S., Frajo-Apor, B., Hoertnagl, C. M., Kemmler, G., & Fleischhacker, W. W. (2019). Self-stigma versus stigma resistance in schizophrenia: Associations with resilience, premorbid adjustment, and clinical symptoms. *Psychiatry Research*, 271, 396–401.

Isaacs, A. N., Beauchamp, A., Sutton, K., & Maybery, D. (2019). Unmet needs of persons with a severe and persistent mental illness and their relationship to unmet accommodation needs. *Health & Social Care in the Community*. https://doi.org/10.1111/hsc.12729

Jacob, S., Munro, I., Taylor, B. J., & Griffiths, D. (2017). Mental health recovery: A review of the peer-reviewed published literature. *Collegian*, 24(1), 53–61. https://doi.org/10.1016/J.COLEGN.2015.08.001

Kidd, S. A., Davidson, L., & McKenzie, K. (2017). Common factors in community mental health intervention: A scoping review. *Community Mental Health Journal*, 53, 1–11.

Mental Health America. (2020). Mental health in American – Access to dare data. https://www.mentalhealthamerica.net/issues/mental-health-america-access-care-data

Morrison, P., Stomski, N. J., Whitely, M., & Brennan, P. (2018). Understanding advocacy practice in mental health: A multidimensional scalogram analysis of case records. *Journal of Mental Health*, 27(2), 127–134.

National Alliance to End Homelessness. (2020). Population at-risk. Homelessness and the COVID-19 crisis. Homelessness Research Institute. https://endhomelessness.org/wp-content/uploads/2020/03/Covid-Fact-Sheet-3.25.2020-2.pdf

National Alliance on Mental Illness. (2016). Engagement: A new standard for mental health care. https://www.nami.org/Support-Education/Publications-Reports/Public-Policy-Reports/Engagement-A-New-Standard-for-Mental-Health-Care/NAMI_Engagement_Web#:~:text=Engagement%20is%20the%20strengths%2Dbased,of%20family%2C%20culture%20and%20community

National Association for Rural Mental Health. (2020). Changes in rural communities in the past twenty-five years. http://www.narmh.org/publications_changes.html

Sarkhel, S., Singh, O. P., & Arora, M. (2020). Clinical Practice Guidelines for Psychoeducation in Psychiatric Disorders General Principles of Psychoeducation. *Indian Journal of Psychiatry*, 62(Suppl 2), S319–S323. https://doi.org/10.4103/psychiatry.IndianJPsychiatry_780_19

Sirgy, M. J. (2019). Positive balance: A hierarchical perspective of positive mental health. *Quality of Life Research*, 28, 1921–1930. https://doi.org/10.1007/s11136-019-02145-5

Sly, K. A., Lewin, T. J., Frost, B. G., Tirupati, S., Turrell, M., & Conrad, A. M. (2020). Care pathways, engagement and outcomes associated with a recovery-oriented intermediate stay mental health program. *Psychiatry Research*, 286, 112889. Advance online publication. https://doi.org/10.1016/j.psychres.2020.112889

Stanhope, V., Ingoglia, C., Schmelter, B., & Marcus, S. (2013). Impact of person-centered and collaborative documentation on treatment adherence. *Psychiatric Services*, 64, 76–79. https://doi.org/10.1176/appi.ps.20110 0489

Substance Abuse and Mental Health Services Administration. (2015). Core competencies for peer workers in behavioral health services. https://www.samhsa.gov/sites/default/files/programs_campaigns/brss_tacs/core-competencies_508_12_13_18.pdf

Sylvestre, J., Notten, G., Kerman, N., Polillo, A., & Czechowki, K. (2018). Poverty and serious mental illness: Toward action on a seemingly intractable problem. *American Journal of Community Psychology*, 61(1–2), 153–165.

Thomas, E. C., Snethen, G., & Salzer, M. S. (2019a). Community participation factors and poor neurocognitive functioning among persons with schizophrenia. *American Journal of Orthopsychiatry*. Advance online publication. https://doi.org/10.1037/ort0000399

Thomas, T. L., Prasad Muliyala, K., Jayarajan, D., Angothu, H., & Thirthalli, J. (2019b). Vocational challenges in severe mental illness: A qualitative study in persons with professional degrees. *Asian Journal of Psychiatry*, 42, 48–54. https://doi.org/10.1016/j.ajp.2019.03.011

Winsper, C., Crawford-Docherty, A., Weich, S., Fenton, S. J., & Singh, S. P. (2020). How do recovery-oriented interventions contribute to personal mental health recovery? A systematic review and logic model. *Clinical Psychology Review*, 76, 101815. https://doi.org/10.1016/j.cpr.2020.101815

World Health Organization. (2015). WHO global strategy on integrated people-centred health services 2016-2026: Executive summary. https://apps.who.int/iris/bitstream/handle/10665/155002/WHO_HIS_SDS_2015.6_eng.pdf;jsessionid=6B9D895F7B9838F2225B4C2A32F7B30E?sequence=1

World Health Organization. (2003). Advocacy for mental health. World Health Organization, 2003 (Mental Health Policy and Service Guidance Package). https://www.who.int/mental_health/policy/services/essentialpackage1v7/en/

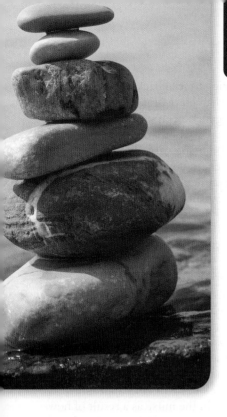

10

Communication and the Therapeutic Relationship

Cheryl Forchuk and Rebecca Luebbert

KEYCONCEPTS

- nurse–patient relationship
- self-awareness
- therapeutic communication

LEARNING OBJECTIVES

After studying this chapter, you will be able to:

1. Identify the importance of self-awareness in nursing practice.

2. Demonstrate the appropriate use of verbal and nonverbal communication skills.

3. Distinguish between active and passive listening.

4. Incorporate therapeutic communication strategies when working with patients.

5. Identify common barriers to therapeutic communication.

6. Explain how the nurse can establish a therapeutic relationship with patients by using rapport and empathy.

7. Understand the physical, emotional, and social boundaries of the nurse–patient relationship.

8. Appreciate the significance of adaptive and maladaptive defense mechanisms.

9. Explain what occurs in each of the three phases of the nurse–patient relationship: orientation, working, and resolution.

10. Describe what characterizes a nontherapeutic or deteriorating nurse–patient relationship.

KEY TERMS

- Active listening • Boundaries • Communication blocks • Content themes • Countertransference • Defense mechanisms
- Deteriorating relationship • Empathy • Empathic linkages • Introspective • Nontherapeutic relationship
- Nonverbal communication • Orientation phase • Passive listening • Process recording • Rapport • Resolution phase
- Self-disclosure • Strength-based communication • Symbolism • Transference • Verbal communication • Working phase

INTRODUCTION

Patients with psychiatric disorders have special communication needs that require advanced therapeutic communication skills. In psychiatric nursing, the nurse–patient relationship is an important tool used to reach treatment goals. The purpose of this chapter is to help the nurse (1) develop self-awareness and communication techniques needed for a therapeutic nurse–patient relationship, (2) examine the specific stages or steps involved in establishing the relationship, (3) explore the specific factors that make a nurse–patient relationship successful and therapeutic, (4) differentiate therapeutic from nontherapeutic relationships, and (5) recognize the significance and impact of a patient's use of **defense mechanisms**.

SELF-AWARENESS

Self-awareness is the process of understanding one's own beliefs, thoughts, motivations, biases, and limitations and recognizing how they affect others. Without self-awareness, nurses will find it impossible to establish and maintain therapeutic relationships with patients. "Know thyself" is a basic tenet of psychiatric–mental health nursing (Box 10.1).

A well-developed sense of self-awareness can only come after nurses carry out self-examination. Self-awareness requires a willingness to be **introspective** and to examine one's own personal beliefs, attitudes, and motivations. While this process may be uncomfortable and time consuming, this objective examination is an essential exercise for a professional nurse. Self-examination should be an ongoing process and involves reflecting on the personal meaning of the current situation. This reflection can relate to the nurse's past situations and issues related to their own personal values. Self-examination without the benefit of another's perspective might lead to a biased view of self. Therefore, conducting self-examinations with a trusted individual who can give objective, but realistic, feedback is best.

> **KEYCONCEPT Self-awareness** is the process of understanding one's own beliefs, thoughts, motivations, biases, and limitations and recognizing how they affect others.

The Biopsychosocial Self

Each nurse brings a biopsychosocial self to nursing practice. The patient perceives the biologic dimension of the nurse in terms of physical characteristics: age, gender, body weight, height, ethnic or racial background, and any other observed physical characteristics. Additionally, the nurse can have a certain genetic composition, an illness, or an unobservable physical disability that may influence the quality or delivery of nursing care. The nurse's psychological state also influences how they analyze patient information and select treatment interventions. An emotional state or behavior can inadvertently influence the therapeutic relationship. For example, a nurse who has just learned that her child is using illegal drugs and who has a patient with a history of drug use may inadvertently project a judgmental attitude toward her patient, which would interfere with the formation of a therapeutic relationship. The nurse needs to examine underlying emotions, motivations, and beliefs and determine how these factors shape behavior.

The nurse's social biases can be particularly problematic for the nurse–patient relationship. Although the nurse may not verbalize these values to patients, some are readily evident in the nurse's behavior and appearance. A patient may perceive biases in the nurse as a result of how the nurse acts or appears at work. Other sociocultural values may not be immediately obvious to the patient, for example, the nurse's religious or spiritual beliefs or feelings about death, divorce, abortion, or homosexuality. These beliefs and thoughts can influence how the nurse interacts with a patient who is dealing with such issues. Similarly, cultural beliefs and patterns of communicating may influence the emerging relationship by each partner's behaviors conforming to or confronting cultural norms.

Understanding Personal Feelings and Beliefs and Changing Behavior

Nurses must understand their own personal feelings and beliefs and try to avoid projecting them onto patients. The development of self-awareness will enhance the nurse's objectivity and foster a nonjudgmental attitude, which is so important for building and maintaining trust throughout the nurse–patient relationship. Soliciting feedback from colleagues and supervisors about how personal beliefs or thoughts are being projected onto others is a useful self-assessment technique. One of the reasons that ongoing clinical supervision is so important is that the supervisor really knows the nurse and can continually observe for inappropriate communication and question assumptions that the nurse may hold. Clinical supervision is different from administrative supervision in that the focus is on the therapeutic development of the helper and it does not generally involve an administrative or a reporting relationship.

After a nurse has identified and analyzed their personal beliefs and attitudes, behaviors that were driven by prejudicial ideas may change. The change process requires introspective analysis that may result in viewing the world differently. Through self-awareness and

---

BOX 10.1

"Know Thyself"

- What physical problems or illnesses have you experienced?
- What significant traumatic life events (e.g., divorce, death of significant person, abuse, disaster) have you experienced?
- What prejudiced or embarrassing beliefs and attitudes about groups different from yours can you identify from your family, significant others, and yourself?
- Which sociocultural factors in your background could contribute to your being rejected by members of other cultures?
- How would the above experiences affect your ability to care for patients?

conscious effort, the nurse can change learned behaviors to engage effectively in therapeutic relationships with patients. Nevertheless, sometimes a nurse realizes that some attitudes are too ingrained to support a therapeutic relationship with a patient with different beliefs. In such cases, the nurse should refer the patient to someone with whom the patient is more likely to develop a successful therapeutic relationship.

EFFECTIVE COMMUNICATION

Effective communication, including verbal and nonverbal techniques, is a building block for all successful relationships. The nurse–patient relationship is built on therapeutic communication, the ongoing process of interaction through which meaning emerges (Box 10.2). **Verbal communication**, which is principally achieved by spoken words, includes the underlying emotion, context, and connotation of what is actually said. **Nonverbal communication** includes gestures, expressions, and body language. Both the patient and the nurse use verbal and nonverbal communication. To respond therapeutically in a nurse–patient relationship, the nurse is responsible for assessing and interpreting all forms of patient communication.

> **NCLEXNOTE** In analyzing patient–nurse communication, nonverbal behaviors and gestures are communicated first. If a patient's verbal and nonverbal communications are contradictory, priority should be given to the nonverbal behavior and gestures.

Verbal Communication

The process of verbal communication involves a sender, a message, and a receiver. The patient is often the sender,

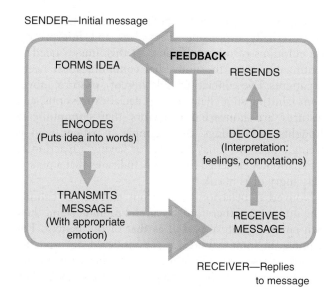
SENDER—Initial message

FIGURE 10.1 The communication process. (Adapted with permission from Boyd, M. [1995]. Communication with patients, families, healthcare providers, and diverse cultures. In M. K. Strader & P. J. Decker [Eds.]. *Role transition to patient care management* [p. 431]. Appleton & Lange.)

and the nurse is often the receiver, but communication is always two way (Fig. 10.1). The patient formulates an idea, encodes that message (puts ideas into words), and then transmits the message with emotion. The patient's words and their underlying emotional tone and connotation communicate the individual's needs and emotional problems. The nurse receives the message, decodes it (interprets the message, including its feelings, connotation, and context), and then responds to the patient.

On the surface, this interaction is deceptively simple; unseen complexities lie beneath. Is the message the nurse receives consistent with the patient's original idea? Did the nurse interpret the message as the patient intended? Is the verbal message consistent with the nonverbal flourishes that accompany it? Validation is essential to ensure that the nurse has received the information accurately.

Nonverbal Communication

Gestures, facial expressions, and body language actually communicate more than verbal messages. Under the best circumstances, body language mirrors or enhances what is verbally communicated. However, if verbal and nonverbal messages conflict, the listener should rely on the nonverbal message. For example, if a patient says that they feel fine but has a sad facial expression and is slumped in a chair away from others, the message of sadness and depression, rather than the patient's report of feeling fine, should be accepted. The same is true of a nurse's behavior. For example, if a nurse tells a patient "I am happy to see you" but the nurse's facial expression communicates indifference, the patient will receive the message that the nurse is bored.

BOX 10.2

Principles of Therapeutic Communication

- The patient should be the primary focus of the interaction.
- A professional attitude sets the tone of the therapeutic relationship.
- Use self-disclosure cautiously and only when the disclosure has a therapeutic purpose.
- Avoid social relationships with patients.
- Maintain patient confidentiality.
- Assess the patient's intellectual competence to determine the level of understanding.
- Implement interventions from a theoretic base.
- Maintain a nonjudgmental attitude. Avoid making judgments about the patient's behavior.
- Avoid giving advice. By the time the patient sees the nurse, they have had plenty of advice.
- Guide the patient to reinterpret their experiences rationally.
- Track the patient's verbal interaction through the use of clarifying statements.
- Avoid changing the subject unless the content change is in the patient's best interest.

People with psychiatric problems often have difficulty verbally expressing themselves and interpreting the emotions of others. Because of this, nurses need to continually assess the nonverbal communication needs of patients. Eye contact (or lack thereof), posture, movement (shifting in a chair, pacing), facial expressions, and gestures are nonverbal behaviors that communicate thoughts and feelings. For example, a patient who is pacing and restless may be upset or having a reaction to medication. A clenched fist usually indicates that a person feels angry or is hostile.

Nonverbal behavior varies from culture to culture. The nurse must, therefore, be careful to understand their own cultural context as well as that of the patient. For example, in some cultures, it is considered disrespectful to look a person straight in the eye. In other cultures, not looking a person in the eye may be interpreted as "hiding something" or as having low self-esteem. Whether one points with the finger, nose, or eyes and how much hand gesturing to use are other examples of nonverbal communication that may vary considerably among cultures. The nurse needs to be aware of cultural differences in communication in the context of each relationship and may need to consult with a cultural interpreter or use other learning opportunities to ensure that their communication is culturally congruent.

Nurses should use positive body language, such as sitting at the same eye level as the patient with a relaxed posture that projects interest and attention. Leaning slightly forward helps engage the patient. Generally, the nurse should not cross their arms or legs during therapeutic communication because such postures pose a barrier to interaction. Uncrossed arms and legs project openness and a willingness to engage in conversation (Fig. 10.2). Any verbal message should be consistent with nonverbal messages.

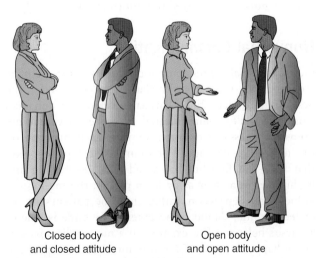

Closed body   Open body
and closed attitude   and open attitude

FIGURE 10.2   Open and closed body language.

THERAPEUTIC COMMUNICATION STRATEGIES AND TECHNIQUES

KEYCONCEPT Therapeutic communication is the ongoing process of interaction through which meaning emerges.

Therapeutic and social interactions are very different. In a therapeutic communication, the nurse focuses on the patient and patient-related issues. Activities should have a definite purpose, and conversation should focus only on the patient. The nurse must not attempt to meet their own social or other needs during the activity.

Limiting Self-Disclosure

One of the most important principles of therapeutic communication for the nurse to follow is to focus the interaction on the patient's concerns. **Self-disclosure**, telling the patient personal information, generally is not a good idea. The conversation should focus on the patient, not the nurse. If a patient asks the nurse personal questions, the nurse should elicit the underlying reason for the request. The nurse can then determine how much personal information to disclose, if any. In revealing personal information, the nurse should be purposeful and have identified therapeutic outcomes. For example, a male patient who was struggling with the implications of marriage and fidelity asked a male nurse if he had ever had an extramarital affair. The nurse interpreted the patient's statement as seeking role-modeling behavior for an adult man and judged self-disclosure in this instance to be therapeutic. He honestly responded that he did not engage in affairs and redirected the discussion back to the patient's concerns.

Nurses sometimes may feel uncomfortable avoiding patients' questions for fear of seeming rude. As a result, they might sometimes disclose too much personal information because they are trying to be "nice." However, being nice is not necessarily therapeutic. As appropriate, redirecting the patient, giving a neutral or vague answer, or saying "Let's talk about you" may be all that is necessary to limit self-disclosure. In some instances, nurses may need to tell the patient directly that the nurse will not share personal information (Table 10.1).

Active Listening

Listening is an ongoing activity by which the nurse attends to the patient's verbal and nonverbal communication. The art of listening is developed through careful attention to the content and meaning of the patient's speech. There are two types of listening: passive and active. **Passive listening** involves sitting quietly and letting the patient talk. A passive listener allows the

TABLE 10.1 SELF-DISCLOSURE IN THERAPEUTIC VERSUS SOCIAL RELATIONSHIPS

Situation	Appropriate Therapeutic Response	Inappropriate Social Response with Rationale
A patient asks the nurse if she had fun over the weekend.	"The weekend was fine. How did you spend your weekend?"	"It was great. My boyfriend and I went to dinner and a movie." (This self-disclosure has no therapeutic purpose. The response focuses the conversation on the nurse, not the patient.)
A patient asks a student nurse if she has ever been to a particular bar.	"Many people go there. I'm wondering if you have ever been there?"	"Oh yes—all the time. It's a lot of fun." (Sharing information about outside activities is inappropriate.)
A patient asks a nurse if mental illness is in the nurse's family.	"Mental illnesses do run in families. I've had a lot of experience caring for people with mental illnesses."	"My sister is being treated for depression." (This self-disclosure has no purpose, and the nurse is missing the meaning of the question.)
While shopping with a patient, the nurse sees a friend, who approaches them.	To her friend: "I know it looks like I'm not working, but I really am. I'll see you later."	"Hi, Bob. This is Jane Doe, a patient." (Introducing the patient to the friend is very inappropriate and violates patient confidentiality.)

patient to ramble and does not focus or guide the thought process. This form of listening does not foster a therapeutic relationship. Body language during passive listening usually communicates boredom or indifference (Fig. 10.3).

Through **active listening**, the nurse focuses on what the patient is saying, interprets the underlying meaning, and responds to the message objectively. The nurse's verbal and nonverbal behaviors indicate active listening. The nurse usually responds indirectly using techniques such as open-ended statements, reflection (see Table 10.2), and questions that elicit additional responses from the patient. In active listening, the nurse should avoid changing the subject and instead follow the patient's lead. At times, however, it is necessary to direct a patient's focus on a specific topic or to clarify their thoughts or beliefs about that topic.

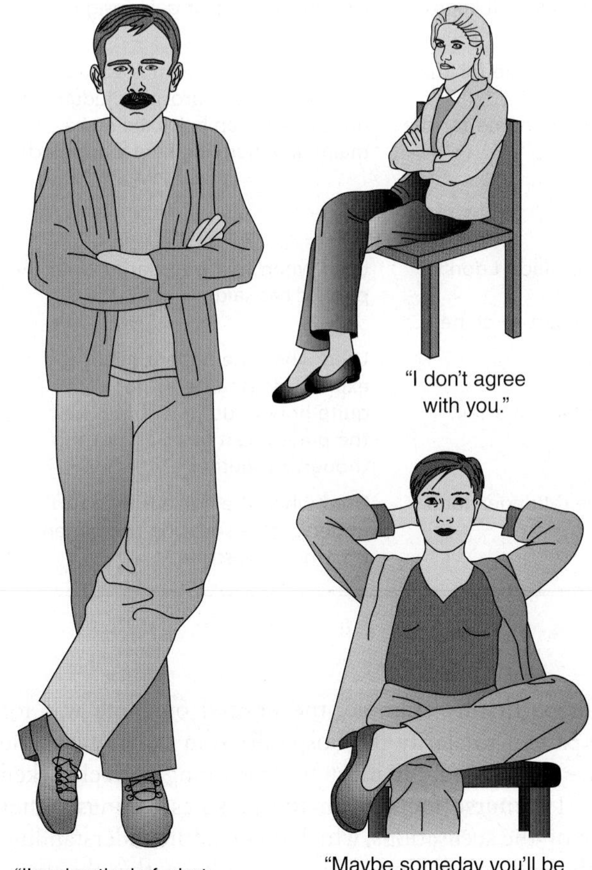

NCLEXNOTE Self-disclosure can be used in very specific situations, but self-disclosure is not the first intervention to consider. In prioritizing interventions, active listening is one of the first to use.

Selection of Communication Techniques

Psychiatric nurses use many therapeutic techniques in establishing relationships and helping patients focus on their problems. Asking a question, restating, and reflecting are examples of such techniques. These techniques may at first seem artificial, but with practice, they can be useful. Table 10.2 lists useful therapeutic techniques along with examples. Choosing the best response begins with assessing and interpreting the meaning of the patient's communication—both verbal and nonverbal. For example, if a patient is angry and upset, should the nurse invite the patient to sit down and discuss the problem, walk quietly with the patient, or simply observe the patient from a distance and not initiate conversation?

Nurses should not necessarily take verbal messages literally, especially when a patient is upset or angry. For example, one nurse walked into the room of a newly admitted patient, who accused, "You locked me up and threw away the key." The nurse could have responded defensively that they had nothing to do with the patient being admitted; however, that response could have

"I don't agree with you."

"I'm skeptical of what you're telling me."

"Maybe someday you'll be as smart as I am."

FIGURE 10.3 Negative body language.

TABLE 10.2	VERBAL COMMUNICATION TECHNIQUES		
Technique	Definition	Example	Use
Acceptance	Encouraging and receiving information in a nonjudgmental and interested manner	*Patient:* I have done something terrible. *Nurse:* I would like to hear about it. It's OK to discuss it with me.	Used in establishing trust and developing empathy
Confrontation	Presenting the patient with a different reality of the situation	*Patient:* My doctor won't talk to me. *Nurse:* I was in the room yesterday when you refused to speak with him.	Used cautiously to immediately redefine the patient's reality. However, it can alienate the patient if used inappropriately. A nonjudgmental attitude is critical for confrontation to be effective.
Doubt	Expressing or voicing doubt when a patient relates a situation	*Patient:* My best friend hates me. She never calls me. *Nurse:* From what you have told me, that does not sound like her. When did she call you last?	Used carefully and only when the nurse feels confident about the details. It is used when the nurse wants to guide the patient toward other explanations.
Interpretation	Putting into words what the patient is implying or feeling	*Patient:* I could not sleep because someone would come into my room and rape me. *Nurse:* It sounds like you were scared last night.	Used in helping the patient identify underlying thoughts or feelings
Observation	Stating to the patient what the nurse is observing	*Nurse:* You are trembling and perspiring. When did this start?	Used when a patient's behaviors (verbal or nonverbal) are obvious and unusual for that patient
Open-ended statements	Introducing an idea and letting the patient respond	*Nurse:* Trust means… *Patient:* That someone will keep you safe.	Used when helping the patient explore feelings or gain insight
Reflection	Redirecting the idea back to the patient for classification of important emotional overtones, feelings, and experiences; it gives patients permission to have feelings they may not realize they have	*Patient:* Should I go home for the weekend? *Nurse:* Should you go home for the weekend?	Used when the patient is asking for the nurse's approval or judgment; use of reflection helps the nurse maintain a nonjudgmental approach
Restatement	Repeating the main idea expressed lets the patient know what was heard	*Patient:* I hate this place. I don't belong here. *Nurse:* You don't want to be here.	Used when trying to clarify what the patient has said
Silence	Remaining quiet but nonverbally expressing interest during an interaction	*Patient:* I am angry! *Nurse:* (Silence) *Patient:* My wife had an affair.	Used when the patient needs to express ideas but may not know quite how to do it; with silence, the patient can focus on putting thoughts together
Validation	Clarifying the nurse's understanding of the situation	*Nurse:* Let me see if I understand.	Used when the nurse is trying to understand a situation the patient is trying to describe

ended in an argument, and communication would have been blocked. Fortunately, the nurse recognized that the patient was communicating frustration at being in a locked psychiatric unit and did not take the accusation personally.

The next step is identifying the desired patient outcome. To do so, the nurse should engage the patient with eye contact and quietly try to interpret the patient's feelings. In this example, the desired outcome was for the patient to clarify the hospitalization experience. The nurse responded, "It must be frustrating to feel locked up." The nurse focused on the patient's feelings rather than on the accusations, which reflected an understanding of the patient's feelings. The patient knew that the nurse accepted these feelings, which led to further discussion. It may seem impossible to plan reactions for each situation, but with practice, the nurse will begin to respond automatically in a therapeutic way.

Silence

Silence consists of deliberate pauses to encourage the patient to reflect and eventually respond. One of the most difficult but often most effective communication techniques is the use of silence during verbal interactions. By maintaining silence, the nurse allows the patient to gather thoughts and to proceed at their own pace. It is important that the nurse not interrupt periods of silence because of their own anxiety or concern of "not doing anything" if sitting quietly with a patient.

Validation

Another important technique is *validation*, which means explicitly checking one's own thoughts or feelings with another person. To do so, the nurse must own their own thoughts or feelings by using "I" statements (Orlando, 1961). Validation generally refers to observations, thoughts, or feelings and seeks explicit feedback. For example, a nurse who sees a patient pacing the hallway before a planned family visit may conclude that the patient is anxious. Validation may occur with a statement such as, "I notice you pacing the hallway. I wonder if you are feeling anxious about the family visit." The patient may agree, "Yes. I keep worrying about what is going to happen!" or disagree, "No. I have been trying to get into the bathroom for the last 30 minutes, but my roommate is still in there!"

Strength-Based Communication

Strength-based communication should be supportive, focusing on the patient's strengths instead of potential deficits. Language that promotes acceptance and respect should be favored over language that distracts from acceptance of the person. For example, instead of stating that a patient is "manipulative," an alternate consideration is that the person is "resourceful; trying to get help." An "entitled" person might be viewed instead as someone who is "aware of their rights." Instead of noting that a patient is "resistant to treatment," it may be that the person is instead "choosing a different treatment." The nurse should incorporate language that promotes the strengths and unique characteristic of their patients (Ashcraft & Anthony, 2014).

Avoiding Blocks to Communication

Some verbal techniques block interactions and inhibit therapeutic communication (Table 10.3). One of the biggest blocks to communication is giving advice, particularly when others have already given the same advice. Giving advice is different from supporting a patient through decision-making. The therapeutic dialogue presented in Box 10.3 differentiates between advice (telling the patient what to do or how to act) and therapeutic communication, through which the nurse and patient explore alternative ways of viewing the patient's world. The patient can then reach their own conclusions about the best approaches to use.

TABLE 10.3	TECHNIQUES THAT INHIBIT COMMUNICATION		
Technique	Definition	Example	Problem
Advice	Telling a patient what to do	*Patient:* I am struggling at work. *Nurse:* You should probably find a new job.	The nurse solves the patient's problem, which implies that the nurse knows best and may not be the appropriate solution; it also encourages dependency on the nurse.
Agreement	Agreeing with a particular viewpoint of a patient	*Patient:* Abortions are sinful. *Nurse:* I agree.	The patient is denied the opportunity to change their view now that the nurse agrees.
Challenges	Disputing the patient's beliefs with arguments, logical thinking, or direct order	*Patient:* I'm a cowboy. *Nurse:* If you are a cowboy, what are you doing in the hospital?	The nurse belittles the patient and decreases the patient's self-esteem. The patient will avoid relating to the nurse who challenges.
Reassurance	Telling a patient that everything will be OK	*Patient:* I don't think I will ever get better. *Nurse:* Hang in there. Everything will turn out just fine.	The nurse makes a statement that may not be true. The patient is blocked from exploring their feelings.
Disapproval	Judging the patient's situation and behavior	*Patient:* I'm so sorry. I did not mean to kill my mother. *Nurse:* You should be. How could anyone kill their mother?	The nurse belittles the patient. The patient will avoid the nurse.

BOX 10.3 • GIVING ADVICE VERSUS RECOMMENDATIONS

Ms. J has just received a diagnosis of phobic disorder and has been given a prescription for fluoxetine (Prozac). She was referred to the home health agency because she does not want to take her medication. She is fearful of becoming suicidal. Two approaches are given in the following section.

INEFFECTIVE COMMUNICATION (ADVICE)

Nurse: Ms. J, the doctor has ordered the medication because it will help with your anxiety.

Ms. J: Yes, but I don't want to take the medication. I'm afraid it will make me suicidal. Some psychiatric medication does that. I haven't had any attacks for 2 weeks, and it seems too risky since I'm doing better. I'm scared of the side effects.

Nurse: This medication has rarely had that side effect. You should try it and see if you have any suicidal thoughts.

Ms. J: [Remains silent for a while, crosses her legs, and looks away from the nurse and down at her feet] Okay.

(The nurse leaves, and Ms. J decides not to take the medication. Within 1 week, Ms. J is taken to the emergency room with a panic attack.)

EFFECTIVE COMMUNICATION

Nurse: Ms. J, how have you been doing?

Ms. J: So far, so good. I haven't had any attacks for 2 weeks.

Nurse: I understand that the doctor gave you a prescription for medication that may help with the panic attacks.

Ms. J: Yes, but I don't want to take it. I'm afraid of becoming suicidal. Some of this psychiatric medication does that. I don't really want to take a needless risk since I've been feeling better.

Nurse: Those worries are understandable. Have you ever had feelings of hurting yourself?

Ms. J: Not yet.

Nurse: If you took the medication and had thoughts like that, what would you do?

Ms. J: I don't know, that's why I'm scared.

Nurse: I think I see your dilemma. This medication may help with your panic attacks, but if the medication produces suicidal thoughts, then it might compromise your progress and that's a pretty serious risk. Is that correct?

Ms. J: Yeah, that's it.

Nurse: What are the circumstances under which you would feel more comfortable trying the medication?

Ms. J: If I knew that I would not have suicidal thoughts. If I could be assured of that.

Nurse: I can't guarantee that, but perhaps we could create an environment in which you would feel safe. I could call you every few days to see if you are having any of these thoughts and, if so, I could help you deal with them and make sure you see the doctor to review the medication.

Ms. J: Oh, that helps. If you do that, then I think that I will be alright.

(Ms. J successfully takes the medication.)

CRITICAL THINKING CHALLENGE

• Contrast the communication in the first scenario with that in the second.

• What therapeutic communication techniques did the second nurse use that may have contributed to a better outcome?

• Are there any cues in the first scenario that indicate that the patient will not follow the nurse's advice? Explain.

CONSIDERATIONS FOR EFFECTIVE COMMUNICATION AND RELATIONSHIPS

When the nurse is interacting with patients, additional considerations can enhance the quality of communication. This section describes the importance of **rapport**, **empathy**, recognition of **empathic linkages**, the role of **boundaries** and body space, and recognition of defense mechanisms in nurse–patient interactions.

Rapport

Rapport, interpersonal harmony characterized by understanding and respect, is important in developing a trusting, therapeutic relationship. Nurses establish rapport through interpersonal warmth, a nonjudgmental attitude, and a demonstration of understanding. A skilled nurse will establish rapport that will alleviate the patient's anxiety in discussing personal problems.

People with psychiatric problems often feel alone and isolated. Establishing rapport helps lessen feelings of being alone. When rapport develops, a patient feels comfortable with the nurse and finds self-disclosure easier. The nurse also feels comfortable and recognizes that an interpersonal bond or alliance is developing. All of these factors—comfort, sense of sharing, and decreased anxiety—are important in establishing and building the nurse–patient relationship.

Empathy

The use of empathy in a therapeutic relationship is central to psychiatric–mental health nursing. Empathy is sometimes confused with sympathy, which is the expression of compassion and kindness. Empathy is the ability to experience, in the present, a situation as another did at some time in the past. It is the ability to put oneself in another person's circumstances and to imagine what it would be like to share their feelings. The nurse does not actually have to have had the experience but has to be able to imagine the feelings associated with it. For empathy to develop, there must be a giving of self to the other individual and a reciprocal desire to know each other personally. The process involves the nurse receiving information from the patient with open, nonjudgmental acceptance and communicating this understanding of the experience and feelings so that the patient feels understood.

Recognition of Empathic Linkages

While empathy is essential, it is important for the nurse to be aware of empathic linkages, the direct communication of feelings (Peplau, 1952, 1992). This commonly occurs with anxiety. For example, a nurse may be speaking with a patient who is highly anxious, and the nurse may notice their own speech becoming more rapid in tandem with the patient's. The nurse may also become aware of subjective feelings of anxiety. It may be difficult for the nurse to determine if the anxiety was communicated interpersonally or if the nurse is personally reacting to some of the content of what the patient is communicating. However, being aware of one's own feelings and analyzing them are crucial to determining the source of the feeling and addressing associated problems.

Biopsychosocial Boundaries and Body Space Zones

Boundaries are the defining limits of individuals, objects, or relationships. Boundaries mark territory, distinguishing what is "mine" from what is "not mine." Human beings have many different types of boundaries. Material boundaries, such as fences around property, artificially imposed state lines, and bodies of water, define territory

as well as provide security and order. Personal boundaries can be conceptualized within the biopsychosocial model as including physical, psychological, and social dimensions. Physical boundaries are those established in terms of physical closeness to others—who we allow to touch us or how close we want others to stand near us.

Psychological boundaries are established in terms of emotional distance from others—how much of our innermost feelings and thoughts we want to share. Social boundaries, such as norms, customs, and roles, help us establish our closeness and place within the family, culture, and community. Boundaries are not fixed but dynamic. When boundaries are involuntarily infringed upon, the individual feels threatened and responds to the perceived threat. The nurse must elicit permission before implementing interventions that invade the patient's personal space.

Personal Boundaries

Every individual is surrounded by four different body zones that provide varying degrees of protection against unwanted physical closeness during interactions. These were identified by Hall (1990) as the intimate zone (e.g., for whispering and embracing), the personal zone (e.g., for close friends), the social zone (e.g., for acquaintances), and the public zone (usually for interacting with strangers) (Fig. 10.4). The actual sizes of the different zones vary according to culture. Some cultures define the intimate zone narrowly and the personal zones widely. Thus, friends in these cultures may stand and sit close while interacting. People of other cultures define the intimate zone widely and are uncomfortable when others stand close to them.

The variability of intimate and personal zones has implications for nursing. For a patient to be comfortable

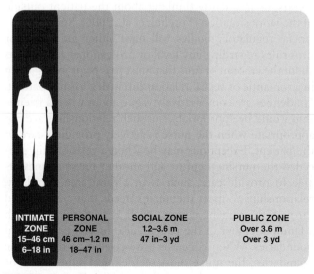

FIGURE 10.4 Body space zones.

with a nurse, the nurse needs to protect the intimate zone of that individual. The patient usually will allow the nurse to enter the personal zone but will express discomfort if the nurse breaches the intimate zone. For the nurse, the difficulty lies in differentiating the personal zone from the intimate zone for each patient.

The nurse's awareness of their own need for intimate and personal space is another prerequisite for therapeutic interaction with the patient. It is important that a nurse feel comfortable while interacting with patients. Establishing a comfort zone may well entail fine-tuning the size of body zones. Recognizing this will help the nurse understand occasional inexplicable reactions to the proximity of patients.

Professional Boundaries and Ethics

For nurses, professional boundaries are also essential to consider in the context of the nurse–patient relationship. Patients often enter such relationships at a very vulnerable point, and nurses need to be aware of professional boundaries to avoid exploitation of the patient. For example, in a friendship, there is a two-way sharing of personal information and feelings, but as mentioned previously, in a nurse–patient relationship, the focus is on the patient's needs, and the nurse generally does not share personal information or attempt to meet their own needs through the relationship. The patient may seek a friendship or sexual relationship with the nurse (or vice versa), but this would be inconsistent with the professional role and is usually considered unethical.

Indicators that the relationship may be moving outside the professional boundaries are gift giving on either party's part, spending more time than usual with a particular patient, strenuously defending or explaining the patient's behavior in team meetings, the nurse feeling that they are the only one who truly understands the patient, keeping secrets, or frequently thinking about the patient outside of the work situation (Forchuk et al., 2006). State or provincial regulatory bodies will have either guidelines or firm rules regarding any legal or professional restrictions about the amount of time that must pass prior to engaging in a romantic or sexual relationship with a former patient. Guidelines are comparatively vague about when a friendship would be appropriate, but such relationships are not appropriate when the nurse is actively providing care to the patient. Exceptions may be when a relationship preceded the nursing context and another nurse is unavailable to provide care, such as in a rural area. Similarly, relationships to meet the nurse's needs that are acquired through the nursing context, such as a relationship with a family member of the patient, also breach professional boundaries. When concerns arise related to therapeutic boundaries, the nurse must seek clinical supervision or transfer the care of the patient immediately.

Defense Mechanisms

When communicating with patients, it is also important for the nurse to be aware of the defense mechanisms that patients may use. Defense mechanisms (also known as coping styles) are psychological mechanisms that help an individual respond to and cope with difficult situations, emotional conflicts, and external stressors. While defense mechanisms might seem to indicate the existence of problematic mental state, this is not true. Healthy individuals in many different contexts use defense mechanisms. The use of defense mechanisms may be conscious or unconscious. Some defense mechanisms (e.g., projection, splitting, acting out) are mostly maladaptive. Others (e.g., suppression, denial) may be either maladaptive or adaptive depending on the context in which they occur. The use of defense mechanisms becomes maladaptive when its persistent use interferes with the person's ability to function and their quality of life (see Table 10.4).

For example, responding to a difficult life event altruistically is very often a healthy way to recover. On the other hand, defense mechanisms such as acting out, autistic fantasies, projection, and splitting are rarely adaptive. A defense mechanism such as repression can be a natural way to react to a traumatic experience, specifically when used in appropriate moderation. However, the unchecked repression of difficult thoughts or feelings can keep someone from coming to terms with their experiences. In developing a successful therapeutic relationship, and in establishing open communication, such knowledge of defense mechanisms will prove itself invaluable.

As nurses develop therapeutic relationships, they will recognize their patients using defense mechanisms. With experience, the nurse will evaluate the purpose of a defense mechanism and then determine whether or not it should be discussed with the patient. For example, if a patient is using humor to alleviate an emotionally intense situation, that may be very appropriate. On the other hand, if someone continually rationalizes antisocial behavior, the use of the defense mechanism should be discussed.

NCLEXNOTE When studying defense mechanisms, focus on mechanisms and coping styles that are similar. For example, displacement versus devaluation versus projection should be differentiated. Identify these mechanisms in your process recordings.

COMMUNICATION CONSIDERATIONS FOR PATIENTS WITH MENTAL HEALTH CHALLENGES

For patients with specific, known mental health problems or illnesses, the nurse must consider how these issues may impact communication and be prepared to analyze the content of nurse–patient interactions.

TABLE 10.4	SPECIFIC DEFENSE MECHANISMS AND COPING STYLES	

The following defense mechanisms and coping styles are commonly used when the individual deals with emotional conflict or stressors (either internal or external).

Defense Mechanism	Definition	Example
Acting out	Using actions rather than reflections or feelings during periods of emotional conflict	A teenager gets mad at his parents and begins staying out late at night.
Affiliation	Turning to others for help or support (sharing problems with others without implying that someone else is responsible for them)	An individual has a fight with her spouse and turns to her best friend for emotional support.
Altruism	Dedicating life to meeting the needs of others (receives gratification either vicariously or from the response of others)	After being rejected by her boyfriend, a young girl joins the Peace Corps.
Anticipation	Experiencing emotional reactions in advance or anticipating consequences of possible future events and considering realistic, alternative responses or solutions	A mother cries for 3 weeks before her last child leaves for college.
Autistic fantasy	Excessive daydreaming as a substitute for human relationships, more effective action, or problem-solving	A young man sits in his room all day and dreams about being a rock star instead of attending a baseball game with a friend.
Denial	Refusing to acknowledge some painful aspect of external reality or subjective experience that would be apparent to others (*Psychotic denial* is used when there is gross impairment in reality testing.)	A teenager's best friend moves away, but the adolescent says he does not feel sad.
Devaluation	Attributing exaggerated negative qualities to self or others	A boy has been rejected by his long-time girlfriend. He tells his friends that he realizes that she is stupid and ugly.
Displacement	Transferring a feeling about, or a response to, one object onto another (usually less threatening) substitute object	A woman has an argument with her boss. She comes home from work and yells at her children.
Dissociation	Experiencing a breakdown in the usually integrated functions of consciousness, memory, perception of self or the environment, or sensory and motor behavior	An adult relates severe sexual abuse experienced as a child but does it without feeling. She says that the experience was as if she were outside her body watching the abuse.
Help-rejecting complaining	Complaining or making repeated requests for help that disguise covert feelings of hostility or reproach toward others, which are then expressed by rejecting the suggestions, advice, or help that others offer (Complaints or requests may involve physical or psychological symptoms or life problems.)	A college student asks a teacher for help after receiving a bad grade on a test. Every suggestion the teacher has is rejected by the student.
Humor	Emphasizing the amusing or ironic aspects of the conflict or stressor	A person makes a joke right after experiencing an embarrassing situation.
Idealization	Attributing exaggerated positive qualities to others	An adult falls in love and fails to see the negative qualities in the other person.
Intellectualization	Excessive use of abstract thinking or the making of generalizations to control or minimize disturbing feelings	After rejection in a romantic relationship, the rejected explains the relationship dynamics to a friend.
Isolation of affect	Separation of ideas from the feelings originally associated with them	The individual loses touch with the feelings associated with a rape while remaining aware of the details.
Omnipotence	Feeling or acting as if one possesses special powers or abilities and is superior to others	An individual tells a friend about personal expertise in the stock market and the ability to predict the best stocks.
Passive aggression	Indirectly and unassertively expressing aggression toward others. There is a facade of overt compliance masking covert resistance, resentment, or hostility.	One employee doesn't like another, so he secretly steals her milk from the office refrigerator. She is unaware of his hostile feelings.

(Continued)

TABLE 10.4   SPECIFIC DEFENSE MECHANISMS AND COPING STYLES (*Continued*)

Defense Mechanism	Definition	Example
Projection	Falsely attributing to another one's unacceptable feelings, impulses, or thoughts	A child is very angry at a parent but accuses the parent of being angry.
Projective identification	Falsely attributing to another one's unacceptable feelings, impulses, or thoughts. Unlike simple projection, the individual does not fully disavow what is projected. Instead, the individual remains aware of their own affect or impulses but misattributes them as justifiable reactions to the other person. Frequently, the individual induces the very feelings in others that were first mistakenly believed to be there, making it difficult to clarify who did what to whom first.	A child is mad at a parent, who in turn becomes angry at the child but may be unsure of why. The child then feels justified at being angry with the parent.
Rationalization	Concealing the true motivations for one's own thoughts, actions, or feelings through the elaboration of reassuring or self-serving but incorrect explanations	A man is rejected by his girlfriend but explains to his friends that her leaving was best because she was beneath him socially and would not be liked by his family.
Reaction formation	Substituting behavior, thoughts, or feelings that are diametrically opposed to one's own unacceptable thoughts or feelings (this usually occurs in conjunction with their repression)	A wife finds out about her husband's extramarital affairs and tells her friends that she thinks his affairs are perfectly appropriate. She truly does not feel, on a conscious level, any anger or hurt.
Repression	Expelling disturbing wishes, thoughts, or experiences from conscious awareness (The feeling component may remain conscious, detached from its associated ideas.)	A woman does not remember the experience of being raped in the basement but does feel anxious when going into that house.
Self-assertion	Expressing feelings and thoughts directly in a way that is not coercive or manipulative	An individual reaffirms that going to a ball game is not what she wants to do.
Self-observation	Reflecting feelings, thoughts, motivation, and behavior and responding to them appropriately	An individual notices an irritation at his friend's late arrival and decides to tell the friend of the irritation.
Splitting	Compartmentalizing opposite affect states and failing to integrate the positive and negative qualities of the self or others into cohesive images	Self and object images tend to alternate between polar opposites: exclusively loving, powerful, worthy, nurturing, and kind or exclusively bad, hateful, angry, destructive, rejecting, or worthless. One friend is wonderful and another former friend, who was at one time viewed as being perfect, is now believed to be an evil person.
Sublimation	Channeling potentially maladaptive feelings or impulses into socially acceptable behavior	An adolescent boy is very angry with his parents. On the football field, he tackles someone very forcefully.
Suppression	Intentionally avoiding thinking about disturbing problems, wishes, feelings, or experiences	A student is anxiously awaiting test results but goes to a movie to stop thinking about it.
Undoing	Words or behavior designed to negate or to make amends symbolically for unacceptable thoughts, feelings, or actions	A man has sexual fantasies about his wife's sister. He takes his wife away for a romantic weekend.

Considering Specific Mental Health Issues

It is important to consider the individual's mental health challenges when selecting specific communication strategies. For example, patients with increased levels of anxiety may have poor communication, requiring the nurse to use shorter and simpler statements or questions.

Patients who are experiencing depression may have difficulty articulating their feelings, or their thinking and responses may be slowed. The nurse will frequently use silence and empathic techniques throughout this interaction. The person who is depressed may also use communication styles such as overgeneralizing ("This always happens to me. … Everything always turns out for the worse."). The nurse can assist the patient and ask them to be more specific (e.g., asking about a specific time or a specific exception).

Patients with schizophrenia may exhibit symptoms such as hallucinations or delusions. If a person is having auditory hallucinations (hearing sounds that are imagined), the nurse's voice may be one of several the patient is hearing. Clear, short sentences may assist in getting the patient's attention on the nurse's voice. A person experiencing delusions may use pronouns vaguely ("they" did it) or other forms of vague or unclear communication. Clarifying and assisting the patient to be more specific may assist the patient's thinking as well as communication.

As you read through the chapters on various psychiatric disorders, consider how the signs and symptoms of each illness could have an impact on communication and the evolving therapeutic relationship.

Analyzing Interactions

Many patients with psychiatric disorders have difficulty communicating. They may have perceptual, cognitive, and information-processing deficits that interfere with their ability to express ideas, understand concepts, and accurately perceive the environment (Pounds, 2017).

Because of the complexity of communication, mental health professionals monitor their interactions with patients using various methods, including audio recording, video recording, and **process recording**, which entails writing a verbatim transcript of the interaction. A video or audio recording of an interaction provides the most accurate monitoring but is cumbersome to use. Process recording, one of the easiest methods to use, is adequate in most situations. Nurses should use it when first learning therapeutic communication and during times when communication becomes a problem. In a process recording, the nurse records, from memory, the verbatim interaction immediately after the communication (Table 10.5). Nonverbal communication, by both the patient and the nurse, should also be recorded.

The nurse then analyzes the content of the interaction in terms of the words and their meaning for both the patient and the nurse. The analysis is especially important because the ability to communicate is often compromised in people with mental disorders. Because words may not have the same meaning for the patient as they do for the nurse, clarification of meaning becomes especially important. The analysis can identify symbolic meanings, **content themes**, and blocks in communication.

TABLE 10.5   PROCESS RECORDING

Setting: The living room of Mr. S's home. Mr. S is 23 years old and was hospitalized for 2 weeks. His diagnosis is a bipolar mood disorder, and he is recovering from a depressive episode. His parents are in the room but cannot hear the conversation. Mr. S is sitting on the couch, and the nurse is sitting on a chair. This is the nurse's first visit after Mr. S's discharge from the hospital.

Patient	Nurse	Interpretation/Analysis
	How are you doing, Mr. S? (smiles and offers hand to shake)	*Plan:* Initially develop a sense of trust and initiate a therapeutic relationship.
I'm fine. It's good to be home (looking at floor, takes nurse's hand to briefly shake). I really don't like the hospital (shakes his head while still looking at floor).	You didn't like the hospital?	Interpretation: Validating assumption that Mr. S does not want to return to hospital. Nonverbal communication may indicate sadness or low self-esteem. This needs further exploration.
No. The nurses lock you up (maintains eye contact with nurse, frowning, arms crossed). Are you a nurse?		Patient validates assumption regarding hospital, but nonverbal behavior indicates there may be further concerns.
	I'm a nurse. I'm wondering if you think that I will lock you up (maintains eye contact and open posture).	Interpretation: Mr. S may be wondering what my role is and whether I will put him back in the hospital. This assumption needs to be validated, and my role needs clarification.
You could tell my mom to put me back in the hospital (maintains eye contact with nurse).	Any treatment that I recommend will be thoroughly discussed with you first. I am here to help you stay out of the hospital. I will not discuss anything with your mother unless you give me permission to do so (nurse maintains eye contact and open posture).	Use interpretation to clarify Mr. S's thinking. Mr. S is wondering about my relationship with his mother. Explain my role and confidentiality.
(Patient maintains eye contact and uncrosses arms.)		Patient's nonverbal communication appears to indicate he is more comfortable with this clarification.

Symbolism

Symbolism, the use of a word or phrase to represent an object, event, or feeling, is used universally. For example, automobiles are named for wild animals that represent speed, prowess, and beauty. In people with mental disorders, the use of words to symbolize events, objects, or feelings is often idiosyncratic, and they cannot explain their choices. For example, a person who is feeling scared and anxious may tell the nurse that bombs and guns are exploding. It is up to the nurse to make the connection between the bombs and guns and the patient's feelings and then validate this with the patient. Because of the patient's cognitive limitations, the individual may express feelings only symbolically. Another example is found in Table 10.6.

Some patients, for example, those with developmental disabilities or organic brain difficulties, may have difficulty with abstract thinking and symbolism. Conversations may be interpreted literally. For example, in response to the question "What brings you to the hospital?" a patient might reply, "The ambulance." In these situations, the nurse must be cautious to avoid using symbols or metaphors. Concrete language, that is, language reflecting what can be observed through the senses, will be more easily understood.

Content Themes

Verbal behavior is also interpreted by analyzing content themes. Patients often express concerns or feelings repeatedly in several different ways. After a few sessions, a common theme emerges. Themes may emerge symbolically,

---

BOX 10.4

Themes and Interactions

Session 1: Patient discusses the death of his mother at a young age.
Session 2: Patient explains that his sister is now married and never visits him.
Session 3: Patient says that his best friend in the hospital was discharged and he really misses her.
Session 4: Patient cries about a lost kitten.
Interpretation: Theme of loss is pervasive in several sessions.

---

as in the case with the patient who constantly talks about the "guns and bombs." Alternatively, a theme may simply be identified as a recurrent thread of a story that a patient retells at each session. For example, one patient often discussed his early abandonment by his family. This led the nurse to hypothesize that he had an underlying fear of rejection. The nurse was then able to test whether there was an underlying fear and to develop strategies to help the patient explore the fear (Box 10.4). It is important to involve patients in analyzing themes so they may learn this skill. Within the therapeutic relationship, the person who does the work is the one who develops the competencies, so the nurse must be careful to share this opportunity with the patient (Peplau, 1952, 1992).

Communication Blocks

Communication blocks are identified by topic changes that either the nurse or the patient makes. Topics are

---

TABLE 10.6	USE OF SYMBOLISM

Setting: Mr. A has been diagnosed with schizophrenia and expresses himself through the use of television characters. A nurse observed another patient shoving him against the wall. As the nurse approached the two patients, the other patient ran, leaving Mr. A noticeably shaking. The nurse checked to see if Mr. A was all right.

Patient	Nurse	Interpretation/Analysis
	Mr. A, are you OK? (approaches patient)	
Robin Hood saved the day. (trembling, arms crossed)		Mr. A could not say, "Thank you for helping me." Instead, he could only describe a fictional character's response.
	You feel that you are saved?	The nurse focused on what Mr. A must be feeling if he felt that he had been rescued.
It's a glorious day in Sherwood Forest! (trembling decreases; smiles at nurse)		He seems to be happy now.
	Mr. A, are you hurting anywhere? (Eyes scan over patient, using concerned tone of voice.)	The nurse wanted to check whether the patient had been hurt when pushed against the wall.
The angel of mercy put out the fire (continues to smile and extends hand to shake hands with nurse).		The patient is apparently not hurting now.

changed for various reasons. A patient may change the topic from one that does not interest him to one that he finds more meaningful. However, an individual usually changes the topic because they are uncomfortable with a particular subject. When a topic change is identified, the nurse or patient hypothesizes the reason for it. If the nurse changes the topic, they need to determine why. The nurse may find that they are uncomfortable with the topic or may not be listening to the patient. Novice mental health nurses, who are uncomfortable with silences or trying to elicit specific information from the patient, often change topics. When communication blocks are recognized, the nurse should attempt to redirect the conversation back to the topic at hand unless the particular topic is too uncomfortable for the patient at that point in time.

The nurse must also record and interpret the patient's nonverbal behavior in light of the verbal behavior. Is the patient communicating one thing verbally and another nonverbally? The nurse must consider the patient's cultural background. Is the behavior consistent with cultural norms? For example, if a patient denies any problems but is affectionate and physically demonstrative (which is antithetical to their naturally stoic cultural beliefs and behaviors), the nonverbal behavior is inconsistent with what is normal behavior for that person. Further exploration is needed to determine the meaning of the culturally atypical behavior.

THE NURSE–PATIENT RELATIONSHIP

The nurse–patient relationship is a dynamic process that changes with time. It can be viewed in steps or phases with characteristic behaviors for both patient and nurse. This text uses an adaptation of Hildegarde Peplau's model, which she introduced in her seminal work, *Interpersonal Relations in Nursing* (1952, 1992). Emerging evidence suggests that a well-developed nurse–patient relationship positively affects patient care.

Introduction

The nurse–patient relationship begins with the initial introduction. Nurses initiate the introduction by simply explaining their role and their task—an initial assessment or an invitation to a group. It is very important to introduce oneself. The language used is also very important. The nurse should be sensitive to using patient-centered and gender-neutral language. When first meeting a patient, do not assume gender or sexual orientation by the clothing or appearance. If you are unsure of the patient's gender but must use pronouns, the terms "they/them/their" are preferable to terms that make patients select a male or female category (Sullivan et al., 2017).

Phases

The nurse–patient relationship is conceptualized in three overlapping phases that evolve with time: **orientation phase**, **working phase**, and **resolution phase**. The orientation phase is the phase during which the nurse and patient get to know each other. During this phase, which can last from a few minutes to several months, the patient develops a sense of trust in the nurse. The second is the working phase, in which the patient uses the relationship to examine specific problems and learn new ways of approaching them. The final stage, resolution phase, is the termination stage of the relationship and lasts from the time the problems are actually resolved to the close of the relationship. The relationship does not evolve as a simple linear relationship. Instead, the relationship may be predominantly in one phase, but reflections of all phases can be seen in each interaction (Table 10.7).

TABLE 10.7	PHASES OF THE NURSE–PATIENT RELATIONSHIP		
	Orientation	Working	Resolution
Patient	Seeks assistance Identifies needs Commits to a therapeutic relationship During the later part, begins to test relationship	Discusses problems and underlying needs Uses emotional safety of relationship to examine personal issues Tests new ways of solving problems Feels comfortable with nurse May use transference	May express ambivalence about the relationship and its termination Uses personal style to say "good-bye"
Nurse	Actively listens Establishes boundaries of the relationship Clarifies expectations Identifies countertransference issues Uses empathy Establishes rapport	Supports development of healthy problem-solving Encourages patient to prepare for the future	Avoids returning to patient's initial problems Encourages independence Promotes positive family interactions

> **KEYCONCEPT The nurse–patient relationship** is a dynamic process that changes with time. It can be viewed in steps or phases with characteristic behaviors for both the patient and the nurse.

Orientation Phase

The orientation phase begins when the nurse and patient meet and ends when the patient begins to identify the problems to be examined. During the orientation phase, the nurse discusses the patient's expectations, explains the purpose of the relationship and its boundaries, and facilitates the development of the relationship. It is natural for the nurse to be nervous during the first few sessions. The goal of the orientation phase is to develop trust and security within the nurse–patient relationship. During this initial phase, the nurse listens intently to the patient's history and perception of problems and begins to understand the patient and identify themes. The use of empathy facilitates the development of a positive therapeutic relationship.

First Meeting

During the first meeting, outlining both nursing and patient responsibilities is important. The nurse is responsible for providing guidance throughout the therapeutic relationship, protecting confidential information, and maintaining professional boundaries. The patient is responsible for attending agreed-upon sessions, interacting during the sessions, and participating in the nurse–patient relationship. The nurse should also explain clearly to the patient meeting times, handling of missed sessions, and the estimated length of the relationship. Issues related to recording information and how the nurse will work within the interdisciplinary team should also be made explicit.

Usually, both the nurse and the patient feel anxious at the first meeting. The nurse should recognize the anxieties and attempt to alleviate them before the meeting. The patient's behavior during this first meeting may indicate to the nurse some of the patient's problems in interpersonal relationships. For example, a patient may talk nonstop for 15 minutes or may brag of sexual conquests. What the patient chooses to tell or not to tell is significant. What a patient first does or says may not accurately indicate their true feelings or the situation. In the beginning, patients may deny problems or employ various forms of defense mechanisms or prevent the nurse from getting to know them. The patient is usually nervous and insecure during the first few sessions and may exhibit behavior reflective of these emotions, such as rambling. Typically, by the third session, the patient can focus on a topic.

Confidentiality in Treatment

Ideally, nurses include people who are important to the patient in planning and implementing care. The nurse and patient should discuss the issue of confidentiality in the first session. The nurse should be clear about any information that is to be shared with anyone else. The nurse shares significant assessment data and patient progress with a supervisor, team members, and a physician. Most patients expect the nurse to communicate with other mental health professionals and are comfortable with this arrangement. Restrictions regarding what can be shared and with whom are also covered by state or provincial mental health acts and health information acts.

Testing the Relationship

This first part of the orientation phase, called the "honeymoon phase," is usually pleasant. However, the therapeutic team typically hits rough spots before completing this phase. The patient begins to test the relationship to become convinced that the nurse will really accept them. Typical "testing behaviors" include forgetting a scheduled session or being late. Patients may also express anger at something a nurse says or accuse the nurse of breaking confidentiality. Another common pattern is for the patient to first introduce a relatively superficial issue as if it is the major problem. The nurse must recognize that these behaviors are designed to test the relationship and establish its parameters, not to express rejection or dissatisfaction with the nurse. The student nurse often feels personally rejected during the patient's testing and may even become angry with the patient. If the nurse simply accepts the behavior and continues to be available and consistent to the patient, these behaviors usually subside. Testing needs to be understood as a normal way that human beings develop trust.

Working Phase

When the patient begins identifying problems to work on, the working phase of the relationship has started. Problem identification can yield a wide range of issues, such as managing symptoms of a mental disorder, coping with chronic pain, examining issues related to sexual abuse, or dealing with problematic interpersonal relationships. Through the relationship, the patient begins to explore the identified problems and develop strategies to resolve them. By the time the working phase is reached, the patient has developed enough trust that they can examine the identified problems within the security of the therapeutic relationship. In the working phase, the nurse can use various verbal and nonverbal techniques to help the patient examine problems and to support the patient through the healing process.

Transference (unconscious assignment to others of the feelings and attitudes that the patient originally associated with important figures) and **countertransference** (the provider's emotional reaction to the patient based on personal unconscious needs and conflicts) become important issues in the working phase. For example, a patient could be hostile to a nurse because of underlying resentment of authority figures; the nurse, in turn, could respond defensively because of earlier experiences of anger. The patient uses transference to examine problems. During this phase, the patient is psychologically vulnerable and emotionally dependent on the nurse. The nurse needs to recognize countertransference and prevent it from eroding professional boundaries.

Often, nurses are eager to implement rehabilitation plans. However, this cannot be done until the patient trusts the nurse and identifies what issues they wish to work on in the context of the relationship.

Resolution Phase

The final stage of the nurse–patient relationship is resolution, which begins when the actual problems are resolved and ends with the termination of the relationship. During this phase, the patient is redirected toward a life without this specific therapeutic relationship. The patient connects with community resources, solidifies a newly found understanding, and practices new behaviors. The patient takes responsibility for follow-up appointments and interacts with significant others in new ways. New problems are not addressed during this phase except in terms of what was learned during the working stage. The nurse assists the client in strengthening relationships, making referrals, and recognizing and understanding signs of future relapse.

Termination begins on the first day of the relationship, when the nurse explains that this relationship is time limited and has been established to resolve the patient's problems and help them handle their problems. Because a therapeutic relationship is dependent, the nurse must constantly evaluate the patient's level of dependence and continually support the patient's move toward independence. Termination is usually stressful for the patient, who must sever ties with the nurse who has shared thoughts and feelings and given guidance and support over many sessions.

Depending on previous experiences with terminating relationships, some patients may not handle their emotions well during termination. Some may not show up for the last session at all to avoid their feelings of sadness and separation. Many patients display anger about the relationship's ending. Patients may express anger toward the nurse or displace it onto others. For example, a patient may shout obscenities at another patient after being told that his therapeutic relationship with the nurse would end in a few weeks. One of the best ways to handle the

anger is to help the patient acknowledge it, to explain that anger is a normal emotion when a relationship is ending, and to reassure the patient that it is acceptable to feel angry. The nurse should also reassure the patient that anger subsides after the relationship is over.

Another typical termination behavior is raising old problems that have already been resolved. The nurse may feel frustrated if patients in the termination phase present resolved problems as if they were new. The nurse may feel that the sessions were unsuccessful. In reality, patients are attempting to prolong the relationship and avoid its ending. Nurses should avoid addressing these problems. Instead, they should reassure patients that they already covered those issues and learned methods to control them. They should explain that the patient may be feeling anxious about the relationship's ending and redirect the patient to newly found skills and abilities in forming new relationships, including support groups and social groups. The final meeting should focus on the future (Box 10.5). The nurse can reassure the patient that the nurse will remember them, but the nurse should not agree to see the patient outside the relationship.

Nontherapeutic Relationships

Although it is hoped that all nurse–patient relationships will go through the phases of the relationship described earlier, this is not always the case. In a **nontherapeutic relationship**, the nurse and the patient both feel very frustrated and keep varying their approach with each other in an attempt to establish a meaningful relationship. This is different from a prolonged orientation phase in that the efforts are not sustained; rather, they vary constantly.

The nurse may try longer meetings, shorter meetings, being more or less directive, and varying the therapeutic stance from warm and friendly to aloof. Patients in this phase may try to talk about the past but then change to discussions of the "here and now." They will try talking about their family and in the next meeting talk about their work goals. Both *grapple and struggle* to come to a common ground, and both become increasingly frustrated with each other.

Eventually, the frustration becomes so great that the pair gives up on each other and moves to a phase of *mutual withdrawal*. The nurse may schedule seeing this patient at the end of the shift and "run out of time" so the meeting never happens. The patient will leave the unit or otherwise be unavailable during scheduled meeting times. If a meeting does occur, the nurse will try to keep it short, thinking, "What's the point—we just cover the same old ground anyway." The patient will attempt to keep it superficial and stay on safe topics ("You can always ask about your medications—nurses love to health teach, you know.").

BOX 10.5

Transitional Relationship Model

Forchuk, C., Martin, M. L., Jensen, E., Ouseley, S., Sealy, P., Beal, G., et al. (2013). Integrating an evidence-based intervention into clinical practice: 'Transitional relationship model.' Journal of Psychiatric and Mental Health Nursing, 20(7), 584–594.

THE QUESTION: The Transitional Relationship Model (TRM) facilitates an effective discharge from the hospital to the community. Given this, what is the most effective way of implementing this model? What might facilitate the successful implementation of the TRM? What are the barriers to successful implementation?

METHODS: This study implemented the TRM in three waves, across six wards using a delayed implementation control group design to study how the addition of new information changed the implementation of the TRM. Following the experiences of the wards in which the TRM was initially implemented, recommendations for successful implementation of the model were developed for the subsequent waves of wards. Recommendations were developed using a combination of qualitative methods: monthly summaries, progress reports, meeting minutes, and focus groups.

FINDINGS: The results of this study can be divided into two categories: facilitators and barriers. The successful implementation of the TRM was aided by the use of educational modules (for both staff and peer training), on-site champions, and supportive documentation systems. Barriers included feeling swamped or overwhelmed, "death by process," preexisting conflicts within teams, and changes in champions.

IMPLICATIONS FOR NURSING: The positive health outcomes associated with the TRM require careful preparation and constant attention to education, communication, and the effectiveness of the support given to caregivers.

A **deteriorating relationship** is also nontherapeutic and has been shown to have predictable phases (Coatsworth-Puspoky et al., 2006). This relationship starts in the *withholding* phase, during which the nurse is perceived as "withholding" nursing support. The nurse fails to recognize that the patient is a person with an illness or health needs. The patient feels uncomfortable, anxious, frustrated, and guilty about being ill and does not develop a sense of trust. A barrier exists between the patient and the nurse.

The middle phase of a deteriorating relationship consists of two subphases: *avoiding* and *ignoring*. The patient begins to avoid the nurse and perceives that the nurse is avoiding them. The patient abides by the rules because they do not want to cause problems. The nurse is perceived as rude and condescending. The nurse ignores and avoids the patient's requests for help; in turn, the patient becomes more anxious, frustrated, and fearful. Patients experiencing this phase report feelings of wanting to give up, being rejected, not being cared for, and not being listened to.

The end phase is named *struggling with and making sense of*. In the final phase of a nontherapeutic, deteriorating relationship, the patient struggles with and tries to understand the unsatisfactory relationship. The patient feels hopeless and frustrated as a result of the lack of support received by the nurse. In a deteriorating relationship, the patient and nurse begin as strangers and end as enemies.

Obviously, no therapeutic progress can be made in a nontherapeutic or deteriorating relationship. The nurse may be hesitant to ask for a therapeutic transfer, assuming that a relationship would similarly fail with another nurse. However, each relationship is unique, and difficulties in one relationship do not predict difficulties in the next. Clinical supervision early on may assist the development of the relationship, but often a therapeutic transfer to another nurse is required.

EXAMPLES OF STRATEGIES RELATED TO THERAPEUTIC RELATIONSHIPS

Motivational Interviewing

Motivational interviewing (MI) is a clinical method intended to engage a patient's own decision-making ability. By focusing and reinforcing the client's own arguments for change, MI can be used to achieve positive outcomes. This is a collaborative process involving directed counseling and focused discussions between the care provider and the patient. As a result, MI is inherently exploratory and adaptive.

There is a lot of evidence to suggest that MI produces positive health outcomes; however, more studies that explore the long-term outcomes and cost effectiveness of MI are needed (Frost et al., 2018). A review of other published reviews by DiClemente et al. (2017) indicated that MI and similar interventions can have varying degrees of efficacy. For example, substantial empirical evidence exists for MI in reducing alcohol, marijuana, and tobacco use, but there is limited support regarding its effectiveness in reducing cocaine, opiate, and methamphetamine use and issues with gambling. Because much of the success of MI depends on the quality of interaction between the care provider and the patient, good communication practices are essential for effective implementation of MI. Many of these problems are the result of the assumption that high-risk behaviors are entirely or mostly under the control of the individual (Berg et al., 2011). Careful attention to the effects of this assumption can make clear where MI may or may not be an ideal treatment option.

Because the success of MI is, in part, dependent on contingent factors, care providers require frequent instruction and feedback. Strong communication in the context of therapeutic relationships as discussed in this chapter, especially self-awareness, empathetic linkages, active listening, and the avoidance of unhelpful varieties of defense mechanisms, requires ongoing training and will affect therapeutic outcomes. While challenging to successfully implement, MI has produced positive health outcomes in many different settings (Dean et al., 2016; Ekong & Kavookjian, 2016; Wade et al., 2019; Wong-Anuchit et al., 2019). Every particular use of MI is likely to vary according to patient needs; Miller and Moyers (2006) have identified eight features of MI that should appear in every application of this technique:

1. Openness to collaboration with clients' own expertise,
2. Proficiency in client-centered counseling, including accurate empathy,
3. Recognition of key aspects of client speech that guides the practice of MI,
4. Eliciting and strengthening client change talk,
5. Rolling with resistance,
6. Negotiating change plans,
7. Consolidating client commitment, and
8. Switching flexibly between MI and other intervention styles. (p. 3)

Transitional Relationship Model/ Transitional Discharge Model

The Transitional Relationship Model (TRM) is theoretically grounded in the work of Hildegard Peplau; healing occurs in relationships. Therapeutic relationships can be formed with either professionals or peer supporters. The TRM was first developed to ease the transition from hospital to community, but its use has now been expanded to a variety of transitional care processes. There are two essential components of the TRM:

1. The therapeutic relationship should be extended until a new relationship with another care provider is established (continuing relationships formed in the hospital until new therapeutic relationships in the community are formed).
2. Trained peer support (often through a consumer survivor group) from a psychiatric survivor who has now successfully transitioned to the community.

In addition to producing positive therapeutic outcomes, the TRM also reduces time spent in hospital, the number of readmissions (Reynolds et al., 2004), and costs to the health care system (Forchuk et al., 2019) (see Box 10.6).

Technology and the Therapeutic Relationship

As technology develops and becomes increasingly accessible, traditional face-to-face communication can be replaced with technologic interactions. Situations such as the coronavirus disease 2019 (COVID-19) pandemic have quickly accelerated mental health services moving to a virtual environment. Telehealth modalities can include phone and video conferencing, mental health apps, and internet-delivered programs (Reay et al., 2020). Studies have found telephone or video conferencing to be as effective as standard in-person treatment for a variety of mental health disorders, particularly depression and anxiety disorders (Varker et al., 2019). Telehealth is a useful alternative for individuals living in rural and other underserved areas, those perceiving stigma associated with going to a provider's office, and those lacking reliable transportation (Goldin et al., 2021; Hasselberg, 2020). Patients report many advantages to receiving virtual care, including accessibility, convenience, cost-effectiveness, and privacy (Reay et al., 2020).

There are barriers to telehealth. Establishing a therapeutic relationship can take longer due to a lack of physical presence. Nonverbal communication, such as gestures, mannerisms, and tone, is more difficult to assess when not communicating in person (Reay et al., 2020). Misinterpretation of body language and behavioral manifestations may result in an inaccurate assessment of the patient (Goldin et al., 2021). Telepsychiatry is not appropriate when a patient's safety is an imminent risk. It is also less effective in individuals with severe mental illness who have diminished cognitive abilities and impaired insight (Reay et al., 2020). Lack of technology or unreliable internet access is another barrier. It is critical for communication over the internet to be HIPAA compliant and secure to maintain confidentiality. Many cheaper hardware devices may have "bloatware" that tracks information, and similarly "free" or cheap software may sell information to third parties. Hospital firewalls can be useful in establishing such connections (Forchuk et al., 2012). One must always be aware of a community agency, hospital, or research site's policies and best practices regarding communication online. Some commonly used platforms for online communication, such as Facebook Messenger, cannot meet privacy standards and should not be used in communication with patients. However, the internet is an invaluable resource for educational and research purposes.

SUMMARY OF KEY POINTS

- To deal therapeutically with the emotions, feelings, and problems of patients, nurses must understand their own values and beliefs and interpersonal strengths and limitations.

- The nurse–patient relationship is built on therapeutic communication, including verbal and nonverbal interactions between the nurse and the patient. Some communication skills include active listening, positive body language, appropriate verbal responses, and the ability of the nurse to interpret appropriately and analyze the patient's verbal and nonverbal behaviors.

BOX 10.6 • THE LAST MEETING

INEFFECTIVE APPROACH

Ms. J: Why did the other nurses bring you flowers and cards today?

Nurse: Well, that's because today is my last day; I'm transferring to the new hospital, across town.

Ms. J: Oh, um. I was just thinking, I need to talk to you about something important.

Nurse: What is it?

Ms. J: I have been worrying about my medication again.

Nurse: Oh, have you had any side effects?

Ms. J: No, but I might.

Nurse: I think you should tell the new nurse.

Ms. J: She is too new. She won't understand and you helped me last time. I feel so worried about your leaving. Is there any way you can stay? You said that you would check in, remember?

Nurse: Well, I could check on you tomorrow?

Ms. J: Oh, would you? I would really appreciate it if you would give me your new telephone number and that way I can tell you if anything happens.

Nurse: I don't know what the number will be, but you might be able to find it online.

EFFECTIVE APPROACH

Ms. J: Why did the other nurses bring you flowers and cards today?

Nurse: Oh, hello Ms. J. Do you remember? Today is my last day.

Ms. J: Oh, yes. Well, I need to talk to you about something important.

Nurse: We talked about that. Anything "important" needs to be shared with the new nurse.

Ms. J: But I want to tell you. You really made me feel better last time.

Nurse: Thank you but remember that you improved a lot because you know what to do in order to continue progressing. Saying goodbye can be very hard.

Ms. J: I'll miss you.

Nurse: Your feelings are very normal when relationships are ending. I will remember you in a very special way.

Ms. J: Can I please have your telephone number in case I need to talk to you?

Nurse: No, I can't give that to you. It is important that we say goodbye today. And, remember, you can always talk to the new nurse about your concerns.

Ms. J: Okay, I know. Goodbye. Good luck.

Nurse: Goodbye.

CRITICAL THINKING CHALLENGE

• What were some of the mistakes the nurse in the first scenario made?

• In the second scenario, how does therapeutic communication in the termination phase differ from effective communication in the working phase?

■ Two of the most important communication concepts are empathy and rapport.

■ In the nurse–patient relationship, as in all types of relationships, certain physical, emotional, and social boundaries and limitations need to be observed.

■ The therapeutic nurse–patient relationship consists of three major and overlapping stages or phases: the orientation phase, in which the patient and nurse meet and establish the parameters of the relationship; the working phase, in which the patient identifies and explores problems; and the resolution phase, in which the patient learns to manage the problems and the relationship is terminated.

■ The nontherapeutic relationship consists of three major and overlapping phases: the orientation phase,

Unfolding Patient Stories: Sharon Cole

Part 1

Sharon Cole, a 31-year-old female with bipolar disorder, had a surgical repair of an ankle fracture sustained in a fall during a manic episode. What verbal and nonverbal communication techniques can be used to establish a therapeutic relationship when she arrives on the orthopedic unit following surgery? Why is it important for the nurse to assess both verbal communication and nonverbal behavior? What methods can be used to facilitate a therapeutic interaction when she is manic, talking constantly, expressing grandiose thoughts that she is needed in Washington, DC to solve political issues, and wanting to leave the hospital? What approaches can block effective communication?

the grappling and struggling phase, and the phase of mutual withdrawal. A deteriorating relationship begins with a withholding phase, continues through the phases of avoiding and ignoring, and finally ends unsatisfactorily with a phase named "struggling with and making sense of."

CRITICAL THINKING CHALLENGES

1. Describe how you would do a suicide assessment on a distraught patient who comes to the physician's office expressing concerns about her ability to cope with her current situation. Describe how you would approach this patient if you determined she was suicidal. How might this assessment look different depending on the phase of the therapeutic relationship?

2. Describe how you would communicate with a patient who is concerned that the diagnosis of bipolar disorder will negatively affect their social and work relationships.

3. Your depressed patient does not seem inclined to talk about the depression. Describe the measures you would take to initiate a therapeutic relationship with them.

4. Think of a time that you worked with a patient you did not like. What was behind the dislike? How did you handle the therapeutic relationship? What could you do differently?

Movie Viewing Guides

Joker: 2019. *Joker* is written as a potential origins movie for this popular DC Comics villain. Arthur Fleck, who later in the film becomes known as Joker (Joaquin Phoenix), is a street clown and unsuccessful stand-up comic. He is afflicted with an uncontrollable laughter from an unspecified condition, which has led to institutionalization in the past and ostracization, exclusion, and abuse by society. The movie follows Arthur through a series of events that leads him to cement his identity as Joker.

VIEWING POINTS: A number of critics, including health care professionals, responded to *Joker* with opinion pieces depicting the potentially damaging and stigmatizing portrayal of mental illness and its association with violence. While it is normal for clients and health care professionals to enter the therapeutic relationship with preconceptions of one another, harmful attitudes and stigmatizing beliefs by the provider can create a barrier to therapeutic communication. How are people with mental illness portrayed in this film? What beliefs could be formed or reinforced about people with mental illness? What evidence exists to support or counter those beliefs (e.g., people with mental illness are violent)? How might your attitudes, beliefs, and preconceptions impact therapeutic communication with a client who has mental illness or a history of violence?

The King's Speech: 2010. This movie centers on the Duke of York/King George VI (Colin Firth), who has experienced incredible frustration with unsuccessful therapies to control his childhood stammer. His wife, the Duchess of York/Queen Elizabeth (Helena Bonham Carter), arranges services with Australian speech therapist and actor Lionel Logue (Geoffrey Rush), with resistance of the duke. Logue demonstrates results in the very first meeting, and over time, creates an atmosphere of trust that permits the Duke to disclose a deep-rooted secret related to his condition.

VIEWING POINTS: Although many differences exist in this relationship, including power, social status, and culture, Logue creates a dynamic of equity and trust from the start. How does Logue close the gap on these differences? What factors contribute to the development of rapport, trust, and safety in the relationship?

Call Me Crazy: A Five Film: 2013. This made-for-TV film follows five individuals and their experience with mental illness. Lucy (Brittney Snow) is a law student who experiences an episode of psychosis after stopping her medication to prove she does not have schizophrenia. She is admitted to a hospital, where she receives individual and group therapy and befriends Bruce (Jason Ritter). The focus turns to another character, Grace (Sarah Hyland), a youth who has been hiding her mother's (Melissa Leo) experience of bipolar disorder from friends but finds support from an unlikely place. The segment on Allison (Sofia Vassilieva) further demonstrates the impact of mental illness on family as she expresses her experience with her sister. Eddie (Mitch Rouse) is a comedian who has been hiding his increasing feelings of depression from his wife, Julia (Lea Thompson). The final individual is Maggie (Jennifer Hudson), a war veteran who has returned home but has recurrent nightmares following trauma she endured.

VIEWING POINTS: Throughout the film, each character displays defense mechanisms to cope with personal challenges. Identify these coping strategies and determine whether they are healthy or unhealthy. How would the signs and symptoms of each illness impact communication and the therapeutic relationship?

Love and Mercy: 2014. This film details the life of Brian Wilson in two time points: a young Brain Wilson (Paul Dano) in the 1960s as he begins to experience symptoms of auditory hallucinations and mania and an older Brian Wilson (John Cusak) in the 1980s as he was heavily exploited by psychotherapist Dr. Eugene Lundy (Paul Giamatti). A chance encounter with Melinda Ledbetter (Elizabeth Banks) when Brian was purchasing a car leads to a romantic relationship between the two. Melinda is distrustful of Dr. Lundy, who exhibits angry outbursts toward Brian and has him under 24-hour surveillance. With the help of housekeeper Gloria (Diana Maria

Riviera) and Brian's brother, Carl Wilson (Brett Davern), Melinda is able to release Brian from Dr. Lundy's control and help him access the care he needs to live a quality life.

VIEWING POINTS: This film demonstrates gross ethical and boundary crossings by a health care professional. What professional boundaries and ethics did Dr. Lundy violate? What guidelines are available in your jurisdiction that describe professional boundaries and ethics in the therapeutic relationship and how would you incorporate these in your care?

Good Will Hunting: 1997. Robin Williams plays a therapist, Dr. Sean Maguire. His patient, Will Hunting (Matt Damon), is a janitor at MIT who is a troubled genius. Through a strong relationship, Will begins to realize his potential. This film deals with intense blocks to communication, as well as issues around justice system use and class.

VIEWING POINTS: Watch closely how the relationship develops between the characters played by Williams and Damon. How does the relationship change as the characters move through different stages of their relationship? Do you think that the level of self-disclosure depicted is therapeutic?

Silver Linings Playbook: 2012. This film portrays one man's struggle to return to society after he is released from a psychiatric inpatient hospital. Patrick (Bradley Cooper), who is trying to reconnect with his ex-wife and manage bipolar disorder, meets Tiffany (Jennifer Lawrence), who is struggling with depression following the death of her husband. Throughout the film, issues relating to stigma, establishing a therapeutic relationship, and how individuals suffering from mental illness may mutually support each other are dealt with.

VIEWING POINTS: As part of Patrick's release, he is mandated to continue meeting with a therapist. Think of this in relation to the Transitional Discharge Model discussed earlier. How is it similar and how is it different? Others often stigmatize Patrick and Tiffany. Can you identify where this happens and how such treatment might be avoided? Reflect on the fact that many other characters seem to have undiagnosed mental illnesses (such as obsessive-compulsive disorder and anxiety). How do the characters help and hurt each other as they deal with the challenges of mental illness?

REFERENCES

Ashcraft, L., & Anthony, W. (2014). Tools for transforming language into therapeutic strength-based communication. (Person-centered alternatives to commonly used words and phrases). Presentation at Annual APNA Conference. https://www.apna.org/i4a/pages/index.cfm?pageid=6025

Berg, R. C., Ross, M. W., & Tikkanen, R. (2011). The effectiveness of MI4MSM: How useful is motivational interviewing as an HIV risk prevention program for men who have sex with men? A systematic review. *AIDS Education and Prevention, 23*(6), 533–549.

Boyd, M. (1995). Communication with patients, families, healthcare providers, and diverse cultures. In M. Strader & P. Decker (Eds.), *Role transition to patient care management* (p. 431). Appleton & Lange.

Coatsworth-Puspoky, R., Forchuk, C., & Ward-Griffin, C. (2006). Nurse–client processes in mental health: Recipient's perspectives. *Journal of Psychiatric and Mental Health Nursing, 13*(3), 347–355.

Dean, S., Britt, E., Bell, E., & Stanley, J. (2016). Motivational interviewing to enhance adolescent mental health treatment engagement: A randomized clinical trial. *Psychological Medicine, 46*(9), 1961–1969.

DiClemente, C. C., Corno, C. M., Graydon, M. M., Wiprovnick, A. E., & Knoblach, D. J. (2017). Motivational interviewing, enhancement, and brief interventions over the last decade: A review of reviews of efficacy and effectiveness. *Psychology of Addictive Behaviors, 31*(8), 862–887.

Ekong, G., & Kavookjian, J. (2016). Motivational interviewing and outcomes in adults with type 2 diabetes: A systematic review. *Patient Education and Counseling, 99*(6), 944–952.

Forchuk, C., Carmichael, K., Golea, G., Johnston, N., Martin, M. L., Patterson, P., Ray, K., Robinson, T., Sogbein, S. A., Srivastava, R., & Skov, T. (2006). *Nursing best practice guideline: Establishing therapeutic relationships (revision).* Registered Nurses Association of Ontario.

Forchuk, C., Martin, M. L., Corring, D., Sherman, D., Srivastava, R., Harerimana, B., & Cheng, R. (2019). Cost-effectiveness of the implementation of a transitional discharge model for community integration of psychiatric clients. Practice insights and policy implications. *International Journal of Mental Health, 48*(3), 236–249.

Forchuk, C., Martin, M. L., Jensen, E., Ouseley, S., Sealy, Pl, Beal, G., Reynolds, W., Sharkey, S. (2013). Integrating an evidence-based intervention into clinical practice: 'Transitional relationship model.' *Journal of Psychiatric and Mental Health Nursing, 20*(7), 584–594.

Forchuk, F., Martin, M. L., Jensen, E., Ouseley, S., Sealy, P., Beal, G., Reynolds, W., Sharkey, S. (2012). Integrating the transitional relationship model into clinical practice. *Archives of Psychiatric Nursing, 26*(5), 374–381.

Frost, H., Campbell, P., Maxwell, M., O'Carroll, R. E., Dombrowski, S. U., Williams, B., Cheyne, H., Coles, E., Pollock, A. (2018). Effectiveness of motivational interviewing on adult behaviour change in health and social care settings: A systematic review of reviews. *PLOS One, 13*(10), 1–39.

Goldin, D., Maltseva, T., Scaccianoce, M., & Brenes, F. (2021). Cultural and practical implications for psychiatric telehealth services: A response to COVID-19. *Journal of Transcultural Nursing, 32*(2), 186–190.

Hall, E. T. (1990). *The hidden dimension.* Anchor Books.

Hasselberg, M. J. (2020). The digital revolution in behavioral health. *Journal of the American Psychiatric Nurses Association, 26*(1), 102–111.

Miller, W. R., & Moyers, T. B. (2006). Eight stages in learning motivational interviewing. *Journal of Teaching in the Addictions, 5*(1), 3–17.

Orlando, I. (1961). *Orlando's dynamic nurse-patient relationship: Function, process and principles.* G. P. Putman's Sons.

Peplau, H. E. (1952, 1992). *Interpersonal relations in nursing.* G. P. Putnam's Sons.

Pounds, K. G. (2017). A theoretical and clinical perspective on social relatedness and the patient with serious mental illness. *Journal of the American Psychiatric Nurses Association, 23*(3), 193–199.

Reay, R. E., Looi, J. C. L., & Keightley, P. (2020). Telehealth mental health services during COVID-19: Summary of evidence and clinical practice. *Australasian Psychiatry, 28*(5), 514–516.

Reynolds, W., Lauder, W., Sharkey, S., Maciver, S., Veitch, T., & Cameron, D. (2004). The effects of transitional discharge model for psychiatric patients. *Journal of Psychiatric and Mental Health Nursing, 11*(1), 82–88.

Sullivan, K., Guzman, A., & Lancellotti, D. (2017). Nursing communication and the gender identity spectrum. *American Nurse Today, 12*(5), 6–11.

Varker, T., Brand, R. M., Ward, J., Terhaag, S., & Phelps, A. (2019). Efficacy of synchronous telepsychology for people with anxiety, depression, posttraumatic stress disorder, and adjustment disorder: A rapid evidence assessment. *Psychological Services, 16*(4), 621–635.

Wade, M., Brown, N., Winter, S., Dancy, S., & Majumdar, A. (2019). Effects of disability or medical condition on physical activity and mental wellbeing: A community-based motivational interviewing physical activity intervention. *The Lancet, 394*(2), S95–S95.

Wong-Anuchit, C., Chantamit-o-pas, C., Schneider, J., & Mills, A. C. (2019). Motivational interviewing-based compliance/adherence therapy interventions to improve psychiatric symptoms of people with severe mental illness: Meta-analysis. *Journal of the American Psychiatric Nurses Association, 25*(2), 122–133.

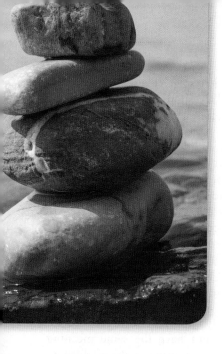

11
The Psychiatric–Mental Health Nursing Process

Mary Ann Boyd

KEYCONCEPTS

- assessment
- clinical Judgment
- mental status examination
- outcomes
- recovery-oriented nursing interventions
- spirituality

LEARNING OBJECTIVES

After studying this chapter, you will be able to:

1. Define the recovery-oriented nursing process in psychiatric–mental health nursing.

2. Conduct a psychiatric–mental health nursing assessment.

3. Apply clinical judgment in recognizing, analyzing, and prioritizing assessment data.

4. Develop recovery-oriented goals in collaboration with the patient.

5. Apply recovery-oriented psychiatric–mental health nursing interventions by supporting patient strengths and addressing mental health problems and mental disorders.

6. Collaborate with the patient in evaluating outcomes.

KEY TERMS

- Affect • Asynchronous communication • Behavior modification • Bibliotherapy • Body image • Cognition • Conflict resolution • Containment • Counseling • Cultural brokering • De-escalation • Distraction • Dysphoric • Emotional well-being • Environmental well-being • Euphoric • Euthymic • Financial well-being • Guided imagery • Home visits • Insight • Intellectual well-being • Labile • Milieu therapy • Mood • Occupational well-being • Open communication • Patient observation • Personal identity • Physical well-being • Psychoeducation • Reminiscence • Risk factors • Self-care • Self-concept • Self-esteem • Social well-being • Spiritual care assessment • Spiritual support • Structured interaction • Synchronous communication • Token economy • Validation

INTRODUCTION

The psychiatric–mental health nursing process is approached from the perspectives of wellness and strength as well as mental health problems. The process is guided by recovery principles and practices (see Chapters 1 and 9). In this text, the nursing process is built by recognizing and analyzing patient's data and cues,

prioritizing problems or concerns, generating a plan in collaboration with the patient, using clinical judgment, applying interventions, and evaluating outcomes. This chapter describes some, but not all, of the commonly applied interventions. The nursing process targeting specific psychiatric disorders and emotional problems is discussed in later chapters.

RECOVERY-ORIENTED PSYCHIATRIC– MENTAL HEALTH NURSING ASSESSMENT

Assessment is the collection and interpretation of information related to health, wellness, strengths, functional status, and human responses to mental health problems. Assessment involves recognizing cues and analyzing the information for significance to the patient's health status. These data are collected within a collaborative relationship with the person seeking nursing care.

Assessment is not an isolated activity. Rather, it is a systematic and ongoing process that occurs throughout the nurse's care of the patient. The psychiatric–mental health nursing assessment (Box 11.1) is a basic guide to collecting assessment data. Assessment information is entered into the patient's written or computerized record, which may be presented in several different formats, including forms, checklists, narratives, and problem-oriented notes.

> **KEYCONCEPT Assessment** is the deliberate and systematic collection and interpretation of information or data to determine current and past health, wellness, strengths, functional status, and mental health problems, both actual and potential.

Assessment begins with the first contact with the patient when a collaborative relationship is initiated. Legal consent must be given by the patient, and the nurse must follow the Health Insurance Portability and Accountability Act of 1996 guidelines (see Chapter 4). The patient must develop a sense of trust before they will be comfortable revealing intimate life details. It is of paramount importance that the nurse have a healthy knowledge of themselves as well (Box 11.2). The nurse's own biases and values, which may be different from those of the patient, can influence the nurse's interpretation of assessment data. A careful self-assessment helps the nurse interpret the data objectively.

Patient Interviews

An assessment interview usually involves direct questions to obtain facts, clarify perceptions, validate observations, interpret the meanings of facts, or compare information. The specific questions may take different forms. The nurse must clearly state the purpose of the interview and, if necessary, modify the interview process, so that both the patient and nurse agree on its purpose. The nurse may choose to use open- or closed-ended questions. Open-ended questions are most helpful when beginning the interview because they allow the nurse to observe how the patient responds verbally and nonverbally. They also convey caring and interest in the person's well-being, which helps to establish rapport. Nurses should use closed-ended questions when they need specific information. For example, "How old are you?" asks for specific

information about the patient's age. These types of questions limit the individual's response but often serve as good follow-up questions for clarification of thoughts or feelings expressed.

Questions such as "How did you come to this clinic today?" allow patients to describe their experience in their own way. Some patients may answer this question concretely by saying, "I took a taxi" or "I came by car." Others may address this question by responding, "My family thought I should come, so they brought me" or "Well, I got up this morning … I took a shower, got dressed … and then, well you know, it's difficult sometimes to decide." Each of these answers helps the nurse assess the patient's thinking process as well as evaluate the content of the response.

Clarification is extremely important during the assessment process. Words do not have the same meaning to all people. Education, language, culture, history, and experience may influence the meaning of words. Sometimes, simple and direct questioning provides clarification. In other situations, the nurse may clarify by providing a specific example for a more global thought the patient is trying to express. For example, a patient may say, "Things have been so strange since the children left." The nurse may respond with, "Sometimes, parents feel sad and empty when their children leave home. They don't know what to do with their time." Frequently summarizing what has been said allows the patient the opportunity to correct the nurse's interpretation. For example, verbalizing a sequence of events that the patient has reported may help to identify omissions or inconsistencies. Restating information or reflecting feelings that the patient has described also allows opportunity for clarification. It is essential that nurses understand exactly what patients are attempting to communicate before beginning to intervene. Box 11.3 provides a summary of other behaviors that enhance the effectiveness of an assessment interview.

Many psychiatric symptoms are beyond a patient's awareness. Family members, friends, and other health care professionals are important sources of information. Before seeking information from others, the nurse must obtain permission from the patient. The nurse needs to provide the patient with a clear explanation of why the information is needed and how it will be used. The nurse should explain that the strength-based assessment will include questions about wellness and strengths as well as mental health problems because these are all related to well-being.

Assessment of Trauma

During the assessment, the nurse should listen for any clues of trauma including physical, emotional, or social events. If a person has been hospitalized for any mental health problem, it is important to understand the meaning

BOX 11.1

Psychiatric–Mental Health Nursing Assessment

I. **Major reason for seeking help** _____

II. **Initial information**
   Name _____
   Age _____ Marital status _____ Gender _____ Ethnic identification _____

III. **Present and past health status** _____ (Include ht., wt., BMI)
   Summary of strengths and wellness related to physical health

	Normal	Treated	Untreated
Physical functions: System review	☐	☐	☐
Elimination	☐	☐	☐
Activity/exercise	☐	☐	☐
Sleep	☐	☐	☐
Appetite and nutrition	☐	☐	☐
Hydration	☐	☐	☐
Sexuality	☐	☐	☐
Self-care	☐	☐	☐
Neurological status (head trauma, movement disorder)	☐	☐	☐
Existing physical illnesses	☐	☐	☐
Medications (prescription and over the counter)	Dosage	Side effects	Frequency
Significant laboratory tests	Values	Normal range	

IV. **Mental health problems**
   Major concerns regarding mental health problem _____
   Major loss/change in past year: No _____ Yes _____
   Fear of violence: No _____ Yes _____
   Past abuse or trauma: No _____ Yes _____
   Strategies for managing problems/disorder _____

V. **Mental status examination**
   General observations (appearance, psychomotor activity, attitude) _____
   Orientation (time, place, person) _____
   Mood, affect, emotions _____
   Speech (verbal ability, speed, use of words correctly) _____
   Thought processes (tangential, logic, repetition, rhyming of words, loose connections, disorganized) _____
   Cognition and intellectual performance _____
   Attention and concentration _____
   Abstract reasoning and comprehension _____
   Memory (recall, short-term, recent, and remote) _____
   Judgment and insight _____

VI. **Significant behaviors (psychomotor, agitation, aggression, withdrawn)** _____

VII. **Self-concept (body image, self-esteem, personal identity)** _____

VIII. **Stress and coping patterns** _____

IX. **Risk assessment**
   Suicide: High _____ Low _____ Assault/homicide: High _____ Low _____
   Suicidal thoughts or ideation: No _____ Yes _____
   Current thoughts of harming self _____
   Intention _____
   Behavior _____
   Lethality _____
   Assault/homicide thoughts: No _____ Yes _____
   What do you do when angry with a stranger? _____
   What do you do when angry with family or partner? _____
   Have you ever hit or pushed anyone? No _____ Yes _____
   Have you ever been arrested for assault? No _____ Yes _____
   Current thoughts of harming others _____

X. **Functional status**
   Changes in functioning (work, school, home) _____

XI. **Social systems**
   Family assessment
      Family members _____
      Members important to patient _____
      Decision makers, family roles, supportive members _____
   Cultural assessment
      Cultural group _____
      Cultural group's view of health and mental illness _____
      What cultural rules do you try to live by? _____
      Important cultural foods _____
      Community resources _____

XII. **Spiritual assessment**

XIII. **Economic status**

XIV. **Legal status**

XV. **Quality of life**

XVI. **Spiritual Care Assessment**

XVII. **SUMMARY OF PSYCHOSOCIAL STRENGTHS:**
Summary of significant data that can be used in prioritizing patient needs.
SIGNATURE/TITLE _____ Date _____

BOX 11.2

Self-Concept Awareness

Self-awareness is important in any interaction. To understand a patient's self-concept, the nurse must be aware of their own self-concept. By answering these questions, nurses can evaluate self-concept components and increase their self-understanding. The more comfortable nurses are with themselves, the more effective they can be in each patient interaction.

BODY IMAGE

- How do I feel about my body?
- How important is my physical appearance?
- How does my body measure up to my ideal body? (How would I like to appear?)
- What is positive about my body?
- What would I like to change about my body?
- How does my body image affect my self-esteem?

SELF-ESTEEM

- When do I feel confident and good about myself?
- When do I feel unimportant?
- What do I do when I feel good about myself? (Call friends, socialize?)
- What do I do when I have negative feelings about myself? (Withdraw, dress poorly?)
- When do I make negative statements?
- Am I able to correct my negative self-statements?

PERSONAL IDENTITY

- How do I describe myself?
- What three adjectives describe who I am?
- Do I identify with a particular cultural group, family role, or place of residence?
- What would I like to have on my tombstone?

BOX 11.3

Assessment Interview Behaviors

The following behaviors carried out by the nurse will enhance the effectiveness of the assessment interview:

- *Exhibiting empathy*—to show empathy to the patient, the nurse uses phrases such as "That must have been upsetting for you" or "I can understand your hurt feelings."
- *Giving recognition*—the nurse gives recognition by listening actively: verbally encouraging the patient to continue and nonverbally presenting an open, interested demeanor.
- *Demonstrating acceptance*—note that acceptance does not mean agreement or nonagreement with the patient but is a neutral stance that allows the patient to continue.
- *Restating*—the nurse tries to clarify what the patient is trying to say by restating it.
- *Reflecting*—the nurse presents the patient's last statement as a question. This gives the patient a chance to expand on the information.
- *Focusing*—the nurse attempts to bring the conversation back to the questions at hand when the patient goes off on a tangent.
- *Using open-ended questions*—general questions give the patient a chance to speak freely.
- *Presenting reality*—the nurse presents reality when the patient makes unrealistic or exaggerated statements.
- *Making observations*—the nurse says aloud what patient behaviors are observed to give the patient a chance to speak to those behaviors. For example, the nurse may say, "I notice you are twisting your fingers; are you nervous about something?"

---

of the experience to the individual. Psychiatric hospitalizations can be traumatic and can contribute to posttraumatic stress disorders. Any abuse or mistreatment should be identified in the assessment (see Chapters 23 and 29).

Virtual Mental Health Assessment

There is an emerging trend to use virtual health technology (i.e., telehealth) in assessment and treatment of mental health problems. The need for social distancing due to the COVID-19 pandemic escalated the use of digital tools. Limiting face-to-face contact is especially important for vulnerable populations such as the older adult. Virtual health care increases access to care in those areas where there is a shortage of services.

There are two types of telehealth used in mental health. **Synchronous communication**, real-time telehealth interactions between nurse and patient, and asynchronous or stored-and-forward telehealth. In asynchronous communication, clinical information is transmitted from patient to clinician or clinician to patient and stored for review at a later point. **Asynchronous communication** can include emails, text message, and video recordings. Mobile technologies, cell phones, and other devices are becoming increasingly popular and useful throughout the care process. Consistent with patient-centered care, use of mobile health applications (*mHealth*) is useful for history taking, interviewing, assessment, and treatment as well as clinician support for decision-making and up-to-date treatment (Tsanas et al., 2021).

It is important that nurses assess their patients' use of virtual devices (Smahel et al., 2019). These devices can be incorporated into their care based on patient preference, skill, and need. There are some risks related to using virtual technology, such as privacy breaches, unnecessary self-disclosure, and cyberbullying.

Assessment of Physical Health

Many mental disorders produce physical symptoms, such as the lack of appetite and weight loss associated with depression. Physical health can also affect mental health and illness, producing a recurrence or increase in symptoms. Many physical disorders may present first with symptoms considered to be psychiatric. For example, hypothyroidism often presents with feelings of lethargy, decreased concentration, and depressed mood. For these reasons, physical health information about the patient is always considered.

Current and Past Health Status

Beginning with a history of the patient's general medical condition, the nurse should consider the following:

- Availability of, frequency of, and most recent medical evaluation, including test results
- Past hospitalizations and surgical procedures
- Vision and hearing impairments
- Cardiac problems, including cerebrovascular accidents (strokes), myocardial infarctions (heart attacks), and childhood illnesses
- Respiratory problems, particularly those that result in a lack of oxygen to the brain
- Neurologic problems, particularly head injuries, seizure disorders, or any losses of consciousness
- Endocrine disorders, particularly unstable diabetes or thyroid or adrenal dysfunction
- Immune disorders, particularly human immunodeficiency virus (HIV) and autoimmune disorders
- Use, exposure, abuse, or dependence on substances, including alcohol, tobacco, prescription drugs, illicit drugs, and herbal preparations

Physical Examination

Body Systems Review

After the nurse obtains historical information, they should examine physiologic systems to evaluate the patient's current physical condition. The psychiatric nurse should pay special attention to various systems that treatment may affect. For example, if a patient is being treated with antihypertensive medication, the dosage may need to be adjusted if an antipsychotic medication is prescribed. If a patient is overweight or has diabetes, some psychiatric medications can affect these conditions. Patients with compromised immune function (HIV, cancer) may experience mood alterations.

Neurologic Status

Particular attention is paid to recent head trauma; episodes of hypertension; and changes in personality, speech, or the ability to handle activities of daily living (ADLs). Cranial nerve dysfunction, reflexes, muscle strength, and balance are included in a thorough assessment. The nurse routinely assesses and documents movement disorders using such tools as the Abnormal Involuntary Movement Scales (see Chapter 24 and Appendix B).

Laboratory Results

The nurse reviews and documents any available laboratory data, especially any abnormalities. Hepatic, renal, or urinary abnormalities are particularly important to document because these systems metabolize or excrete many psychiatric medications. In addition, the nurse notes abnormal white blood cell and electrolyte levels. Laboratory data are especially important, particularly if the nurse is the only person in the mental health team who has a "medical" background (Table 11.1).

TABLE 11.1	**SELECTED HEMATOLOGIC MEASURES AND THEIR RELEVANCE TO PSYCHIATRIC DISORDERS**	
Test	**Possible Results**	**Possible Cause or Meaning**
Complete Blood Count		
Leukocyte (WBC) count	Leukopenia—decrease in leukocytes (WBCs)	May be produced by phenothiazine, clozapine, carbamazepine
		Lithium causes a benign mild to moderate increase (11,000–17,000/mcL)
	Agranulocytosis—decrease in number of granulocytic leukocytes	NMS can be associated with increases of 15,000–30,000/mm3 in about 40% of cases
	Leukocytosis—increase in leukocyte count above normal limits	
WBC differential	"Shift to the left"—from segmented neutrophils to band forms	Shift often suggests a bacterial infection but has been reported in about 40% of cases of NMS
RBC count	Polycythemia—increased RBCs	Primary form—true polycythemia caused by several disease states
		Secondary form—compensation for decreased oxygenation, as in chronic pulmonary disease
		Blood is more viscous, and the patient should not become dehydrated

(Continued)

TABLE 11.1   SELECTED HEMATOLOGIC MEASURES AND THEIR RELEVANCE TO PSYCHIATRIC DISORDERS (Continued)

Test	Possible Results	Possible Cause or Meaning
	Decreased RBCs	Decrease may be related to some types of anemia, which requires further evaluation
Hct	Elevations	Elevation may be caused by dehydration
	Decreased Hct	Anemia may be associated with a wide range of mental status changes, including asthenia, depression, and psychosis
		20% of women of childbearing age in the United States have iron-deficiency anemia
Hb	Decreased	Another indicator of anemia; further evaluation of source requires review of erythrocyte indices
Erythrocyte indices, such as RDW	Elevated RDW	Finding suggests a combined anemia, as in that from chronic alcoholism, resulting from both vitamin B_{12} and folate acid deficiencies and iron deficiency
		Oral contraceptives also decrease vitamin B_{12}

Other Hematologic Measures

Test	Possible Results	Possible Cause or Meaning
Vitamin B_{12}	Deficiency	Neuropsychiatric symptoms, such as psychosis, paranoia, fatigue, agitation, marked personality change, dementia, and delirium may develop
Folate	Deficiency	The use of alcohol, phenytoin, oral contraceptives, and estrogens may be responsible
Platelet count	Thrombocytopenia—decreased platelet count	Some psychiatric medications, such as carbamazepine, phenothiazine, or clozapine, or other nonpsychiatric medications may cause thrombocytopenia
		Several medical conditions are other causes

Serum Electrolytes

Test	Possible Results	Possible Cause or Meaning
Sodium	Hyponatremia—low serum sodium	Significant mental status changes may ensue. Condition is associated with Addison disease, the SIADH, and polydipsia (water intoxication) as well as carbamazepine use
Potassium	Hypokalemia—low serum potassium	Produces weakness, fatigue, ECG changes; paralytic ileus and muscle paresis may develop
		Common in individuals with bulimic behavior or psychogenic vomiting and use or abuse of diuretics; laxative abuse may contribute; can be life threatening
Chloride	Elevation	Chloride tends to increase to compensate for lower bicarbonate
	Decrease	Binging–purging behavior and repeated vomiting may be causes
Bicarbonate	Elevation	Causes may be binging and purging in eating disorders, excessive use of laxatives, or psychogenic vomiting
	Decrease	Decrease may develop in some patients with hyperventilation syndrome and panic disorder

Renal Function Tests

Test	Possible Results	Possible Cause or Meaning
BUN	Elevation	Increase is associated with mental status changes, lethargy, and delirium
		Cause may be dehydration
		Potential toxicity of medications cleared via the kidney, such as lithium and amantadine, may increase
Serum creatinine	Elevation	Level usually does not become elevated until about 50% of nephrons in the kidney are damaged

Serum Enzymes

Test	Possible Results	Possible Cause or Meaning
Amylase	Elevation	Level appears to increase after binging and purging behavior in eating disorders and declines when these behaviors stop

TABLE 11.1	SELECTED HEMATOLOGIC MEASURES AND THEIR RELEVANCE TO PSYCHIATRIC DISORDERS (*Continued*)	
Test	**Possible Results**	**Possible Cause or Meaning**
ALT—formerly SGPT	ALT > AST	Disparity is common in acute forms of viral and drug-induced hepatic dysfunction
	Elevation	Mild elevations are common with use of sodium valproate
AST—formerly SGOT	AST > ALT	Severe elevations in chronic forms of liver disease and postmyocardial infarction may develop
CPK	Elevations of the isoenzyme related to muscle tissue	Muscle tissue injury is the cause
		Level is elevated in NMS
		Level is also elevated by repeated intramuscular injections (e.g., antipsychotics)
Thyroid Function		
Serum triiodothyronine (T_3)	Decrease	Hypothyroidism and nonthyroid illness cause decrease
		Individuals with depression may convert less T_4 to T_3 peripherally but not out of the normal range
		Medications such as lithium and sodium valproate may suppress thyroid function, but clinical significance is unknown
	Elevations	Hyperthyroidism, T_3, and toxicosis may produce mood changes, anxiety, and symptoms of mania
Serum thyroxine (T_4)	Elevations	Hyperthyroidism is a cause
TSH or thyrotropin	Elevations	Hypothyroidism—symptoms may appear very much like those of depression except for additional physical signs of cold intolerance, dry skin, hair loss, bradycardia, and so on
		Lithium—may also cause elevations
	Decrease	Considered nondiagnostic—may be hyperthyroidism, pituitary hypothyroidism, or even euthyroid status

Note. ALT = alanine aminotransferase; AST = aspartate aminotransferase; BUN = blood urea nitrogen; CPK = creatine phosphokinase; ECG = electrocardiogram; Hb = hemoglobin; Hct = hematocrit; NMS = neuroleptic malignant syndrome; RBC = Red blood cell; RDW = red cell distribution width; SIADH = syndrome of inappropriate secretion of antidiuretic hormone; SGPT = serum glutamic pyruvic transaminase; SGOT = serum glutamic oxaloacetic transaminase; TSH = thyroid-stimulating hormone; WBC = white blood cell.

Physical Functions

Elimination

The nurse should inquire about and document the patient's daily urinary and bowel habits. Various medications can affect bladder and bowel functioning, so a baseline must be noted. For example, diarrhea and frequency of urination can occur with the use of lithium carbonate. Anticholinergic effects of antipsychotic medication can cause constipation and urinary hesitancy or retention.

Activity and Exercise

The patient's daily methods and levels of activity and exercise must be queried and documented. Activities are important interventions, and baseline information is needed to determine what the patient already enjoys or dislikes and whether they are getting sufficient exercise or adequate recreation. A patient may have altered activity or exercise in response to medication or therapies. In addition, many psychiatric medications cause weight gain, and nurses need to develop interventions that assist the patient in increasing activities to counteract the weight gain.

Sleep

Changes in sleep patterns often reflect changes in a patient's emotions and are symptoms of disorders. If the patient responds positively to a question about changes in sleep patterns, it is important to clarify just what those changes are. For example, "difficulty falling asleep" means different things to different people. For a person who usually falls right to sleep, it could mean that it takes 10 extra minutes to fall asleep. For a person who normally takes 35 minutes to fall asleep, it could mean that it takes 90 minutes to do so.

Appetite and Nutrition

Changes in appetite and nutritional intake are assessed and documented because they can indicate changes in moods or relapse. For example, a patient who is depressed may not notice hunger or even that they do not have the energy to prepare food. Others may handle stressful emotions through eating more than usual. This information also provides valuable clues to possible eating disorders and problems with body image.

Obesity is one of the major health problems of many Americans, but it is particularly problematic for persons with psychiatric disorders. Many of the medications are associated with weight gain. A baseline body mass index should be determined as treatment is initiated.

Hydration

Gaining perspective on how much fluid patients normally drink and how much they are drinking now provides important data. Some medications can cause retention of fluids, and others can cause diuresis; thus, the patient's current fluid status must be understood.

Sexuality

Questioning a patient on issues involving sexuality requires comfort with one's own sexuality. Changes in sexual activity as well as comfort with sexual orientation are important to assess. Issues involving sexual orientation that are unsettled in a patient or between a patient and family member may cause anxiety, shame, or discomfort. It is necessary to explore how comfortable the patient is with their sexuality and sexual functioning. These questions should be asked in a matter of fact but gentle and nonjudgmental manner. Initiating the topic of sexuality may begin with a question such as "Are you sexually active?" Birth control medications may also alter mood.

Self-Care

Self-care is the ability to perform ADLs successfully. Often, a patient's ability to care for themselves or carry out ADLs, such as washing and dressing, are indicative of their psychological state. For example, a depressed patient may not have the energy to change into clean clothes. This information may also help the nurse to determine actual or potential obstacles to a patient's compliance with a treatment plan.

Pharmacologic Assessment

The review of systems serves as a baseline from which the nurse may judge whether the initiation of a medication exacerbates symptoms or causes new ones to develop. It is important to determine which medications the patient takes now or has taken in the past. These include over-the-counter, herbal, or nonprescription medications as well as prescribed medications. This assessment is important for reasons other than serving as a baseline. It helps target possible drug interactions, determines whether the patient has already used medications that are being considered, and identifies whether medications may be causing psychiatric symptoms.

Strengths and Wellness Assessment

During the assessment, the nurse should identify areas of strength and wellness including **physical well-being** or positive sleep patterns, healthy diet, or motivation to engage in healthy behaviors. Does the patient recognize the need for physical activity, diet, and nutrition? Recognition of this wellness dimension can help motivate the individual to improve these behaviors.

Psychological Assessment

Psychological concerns are the traditional emphasis of the psychiatric–mental health nursing assessment. By definition, mental disorders and emotional problems are manifested through psychological symptoms related to mental status, moods, thoughts, behaviors, and interpersonal relationships. Psychological strengths, psychological growth, and development are important parts of this assessment as well as wellness and emotional and intellectual well-being.

Mental Health Problems

Individual concerns regarding a mental health problem or its consequences are included in the mental health assessment. A mental disorder, like any other illness, affects patients and families in many ways. It is safe to say that a mental illness changes a person's life, and the nurse should identify what the changes are and their meaning to the patient and family members. Many patients experience specific fears, such as losing their job, family, or safety. Because the nurse will be supporting coping strategies, it is important to identify current strategies or behaviors the patient uses. A simple question such as "How do you deal with your voices when you are with other people?" may initiate a discussion about responses to the mental disorder or emotional problem.

Mental Status Examination

The mental status examination establishes a baseline, provides a snapshot of where the patient is at a moment, and creates a written record. Areas of assessment include general observations, orientation, mood and affect, speech, thought processes, and cognition. Box 11.4 provides a narrative note of the results from a patient's mental status examination.

KEYCONCEPT The mental status examination is an organized systematic approach to assessment of an individual's current psychiatric condition.

General Observations

At the beginning of the interview, the nurse should record their initial impressions of the patient. These general observations include the patient's appearance, affect, psychomotor activity, and overall behavior. How is the patient dressed? Is the dress appropriate for the weather and setting? What is the patient's affect (emotional expression)? What behaviors is the patient displaying? For example, the same nurse assessed two male patients with depression. At the beginning of the mental status examination, the differences between these two men were very clear. The nurse described the first patient as "a large, well-dressed man who is agitated and appears angry, shifts in his seat, and does not maintain eye contact. He interrupts often in the initial explanation of mental status." The nurse described the other patient as a "small, unshaven, disheveled man with a strong body odor who appears withdrawn. He shuffles as he walks, speaks very softly, appears sad, and avoids direct eye contact."

Orientation

The nurse can determine the patient's orientation by asking the date, time, and current location of the interview setting. If a patient knows the year but not the exact date, the interviewer can ask the season. A person's orientation tells the nurse the extent of confusion. If a patient does not know the year or the place of the interview, they are exhibiting considerable confusion.

Mood and Affect

Mood refers to the prominent, sustained, overall emotions that the person expresses and exhibits. Mood may

be sustained for days or weeks, or it may fluctuate during the course of a day. For example, some patients with depression have a diurnal variation in their mood. They experience their lowest mood in the morning, but as the day progresses, their depressed mood lifts and they feel somewhat better in the evening. Terms used to describe mood include **euthymic** (normal), **euphoric** (elated), **labile** (changeable), and **dysphoric** (depressed, disquieted, and restless).

Affect refers to the person's capacity to vary outward emotional expression. Affect fluctuates with thought content and can be observed in facial expressions, vocal fluctuations, and gestures. During the assessment, the patient may exhibit anger, frustration, irritation, apathy, and helplessness while their overall mood remains unchanged.

Affect can be described in terms of range, intensity, appropriateness, and stability. Range can be full or restricted. An individual who expresses several different emotions consistent with the stated feelings and content being expressed is described as having a *full range* of affect that is congruent with the situation. An individual who expresses few emotions has a restricted affect. For example, a patient could be describing the recent tragic death of a loved one in a monotone with little expression. In determining whether this response is normal, the nurse compares the patient's emotional response with the cultural norm for that particular response. *Intensity* can be increased, flat, or blunted. The nurse determines whether the emotional response is *appropriate* for the situation. For example, an inappropriate response is shown by a patient who has an extreme reaction to the death of the victims of the September 11 tragedy, as if the victims were personal friends. Another patient said that his life stopped when the World Trade Center towers came down. He could not eat or sleep for weeks afterward. *Stability* can be mobile (normal) or labile. If a patient reports feeling happy one minute and reduced to tears the next, the person probably has an unstable mood. During the interview, the nurse should look for rapid mood changes that indicate lability of mood. A patient who exhibits intense, frequently shifting emotional extremes has a labile affect.

Speech

Speech provides clues about thoughts, emotional patterns, and cognitive organization. Speech may be pressured, fast, slow, or fragmented. Speech patterns reflect the patient's thought patterns, which can be logical or illogical. To check the patient's comprehension, the nurse can show a patient an object (e.g., pen, watch) and ask the person to name them. During conversation, the nurse assesses the fluency and quality of the patient's speech. The nurse listens for repetition or rhyming of words.

Thought Processes

The nurse assesses the patient for rapid change of ideas; inability or taking a long time to get to the point; loose or no connections among ideas or words; rhyming or repetition of words, questions, or phrases; or use of unheard-of words. Any of these observations indicates abnormal thought patterns. The content of what the patient says is also important. What thought is the patient expressing? The nurse listens for unusual and unlikely stories, fears, or behaviors, for example, "The FBI is tracking me" or "I am afraid to leave my house."

Cognition and Intellectual Performance

The nurse can assess for **intellectual well-being** by determining the extent that the patient recognizes their creative abilities and is able to learn new knowledge and skills. To assess the patient's cognition, that is, the ability to think and know, the nurse uses memory, calculation, and reasoning tests to identify specific areas of impairment. The cognitive areas include (1) attention and concentration, (2) abstract reasoning and comprehension, (3) memory, and (4) insight and judgment.

Attention and Concentration

To test attention and concentration, the nurse asks the patient, without pencil or paper, to start with 100 and subtract 7 until reaching 65 or to start with 20 and subtract 3. The nurse must decide which is most appropriate for the patient considering education and understanding. Subtracting 3 from 20 is the easier of the two tasks. Asking a patient to spell "world" backward is also useful in determining attention and concentration.

Abstract Reasoning and Comprehension

To test abstract reasoning and comprehension, the nurse gives the patient a proverb to interpret. Examples include "People in glass houses shouldn't throw stones," "A rolling stone gathers no moss," and "A penny saved is a penny earned."

Recall, Short-Term, Recent, and Remote Memory

There are four spheres of memory to check: recall, or immediate, memory; short-term memory; recent memory; and long-term, or remote, memory. To check immediate and short-term memory, the nurse gives the patient three unrelated words to remember and asks them to recite them right after telling them and at 5- and 15-minute intervals during the interview. To test recent memory, the nurse may question about a holiday or world event within the past few months. The nurse tests long-term or remote memory by asking about events years ago. If they are personal events and the answers seem incorrect, the nurse may check them with a family member.

Insight and Clinical Judgment

Insight and judgment are related concepts that involve the ability to examine thoughts, conceptualize facts, solve problems, think abstractly, and possess self-awareness. **Insight** is a person's awareness of their own thoughts and feelings and ability to compare them with the thoughts and feelings of others. It involves an awareness of how others view one's behavior and its meaning. For example, many patients do not believe that they have mental illness. They may have delusions and hallucinations or be hospitalized for bizarre and sometimes dangerous behavior, but they are completely unaware that their behavior is unusual or abnormal. During an interview, a patient may adamantly proclaim that nothing is wrong or that they do not have a mental illness. Even if a problem is recognized, the patient may lack insight regarding issues related to care.

Clinical judgment is the ability to reach a logical decision about a situation and to choose a course of action after examining and analyzing various possibilities. Throughout the interview, the nurse evaluates the patient's ability to make logical decisions. For example, some patients may continually choose partners who are abusive. The nurse could logically conclude that these patients have poor judgment in selecting partners. Another way to examine a patient's judgment is to give a simple scenario and ask the person to identify the best response. An example of such a scenario is asking, "What would you do if you found a bag of money outside a bank on a busy street?" If the patient responds with "Run with it," their judgment is questionable.

Behavior

Throughout the assessment, the nurse observes any behavior that may have significance in understanding the patient's response or symptoms of the mental disorder or emotional problem. For example, a depressed patient may be tearful throughout the session, whereas an anxious patient may twist or pull their hair, shift in the chair, or be unable to maintain eye contact. The nurse may find that whenever a topic is addressed, the patient's behavior changes. The nurse needs to relate patterned behaviors to significant events by connecting behaviors with the assessment data. For example, a patient may change jobs frequently, causing family distress and financial problems. Exploration of the events leading up to job changes may elicit important information regarding the patient's ability to solve problems.

Self-Concept

Self-concept, which develops over a lifetime, represents the total beliefs about three interrelated dimensions of the self: body image, self-esteem, and personal identity. The importance of each of these dimensions varies among individuals. For some, beliefs about themselves are strongly tied to body image; for others, personal identity is most important. Still others develop personal identity from what others have told them over the years. The nurse carrying out an assessment must keep in mind that self-concept and its components are dynamic and variable. For example, a woman may have a consistent self-concept until her first pregnancy. At that time, the many physiologic changes of pregnancy may cause her body image to change. She may be comfortable and enjoy the "glow of pregnancy," or she may feel like a "bloated cow." Suddenly, her body image is the most important part of her self-concept, and how she handles it can increase or decrease her self-esteem or sense of personal identity. Thus, all the components are tied together, and each one affects the others.

Self-concept is assessed through eliciting patients' thoughts about themselves, their ability to navigate in the world, and their nonverbal behaviors. A disheveled sloppy physical appearance outside cultural norms is an indication of poor self-concept. Negative self-statements, such as, "I could never do that," "I have no control over my life," and "I'm so stupid," reveal poor views of self. The nurse's own self-concept can shape the nurse's view of the patient. For example, a nurse who is self-confident and feels inwardly scornful of a patient who lacks such confidence may intimidate the patient through unconscious, judgmental behaviors or inconsiderate comments.

A useful approach to measuring self-concept is asking the patient to draw a self-portrait. For many patients, drawing is much easier than writing and serves as an excellent technique for monitoring changes. Interpretation of self-concept from drawings focuses on size, color, level of detail, pressure, line quality, symmetry, and placement. Low self-esteem is expressed by small size, lack of color variation, and sparse details in the drawing. Powerlessness and feelings of inadequacy are expressed through a lack of a head, a mouth, arms, feet, or in the drawing. A lack of symmetry (placement of figure parts or entire drawings off center) represents feelings of insecurity and inadequacy. As self-esteem builds, size increases, color tends to become more varied and brighter, and more details appear. Figure 11.1 shows a self-portrait of a patient at the beginning of treatment for depression and another drawn 3 months later.

Body Image

Body image represents a person's beliefs and attitudes about their body and includes such dimensions as size (large or small) and attractiveness (pretty or ugly). People who are satisfied with their body have a more positive body image than those who are not satisfied. Generally, women attach more importance to their body image than do men and may even define themselves in terms of their body.

Patients express body image beliefs through statements about their bodies. Statements such as "I feel so ugly," "I'm so fat," and "No one will want to have sex with me" express negative body images. Nonverbal behaviors

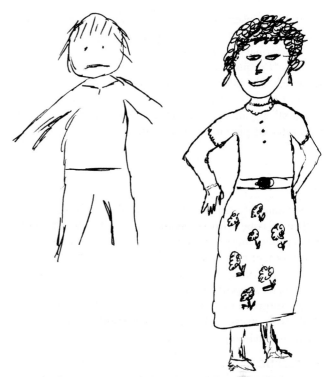

FIGURE 11.1 *Left:* Self-portrait of a 52-year-old woman at first group session following discharge from hospital for treatment of depression. *Right:* Self-portrait after 3 months of weekly group interventions.

indicating problems with body image include avoiding looking at or touching a body part; hiding the body in oversized clothing; or bandaging a particularly sensitive area, such as a mole on the face. Cultural differences must be considered when evaluating behavior related to body image. For example, the expectation of some cultures is that women and girls will keep their bodies completely covered and wear loose-fitting garments.

NCLEXNOTE Be prepared to assess reactions to a body image change (e.g., loss of vision, paralysis, colostomy, amputation).

Self-Esteem

Self-esteem is the person's attitude about the self. Self-esteem differs from body image because it concerns satisfaction with one's overall self. People who feel good about themselves are more likely to have the confidence to try new health behaviors. They are also less likely to be depressed. Negative self-esteem statements include "I'm a worthless person" and "I never do anything right."

Personal Identity

Personal identity is knowing "who I am." Every life experience and interaction contribute to knowing oneself better. Personal identity allows people to establish boundaries and understand personal strengths and limitations. In some psychiatric disorders, individuals cannot separate themselves from others, which shows that their personal identity is not strongly developed. A problem with personal identity is difficult to assess. Statements such as "I'm just like my mother, and she was always in trouble," "I become whatever my current boyfriend wants me to be," and "I can't make a decision unless I check it out first" are all statements that require further exploration into the person's view of self.

Stress and Coping Patterns

Everyone has stress (see Chapter 19). One of the dimensions of wellness is **emotional well-being** or the ability to cope with stress through skills and strategies. Sometimes, the experience of stress contributes to the development of mental disorders. Identification of major stresses in a patient's life helps the nurse understand the person and support the use of successful coping behaviors in the future. The nurse should explore how the patient deals with stress and identify successful coping mechanisms to encourage their use.

> **NCLEXNOTE** Every assessment should focus on stress and coping patterns. Identifying how a patient copes with stress can be used as a basis of care in all nursing situations. Include content from Chapter 19 when studying these concepts.

Risk Assessment

Risk factors are characteristics, conditions, situations, or events that increase the patient's vulnerability to threats to safety or well-being. Throughout this text, the sections concerning risk factors focus on the following:

- Risks to the patient's safety
- Risks for developing psychiatric disorders
- Risks for increasing, or exacerbating, symptoms and impairment in an individual who already has a psychiatric disorder

Consideration of risk factors involving patient safety should be included in each assessment. Examples of these risks include the risk for suicide and violence toward others or the risk for events, such as falling, seizures, allergic reactions, or elopement (unauthorized absence from health care facility). Nurses assess factors on a priority basis. For example, threats of violence or suicide take priority.

Suicide Screening

Every mental health nursing assessment should include a suicide screening. During the assessment, the nurse needs to listen closely to whether the patient describes or mentions thinking about self-harm. If the patient does not openly express ideas of self-harm, it is necessary to ask straightforward questions related to suicide.

The Columbia Suicide Severity Rating Scale (C-SSRS) is a commonly used, evidence-based measure used to identify and assess individuals at risk for suicide (Posner et al., 2011). This instrument measures severity of suicidal ideation, intensity of ideation, suicidal behavior, and lethality. It is appropriate for use over the telephone or in telehealth. C-SSRS screening toolkits are available for specific settings such as health care, correctional facilities, primary care, and police officers. All the screening tools consist of six questions. The C-SSRS for health care providers is a good place for nurses to learn the questions and how to respond (see Box 11.5).

Two questions should be included in the screening. "Have you wished you were dead or wished you could go to sleep and not wake up?" and "Have you actually had any thoughts about killing yourself?" If the answer is "no" to both questions, the nurse should ask one more. "Have you done anything, started to do anything, or prepared to do anything to end your life?" If the answer is "no" to the third question, the nurse can assume that the person most likely is not suicidal.

If the answer is "yes" to any of these three questions, the nurse should ask the following three questions. "Have you thought about how you might do this?" "Have you had any intention of acting on these thoughts of killing yourself, as opposed to you have the thoughts but you would definitely would not act on them?" and "Have you done anything, started to do anything, or prepared to do anything to end your life?" If the answer is "yes" to any of these questions, the nurse should seek a referral to advanced practice nurse, psychologist, or other mental health clinicians trained to complete a comprehensive assessment. The nurse should notify the supervisor and clearly document the patient responses and nursing follow-up. The nurse should not leave the patient alone and should explore the details of the intention and behavior. If a nurse and patient are not face to face, but on the telephone or other virtual means, the nurse should keep the patient talking and follow agency policy. The National Suicide Prevention Lifeline (1-800-273-8255) is a resource that can provide support and direction to the nurse as well as the patient.

To assess patient ability to coping suicidal thoughts, the nurse can ask the patient to identify strategies that were used in resisting suicidal urges and actions. For example, one patient reported calling a family member to talk when the suicidal urges were strong. The nurse can encourage the patient to use these strategies in the future. This information will be helpful in the development of a safety plan (see Chapter 22).

Assaultive or Homicidal Ideation

When assessing a patient, the nurse also needs to listen carefully to any delusions or hallucinations that the patient shares. If the patient gives any indication that they must or are being told to harm someone, the nurse must first think of self-safety and institute assaultive precautions as indicated by the facility protocols.

BOX 11.5

The Columbia Suicide Severity Rating Scale

	Past Month	
1) Have you wished you were dead or wished you could go to sleep and not wake up?		
2) Have you actually had any thoughts about killing yourself?		
If **YES** to 2, answer questions 3, 4, 5 and 6 If **NO** to 2, go directly to question 6		
3) Have you thought about how you might do this?		
4) Have you had any intention of acting on these thoughts of killing yourself, as opposed to you have the thoughts but you definitely would not act on them?	**High Risk**	

5) Have you started to work out or worked out the details of how to kill yourself? Do you intend to carry out this plan?	**High Risk**	

	Life-time	Past 3 Months
Always Ask Question 6		
6) Have you done anything, started to do anything, or prepared to do anything to end your life? *Examples:* Collected pills, obtained a gun, gave away valuables, wrote a will or suicide note, held a gun but changed your mind, cut yourself, tried to hang yourself, etc.		**High Risk**

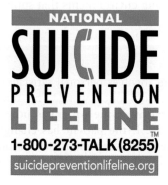

NATIONAL SUICIDE PREVENTION LIFELINE
1-800-273-TALK(8255)
suicidepreventionlifeline.org

Any YES indicates that someone should seek a behavioral health referral. However, if the answer to 4, 5 or 6 is YES, seek immediate help: go to the emergency room, call 1-800-273-8255, text 741741 or call 911 and STAY WITH THEM until they can be evaluated.

General questions to ascertain assaultive or homicidal ideation follow:

- Do you intend to harm someone? If yes, who?
- Do you have a plan? If yes, what are the details of the plan?
- Do you have the means to carry out the plan? (If the plan requires a weapon, is it readily available?)

Social Assessment

The nurse collects information on the patient's social support and networks. The nurse elicits cues about interactions with others in the family and community (work, church, or other organizations); parents and their marital relationship; place in birth order; and relationships with spouse, siblings, and children. The nurse also assesses work and education history and community activities. The nurse observes how the patient relates to any family or friends who may be in attendance. This component of the assessment helps the nurse anticipate how the patient may get along with other patients in an inpatient setting. It also allows the nurse to plan for any anticipated difficulties.

Functional Status

An important aspect of the assessment is determining the functioning of the patient (i.e., Is an adult working and living independently? Is a student attending classes?). How the patient copes with strangers and those with whom they do not get along is also important information.

Social Systems

A significant component of the patient's life involves the social systems in which they may be enmeshed. **Social well-being** involves developing a sense of connection and a well-developed support system. The social systems to examine include the family, the culture to which the patient belongs, and the community in which they live.

Family Assessment

How the patient fits in with and relates to their family is important to know. General questions to ask include the following:

- Who do you consider family?
- How important to you is your family?
- How does your family make decisions?
- What are the roles in your family, and who fills them?
- Where do you fit in your family?
- With whom in your family do you get along best?

- With whom in your family do you have the most conflict?
- Who in your family is supportive of you?

Cultural Assessment

Culture can profoundly affect a person's worldview (see Chapter 3). Culture helps a person frame beliefs about life, death, health and illness, and roles and relationships. During cultural assessment, the nurse must consider factors that influence the manifestations of the current mental disorder. For example, a patient mentions "speaking in tongues." The nurse may identify this experience as a hallucination when, in fact, the patient was having a religious experience common within some branches of Christianity. In this instance, knowing and understanding such religious practices will prevent a misinterpretation of the symptoms.

The nurse can elicit important cultural information by asking the following questions:

- To what cultural group do you belong?
- Were you raised in an ethnic community?
- How do you define health?
- How do you define illness?
- How do you define good and evil?
- What do you do to get better when you are physically ill? Mentally ill?
- Whom do you see for help when you are physically ill? Mentally ill?
- By what cultural rules or taboos do you try to live?
- Do you eat special foods?

Community Support and Resources

Many patients are connected to community resources, and the nurse needs to assess what they are and the patterns of usage. For example, a patient who is homeless may know of a church where they can sleep but may go there only on cold nights. Or a patient may go to the community center daily for lunch to be with other people. Examining the environment is a part of the individual's assessment. **Environmental well-being** involves living in pleasant, stimulating environments that support a healthy lifestyle.

Occupational Status

Occupational well-being involves personal satisfaction and enrichment derived from one's work. The nurse should document the occupation the patient is now in as well as a history of jobs. If the patient has changed jobs frequently, the nurse should ask about the reasons. Perhaps the patient has faced such problems as an inability to focus on the job at hand or to get along with others. If so, such issues require further exploration.

Economic Status

Finances are very private for many people; thus, the nurse must ask questions about economic status carefully. However, **financial well-being** is satisfaction with present and future situations. What the nurse needs to ascertain is not specific dollar amounts but whether the patient feels stressed by finances and has enough for basic needs.

Legal Status

Because of laws governing people with mental illness, ascertaining the patient's correct age, marital status, and any legal guardianship is important. The nurse may need to check the patient's medical records for this information.

Quality of Life

The patient's perspective on quality of life means how the patient rates their life. Does a patient feel his life is poor because he cannot purchase everything he wants? Does another patient feel blessed because the sun is shining today? Listening carefully to the patient's discussion of their life and how they measure the quality of that life provides important information about self-concept, coping skills, desires, and dreams.

Psychosocial Strengths and Wellness Assessment

Throughout the assessment, the nurse should be able to identify areas of strength and wellness. A description of these areas should be validated with the patient and documented in the person's record.

Spiritual Assessment

> **KEYCONCEPT Spirituality** "is a way of being in the world in which a person feels a sense of connectedness to self, others, and/or a higher power or nature: a sense of meaning in life; and transcendence beyond self, everyday living, and suffering" (Weathers et al., 2015, 93).

Several studies show that spirituality and religion are important in coping with mental disorders through providing hope, comfort, and meaning of life and serve as a resource for coping with symptoms, substance abuse, and protection against suicide (Das et al., 2018; Paul et al., 2018). Nurses must be clear about their own spirituality to be sure it does not interfere with assessment of the patient's spirituality. Nurses also need to work within their area of competence and recognize the importance of referring patients to a health care chaplain or other spiritual care support.

The purpose of a **spiritual care assessment**, which is often the responsibility of the nurse, is to identify specific spiritual care needs and to formulate a care plan. A nursing spiritual assessment is usually included in the general nursing assessment, even when there are chaplains available (Timmins & Caldeira, 2017). The Joint Commission requires that spiritual care assessment and spiritual care delivery be directed to the patient or the patient's family but does not identify specific disciplines of the personnel who will conduct the assessment (The Joint Commission, 2020).

The spiritual assessment is based an individual's needs, which are discovered within an open, trusting dialogue. It is important that the nurse does not self-disclose personal values and beliefs during the assessment. The following questions can serve to initiate the assessment:

- How important is spirituality and/or religion in your life and coping with an illness?
- Are you involved in a religious or faith community?
- Would you like to address these issues in your mental health care?
- If yes, with whom would you like to address these issues?

Spiritual assessment questions need to correspond to the patient's readiness to discuss this topic. Patients and clinicians agree that it may take time for the patient to feel comfortable and ready to discuss spirituality. It is essential that questions are asked that focus on a patient's strengths. For example, asking the question "Was there a time in your life where you felt great peace and joy and maybe not so stressed out?" is less judgmental than the question "What were your sources of deep meaning, peace, joy, and strength during your times of stress?" The latter statement has an implied expectation that there should be sources (religious, spiritual) that exist.

Examples of questions that could help patients examine past or current spiritually related strengths and resources include the following (Gomi et al., 2014):

- Was there a time in your life when you really felt at peace?
- What do you do to get through the tough times (pray, meditate, visit nature, family)?
- When do you feel most positive about yourself?
- What brings inspiration to your life?

Questions that can help the individual connect to spiritual goals to recovery goals (if that is a goal of the person) include the following (Gomi et al., 2014):

- What helps you feel good or hopeful about your life?
- Is spirituality something you want to connect with in your recovery?
- Based on what you said, how would you say your spirituality could support your recovery?

KEYCONCEPT: Clinical judgment is an iterative decision-making process that uses nursing knowledge to observe and assess presenting situations; identify a prioritized client concern; and generate the best possible evidence-based solutions to deliver safe client care.

USING CLINICAL JUDGMENT

One of the challenges of conducting an assessment is keeping track of important health and mental health cues and differentiating significant signs and symptoms from those that may not be relevant to the patient's area of concern. In a collaborative process, the patient and nurse prioritize the patient's concerns and generate solutions. There will be times when the patient and nurse are at odds about the top priority. For example, a nurse may identify treatment of psychosis as a priority and the patient may want a place to stay. Using evidence that supports the patient's request, the nurse generates a plan to find housing before the patient will consider medications. In another instance, a patient has a credible suicide plan, and the nurse insists that safety is the top priority and is a life-or-death situation.

With experience, the nurse can cluster the assessment data to identify two or three immediate health or mental health problem issues related to promotion of health and well-being, prevention of illness, reduction of risks, or treat health care problems.

DEVELOPING RECOVERY GOALS AND OUTCOMES

Mutually agreed-upon goals flow from the prioritization of needs and provide guidance in determining appropriate interventions. Initial goals are determined and then are monitored and evaluated throughout the care process.

Measuring outcomes not only demonstrates clinical effectiveness but also helps to promote rational clinical decision-making and is reflective of the nursing interventions.

KEYCONCEPT Outcomes are health experiences and evaluations reported by the patient or observed by the nurse related to symptoms, functioning, well-being, health perceptions, and satisfaction with care that can be attributed to nursing care at a given point in time (Broderick et al., 2013).

An expected outcome is concise, stated in few words and in neutral terms (Table 11.2).

Expected outcomes are developed mutually with the patient. Nurses are accountable for documenting patient outcomes, nursing interventions, and any changes in health status or care plan or both. Outcomes can be expressed in terms of the patient's actual responses (no longer reports hearing voices) or the health or mental health changes after implementation of nursing interventions.

TABLE 11.2 EXAMPLE OF OUTCOMES

Issue	Outcome	Intervention
Social isolation	Social involvement Indicators: a. Interact with other patients b. Attend group meetings	Using a contract format, explain role and responsibility of patients

RECOVERY-ORIENTED NURSING INTERVENTIONS

Recovery-oriented patient/nurse-initiated treatment is an autonomous action within the scope of nursing practice. It can also be physician-initiated treatment through an order written in the patient's record. In both instances, the nurse is held to a standard of nursing care.

KEYCONCEPT Recovery-oriented nursing interventions are nursing actions or treatment, selected based on clinical judgment and mutual decision-making with the patient, that are designed to achieve patient, family, or community outcomes. Interventions can be direct or indirect and can target specific symptoms, health needs, and strengths (see Box 11.6).

There are several nursing interventions systems, including the Nursing Interventions Classification (Butcher et al., 2019), the Clinical Care Classification system (Saba, 2017), and the Omaha nursing model (Martin, 2005; Martin & Kessler, 2017). All these systems are recognized by the American Nurses Association. In this text, the *Psychiatric-Mental Health Nursing: Scope and Standards of Practice* guides the use of interventions (American Nurses Association [ANA], American Psychiatric Nurses Association [APNA], & International Society of Psychiatric-Mental Health Nurses [ISPN], 2014). Some are adapted from classification systems and others from the psychiatric–mental health nursing literature.

Physical Interventions

Biologic interventions focus on physical functioning and are directed toward the patient's self-care, activities and exercise, sleep, nutrition, relaxation, hydration, and thermoregulation as well as pain management and medication management.

Promotion of Self-Care Activities

Many patients with psychiatric–mental health problems can manage ADLs or self-care activities such as bathing, dressing appropriately, selecting adequate nutrition, and sleeping regularly. Others cannot manage such self-care activities, either because of their symptoms or because of the side effects of medications.

BOX 11.6

Recovery-Oriented Intervention in Inpatient Unit

Molin, J., Hällgren Graneheim, U., Ringnér, A., & Lindgren, B. M. (2020). Time Together as an arena for mental health nursing-staff experiences of introducing and participating in a nursing intervention in psychiatric inpatient care. International Journal of Mental Health Nursing, 10.1111/inm.12759. Advance online publication. https://doi.org/10.1111/inm.12759

THE QUESTION: What are the experiences of the staff when a recovery-oriented intervention, Time Together (TT), is implemented in inpatient mental health unit?

METHODS: In this qualitative study, staff were interviewed and data analyzed after implementing TT, a regularly scheduled time the patients every day for a minimum of one hour. In the relationship-building intervention, patients and staff would engage in joint activities, that is, board games, and bingo, preferably chosen by the patients. Staff (N = 17) were asked to talk about what TT

meant to them and how they had experienced introducing and participating is TT. The interviews lasted between 16 and 55 minutes. Interviews were recorded. Data were analyzed using a qualitative content analysis.

FINDINGS: Staff prepared for the introduction of the intervention by laying a framework for success by making joint decisions, providing structure and taking responsibility, and being flexible. Even though the implementation let to feeling burdened, they found that TT fostered relationship between patients and staff.

IMPLICATIONS FOR NURSING: Nurses can easily be consumed with nonpatient responsibilities leading to dissatisfaction. To support the development of therapeutic relationships, nurses must advocate for interventions that are critical components of recovery-oriented practice.

In the inpatient setting, the psychiatric nurse structures the patient's activities, so that basic self-care activities are completed. During acute phases of psychiatric disorders, the inability to attend to basic self-care tasks, such as getting dressed, is very common. Thus, the ability to complete personal hygiene activities (e.g., dental care, grooming) is monitored, and patients are assisted in completing such activities. In a psychiatric facility, patients are encouraged and expected to develop independence in completing these basic self-care activities. In the community, monitoring these basic self-care activities is always a part of the nursing visit or clinic appointment.

Activity and Exercise Interventions

In some psychiatric disorders (e.g., schizophrenia), people become sedentary and appear to lack the motivation to complete ADLs. This lack of motivation is part of the disorder and requires nursing intervention. In addition, side effects of medication often include sedation and lethargy. Encouraging regular activity and exercise can improve general well-being and physical health. In some instances, exercise behavior becomes an abnormal focus of attention, as may be observed in some patients with anorexia nervosa.

When assuming the responsibility of direct care provider, the nurse can help patients identify realistic activities and exercise goals. As leader or manager of a psychiatric unit, the nurse can influence ward routine. Alternatively, the nurse can delegate activity and exercise interventions to nurses' aides. Some institutions have other professionals (e.g., recreational therapists) available for the implementation of exercise programs. As a case manager, the nurse should consider the activity needs of individuals when coordinating care.

Sleep Interventions

Many psychiatric disorders and medications are associated with sleep disturbances. Sleep is also disrupted in patients with dementia; such patients may have difficulty falling asleep or may frequently awaken during the night. In dementia of the Alzheimer type, individuals may reverse their sleeping patterns by napping during the day and staying awake at night.

Nonpharmacologic interventions are always used first because of the side-effect risks associated with the use of sedatives and hypnotics (see Chapter 12). Sleep interventions to communicate to patients include the following:

- Go to bed only when tired or sleepy.
- Establish a consistent bedtime routine.
- Avoid stimulating foods, beverages, or medications.
- Avoid naps in the late afternoon or evening.
- Eat lightly before retiring and limit fluid intake.
- Use your bed only for sleep or intimacy.
- Avoid emotional stimulation before bedtime.
- Use behavioral and relaxation techniques.
- Limit distractions.

Nutrition Interventions

Psychiatric disorders and medication side effects can affect eating behaviors. For varying reasons, some patients eat too little, but others eat too much. For instance, homeless patients with mental illnesses have difficulty maintaining adequate nutrition because of their deprived lifestyle. Substance abuse also interferes with maintaining adequate nutrition, either through stimulation or suppression of appetite or through neglecting nutrition because of drug-seeking behavior. Thus, nutrition interventions should be specific and relevant to the individual's circumstances and mental health. In addition, recommended daily nutritional allowances are important in the promotion of physical and mental health, and nurses should consider them when planning care.

Some psychiatric symptoms involve changes in perceptions of food, appetite, and eating habits. If a patient believes that food is poisonous, they may eat sparingly or not at all. Interventions are then necessary to address the suspiciousness as well as to encourage adequate intake of recommended daily allowances. Allowing patients to examine foods, participate in preparations, and test the safety of the meal by eating slowly or after everyone else may be necessary. For patients who are paranoid, it is sometimes helpful to serve prepackaged foods.

Relaxation Interventions

Relaxation promotes comfort, reduces anxiety, alleviates stress, eases pain, and prevents aggression. It can diminish the effects of hallucinations and delusions. The many different relaxation techniques used as mental health interventions range from simple deep breathing to biofeedback to hypnosis. Although some techniques, such as biofeedback, require additional training and, in some instances, certification, nurses can easily apply simple relaxation, distraction, and imagery techniques.

Simple relaxation techniques encourage and elicit relaxation to decrease undesirable signs and symptoms. **Distraction** is the purposeful focusing of attention away from undesirable sensations, and **guided imagery** is the purposeful use of imagination to achieve relaxation or direct attention away from undesirable sensations (Box 11.7).

Relaxation techniques that involve physical touch (e.g., back rubs) usually are not used for people with mental disorders. Touching and massaging usually are not appropriate, especially for those who have a history of physical or sexual abuse. Such patients may find touching too stimulating or misinterpret it as being sexual or aggressive.

Hydration Interventions

Assessing fluid status and monitoring fluid intake and output are often important interventions. Overhydration or underhydration can be a symptom of a disorder. For example, some patients with psychotic disorders experience chronic fluid imbalance. Many psychiatric medications affect fluid and electrolyte balance (see Chapter 12).

BOX 11.7

Relaxation Techniques: Descriptions and Implementation

RELAXED BREATHING
The goal of this exercise is to slow down your breathing, especially your exhaling.

Steps
1. Choose a word that you associate with relaxation, such as calm, relax, or peaceful.
2. Inhale through your nose and exhale slowly through your mouth. Take normal breaths, not deep ones.
3. While you exhale, say the relaxing word you have chosen. Say it very slowly, like this: "c-a-a-a-a-a-a-l-m" or "r-e-e-e-l-a-a-a-x."
4. Pause after exhaling before taking your next breath. If it is not too distracting, count to 4 before inhaling each new breath.
5. Repeat the entire sequence 10 to 15 times.

MUSCLE RELAXATION
The goal of this technique is to gently stretch your muscles to reduce stiffness and tension. The exercises start at your head and work down to your feet. You can do these exercises while sitting in a chair.

Steps
1. *Neck rolls.* Drop your head to one side. Gently roll it around in a wide circle. Repeat three to five times.

Then reverse directions, and gently roll your head in a wide circle the other way. Repeat three to five times.
2. *Shoulder shrugs.* Lift both shoulders in a shrugging motion. Try to touch your ears with your shoulders. Let your shoulders drop down after each shrug. Repeat three to five times.
3. *Overhead arm stretches.* Raise both arms straight above your head. Interlace your fingers, like you are making a basket, with your palms facing down (toward the floor). Stretch your arms toward the ceiling. Then, keeping your fingers interlaced, rotate your palms to face upward (toward the ceiling). Stretch toward the ceiling. Repeat three to five times. If it is not comfortable to do this step with your arms overhead, try it with your arms reaching out in front of you.
4. *Knee raises.* Reach down and grab your right knee with one or both hands. Pull your knee up toward your chest (as close to your chest as is comfortable). Hold your knee there for a few seconds, before returning your foot to the floor. Reach down and grab your left knee with one or both hands and bring it up toward your chest. Hold it there for a few seconds. Repeat the sequence three to five times.
5. *Foot and ankle rolls.* Lift your feet and stretch your legs out. Rotate your ankles and feet, three to five times in one direction, then three to five times in the other direction.

Reprinted from Substance Abuse and Mental Health Services Administration. (2009). Illness management and recovery: Practitioner guides and handouts. HHS Pub. No. SMA-09-4462, Center for Mental Health Services, Substance Abuse and Mental Health Services Administration, U.S. Department of Health and Human Services.

For example, when taking lithium carbonate, patients must have adequate fluid intake and pay special attention to testing serum sodium levels. Interventions that help patients understand the relationship of medications to fluid and electrolyte balance are important in their overall care.

Thermoregulation Interventions

Many psychiatric disorders can disturb the body's normal temperature regulation. Thus, patients cannot sense temperature increases or decreases and consequently cannot protect themselves from extremes of hot or cold. This problem is especially difficult for people who are homeless or live outside the protected environments of institutions and boarding homes. In addition, many psychiatric medications affect the ability to regulate body temperature.

Interventions include educating patients about the problem of thermoregulation, identifying potential extremes in temperatures, and developing strategies to protect the patient from the adverse effects of temperature changes. For example, reminding patients to wear coats and sweaters in the winter or to wear loose, lightweight garments in the summer may prevent frostbite or heat exhaustion, respectively.

Pain Management

Psychiatric nurses are more likely to provide care to patients experiencing chronic pain than acute pain. However, a single intervention is seldom successful for relieving chronic pain. In some instances, pain is managed by medication; in other instances, nonpharmacologic strategies, such as simple relaxation techniques, distraction, or imagery, are used. Indeed, relaxation is one of the most widely used cognitive and behavioral approaches to pain. Education, stress management techniques, hypnosis, and biofeedback are also used in pain management. Physical agents include heat and cold therapy, exercise, and transcutaneous nerve stimulation.

The key to managing pain is identifying how it disrupts the patient's personal, social, professional, and family life. Education focusing on the pain, use of medications for treatment, and development of cognitive skills are important pain management components. In some cases, redefining treatment success as improvement in functioning, rather than alleviation of pain, may be necessary. The interaction between stress and pain is important; that is, increased stress leads to increased pain. Patients can better manage their pain when stress is reduced.

Medication Management

The psychiatric–mental health nurse uses many medication management interventions to help patients maintain therapeutic regimens. Medication management involves more than the actual administration of medications. Nurses also assess medication effectiveness and side effects and consider drug–drug interactions. Monitoring the amount of lethal prescription medication is particularly important. For example, check if patients have old prescriptions of tricyclic antidepressants in their medicine cabinets. Treatment with psychopharmacologic agents can be lengthy because of the chronic nature of many disorders; many patients remain on medication regimens for years, never becoming free of medication. Thus, medication education is an ongoing intervention that requires careful documentation. Medication follow-up may include home visits as well as telephone calls.

Psychological Interventions

A major emphasis in psychiatric–mental health nursing is the psychological domain: emotion, behavior, and cognition. The basis of nursing care is establishing a therapeutic relationship with the patient. Because the therapeutic relationship was extensively discussed in Chapter 10, it is not covered in this chapter. This section does cover cognitive interventions, counseling, conflict resolution, bibliotherapy, reminiscence, behavior therapy, psychoeducation, health teaching, and spiritual interventions. Chapter 7 presents the theoretic basis for many of these interventions.

Cognitive Interventions

Evidence-based cognitive interventions are used in a variety of practice settings (inpatient and outpatient). The knowledge and skills inherent in cognitively based interventions have been extensively studied, and their effectiveness has been demonstrated for a variety of psychiatric disorders, especially depression (see Chapter 25) and anxiety and related disorders (see Chapters 26–28).

Cognitive interventions are based on the concept of cognition. **Cognition** can be defined as an internal process of perception, memory, and judgment through which an understanding of self and the world is developed.

Cognitive interventions aim to change or reframe an individual's automatic thought patterns that have developed over time and that interfere with the individual's ability to function optimally. The skills and techniques developed based on cognitive theory result in a new view of self and the environment.

Counseling Interventions

Counseling interventions are interactions between a nurse and a patient, family, or group experiencing immediate or ongoing difficulties related to their health or well-being. Counseling is usually short term and focuses on stabilizing symptoms, supporting personal recovery goals, improving coping abilities, reinforcing healthy behaviors, fostering positive interactions, or preventing illness and disability. Counseling strategies are discussed throughout the text. Psychotherapy, which differs from counseling, is generally a long-term approach aimed at improving or helping patients regain previous health status and functional abilities. Mental health specialists, such as advanced practice nurses, use psychotherapy.

Conflict Resolution and Cultural Brokering

Conflict resolution is a process of helping an individual or family identify a problem underling a disagreement or dispute and developing alternative possibilities for solving the conflict (Weitzman & Weitzman, 2014). Conflict can be positive if individuals see the problem as solvable and providing an opportunity for growth and interpersonal understanding. The nurse may be in the position of teaching family members how to resolve their own conflicts positively. Key elements of any conflict resolution process are collaboration, motivation to seek a solution, and the ability to see the other person's point of view. Conflict resolution strategies are commonly taught to adolescents who are experiencing cyberbullying and to adults in marital or romantic relationships (Courtain & Glowacz, 2019; Garaigordobil & Martínez-Valderrey, 2018; Özgüç & Tanriverdi et al., 2018). Nurses are often in leadership positions and use conflict resolution skills to settle employee disputes.

At times, patients who are politically and economically powerless find themselves in conflict with the health care system. Differences in cultural values and languages among patients and health care organizations contribute to feelings of powerlessness. For example, immigrant families, migrant farm workers, people who are homeless, and people who need to make informed decisions under stressful conditions may be unable to navigate the health care system. The nurse can help to resolve such conflicts through **cultural brokering**, the act of bridging, linking, or mediating messages, instructions, and belief systems between groups of people of differing cultural systems to reduce conflict or produce change (Lazarevic, 2017).

For the "nurse as broker" to be effective, the nurse establishes and maintains a sense of connectedness or relationship with the patient. In turn, the nurse also establishes and cultivates networks with other health care facilities and resources. Cultural sensitivity enables the nurse to be aware of and sensitive to the needs of patients from a variety of cultures. Cultural competence is necessary for the brokering process to be effective.

Bibliotherapy and Social Media

Bibliotherapy, sometimes referred to as bibliocounseling, is the reading of selected written materials to express feelings or gain insight under the guidance of a health care provider. The provider assigns and discusses with the patient a book, story, or article. The provider makes the assignment because they believe that the patient can receive therapeutic benefit from the reading. (It is assumed that the provider who assigned the reading has also read it.) The provider needs to consider the patient's reading level before making an assignment. If a patient has limited reading ability, the provider should not use bibliotherapy.

Literary works serve as a projective screen through which people see themselves in the story. Literature can help patients identify with characters and vicariously experience their reality. The use of bibliotherapy has been shown to improve depression when used with cognitive behavioral therapy (Yuan et al., 2018). It can also expose patients to situations that they have not personally experienced—the vicarious experience allows growth in self-knowledge and compassion (Escovar et al., 2019). Bibliotherapy can also support recovery in inpatient units through reading books written in first person (Eisen et al., 2018). Through reading, patients can enrich their lives in the following ways:

- *Catharsis:* expression of feelings stimulated by parallel experiences
- *Problem-solving:* development of solutions to problems in the literature from practical ideas about problem-solving
- *Insight:* increased self-awareness and understanding as the reader explores personal meaning from what is read
- *Anxiety reduction:* use of self-help written materials that can reduce concerns about a diagnosed problem and treatment

Using the internet can be helpful to patients, but it also has drawbacks. Some websites can help patients gain insight into their problems through acquiring new knowledge and interacting with others in the privacy of their own surroundings. Web materials and chat groups are variable in quality and accuracy. Nurses should carefully evaluate the quality of the website.

Reminiscence

Reminiscence, the thinking about or relating of past experiences, is used as a nursing intervention to enhance life review in older patients. Reminiscence encourages patients, either in individual or in group settings, to discuss their past and review their lives. Through reminiscence, individuals can identify past coping strategies that can support them in current stressful situations. Patients can also use reminiscence to maintain self-esteem, stimulate thinking, and support the natural healing process of life review. Activities that facilitate reminiscence include writing an account of past events, making an audio recording and playing it back, explaining pictures in old family albums, drawing a family tree, and writing to old friends.

Behavior Therapy

Behavior therapy interventions focus on reinforcing or promoting desirable behaviors or altering undesirable ones. The basic premise is that because most behaviors are learned, new functional behaviors can also be learned. Behaviors—not internal psychic processes—are the targets of the interventions. The models of behavioral theorists serve as a basis for these interventions (see Chapter 7).

Behavior Modification

Behavior modification is a specific, systematized behavior therapy technique that can be applied to individuals, groups, or systems. The aim of behavior modification is to reinforce desired behaviors and extinguish undesired ones. Desired behavior is rewarded to increase the likelihood that patients will repeat it, and over time, replace the problematic behavior with it. Behavior modification is used for various problematic behaviors, such as dysfunctional eating, addictions, anger management, and impulse control and often is used in the care of children and adolescents.

Token Economy

Used in inpatient settings and in group homes, a **token economy** applies behavior modification techniques to multiple behaviors. In a token economy, patients are rewarded with tokens for selected desired behaviors. They can use these tokens to purchase meals, leave the unit, watch television, or wear street clothes. In less restrictive environments, patients use tokens to purchase additional privileges, such as attending social events.

Token economy systems have been especially effective in reinforcing positive behaviors in people who are developmentally disabled or have severe and persistent mental illnesses. There is good evidence that the use of token economy for behavior and symptom management is effective in adults who are hospitalized, but there is little evidence to support transfer of the new behaviors outside the inpatient settings (Glowacki et al., 2016). The strategy has been expanded to treatment programs for children (Hickey et al., 2018) and cocaine addiction (Pirnia et al., 2016).

Psychoeducation

Psychoeducation uses educational strategies to teach patients the skills they lack because of a psychiatric disorder. The goal of psychoeducation is a change in knowledge and behavior. Nurses use psychoeducation to meet the educational needs of patients by adapting teaching strategies to their disorder-related deficits (Box 11.8). As patients gain skills, functioning improves. Some patients may need to learn how to maintain their morning hygiene. Others may need to understand their illness and cope with hearing voices that others do not hear.

Specific psychoeducation techniques are based on adult learning principles, such as beginning at the point where the learner is currently and building on their current experiences. Thus, the nurse assesses the patient's current skills and readiness to learn. From there, the nurse individualizes a teaching plan for each patient. They can conduct such teaching in a one-to-one situation or in a group format.

Psychoeducation is a continuous process of assessing, setting goals, developing learning activities, and evaluating for changes in knowledge and behavior. Nurses use it with individuals, groups, families, and communities. Psychoeducation serves as a basis for psychosocial rehabilitation, a service delivery approach for those with severe and persistent mental illness (see Chapter 24).

BOX 11.8

Psychoeducation Program for Parents of Children with Attention-Deficit/Hyperactivity Disorder (ADHD)

Gümüş, F., Ergün, G., & Dikeç, G. (2020). Effect of psychoeducation on stress in parents of children with attention-deficit/hyperactivity disorder: A randomized controlled study. Journal of Psychosocial Nursing and Mental Health Services, 58(7), 34–41. https://doi.org/10.3928/02793695-20200506-01

THE QUESTION: Does a psychoeducation program reduce the stress of parents of children with attention-deficit/hyperactivity disorder?

METHODS: A randomized controlled study was performed using pre-/posttest scores in experimental and control groups (*N* = 172). There was no significant difference between mean pretest scores of parents in the experimental and control groups on the Caregiver Stress Scale. The intervention consisted of four psychoeducation sessions for the experimental group, and the control group parents attended two meetings with no intervention.

FINDINGS: Psychoeducation decreased parents' stress immediately and 6 months after compared to the control group.

IMPLICATIONS FOR NURSING: Psychiatric–mental health nurses can use psychoeducation programs to support families of children with attention-deficit/hyperactivity disorder to reduce their stress levels.

NCLEXNOTE Apply knowledge from social sciences to help patients manage responses to psychiatric disorders and emotional problems.

Health Teaching

Health teaching is one of the standards of care for the psychiatric nurse. Teaching methods should be appropriate to the patient's development level, learning needs, readiness, ability to learn, language preference, and culture. Based on principles of learning, health teaching involves transmitting new information to the patient and providing constructive feedback and positive rewards, practice sessions, homework, and experimental learning. Health teaching is the integration of principles of teaching and learning with the knowledge of health and illness (Fig. 11.2).

Thus, in health teaching, the psychiatric nurse attends to potential health care problems other than mental disorders and emotional problems. For example, if a person has diabetes mellitus and is taking insulin, the nurse provides health care teaching related to diabetes and the interaction of this problem with the mental disorder.

Spiritual Interventions

Spiritual care is based on an assessment of the patient's spiritual needs. Some interventions require actions such as listening, requesting a chaplain's presence, or providing readings; other interventions involve use of personal abilities and characteristics such as the use of the therapeutic relationship in supporting patient well-being. A nonjudgmental relationship and just "being with" (not doing for) the patient are key spiritual interventions. To assist people in spiritual distress, the nurse should know and understand the beliefs and practices of various spiritual groups. **Spiritual support**, assisting patients to feel balance and connection within their relationships, involves listening to expressions of loneliness, using empathy, and providing patients with desired spiritual articles (Caldeira & Timmons, 2017).

Social Interventions

The social domain includes the individual's environment and its effect on their responses to mental disorders and distress. Interventions within the social domain are geared toward couples, families, friends, and large and small social groups, with special attention given to ethnicity and community interactions. In some instances, nurses design interventions that affect a patient's environment, such as helping a family member decide to admit a loved one to a long-term care facility. In other instances, the nurse modifies the environment to promote positive behaviors. Group interventions are discussed in Chapter 14.

Social Behavior and Privilege Systems in Inpatient Units

In psychiatric units, unrelated strangers who have problems interacting live together in close quarters, sometimes with two to four people sharing bedrooms and bathrooms. For this reason, most psychiatric units develop a list of behavioral expectations called unit rules that staff members post and explain to patients upon admittance. Their purpose is to facilitate a comfortable and safe environment; they have little to do with the patients' reasons for admission. Getting up at certain times, showering before

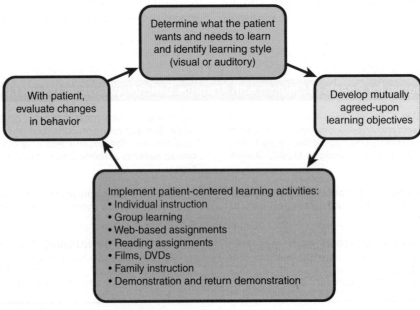

FIGURE 11.2   Teaching evaluation model.

breakfast, making the bed, and not visiting others' rooms are typical expectations. It is usually the nurse manager who oversees the operation of the unit and implementation of privilege systems.

Most psychiatric facilities use a privilege system to protect patients and to reinforce unit rules and other appropriate behavior (also see the previous section discussing token economies). The more appropriate the behavior, the more privileges of freedom the person has. Privileges are based on the assessment of a patient's risk to harm themselves or others and ability to follow treatment regimens. For example, a patient with few privileges may be required to stay on the unit and eat only with other patients. A patient with full privileges may have freedom to leave the unit and go outside the hospital and into the community for short periods.

Milieu Therapy

Milieu therapy provides a stable and coherent social organization to facilitate an individual's treatment. (The terms *milieu therapy* and *therapeutic environment* are often used interchangeably.) In **milieu therapy**, the design of the physical surroundings, structure of patient activities, and promotion of a stable social structure and cultural setting enhance the setting's therapeutic potential. A therapeutic milieu facilitates patient interactions and promotes personal growth. Milieu therapy is the responsibility of the nurse in collaboration with the patient and other health care providers. The key concepts of milieu therapy include containment, validation, structured interaction, and open communication.

Containment

Containment is the process of providing safety and security and involves the patient's access to food and shelter. In a well-contained milieu, patients feel safe from their illnesses and protected against social stigma. The physical surroundings are also important in this process and should be clean and comfortable, with special attention paid to promoting a noninstitutionalized environment. Pictures on walls, comfortable furniture, and soothing colors help patients relax. Most facilities encourage patients and nursing staff to wear street clothes, which help decrease the formalized nature of hospital settings and promote nurse–patient relationships.

Therapeutic milieus emphasize patient involvement in treatment decisions and operation of the unit; nurses should encourage freedom of movement within the contained environment. Patients participate in maintaining the quality of the physical surroundings, assuming responsibility for making their own beds, attending to their own belongings, and keeping an acceptable living area. Families are viewed as a part of the patient's life, and ties are maintained. In most inpatient settings, specific times are set for family interaction, education, and treatment. Family involvement is often a criterion

for admission for treatment, and the involvement may include regular family attendance at therapy sessions.

Validation

In a therapeutic environment, **validation** is another process that affirms patient individuality. Staff–patient interactions should constantly reaffirm the patient's humanity and human rights. All interaction a staff member initiates with a patient should reflect their respect for that patient. Patients must believe that staff members truly like and respect them.

Structured Interaction

One of the most interesting milieu concepts is **structured interaction**, which is purposeful interaction that allows patients to interact with others in a useful way. For instance, the daily community meeting provides structure to explain unit rules and consequences of violations. Ideally, patients who either are elected or volunteer for the responsibility assume leadership for these meetings. In the meeting, the group discusses behavioral expectations, such as making beds daily, appropriate dress, and rules for leaving the unit. Usually, there are other rules, such as no fighting or name calling.

In some instances, the treatment team assigns structured interactions to specific patients as part of their treatment. Specific attitudes or approaches are directed toward individual patients who benefit from a particular type of interaction. Nurses consistently assume indulgence, flexibility, passive or active friendliness, matter-of-fact attitude, casualness, watchfulness, or kind firmness when interacting with specific patients. For example, if a patient is known to overreact and dramatize events, the staff may provide a matter-of-fact attitude when the patient engages in dramatic behavior.

Open Communication

In **open communication**, the staff and patient willingly share information. Staff members invite patient self-disclosure within the support of a nurse–patient relationship. In addition, they provide a model of effective communication when interacting with one another as well as with patients. They arrange an environment to facilitate optimal interaction and resocialization. Support, attention, praise, and reassurance given to patients improve self-esteem and increase confidence. Patient education is also a part of this support, as are directions to foster coping skills.

Milieu Therapy in Different Settings

Milieu therapy is applied in various settings. In long-term care settings, the therapeutic milieu becomes essential because patients may reside there for months or years. These patients typically have schizophrenia or developmental disabilities. Structure in daily living is important to the successful functioning of the individuals and the overall group but must be applied within the context of individual needs. For example, if a patient cannot get up one morning in time to complete assigned tasks (e.g., showering or making a bed) because of a personal crisis the night before, the nurse should consider the situation compassionately and flexibly, not applying the "consequences" rule or taking away the patient's privileges. In turn, the nurse must weigh individual needs against the collective needs of all the patients. For a patient who is consistently late for treatment activities, the nurse should apply the rules of the unit even if it means taking away privileges.

Recently, concepts of milieu therapy have been applied to short-term inpatient and community settings. In acute care inpatient settings, nursing actions provide limits to and controls on patient behavior and provide structure and safety for the patients. Milieu treatments are based on the individual needs of the patients and include relaxation groups, discussion groups, and medication groups. Spontaneous and planned activities are possible on a short-term unit as well as in a long-term setting. In the community, it is possible to apply milieu therapy approaches in day treatment centers, group homes, and single dwellings.

Promotion of Patient Safety

Although the use of social rules of conduct and privilege systems can enhance smooth operation of a unit, some potentially serious problems can be associated with these practices. A most critical aspect of psychiatric–mental health nursing is the promotion of patient safety, especially in inpatient units.

Observation

Patient observation is the ongoing assessment of the patient's mental status to identify and subvert any potential problem. An important process in all nursing practice, observation is particularly important in psychiatric nursing. In psychiatric settings, patients are ambulatory and thus more susceptible to environmental hazards. In addition, judgment and cognition impairment are symptoms of many psychiatric disorders. Often, patients are admitted because they pose a danger to themselves or others. In psychiatric nursing, observation is more than just "seeing" patients. It means continually monitoring them for any indication of harm to themselves or others.

All patients who are hospitalized for psychiatric reasons are continually monitored. The intensity of the observation depends on their risk to themselves and others. Some patients are merely asked to "check in" at different times of the day, but others have a staff member assigned to only them, as in instances of potential suicide. Often "sharps," such as razors, are locked up and given to patients at specified times. Mental health facilities and units all have policies that specify levels of observation for patients of varying degrees of risk.

De-escalation

De-escalation is an interactive process of calming and redirecting a patient who has an immediate potential for violence directed toward self or others. This intervention involves assessing the situation and preventing it from escalating to one in which injury occurs to the patient, staff, or other patients. After the nurse has assessed the situation, the nurse calmly calls to the patient and asks the individual to leave the situation. The nurse must avoid rushing toward the patient or giving orders (see Chapter 20). Nurses can use various interventions in this situation, including distraction, conflict resolution, and cognitive interventions.

Home Visits

Patients usually have been hospitalized or have received treatment for acute psychiatric symptoms before they are referred to psychiatric home service. The goal of **home visits**, the delivery of nursing care in the patient's living environment, is to maximize the patient's functional ability within the nurse–patient relationship and with the family or partner as appropriate. The psychiatric nurse who makes home visits needs to be able to work independently, is skilled in teaching patients and families, can administer and monitor medications, and uses community resources for the patient's needs.

Home visits are especially useful in certain situations, including helping reluctant patients enter therapy, conducting a comprehensive assessment, strengthening a support network, and maintaining patients in the community when their condition deteriorates. Home visits are also useful in helping individuals comply with taking medication. The home visit process consists of three steps: the previsit phase, the home visit, and the postvisit phase. During previsit planning, the nurse sets goals for the home visit based on data received from other health care providers or the patient. In addition, the nurse and patient agree on the time of the visit. As the nurse travels to the home, the nurse should assess the neighborhood for access to services, socioeconomic factors, and safety.

The actual visit can be divided into four parts. The first is the greeting phase, in which the nurse establishes rapport with family members. Greetings, which are usually brief, establish the communication process and the atmosphere for the visit. Greetings should be friendly but professional. In cultures that consider greetings important, this phase may involve more formal interactions, such as eating food or drinking tea with family members. The next phase establishes the focus of the visit. Sometimes, the purpose of the visit is medication administration, health teaching, or counseling. The patient and family must be clear regarding the purpose. The implementation of the service is the next phase and should use most of the visit time. If the purpose of the visit is problem-solving or decision-making, the family's cultural values may determine the types of interaction and decision-making approaches. Closure is the last phase, the end of the home visit. It is a time to summarize and clarify important points. The nurse should also schedule any additional visits and reiterate patient expectations between visits. Usually, the nurse is the only provider to see the patient regularly. The nurse should acknowledge family members on leaving if they were not a part of the visit.

The postvisit phase includes documentation, reporting, and follow-up planning. This is also when the nurse meets with the supervisor and presents data from the home visit at the team meeting.

Community Action

Nurses have a unique opportunity to promote mental health awareness and support humane treatment for people with mental disorders. Activities range from being an advisor to support groups to participating in the political process through lobbying efforts and serving on community mental health boards. These unpaid activities are usually outside the realm of a job. However, an important role of professionals is to provide community service in addition to service through income-generating positions.

EVALUATING OUTCOMES

Evaluation of patient outcomes involves answering the following questions:

- What is the cost effectiveness of the intervention?
- What benefits did the patient receive?
- What was the patient's level of satisfaction?
- Was the outcome specific or nonspecific to the patient's need?

Outcomes can be measured immediately after the nursing intervention or after time passes. For example, a patient may be able to resolve the acute depression and demonstrate confidence and improved self-esteem during a hospital stay. In various cases, it may be several months before the person can engage in positive interpersonal relationships.

SUMMARY OF KEY POINTS

- Assessment is the deliberate and systematic collection of information or data to determine current and past health, mental health, wellness, strengths, functional status, and present and past coping patterns.
- The assessment of the physical domain includes current and past health status; physical examination with review of body systems; review of physical functions; and pharmacologic, strength, and wellness assessment.

- The psychological assessment includes the mental status examination, behavioral responses, and risk factor assessment.
- The mental status examination includes general observation of appearance, psychomotor activity, and attitude; orientations; mood; affect; emotions; speech; and thought processes.
- Behavioral responses are assessed, as are self-concept and current and past coping patterns.
- Risk factor assessment includes ascertaining whether the patient has any suicidal, assaultive, or homicidal ideation.
- Psychological strengths and wellness attributes are summarized.
- The social assessment includes functional status; social systems; spirituality; occupational, economic, and legal status; quality of life; social strengths; and wellness attributes.
- The nursing assessment provides the data for nursing diagnoses and planning with the patient for mutually agreeable outcomes. Anticipated patient outcomes provide direction for psychiatric–mental health nursing interventions.
- Nursing interventions that are implemented for each domain include biologic (self-care, activity and exercise, sleep, nutrition, thermoregulation, and pain and medication management); psychological (counseling, conflict resolution, bibliotherapy, reminiscence, behavior therapy, psychoeducation, health teaching, and spiritual interventions); and social (behavior therapy and modification, milieu therapy, and various home and community interventions).
- Evaluation of patient outcomes involves assessing cost effectiveness of the interventions, benefits to the patient, and the patient's level of satisfaction. Outcomes should be measurable, either immediately after intervention or after some time.

CRITICAL THINKING CHALLENGES

1. A 23-year-old White woman is admitted to an acute psychiatric setting for depression and suicidal gestures. This admission is her first, but she has experienced bouts of depression since early adolescence. She and her fiancé have just broken their engagement and moved into separate apartments. She has not yet told anyone that she is pregnant. She said that her mother had told her that she was "living in sin" and that she would "pay for it." The patient wants to "end it all!" From this scenario, develop three important assessment questions related to her physical health and safety.

2. Identify normal laboratory values for sodium, blood urea nitrogen, liver enzymes, leukocyte count, and differential and thyroid functioning. Why are these values important to know?

3. Write a paragraph on your self-concept, including all three components: body image, self-esteem, and personal identity. Explore the type of patient situations in which your self-concept can help your interactions with patients. Explore the types of patient situations in which your self-concept can hinder your interactions with patients.

4. Tom, a 25-year-old man with schizophrenia, lives with his parents, who want to retire to Florida. Tom goes to work each day but relies on his mother for meals, laundry, and reminders to take his medication. Tom believes that he can manage the home, but his mother is concerned. She asks the nurse for advice about leaving her son to manage on his own. What approach would you use?

5. Joan, a 35-year-old married woman, is admitted to an acute psychiatric unit for stabilization of her mood disorder. She is extremely depressed but refuses to consider a recommended medication change. She asks the nurse what to do. Using a nursing intervention, explain how you would approach Joan's problem.

6. A nurse reports to work for the evening shift. The unit is chaotic. The television in the day room is loud; two patients are arguing about the program. Visitors are mingling in patients' rooms. The temperature of the unit is high. One patient is running up and down the hall yelling, "Help me, help me." Using a milieu therapy approach, what would you do to calm the unit?

REFERENCES

American Nurses Association, American Psychiatric Nurses Association, & International Society of Psychiatric-Mental Health Nurses. (2014). *Psychiatric-mental health nursing: Scope and standards of practice* (2nd ed.). Nursebooks.org

Broderick, J. E., DeWitt, E. M., Rothrock, N., Crane, P. K., & Forrest, C. B. (2013). Advances in patient-reported outcomes: The NIH PROMIS Measures. *EGEMS (Wash DC) (Generating Evidence & Methods to improve patient outcomes)*, 1(1), 1015.

Butcher, H. K., Bulechek, G. M., McCloskey, J. M., & Wagner, C. M. (2019). *Nursing interventions classification (NIC)* (7th ed.). St. Louis.

Clarke, J., & Baume, K. (2019). Embedding spiritual care into everyday nursing practice. *Nursing Standard (Royal College of Nursing (Great Britain): 1987)*, 10.7748/ns.2019.e11354. Advance online publication. https://doi.org/10.7748/ns.2019.e11354

Courtain, A., & Glowacz, F. (2019). 'Youth's conflict resolution strategies in their dating relationships.' *Journal of Youth and Adolescence*, 48(2), 256–268. https://doi.org/10.1007/s10964-018-0930-6

Das, S., Punnoose, V. P., Doval, N., & Nair, V. Y. (2018). Spirituality, religiousness and coping in patients with schizophrenia: A cross sectional study in a tertiary care hospital. *Psychiatry Research*, 265, 238–243. https://doi.org/10.1016/j.psychres.2018.04.030

Eisen, K., Lawlor, C., Wu, C. D., & Mason, D. (2018). Reading and recovery expectations: Implementing a recovery-oriented bibliotherapy program in an acute inpatient psychiatric setting. *Psychiatric Rehabilitation Journal*, 41(1), 241–245.

Escovar, E. L., Drahota, A., Hitchcock, C., Chorpita, B. F., & Chavira, D. A. (2019). Vicarious improvement among parents participating in child-focused cognitive-behavioral therapy for anxiety. *Child & Family Behavior Therapy*, 41(1), 16–31. https://doi.org/10.1080/07317107.2019.1571770

Garaigordobil, M., & Martínez-Valderrey, V. (2018). Technological resources to prevent cyberbullying during adolescence: The Cyberprogram 2.0 Program and the Cooperative Cybereduca 2.0 Videogame. *Frontiers in Psychology*, 9, 745. https://doi.org/10.3389/fpsyg.2018.00745

Glowacki, K., Warner, G., & White, C. (2016). The use of a token economy for behavior and symptom management in adult psychiatric inpatients: A critical review of the literature. *Journal of Psychiatric Intensive Care*, 12(2), 119–127.

Gomi, S., Starnino, V. R., & Canda, E. R. (2014). Spiritual assessment in mental health recovery. *Community Mental Health Journal*, 50(4), 447–453.

Gümüs, F., Ergün, G., & Dikeç, G. (2020). Effect of psychoeducation on stress in parents of children with attention-deficit/ hyperactivity disorder: Arandomized controlled study. Journal of Psychosocial Nursing and Mental Health Services, 58(7), 34–41. https://doi.org/10.3928/02793695-20200506-01

Hickey, V., Flesch, L., Lane, A., Pai, A., Huber, J., Badia, P., Davies, S. M., & Dandoy, C. E. (2018). Token economy to improve adherence to activities of daily living. *Pediatric Blood & Cancer*, 65(11), e27387. https://doi.org/10.1002/pbc.27387

Lazarevic, V. (2017). Effects of cultural brokering on individual wellbeing and family dynamics among immigrant youth. *Journal of Adolescence*, 55, 77–87. https://doi.org/10.1016/j.adolescence.2016.12.010

Martin, K. S. (2005). *The Omaha system: A key to practice, documentation, and information, management* (2nd ed.). Elsevier Saunders.

Martin, K. S., & Kessler, P. D. (2017). Omaha system: Improving the quality of practice and decision-support. In M. D. Harris (Ed.), *Handbook of home health care administration* (6th ed., pp. 235–248). Jones and Bartlett.

Özgüç, S., & Tanriverdi, D. (2018). Relations between depression level and conflict resolution styles, marital adjustments of patients with major depression and their spouses. *Archives of Psychiatric Nursing*, 32(3), 337–342.

Paul, S., Corneau, S., Boozary, T., & Stergiopoulos, V. (2018). Coping and resilience among ethnoracial individuals experiencing homelessness and mental illness. *International Journal Social Psychiatry*, 64(2), 189–197.

Pirnia, B., Tabatabaei, S. K., Tavallaii, A., Soleimani, A. A., & Pirnia, K. (2016). The efficacy of contingency management on cocaine craving, using prize-based reinforcement of abstinence in cocaine users. *Electronic Physician*, 8(11), 3214–3221. https://doi.org/10.19082/3214

Posner, K., Brown, G. K., Stanley, B., Brent, D. A., Yershova, K. V., Oquendo, M. A., Currier, G. W., Melvin, G. A., Greenhill, L., Shen, S., & Mann, J. J. (2011). The Columbia-Suicide Severity Rating Scale: Initial validity and internal consistency findings from three multisite studies with adolescents and adults. *The American Journal of Psychiatry*, 168(12), 1266–1277. https://doi.org/10.1176/appi.ajp.2011.10111704

Saba, V. K. (2017). *Clinical care classification (CCC) system (version 2.1) (User's Guide)* (2nd ed.). Springer Publishing Company.

Smahel, D., Elavsky, S., & Machackova, H. (2019). Functions of mHealth applications: A user's perspective. *Health Informatics Journal*, 25(3), 1065–1075. https://doi.org/10.1177/1460458217740725

Substance Abuse and Mental Health Services Administration. (2009). *Illness management and recovery: Practitioner guides and handouts*. HHS Pub. No. SMA-09-4462, Center for Mental Health Services, Substance Abuse and Mental Health Services Administration, U.S. Department of Health and Human Services.

The Joint Commission Standards. (2020). Medical record - Spiritual assessment. https://www.jointcommission.org/standards/standard-faqs/home-care/provision-of-care-treatment-and-services-pc/000001669/.

Tsanas, A., Little, M. A., & Ramig, L. O. (2021). Remote assessment of Parkinson's Disease symptom severity using the simulated cellular mobile telephone network. *IEEE Access: Practical Innovations, Open Solutions*, 9, 11024–11036. https://doi.org/10.1109/ACCESS.2021.3050524

Timmins, F., & Caldeira, S. (2017). Assessing the spiritual needs of patients. *Nursing Standard*, 31(29), 47–53.

Weathers, E., McCarthy, G., & Goffey, A. (2015). Concept analysis of spirituality: An evolutionary approach, *Nursing Forum*, 51(2), 79–96.

Weitzman, E. A., & Weitzman, P. F. (2014). In P. T. Coleman, M. Deutcsh, & E. Marcus (Eds.), *The handbook of conflict resolution: Theory and practice* (3rd ed., pp. 203–229). Jossey-Bass.

Yuan, S., Zhou, X., Zhang, Y., Zhang, H., Pu, J., Yang, L., Liu, L., Jiang, X., & Xie, P. (2018). Comparative efficacy and acceptability of bibliotherapy for depression and anxiety disorders in children and adolescents: A meta-analysis of randomized clinical trials. *Neuropsychiatric Disease and Treatment*, 14, 353–365. https://doi.org/10.2147/NDT.S152747

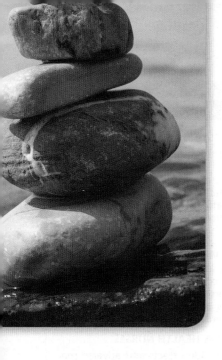

12

Psychopharmacology, Dietary Supplements, and Biologic Interventions

Mary Ann Boyd

KEYCONCEPTS

- agonists
- antagonists
- pharmacokinetics
- pharmacodynamics

LEARNING OBJECTIVES

After studying this chapter, you will be able to:

1. Differentiate target symptoms from side effects.
2. Identify nursing interventions for common side effects of psychiatric medications.
3. Explain the role of the governmental regulatory process in the approval of medication and the use of other biologic interventions.
4. Discuss the pharmacodynamics of psychiatric medications.
5. Discuss the pharmacokinetics of psychiatric medications.
6. Explain the major classifications of psychiatric medications.
7. Identify typical nursing interventions related to the administration of psychiatric medications.
8. Analyze the potential benefits of other forms of somatic treatments, including herbal supplements, nutrition therapies, electroconvulsive therapy, light therapy, transcranial magnetic stimulation, and vagus nerve stimulation.
9. Evaluate the significance of nonadherence and discuss strategies supportive of medication adherence.

KEY TERMS

- Absorption • Adherence • Adverse reactions • Affinity • Akathisia • Atypical antipsychotics • Augmentation
- Bioavailability • Biotransformation • Boxed warning • Carrier protein • Chronic syndromes • Clearance
- Compliance • Conventional antipsychotics • Cytochrome P450 (CYP450) system • Desensitization • Distribution
- Dosing • Drug–drug interaction • Dystonia • Efficacy • Enzymes • Ethnopsychopharmacology • Excretion
- Extrapyramidal symptoms • First-pass effect • Half-life • Hypnotics • Inducer • Inhibitor • Intrinsic activity
- Metabolism • Metabolites • Partial agonists • Pharmacogenomics • Phototherapy • Polypharmacy • Potency
- Prescribing Information • Protein binding • Pseudoparkinsonism • Relapse • Transcranial magnetic stimulation
- Sedative–hypnotics • Sedatives • Selectivity • Serotonin syndrome • Side effects • Solubility • Steady state • Substrate
- Tardive dyskinesia • Target symptoms • Therapeutic index • Tolerance • Toxicity • Uptake receptors

INTRODUCTION

Recent scientific and technologic developments have opened the door for the development of new medications that treat mental disorders. Nurses administer these medications, monitor their effectiveness, and manage side effects; they also have an important role in educating patients about their medications. Psychiatric medications are increasingly prescribed in primary care settings, and nurses practicing in nonpsychiatric settings now need an in-depth knowledge of them.

This chapter focuses on the pharmacodynamics and pharmacokinetics of psychiatric medications. Included in this chapter is an overview of the major classes of psychopharmacologic drugs used in treating patients with mental disorders and the role of herbal supplements and nutritional therapies. In addition, other biologic treatments are discussed, including electroconvulsive therapy (ECT), light therapy, transcranial magnetic stimulation (rTMS), and vagus nerve stimulation (VNS).

PSYCHIATRIC MEDICATIONS

As with any drug, psychiatric medications are designated for use in certain conditions for specific symptoms. The nurse quickly realizes that these symptoms are present in several conditions, leading to many medications being prescribed for different diagnoses. Because medications can have both desirable and undesirable effects, it is important for the nurse to understand these factors to help ensure patient safety.

Target Symptoms and Side Effects

Psychiatric medications and other biologic interventions are indicated for **target symptoms** , which are specific measurable symptoms expected to improve with treatment. Standards of care guide nurses in monitoring and documenting the effects of medications and other biologic treatments on target symptoms.

As yet, no drug has been developed that is so specific it affects only its target symptoms; instead, drugs typically act on several other organs and sites within the body. Even drugs with a high affinity and selectivity for a specific neurotransmitter will cause some responses in the body that are not related to the target symptoms. These unwanted effects of medications are called **side effects**. If unwanted effects have serious physiologic consequences, they are considered **adverse reactions**. The nurse monitors, documents, and reports the appearance of side effects and adverse reactions and implements nursing interventions for relief of medication side effects (Table 12.1).

BOX 12.1

Testing New Drugs for Safety and Efficacy

PHASES OF NEW DRUG TESTING

- Phase I: Testing defines the range of dosages tolerated in healthy individuals.
- Phase II: Effects of the drug are studied in a limited number of persons with the disorder. This phase defines the range of clinically effective dosage.
- Phase III: Extensive clinical trials are conducted at multiple sites throughout the country with larger numbers of patients. Efforts focus on corroborating the efficacy identified in phase II. Phase III concludes with a new drug application being submitted to the FDA.
- Phase IV: Drug studies continue after FDA approval to detect new or rare adverse reactions and potentially new indications. During this period, adverse reactions from the new medication should be reported to the FDA.

IMPLICATIONS FOR MENTAL HEALTH NURSES

- Throughout the phases, side effects and adverse reactions are monitored closely. The studies are tightly controlled, and strict regulations are enforced at each step.
- To prove drug effectiveness, diagnoses must be accurate, strict guidelines are followed, and subjects usually are not taking other medications and do not have complicating illnesses.
- A newly approved drug is approved only for the indications for which it has been tested.

Drug Regulation and Use

The U.S. Food and Drug Administration (FDA) is responsible for ensuring the safety, efficacy, and security of human and veterinary drugs, biologic products, medical devices, nation's food supply, cosmetics, and products that emit radiation (www.FDA.gov). The FDA approves the labeling of medications and other biologic treatments after a thorough review of efficacy and safety data (Box 12.1). Nurses administering medications are responsible for knowing the labeling content, which is found in each medication's package insert or **Prescribing Information (PI)** and includes approved indications for the medication, side effects, adverse reactions, contraindications, and other important information. If the FDA identifies serious adverse reactions that can occur with the use of a specific medication, it may issue a warning found in a **boxed warning** in the PI. The nurse should be aware of these boxed warnings and monitor for the appearance of the adverse reactions. If a PI is not readily available, the labeling information is easily found on the FDA's website and in most pharmacy departments.

PSYCHOPHARMACOLOGY

A comparatively small amount of medication can have a significant and large impact on cell function and resulting behavior. When tiny molecules of medication are compared with the vast amount of cell surface in the

TABLE 12.1 MANAGING COMMON SIDE EFFECTS OF PSYCHIATRIC MEDICATIONS

Side Effect or Discomfort	Intervention
Blurred vision	Reassurance (generally subsides in 2–6 wk).
Dry eyes	Artificial tears may be required; increased use of wetting solutions for those wearing contact lens. Alert ophthalmologist; no eye examination for new glasses for at least 3 wk after a stable dose.
Dry mouth and lips	Frequent rinsing of mouth, good oral hygiene, sucking sugarless candies or lozenges, lip balm, lemon juice, and glycerin mouth swabs.
Constipation	High-fiber diet; encourage bran, fresh fruits, and vegetables. Metamucil (must consume at least 16 oz of fluid with dose). Increase hydration. Exercise; increase fluids. Mild laxative.
Urinary hesitancy or retention	Monitor frequently for difficulty with urination, including changes in starting or stopping stream. Notify prescriber if difficulty develops. A cholinergic agonist, such as bethanechol, may be required.
Nasal congestion	Nose drops, moisturizer, *not* nasal spray
Sinus tachycardia	Assess for infections. Monitor pulse for rate and irregularities. Withhold medication and notify prescriber if resting rate exceeds 120 bpm.
Decreased libido, anorgasmia, ejaculatory inhibition	Reassurance (reversible); change to another medication.
Postural hypotension	Frequently monitor lying-to-standing blood pressure during dosage adjustment period, immediate changes and accommodation, and measure pulse in both positions; consider change to less antiadrenergic drug. Advise patient to get up slowly, sit for at least 1 min before standing (dangling legs over side of bed), and stand for 1 min before walking or until lightheadedness subsides. Increase hydration, avoid caffeine. Elastic stockings if necessary. Notify prescriber if symptoms persist or significant blood pressure changes are present; medication may have to be changed if patient does not have impulse control to get up slowly.
Photosensitivity	Protective clothing. Dark glasses. Use of sun block; remember to cover all exposed areas.
Dermatitis	Stop medication usage. Consider medication change; may require a systemic antihistamine. Initiate comfort measures to decrease itching.
Impaired psychomotor functions	Advise patient to avoid dangerous tasks, such as driving. Avoid alcohol, which increases this impairment.
Drowsiness or sedation	Encourage activity during the day to increase accommodation. Avoid tasks that require mental alertness, such as driving. May need to adjust dosing schedule or, if possible, give a single daily dose at bedtime. May need a cholinergic medication if sedation is the problem. Avoid driving or operating potentially dangerous equipment. May need change to less sedating medication. Provide quiet and decreased stimulation when sedation is the desired effect.
Weight gain and metabolic changes	Exercise and diet teaching. Caloric control.
Edema	Check fluid retention. Reassurance. May need a diuretic.
Irregular menstruation or amenorrhea	Reassurance (reversible). May need to change class of drug. Reassurance and counseling (does not indicate lack of ovulation). Instruct patient to continue birth control measures.
Vaginal dryness	Instruct in use of lubricants.

human body, the fraction seems disproportionate. Yet, the drugs used to treat mental disorders often have profound effects on behavior. To understand how this occurs, one needs to understand both where and how drugs work. The following discussion highlights important concepts relevant to psychiatric medications.

Pharmacodynamics: Where Drugs Act

Drug molecules act at specific sites, not on the entire cell surface. Psychiatric medications primarily target the central nervous system (CNS) at the cellular, synaptic level at four sites: receptors, ion channels, enzymes, and carrier proteins.

> **KEYCONCEPT Pharmacodynamics** is the action or effect of drugs on living organisms.

Receptors

Receptors are specific proteins intended to respond to a chemical (i.e., neurotransmitter) normally present in blood or tissues (see Chapter 8). Receptors also respond to drugs with similar chemical structures. When drugs attach to a receptor, they can act as **agonists**—substances that initiate the same response as the chemical normally present in the body—or as **antagonists**—substances that block the response of a given receptor. Figure 12.1 illustrates the action of an agonist and an antagonist drug at a receptor site. A drug's ability to interact with a

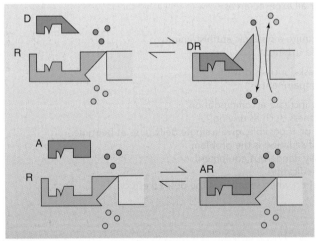

FIGURE 12.1 Agonist and antagonist drug actions at a receptor site. This schematic drawing represents drug–receptor interactions. At the *top*, drug D has the correct shape to fit receptor R, forming a drug–receptor complex, which results in a conformational change in the receptor and the opening of a pore in the adjacent membrane. Drug D is an agonist. At the *bottom*, drug A also has the correct shape to fit the receptor, forming a drug–receptor complex, but in this case, there is no conformational change and therefore no response. Drug A is, therefore, an antagonist.

given receptor type may be judged by three properties: selectivity, affinity, and **intrinsic activity**.

> **KEYCONCEPT Agonists** (mimic the neurotransmitter) have all three properties: selectivity, affinity, and intrinsic activity.
> **Antagonists** (block the receptor) have only selectivity and affinity properties; they do not have intrinsic activity because they produce no biologic response by attaching to the receptor.

Some drugs are referred to as **partial agonists** because they have some intrinsic activity (although weak). Because there are no "pure" drugs affecting only one neurotransmitter, most drugs have multiple effects. A drug may act as an agonist for one neurotransmitter and an antagonist for another. Medications that have both agonist and antagonist effects are called mixed agonist–antagonists.

Selectivity

Selectivity is the ability of a drug to be specific for a receptor. If a drug is highly selective, it will interact only with its specific receptors in the areas of the body where these receptors occur and therefore not affect tissues and organs where its receptors do not occur. Using a "lock-and-key" analogy, only a specific, highly selective key will fit a given lock. The more selective or structurally specific a drug is, the more likely it will affect only the specific receptor for which it is meant. The less selective the drug, the more receptors are affected and the more likely there will be unintended effects or side effects.

Affinity

Affinity is the degree of attraction or strength of the bond between the drug and its biologic target. Affinity is strengthened when a drug has more than one type of chemical bond with its target. If a cell membrane contains several receptors to which a drug will adhere, the affinity is increased. The weaker the chemical bond, the more likely a drug's effects are reversible. Most drugs used in psychiatry adhere to receptors through weak chemical bonds, but some drugs, specifically the monoamine oxidase inhibitors (MAOIs; discussed later), have a different type of bond, called a covalent bond. A covalent bond is formed when two atoms share a pair of electrons. This type of bond is stronger and irreversible at normal temperatures. The effects of the drugs that form covalent bonds are often called "irreversible" because they are long lasting, taking several weeks to resolve. Knowledge of a medication's affinity for receptors and subtypes of receptors may give some indication of the likelihood that specific target symptoms might improve and what side effects might be predicted.

Intrinsic Activity

A drug's ability to interact with a given receptor is its intrinsic activity, or the ability to produce a response after it becomes attached to the receptor. Some drugs have selectivity and affinity but produce no response. An important measure of a drug is whether it produces a change in the cell containing the receptor.

Ion Channels

Some drugs directly block the ion channels of the nerve cell membrane. For example, the antianxiety benzodiazepine drugs, such as diazepam (Valium), bind to a region of the gamma aminobutyric acid (GABA) receptor–chloride channel complex, which helps to open the chloride ion channel. In turn, the activity of GABA is enhanced.

Enzymes

Enzymes are usually proteins that act as catalysts for physiologic reactions and can be targets for drugs. For example, monoamine oxidase (MAO) is an enzyme required to break down neurotransmitters associated with depression (norepinephrine, serotonin, and dopamine). The MAOI antidepressants inhibit this enzyme, resulting in more neurotransmitter activity.

Carrier Proteins: Uptake Receptors

A **carrier protein** is a membrane protein that transports a specific molecule across the cell membrane. Carrier proteins (also referred to as **uptake receptors**) recognize sites specific for the type of molecule to be transported. When a neurotransmitter is removed from the synapse, specific carrier molecules return it to the presynaptic nerve, where most of it is stored to be used again. Medications specific for this site block or inhibit this transport and therefore increase the activity of the neurotransmitter in the synapse. Figure 12.2 illustrates the reuptake blockade.

Clinical Concepts

Efficacy is the ability of a drug to produce a response and is considered when a drug is selected. The degree of receptor occupancy contributes to the drug's efficacy, but a drug may occupy many receptors and not produce a response. Table 12.2 provides a brief summation of possible physiologic effects from drug actions on specific neurotransmitters. This information should serve only as a guide in predicting side effects because many physical outcomes or behaviors resulting from neural transmission are controlled by multiple receptors and neurotransmitters.

Potency refers to the dose of drug required to produce a specific effect. One drug may be able to achieve the same clinical effect as another drug but at a lower dose, making it more potent. Although the drug given at the lower dose is more potent because both drugs achieve similar effects, they may be considered to have equal efficacy.

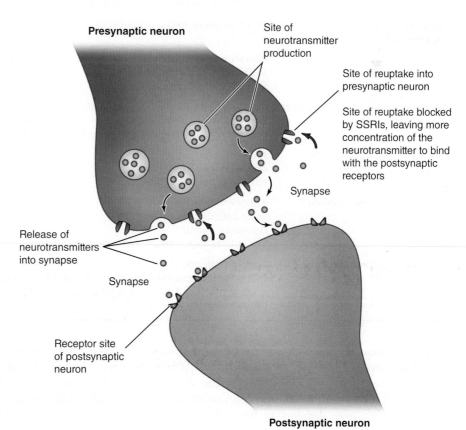

FIGURE 12.2 Reuptake blockade of a carrier molecule for serotonin by a selective serotonin reuptake inhibitor.

Note. SSRI = selective serotonin reuptake inhibitor.

TABLE 12.2 DRUG ACTIONS ON NEUROTRANSMITTERS

Action by Drug on Neurotransmitter	Physiologic Effects	Example of Drugs
Reuptake Inhibition		
Norepinephrine reuptake inhibition	Antidepressant action Potentiation of pressor effects of norepinephrine Interaction with guanethidine Side effects: tachycardia, tremors, insomnia, erectile, and ejaculation dysfunction	Desipramine Venlafaxine
Serotonin reuptake inhibition	Antidepressant action Antiobsessional effect Increase or decrease in anxiety (dose dependent) Side effects: gastrointestinal distress; nausea; headache; nervousness; motor restlessness; and sexual side effects, including anorgasmia	Fluoxetine Fluvoxamine
Dopamine reuptake inhibition	Antidepressant action Antiparkinsonian effect Side effects: increase in psychomotor activity, aggravation of psychosis	Bupropion
Receptor Blockade		
Histamine receptor blockade (H$_1$)	Side effects: sedation, drowsiness, hypotension, and weight gain	Quetiapine Imipramine Clozapine Olanzapine
Acetylcholine receptor blockade (muscarinic)	Side effects: anticholinergic (dry mouth, blurred vision, constipation, urinary hesitancy and retention, memory dysfunction) and sinus tachycardia	Imipramine Amitriptyline Olanzapine
Norepinephrine receptor blockade (α$_1$ receptor)	Potentiation of antihypertensive effect of prazosin and terazosin	Amitriptyline Clomipramine
	Side effects: postural hypotension, dizziness, reflex tachycardia, sedation	Clozapine
Norepinephrine receptor blockade (α$_2$ receptor)	Increased sexual desire (yohimbine)	Amitriptyline Clomipramine
	Interactions with antihypertensive medications, blockade of the antihypertensive effects of clonidine Side effect: priapism	Clozapine Trazodone Yohimbine
Norepinephrine receptor blockade (β$_1$ receptor)	Antihypertensive action (propranolol) Side effects: orthostatic hypotension, sedation, depression, sexual dysfunction (including impotence and decreased ejaculation)	Propranolol
Serotonin receptor blockade (5-HT$_{1a}$)	Antidepressant action Antianxiety effect Possible control of aggression	Trazodone Risperidone Ziprasidone
Serotonin receptor blockade (5-HT$_2$)	Antipsychotic action Some antimigraine effect Decreased rhinitis Side effects: hypotension, ejaculatory problems	Risperidone Clozapine Olanzapine Ziprasidone
Dopamine receptor blockade (D$_2$)	Antipsychotic action Side effects: extrapyramidal symptoms, such as tremor, rigidity (especially acute dystonia and parkinsonism); endocrine changes, including elevated prolactin levels	Haloperidol Ziprasidone

In some instances, the effects of medications diminish with time, especially when they are given repeatedly, as in the treatment of chronic psychiatric disorders. This loss of effect is most often a form of physiologic adaptation that may develop as the cell attempts to regain homeostatic control to counteract the effects of the drug. There are many reasons for decreased drug effectiveness (Box 12.2).

Desensitization is a rapid decrease in drug effects that may develop in a few minutes of exposure to a drug. This

---

BOX 12.2
Mechanisms Causing Decreases in Medication Effects
• Change in receptors
• Loss of receptors
• Exhaustion of neurotransmitter supply
• Increased metabolism of the drug
• Physiologic adaptation

reaction is rare with most psychiatric medications but can occur with some medications used to treat serious side effects (e.g., physostigmine, sometimes used to relieve severe anticholinergic side effects). A rapid decrease can also occur with some drugs because of immediate transformation of the receptor when the drug molecule binds to the receptor. Other drugs cause a decrease in the number of receptors or exhaust the mediators of neurotransmission.

Tolerance is a gradual decrease in the action of a drug at a given dose or concentration in the blood. This decrease may take days or weeks to develop and results in loss of therapeutic effect of a drug. For therapeutic drugs, this loss of effect is often called *treatment refractoriness*. In the abuse of substances such as alcohol or cocaine, tolerance is a part of the addiction (see Chapter 31).

Toxicity generally refers to the point at which concentrations of the drug in the bloodstream are high enough to become harmful or poisonous to the body. Individuals vary widely in their responses to medications. Some patients experience adverse reactions more easily than others. The **therapeutic index** is the ratio of the maximum nontoxic dose to the minimum effective dose. A high therapeutic index means that there is a large range between the dose at which the drug begins to take effect and a dose that would be toxic to the body. Drugs with a low therapeutic index have a narrow range.

This concept of toxicity has some limitations. The range can be affected by drug tolerance. For example, when tolerance develops, the person increases the dosage, which makes them more susceptible to an accidental suicide. The therapeutic index of a medication also may be greatly changed by the coadministration of other medications or drugs. For example, alcohol consumed with most CNS-depressant drugs will have added depressant effects, greatly increasing the likelihood of toxicity or death.

Pharmacokinetics: How the Body Acts on the Drugs

The field of pharmacokinetics studies the process of how drugs are acted on by the body through absorption, distribution, metabolism (biotransformation), and excretion. Pharmacokinetics for specific medications is always explained in a drug's PI. Together with the principles of

pharmacodynamics, this information is helpful in monitoring drug effects and predicting behavioral response.

KEYCONCEPT Pharmacokinetics is the process by which a drug is absorbed, distributed, metabolized, and eliminated by the body.

Absorption and Routes of Administration

The first phase of **absorption** is the movement of the drug from the site of administration into the plasma. The typical routes of administration of psychiatric medications include oral (tablet, capsule, and liquid), deltoid and gluteal intramuscular (IM; short- and long-acting agents), and intravenous (IV; rarely used for treatment of the primary psychiatric disorder but instead for rapid treatment of adverse reactions). A transdermal patch antidepressant and oral inhalation are also available. The advantages and disadvantages of each route and the subsequent effects on absorption are listed in Table 12.3.

Drugs taken orally are usually the most convenient for the patient; however, this route is also the most variable because absorption can be slowed or enhanced by several factors. Taking certain drugs orally with food or antacids may slow the rate of absorption or change the amount of the drug absorbed. For example, antacids containing aluminum salts decrease the absorption of most antipsychotic drugs; thus, antacids must be given at least 1 hour before administration or 2 hours after.

Oral preparations are absorbed from the gastrointestinal tract into the bloodstream through the portal vein and then to the liver. They may be metabolized within the gastrointestinal wall or liver before reaching the rest of the body. This is called the **first-pass effect**. The consequence of first-pass effect is that only a fraction of the drug reaches systemic circulation. Oral dosages are adjusted for the first-pass effect. That is, the dose of the oral form is significantly higher than the IM or IV formulations.

Bioavailability describes the amount of the drug that reaches systemic circulation unchanged. The route by which a drug is administered significantly affects bioavailability. With some oral drugs, the amount of drug entering the bloodstream is decreased by first-pass metabolism, and bioavailability is lower. On the other hand, some rapidly dissolving oral medications have increased bioavailability.

 Concept Mastery Alert

First-pass effect refers to the metabolism that a drug undergoes within the gastrointestinal wall or liver before reaching the rest of the body. Bioavailability describes the amount of a drug that reaches the systemic circulation unchanged.

TABLE 12.3 SELECTED FORMS AND ROUTES OF PSYCHIATRIC MEDICATIONS

Preparation and Route	Examples	Advantages	Disadvantages
Oral tablet	Basic preparation for most psychopharmacologic agents, including antidepressants, antipsychotics, mood stabilizers, anxiolytics, and so on	Usually most convenient	Variable rate and extent of absorption, depending on the drug May be affected by the contents of the intestines May show first-pass metabolism effects May not be easily swallowed by some individuals
Oral liquid	Also known as concentrates The antipsychotic risperidone The antidepressant fluoxetine Antihistamines, such as diphenhydramine Mood stabilizers, such as lithium citrate	Ease of incremental dosing Easily swallowed In some cases, more quickly absorbed	More difficult to measure accurately Depending on drug: • Possible interactions with other liquids such as juice, forming precipitants • Possible irritation to mucosal lining of mouth if not properly diluted
Rapidly dissolving tablet	Atypical antipsychotics, such as olanzapine, risperidone, asenapine	Dissolves almost instantaneously in mouth	Patient needs to remember to have completely dry hands and to place tablet in mouth immediately. Tablet should not linger in the hand. Handy for people who have trouble swallowing or for patients who let medication linger in the cheek for later expectoration Can be taken when water or other liquid is unavailable
Intramuscular	Some antipsychotics, such as ziprasidone, olanzapine, haloperidol, and chlorpromazine Anxiolytics, such as lorazepam Anticholinergics, such as benztropine mesylate No antidepressants No mood stabilizers	More rapid acting than oral preparations No first-pass metabolism	Injection-site pain and irritation Some medications may have erratic absorption if heavy muscle tissue at the site of injection is not in use.
Intramusculardepot (or long acting)	Risperidone (Risperdal Consta), paliperidone palmitate (Invega Sustenna), olanzapine (Zyprexa Relprevv), aripiprazole (Abilify Maintena), aripiprazole lauroxil (Aristada), haloperidol decanoate, fluphenazine decanoate	May be more convenient for some individuals who have difficulty following medication regimens	Pain at injection site
Intravenous	Anticholinergics, such as diphenhydramine, benztropine mesylate Anxiolytics, such as diazepam, lorazepam, and chlordiazepoxide	Rapid and complete availability to systemic circulation	Inflammation of tissue surrounding site Often inconvenient for patient and uncomfortable Continuous dosage requires use of a constant rate IV infusion
Subcutaneous (abdominal)	Risperidone (Perseris)	More convenient than oral regime; injection in abdomen may be preferable to the gluteus.	Pain at injection site
Transdermal patch	Antidepressant, selegiline	Avoid daily oral ingestion of medication.	Skin irritation
Oral inhalation	Conventional antipsychotic, loxapine	Rapidly absorbed to treat psychomotor agitation	Bronchospasm
Intranasal spray	Antidepressant, esketamine	Rapidly absorbed to treat severe depression	Nasal discomfort Oropharyngeal pain Throat irritation

Note. IV = intravenous.

Distribution

Distribution of a drug is the amount of the drug found in various tissues, particularly the target organ at the site of drug action. Factors that affect distribution include the size of the organ; amount of blood flow or perfusion within the organ; solubility of the drug; plasma protein binding (the degree to which the drug binds to plasma proteins); and anatomic barriers, such as the blood–brain barrier, that the drug must cross. A psychiatric drug may have rapid absorption and high bioavailability, but if it does not cross the blood–brain barrier to reach the CNS, it is of little use. Table 12.4 provides a summary of how some significant factors affect distribution. Two of these factors, solubility (ability of a drug to dissolve) and protein binding, warrant additional discussion about how they relate to psychiatric medications.

Solubility

Substances may cross a membrane in several ways, but passive diffusion is by far the simplest. To do this, the drug must dissolve in the structure of the cell membrane. Therefore, the **solubility** of a drug is an important characteristic. Being soluble in lipids allows a drug to cross most of the membranes in the body, and the tissues of the CNS are less permeable to water-soluble drugs than are other areas of the body. Most psychopharmacologic agents are lipid soluble and easily cross the blood–brain barrier. However, this characteristic means that psychopharmacologic agents also cross the placenta; consequently, most are contraindicated during pregnancy.

TABLE 12.4	FACTORS AFFECTING DISTRIBUTION OF A DRUG
Factor	**Effect on Drug Distribution**
Size of the organ	Larger organs require more drug to reach a concentration level equivalent to other organs and tissues.
Blood flow to the organ	The more blood flow to and within an organ (perfusion), the greater the drug concentration. The brain has high perfusion.
Solubility of the drug	The greater the solubility of a drug within a tissue, the greater its concentration.
Plasma protein binding	If a drug binds well to plasma proteins, particularly to albumin, it will stay in the body longer but have a slower distribution.
Anatomic barriers	Both the gastrointestinal tract and the brain are surrounded by layers of cells that control the passage or uptake of substances. Lipid-soluble substances are usually readily absorbed and pass the blood–brain barrier.

Protein Binding

Of considerable importance is the degree to which a drug binds to plasma proteins. Only unbound or "free" drugs act at the receptor sites. High **protein binding** reduces the concentration of the drug at the receptor sites. However, because the binding is reversible, as the unbound drug is metabolized, more drug is released from the protein bonds. Drugs are also released from storage in the fat depots. These processes can prolong the duration of action of the drug. When patients stop taking their medication, they often do not experience an immediate return of symptoms because they continue to receive the drug as it is released from storage sites in the body.

Metabolism

Metabolism, also called **biotransformation**, is the process by which a drug is altered and broken down into smaller substances, known as metabolites. Most metabolism occurs in the liver, but it can also occur in the kidneys, lungs, and intestines. Phase I includes oxidation, hydrolysis, and reduction reactions. In most cases, **metabolites** are inactive but in some psychiatric drugs, such as norfluoxetine (metabolite of fluoxetine [Prozac]), they are also active. Phase II reactions or conjugation combines a drug or metabolite with other chemicals. Through the phases of biotransformation, lipid-soluble drugs eventually become more water soluble so they may be readily excreted.

Phase I oxidation reactions are carried out by the **cytochrome P450 (CYP450) system**, a set of microsomal enzymes (usually hepatic) referred to as CYP1, CYP2, and CYP3. Within each CYP family, there are enzyme subgroups identified by a number–letter sequence (i.e., 1A2 or 3A4). There are more than 50 enzymes, but most of the metabolism occurs in only a few of them. A **substrate** is the drug or compound that is identified as a target of an enzyme. For example, clozapine is the substrate for the CYP1A2 enzyme.

The functioning of these enzymes is influenced by drugs and other chemical substances. An **inhibitor** of a CYP enzyme slows down metabolism, which in turn decreases the clearance of the substrate and elevates its plasma level. An **inducer** speeds up metabolism, which in turn increases the clearance of the substrate and decreases its plasma level. For example, cigarette smoke is a potent inducer of CYP1A2, which in turn speeds up the clearance of clozapine and decreases its plasma level. A smoker will clear clozapine faster than a nonsmoker even though both take the same dose.

A **drug–drug interaction** can occur if one substance inhibits an enzyme system. For example, nortriptyline (an antidepressant with a narrow therapeutic index) is the substrate of the CYP2D6 enzyme. By adding paroxetine (a selective serotonin reuptake inhibitor [SSRI] antidepressant and an inhibitor of the CYP2D6 enzyme), the 2D6 enzyme is inhibited, and the level of nortriptyline in the blood increases. Toxicity can easily develop because of a low therapeutic index. The PI informs the nurse which drugs should not be given together.

Each human CYP450 enzyme is an expression of a unique gene. The science of pharmacogenomics blends pharmacology with genetic knowledge and is concerned with understanding and determining an individual's specific CYP450 makeup and then individualizing medications to match the person's CYP450 profile. Genetically (inherited as an autosomal recessive trait), some individuals are poor metabolizers, and others may be rapid metabolizers. Whereas poor metabolizers are more likely to have adverse reactions, rapid metabolizers may not allow certain drugs to reach therapeutic levels. Research has suggested that there are variations among ethnic groups with poor metabolizers accounting for up to 7% of White individuals for CYP2D6 and up to 25% of East Asians for CYP2C19. Knowing whether patients are poor or rapid metabolizers is important because most psychiatric medications are metabolized by these enzymes. DNA laboratory tests are available for patients who have a personal or family history of adverse drug reactions to medications metabolized by 2D6 and 2D19 to confirm the presence of genotypes that affect metabolism. Enzyme CYP2D6 is important in the metabolism of many antidepressants and antipsychotics, and CYP2C19 is important for some antidepressant metabolism (Walden et al., 2019).

Excretion

Excretion refers to the removal of drugs from the body either unchanged or as metabolites. **Clearance** refers to the total volume of blood, serum, or plasma from which a drug is completely removed per unit of time to account for the excretion. The half-life of a drug provides a measure of the expected rate of clearance. **Half-life** refers to the time required for plasma concentrations of the drug to be reduced by 50%. For most drugs, the rate of excretion slows, but the half-life remains unchanged. It usually takes four half-lives or more of a drug in total time for more than 90% of a drug to be eliminated.

Drugs bound to plasma proteins do not cross the glomerular filter freely. These lipid-soluble drugs are passively reabsorbed by diffusion across the renal tubule and thus are not rapidly excreted in the urine. Because many psychiatric medications are protein bound and lipid soluble, most of their excretion occurs through the liver, where they are excreted in the bile and delivered into the intestine. Lithium and gabapentin, mood stabilizers, are notable examples of renal excretion. Any impairment in renal function or renal disease may lead to toxic symptoms.

Dosing refers to the administration of medication over time so that therapeutic levels may be achieved or maintained without reaching toxic levels. In general, it is necessary to give a drug at intervals no greater than the half-life of the medication to avoid excessive fluctuation of concentration in the plasma between doses. With repeated dosing, a certain amount of the drug is accumulated in the body.

Steady-state plasma concentration, or simply **steady state**, occurs when absorption equals excretion and the therapeutic level plateaus. The rate of accumulation is determined by the half-life of the drug. Drugs generally reach steady state in four to five times the elimination half-life. However, because elimination or excretion rates may vary significantly in any individual, fluctuations may still occur, and dose schedules may need to be modified.

Individual Variations in Drug Effects

Many factors affect drug absorption, distribution, metabolism, and excretion. These factors may vary among individuals, depending on their age, genetics, and ethnicity.

Age

Pharmacokinetics is significantly altered at the extremes of the life cycle. Gastric absorption changes as individuals' age. Gastric pH increases, and gastric emptying decreases. Gastric motility slows and splanchnic circulation is reduced. Normally, these changes do not significantly impair oral absorption of a medication, but addition of common conditions, such as diarrhea, may significantly alter and reduce absorption. Malnutrition, cancer, and liver disease decrease the production of the primary protein albumin. More free drug is acting in the system, producing higher blood levels of the medication and potentially toxic effects. The activity of hepatic enzymes also slows with age. As a result, the ability of the liver to metabolize medications may slow as much as a fourfold decrease between the ages of 20 and 70 years. Production of albumin by the liver generally declines with age. Changes in the parasympathetic nervous system produce a greater sensitivity in older adults to anticholinergic side effects, which are more severe with this age group.

Renal function also declines with age. Creatinine clearance in a young adult is normally 100 to 120 mL/min, but after age 40, this rate declines by about 10% per decade (Delanaye et al., 2019). Medical illnesses, such as diabetes and hypertension, may contribute to further decline of renal function. When creatinine clearance falls below 30 mL/min, the excretion of drugs by the kidneys is significantly impaired, and potentially toxic levels may accumulate.

Pharmacogenetics and Ethnopsychopharmacology

Pharmacogenomics is the study of how a person's genetic makeup affects their response to drugs. There are important genetic variations that influence the metabolism and action of psychotropic drugs in different ethnic groups. Various tests are used to predict genetic responses to drugs and the potential for adverse effects. For example, studies show that selecting antidepressants according to genetic profile can improve treatment outcomes for people with depression and anxiety (Bradley et al., 2018).

Overlapping pharmacogenetics is the field of **ethnopsychopharmacology**, the study of how culture and genetic differences in human groups determine and influence the response to medications. Ethnopsychopharmacology focuses on the impact of cultural practices, such as consuming foods or ingesting beverages, on genetic variations in metabolism, on complementary and alternate health care practices, and on herbal substances.

Although ethnic and racial groups are genetically heterogeneous, there are population differences in disease susceptibility (Roberts & Erdei, 2020). For example, some individuals of Asian descent produce higher concentrations of acetaldehyde with alcohol use than do those of European descent, resulting in a higher incidence of adverse reactions such as flushing and palpitations. Asians often require one half to one third the dose of antipsychotic medications and lower doses of antidepressants than Whites require (Matsushita & Higuchi, 2017). In the African populations, there is a high degree of variability in the dosage of many medications (Nievergelt et al., 2019).

PHASES OF DRUG TREATMENT AND THE NURSE'S ROLE

Phases of drug treatment include initiation, stabilization, maintenance, and discontinuation of the medication. The following explains the role of the nurse in these phases.

Initiation Phase

Before the initiation of medications, patients must undergo several assessments.

- A psychiatric evaluation to determine the diagnosis and target symptoms
- A nursing assessment that includes cultural beliefs and practices (see Chapter 12)
- Physical examination and indicated laboratory tests, often including baseline determinations such as a complete blood count (CBC), liver and kidney function tests, electrolyte levels, urinalysis, and possibly thyroid function tests and electrocardiography (ECG), to determine whether a physical condition may be causing the symptoms and to establish that it is safe to initiate use of a particular medication

During the initiation of medication, the nurse assesses, observes, and monitors the patient's response to the medication; teaches the patient about the action, dosage, frequency of administration, and side effects; and develops a plan for ongoing contact with clinicians. The first medication dose should be treated as if it were a "test" dose. Patients should be monitored for adverse reactions such as changes in blood pressure, pulse, or temperature; changes in mental status; allergic reactions; dizziness; ataxia; or gastric distress. If any of these symptoms develop, they should be reported to the prescriber.

Stabilization Phase

During stabilization, the prescriber adjusts or titrates the medication dosage to achieve the maximum amount of improvement with a minimum of side effects. Psychiatric–mental health nurses assess for improvements in the target symptoms and for the appearance of side effects. If medications are being increased rapidly, such as in a hospital setting, nurses must closely monitor temperature, blood pressure, pulse, mental status, common side effects, and unusual adverse reactions.

In the outpatient setting, nurses focus on patient education, emphasizing the importance of taking the medication, expected outcomes, and potential side effects. Patients need to know how and when to take their medications, how to minimize any side effects, and which side effects require immediate attention. A plan should be developed for patients and their families to clearly identify what to do if adverse reactions develop. The plan, which should include emergency telephone numbers or available emergency treatment, should be reviewed frequently.

Therapeutic drug monitoring is most important in this phase of treatment. Many medications used in psychiatry improve target symptoms only when a therapeutic level of medication has been obtained in the individual's blood. Some medications, such as lithium, have a narrow therapeutic range and must be monitored frequently and accurately. Nurses must be aware of when and how these levels are to be determined and assist patients in learning these procedures. Because of protein binding and lipid solubility, most medications do not have obtainable plasma levels that are clinically relevant. However, plasma levels of these medications may still be requested to evaluate further such issues as absorption and adverse reactions.

Sometimes, the first medication chosen does not adequately improve the patient's target symptoms. In such cases, use of the medication will be discontinued, and treatment with a new medication will be started. Medications may also be changed when adverse reactions or seriously uncomfortable side effects occur, or these effects substantially interfere with the individual's quality of life. Nurses should be familiar with the pharmacokinetics of both drugs to be able to monitor side effects and possible drug–drug interactions during this change.

At times, an individual may show only partial improvement from a medication, and the prescriber may try an **augmentation** strategy by adding another medication. For example, a prescriber may add a mood stabilizer, such as lithium, to an antidepressant to improve the effects of the antidepressant. **Polypharmacy**, using more than one group from a class of medications, is increasingly being used as an acceptable strategy with most psychopharmacologic agents to match the drug action to the neurochemical needs of the patient. Nurses must be familiar with the potential effects, side effects, drug interactions, and rationale for the treatment regimen.

Maintenance Phase

After the individual's target symptoms have improved, medications are usually continued to prevent **relapse** or return of the symptoms. In some cases, this may occur despite the patient's continued use of the medication. Patients must be educated about their target symptoms and have a plan of action if the symptoms return. In other cases, the patient may experience medication side effects. The psychiatric–mental health nurse has a central role in assisting individuals to monitor their own symptoms, identify emerging side effects, manage psychosocial stressors, and avoid other factors that may cause the medications to lose effect.

Discontinuation Phase

Some psychiatric medications will be discontinued; others will not. Some require a tapered discontinuation, which involves slowly reducing dosage while monitoring closely for reemergence of the symptoms. Some psychiatric disorders, such as mild depression, respond to treatment and do not recur. Other disorders, such as schizophrenia, usually require lifetime medication. Discontinuance of some medications, such as controlled substances, produces withdrawal symptoms; discontinuance of others does not.

MAJOR PSYCHOPHARMACOLOGIC DRUG CLASSES

Major classes of psychiatric drugs include antipsychotics, mood stabilizers, antidepressants, antianxiety and sedative–hypnotic medications, and stimulants.

Antipsychotic Medications

Antipsychotic medications can be thought of as "newer" and "older" medications. Newer or **atypical antipsychotics** appear to be equally or more effective but have fewer side effects than the traditional older agents. The term *typical* or **conventional antipsychotics** identifies the older antipsychotic drugs. Table 12.5 provides a list of selected antipsychotics.

Indications and Mechanism of Action

Antipsychotic medications are indicated for schizophrenia, mania, and autism and to treat the symptoms of psychosis, such as hallucinations, delusions, bizarre behavior, disorganized thinking, and agitation. (These symptoms are described more fully in later chapters.) These medications also reduce aggressiveness, and inappropriate behavior associated with psychosis. Within the typical antipsychotics, haloperidol and pimozide are approved for treating patients with Tourette syndrome, reducing the frequency and severity of vocal tics. Some of the typical antipsychotics, particularly chlorpromazine, are used as antiemetics or for postoperative intractable hiccoughs.

The atypical antipsychotic medications differ from the typical antipsychotics in that they block serotonin receptors more potently than the dopamine receptors. The difference between the mechanism of action of the typical and atypical antipsychotics helps to explain their differences in terms of effect on target symptoms and in the degree of side effects they produce.

Pharmacokinetics

Antipsychotic medications administered orally have a variable rate of absorption complicated by the presence of food, antacids, smoking, and even the coadministration of anticholinergics, which slow gastric motility. Clinical effects begin to appear in about 30 to 60 minutes. Absorption after IM administration is less variable because this method avoids the first-pass effects. Therefore, IM administration produces greater bioavailability. It is important to remember that IM medications are absorbed more slowly when muscles are not used. Typically, the deltoid is used more than the gluteal muscles, which may account for faster absorption of medication and which has better blood perfusion.

Metabolism of these drugs occurs almost entirely in the liver with the exception of paliperidone (Invega, Sustenna), which is not extensively metabolized by the liver but is excreted largely unchanged through the kidney, and Lurasidone (Latuda), which is excreted through the urine and feces. Most antipsychotics are subject to the effects of other drugs that induce or inhibit the liver enzymes described earlier (see Table 12.6). Careful

TABLE 12.5 ANTIPSYCHOTIC MEDICATIONS			
Generic (Trade) Drug Name	Usual Dosage Range	Half-Life	Route of Administration
Atypical Antipsychotics			
Aripiprazole (Abilify)	10–30 mg/day	75–94 h	Oral tablets, injection, disintegrating tablet
Aripiprazole (Abilify MyCite)	10–30 mg/day	75–49 h	Oral tablet embedded with an ingestible event marker sensor intended to track drug ingestion
Aripiprazole (Maintena)	200–400 mg	29.9–46.6 days	Injection
Aripiprazole lauroxil (Aristada)	441–882 mg monthly	29.2–34.9 days	Injection
Asenapine (Saphris)	5–10 mg BID	24 h	Sublingual tablet
Brexpiprazole (Rexulti)	0.5–1.0 mg/day	86–91 h	Oral tablet
Cariprazine (Vraylar)	1.5–6.0 mg/day	2–4 days 1–3 wk (metabolite)	Oral capsule
Clozapine (Clozaril, Fazaclo, Versacloz)	300–900 mg/day	4–12 h	Oral tablet, disintegrating tablet, oral suspension
Iloperidone (Fanapt)	6–12 mg BID	18–33 h	Oral tablet
Lurasidone (Latuda)	40 mg/day	18 h	Oral tablet
Olanzapine (Zyprexa)	5–15 mg/day 2.5–10 mg/day IM	21–54 h	Oral tablet, disintegrating tablet Injection
Olanzapine (Relprevv)	150–300 mg q2–4wk	30 days	Injection
Paliperidone (Invega Extended Release)	3–12 mg once daily in AM	23 h	Oral
Paliperidone (Invega Sustenna)	117 mg monthly	29–49 days	Injection
Pimavanserin (Nuplazid)	34 mg once daily	5 h for 17 mg	Oral tablet
Quetiapine fumarate (Seroquel)	150–750 mg/day	7 h	Oral tablet
Risperidone (Risperdal)	2–8 mg/day	20 h	Oral tablet, oral solution, disintegrating tablet
Risperdal (Consta)	25–50 mg q2wk	3–6 days	IM Injection
Risperidone (Perseris)	90 or 120 mg once monthly	9–11 days	Abdominal subcutaneous injection
Ziprasidone HCl (Geodon)	40–160 mg/day 10–20 mg/day IM	7 h	Oral capsule, oral suspension Injection
Lurasidone HCl (Latuda)	40–80 mg	18 h	Oral tablet
Conventional (Typical) Antipsychotics			
Chlorpromazine	50–1200 mg/day	2–30 h	Oral tablet
Fluphenazine	2–20 mg/day	4.5–15.3 h	Oral elixir, oral tablet, injection
Fluphenazine decanoate	12.5–25 mg q3wk		Injection
Perphenazine	12–64 mg/day	Unknown	Oral tablet
Trifluoperazine	5–40 mg/day	47–10 h	Oral tablet
Thiothixene (Navane)	5–60 mg/day	3 h	Oral capsule
Loxapine (Adasuve)	10 mg/day	7 h	Oral inhalation with inhaler
Haloperidol (Haldol)	2–20 mg/day	21–2 h	Oral tablet, oral concentration, injection
Haloperidol decanoate (Haldol D)	50–100 mg q3wk	3 wk	Injection
Molindone	50–400 mg/day	1.5 h	Oral tablets
Pimozide (ORAP)	10 mg/day	55 h	Oral tablets

Note. IM = intramuscular.

TABLE 12.6 CYP450 METABOLISM OF COMMONLY USED ANTIPSYCHOTICS

Drug	How Metabolized	Induces	Inhibits
Aripiprazole	2D6, 3A4	None	None
Clozapine	1A2, 2C19, 2D6, 3A4	None	None
Haloperidol	1A2, 2D6, 3A4	None	2D6
Iloperidone	3A4, 2D6	None	3A
Lurasidone	3A4 Eliminated in urine and feces	None	None
Olanzapine	1A2, 2D6	None	None
Paliperidone	<10% 2D6, 3A4; primarily renal elimination	None	None
Quetiapine	3A4	None	None
Risperidone	2D6	None	Mild 2D6
Ziprasidone	1A2, 3A4	None	None

Note. Information based on Prescribing Information of each medication.

observance of concurrent medication use, including prescribed, over the counter, and substances of abuse, is required to avoid drug–drug interactions. For example, atypical antipsychotic concentrations may be affected by CYP450-inhibiting drugs such as paroxetine and fluoxetine.

Excretion of these substances tends to be slow. Most antipsychotics have a half-life of 24 hours or longer, but many also have active metabolites with longer half-lives. These two effects make it difficult to predict elimination time, and metabolites of some of these agents may be found in the urine months later. When a medication is discontinued, the adverse reactions may not immediately subside. The patient may continue to experience and sometimes need treatment for the adverse reactions for several days. Similarly, patients who discontinue their antipsychotic drugs may still derive therapeutic benefit for several days to weeks after drug discontinuation.

High lipid solubility, accumulation in the body, and other factors have also made it difficult to correlate blood levels with therapeutic effects. Table 12.5 shows the therapeutic ranges available for some of the antipsychotic medications. The potency of the antipsychotics also varies widely and is of specific concern when considering typical antipsychotic drugs.

Long-Acting Preparations

Currently, in the United States, atypical and conventional antipsychotics are available in long-acting forms. These antipsychotics are administered by injection once every 2 weeks to 3 months. Whereas the long-acting injectable atypical antipsychotics (risperidone, paliperidone, olanzapine, and aripiprazole) are water-based suspensions, the conventional antipsychotics are oil-based solutions.

Long-acting injectable medications maintain a constant blood level between injections. Because they bypass problems with gastrointestinal absorption and first-pass metabolism, this method may enhance therapeutic outcomes for the patient. The use of these medications is expected to increase the likelihood of adhering to a prescribed medication regimen.

Nurses should be aware that the injection site may become sore and inflamed if certain precautions are not taken. The oil-based injections (fluphenazine and haloperidol) are viscous liquids. For these injections, a large gauge needle (at least 21 gauge) should be used. Because the medication is meant to remain in the injection site, the needle should be dry, and a deep IM injection should be given by the Z-track method. (Note: Do not massage the injection site. Rotate sites and document in the patient's record.) Manufacturer recommendations should be followed.

Side Effects, Adverse Reactions, and Toxicity

Various side effects and interactions can occur with antipsychotics, with the conventional (typical) antipsychotics producing different side effects than the atypical antipsychotics. The side effects vary largely based on their degree of attraction to different neurotransmitter receptors and their subtypes.

Cardiovascular Side Effects

Cardiovascular side effects include orthostatic hypotension and prolongation of the QTc interval (a marker indicating an abnormal electrocardiogram that could cause serious irregular heart rhythms). Orthostatic hypotension is very common and depends on the degree of blockade of α-adrenergic receptors. Typical and atypical antipsychotics have been associated with prolonged QTc intervals and should be used cautiously in patients who have increased QTc intervals or are taking other medications that may prolong the QTc interval (Das et al., 2019). Other cardiovascular side effects from typical antipsychotics have been rare, but occasionally they cause ECG changes that have a benign or undetermined clinical effect.

Anticholinergic Side Effects

Anticholinergic side effects resulting from blockade of acetylcholine are another common side effect associated with antipsychotic drugs. Dry mouth, slowed gastric motility, constipation, urinary hesitancy or retention, vaginal dryness, blurred vision, dry eyes, nasal congestion, and confusion or decreased memory are examples of these side effects. Interventions for decreasing the impact of these side effects are outlined in Table 12.1.

This group of side effects occurs with many of the medications used for psychiatric treatment. Using more than one medication with anticholinergic effects often increases the symptoms. Older patients are often most susceptible to a potential toxicity that results from high blockade of acetylcholine. This toxicity is called an *anticholinergic crisis* and is described more fully, along with its treatment, in Chapter 24.

Weight Gain

Weight gain is a common side effect of the atypical antipsychotics, particularly clozapine and olanzapine (Zyprexa), which can cause a weight gain of up to 20 lb within 1 year. Ziprasidone (Geodon), aripiprazole (Abilify), and lurasidone (Latuda) are associated with little to no weight gain. If a patient becomes overweight or obese, switching to another antipsychotic should be considered and weight control interventions implemented.

Diabetes

One of the more serious side effects is the risk of type II diabetes. The FDA has determined that all atypical antipsychotics increase the risk for type II diabetes. Nurses should routinely assess for emerging symptoms of diabetes and alert the prescriber of these symptoms (see Box 12.3).

Sexual Side Effects

Sexual side effects result primarily from the blockade of dopamine in the tuberoinfundibular pathways of the hypothalamus. As a result, blood levels of prolactin may increase, particularly with risperidone and the typical antipsychotics. Increased prolactin causes breast

---

> **BOX 12.3**
>
> **Recommended Assessments Before and During Antipsychotic Therapy**
>
> - Weigh all patients and track BMI during treatment.
> - Determine if overweight (BMI 25–29.9) or obese (BMI ≥30).
> - Monitor BMI monthly for first 3 months; then quarterly.
> - Obtain baseline personal and family history of diabetes, obesity, dyslipidemia, hypertension, and cardiovascular disease.
> - Get waist circumference (at umbilicus).
> - Men: >40 in. (102 cm).
> - Women: >35 in. (88 cm).
> - Monitor BP, fasting plasma glucose, and fasting lipid profile within 3 months and then annually (more frequently for patients with diabetes or who have gained >5% of initial weight).
> - Prediabetes (fasting plasma glucose 100–125 mg/dL).
> - Diabetes (fasting plasma glucose >126 mg/dL).
> - Hypertension (BP >140/90 mm Hg).
> - Dyslipidemia (increased total cholesterol [>200 mg], decreased HDL, and increased LDL).
>
> BMI, body mass index; BP, blood pressure; HDL, high-density lipoprotein; LDL, low-density lipoprotein.

---

enlargement and rare but potential galactorrhea (milk production and flow), decreased sexual drive, amenorrhea, menstrual irregularities, and increased risk for growth in preexisting breast cancers. Other sexual side effects include retrograde ejaculation (backward flow of semen), erectile dysfunction, and anorgasmia.

Blood Disorders

Blood dyscrasias are rare but have received renewed attention since the introduction of clozapine (Clozaril). Agranulocytosis is an acute reaction that causes the individual's white blood cell count to drop to very low levels often related to neutropenia, a drop in neutrophils. In the case of the antipsychotics, the medication suppresses the bone marrow precursors to blood factors. The exact mechanism by which the drugs produce this effect is unknown. The most notable symptoms of this disorder include high fever, sore throat, and mouth sores. Although benign elevations in temperature have been reported in individuals taking clozapine, no fever should go uninvestigated. Untreated neutropenia can be life threatening. Although severe neutropenia can occur with any of the antipsychotics, the risk with clozapine is greater than with the other antipsychotics. Therefore, prescription of clozapine requires weekly blood samples for the first 6 months of treatment and then every 2 weeks after that for as long as the drug is taken. Drawing of these samples must continue for 4 weeks after clozapine use has been discontinued. If sore throat or fever develops, medications should be withheld until a leukocyte count can be obtained. Hospitalization, including reverse isolation to prevent infections, is usually required. Severe neutropenia is more likely to develop during the first 18 weeks of treatment (Novartis, 2020).

Neuroleptic Malignant Syndrome

Neuroleptic malignant syndrome (NMS) is a serious complication that may result from antipsychotic medications. Characterized by rigidity and high fever, NMS is a rare condition that may occur abruptly with even one dose of medication. Temperature must always be monitored when administering antipsychotics, especially high-potency medications. This condition is discussed more fully in Chapter 24.

Other Side Effects

Photosensitivity reactions to antipsychotics, including severe sunburns or rash, most commonly develop with the use of low-potency typical medications. Sun block must be worn on all areas of exposed skin when taking these drugs. In addition, sun exposure may cause pigmentary deposits to develop, resulting in discoloration of exposed areas, especially the neck and face. This discoloration may progress from a deep orange color to a blue gray. Skin exposure should be limited, and skin tone changes reported to the prescriber. Pigmentary deposits, retinitis pigmentosa, may also develop on the retina of the eye.

Antipsychotics may also lower the seizure threshold. Patients with an undetected seizure disorder may experience seizures early in treatment. Those who have a preexisting condition should be monitored closely.

Medication-Related Movement Disorders

Medication-related movement disorders are side effects or adverse reactions that are commonly caused by typical antipsychotic medications but less commonly with atypical antipsychotic drugs. These disorders of abnormal motor movements can be divided into two groups: acute **extrapyramidal symptoms (EPS)**, which develop early in the course of treatment (sometimes after just one dose), and chronic syndromes, which develop from longer exposure to antipsychotic drugs.

Acute Extrapyramidal Symptoms

Acute EPS are acute abnormal movements that include dystonia, pseudoparkinsonism, and akathisia. They develop early in treatment, sometimes from as little as one dose. Although the abnormal movements are treatable, they are at times dramatic and frightening, causing physical and emotional impairments that often prompt patients to stop taking their medication. EPS occur when there is an imbalance of acetylcholine, dopamine, and GABA in the basal ganglia because of blocking dopamine.

Dystonia, sometimes referred to as an *acute dystonic reaction*, is impaired muscle tone that generally is the first EPS to occur, usually within a few days of initiating use of an antipsychotic. Acetylcholine is overactive because one of its modulators, dopamine, is blocked. Dystonia is characterized by involuntary muscle spasms that lead to abnormal postures especially of the head and neck muscles. Acute dystonia occurs most often in young men, adolescents, and children. Patients usually first report a thick tongue, tight jaw, or stiff neck. Dystonia can progress to a protruding tongue, oculogyric crisis (eyes rolled up in the head), torticollis (muscle stiffness in the neck, which draws the head to one side with the chin pointing to the other), and laryngopharyngeal constriction. Abnormal postures of the upper limbs and torso may be held briefly or sustained. In severe cases, the spasms may progress to the intercostal muscles, producing more significant breathing difficulty for patients who already have respiratory impairment from asthma or emphysema. The treatment is the administration of a medication such as the anticholinergic agents that inhibit acetylcholine and thereby restore the balance of neurotransmitters (Table 12.7).

Drug-induced parkinsonism is sometimes referred to as **pseudoparkinsonism** because its presentation is identical to Parkinson disease. The difference is that the activity of dopamine is blocked in pseudoparkinsonism, and in Parkinson disease, the cells of the basal ganglia are destroyed. Older patients are at the greatest risk for experiencing pseudoparkinsonism (Factor et al., 2020). Symptoms include the classic triad of rigidity, slowed movements (akinesia), and tremor. The rigid muscle stiffness is usually seen in the arms. Akinesia can be observed by the loss of spontaneous movements, such as the absence of the usual relaxed swing of the arms while walking. In addition, mask-like facies or loss of facial expression and a decrease in the ability to initiate movements also are present. Usually, tremor is more pronounced at rest, but it can also be observed with intentional movements, such as eating. If the tremor becomes severe, it may interfere with the patient's ability to eat or maintain adequate fluid intake. Hypersalivation is possible as well. Pseudoparkinsonism symptoms may occur on one or both sides of the body and develop abruptly or subtly but usually within the first 30 days of treatment. The treatment is the reduction in dosage or a change of antipsychotic that has less affinity for the dopamine receptor. Anticholinergic medication is sometimes given.

Akathisia is characterized by an inability to sit still or restlessness and is more common in middle-aged patients. The person will pace, rock while sitting or standing, march in place, or cross and uncross the legs. All these repetitive motions have an intensity that is

TABLE 12.7	DRUG THERAPIES FOR ACUTE MEDICATION-RELATED MOVEMENT DISORDERS		
Agents	Typical Dosage Ranges	Routes Available	Common Side Effects
Anticholinergics			
Benztropine (Cogentin)	2–6 mg/day	PO, IM, IV	Dry mouth, blurred vision, slowed gastric motility causing constipation, urinary retention, increased intraocular pressure; overdose produces toxic psychosis.
Trihexyphenidyl (Artane)	4–15 mg/day	PO	Same as benztropine, plus gastrointestinal distress. Older adults are most prone to mental confusion and delirium.
Biperiden (Akineton)	2–8 mg/day	PO	Fewer peripheral anticholinergic effects. Euphoria and increased tremor may occur.
Antihistamines			
Diphenhydramine (Benadryl)	25–50 mg QID to 400 mg daily	PO, IM, IV	Sedation and confusion, especially in older adults.
Dopamine Agonists			
Amantadine (Symmetrel)	100–400 mg daily	PO	Indigestion, decreased concentration, dizziness, anxiety, ataxia, insomnia, lethargy, tremors, and slurred speech may occur with higher doses. Tolerance may develop on fixed dose.
α-Blockers			
Propranolol (Inderal)	10 mg TID to 120 mg daily	PO	Hypotension and bradycardia. Must monitor pulse and blood pressure. Do not stop abruptly because doing so may cause rebound tachycardia.
Benzodiazepines			
Lorazepam (Ativan)	1–2 mg IM		
	0.5–2 mg PO	PO, IM	All may cause drowsiness, lethargy, and general sedation or paradoxical agitation. Confusion and disorientation in older adults.
Diazepam (Valium)	2–5 mg TID	PO, IV	Most side effects are rare and will disappear if dose is decreased.
Clonazepam (Klonopin)	1–4 mg/day	PO	Tolerance and withdrawal are potential problems.

Note. IM = intramuscular; IV = intravvenous.

frequently beyond the explanation of the individual. In addition, akathisia may be present as a primarily subjective experience without obvious motor behavior. This subjective experience includes feelings of anxiety, jitteriness, or the inability to relax, which the individual may or may not be able to communicate. It is extremely uncomfortable for a person experiencing akathisia to be forced to sit still or be confined. These symptoms are sometimes misdiagnosed as agitation or an increase in psychotic symptoms. If an antipsychotic medication is given, the symptoms will not abate and will often worsen. Differentiating akathisia from agitation may be aided by knowing the person's symptoms before the introduction of medication. Whereas psychotic agitation does not usually begin abruptly after antipsychotic medication use has been started, akathisia may occur after administration. In addition, the nurse may ask the patient if the experience is felt primarily in the muscles (akathisia) or in the mind or emotions (agitation).

Akathisia is the most difficult acute medication-related movement disorder to relieve. It does not usually respond well to anticholinergic medications. Rapid initiation of antipsychotics can increase the onset of akathisia (Yoshimura et al., 2018). The pathology of akathisia may involve more than just the extrapyramidal motor system. It may include serotonin changes that also affect the dopamine system. The usual approach to treatment is to change or reduce the antipsychotic. Several medications are used to reduce symptoms, including β-adrenergic blockers, anticholinergics, antihistamines, and low-dose antianxiety agents with limited success. Frequently, combinations of these medication are used (Poyurovsky & Weizman, 2020).

Several nursing interventions reduce the impact of these syndromes. Individuals with acute EPS need frequent reassurance that this is not a worsening of their psychiatric condition but instead is a treatable side effect of the medication. They also need validation that what they are experiencing is real and that the nurse is concerned and will be responsive to changes in these symptoms. Physical and psychological stress appears to increase the symptoms and further frighten the patient; therefore, decreasing stressful situations becomes important. These symptoms are often physically exhausting for the patient, and the nurse should ensure that the patient receives adequate rest and hydration. Because tremors, muscle rigidity, and motor restlessness may interfere with the individual's ability to eat, the nurse may need to assist the patient with eating and drinking fluids to maintain nutrition and hydration.

Risk factors for acute EPS include previous episodes of EPS. The nurse should listen closely when patients say they are "allergic" or have had "bad reactions" to antipsychotic medications. Often, they are describing one of the medication-related movement disorders, particularly dystonia, rather than a rash or other allergic symptom.

Chronic Syndromes: Tardive Dyskinesia

Chronic syndromes develop from long-term use of antipsychotics. They are serious and affect about 20% of the patients who receive typical antipsychotics for an extended period. These conditions are typically irreversible and cause significant impairment in self-image, social interactions, and occupational functioning. Early symptoms and mild forms may go unnoticed by the person experiencing them.

Tardive dyskinesia, the most well-known of the chronic syndromes, involves irregular, repetitive involuntary movements of the mouth, face, and tongue, including chewing, tongue protrusion, lip smacking, puckering of the lips, and rapid eye blinking. Abnormal finger movements are common as well. In some individuals, the trunk and extremities are also involved, and in rare cases, irregular breathing and swallowing lead to belching and grunting noises. These symptoms usually begin no earlier than after 6 months of treatment or when the medication is reduced or withdrawn. Once thought to be irreversible, considerable controversy now exists as to whether this is true.

The risk for experiencing tardive dyskinesia increases with age. Although the prevalence of tardive dyskinesia averages 15% to 20%, the rate rises to 50% to 70% in older patients receiving antipsychotic medications. The risk of probable tardive dyskinesia is three times lower in older adults receiving atypical antipsychotics compared to conventional antipsychotics (O'Brien, 2016). Women are at higher risk than men. Anyone receiving antipsychotic medication can develop tardive dyskinesia. Risk factors

> **BOX 12.4**
> **Risk Factors for Tardive Dyskinesia**
> - Age older than 50 years
> - Female
> - Affective disorders, particularly depression
> - Brain damage or dysfunction
> - Increased duration of treatment
> - Standard antipsychotic medication
> - Possible higher doses of antipsychotic medication

are summarized in Box 12.4. The causes of tardive dyskinesia remain unclear, but the most widely accepted theory is that dopamine antagonists block dopamine receptors, and evidence does suggest that imbalances of other neurotransmitters may be involved (Cornett et al., 2017).

Two medications recently approved by the FDA have shown promising results. Valbenazine (INGREZZA), a vesicular monoamine transporter 2 (VAMT2), was approved for the treatment of tardive dyskinesia. A related medication, deutetrabenazine (AUSTEDO), has a longer half-life than valbenazine, but twice-daily dosing with food is recommended (Citrome, 2020). Dietary precursors of acetylcholine, such as lecithin and vitamin E supplements, may prove to be beneficial.

The best approach to treatment remains avoiding the development of the chronic syndromes. Preventive measures include use of atypical antipsychotics, using the lowest possible dose of typical medication, minimizing use of as-needed (PRN) medication, and closely monitoring individuals in high-risk groups for development of the symptoms of tardive dyskinesia. All members of the mental health treatment team who have contact with individuals taking antipsychotics for longer than 3 months must be alert to the risk factors and earliest possible signs of chronic medication-related movement disorders.

Monitoring tools, such as the Abnormal Involuntary Movement Scale (see Appendix B), should be used routinely to standardize assessment and provide the earliest possible recognition of the symptoms. Standardized assessments should be performed at a minimum of 3- to 6-month intervals. The earlier the symptoms are recognized, the more likely they will resolve if the medication can be changed or its use discontinued. Newer, atypical antipsychotic medications have a much lower risk of causing tardive dyskinesia and are increasingly being considered first-line medications for treating patients with schizophrenia. Other medications are under development to provide alternatives that limit the risk for tardive dyskinesia.

Mood Stabilizers (Antimanic Medications)

Mood stabilizers, or antimanic medications, are psychopharmacologic agents used primarily for stabilizing mood swings, particularly those of mania in bipolar disorders. Lithium, the oldest, is the gold standard of treatment for acute mania and maintenance of bipolar disorders. Not all respond to lithium, and increasingly, other drugs are being used as first-line agents. Anticonvulsants, calcium channel blockers, adrenergic blocking agents, and atypical antipsychotics are used for mood stabilization.

Lithium

Lithium, a naturally occurring element, is effective in about 40% of patients with bipolar disorder. Although lithium is not a perfect drug, a great deal is known regarding its use—it is inexpensive, it has restored stability to the lives of thousands of people, and it remains the gold standard of bipolar pharmacologic treatment.

Indications and Mechanisms of Action

Lithium is indicated for symptoms of mania characterized by rapid speech, flight of ideas (jumping from topic to topic), irritability, grandiose thinking, impulsiveness, and agitation. Because it has mild antidepressant effects, lithium is used in treating depressive episodes of bipolar illness. It is also used as augmentation in patients experiencing major depression that has only partially responded to antidepressants alone. Lithium also has been shown to be helpful in reducing impulsivity and aggression in certain psychiatric patients.

The exact action by which lithium improves the symptoms of mania is unknown, but it is thought to exert multiple neurotransmitter effects, including enhancing serotonergic transmission, increasing synthesis of norepinephrine, and blocking postsynaptic dopamine. It has also been suggested that lithium's mood-stabilizing effects are related to the fact that it acts on cellular targets and exerting neuroprotective effects (Van Gestel et al., 2019).

Lithium is actively transported across cell membranes, altering sodium transport in both nerve and muscle cells. It replaces sodium in the sodium–potassium pump and is retained more readily than sodium inside the cells. Conditions that alter sodium content in the body, such as vomiting, diuresis, and diaphoresis, also alter lithium retention. The results of lithium influx into the nerve cell lead to increased storage of catecholamines within the cell, reduced dopamine neurotransmission, increased norepinephrine reuptake, increased GABA activity, and increased serotonin receptor sensitivity. Lithium also alters the distribution of calcium and magnesium ions and inhibits second messenger systems within the neuron. The mechanisms by which lithium improves the symptoms of mania are complex and interrelated, involving the sum of all or part of these actions and more.

Pharmacokinetics

Lithium carbonate is available orally in capsule, tablet, and liquid forms. Slow-release preparations are also available. Lithium is readily absorbed in the gastric system and may be taken with food, which does not impair absorption. Peak blood levels are reached in 1 to 4 hours, and the medication is usually completely absorbed in 8 hours. Slow-release preparations are absorbed at a slower, more variable rate.

Lithium is not protein bound, and its distribution into the CNS across the blood–brain barrier is slow. The onset of action is usually 5 to 7 days and may take as long as 2 weeks. The elimination half-life is 8 to 12 hours and is 18 to 36 hours in individuals whose blood levels have reached steady state and whose symptoms are stable. Lithium is almost entirely excreted by the kidneys but is present in all body fluids. Conditions of renal impairment or decreased renal function in older patients decrease lithium clearance and may lead to toxicity. Several medications affect renal function and therefore change lithium clearance. See Chapter 26 for a list of these and other medication interactions with lithium. About 80% of lithium is reabsorbed in the proximal tubule of the kidney along with water and sodium. In conditions that cause sodium depletion, such as dehydration caused by fever, strenuous exercise, hot weather, increased perspiration, and vomiting, the kidneys attempt to conserve sodium. Because lithium is a salt, the kidneys retain lithium as well, leading to increased blood levels and potential toxicity. Significantly increasing sodium intake causes lithium levels to fall.

Lithium is usually administered in doses of 300 mg two to three times daily. Because it is a drug with a narrow therapeutic range or index, blood levels are monitored frequently during acute mania, and the dosage is increased every 3 to 5 days. These increases may be slower in older adult patients or patients who experience uncomfortable side effects. Blood levels should be monitored 12 hours after the last dose of medication. In the hospital setting, nurses should withhold the morning dose of lithium until the serum sample is drawn to avoid falsely elevated levels. Individuals who are at home should be instructed to have their blood drawn in the morning about 12 hours after their last dose and before they take their first dose of medication. During the acute phases of mania, blood levels of 0.8 to 1.4 mEq/L are usually attained and maintained until symptoms are under control. The therapeutic range for lithium is narrow, and patients in the higher end of that range usually experience more uncomfortable side effects. During maintenance, the dosage is reduced, and dosages are adjusted to maintain blood levels of 0.4 to 1 mEq/L.

Lithium clears the body relatively quickly after discontinuation of its use. Withdrawal symptoms are rare, but occasional anxiety and emotional lability have been reported. It is important to remember that almost half of the individuals who discontinue lithium treatment abruptly experience a relapse of symptoms within a few weeks. Some research suggests that if a person stops taking lithium, the drug will be less effective when the medication is restarted. Patients should be warned of the risks in abruptly discontinuing their medication and should be advised to consider the options carefully in consultation with their prescriber.

Side Effects, Adverse Reactions, and Toxicity

At lower therapeutic blood levels, side effects from lithium are relatively mild. These reactions correspond with peaks in plasma concentrations of the medication after administration and most subside during the first few weeks of therapy. Frequently, individuals taking lithium complain of excessive thirst and an unpleasant metallic-like taste. Sugarless throat lozenges may be useful in minimizing this side effect. Other common side effects include increased frequency of urination, fine head tremor, drowsiness, and mild diarrhea. Weight gain occurs in about 20% of the individuals taking lithium. Nausea may be minimized by taking the medication with food or by use of a slow-release preparation. However, slow-release forms of lithium increase diarrhea. Muscle weakness, restlessness, headache, acne, rashes, and exacerbation of psoriasis have also been reported. See Chapter 26 for a summary of selected nursing interventions to minimize the impact of common side effects associated with lithium treatment. Patients most frequently discontinued their own medication use because of concerns with mental slowness, poor concentration, and memory problems.

As blood levels of lithium increase, the side effects of lithium become more numerous and severe. Early signs of lithium toxicity include severe diarrhea, vomiting, drowsiness, muscular weakness, and lack of coordination. Lithium should be withheld, and the prescriber consulted if these symptoms develop. Lithium toxicity can easily be resolved in 24 to 48 hours by discontinuing the medication, but hemodialysis may be required in severe situations. See Chapter 26 for a summary of the side effects and symptoms of toxicity associated with various blood levels of lithium.

Monitoring of creatinine concentration, thyroid hormones, and CBC every 6 months during maintenance therapy helps to assess the occurrence of other potential adverse reactions. Kidney damage is considered an uncommon but potentially serious risk of long-term lithium treatment. This damage is usually reversible after discontinuation of the lithium use. A gradual rise in serum creatinine and decline in creatinine clearance indicate the development of renal dysfunction. Individuals

with preexisting kidney dysfunction are susceptible to lithium toxicity.

Lithium may alter thyroid function, usually after 6 to 18 months of treatment. About 30% of the individuals taking lithium exhibit elevations in thyroid-stimulating hormone, but most do not show suppression of circulating thyroid hormone. Thyroid dysfunction from lithium treatment is more common in women, and some individuals require the addition of thyroxine to their care. During maintenance, thyroid-stimulating hormone levels may be monitored. Nurses should observe for dry skin, constipation, bradycardia, hair loss, cold intolerance, and other symptoms of hypothyroidism. Other endocrine system effects result from hypoparathyroidism, which increases parathyroid hormone levels and calcium. Clinically, this change is not significant, but elevated calcium levels may cause mood changes, anxiety, lethargy, and sleep disturbances. These symptoms may erroneously be attributed to depression if hypercalcemia is not investigated.

Lithium use must be avoided during pregnancy because it has been associated with birth defects, especially when administered during the first trimester. If lithium is given during the third trimester, toxicity may develop in a newborn, producing signs of hypotonia, cyanosis, bradykinesia, cardiac changes, gastrointestinal bleeding, and shock. Diabetes insipidus may persist for months. Lithium is also present in breast milk, and women should not breastfeed while taking lithium. Women expecting to become pregnant should be advised to consult with a physician before discontinuing use of birth control methods.

Anticonvulsants

In the psychiatric–mental health area, anticonvulsants are commonly used to treat patients with bipolar disorder and are considered mood stabilizers. The following discussion highlights the use of anticonvulsants as mood stabilizers in the treatment of bipolar disorder.

Indications and Mechanisms of Action

Valproate (valproic acid; Depakote), carbamazepine (Equetro), and lamotrigine (Lamictal) have FDA approval for the treatment of bipolar disorder, mania, or mixed episodes (see Chapter 26). In general, the anticonvulsant mood stabilizers have many actions, but their effects on ion channels, reducing repetitive firing of action potentials in the nerves, most directly decrease manic symptoms. No one action has successfully accounted for the anticonvulsants' ability to stabilize mood (Landgraf et al., 2016).

Pharmacokinetics

Valproic acid is rapidly absorbed, but the enteric coating of divalproex sodium adds a delay of as long as 1 hour.

Peak serum levels occur in about 1 to 4 hours. The liquid form (sodium valproate) is absorbed more rapidly and peaks in 15 minutes to 2 hours. Food appears to slow absorption but does not lower bioavailability of the drug.

Carbamazepine is absorbed in a somewhat variable manner. The liquid suspension is absorbed more quickly than the tablet form, but food does not appear to interfere with absorption. Peak plasma levels occur in 2 to 6 hours. Because high doses influence peak plasma levels and increase the risk for side effects, carbamazepine should be given in divided doses two or three times a day. The suspension, which has higher peak plasma levels and lower trough levels, must be given more frequently than the tablet form.

These medications cross easily into the CNS, move into the placenta as well, and are associated with an increased risk for birth defects. Carbamazepine, valproic acid, and lamotrigine are metabolized by the CYP450 system. However, one of the metabolites of carbamazepine is potentially toxic. If other concurrent medications inhibit the enzymes that break down this toxic metabolite, severe adverse reactions are often the result. Medications that inhibit this breakdown include erythromycin, verapamil, and cimetidine (now available in nonprescription form).

Teaching Points

Nurses need to educate patients about potential drug interactions, especially with nonprescription medications. Nurses can also inform other health care practitioners who may be prescribing medication that these patients are taking carbamazepine. It is important to note that oral contraceptives may become ineffective, and female patients should be advised to use other methods of birth control.

Side Effects, Adverse Reactions, and Toxicity of Anticonvulsants

The most common side effects of carbamazepine are dizziness, drowsiness, tremor, visual disturbance, nausea, and vomiting. These side effects may be minimized by initiating treatment in low doses. Patients should be advised that these symptoms will diminish, but care should be taken when changing positions or performing tasks that require visual alertness. Giving the drug with food may diminish nausea. Adverse reactions include rare aplastic anemia, agranulocytosis, severe rash, rare cardiac problems, and syndrome of inappropriate secretion of the diuretic hormone caused by hyponatremia.

Valproic acid also causes gastrointestinal disturbances, tremor, and lethargy. In addition, it can produce weight gain and alopecia (hair loss). These symptoms are transient and should diminish with the course of treatment. Dietary supplements of zinc and selenium may be helpful to patients experiencing hair loss. Constipation and urinary retention occur in some individuals. Nurses should monitor urinary output and assist patients to increase fluid consumption to decrease constipation.

Benign skin rash, sedation, blurred or double vision, dizziness, nausea, vomiting, and other gastrointestinal symptoms are side effects of lamotrigine. In rare cases, lamotrigine (Lamictal) produces severe, life-threatening rashes that usually occur within 2 to 8 weeks of treatment. This risk is highest in children. Use of lamotrigine should be immediately discontinued if a rash is noted.

Transient elevations in liver enzymes occur with both carbamazepine and valproic acid but symptoms of hepatic injury rarely occur. If the patient reports abnormal pain or shows signs of jaundice, the prescriber should be notified immediately. Several blood dyscrasias are associated with carbamazepine, including aplastic anemia, agranulocytosis, and leukopenia. Patients should be advised to report fever, sore throat, rash, petechiae, or bruising immediately. In addition, patients should be advised of the importance of completing routine blood tests throughout treatment. The risks for aplastic anemia and agranulocytosis with carbamazepine use still require close monitoring of CBCs during treatment. Valproate and its derivatives have had a similar course of development.

Antidepressant Medications

Medications classified as antidepressants are used not only for the treatment of depression but also in the treatment of anxiety disorders, eating disorders, and other mental health states (Table 12.8). They are used very cautiously in persons with bipolar disorder because of the possibility of precipitating a manic episode. The exact neuromechanism for the antidepressant effect is unknown in all of them. The onset of action also varies considerably and appears to depend on factors outside of steady-state plasma levels. Initial improvement with some antidepressants, such as the SSRIs, may appear within 7 days, but complete relief of symptoms may take several weeks. Antidepressants should not be discontinued abruptly because of uncomfortable symptoms that result. Discontinuance of use of these medications requires slow tapering. Individuals taking these medications should be cautioned not to abruptly stop using them without consulting their prescriber. Antidepressant medications are well absorbed from the gastrointestinal system; however, some individual variations exist. Most of the antidepressants are metabolized by liver enzymes so that other drugs metabolized by these enzymes may increase or decrease blood levels of the antidepressants (see Table 12.9). All these medications have a "boxed warning" for increased risk of suicidal behavior in children, adolescents, and young adults.

TABLE 12.8 ANTIDEPRESSANT MEDICATIONS

Generic (Trade) Drug Name	Usual Dosage Range (mg/day)	Half-Life (h)	Therapeutic Blood Level (ng/mL)
Selective Serotonin Reuptake Inhibitors			
Citalopram (Celexa)	20–50	35	Not available
Escitalopram (Lexapro)	10–20	27–32	Not available
Fluoxetine (Prozac)	20–80	2–9 days	72–300
Fluvoxamine (Luvox)	50–300	17–22	Not available
Paroxetine (Paxil)	10–50	10–24	Not available
Sertraline (Zoloft)	50–200	24	Not available
Serotonin Norepinephrine Reuptake Inhibitors			
Desvenlafaxine (Pristiq Extended Release)	50	11	Not available
Duloxetine (Cymbalta)	40–60	8–17	Not available
Levomilnacipran (Fetzima)	40–120	12	Not available
Nefazodone	100–600	2–4	Not available
Venlafaxine (Effexor)	75–375	5–11	100–500
Norepinephrine Dopamine Reuptake Inhibitor			
Bupropion (Wellbutrin)	200–450	8–24	10–29
α_2 blocker-Antagonist			
Mirtazapine (Remeron)	15–45	20–40	Not available
NMDA Antagonist			
Esketamine (Spravato)	56–84 titrated from twice a week to every other week	2–12 hours	Not available
Others			
Trazodone (Desyrel)	150–600	4–9	650–1600
Vilazodone (Viibryd)	10–40	25	Not available
Vortioxetine (Brintellix)	5–20	66	Not available
Tricyclic Antidepressants			
Amitriptyline (Elavil)	50–300	31–46	110–250
Amoxapine	50–600	8	200–500
Clomipramine (Anafranil)	25–250	19–37	80–100
Imipramine (Tofranil)	30–300	11–25	200–350
Desipramine (Norpramin)	25–300	12–24	125–300
Doxepin	25–300	8–24	100–200
Nortriptyline (Aventyl, Pamelor)	30–100	18–44	50–150
Protriptyline (Vivactil)	15–60	67–89	100–200
Tetracyclic			
Maprotiline (Ludiomil)	50–225	21–25	200–300
Monoamine Oxidase Inhibitors			
Isocarboxazid (Marplan)	20–60	Not available	Not available
Phenelzine (Nardil)	15–90	24 (effect lasts 3–4 days)	Not available
Tranylcypromine (Parnate)	10–60	24 (effect lasts 3–10 days)	Not available
Selegiline (Emsam)	6–12 mg/24 h	25%–50% delivered in 24 h	Not available

Note. IM = intramuscular; IV = intravenous; NMDA = N-methyl D-aspartate.

TABLE 12.9	CYP450 METABOLISM OF COMMON ANTIDEPRESSANTS		
Drug	How Metabolized	Induces	Inhibits
Bupropion	2B6	None	2D6
Citalopram	2C19, 2D6, 3A4	None	Mild 2D6
Desvenlafaxine	3A4	None	Mild 2D6
Duloxetine	1A2, 2D6	None	2D6
Escitalopram	2C19, 2D6, 3A4	None	Mild 2D6
Esketamine	2B6, 3A4, 2C9, 2C19	2B	3A4, 2D1
Fluoxetine	2C9, 2C19, 2D6, 3A4	None	2C19, 2D6 3A4, norfluoxetine
Fluvoxamine	1A2, 2D6	None	1A2, 2C9, 2C19, 3A4
Mirtazapine	1A2, 2D6, 3A4	None	None
Nefazodone	2D6, 3A4	None	3A4
Paroxetine	2D6	None	2D6, 2B6
Selegiline	2A6, 2C9, 3A4/5	None	2D6, 3A4/5
Sertraline	2B6, 2C9, 2D6, 3A4	None	2B6, 2C9, 2C19, 2D6, 3A4 (dosage >200 mg)
St. John's Wort*	3A4	3A4	None
Trazodone	2D6, 3A4	None	None
Tricyclic antidepressants	2D6, others depending on drug	None	Mild 2D6
Venlafaxine	2D6	None	Mild 2D6
Vilazodone	3A4, 2C19, 2D6	None	2C8
Vortioxetine	2D6, 3A4/5, 2C9, 2A6, 2C8, 2B6	None	None

*Not a U.S. Food and Drug Administration–approved antidepressant.
Note. Information from the Prescribing Information of each medication.

Serotonin syndrome, or serotonin intoxication syndrome, can occur if there is an overactivity of serotonin or an impairment of the serotonin metabolism. Concomitant medications such as triptans used to treat migraines also can increase the serotonergic activity. With the advent of widely used antidepressants targeting the serotonergic systems, symptoms of this serious side effect should be assessed. Symptoms include mental status changes (hallucinations, agitation, coma), autonomic instability (tachycardia, hyperthermia, changes in blood pressure), neuromuscular problems (hyperreflexia, incoordination), and gastrointestinal disturbance (nausea, vomiting, diarrhea). Serotonin syndrome can be life threatening. The treatment for serotonin syndrome is discontinuation of the medication and symptom management.

Selective Serotonin Reuptake Inhibitors

The serotonergic system is associated with mood, emotion, sleep, and appetite and is implicated in the control of numerous emotional, physical, and behavioral functions (see Chapter 8). Decreased serotonergic neurotransmission has been proposed to play a key role in depression. In 1988, fluoxetine (Prozac) was the first of a class of drugs that acted "selectively" on serotonin, one group of neurotransmitters associated with depression. Other similarly selective medications, sertraline (Zoloft), paroxetine (Paxil), and fluvoxamine (Luvox), soon followed. The newest SSRI is escitalopram oxalate (Lexapro).

All the SSRIs inhibit the reuptake of serotonin by blocking its transport into the presynaptic neuron, which in turn increases the concentration of synaptic serotonin. The concentration of synaptic serotonin is controlled directly by its reuptake; thus, drugs blocking serotonin transport have been successfully used for the treatment of depression and other conditions associated with serotonergic activity.

The SSRIs also have other properties that account for the common side effects, which include headache, anxiety, insomnia, transient nausea, vomiting, and diarrhea. Sedation may also occur, especially with paroxetine. Most often, these medications are given in the morning, but if daytime sedation occurs, they may be given in the evening. Higher doses, especially of fluoxetine, are more likely to produce sedation. Nausea and dizziness are common side effects which may subside within a few weeks. These side effects, along with sexual dysfunction, sedation, diastolic hypertension, and increased perspiration, tend to be dose dependent, occurring more frequently at higher doses. Other common side effects include insomnia, constipation, dry mouth, tremors, blurred vision, and asthenia or muscle weakness.

Sexual dysfunction is a relatively common side effect with most antidepressants. Erectile and ejaculation disturbances occur in men and anorgasmia in women. This side effect is often difficult to assess if the nurse has not obtained a sexual history before initiation of use of the medication. Anorgasmia is particularly common with the SSRIs and often goes unreported, frequently because nurses and other health care providers do not ask.

Serotonin Norepinephrine Reuptake Inhibitors

Decreased activity of the neurotransmitter norepinephrine is also associated with depression and anxiety disorders. Venlafaxine (Effexor), nefazodone, duloxetine (Cymbalta), and desvenlafaxine (Pristiq) prevent the reuptake of both serotonin and norepinephrine at the presynaptic site and are classified as serotonin norepinephrine reuptake inhibitors (SNRIs). Desipramine (Norpramin) is technically a tricyclic antidepressant (TCA) and is usually categorized as such. It works, however, on both serotonin and norepinephrine, so it can also be considered an SNRI.

The side effects are like those of the SSRIs; there is also a risk for an associated increase in blood pressure. Elevations in blood pressure have been described, and nurses should monitor blood pressure, especially in patients who have a history of hypertension. Venlafaxine (Effexor) has little effect on acetylcholine and histamine; thus, it creates only mild sedation and anticholinergic symptoms. This medication is often used if a depressed patient is sleeping excessively and reports little energy. The most common side effects of nefazodone (Serzone) include dry mouth, nausea, dizziness, muscle weakness, constipation, and tremor. It is unlikely to cause sexual disturbance. Nefazodone also has a "boxed warning" for hepatic failure and should not be used in those with acute liver disease.

Norepinephrine Dopamine Reuptake Inhibitors

Bupropion (Wellbutrin, Zyban) inhibits reuptake of norepinephrine, serotonin, and dopamine. Wellbutrin is indicated for depression and Zyban for nicotine addiction. The smoking cessation medication, Zyban, is given at a lower dose than Wellbutrin. Patients should not take Zyban if they are taking Wellbutrin. Bupropion has a chemical structure unlike any of the other antidepressants and somewhat resembles a few

of the psychostimulants. Bupropion's activating effects may be experienced as agitation or anxiety by some patients. Others also experience insomnia and appetite suppression. For a few individuals, bupropion has produced psychosis, including hallucinations and delusions. Most likely, this is secondary to overstimulation of the dopamine system. Bupropion is contraindicated for people with seizure disorders and those at risk for seizures. The rate of seizures is similar to that with the SSRIs and mirtazapine but is lower than the rate associated with the older antidepressants. Most importantly, bupropion has a lower incidence of sexual dysfunction and often is used in individuals who are experiencing these side effects with other antidepressants (GlaxoSmithKline, 2019; Montejo et al., 2019).

α₂-Antagonist

Mirtazapine (Remeron) boosts norepinephrine or noradrenaline and serotonin by blocking α_2-adrenergic presynaptic receptors on a serotonin receptor (5-HT$_{2A}$, 5-HT$_{2C}$, 5-HT$_3$). This is a different action than the other antidepressants. A histamine receptor is also blocked, which may explain its sedative side effect. Mirtazapine is indicated for depression. Side effects include sedation (at lower doses), dizziness, weight gain, dry mouth, constipation, and change in urinary functioning.

N-methyl D-aspartate Receptor Antagonist

In March 2019, the FDA approved a nasal spray formulation of esketamine (Spravato) for treatment resistant depression. Esketamine is a similar formulation to ketamine, an FDA-approved anesthetic. Esketamine is not approved as an anesthetic agent and ketamine is not approved for the treatment of depression, but it has been used off-label for rapid relief of severe depression. Ketamine also produces euphoria, dissociation, and hallucinations, has a high risk of abuse, and is a well-known street drug, Special K (see Chapter 31).

Esketamine is a nonselective, noncompetitive antagonist of N-methyl D-aspartate receptor, blocking glutamate. Esketamine reaches maximum plasma concentration in 20 to 24 minutes. Once administered, there is a rapid decline in plasma concentration within 4 to 8 hours. It is metabolized primarily in the liver and excreted in the urine (Dinis-Oliveira, 2017; Janssen Pharmaceutical Companies, 2019).

Esketamine is given under direct supervision of a health care provider. The FDA recommends that esketamine be given in conjunction with an oral antidepressant. A treatment session consists of a nasal administration and post-administration observation. Blood pressure is assessed before and after treatment. The medication is given in two phases. During the induction phase (weeks 1–4), the medication is given twice a week; during maintenance phase (weeks 5–8), esketamine is given weekly, and after 9 weeks, it is given every 2 weeks. The medication has a boxed warning for sedation, dissociation, abuse and misuse, and suicidal thoughts and behavior. Other side effects include increase in blood pressure, short- and long-term cognitive impairment, impaired ability to drive and operate machinery, ulcerative or interstitial cystitis, and embryo–fetal toxicity (Gastaldon et al., 2020, Janssen Pharmaceutical Companies, 2019). Due to the possibility of nausea and vomiting after administration, patient should avoid food for at least 2 hours before administration and avoid drinking liquids at least 30 minutes prior to administration.

Other Antidepressants

Trazodone (Desyrel) blocks serotonin 2A receptor potently and blocks the serotonin reuptake pump less potently. It is indicated for depression but is often used off-label for insomnia and anxiety. Sedation is a very common side effect. Other side effects include weight gain, nausea, vomiting, constipation, dizziness, fatigue, incoordination, and tremor.

Other newly FDA-approved antidepressants target other receptor sites. For example, vilazodone (Viibryd) is a serotonin reuptake inhibitor and a partial agonist of 5-HT_{1A}; vortioxetine (Brintellix) inhibits reuptake of serotonin and norepinephrine, but is also a partial agonist to 5-HT_{1A}. These subtle differences translate into subtle clinical effects.

Tricyclic Antidepressants

The TCAs were once the primary medication used for treating depression. With the introduction of the SSRIs and other previously discussed antidepressants, the use of TCAs has significantly declined. In most cases, these medications are as effective as the other drugs, but they have more serious side effects and a higher lethal potential (see Table 12.9). The TCAs act on a variety of neurotransmitter systems, including the norepinephrine and serotonin reuptake systems.

Pharmacokinetics

The TCAs are highly bound to plasma proteins, which make the association between blood levels and therapeutic clinical effects difficult. However, some plasma ranges have been established (see Table 12.7). Most of the TCAs have active metabolites that act in as much the same manner as the parent drug. Most of these antidepressants may be given in a once-daily single dose. If the medication causes sedation, this dose should be given at bedtime.

Side Effects, Adverse Reactions, and Toxicity

Because the TCAs act on several neurotransmitters in addition to serotonin and norepinephrine, these drugs have many unwanted effects. With the TCAs, sedation, orthostatic hypotension, and anticholinergic side effects are the most common sources of discomfort for patients receiving these medications. Other side effects of the TCAs include tremors, restlessness, insomnia, nausea and vomiting, confusion, pedal edema, headache, and seizures. Blood dyscrasias may also occur, and any fever, sore throat, malaise, or rash should be reported to the prescriber. Interventions to assist in minimizing these side effects are listed in Table 12.1.

The TCAs have the potential for cardiotoxicity. Symptoms include prolongation of cardiac conduction that may worsen preexisting cardiac conduction problems. The TCAs are contraindicated with second-degree atrioventricular block and should be used cautiously in patients who have other cardiac problems. Occasionally, they may precipitate heart failure, myocardial infarction, arrhythmias, and stroke.

Antidepressants that block the dopamine (D_2) receptor, such as amoxapine, have produced symptoms of NMS. Mild forms of EPS and endocrine changes, including galactorrhea and amenorrhea, may develop.

Monoamine Oxidase Inhibitors

The MAOIs, as their name indicates, inhibit MAO, an enzyme that breaks down the biogenic amine neurotransmitters serotonin, norepinephrine, and others. By inhibiting this enzyme, serotonin and norepinephrine activity is increased in the synapse. In the United States, there are three oral formulations: phenelzine (Nardil), tranylcypromine (Parnate), and isocarboxazid (Marplan) and one available by a transdermal patch: selegiline (Emsam). These are considered MAOIs because they form strong covalent bonds to block the enzyme MAO. The inhibition of this enzyme increases with repeated administration of these medications and takes at least 2 weeks to resolve after discontinuation of use of the medication.

The major problem with the MAOIs is their interaction with tyramine-rich foods and certain medications that can result in a hypertensive crisis. All the MAOIs have dietary modification except the 6 mg/24 hours dose of selegiline. The enzyme monoamine is important in the breakdown of dietary amines (e.g., tyramine). When the enzyme is inhibited, tyramine, a precursor for dopamine, increases in the nerve cells. Tyramine has a vasopressor action that induces hypertension. If the individual ingests food that contains high levels of tyramine while taking MAOIs, severe headaches, palpitation, neck stiffness and soreness, nausea, vomiting, sweating, hypertension, stroke, and, in rare instances, death may result. Patients

TABLE 12.10	EXAMPLE OF A TYRAMINE-RESTRICTED DIET	
Category of Food	**Food with Tyramine**	**Food Allowed**
Nonrefrigerated food	Spoiled foods or foods not refrigerated, handled, or stored properly	Food that is handled and stored properly
Cheese	All aged and mature cheeses, especially strong, aged, or processed cheeses such as American processed cheddar, Colby, blue, brie, mozzarella, and parmesan; yogurt, sour cream	Fresh cottage cheese, cream cheese, ricotta cheese
Meat, fish, and poultry	Air-dried, aged, and fermented meats; sausages and salamis Beef or chicken liver Dried and pickled herring Pepperoni Anchovies, meat extracts, meat tenderizers Meats prepared with tenderizers, improperly stored meat Spoiled or improperly stored animal liver	Fresh meat, poultry, and fish, including fresh processed meats (e.g., lunch meats, hot dogs, breakfast sausage, and cooked sliced ham)
Fruits and vegetables	Broad bean pods (Fava bean pods)	All other vegetables
Alcoholic beverages	All tap beers and other beers that have not been pasteurized; red wine, sherry, liqueurs; some alcohol-free and reduced alcohol beer	White wines may not contain tyramine.
Miscellaneous foods	Marmite concentrated yeast extract Sauerkraut Soy sauce and other soybean condiments	Soy milk Pizzas from commercial chain restaurants prepared with cheeses low in tyramine

Source: U.S. Food & Drug Administration. Avoiding drug interactions. https://www.fda.gov/consumers/consumer-updates/avoiding-drug-interactions; Parke-Davis. (2007). http://www.accessdata.fda.gov/drugsatfda_docs/label/2007/011909s038lbl.pdf

who are taking MAOIs are prescribed a low-tyramine diet (Table 12.10).

In addition to food restrictions, many prescription and nonprescription medications that stimulate the sympathetic nervous system (sympathomimetic) produce the same risk for hypertensive crisis as do foods containing tyramine. The nonprescription medication interactions involve primarily diet pills and cold remedies. Patients should be advised to check the labels of any nonprescription drugs carefully for a warning against use with antidepressants, especially the MAOIs, and then consult their prescriber before consuming these medications. In addition, symptoms of other serious drug–drug interactions may develop, such as coma, hypertension, and fever, which may occur when patients receive meperidine (Demerol) while taking an MAOI. Patients should notify other health care providers, including dentists, that they are taking an MAOI before being prescribed or given any other medication.

The MAOIs frequently produce dizziness, headache, insomnia, dry mouth, blurred vision, constipation, nausea, peripheral edema, urinary hesitancy, muscle weakness, forgetfulness, and weight gain. Older patients are especially sensitive to the side effect of orthostatic hypotension and require frequent assessment of lying and standing blood pressures. They may be at risk for falls and subsequent bone fractures and require assistance in changing position. Sexual dysfunction, including decreased libido, impotence, and anorgasmia, also is common with MAOIs.

Antianxiety and Sedative–Hypnotic Medications

Sometimes called *anxiolytics*, antianxiety medications, such as buspirone and sedative–hypnotic medications, such as lorazepam (Ativan), come from various pharmacologic classifications, including barbiturates, benzodiazepines, nonbenzodiazepines, and nonbarbiturate sedative–hypnotic medications, such as chloral hydrate. These drugs represent some of the most widely prescribed medications today for the short-term relief of anxiety or anxiety associated with depression.

Benzodiazepines

Commonly prescribed benzodiazepines include alprazolam (Xanax), lorazepam (Ativan), diazepam (Valium), chlordiazepoxide (Librium), flurazepam (Dalmane), and triazolam (Halcion). Although benzodiazepines are known to enhance the effects of the inhibitory neurotransmitter GABA, their exact mechanisms of action are not well understood. Of the various benzodiazepines in use to relieve anxiety (and treat insomnia), oxazepam

TABLE 12.11	ANTIANXIETY AND SEDATIVE–HYPNOTIC MEDICATIONS		
Generic (Trade) Drug Name	Usual Dosage Range (mg/day)	Half-Life (h)	Speed of Onset After Single Dose
Benzodiazepines			
Diazepam (Valium)	4–40	30–100	Very fast
Chlordiazepoxide (Librium)	15–100	50–100	Intermediate
Clorazepate (Tranxene)	15–60	30–200	Fast
Prazepam (Centrax)	20–60	30–200	Very slow
Lorazepam (Ativan)	2–8	10–20	Slow intermediate
Oxazepam (Serax)	30–120	3–21	Slow intermediate
Alprazolam (Xanax)	0.5–10	12–15	Intermediate
Halazepam (Paxipam)	80–160	30–200	Slow intermediate
Clonazepam (Klonopin)	1.5–20	18–50	Intermediate
Nonbenzodiazepine			
Buspirone (BuSpar)	15–30	3–11	Very slow

(Serax) and lorazepam (Ativan) are often preferred for patients with liver disease and for older patients because of their short half-lives.

Pharmacokinetics

The variable rate of absorption of the benzodiazepines determines the speed of onset. Table 12.11 provides relative indications of the speed of onset, from very fast to slow, for some of the commonly prescribed benzodiazepines. Whereas chlordiazepoxide (Librium) and diazepam (Valium) are slow, erratic, and sometimes incompletely absorbed when given intramuscularly, lorazepam (Ativan) is rapidly and completely absorbed when given intramuscularly.

All the benzodiazepines are highly lipid soluble and highly protein bound. They are distributed throughout the body and enter the CNS quickly. Other drugs that compete for protein-binding sites may produce drug–drug interactions. The degree to which each of these drugs is lipid soluble affects its duration of action. Most of these drugs have active metabolites, but the degree of activity of each metabolite affects duration of action and elimination half-life. Most of these drugs vary markedly in length of half-life. Oxazepam and lorazepam have no active metabolites and thus have shorter half-lives. Elimination half-lives may also be sustained for obese patients when using diazepam and chlordiazepoxide.

Side Effects, Adverse Reactions, and Toxicity

The most commonly reported side effects of benzodiazepines result from the sedative and CNS depression effects of these medications. Drowsiness, intellectual impairment, memory impairment, ataxia, and reduced motor coordination are common adverse reactions. If prescribed for sleep, many of these medications, especially the long-acting benzodiazepines, produce significant "hangover" effects experienced on awakening. Older patients receiving repeated doses of medications such as flurazepam at bedtime may experience paradoxical confusion, agitation, and delirium, sometimes after the first dose. In addition, daytime fatigue, drowsiness, and cognitive impairments may continue while the person is awake. For most patients, the effects subside as tolerance develops; however, alcohol increases all these symptoms and potentiates the CNS depression. Individuals using these medications should be warned to be cautious when driving or performing other tasks that require mental alertness. If these tasks are part of the person's work requirements, another medication may be chosen. Administered intravenously, benzodiazepines often cause phlebitis and thrombosis at the IV sites, which should be monitored closely and changed if redness or swelling develops.

Because tolerance develops to most of the CNS depressant effects, individuals who wish to experience the feeling of "intoxication" from these medications may be tempted to increase their own dosage. Psychological dependence is more likely to occur when using these medications for a longer period. Abrupt discontinuation of the use of benzodiazepines may result in a recurrence of the target symptoms, such as rebound insomnia or anxiety. Other withdrawal symptoms appear rapidly, including tremors, increased perspiration, palpitations, increased sensitivity to light, abdominal discomfort or pain, and elevations in systolic blood pressure. These symptoms may be more pronounced with the short-acting benzodiazepines, such as lorazepam. Gradual tapering is recommended for discontinuing use of benzodiazepines after long-term treatment. When tapering short-acting medications, the prescriber may switch the patient to a long-acting benzodiazepine before discontinuing use of the short-acting drug.

Individual reactions to the benzodiazepines appear to be associated with sensitivity to their effects. Some patients feel apathy, fatigue, tearfulness, emotional lability, irritability, and nervousness. Symptoms of depression may worsen. The psychiatric–mental health nurse should closely monitor these symptoms when individuals are receiving benzodiazepines as adjunctive treatment for anxiety that coexists with depression. Gastrointestinal disturbances, including nausea, vomiting, anorexia, dry mouth, and constipation, may develop. These medications may be taken with food to ease the gastrointestinal distress.

Older patients are particularly susceptible to incontinence, memory disturbances, dizziness, and increased risk for falls when using benzodiazepines. Pregnant patients should be aware that these medications cross the placenta and are associated with increased risk for birth defects, such as cleft palate, mental retardation, and pyloric stenosis. Infants born addicted to benzodiazepines often exhibit flaccid muscle tone, lethargy, and difficulties sucking. All the benzodiazepines are excreted in breast milk, and breastfeeding women should avoid using these medications. Infants and children metabolize these medications more slowly; therefore, more drug accumulates in their bodies.

Toxicity develops in overdose or accumulation of the drug in the body from liver dysfunction or disease. Symptoms include worsening of the CNS depression, ataxia, confusion, delirium, agitation, hypotension, diminished reflexes, and lethargy. Rarely do the benzodiazepines cause respiratory depression or death. In overdose, these medications have a high therapeutic index and rarely result in death unless combined with another CNS depressant drug, such as alcohol.

Nonbenzodiazepines: Buspirone

Buspirone, a nonbenzodiazepine, is effective in controlling the symptoms of anxiety but has no effect on panic disorders and little effect on obsessive–compulsive disorder.

Indications and Mechanisms of Actions

Nonbenzodiazepines are effective for treating anxiety disorders without the CNS depressant effects or the potential for abuse and withdrawal syndromes. Buspirone is indicated for treating generalized anxiety disorder; therefore, its target symptoms include anxiety

and related symptoms, such as difficulty concentrating, tension, insomnia, restlessness, irritability, and fatigue. Because buspirone does not add to depression symptoms, it has been tried for treating anxiety that coexists with depression. In some instances, it is thought to potentiate the antidepressant actions of other medications.

Buspirone has no effect on the benzodiazepine–GABA complex but instead appears to control anxiety by blocking the serotonin subtype of receptor, 5-HT$_{1a}$, at both presynaptic reuptake and postsynaptic receptor sites. It has no sedative, muscle relaxant, or anticonvulsant effects. It also lacks potential for abuse.

Pharmacokinetics

Buspirone is rapidly absorbed but undergoes extensive first-pass metabolism. Food slows absorption but appears to reduce first-pass effects, increasing the bioavailability of the medication. Buspirone is given on a continual dosing schedule of three times a day because of its short half-life of 2 to 3 hours. Clinical action depends on reaching steady-state concentrations; taking this medication with food may facilitate this process.

Buspirone is highly protein bound but does not displace most other medications. However, it does displace digoxin and may increase digoxin levels to the point of toxicity. It is metabolized in the liver and excreted predominantly by the kidneys but also via the gastrointestinal tract. Patients with liver or kidney impairment should be given this medication with caution.

Buspirone cannot be used on a PRN basis; rather, it takes 2 to 4 weeks of continual use for symptom relief to occur. It is more effective in reducing anxiety in patients who have never taken a benzodiazepine.

Buspirone does not block the withdrawal of other benzodiazepines. Therefore, a switch to buspirone must be initiated gradually to avoid withdrawal symptoms. Nurses should closely monitor patients who are undergoing this change of medication for emergence of withdrawal symptoms from the benzodiazepines and report such symptoms to the prescriber.

Side Effects, Adverse Reactions, and Toxicity

Common side effects from buspirone include dizziness, drowsiness, nausea, excitement, and headache. Most other side effects occur at an incidence of less than 1%. There have been no reports of death from an overdose of buspirone alone. Older patients, pregnant women, and children have not been adequately studied. For now, buspirone can be assumed to cross the placenta and is present in breast milk; therefore, its use should be avoided in pregnant women, and women who are taking this medication should not breastfeed.

Antihistamines

Antihistamine, hydroxyzine (Atarax, Vistaril), is increasingly used for the treatment of anxiety as a substitute for the benzodiazepines which can lead to psychological dependence. Histamine can produce symptoms of itching or hives on the skin.

Indications and Mechanisms of Actions

Even though hydroxyzine is primarily used for itching and nausea, it is also approved for anxiety, tension, and sleep. Hydroxyzine's metabolite, *cetirizine*, blocks the H_1 histamine receptor and prevents symptoms that are caused by histamine activity on capillaries, bronchial smooth muscle, and gastrointestinal smooth muscle. It crosses the blood–brain barrier and acts on the H_1 receptors in the CNS, which results in suppression of certain subcortical regions of the brain causing sedation and anticholinergic action.

Pharmacokinetics

Hydroxyzine is rapidly absorbed and distributed in oral and IM administration and is metabolized in the liver. The effects are observed within 1 hour of administration with a peak effect in 2 hours. The elimination half-life is around 20 hours in adults (Paton & Webster, 1985).

Side Effects, Adverse Reactions, and Toxicity

The side effects include deep sleep, incoordination, sedation, calmness, and dizziness as well as hypotension, tinnitus, and headaches. Due to the anticholinergic property, constipation and dry mouth can occur. There is some evidence that hydroxyzine can prolong the QTc interval. Hydroxyzine should be avoided in older adults (Golembesky et al., 2018).

Sedative–Hypnotics

Sedatives reduce activity, nervousness, irritability, and excitability without causing sleep, but if given in large enough doses, they have a hypnotic effect. **Hypnotics** cause drowsiness and facilitate the onset and maintenance of sleep. These two classifications are usually referred to as **sedative–hypnotics**—drugs that have a calming effect or depress the CNS. These medications include (1) benzodiazepines, (2) GABA enhancers, (3) melatonergic hypnotics, (4) antihistamines, and (5) the orexin receptor antagonist (Table 12.12). The benzodiazepines have been

TABLE 12.12 HYPNOTICS FOR INSOMNIA			
Generic (Trade) Drug Name	Usual Dosage Range (mg/day)	Elimination Half-Life (h)	Speed of Onset After Single Dose
Benzodiazepine Hypnotics			
Flurazepam	15–30	47–100	Fast
Temazepam (Restoril)	15–30	9.5–20	Moderately fast
Triazolam (Halcion)	0.25–0.5	1.5–5	Fast
Quazepam (Doral)	0.75–15	39	Fast
Estazolam (ProSom)	1	10–24	Fast
Nonbenzodiazepine Hypnotics			
Eszopiclone (Lunesta)	2–3	6	Fast
Zaleplon (Sonata)	10	1	Fast
Zolpidem (Ambien)	5–10	2.6	Fast
Zolpidem CR (Ambien CR)	12.5	2.6	Fast
Melatonergic Hypnotics			
Melatonin	0.1–10	0.5–0.75	Fast
Ramelteon (Rozerem)	8	1–2.6	Fast
Antihistamines			
Hydroxyzine (Vistaril)	50–100	20	Fast
Doxylamine (Unisom)	25	10	Fast
Orexin Receptor Antagonist			
Suvorexant (Belsomra)	10–20 mg	12	Fast

previously discussed. The GABA enhancers modulate GABA-A receptors. They do not cause a high degree of tolerance or dependence and are easier to discontinue than the benzodiazepines. Melatonergic hypnotics are melatonin agonists, and antihistamines block histamines, causing sedation (Atkin et al., 2018). The orexin receptor antagonists block the activity of orexins, neurotransmitters involved in wakefulness and arousal. These medications are discussed thoroughly in Chapter 34.

Stimulants and Wakefulness-Promoting Agents

Amphetamines were first synthesized in the late 1800s but were not used for psychiatric disorders until the 1930s. Initially, amphetamines were prescribed for a variety of symptoms and disorders, but their high abuse potential soon became obvious.

Currently, among the medications known as stimulants are methylphenidate (Ritalin, Methylin, Metadate), d-amphetamine (Dexedrine), amphetamine/dextroamphetamine (Adderall), dexmethylphenidate (Focalin), lisdexamphetamine (Vyvanse), and CNS stimulants. Modafinil (Provigil) and armodafinil (Nuvigil) are wakefulness-promoting agents used for narcolepsy and other sleep disorders.

Indications and Mechanisms of Action

Medical use of these stimulants is now restricted to a few disorders, including narcolepsy, attention deficit hyperactivity disorder (ADHD), particularly in children, and obesity unresponsive to other treatments. However, stimulants are increasingly being used as an adjunctive treatment in depression and other mood disorders to address the fatigue and low energy common to these conditions.

Amphetamines indirectly stimulate the sympathetic nervous system, producing alertness, wakefulness, vasoconstriction, suppressed appetite, and hypothermia. Tolerance develops to some of these effects, such as suppression of appetite, but the CNS stimulation continues. Although the exact mechanism of action is not completely understood, stimulants cause a release of catecholamines, particularly norepinephrine and dopamine, into the synapse from the presynaptic nerve cell. They also block reuptake of these catecholamines. Methylphenidate is structurally like the amphetamines but produces a milder CNS stimulation. Psychostimulants should be used very cautiously in individuals who have a history of substance abuse.

Although the stimulant effects of these medications may seem logically indicated for narcolepsy, a disorder in which the individual frequently and abruptly falls asleep, the indications for childhood ADHD seem less obvious. The etiology and neurobiology of ADHD remain unclear,

but psychostimulants produce a paradoxical calming of the increased motor activity characteristic of ADHD. Studies show that medication decreases disruptive activity during school hours, reduces noise and verbal activity, improves attention span and short-term memory, improves ability to follow directions, and decreases distractibility and impulsivity. Although these improvements have been well documented in the literature, the diagnosis of ADHD and subsequent use of psychostimulants with children remain matters of controversy (see Chapter 37).

Modafinil (Provigil) and armodafinil (Nuvigil), wake-promoting agents, are used for treating excessive sleepiness associated with narcolepsy, sleep apnea, and residual sleepiness for shift work sleep disorder. Armodafinil is longer acting than modafinil. The mechanism of action is unclear, but it is hypothesized that they increase glutamate and suppress GABA in the hypothalamus, hippocampus, and thalamus. There is no evidence of direct effects on dopamine, but there may be action on a dopamine transport. These drugs may increase the risk of Stevens–Johnson syndrome (Holfinger et al., 2018; Ogeil et al., 2019).

Pharmacokinetics

Psychostimulants are rapidly absorbed from the gastrointestinal tract and reach peak plasma levels in 1 to 3 hours. Considerable individual variations occur between the drugs in terms of their bioavailability, plasma levels, and half-lives. Table 12.13 compares the primary psychostimulants used in psychiatry. Some of these differences are age dependent because children metabolize these medications more rapidly, producing shorter elimination half-lives.

The psychostimulants appear to be unaffected by food in the stomach and should be given after meals to reduce the appetite suppressant effects when indicated. However, changes in urine pH may affect the rates of excretion. Excessive sodium bicarbonate alkalizes the urine and reduces amphetamine secretion. Increased vitamin C or citric acid intake may acidify the urine and increase its excretion. Starvation from appetite suppression may have a similar effect. All these drugs are highly lipid soluble, crossing easily into the CNS and the placenta. Psychostimulants undergo metabolic changes in the liver, where they may affect, or be affected by, other drugs. They are primarily excreted through the kidneys; therefore, renal dysfunction may interfere with excretion.

Psychostimulants are usually begun at a low dose and increased weekly, depending on the improvement of symptoms and occurrence of side effects. Initially, children with ADHD are given a morning dose so their school performance may be compared from morning to afternoon. Rebound symptoms of excitability and overtalkativeness may occur when use of the medication is withdrawn or

TABLE 12.13 PSYCHOSTIMULANT MEDICATIONS		
Generic (Trade) Drug Name	Usual Dosage Range (mg/day)	Elimination Half-Life
Dextroamphetamine (Dexedrine)	5–40	Highly variable depending on urine pH
Methylphenidate (Ritalin)	10–60	2.4 h (children); 2.1 h (adults)
Amphetamine/dextroamphetamine (Adderall)	2.5 mg (3–5 y) 5 mg (6 y) 5–60 mg for narcolepsy	9–11 h
Dexmethylphenidate extended release (Focalin XR)	5–40 mg	3 h
Lisdexamphetamine (Vyvanse)	30 mg	<1 h

after dose reduction. These symptoms also begin about 5 hours after the last dose of medication, which may affect the dosing regimen for some individuals. The return of symptoms in the afternoon for children with ADHD may require that a second dose be given at school. Prescribers should work with parents to implement other interventions after school and on weekends when the psychostimulants are not used. The severity of symptoms may require that the medications be continued during these times, but this dosing schedule should be determined after careful evaluation on an individual basis. Use of these medications should not be stopped abruptly, especially with higher doses, because the rebound effects may last for several days.

Modafinil (Provigil) is absorbed rapidly and reaches peak plasma concentration in 2 to 4 hours. Armodafinil reaches peak plasma concentration later and is maintained for 6 to 14 hours. Absorption of both may be delayed by 1 to 2 hours if taken with food. Modafinil is eliminated via liver metabolism with subsequent excretion of metabolites through renal excretion. They may interact with drugs that are metabolized by liver enzymes including phenytoin, diazepam, and propranolol. Concurrent use of modafinil or armodafinil and other drugs metabolized by the liver enzyme system may lead to increased circulating blood levels of the other drugs.

Side Effects, Adverse Reactions, and Toxicity

Side effects associated with psychostimulants typically arise within 2 to 3 weeks after use of the medication begins. From most to least common, these side effects include appetite suppression, insomnia, irritability, weight loss, nausea, headache, palpitations, blurred vision, dry mouth, constipation, and dizziness. Because of the effects on the sympathetic nervous system, some individuals experience blood pressure changes (both hypertension and hypotension), tachycardia, tremors, and irregular heart rates. Blood pressure and pulse should be monitored initially and after each dosage change.

Rarely, psychostimulants suppress growth and development in children. These effects are a matter of controversy, and research has produced conflicting results. Although suppression of height seems unlikely to some researchers, others have indicated that psychostimulants may have an effect on cartilage. Height and weight should be monitored several times annually for children taking these medications and compared with prior history of growth. Weight should be monitored, especially closely during the initial phases of treatment. These effects also may be minimized by drug "holidays," such as during school vacations.

Rarely, individuals may experience mild dysphoria, social withdrawal, or mild-to-moderate depression. These symptoms are more common at higher doses and may require discontinuation of use of medication. Abnormal movements and motor tics may also increase in individuals who have a history of Tourette syndrome. Psychostimulants should be avoided by patients with Tourette symptoms or with a positive family history of the disorder. In addition, dextroamphetamine has been associated with an increased risk for congenital abnormalities. Because there is no compelling reason for a pregnant woman to continue to take these medications, patients should be informed and should advise their prescriber immediately if they plan to become pregnant or if pregnancy is a possibility.

Death is rare from overdose or toxicity of the psychostimulants, but a 10-day supply may be lethal, especially in children. Symptoms of overdose include agitation, chest pain, hallucinations, paranoia, confusion, and dysphoria. Seizures may develop, along with fever, tremor, hypertension or hypotension, aggression, headache, palpitations, rashes, difficulty breathing, leg pain, and abdominal pain. Toxic doses of dextroamphetamine are above 20 mg, with potential death resulting from a 400-mg dose. Parents should be warned regarding the potential lethality of these medications and take preventive measures by keeping the medication in a safe place.

Side effects associated with modafinil and armodafinil include nausea, nervousness, headache, dizziness, and trouble sleeping. If the effects continue or are bothersome, patients should consult the prescriber. Modafinil and armodafinil are generally well tolerated with few clinically significant side effects. It is potentially habit forming and must be used with great caution in individuals with a history of substance abuse or dependence (Cephalon, 2017).

INTEGRATIVE AND COMPLEMENTARY HEALTH CARE

Herbal Therapies

Integrative health care expands and incorporates treatment modalities outside the norm of Western medicine. Herbal therapies are often used in addition to or in place of antidepressants and antianxiety medication (Shah et al., 2017). An in depth discussion of herbal therapies is outside the scope of this text, and readers are encouraged to seek additional resources from the National Center for Complementary and Integrative Health within the National Institutes of Health.

This chapter discusses dietary supplements and herbal therapies commonly used by persons receiving mental health care. These are exempt from the FDA's efficacy and safety standards because they are considered food. Lack of regulation does not mean that these supplements are ineffective or unsafe. These substances can be effective but can also have adverse reactions and interact with prescribed medications. Nurses need to understand these potential interactions and assess their patients for the impact of these substances.

St. John's wort (SJW), derived from *Hypericum perforatum L.*, is used for depression, pain, anxiety, insomnia, and premenstrual syndrome. SJW is believed to modulate serotonin, dopamine, and norepinephrine. The risk of developing serotonin syndrome is increased when taken with other serotonergic drugs. It has the potential to interact with other medications (i.e., birth control pills, digoxin) and should not be taken with prescribed antidepressants (National Center for Complementary & Integrative Health, [NCCIH], 2020; Nicolussi et al., 2020).

Kava, derived from the *Piper methysticum* plant, is used for anxiety reduction. Kava interacts with dopaminergic transmission, inhibits the MAO-B enzyme system, and modulates the GABA receptor. It may also inhibit uptake of noradrenaline. Kava is widely used by Pacific Islanders as a social and ceremonial tranquilizing drink. In 2002, the FDA issued warnings about the risk of severe liver injury associated with kava. Several countries have restricted its use. Thrombocytopenia, leukopenia, and hearing impairment have been reported with the use of kava (National Center for Complementary and Integrative Health., 2020; Raziq, 2020).

Valerian (*Valeriana officinalis*), a member of the Valerianaceae family, is a perennial plant native to Europe and Asia and naturalized to North America. Valerian is a common ingredient in products promoted for insomnia and nervousness. The evidence of its effectiveness is inconclusive. The mechanism of action is unclear but appears to be relatively safe. There are some reports that suggest hepatotoxicity in humans (NCCIH, 2018; Hoban et al., 2019).

Vitamin, Mineral, and Other Dietary Supplements

The neurotransmitters necessary for normal healthy functioning are produced from chemical building blocks taken in with the foods we eat. Many nutritional deficiencies may produce symptoms of psychiatric disorders. Fatigue, apathy, and depression are caused by deficiencies in iron, folic acid, pantothenic acid, magnesium, vitamin C, or biotin. Logically, treating these deficiencies with dietary supplements should improve the psychiatric symptoms. The question becomes, Can nutritional supplements improve psychiatric symptoms that are not the result of such deficiencies?

Tryptophan, the dietary precursor for serotonin, is involved in several physiological processes including neuronal function, immunity, and gut homeostasis. Tryptophan is metabolized into biologically active compounds such as serotonin, melatonin, and niacin and has been most extensively investigated as it relates to low serotonin levels and increased aggression. It is involved in diseases in the CNS, malignancy, inflammatory bowel, and cardiovascular disease. Individuals who have low tryptophan levels are prone to have lower levels of serotonin in the brain, resulting in depressed mood and aggressive behavior (Comai et al., 2020).

Dietary supplements such as melatonin and lecithin target CNS functioning. Melatonin, a naturally occurring hormone secreted from the pineal gland, is used for treatment of insomnia and prevention of "jet lag" in air travelers. Lecithin, a precursor to acetylcholine, is used to improve memory and treat dementia. The extent to which the level of acetylcholine is raised by ingestion of lecithin is unknown (Tayebati, 2018).

Medications may also influence the development of nutritional deficiencies that may worsen psychiatric symptoms. For example, drugs with strong anticholinergic activity often produce impaired or enhanced gastric motility, which may lead to generalized malabsorption of vitamins and minerals. In addition, many vitamin and mineral supplements have toxicities of their own when given in excess. For example, daily ingestion of more than 100 mg of pyridoxine (vitamin B_6) can produce neurotoxic symptoms, photosensitivity, and ataxia. More research is needed to identify the underlying mechanisms and relationships of dietary supplements and dietary precursors of the bioamines to mood and behavior and psychopharmacologic medications. For now, it is important for the psychiatric–mental health nurse to recognize that these issues may be potential factors in improvement of the patient's mental status and target symptoms.

OTHER BIOLOGIC TREATMENTS

Although the primary biologic interventions remain pharmacologic, other somatic treatments have gained acceptance, remain under investigation, or show promise for the future. These include neurosurgery, ECT, phototherapy, and (most recently) rTMS and VNS. The use of neurosurgery is very limited and outside the scope of this text.

Electroconvulsive Therapy

For hundreds of years, seizures have been known to produce improvement in some psychiatric symptoms. Camphor-induced seizures were used in the 16th century to reduce psychosis and mania. With time, other substances, such as inhalants, were tried, but most were difficult to control or produced adverse reactions, sometimes even fatalities. ECT was formally introduced in Italy in 1938. It is one of the oldest medical treatments available and remains safely in use today. It is one of the most effective treatments for severe depression but has been used for other disorders, including mania and schizophrenia, when other treatments have failed.

With ECT, a brief electrical current is passed through the brain to produce generalized seizures lasting 25 to 150 seconds. The patient does not feel the stimulus or recall the procedure. A short-acting anesthetic and a muscle relaxant are given before induction of the current. A brief pulse stimulus, administered unilaterally on the nondominant side of the head, is associated with less confusion after ECT. However, some individuals require bilateral treatment for effective resolution of depressive symptoms. Induction of a seizure is necessary to produce positive treatment outcomes. Because individual seizure thresholds vary, the electrical impulse and treatment method also may vary. In general, the lowest possible electrical stimulus necessary to produce seizure activity is used. Blood pressure and the ECG are monitored during the procedure. This procedure is repeated two or three times a week, usually for a total of 6 to 12 treatments. Because there is no difference in treatment efficacy and a twice-weekly regimen produces less accumulative memory loss, this treatment course is often chosen. After symptoms have improved, antidepressant medication may be used to prevent relapse. Some patients who cannot take or do not experience response to antidepressant treatment may continue to have ECT treatment. Usually, once-weekly treatments are gradually decreased in frequency to once monthly. The number and frequency vary depending on the individual's response.

Although ECT produces rapid improvement in depressive symptoms, its exact mechanism of antidepressant action remains unclear. It is known to downregulate β-adrenergic receptors in much the same way as antidepressant medications. However, unlike antidepressant therapy, ECT produces an upregulation in serotonin, especially 5-HT$_2$. ECT also has several other actions on neurochemistry, including increased influx of calcium and effects on second messenger systems.

Brief episodes of hypotension or hypertension, bradycardia or tachycardia, and minor arrhythmias are among the adverse reactions that may occur during and immediately after the procedure but usually resolve quickly. Common aftereffects from ECT include headache, nausea, and muscle pain. Memory loss is the most troublesome long-term effect of ECT. Many patients do not experience amnesia, but others report some memory loss for months or even years. Evidence is conflicting on the effects of ECT on the formation of memories after the treatments and on learning, but most patients experience no noticeable change. Memory loss occurring as part of the symptoms of untreated depression presents a confounding factor in determining the exact nature of the memory deficits from ECT. It is important to remember that patient surveys are positive, with most individuals reporting that they were helped by ECT and would have it again (Brown et al., 2018).

ECT is contraindicated in patients with increased intracranial pressure. Risk also increases in patients with recent myocardial infarction, recent cerebrovascular accident, retinal detachment, or pheochromocytoma (a tumor on the adrenal cortex) and in patients at high risk for complications from anesthesia. Although ECT should be considered cautiously because of its specific side effects, added risks of general anesthesia, possible contraindications, and substantial social stigma, it is a safe and effective treatment.

Psychiatric–mental health nurses are involved in many aspects of care for individuals undergoing ECT. Informed consent is required, and all treating professionals have a responsibility to ensure that the patient's and family's questions are answered completely. Available treatment options, risks, and consequences must be fully discussed. Sometimes, memory difficulties associated with severe depression make it difficult for patients to retain information or ask questions. Nurses should be prepared to restate or explain the procedure as often as necessary. Whenever possible, the individual's family or other support systems should be educated and involved in the consent process. Educational videos are available, but they should not replace direct discussions. Language should be in terms the patient and family members can understand. Other nursing interventions

---

BOX 12.5

Interventions for the Patient Receiving Electroconvulsive Therapy

- Discuss treatment alternatives, procedures, risks, and benefits with patient and family. Make sure that informed consent for ECT has been given in writing.
- Provide initial and ongoing patient and family education.
- Assist and monitor the patient who must take NPO after midnight, the evening before the procedure.
- Make sure that the patient wears loose, comfortable, nonrestrictive clothing to the procedure.
- If the procedure is performed on an outpatient basis, ensure that the patient has someone to accompany them home and stay with them after the procedure.
- Ensure that pretreatment laboratory tests are complete, including a CBC, serum electrolytes, urinalysis, ECG, chest radiography, and physical examination.
- Teach the patient to create memory helps, such as lists and notepads, before the ECT.
- Explain that no foreign or loose objects can be in the patient's mouth during the procedure. Dentures will be removed, and a bite block may be inserted.
- Insert an IV line and provide oxygen by nasal cannula (usually 100% oxygen at 5 L/min).
- Obtain emergency equipment and be sure it is available and ready if needed.
- Monitor vital signs frequently immediately after the procedure, as in every postanesthesia recovery period.
- When the patient is fully conscious and vital signs are stable, assist them to get up slowly, sitting for some time before standing.
- Monitor confusion closely; the patient may need reorientation to the bathroom and other areas.
- Maintain close supervision for at least 12 hours and continue observation for 48 hours after treatment. Advise family members to observe how the patient manages at home, provide assistance as needed, and report any problems.
- Assist the patient to keep or schedule follow-up appointments.

CBC, complete blood count; ECG, electrocardiogram; ECT, electroconvulsive therapy; IV, intravenous; NPO, nothing by mouth.

---

involve preparation of the patient before treatment, monitoring immediately after treatment, and follow-up. Many of these considerations are listed in Box 12.5.

Light Therapy (Phototherapy)

Human circadian rhythms are set by time clues (*Zeitgebers*) inside and outside the body. One of the most powerful regulators of these body patterns is the cycle of daylight and darkness.

Research findings indicate that some individuals with certain types of depression may experience disturbance in these normal body patterns or of circadian rhythms, particularly those who experience a seasonal variation in their depression. These individuals are more depressed during the winter months, when there is less light; they improve spontaneously in the spring (see Chapter 26).

These individuals usually have symptoms that are somewhat different from classic depression, including fatigue, increased need to sleep, increased appetite and weight gain, irritability, and carbohydrate craving. Sometimes, the symptoms appear in the summer, and some individuals have only subtle changes without developing the full pattern. Administering artificial light to these patients during winter months has reduced these depressive symptoms.

Light therapy, sometimes called **phototherapy**, involves exposing the patient to an artificial light source during winter months to relieve seasonal depression. Artificial light is believed to trigger a shift in the patient's circadian rhythm to an earlier time. The light source must be very bright, full-spectrum light, usually 2500 lux, which is about 200 times brighter than normal indoor lighting. Harmful ultraviolet light is filtered out. Exposure to this light source has produced improvement and relief of depressive symptoms for significant numbers of seasonally and nonseasonally depressed individuals. Research remains ongoing (Geoffroy et al., 2019).

Studies have shown that morning phototherapy produces a better response than either evening or morning and evening timing of the phototherapy session. Light banks with full-spectrum light may be put together by the individual or obtained from various companies now producing these light sources. Light visors (visors containing small, full-spectrum light bulbs that shine on the eyelids) have also been developed. The patient is instructed to sit in front of the lights at about 3 ft, engaging in a variety of other activities, but glancing directly into the light every few minutes. This should be done immediately on arising and is most effective before 8 AM. The duration of administration may begin with as little as 30 minutes and increase to 2 to 5 hours. One to 2 hours is usually sufficient, and the antidepressant response begins in 1 to 4 days, with the full effect usually complete after 2 weeks. Full antidepressant effect is usually maintained with daily sessions of 30 minutes (Geoffroy et al., 2019).

Side effects of phototherapy are rare, but eye strain, headache, and insomnia are possible. An ophthalmologist should be consulted if the patient has a preexisting eye disorder. In rare instances, phototherapy has been reported to produce an episode of mania. Irritability is a more common complaint. Follow-up visits with the prescriber or therapist are needed to help manage side effects and assess positive results. Phototherapy should be implemented only by a provider knowledgeable in its use.

Transcranial Magnetic Stimulation

Transcranial magnetic stimulation (TMS) was introduced in 1985 as a noninvasive, painless method to stimulate the cerebral cortex. There are two types of TMS. The repetitive transcranial magnetic stimulation (rTMS) and the deep transcranial magnetic stimulation (dTMS).

Both types are effective. Undergirding this procedure is the hypothesis that a time-varying magnetic field will induce an electrical field, which, in brain tissue, activates inhibitory and excitatory neurons, thereby modulating neuroplasticity in the brain. The low-frequency electrical stimulation from rTMS triggers lasting anticonvulsant effects in rats, and the therapeutic benefits of rTMS in humans are thought to be related to an action like that produced by anticonvulsant medication. The rTMS has been used for both clinical and research purposes. The rTMS stimulation of the brain's prefrontal cortex may help some depressed patients in much the same way as ECT but without its side effects (Trevizol & Blumberger, 2019). Thus, it has been proposed as an alternative to ECT in managing symptoms of depression. The rTMS treatment is administered daily for at least 1 week, much like ECT, except that subjects remain awake. Although proven effective for depression, rTMS does have some side effects, including mild headaches.

Vagus Nerve Stimulation

VNS sends electrical impulses to the brain to improve depression. The vagus nerve has traditionally been considered a parasympathetic efferent nerve that was responsible only for regulating autonomic functions, such as heart rate and gastric tone. However, the vagus nerve (cranial X) also carries sensory information to the brain from the head, neck, thorax, and abdomen, and research has identified that the vagus nerve has extensive projections of its sensory afferent connections to many brain areas. Although the basic mechanism of action of VNS is unknown, incoming sensory, or afferent, connections of the left vagus nerve directly project into many of the very same brain regions implicated in neuropsychiatric disorders. These help us to understand how VNS is helpful in treating psychiatric disorders. VNS connections change levels of several neurotransmitters implicated in the development of major depression, including serotonin, norepinephrine, GABA, and glutamate, in the same way that antidepressant medications produce their therapeutic effect (Redgrave et al., 2018).

Approved by the FDA for the adjunctive treatment of severe depression for adults who are unresponsive to four or more adequate antidepressant treatments, VNS is a permanent implant. VNS is not a cure for depression, and patients must be seen regularly for assessment of mood states and suicidality.

THE ISSUE OF ADHERENCE

Medications and other biologic treatments work only if they are used. On the surface, **adherence**, or **compliance** to a therapeutic routine, seems amazingly simple. However, following therapeutic regimens, self-administering medications as prescribed, and keeping appointments are amazingly complex activities that often prevent successful treatment. In recovery-oriented practice, the patient makes the decision to take medications. It is important that the patient does not feel coerced into taking the medication. The nurse's role is to support the patient's decision-making process and provide honest, evidence-based advice.

Adherence exists on a continuum and can be conceived of as full, partial, or nil. Partial adherence, whereby a patient either attempts to take medications but misses doses or takes more than prescribed, is by far the most common. Recent estimates indicate that on the average, 50% or more of the individuals with schizophrenia taking antipsychotic medications stop taking the medications or do not take them as prescribed. It should be remembered that problems with adherence are an issue with many chronic health states, including diabetes and arthritis, not just psychiatric disorders. Box 12.6 lists some of the common reasons for nonadherence. Psychiatric–mental health nurses should be aware that several factors contribute to the decision to discontinue medications.

The most often cited reasons for not taking medications as prescribed are the side effects. Medication side effects may interfere with work performance or other important aspects of the individual's life. For example, a construction worker cannot afford to be drowsy and sedated while operating a crane at a construction site, and a woman in an intimate relationship may find anorgasmia intolerable. Even though symptom improvement may be observed by health care professionals, they may not be noticed by the patient. Nurses need to be sensitive to the patient's ability to tolerate side effects and to the impact that side effects have on the patient's life. Medication choice, dosing schedules, and prompt treatment of side effects may be crucial factors in helping patients continue with their treatment.

Cognitive deficits associated with some psychiatric disorders may make it difficult for the individual to self-monitor, develop insight, make choices, remember to fill prescriptions, or keep appointments. Forgetfulness, cost, and confusion regarding dosage or timing may also contribute to noncompliance. New advances in medication formulation are designed to address some of these issues. For example,

---

BOX 12.6

Common Reasons for Not Taking Medications as Prescribed

- Uncomfortable side effects and those that interfere with quality of life, such as work performance or intimate relationships
- Lack of awareness or denial of illness
- Stigma
- Feeling better
- Confusion about dosage or timing
- Difficulties in access to treatment
- Substance abuse

long-acting injections are designed to reduce or eliminate the need to remember an oral medication regime. Recently, the FDA approved a tablet formulation of an antipsychotic aripiprazole embedded with a digital adherence-assessment device. The system consists of an ingestible sensor, a wearable sensor, and software applications that confirm adherence. More research is needed to confirm the practicality of using the device and its effectiveness in improving treatment adherence (Papola et al., 2018).

Family members may have similar difficulties that influence the individual not to take the medication. They may misunderstand or deny the illness, thinking, for example, "My wife's better, so she doesn't need that medicine anymore." Family members may be distressed when observable side effects occur. Adherence concerns must not be dismissed as the patient's or family's problem. Psychiatric nurses should actively address this issue. A positive therapeutic relationship between the nurse and patient and family must provide a strong sense of trust that side effects and other difficulties in treatment will be addressed and minimized. When individuals report experiencing distressing side effects, the nurse should immediately respond with assessment and interventions to reduce these effects. It is important to assess compliance often, asking questions in a nonthreatening, nonjudgmental manner. It also may be helpful to seek information from others who are involved with the patient.

Adherence can be improved by psychoeducation. This approach is most helpful if it addresses the individual's specific symptoms and concerns. For example, if the patient is having difficulty with understanding the purpose of the medication, it may be helpful to link taking it to reduction of specific unwanted symptoms or improved functioning, such as continuing to work. Family members should also be included in these discussions.

Other factors that interfere with adherence should also be assessed and plans developed to minimize their effect. For example, an individual who is being considered for clozapine therapy may have missed several appointments in the past. On assessment, the nurse may discover that it takes the individual 2 hours on three different buses each way to reach the clinic. The nurse can then assist with arranging for a home health nurse to visit the patient's apartment, draw blood samples for analysis, and assess side effects, thus decreasing the number of trips the patient must make to the clinic.

SUMMARY OF KEY POINTS

- Target symptoms and side effects of medications should be clearly identified. The FDA approves the use of medications for specific disorders and symptoms.
- Psychiatric medications primarily act on CNS receptors, ion channels, enzymes, and carrier proteins.

Agonists mimic the action of a specific neurotransmitter; antagonists block the response.

- A drug's ability to interact with a given receptor type depends on three qualities: selectivity—the ability to interact with specific receptors while not affecting other tissues and organs; affinity—the degree of strength of the bond between drug and receptor; and intrinsic activity—the ability to produce a certain biologic response.
- Pharmacokinetics refers to how the human body processes the drug, including absorption, distribution, metabolism, and excretion. Bioavailability describes the amount of the drug that reaches circulation throughout the body. The wide variations in the way each individual processes any medication often are related to physiologic differences caused by age, genetic makeup, other disease processes, and chemical interactions.
- Antipsychotic medications are drugs used in treating patients with psychotic disorders, such as schizophrenia. They act primarily by blocking dopamine or serotonin postsynaptically. In addition, they have several actions on other neurotransmitters. Older typical antipsychotic drugs work on positive symptoms and are inexpensive but produce more side effects than the newer atypical antipsychotic drugs which work on positive and negative symptoms.
- Medication-related movement disorders are a particularly serious group of side effects that principally occur with the typical antipsychotic medications and that may be acute syndromes, such as dystonia, pseudoparkinsonism, and akathisia, or chronic syndromes, such as tardive dyskinesia.
- The mood stabilizers, or antimanic medications, are drugs used to control wide variations in mood related to mania, but these agents may also be used to treat patients with other disorders. Lithium and the anticonvulsants are chemically unrelated and act in different ways to stabilize mood.
- Antidepressant medications are drugs used primarily for treating symptoms of depression. They act by blocking reuptake of one or more of the bioamines, especially serotonin and norepinephrine. These medications vary considerably in their structure and action. Newer antidepressants, such as the SSRIs, have fewer side effects and are less lethal in overdose than the older TCAs.
- Antianxiety medications also include several subgroups of medications, but the benzodiazepines and nonbenzodiazepines are those principally used in psychiatry. The benzodiazepines act by enhancing the effects of GABA, and the nonbenzodiazepine buspirone acts on serotonin. Benzodiazepines can be used on a PRN basis, but buspirone, the one available nonbenzodiazepine, must be taken regularly.

- Psychostimulants enhance neurotransmitter activity, acting at several sites in the nerves. These medications are most often used for treating symptoms related to ADHD and narcolepsy.

- ECT uses the application of an electrical pulsation to induce seizures in the brain. These seizures produce several effects on neurotransmission that result in the rapid relief of depressive symptoms.

- rTMS and VNS are two emerging somatic treatments for psychiatric disorders. They are both means to directly affect brain function through stimulation of the nerves that are direct extensions of the brain.

- Phototherapy involves the application of full-spectrum light in the morning hours, which appears to reset circadian rhythm delays related to seasonal affective disorder and other forms of depression. Nutritional therapies are in various stages of investigation.

- Adherence refers to the ability of an individual to self-administer medications as prescribed and to follow other instructions related to medication treatment. It can be full, partial, or nil. Nonadherence is related to factors such as medication side effects, stigma, and family influences. Nurses play a key role in educating patients and helping them to improve adherence.

Unfolding Patient Stories: David Carter

Part 1

David Carter is a 28-year-old male with schizophrenia. He became violent and was brought to the emergency room with paranoid delusions and auditory hallucinations. During admission, he was alternately agitated and withdrawn. Medications ordered include: olanzapine 10 mg orally daily, venlafaxine 75 mg XR orally daily, Lorazepam 2 mg orally every 8 hours as needed for agitation, and haloperidol 5 mg orally every 8 hours as needed for agitation. Describe the classification, action, dosing, and side effects for each medication? What monitoring should the nurse consider for each medication and when administering the as-needed medications? What client teaching should the nurse provide when administering the medications while considering his alternate states of agitation and withdrawal?

CRITICAL THINKING CHALLENGES

1. Discuss how you would go about identifying the target symptoms for a specific patient for the following medications: antipsychotic, antidepressant, and antianxiety drugs.

2. Track the approval process from identification of a potential substance to marketing a medication. Compare at least three psychiatric medications that are in phase III trials (hint: www.FDA.gov).

3. Obtain the PIs for the three atypical antipsychotics, two SSRIs, and one SNRI. Compare their boxed warnings, pharmacodynamics, pharmacokinetics, indications, side effects, and dosages.

4. Compare the oral and IM dose of lorazepam. Why are these doses similar?

5. Mr. J. has schizophrenia and was just prescribed an antipsychotic. His family wants to know the risk–benefits of the medication. How would you answer?

6. Identify the CYP450 enzyme that metabolizes the following medications: risperidone, olanzapine, quetiapine, clozapine, fluoxetine, venlafaxine, trazodone, nefazodone, and bupropion.

7. Find the four medications or substances that induce or inhibit the following CYP450 enzymes: 2D6, 2C19, 3A4, and 1A2.

8. Obtain the PI for clozapine, risperidone, quetiapine, and Risperdal Consta. Compare the half-lives of each drug. Discuss the relationship of the drug's half-life to the dosing schedule. When is steady state reached in each of these medications?

9. Explain the health problems associated with anticholinergic side effects of the antipsychotic medications.

10. Compare the type of movements that characterize tardive dyskinesia with those that characterize akathisia and dystonia and explore which one is easier for a patient to experience.

11. One patient is prescribed the MAOI Emsam, 6 mg/day, and another is taking another MAOI, Nardil, 15 mg/day. Are the dietary restrictions different?

12. A patient who is taking an MAOI asks you to explain what will happen if she eats pizza. Prepare a short teaching intervention beginning with the action of the medication and its consequences.

13. Explain how your nursing care would be different for a male patient taking lithium carbonate than for a female patient.

14. Patient A is taking valproic acid (Depakote) for mood stabilization, and patient B is taking lamotrigine (Lamictal). After comparing notes with each other, they ask you why patient A must have drug blood levels and patient B does not. How are these two drugs alike? How are they different?

15. Two patients are getting their blood drawn. One patient is getting lithium and the other clozapine. What laboratory tests are being ordered?

16. A patient who is depressed has been started on sertraline. During the assessment, she tells you that she is also taking SJW, lecithin, and a multiple vitamin. What is your next step?

17. Compare different approaches that you might use with a patient with schizophrenia who has decided to stop taking their medication because of intolerance to side effects.

REFERENCES

Atkin, T., Comai, S., & Gobbi, G. (2018). Drugs for insomnia beyond benzodiazepines: Pharmacology, clinical applications, and discovery. *Pharmacological Reviews*, 70(2), 197–245. https://doi.org/10.1124/pr.117.014381

Bradley, P., et al. (2018). Improved efficacy with targeted pharmacogenetic-guided treatment of patients with depression and anxiety: A randomized clinical trial demonstrating clinical utility. *Journal of Psychiatric Research*, 96, 100–107. https://doi.org/10.1016/j.jpsychires.2017.09.024

Brown, S. K., et al. (2018). Patient experience of electroconvulsive therapy: A retrospective Review of clinical outcomes and satisfaction. *Journal of ECT*, 34(4), 240–246.

Cephalon. (2017). *Nuvigil (armodafinil) tablets*. https://www.accessdata.fda.gov/drugsatfda_docs/label/2017/021875s023lbl.pdf

Citrome, L. L. (2020). Medication options and clinical strategies for treating tardive dyskinesia. *The Journal of Clinical Psychiatry*, 81(2), TV18059BR2C. https://doi.org/10.4088/JCP.TV18059BR2C

Comai, S., Bertazzo, A., Brughera, M., & Crotti, S. (2020). Tryptophan in health and disease. *Advances in Clinical Chemistry*, 95, 165–218. https://doi.org/10.1016/bs.acc.2019.08.005

Cornett, E. M., Novitch, M., Kaye, A. D., Kata, V., & Kaye, A. M. (2017). Medication-induced tardive dyskinesia: A review and update. *Ochsner Journal*, 17(2), 162–174.

Das, B., Rawat, V. S., Ramasubbu, S. K., & Kumar, B. (2019). Frequency, characteristics and nature of risk factors associated with use of QT interval prolonging medications and related drug-drug interactions in a cohort of psychiatry patients. *Therapie*, 74(6), 599–609. https://doi.org/10.1016/j.therap.2019.03.008

Delanaye, P., Jager, K. J., Bökenkamp, A., Christensson, A., Dubourg, L., Eriksen, B. O., Gaillard, F., Gambaro, G., van der Giet, M., Glassock, R. J., Indridason, O. S., van Londen, M., Mariat, C., Melsom, T., Moranne, O., Nordin, G., Palsson, R., Pottel, H., Rule, A. D., Schaeffner, E., … van den Brand, J. (2019). CKD: A call for an age-adapted definition. *Journal of the American Society of Nephrology: JASN*, 30(10), 1785–1805. https://doi.org/10.1681/ASN.2019030238

Dinis-Oliveira, R. J. (2017). Metabolism and metabolomics of ketamine: A toxicological approach. *Forensic Sciences Research*, 2(1), 2–10. https://doi.org/10.1080/20961790.2017.1285219

Factor, S. A., Burkhard, P. R., Caroff, S., Friedman, J. H., Marras, C., Tinazzi, M., & Comella, C. L. (2019). Recent developments in drug-induced movement disorders: A mixed picture. *The Lancet. Neurology*, 18(9), 880–890. https://doi.org/10.1016/S1474-4422(19)30152-8

Gastaldon, C., Papola, D., Ostuzzi, G., & Barbui, C. (2020). Esketamine for treatment resistant depression: A trick of smoke and mirrors? *Epidemiology and Psychiatric Sciences*, 29, E79. https://doi.org/10.1017/S2045796019000751

Geoffroy, P. A., Schroder, C. M., Reynaud, E., & Bourgin, P. (2019). Efficacy of light therapy versus antidepressant drugs, and of the combination versus monotherapy, in major depressive episodes: A systematic review and meta-analysis. *Sleep Medicine Reviews*, 48, 101213. https://doi.org/10.1016/j.smrv.2019.101213

GlaxoSmithKline. (2019). Wellbutrin prescribing information. https://www.accessdata.fda.gov/drugsatfda_docs/label/2019/020358s061lbl.pdf

Golembesky, A., Cooney, M., Boev, R., Schlit, A. F., & Bentz, J. (2018). Safety of cetirizine in pregnancy. *Journal of Obstetrics and Gynaecology: The Journal of the Institute of Obstetrics and Gynaecology*, 38(7), 940–945. https://doi.org/10.1080/01443615.2018.1441271

Hoban, C. L., Byard, R. W., & Musgrave, I. F. (2019). Analysis of spontaneous adverse drug reactions to echinacea, valerian, black cohosh and ginkgo in Australia from 2000 to 2015. *Journal of Integrative Medicine*, 17(5), 338–343. https://doi.org/10.1016/j.joim.2019.04.007

Holfinger, S., Roy, A., & Schmidt, M. (2018). Stevens-Johnson Syndrome after armodafinil use. *Journal of Clinical Sleep Medicine: JCSM: Official Publication of the American Academy of Sleep Medicine*, 14(5), 885–887. https://doi.org/10.5664/jcsm.7132

Janssen Pharmaceutical Companies. (2019). *Spravato prescribing information*. https://www.accessdata.fda.gov/drugsatfda_docs/label/2019/211243lbl.pdf

Landgraf, D., Joiner, W. J., McCarthy, M. J., Kiessling, S., Barandas, R., Young, J. W., Cermakian, N., & Welsh, D. K. (2016). The mood stabilizer valproic acid opposes the effects of dopamine on circadian rhythms. *Neuropharmacology*, 107, 262–270. https://doi.org/10.1016/j.neuropharm.2016.03.047

Matsushita, S., & Higuchi, S. (2017). Review: Use of Asian samples in genetic research of alcohol use disorders: Genetic variation of alcohol metabolizing enzymes and the effects of acetaldehyde. *The American Journal on Addictions*, 26(5), 469–476. https://doi.org/10.1111/ajad.12477

Montejo, A. L., et al. (2019). Management strategies for antidepressant-related sexual dysfunction: A clinical approach. *Journal of Clinical Medicine*, 8(10), 1640. https://doi.org/10.3390/jcm8101640

National Center for Complementary and Integrative Health. (2020). *Herbs at a glance*. https://www.nccih.nih.gov/health/herbsataglance

Nicolussi, S., Drewe, J., Butterweck, V., & Meyer Zu Schwabedissen, H. E. (2020). Clinical relevance of St. John's wort drug interactions revisited. *British Journal of Pharmacology*, 177(6), 1212–1226. https://doi.org/10.1111/bph.14936

Nievergelt, C. M., et al. (2019). International meta-analysis of PTSD genome-wide association studies identifies sex- and ancestry-specific genetic risk loci. *Nature Communications*, 10(1), 4558. https://doi.org/10.1038/s41467-019-12576-w

Novartis. (2020). *Clozaril (prescribing information)*. https://www.accessdata.fda.gov/drugsatfda_docs/label/2020/019758s095lbl.pdf

Ogeil, R. P., Phillips, J. G., Savic, M., & Lubman, D. I. (2019). Sleep- and wake-promoting drugs: Where are they being sourced, and what is their impact? *Substance Use & Misuse*, 54(12), 1916–1928. https://doi.org/10.1080/10826084.2019.1609040

O'Brien, A. (2016). Comparing the risk of tardive dyskinesia in older adults with first-generation and second-generation antipsychotics: A systematic review and meta-analysis. *International Journal of Geriatric Psychiatry*, 31(7), 683–693.

Papola, D., Gastaldon, C., & Ostuzzi, G. (2018). Can a digital medicine system improve adherence to antipsychotic treatment? *Epidemiology and Psychiatric Sciences*, 27(3), 227–229.

Paton, D. M., & Webster, D. R. (1985). Clinical pharmacokinetics of H_1-receptor antagonists (The antihistamines). *Clinical Pharmacokinetics*, 10, 477–497. https://doi.org/10.2165/00003088-198510060-00002

Poyurovsky, M., & Weizman, A. (2020). Treatment of antipsychotic-induced akathisia: Role of serotonin $5\text{-}HT_{2a}$ receptor antagonists. *Drugs*, 80(9), 871–882. https://doi.org/10.1007/s40265-020-01312-0

Raziq, F. I. (2020). Kava induced acute liver failure. *American Journal of Therapeutics*, 10.1097/MJT.0000000000001180. Advance online publication. https://doi.org/10.1097/MJT.0000000000001180

Redgrave, J., Day, D., Leung, H., Laud, P. J., Ali, A., Lindert, R., & Majid, A. (2018). Safety and tolerability of Transcutaneous Vagus Nerve stimulation in humans; a systematic review. *Brain Stimulation*, 11(6), 1225–1238. https://doi.org/10.1016/j.brs.2018.08.010

Roberts, M. H., & Erdei, E. (2020). Comparative United States autoimmune disease rates for 2010–2016 by sex, geographic region, and race. *Autoimmunity Reviews*, 19(1), 102423. https://doi.org/10.1016/j.autrev.2019.102423

Shah, A. K., Becicka, R., Talen, M. R., Edberg, D., & Namboodiri, S. (2017). Integrative medicine and mood, emotions and mental health. *Primary Care*, 44(2), 281–304. https://doi.org/10.1016/j.pop.2017.02.003

Tayebati, S. K. (2018). Phospholipid and lipid derivatives as potential neuroprotective compounds. *Molecules*, 23(9). pii: E2257. https://doi.org/10.3390/molecules23092257

Trevizol, A. P., & Blumberger, D. M. (2019). An update on Repetitive Transcranial Magnetic Stimulation for the treatment of major depressive disorder. *Clinical Pharmacology and Therapeutics*, 106(4), 747–762. https://doi.org/10.1002/cpt.1550

Van Gestel, H., Franke, K., Petite, J., Slaney, C., Garnham, J., Helmick, C., Johnson, K., Uher, R., Alda, M., & Hajek, T. (2019). Brain age in bipolar disorders: Effects of lithium treatment. *The Australian and New Zealand Journal of Psychiatry*, 53(12), 1179–1188. https://doi.org/10.1177/0004867419857814

Walden, L. M., Brandl, E. J., Tiwari, A. K., Cheema, S., Freeman, N., Braganza, N., Kennedy, J. L., & Müller, D. J. (2019). Genetic testing for CYP2D6 and CYP2C19 suggests improved outcome for antidepressant and antipsychotic medication. *Psychiatry Research*, 279, 111–115. https://doi.org/10.1016/j.psychres.2018.02.055

Yoshimura, B., Sato, K., Sakamoto, S., Tsukahara, M., Yoshimura, Y., & So, R. (2018). Incidence and predictors of acute akathisia in severely ill patients with first-episode schizophrenia treated with aripiprazole or risperidone: Secondary analysis of an observational study. *Psychopharmacology*. 236(2), 723–730. https://doi.org/10.1007/s00213-018-5101-7

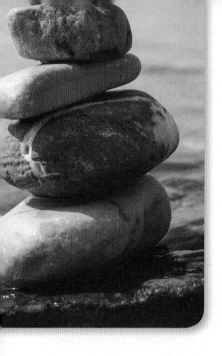

13
Cognitive Interventions in Psychiatric Nursing

Mary Ann Boyd and Jeanne Clement-Alvarez

KEYCONCEPTS

- cognitive behavioral therapy
- rational emotive behavior therapy
- solution-focused brief therapy

LEARNING OBJECTIVES

After studying this chapter, you will be able to:

1. Discuss the history of cognitively based therapeutic interventions.

2. Identify the concepts underlying cognitive interventions.

3. Compare and contrast three forms of cognitively based therapies.

4. Apply cognitive interventions in a clinical setting.

5. Describe the contexts in which psychiatric nurses use cognitive interventions.

KEY TERMS

- ABCDE • Activating event • Belief system • Cognition • Cognitive interventions • Cognitive distortions
- Cognitive triad • Compliments • Dysfunctional consequences • Exception questions • Functional consequences
- Miracle questions • Relationship questions • Scaling questions • Schema

INTRODUCTION

Psychiatric nurses use evidence-based cognitive interventions in a variety of practice settings (inpatient and outpatient). The knowledge and skills inherent in cognitively based interventions have been extensively studied and their effectiveness has been demonstrated for a variety of psychiatric disorders, especially depression (see Chapter 23) and anxiety disorders (see Chapter 25). Cognitive interventions are based on the concept of cognition.

Cognition can be defined as an internal process of perception, memory, and judgment through which an understanding of self and the world is developed. **Cognitive interventions** aim to change or reframe an individual's automatic thought patterns that have developed over time and which interfere with the individual's ability to function optimally. The skills and techniques that were developed on the basis of cognitive theory result in a new view of self and the environment.

Cognitive interventions had their beginnings in the long-term inpatient environment, but today they are a mainstay of psychiatric care in all settings and are used by all disciplines and at all levels of practice. Evidence from several studies, and as reinforced by meta-analysis of groups in the past decade, supports the use of cognitive therapies with a wide variety of psychological and psychiatric conditions, and it has been shown to be effective with diverse individuals in diverse settings (Olthuis, 2016; Shepardson et al., 2020). Cognitive therapies are incorporating additional therapeutic modalities such as mindfulness and targeting for persons with anxiety and depressive disorders (Cladder-Micus et al., 2018). The current chapter explains the theoretical perspectives and application of cognitive interventions.

DEVELOPMENT OF COGNITIVE THERAPIES

Cognitive therapy was first developed and implemented in the 1950s by Albert Ellis (1913–2007), a psychologist, who was uncomfortable with the nondirective Freudian and neo-Freudian approaches. According to Ellis, cognition, emotions, and behavior are integrated and holistic. From the 1950s until his death, Ellis continued to develop and refine his theory and therapeutic approach into what he calls rational emotive behavior therapy (REBT; Ellis et al., 2008).

Beginning in the 1960s, other cognitively based theories and therapeutic approaches were developed, the most prominent being cognitive behavioral therapy (CBT) by Aaron Beck (see Chapter 7) (Beck, 2008). Steven de Shazer (1940–2005) and Insoo Kim Berg (1934–1997) developed solution-focused brief therapy (SFBT), an approach that is useful with persons who have diagnoses such as depression, obsessive–compulsive disorder, schizophrenia, and other psychiatric disorders (Franklin et al., 2017). These models will be discussed in the current chapter.

COGNITIVE THERAPY MODELS

Cognitive approaches are congruent with the standards of practice and are particularly effective in challenging care environments. Brief cognitive therapies offer approaches that can be applied within the therapeutic patient–nurse relationship and the nursing process. Patients undergoing cognitively based psychotherapy are frequently treated by an interdisciplinary team that supports this approach.

Cognitive Behavioral Therapy

> **KEYCONCEPT Cognitive behavioral therapy (CBT)** is a highly structured psychotherapeutic method used to alter distorted beliefs and problem behaviors by identifying and replacing negative inaccurate thoughts and changing the rewards for behaviors.

In CBT, the relationship between thoughts, feelings, and behavior is examined and identified. CBT operates on the following assumptions:

• People are disturbed not by an event but by the perception of that event.

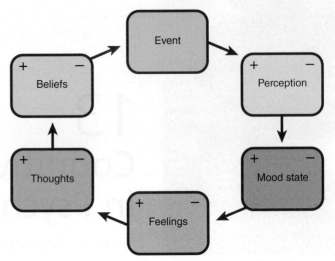

FIGURE 13.1 Model of perception, thoughts, and mood states: the cycle of cognition.

• Whenever and however a belief develops, the individual believes it.

• Work and practice can modify beliefs that create difficulties in living.

Figure 13.1 depicts the interaction of individual experiences, perception of these experiences, and the unique thoughts attached to these experiences that influence the development of beliefs (functional or dysfunctional). The person develops an explanation of their relationship to their environment and to other people from these beliefs. Dysfunctional thinking develops from a variety of human experiences and can become the predominant way the world is viewed. To quote from Shakespeare's *Hamlet*, "For there is nothing either good or bad but thinking makes it so."

Thoughts have a powerful effect on emotion and behavior. By changing dysfunctional thinking, a person can alter their emotional reaction to a situation and reinterpret the meaning of an event. That is, by identifying, analyzing, and changing thoughts and behaviors that are counterproductive, feelings such as helplessness, anxiety, and depression can be reduced. The goal of CBT is to restructure how a person perceives events in their life to facilitate behavioral and emotional change.

Cognitive Processes

Three cognitive processes are involved in the development of common mental disorders such as depression. These processes include the cognitive triad, cognitive distortions, and schema.

The **cognitive triad** includes thoughts about oneself, the world, and the future. Accumulation of thoughts about oneself is reflected in spoken and unspoken beliefs and moods that grow out of these beliefs. Emotions and behavior reflect the strength of the accumulated beliefs. Dysfunctional thoughts about the self are usually overly negative or overly positive whereas functional thoughts more closely reflect the reality of the perceived situation. For example, one student has the belief that learning is very difficult for them and that they will fail the examination no matter how hard they study. He does not study for the examination because he believes that he will fail anyway. A second student believes that she is very bright, understands the material, and does not need to study. She attends a concert the night before the test. A third student believes that he has a grasp of the material to be covered on the test but ensures this by studying notes and the text before the examination. The first two students fail the examination. Failure for the first student reinforces the dysfunctional belief that no matter what, he will fail. The second student argues that the test was unfair, which also reinforces her dysfunctional belief that she is bright and understands the material. The third student earned a good grade. His functional thoughts and behaviors are also reinforced.

Students one and two mentioned earlier both hold distinctive views that are not supported by empirical evidence but are generated automatically in response to a given situation. These automatic thoughts are called **cognitive distortions** and are generated by organizing distorted information and/or inaccurate interpretation of a situation. Cognitive distortions or "twisted thinking" occurs in a variety of ways such as *overgeneralization* (asserting that something general is always true about an event, situation or group of people), *personalizing* (applying a general statement to oneself), *catastrophizing* (viewing or talking about an event as worse than it actually was), and *selective abstraction* (selectively abstracting negative information from stressful events) (see Box 13.1) (Del Pozo et al., 2018).

Schemas are the individual's life rules that act as a sieve or filter. They allow only information compatible with the internal picture of self and the world to be brought to the person's awareness. Schemas develop in early childhood and become relatively fixed by middle childhood. Schemas are an accumulation of learning and experience from the individual's genetic makeup, family and school environments, peer relationships, and society as a whole. Ethnicity, culture, gender, and religious affiliation influence schema development, as well as the age of the individual at the time a given event occurs, the influence of the persons or circumstances involved on how that event is perceived, and the relative strength of that influence. In the example, student number one believes that he is not intelligent. This belief could have initiated in early childhood if the student was constantly unfavorably compared with an older sibling. This schema increases vulnerability in a host of interpersonal situations, particularly those that relate to scholarly endeavors. Student number two was overly praised by parents and other relatives and developed a schema of being more accomplished than most.

Implementing Cognitive Behavioral Therapy

The use of CBT is based on a collaborative therapeutic relationship in which a mutual trust develops through promoting patients' strengths and control over their own lives. CBT assumes that individuals have the innate ability to solve their own problems; thus, the overarching treatment goal is for the patient to be able to engage in self-care, independent of professional assistance.

In CBT, goals are developed in partnership and supply a forward-looking focus for what "can be" in the future as opposed to "what happened" in the past. The present serves as a platform from which current perceptions of earlier events can be reexamined. Movement toward goals is facilitated by strategies designed to engage the patient in the service of their own mental health. Strategies emerge when nurse and patient develop a working conceptualization of the issue or problem as the patient sees it. The nurse educates the patient about the therapeutic approach. An agenda is mutually established for each therapeutic interaction. Techniques that focus on both cognition and behavior are used to promote patient growth.

Engagement and Assessment

The first step in CBT is engagement and assessment. In this phase, the therapist establishes rapport with the patient and develops the theme that problems are manageable. The patient's definition of the problem that brought them into treatment is explored through a series of open-ended questions. A problem list is developed and reframed into manageable goals that are prioritized. The prioritized list forms the agenda for the treatment plan and structures the content of each individual session. A contract is developed

BOX 13.1 CLINICAL VIGNETTE

Cognitive Distortions

Amy has been working on a group project with her classmates in a psychiatric nursing course. Part of the process for the group project is to provide anonymous peer evaluation of the work of each of the six group members. Amy received a score of 10/10 from four of the members, a 7/10 from another, and 5/10 from the sixth. Amy thinks, "I guess I didn't do a good job on this project. I never do anything right. My classmates look down on me."

What Do You Think?
• What cognitive distortions does Amy exhibit?

for a number of sessions (frequently 10–12). The therapist seeks information about the patient's strengths and successes on which to base reexamination and reframing of negative beliefs and to design interventions. During all sessions, the therapist summarizes issues identified and develops homework assignments that enhance and expand the work done during the sessions.

Intervention Framework

Specific interventions used with CBT, in addition to the interaction that takes place in the therapy sessions, revolve around carefully crafted homework assignments that the patient works on in the time between sessions. Subsequently, sessions may be scheduled regularly once or twice a month. Typical homework assignments include evaluating the accuracy of automatic thoughts and beliefs. It is important for the therapist to realize that the thoughts a person has about a problem are not beliefs. In CBT, the therapist helps the patient identify the underlying belief, and then they

- explore the evidence that supports or refutes the belief about the event,
- identify alterative explanations for the event, and
- examine the real implications if the belief is true. (e.g., "What is the worst thing that could happen?")

In the sessions, the therapist challenges negative beliefs and helps the patient examine the "self-talk" that helps to sustain these beliefs. Cognitive techniques focus on the patient's patterns of automatic thinking, first identifying what they are by examining the patient's recurrent patterns in everyday life and then testing the validity of these automatic thoughts.

Other tools that are used to help change the patient's self-perception include bibliotherapy (the use of books that offer alternative thoughts and responses), journaling, and keeping a diary focused on emotional and behavioral responses to upsetting situations that documents small changes that might otherwise go unnoticed. The patient is also encouraged to make note of positive events and positive thoughts about themselves and their ability to cope with negative events. These positive thoughts and effective coping responses are reinforced in interactions with the therapist. As goals are developed at the beginning of each therapy session, the last few minutes are spent reviewing the progress toward the goals for that day.

Evaluation and Termination

Evaluation and termination begin with the original contract when patient and therapist determined the number of sessions. The patient's progress toward treatment goals is continually evaluated, and the patient is urged to

become more self-reliant and independent. As progress is never a continuous upward process, therapists prepare the patient for setbacks by acknowledging that setbacks are normal and expected and crafting ways in which the patient can deal with them. It is not uncommon for the time between sessions to lengthen as the final session approaches. At the final session, the use of "booster" sessions is discussed. Frequently, a session is scheduled in 6 months to do a quick "check-up" and review continuing progress.

Strengths and Limitations of Cognitive Behavioral Therapy

One of the strengths of CBT lies in the body of empirical evidence supporting the effectiveness of these interventions (Possemato et al., 2018; Spoelstra et al., 2015). Many studies show positive, sustained improvement in people treated with this form of intervention. Critics, however, identify some limitations. Chief among the limitations identified is the concern that the therapeutic relationship, long believed to be the main factor in patient improvement, may be forgotten in the rigid adherence to specific techniques. Others believe that change is dependent on the patient developing a clear understanding of their belief system and the origin of that system; thus, CBT is not effective with persons who have thought disorders and other issues that interfere with the ability to do so.

Rational Emotive Behavior Therapy

> **KEYCONCEPT Rational emotive behavior therapy (REBT)** is a psychotherapeutic approach that proposes that unrealistic and irrational beliefs cause many emotional problems. It is a form of CBT with a primary emphasis on changing irrational beliefs that cause emotional distress into thoughts that are more reasonable and rational.

REBT is based on the assumptions that people are born with the potential to be rational (self-constructive) and irrational (self-defeating). Ellis believes that highly cognitive, active, directive homework assignments and structured therapies are likely to be more effective in a shorter time than other therapies. Irrational thinking, self-damaging habituations, wishful thinking, and intolerance are exacerbated by culture and family groups (Ellis et al., 2008).

Rational Emotive Behavior Therapy Framework

The basic framework for REBT uses the acronym **ABCDE** (see Box 13.2).

The **activating event** may be either external or internal and not necessarily an actual event, but it may also

---

BOX 13.2

The Rational Emotive Behavior Therapy Framework

A. Activating event that triggers automatic thoughts and emotions
B. Beliefs that underlie the thoughts and emotions
C. Consequences of this automatic process
D. Dispute or challenge unreasonable expectations
E. Effective outlook developed by disputing or challenging negative belief systems

---

be an emotion or a thought/expectation. For example, a person who is lonely and feels isolated but is uncomfortable in interpersonal situations may see a flyer advertising a gathering of people who are interested in discussing solutions to global warming and would really like to attend (**A**ctivating event). However, when this person thinks about going to the gathering, they imagine going into the room where they do not know anybody and someone trying to engage them in conversation. Their imagination provides a picture of not being able to respond and leaving the room after suffering great embarrassment (**B**elief system: "I am a failure in social situations, and everybody can see what a loser I am."). Of course, he decides not to go (**C**onsequences of his belief system).

Belief systems are shaped by rationality, which is self-constructive, and irrationality, which is self-defeating. Rational beliefs are flexible and lead to reasonable evaluations of negative activating events. For example, after a low grade on an examination, instead of believing "I am stupid" or "that instructor is out to get me," student might conclude that "I earned a low grade on the test; I really need to work to develop a better understanding of the content," or "I think I need to get help with my test-taking skills." Other rational beliefs might be "I really didn't have time to study; so, I can accept this grade and just move on." In other words, "I don't like it, but I can live with it." Rational beliefs accept that human beings are fallible and reject absolutes such as always and never.

Irrational beliefs promote dysfunctional negative emotions that in turn lead to psychic pain and discomfort. Behaviors directed at relief of this pain tend to be self-defeating: "I can't fight the system; I will never succeed in this class." There are five themes common in irrational beliefs:

1. A demand: "This *must* happen."

2. Absolute thinking: "All or nothing at all."

3. Catastrophizing: Exaggerating negative consequences of an event.

4. Low frustration tolerance: Everything should be easy.

5. Global evaluations of human worth: "People can be rated, and some are better than others."

Dysfunctional consequences of the interaction between A (activating event) and B (belief system) follow from absolute, rigid, and irrational beliefs whereas **functional consequences** follow from flexible and rational beliefs. For example, demands about self based on "musts" reinforce dysfunctional beliefs such as, "I must do well and be approved by significant others, and if I'm not, then it's awful." The consequences of these beliefs are often anxiety, depression, shame, and guilt that lead to the inability to develop or achieve life's goals or to develop satisfying interpersonal relationships. Self-regard that is dependent on the approval of others demands that others "treat me fairly and considerately; it's terrible I can't bear it when you don't." Thus, when fairness and consideration are not forthcoming, passive-aggressiveness, anger, rage, and violence may erupt. Demands that the world or life be exactly as one wants can also lead to self-pity as well as problems of self-discipline and addictive behaviors.

Rational Emotive Behavior Therapy Interventions

REBT uses role-playing, assertion training, desensitization, humor, operant conditioning, suggestion, support, and other interventions. According to Ellis, there are two basic forms of REBT: general and preferential. General REBT is synonymous with CBT and teaches patients rational and healthy behavior. Preferential REBT includes general REBT but also emphasizes a profound philosophic change. It teaches patients how to dispute irrational ideas and unhealthy behaviors and to become more creative, scientific, and skeptical thinkers (Ellis et al., 2008). The therapist uses the ABCDE model in a structured manner (Box 13.2). A major challenge for the therapist is to teach the patient the difference between thoughts and beliefs. Automatic thoughts are not irrational beliefs but are inferences about the belief. The focus of interventions during the therapy sessions (frequently several weeks or months apart) is on developing rational beliefs to replace those that are irrational and interfere with the patient's quality of life. Figure 13.2 examines the sequence of treatment used in REBT.

Solution-Focused Brief Therapy

KEYCONCEPT Solution-focused brief therapy (SFBT) focuses on solutions rather than problems. This approach does not challenge the existence of problems but proposes that problems are best understood in relation to their solutions. Solution-focused therapy assists the client in exploring life without the problem (De Shazer, 1985; Miller & Berg, 1995).

SFBT, although basically a cognitive approach, differs in philosophy and approach from other cognitively based approaches. The primary difference is the de-emphasis

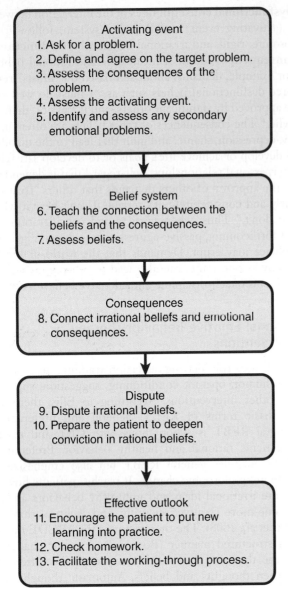

FIGURE 13.2 Rational emotive behavior therapy sequence of treatment.

of the individual and their capacity to make changes or to deal with their day-to-day lives despite what may seem to be the predominant pathology (Bond et al., 2014).

Solution-Focused Behavior Therapy Assumptions

SFBT assumes that change is constant and inevitable. Essentially, everyone changes constantly and is never the same from 1 minute to the next. A person interacts, if only in a minute way, with a constantly changing environment. Very small changes can lead to larger changes, and the stimulus to change comes from a variety of sources. Constant change and its "ripple effect" direct the strategies and interventions used by the therapist. Both assumptions and strategies point the patient toward a positive, future-oriented change. Box 13.3 lists the assumptions that underlie this approach.

Solution-Focused Behavior Therapy Interventions

In SFBT, the therapist takes a position of curiosity in learning about the patient, as opposed to an expert to whom the person has come to be helped. This curiosity is manifested in the questions and techniques that are

on the patient's "problems," or symptoms, and an emphasis on what is functional and healthful. SFBT assists the patient in exploring life without the problem, and it asserts that what is expected to happen influences what the patient does. By discovering what future the client sees as worth striving for, the present becomes important to that future. Otherwise, there is no sense in the patient doing something different or seeing something in a different light. Empirical evidence exists that supports the use of solution-focused approaches (Franklin et al., 2017).

Solution-focused theory views the patient as an individual with a collection of strengths and successes as opposed to a diagnosis and collection of symptoms. Solution-focused approaches emphasize the uniqueness

---

BOX 13.3

Solution-Focused Behavior Therapy Assumptions

1. People have the strengths and resources needed to solve their problems; therefore, the therapist's role is to recognize and emphasize these by amplifying them primarily through asking questions that enable a collaborative approach to constructing solutions.
2. It isn't necessary to know a lot about the complaint and its origins or functions in order to resolve it.
3. Define and dissect the "problem" from the perspective of the patient and look for exceptions to the "problem" in the patient's life.
4. Even long-standing issues can be resolved in a relatively short period of time.
5. There is no right or wrong way to see things.
6. Change is most likely to occur when the focus is on what is changeable.
7. The job of the therapist is to identify and amplify change and maintain a focus on the present and the future.
8. The therapist and patient cocreate reality, utilizing what the patient perceives is "truth," and develop small, concrete, specific, and reality-based goals that are realistic in the context of the patient's life.
9. The therapist expects change and movement and that expectation is inherent in the questions used and the attitude of the therapist.

Based on O'Hanlon, W. H., & Weiner-Davis, M. (2003). *In search of solutions: A new direction in psychotherapy.* W. W. Norton & Company.

integral to this approach and enable the development of realistic goals at each session. Questions used in eliciting the "problem" (frequently referred to as the "issue(s)" to avoid focusing on the "problem") seek very specific information. Examples of questioning in the initial session might include the following:

1. What brought you here today?
   What is going on that made you choose to seek help?
2. Give me a recent example of how that was demonstrated in your life.
3. Who was present when this happened? What did they say and do, and what did you say or do?
   And then what happened?
4. When does this kind of thing happen most often?
5. Where is it likely to occur?
6. Where is it least likely to occur?
7. Is there a particular time (of day, month, and year) when this is **un**likely to happen?
8. How does this interfere with your life, your relationships, self-image, etc.?

If your partner/significant other/coworker were here now, how would they say that you were trying to solve the issue or problem?

Interventions in SFBT focus on achievement of specific, concrete, and achievable goals developed in the collaboration between therapist and patient. These goals, formed using the patient's language, are specific and focus on strengths. Primary techniques used to facilitate progress toward goal attainment are skillfully crafted questions that include the use of the "miracle question," exceptions, scaling, relationship questions, as well as the use of feedback, with an emphasis on complimenting any small, goal-oriented change the patient makes. Feedback conveys to the patient that the therapist has listened carefully and recognizes that working toward a goal of change is difficult and requires hard work.

In **miracle questions**, the therapist structures a scenario that the patient is asked to think about carefully (even though it sounds strange) and to use their imagination in crafting the response, again to very specific questions (see Box 13.4 for a sample scenario and questions).

Other ways of facilitating a similar focus on what the solution would look like are to ask the patient to keep track of what goes well in their life that they would like to see happen again. The patient is encouraged to keep a written list of what they have noticed and bring it to the next session.

Exception questions are rooted in the belief that nothing is constantly present at the same level of intensity, so that there are fluctuations on how the patient experiences "the problem." Exception questions are used to help the patient identify times when they are not bothered by

---

BOX 13.4

Miracle Questions

"I want you to pretend that tonight after you go to bed and are soundly asleep a miracle occurs. The miracle is that the issues that have been bothering you and interfering in your life disappear. Since you have been asleep, you are not aware that the miracle has occurred when you wake up in the morning."

1. What would be your first clue that something was different for you?
2. How will your life be different?
3. What will you be doing instead of _____?
4. How will you be doing this?
5. Beside yourself, who will be the first to notice that there is something different about you?
6. What will that person say or do?
7. How will you respond differently than you might if the issue or problem was still present?

---

the issue or it causes less distress. The role of the therapist is then to amplify these times for the patient. Questions used to elicit exceptions may be as follows:

1. When do you not have that problem/issue?
2. How do you explain that the problem/issue doesn't happen then?
3. What is different in those times, and what are you doing differently?
4. What has occurred that causes the problem/issue to happen more often?

Scaling questions are useful in making the patient's problem or issue more specific, in quantifying the exceptions noted in intensity, and in tracking change over time. Scaling questions ask the patient to rate the issue or problem on a scale of 1 to 10, with 1 being the worst, or greatest intensity, and 10 being the complete absence of the issue. The therapist notes any change on the scale toward 10, asking the patient what was done to make that happen.

Relationship questions are used to amplify and reinforce positive responses to the other questions (see Box 13.4). Patients are asked to consider the point of view of the significant others in their lives. The use of relationship questions can expand the patient's world and help to develop and maintain empathic relationships with others.

Compliments are affirmations of the patient. They reinforce the patient's successes and the strengths needed to achieve those successes. For example, a patient who has frequently gotten into trouble because of a "bad" temper reports in a session that he almost got into an argument while standing in a supermarket checkout lane but instead walked away. An appropriate compliment by the therapist might be "Wow! That's great. That must have been very difficult for you." Compliments can create hope in the patient.

| **NCLEXNOTE** Application of knowledge from the social sciences such as psychology will underlie many of the psychosocial questions. Familiarity with the basic cognitive therapy models will strengthen the application of these concepts to patient situations.

USE OF COGNITIVE THERAPIES IN PSYCHIATRIC NURSING

The context of practice has changed considerably for psychiatric nurses. Length of stay for patients in inpatient settings is becoming shorter every year. The patients admitted to inpatient settings are acutely ill and dealing with more complex issues than ever before. More psychiatric care occurs in prisons than in psychiatric hospitals. More and more the focus of practice is in the community, private homes, and primary care settings rather than in specialty hospitals.

Inpatient Settings

Solution-focused therapy is one of the brief cognitive therapies used by psychiatric nurses in acute inpatient psychiatric settings. SFBT's emphasis on strengths fits well with the values of psychiatric nurses, and the techniques used are well within their scope of practice. Solution-focused approaches have been effective with hospitalized people who were experiencing delusions, hallucinations, and/or loosening of associations (see Box 13.5).

Other cognitive therapeutic techniques used in inpatient settings include journaling and "homework" assignments that focus on education about diagnoses and medications, as well as on group process. These interventions seem to work well in conjunction with shortened length of stay in inpatient settings.

Primary Care Settings

Cognitive interventions in primary care settings are useful and cost-effective. For example, insomnia in breast cancer survivors, depression, chronic pain, and anxiety has been successfully treated with CBT (Bélanger et al., 2016; Gudenkauf et al., 2015; Shepardson et al., 2020). Researchers in the United Kingdom have reported 10% to 20% of hospital patients suffer from "health anxiety" that has responded well to interventions by nurses who were trained in 2-day workshops in the application of CBT skills. These positive results were sustained over a period of 2 years (Tyrer et al., 2014). Nurses in nonpsychiatric settings can learn the techniques of CBT that can be easily applied in hospital settings. Patient education about sleep hygiene and relaxation training can be used by nurses in any setting.

BOX 13.5

Trauma-Informed Care and Brief Solution-Focused Therapy

Aremu, B., Hill, P. D., McNeal, J. M., Petersen, M. A., Swanberg, D., & Delaney, K. R. (2018). Implementation of trauma-informed care and brief solution-focused therapy: A quality improvement project aimed at increasing engagement on an inpatient psychiatric unit. Journal of Psychosocial Nursing and Mental Health Services, 56(8), 16–22.

THE QUESTION: After receiving training on trauma-informed care and brief solution-focused therapy approach, are nurses able to use patient engagement techniques in brief solution-focused therapy, and will the use of PRN medications for de-escalation be reduced?

METHODS: This quality improvement project occurred on a 25-bed acute psychiatric unit. Staff received education on patient engagement and new staff were educated on their role in creating and maintaining a trauma-informed care organization, building trusting relationships, and creating a safe, healing environment. A total of 33 staff participated in one of two educational sessions. The Management of Aggression and Violence Attitude Scale measured staff comfort when handling aggression and engaging clients during de-escalation. The Combined Assessment of Psychiatric Environments–brief version measured staff engagement and patient experience of care on inpatient psychiatric units. These tools were administered pre- and post (1 and 3 months) education for a change in engagement and knowledge. PRN usage was measured at pre- and post-education. Patient records were audited for use of SBFT techniques.

FINDINGS: While there was improvement in all of the measures, the use of PRN medications declined, and the patient records showed that SBFT approaches were being used, the measures did not reach the level of significance.

IMPLICATIONS FOR NURSING: Changing nursing practice takes time. Quality improvement projects can be useful in shaping nursing practices even though the results may not reach the level of significance.

Community Settings

In community settings, cognitive approaches are used in combination with a broad array of interpersonal, behavioral, educational, and pharmacologic interventions. Cognitive interventions are used within a holistic evaluation of patients that includes a complete health history and physical examination and evaluation of possible co-occurring disorders such as depression and alcohol and other drug use or abuse. In particular, the use of questioning such as that integral to solution-focused approaches elicits strengths in a relatively short time and can provide a means for the nurse to support positive coping. The focus on realistic goal development provides a means of evaluation of patient progress.

Home settings are also conducive to the implementation of cognitive techniques. Small, concrete, specific goals developed in a naturalistic setting such as the home can create significant change for the whole family. CBT and SFBT approaches are very useful in primary care settings where time with patients is very short. Goal setting, use of scaling questions, and compliments can be done in the course of a 15-minute interaction.

SUMMARY OF KEY POINTS

- Cognitive therapies have a long history in mental health care and have support as evidence-based interventions effective in several mental disorders.

- Psychiatric nurses use cognitive interventions in a variety of settings. Cognitive therapies serve as the framework for psychotherapy as well as interdisciplinary treatment.

- CBT focuses on dysfunctional thinking through the examination of the cognitive triad, cognitive distortions, and schema.

- REBT assumes that people are born with the tendency to be rational and irrational. Using the ABCDE framework, REBT focuses on identifying and changing irrational beliefs that lead to negative consequences.

- SFBT identifies the possible solutions before addressing the problem.

CRITICAL THINKING CHALLENGES

1. Compare and contrast the three cognitive therapies in terms of assumptions and interventions.

2. A patient has recently been fired from her job, which is the third job that she has had within 1 year. She is depressed but denies suicidal thoughts. She tells you that she is a failure and can never get and keep a job. Discuss how CBT, REBT, and SFBT would view and treat this patient.

3. A nurse manager plans to use CBT as a theoretical model for an inpatient unit. Discuss the interventions that should be used on an inpatient unit that applies the CBT model.

REFERENCES

Beck, A. T. (2008). The evolution of the cognitive model of depression and its neurobiological correlates. *American Journal of Psychiatry, 165*(8), 969–977.

Bélanger, L., Harvey, A. G., Fortier-Brochu, É., Beaulieu-Bonneau, S., Eidelman, P., Talbot, L., Ivers, H., Hein, K., Lamy, M., Soehner, A. M., Mérette, C., & Morin, C. M. (2016). Impact of comorbid anxiety and depressive disorders on treatment response to cognitive behavior therapy for insomnia. *Journal of Consulting and Clinical Psychology, 84*(8), 659–667.

Bond, C., Woods, K., Humphrey, N., Symes, W., & Green, L. (2014). Practitioner review: The effectiveness of solution focused brief therapy with children and families: A systematic and critical evaluation of the literature from 1990–2010. *Journal of Child Psychology & Psychiatry, 54*(7), 707–723.

Cladder-Micus, M. B., Speckens, A., Vrijsen, J. N., T Donders, A. R., Becker, E. S., & Spijker, J. (2018). Mindfulness-based cognitive therapy for patients with chronic, treatment-resistant depression: A pragmatic randomized controlled trial. *Depression and Anxiety, 35*(10), 914–924. https://doi.org/10.1002/da.22788

De Shazer, S. (1985). *Keys to solution in brief therapy*. W. W. Norton & Company.

Del Pozo, M. A., Harbeck, S., Zahn, S., Kliem, S., & Kröger, C. (2018). Cognitive distortions in anorexia nervosa and borderline personality disorder. *Psychiatry Research, 260*, 164–172. https://doi.org/10.1016/j.psychres.2017.11.043

Ellis, A., Abrams, M., & Lidia, D. A. (2008). *Personality theories: Critical perspectives*. Sage.

Franklin, C., Zhang, A., Froerer, A., & Johnson, S. (2017). Solution focused brief therapy: A systematic review and meta-summary of process research. *Journal of Marital and Family Therapy, 43*(1), 16–30. https://doi.org/10.1111/jmft.12193

Gudenkauf, L. M., Antoni, M. H., Stagl, J. M., Lechner, S. C., Jutagir, D. R., Bouchard, L. C., Blomberg, B. B., Glück, S., Derhagopian, R. P., Giron, G. L., Avisar, E., Torres-Salichs, M. A., & Carver, C. S. (2015). Brief cognitive-behavioral and relaxation training interventions for breast cancer: A randomized controlled trial. *Journal of Consulting and Clinical Psychology, 83*(4), 677–688.

Miller, S. D., & Berg, I. K. (1995). *The miracle method: A radically new approach to problem drinking*. W. W. Norton & Company.

Olthuis, J. V. (2016). Therapist-supported internet cognitive behavioural therapy for anxiety disorders in adults. *(Protocol) Cochrane Database of Systematic Reviews, 3*(CD011565). https://doi.org/10.1002/14651858.CD011565.pub2

Possemato, K., Johnson, E. M., Beehler, G. P., Shepardson, R. L., King, P., Vair, C. L., Funderburk, J. S., Maisto, S. A., & Wray, L. O. (2018). Patient outcomes associated with primary care behavioral health services: A systematic review. *General Hospital Psychiatry, 53*, 1–11. https://doi.org/10.1016/j.genhosppsych.2018.04.002

Shepardson, R. L., Minnick, M. R., & Funderburk, J. S. (2020). Anxiety interventions delivered in primary care behavioral health routine clinical practice. *Families, Systems & Health: The Journal of Collaborative Family Healthcare, 38*(2), 193–199. https://doi.org/10.1037/fsh0000493

Spoelstra, S. L., Schueller, M., Hilton, M., & Ridenour, K. (2015). Interventions combining motivational interviewing and cognitive behaviour to promote medication adherence: A literature review. *Journal of Clinical Nursing, 24*(9–10), 1163–1173.

Tyrer, P., Cooper, S., Salkovskis, P., Tyrer, H., Crawford, M., Byford, S., Dupont, S., Finnis, S., Green, J., McLaren, E., Murphy, D., Reid, S., Smith, G., Wang, D., Warwick, H., Petkova, H., & Barrett, B. (2014). Clinical and cost-effectiveness of cognitive behavior therapy for health anxiety in medical patients: A multicenter randomized controlled trial. *Lancet, 383*(9913), 219–225.

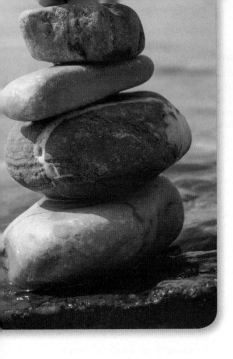

14
Group Interventions

Mary Ann Boyd

KEYCONCEPTS

- group
- group dynamics
- group process

LEARNING OBJECTIVES

After studying this chapter, you will be able to:

1. Discuss concepts used in leading groups.

2. Compare the roles that group members can assume.

3. Identify important aspects of leading a group, such as member selection, leadership skills, seating arrangements, and ways of dealing with challenging behaviors of group members.

4. Distinguish types of groups: psychoeducation, support, psychotherapy, and self-help.

5. Describe common nursing intervention groups.

KEY TERMS

• Closed group • Cohesion • Coleadership • Communication pathways • Direct leadership • Dyad • Formal group roles • Group themes • Groupthink • Indirect leadership • Individual roles • Informal group roles • Maintenance roles • Open group • Task roles • Triad

INTRODUCTION

Group interventions are a key nursing strategy in mental health promotion and recovery. A group experience can help an individual enhance self-understanding, conquer unwanted thoughts and feelings, and learn new behaviors. In a group, members learn from each other as well as the leader. Group interventions are efficient because several patients can participate at one time, and they can be used in most settings. Groups can vary in purpose from being a social group attending a local ball game to an intensive psychotherapy group.

Group interventions are not unique to mental health but are used universally in all aspects of the health care system. For example, web-based psychoeducational groups were used with first-time mothers (Jiao et al.,

2019); persons with head and neck cancer (Richardson et al., 2019); and caregivers (Frias et al., 2020). Group interventions are delivered in several formats including face-to-face, virtual, and mobile applications. Digital group interventions are being tested and are expected to stay mainstream even after the coronavirus threat decreases. Digital reminiscence therapy can help people with dementia improve their mood and increase opportunities to engage with other people (Moon & Park, 2020).

> **KEYCONCEPT A group** is two or more people who develop interactive relationships and share at least one common goal or issue. *A group is more than the sum of its parts.* A group develops its own personality, patterns of interaction, and rules of behavior.

Nurses in various roles and settings use group interventions, such as when conducting patient education or leading support groups. This chapter discusses group concepts, considerations in group leadership, and types of groups that nurses commonly lead.

PREPARING TO LEAD A GROUP

Psychiatric nurses lead a wide range of groups (see later discussion of Types of Groups). Some are structured such as a psychoeducation group, and others are unstructured (e.g., a social group). Groups can be face-to-face groups or virtual groups. The virtual groups may be synchronous or asynchronous. The purpose of the group will dictate the amount of structure and types of activities. In all groups, nurses maintain professional boundaries. Because some group activities are social in nature (unit parties, community trips), it is easy to forget that socialization is a treatment intervention. Nurses should avoid meeting personal social needs within this context.

Thoughtful planning and preparation make for a successful group. Confidentiality is important in all groups. The following sections discuss important considerations when planning for a group.

Virtual Group Interventions

Offering a virtual group has the advantage of being efficient and convenient, but there are also real challenges when planning the group. For example, is the software new or is the person already using it? Software should be Health Insurance Portability and Accountability Act compliant, which may necessitate purchase of new software. Do all of the potential group members have access to the internet recognizing that the strength varies by location? What will it cost, and will the virtual group fit in with your workflow? For example, face-to-face inpatient group require less preparation time.

During the COVID-19 nationwide public health emergency, the social distancing requirements have increased the use of virtual groups replacing in-person, face-to-face groups such as support and substance use groups. The importance of engagement becomes more challenging as members may not be as actively engaged in the virtual groups as the face-to-face groups (Colditz et al., 2020). The leader must additional strategies to engage and motivate the members to engage and participate in the group.

Selecting Members

Individuals can self-refer or be referred to a group by treatment teams or clinicians, but the leader is responsible for assessing each individual's suitability for the group. One factor to consider is sociodemographic similarity, especially when forming a larger group. Research shows that there is a higher probability of attendance in larger groups, when members were similar in age and ethnicity (Firth et al., 2020). The individual's suitability for the group can be based on the following criteria:

- Does the purpose of the group match the needs of the potential member?
- Does the potential member have the social skills to function comfortably in the group?
- Will the other group members accept the new group member?
- Can the potential member make a commitment to attending group meetings?

Forming an Open or Closed Group

In planning for a group, one of the early decisions is whether the group will be open or closed. In an **open group**, new members may join, and old members may leave the group at different sessions. Because length of patient hospitalization is relatively short, open groups are typical of inpatient units. For example, a newly admitted patient may join an anger management group that is part of an ongoing program in an inpatient unit.

In a **closed group**, members begin the group at one time, and no new members are admitted. If a member leaves, no replacement member joins. In a closed group, participants get to know one another very well and can develop close relationships. Closed groups are more typical of outpatient groups that have a sequential curriculum or psychotherapy groups. These groups usually meet weekly for a specified period. Outpatient smoking cessation, psychotherapy, and psychoeducation groups are examples.

Determining Composition

Another decision is the group size. The size of a group will depend on the overall group goals and patients' abilities. Patients with challenging behaviors should be carefully screened and may be able to function in smaller rather than larger groups.

Small groups (usually no more than seven to eight members) become more cohesive, are less likely to form subgroups, and can provide a richer interpersonal experience than large groups (Yalom & Leszcz, 2005). A very small group is two people (**dyad**) or three (**triad**). Small groups function nicely with one group leader although many small groups are led by two people. Although small groups cannot easily withstand the loss of members, they are ideal for patients who are highly motivated to deal with complex emotional problems, such as sexual abuse, eating disorders, or trauma or for those who have cognitive dysfunction and require a more focused group environment with minimal distractions.

In leading a small group, the leader gets to know the members very well but maintains objectivity. The nurse observes for transference of participants toward the leader or other member. If a member becomes a "favorite patient," the leader should reflect upon any underlying personal countertransference issues (see Chapter 10).

> **NCLEXNOTE** Be prepared to select members and plan for a patient or family support group to help deal with the impact of mental illnesses on the family lifestyle.

Large groups (more than 8–10 members) are effective for specific problems or issues, such as smoking cessation or medication information. Large groups are often used in the workplace for health promotion activities such as smoking cessation, healthy eating, and meditation. A large group can be ongoing and open ended. Usually, transference and countertransference issues do not develop.

However, leading a large group is challenging because of the number of potential interactions and relationships that can form and the difficulty in determining the feelings and thoughts of the participants. As the size of the group increases, the level of engagement decreases and conflict increases (Wu et al., 2020). It may be difficult to get everyone's attention to begin a group session. Subgroups can form, making it difficult to develop a cohesive group. If subgroups form that are detrimental to the group, the nurse can change the structure and function of communication within the subgroups by rearranging seating and encouraging the subgroup to interact with the rest of the group. Gender mix is also a consideration and can make a difference in the success of the group. It is important to avoid making assumptions about the gender of your group members. Asking members for their personal pronouns will set the stage for using gender-inclusive interactions.

Selecting a Leadership Style

A group is led within the context of the group leader's theoretic background and the group's purpose. For example, a leader with training in cognitive-behavioral therapy may focus on treating depression by asking members to think differently about situations, which in turn lead to feeling better. A leader with a psychodynamic orientation may focus on the feelings of depression by examining situations that generate the same feelings. Whatever the leader's theoretic background, their leadership behavior can be viewed on a continuum of direct to indirect.

Direct leadership behavior enables the leader to control the interaction by giving directions and information and allowing little discussion. The leader literally tells the members what to do. On the other end of the continuum is **indirect leadership**, in which the leader primarily reflects the group members' discussion and offers little guidance or information to the group. Sometimes, the group needs a more direct approach, such as in a psychoeducation class; other times, it needs a leader who is indirect. The challenge of providing leadership is to give sufficient direction to help the group meet its goals and develop its own group process

but enough freedom to allow members to make mistakes and recover from their thinking errors in a supportive, caring, and learning environment.

Coleadership, when two people share responsibility for leading the group, is useful in most groups if the coleaders attend all sessions and maintain open communication. Coleadership works well when the coleaders plan together and meet before and after each session to discuss the group process.

Setting the Stage: Arranging Seating in a Face-to-Face Group

Group sessions should be held in a quiet, pleasant room with adequate space and privacy. Holding a session in too large or too small room inhibits communication. The sessions should be held in private rooms that nonmembers cannot access. Interruptions are distracting and can potentially compromise confidentiality. Arrangement of chairs should foster interaction and reduce communication barriers. Communication flows better when no physical barriers, such as tables, are between members. Group members should be able to see and hear each other. Arranging a group in a circle with chairs comfortably close to one another without a table enhances group work. No one should sit outside the group. If a table is necessary, a round table is better than a rectangular one, which implicitly increases the power of those who sit at the ends.

Group members tend to sit in the same places. Those who sit close to the group leader are more likely to have more power in the group than those who sit far away.

Setting the Stage: Arranging for a Virtual Group

Virtual groups are becoming common as the availability and accessibility of platforms (e.g., Microsoft Teams, Zoom, etc.) increases. To participate, patients must have internet access and devices that are compatible with the platform. Ideally, group members who are in synchronous groups have video, as well as audio capability. Groups members should be able to see each other. In asynchronous groups, the members respond to discussion usually through typing their responses. The group leader provides specific directions related to time and date of meeting and accessing the group.

Planning the First Meeting

The leader sets the tone of the group at the first meeting. The leader and members introduce themselves. The leader may ask participants to share some introductory information such as why they joined the group and what do they hope to gain from the experience. The leader can share name, credentials for leading group, and a brief statement about experience. The leader should avoid self-disclosing personal information.

The first session is the time to explain the structure of group, including the purpose and group rules (Box 14.1). It is important the group starts and ends at scheduled times; otherwise, members who tend to be late will not change their behavior, and those who are on time will resent waiting for the others. The leader also explains when and if new members can join the group.

LEADING A GROUP

During the first session, the leader begins to assess the group dynamics or interactions—both verbal and nonverbal. During the group sessions, these interactions will be important in understanding the group process and may determine the success of the group.

Group Dynamics

| **KEYCONCEPT Group dynamics** are the verbal and nonverbal interactions that occur in the group.

The theoretical basis of group dynamics is attributed to Kurt Lewin (1939) and proposes that by joining a group, one's interactions with fellow members change the individual and the other group members; in addition, a highly attractive group can exert influence on its members, and a weak group does not have the same ability (Leach et al., 2019).

As a group develops its unique characteristics, individual members become connected to each other and are included in the group. The group's personality, pattern of interaction, and behavior become primary. Whether individual members are included in the group will depend on how the group treats that individual. Inclusion is also dependent upon whether the individual is motivated to be included. That is, inclusion is a two-way street. If the group's goals are consistent with individual members' goals and members are motivated to participate in the group, the group is more likely to be well attended and successful (Jansen et al., 2020).

Group Process

A group leader is responsible for monitoring and shaping the group process, as well as focusing on the group content. Although models of group development differ, most follow a pattern of a beginning, middle, and ending phase (Table 14.1) (Corey et al., 2018). These stages should not be viewed as a linear progression with one preceding another but as a dynamic process that is constantly revisiting and reexamining group interactions and behaviors, as well as progressing forward. The group leader needs to be aware of the group's stage of development as well as leadership responsibilities.

| **KEYCONCEPT Group process** is the development and culmination of the session-to-session interactions of the members that move the group toward its goals.

Stages of Group Development

Beginning Stage: The Honeymoon

In the beginning, the group leader acknowledges each member; constructs a working environment; develops rapport with the members; begins to build a therapeutic relationship; and clarifies outcomes, processes, and skills related to the group's purpose (Corey et al., 2018). To carry

TABLE 14.1	**COMPARISON OF MODELS OF GROUP DEVELOPMENT**		
Phase	**Robert Bales (1955)**	**William Schutz (1960)**	**Bruce Tuckman (1965)**
Beginning	• *Orientation:* What is the problem?	• *Inclusion:* Deal with issues of belonging and being in and out of the group.	• *Forming:* Get to know one another and form a group.
Middle	• *Evaluation:* How do we feel about it?	• *Control:* Deal with issues of authority (who is in charge?), dependence, and autonomy.	• *Storming:* Tension and conflict occur; subgroups form and clash with one another. • *Norming:* Develop norms of how to work together.
Ending	• *Control:* What should we do about it?	• *Affection:* Deal with issues of intimacy, closeness, and caring versus dislike and distancing.	• *Performing:* Reach consensus and develop cooperative relationships.

Source: Bales, R. (1955). A set of categories for the analysis of small group interaction. *American Sociological Review, 15,* 257–263; Schutz, W. (1960). *FIRO: A three-dimensional theory of interpersonal behavior.* Holt, Rinehart & Winston; Tuckman, B. (1965). Developmental sequence in small groups. *Psychological Bulletin, 63*(6), 384–399.

out these functions, the leader processes group interactions by staying objective and observing members' interactions as well as participating in the group. The leader reflects on, evaluates, and responds to interactions. The use of various techniques enhances the leader's ability to lead the group effectively and to help the group meet its goals (Table 14.2).

During beginning sessions, group members get to know one another and the group leader. The length of the beginning stage depends on the purpose of the group, the number of members, and the skill of the leader. It may last for only a few sessions or several. Members often exhibit polite, congenial behavior typical of those in new social situations. They are "good patients" and often intellectualize their problems; that is, these patients deal with emotional conflict or stress by excessively using abstract thinking or generalizations to minimize disturbing feelings. Members are usually anxious and sometimes display behavior that does not truly represent their feelings.

In this phase, members begin to test whether they can trust one another and the leader. Members may come late to group or try to extend group time. Sometime after the initial sessions, group members usually experience a period of conflict, either among themselves or with the leader. This conflict is a normal part of group development, and many believe that conflict is necessary to move into any working phase. Sometimes, one or more group members become the scapegoat. Such situations challenge the leader

TABLE 14.2   TECHNIQUES IN LEADING GROUPS

Technique	Purpose	Example
Support: giving feedback that provides a climate of emotional support	Helps a person or group continue with ongoing activities Informs group about what the leader thinks is important Creates a climate for expressing unpopular ideas Helps the more quiet and fearful members speak up	"We really appreciate your sharing that experience with us. It looked like it was quite painful."
Confrontation: challenging a participant (needs to be done in a supportive environment)	Helps individuals learn something about themselves Helps reduce some forms of disruptive behavior Helps members deal more openly and directly with one another	"Tom, this is the third time you have changed the subject when we have talked about spouse abuse. Is something going on?"
Advice and suggestions: sharing expertise and knowledge that the members do not have	Provides information that members can use after they have examined and evaluated it Helps focus the group's task and goals	"The medication you are taking may be causing you to be sleepy."
Summarizing: statements at the end of sessions that highlight the session's discussion, any problem resolution, and unresolved problems	Provides continuity from one session to the next Brings to focus still unresolved issues Organizes the past in ways that clarify; brings into focus themes and patterns of interaction	"This session, we discussed Sharon's medication problems, and she will be following up with her physicians."
Clarification: restatement of an interaction	Checks on the meanings of the interaction and communication Avoids faulty communication Facilitates focus on substantive issues rather than allowing members to be sidetracked into misunderstandings	"What I heard you say was that you are feeling very sad right now. Is that correct?"
Probing and questioning: a technique for the experienced group leader that asks for more information	Helps members expand on what they were saying (when they are ready to) Gets at more extensive and wider range of information Invites members to explore their ideas in greater detail	"Could you tell us more about your relationship with your parents?"
Repeating, paraphrasing, highlighting: a simple act of repeating what was just said	Facilitates communication among group members Corrects inaccurate communication or emphasizes accurate communication	*Member:* "I forgot about my wife's birthday." *Leader:* "You forgot your wife's birthday."
Reflecting feelings: identifying feelings that are being expressed	Orients members to the feelings that may lie behind what is being said or done Helps members deal with issues they might otherwise avoid or miss	"You sound upset."
Reflecting behavior: identifying behaviors that are occurring	Gives members an opportunity to see how their behavior appears to others and to evaluate its consequences Helps members to understand others' perceptions and responses to them	"I notice that when the topic of sex is brought up, you look down and shift in your chair."

to guide the group during this period by avoiding taking sides and treating all members respectfully.

Working Stage

The working stage of groups involves a real sharing of ideas and the development of closeness. A group personality may emerge that is distinct from the individual personalities of its members. The group develops norms, which are rules and standards that establish acceptable behaviors. Some norms are formalized, such as beginning group on time, but others are never really formalized, such as sitting in the same place each session. These normative standards encourage conformity and discourage behavioral deviations from the established norms. A member quickly learns the norms or is ostracized.

During this stage, the group realizes its purpose. If the purpose is education, the participants engage in learning new content or skills. If the aim of the group is to share feelings and experiences, these activities consume group meetings. During this phase, the group starts on time, and the leader often needs to remind members when it is time to stop.

Termination Stage or Saying Goodbye

Termination can be difficult for a group, especially an effective one. During the final stages, members begin to grieve for the loss of the group's closeness and begin to reestablish themselves as individuals. Individuals terminate from groups as they do from any relationship. One person may not attend the last session, another person may bring up issues that the group has already addressed, and others may demonstrate anger or hostility. Most members of successful groups are sad as the group terminates. During the last meetings, members may make arrangements for meeting after group. These plans rarely materialize or continue. Leaders should recognize these plans as part of the farewell process—saying goodbye to the group.

In terminating a group, the nurse discusses and summarizes the work of the group, including the accomplishments of members and their future plans. The nurse focuses on ending the group and avoids being pulled into working stage issues. For example, when a patient brings up an issue that was once resolved, the nurse reinforces the skills and then reminds the member of the actions that will be taken after the group has ended.

Facilitating Group Communication

One of the responsibilities of the group leader is to facilitate both verbal and nonverbal communication to meet the treatment goals of the individual members and the entire group. Because of the number of people involved, developing trusting relationships within groups is more complicated than developing a single relationship with a patient. The communication techniques used in establishing and maintaining individual relationships are the same for groups, but the leader also attends to the communication patterns among the members.

Encouraging Interaction

The nurse leads the group during this phase by encouraging interaction among members and being responsive to their comments. Active listening enables the leader to process events and track interactions. The nurse can then formulate responses based on a true understanding of the discussion. A group leader who listens also models listening behavior for others, helping them improve their skills. Members may need to learn to listen to one another, track discussions without changing the subject, and not speak while others are talking. At the end of the session, the nurse summarizes the work of the session and projects the work for the next meeting.

The leader maintains a neutral, nonjudgmental style and avoids showing preference to one member over another. This may be difficult because some members may naturally seek out the leader's attention or ask for special favors. These behaviors are divisive to the group, and the leader should discourage them. Other important skills include providing everyone with an opportunity to contribute and respecting everyone's ideas. A leader who truly wants group participation and decision-making does not reveal their beliefs.

Monitoring Verbal Communication

Group interaction can be viewed as a communication network that becomes patterned and predictable. In a group, verbal comments are linked in a chain formation. Monitoring verbal interactions and leading a group at the same time is difficult for one person. If there are two leaders, one may be the active leader of the group, and the other may sit outside the group and observe and record rather than participating. If all members agree, the leader can use an audio or video recorder for reviewing interaction after the group session.

Interesting interaction patterns can be observed and analyzed (Fig. 14.1). By analyzing the content and patterns, the leader can determine the existence of **communication pathways**—who is most liked in the group, who occupies a position of power, what subgroups have formed, and who is isolated from the group. People who sit next to each other tend to communicate among themselves. Usually, those who are well liked, or display leadership abilities, tend to be chosen for interactions more often than do those who are not. The leader can also determine if there is a change of subject when a sensitive topic is introduced.

Deciphering Content Themes

Group themes are the collective conceptual underpinnings of a group and express the members' underlying

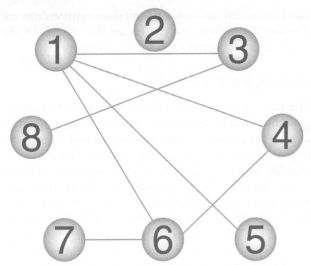

FIGURE 14.1 Sociometric analysis of group behavior. In this sociometric structure, response pattern was recorded during member interaction. Group members interacted with number 1 the most. Therefore, number 1 is the over-chosen person. Numbers 5 and 7 are under chosen. Number 2 is never chosen and is determined to be the isolate.

concerns or feelings regardless of the group's purpose. Themes that emerge in groups help members to understand group dynamics. Different groups have different themes. A grief group most likely would have a theme of loss or new beginnings and an adolescent group may have a theme of independence. Although some predictable themes occur in groups, the obvious or assumed themes at the beginning may actually wind up differing from reality as the process continues. In one hospice support group, the members seemed to be focusing on the memories of their loved ones. However, upon examination of the content of their interactions, discussions were revolving around financial planning for the future (Box 14.2).

Monitoring Nonverbal Communication

Observing nonverbal communication contributes to understanding the group dynamics. Members communicate nonverbally with each other, not only the group leader. Eye contact, posture, and body gestures of one member impact other members. For example, if one member is explaining a painful experience and another member looks away and tries to engage still another, the self-disclosing member may feel devalued and rejected because the disruptive behavior is interpreted as disinterest. However, if the leader interprets the disruptive behavior as anxiety over the topic, they may try to engage the other member in discussing the source of the anxiety.

The leaders should monitor the nonverbal behavior of group members during each session. Often, one or two people can set the overall mood of the group. Someone

who comes to a session very sad or angry can set a tone of sadness or anger for the whole group. An astute group leader recognizes the effects of an individual's mood on the total group. If the purpose of the group is to deal with emotions, the group leader may choose to discuss the member's problem at the beginning of the session. The leader, thus, limits the mood to the one person experiencing it. If the group's purpose is inconsistent with self-disclosure of personal problems, the nurse should acknowledge the individual member's distress and offer a private session after the group. In this instance, the nurse would not encourage repeated episodes of self-disclosure from that member or others.

Tracking Group Communication

The leader tracks the verbal and nonverbal interactions throughout the group sessions. Depending on the group's purpose, the leader may or may not share the observations with the group. For example, if the purpose of the group is psychoeducation, the leader may incorporate the information into a lesson plan without identifying any one individual. If the purpose of the group is to improve the self-awareness and interaction skills of members, the leader may point out the observations. The leader needs to be clear about the purpose of the group and tailor leadership strategies accordingly.

Determining Roles of Group Members

There are two official or **formal group roles**, the leader and the members; however, there are also important **informal group roles** or positions with implicit rights and duties that can either help or hinder the group's process. Ideally, one or more members assume **task roles** or functions. These individuals are concerned about the purpose of the group and "keep things on task." For example, *information seeker* is the member who asks for clarification; the *coordinator* spells out relationships among ideas, and the *recorder* keeps the minutes.

Maintenance roles or functions are assumed by those who help keep the group together. Other members assume maintenance roles and make sure that the group members get along with each other and try to make peace if conflict erupts. These individuals are as interested in maintaining the group's cohesiveness as focusing on the group's tasks. The *harmonizer*, *compromiser*, and *standard setter* are examples of maintenance roles.

Both task and maintenance functions are needed in an effective group. In selecting members and analyzing the progress of the group, the leader pays attention to the balance between the task and maintenance functions. If too many group members assume task functions and too few assume maintenance functions, the group may have difficulty developing **cohesion**, or sticking together. If too many members assume maintenance functions, the group may never finish its work.

Individual roles are played by members to meet personal needs, such as feeling important or being an expert on a subject. These roles have nothing to do with the group's purpose or cohesion and can detract from the group's functioning (Box 14.3). If individual roles predominate, the group may be ineffective.

Dealing with Challenging Group Behaviors

Problematic behaviors occur in all groups. They can be challenging to the most experienced group leaders and frustrating to new leaders. In dealing with any problematic behavior or situation, the leader must remember to

---

BOX 14.3

Roles and Functions of Group Members

TASK ROLES

- *Initiator–contributor* suggests or proposes new ideas or a new view of the problem or goal.
- *Information seeker* asks for clarification of the values pertinent to the group activity.
- *Information giver* offers "authoritative" facts or generalizations or gives own experiences.
- *Opinion giver* states belief or opinions with emphasis on what should be the group's values.
- *Elaborator* spells out suggestions in terms of examples, develops meanings of ideas and rationales, and tries to deduce how an idea would work.
- *Coordinator* shows or clarifies the relationships among various ideas and suggestions.
- *Orienter* defines the position of the group with respect to its goals.
- *Evaluator–critic* measures the outcome of the group against some standard.
- *Energizer* attempts to stimulate the group to action or decision.
- *Procedural technician* expedites group movement by doing things for the group such as distributing copies and arranging seating.
- *Recorder* writes suggestions, keeps minutes, and serves as group memory.

MAINTENANCE ROLES

- *Encourager* praises, agrees with, and accepts the contributions of others.
- *Harmonizer* mediates differences among members and relieves tension in conflict situations.
- *Compromiser* operates from within a conflict and may yield status or admit error to maintain group harmony.

- *Gatekeeper* attempts to keep communication channels open by encouraging or facilitating the participation of others or proposes regulation of the flow of communication through limiting time.
- *Standard setter* expresses standards for the group to achieve.
- *Group observer* keeps records of various aspects of group processes and interprets data to group.
- *Follower* goes along with the movement of the group.

INDIVIDUAL ROLES

- *Aggressor* deflates the status of others; expresses disapproval of the values, acts, or feelings of others; attacks the group or problem; jokes aggressively; and tries to take credit for the work.
- *Blocker* tends to be negative and resistant, disagrees and opposes without or beyond "reason," and attempts to bring back an issue after group has rejected it.
- *Recognition seeker* calls attention to self through such activities as boasting, reporting on personal achievements, or acting in unusual ways.
- *Self-confessor* uses group setting to express personal, non–group-oriented feelings or insights.
- *Playboy* makes a display of lack of involvement in group's processes.
- *Dominator* tries to assert authority or superiority in manipulating the group or certain members of the group through flattery, being directive, or interrupting others.
- *Help-seeker* attempts to call forth sympathy from other group members through expressing insecurity, personal confusion, or depreciation of self beyond reason.
- *Special interest pleader* speaks for a special group, such as "grass roots," usually representing personal prejudices or biases.

Benne, K. D., & Sheats, P. (1948). Functional roles of group members. *Journal of Social Issues, 4*(2), 41–49. Copyright © 1948 The Society for the Psychological Study of Social issues. Reprinted by permission of John Wiley & Sons, Inc.

support the integrity of the individual members and the group as a whole.

Monopolizer

Some people tend to monopolize a group by constantly talking or interrupting others. This behavior is common in the beginning stages of group formation and usually represents anxiety that the member displaying such behavior is experiencing. Within a few sessions, this person usually relaxes and no longer attempts to monopolize the group. However, for some people, monopolizing discussions is part of their normal personality and will continue. Other group members usually find the behavior mildly irritating in the beginning and extremely annoying as time passes. Members may drop out of the group to avoid that person. The leader needs to decide if, how, and when to intervene. The best-case scenario is when savvy group members remind the monopolizer to let others speak. The leader can then support the group in establishing rules that allow everyone the opportunity to participate. However, the group often waits for the leader to manage the situation. There are a couple of ways to deal with the situation. The leader can interrupt the monopolizer by acknowledging the member's contribution but redirecting the discussion to others, or the leader can become more directive and limit the discussion time per member.

"Yes, But ..."

Some people have a patterned response to any suggestions from others. Initially, they agree with suggestions others offer them, but then they add "yes, but ..." and give several reasons why the suggestions will not work for them. Leaders and members can easily identify this patterned response. In such situations, it is best to avoid problem-solving for the member and encourage the person to develop their own solutions. The leader can serve as a role model of the problem-solving behavior for the other members and encourage them to let the member develop a solution that would work specifically for them.

Disliked Member

In some groups, members clearly dislike one member. This situation can be challenging for the leader because it can result in considerable tension and conflict. This person could become the group's scapegoat. The group leader may have made a mistake by placing the person in this group, and another group may be a better match. One solution may be to move the person to a better matched group. Whether the person stays or leaves, the group leader must stay neutral and avoid displaying negative verbal and nonverbal behaviors that indicate that they too dislike the group member or are displeased with the other members for their behavior. Often, the group leader can manage the situation by showing respect for the disliked member and acknowledging

their contribution. In some instances, getting supervision from a more experienced group leader is useful. Defusing the situation may be possible by using conflict resolution strategies and discussing the underlying issues.

The Silent Member

The engagement of a member who does not participate in group discussion can be challenging. This member has had a lifetime of being "the quiet one" and is usually comfortable in the silent role. The leader should respect the person's silent nature. Like all the other group members, the silent member often gains a considerable amount of information and support without verbally participating. It is best for the group leader to get to know the member and understand the meaning of the silence before encouraging interaction.

Group Conflict

Most groups experience periods of conflict. The leader first needs to decide whether the conflict is a natural part of the group process or whether the group needs to address some issues. Member-to-member conflict can be handled through conflict resolution. Leader-to-member conflict is more complicated because the leader has the formal position of power. In this instance, the leader can use conflict resolution strategies but should be sensitive to the power differential between the leader's role and the member's role.

TYPES OF GROUPS

Psychoeducation Groups

The purposes of psychoeducation groups are to enhance knowledge, improve skills, and solve problems. The intervention strategies used in psychoeducation groups focus on transmission of information necessary for making some type of change and providing a process for making the change. Psychoeducation groups are formally planned, and members are purposefully selected. The group leader develops a lesson plan for each session that usually includes objectives, content outline, references, and evaluation tools. These groups are time limited and usually last for only a few sessions. If the group lasts longer than a few sessions, cohesiveness usually enhances outcomes, especially in those that teach health maintenance behaviors such as exercise and weight control (Brown, 2018).

There are a variety of psychoeducation groups, including recovery-oriented and mindfulness groups. Recovery-oriented groups facilitate consumer involvement in the educational process and build on the recovery principles (see Chapters 2 and 9). Examples of recovery-oriented groups include those that focus on how to manage a medication regimen or control angry outbursts. Group psychoeducation has changed perception of illness in persons with bipolar disorder, leading to an improvement in social functioning and improved self-esteem (Etain et al., 2018). Mindfulness groups are helpful in stress reduction.

Task Groups

Task groups focus on completion of specific activities, such as planning a week's menu. When members are strongly committed to completing a task and the leader encourages equal participation, cohesiveness promotes satisfaction and higher performance (Lockhart, 2017). To complete a task, group cohesiveness is especially important. Leaders can encourage cohesiveness by placing participants in situations that promote social interaction with minimal supervision, such as refreshment periods and team-building exercises.

Without cohesiveness, the group's true existence is questionable. In cohesive groups, members are committed to the existence of the group. In large groups, cohesiveness tends to be decreased, with subsequent poorer performance among group members in completing tasks. However, cohesiveness can be a double-edged sword. In very cohesive groups, members are more likely to transgress personal boundaries. Dysfunctional relationships may develop that are destructive to the group process and ultimately not in the best interests of individual members.

Decision-Making Groups

The psychiatric nurse often leads decision-making groups that plan activities, develop unit rules, and select learning materials. The nurse who is leading a decision-making group should observe the process for any signs of **groupthink**, the tendency of group members to avoid conflict and adopt a normative pattern of thinking that is often consistent with the ideas of the group leader (Janis, 1972, 1982). Group members form opinions consistent with the group consensus rather than critically evaluating the situation. Groupthink is more likely to occur if the leader is respected or persuasive. It can also occur if a closed leadership style is used and external threat is present, particularly with time pressure (Cleary et al., 2019). Many catastrophes, such as the *Challenger* explosion and Bay of Pigs invasion, have been attributed to groupthink.

There may be instances in which groupthink can lead to a reasonable decision: for example, a group decides to arrange a going-away party for another patient. In other situations, groupthink may inhibit individual thinking and problem-solving: for example, a team is displaying groupthink if it decides that a patient should lose privileges based on the assumption that the patient is deliberately exhibiting bizarre behaviors. In this case, the team is failing to consider or examine other evidence that suggests the bizarre behavior is really an indication

of psychosis. Another commonly occurring instance of groupthink occurs when a decision is made that is recommended by a charismatic leader who is held in high regard by staff members without the evidence to support the approach (Christensen, 2019).

 Concept Mastery Alert

Groupthink is the tendency of group members to avoid conflict and adopt a normative pattern of thinking that is often consistent with the ideas of the group leader. Group cohesion is the ability of the group to stick together.

Support Groups

Support groups are usually less intense than psychotherapy groups and focus on helping individuals cope with their illnesses and problems. Implementing support groups is one of the basic functions of the psychiatric nurse. In conducting this type of group, the nurse focuses on helping members cope with situations that are common for other group members. Counseling strategies are used. Leadership of the group requires group management, understanding the impact of the group process, role modeling, awareness, willingness, agreeableness, and openness (Pomeroy et al., 2016). For example, a group of patients with bipolar illness whose illness is stable may discuss at a monthly meeting how to tell other people about the illness or how to cope with a family member who seems insensitive to the illness. Family caregivers of persons with mental illnesses benefit from the support of the group, as well as additional information about providing care for an ill family member.

Psychotherapy Groups

Psychotherapy groups treat individuals' emotional problems and can be implemented from various theoretic perspectives, including psychoanalytic, behavioral, and cognitive. These groups focus on examining emotions and helping individuals face their life situations. At times, these groups can be extremely intense. Psychotherapy groups provide an opportunity for patients to examine and resolve psychological and interpersonal issues within a safe environment. Mental health specialists who have a minimum of a master's degree and are trained in group psychotherapy lead such groups. Patients can be treated in psychotherapy and still be members of other nursing groups. Communication with the therapists is important for continuity of care.

One of the most respected approaches is Irvin D. Yalom's model of group psychotherapy. According to Yalom and Leszcz (2005), there are 11 primary factors through which therapeutic changes occur (Table 14.3). In this model, interpersonal relationships are very important because change occurs through a corrective emotional

TABLE 14.3	YALOM'S THERAPEUTIC FACTORS
Therapeutic Factors	**Definition**
Instillation of hope	Hope is required to keep patients in therapy
Universality	Finding out that others have similar problems
Imparting information	Didactic instruction about mental health, mental illness, and so on
Altruism	Learning to give to others
Corrective recapitulation of the primary family group	Reliving and correcting early family conflicts within the group
Development of socializing techniques	Learning basic social skills
Imitative behavior	Assuming some of the behaviors and characteristics of the therapist
Interpersonal learning	Analogue of therapeutic factors in individual therapy, such as insight, working through the transference, and corrective emotional experience
Group cohesiveness	Group members' relationship to therapist and other group members
Catharsis	Open expression of affect to purge or "cleanse" self
Existential factors	Patients' ultimate concerns of existence: death, isolation, freedom, and meaninglessness

Source: Yalom, I., & Leszcz, M. (2005). *The theory and practice of group psychotherapy*. Basic Books.

experience within the context of the group. The group is viewed as a social microcosm of the patients' psychosocial environment (Yalom & Leszcz, 2005).

Self-Help Groups

Self-help groups are led by people who are concerned about coping with a specific problem or life crisis. These groups do not explore psychodynamic issues in depth. Professionals usually do not attend these groups or serve as consultants. Alcoholics Anonymous, Overeaters Anonymous, and One Day at a Time (a grief group) are examples of self-help groups.

Age-Related Groups

Group interventions for specific age groups require attention to the developmental needs of the group members, any physical and mental impairments, social ability, and cognitive level. Children's groups should be structured to accommodate their intellectual and developmental functioning. Groups for older people should be adapted for age-related changes of the members (Box 14.4).

BOX 14.4

Working with Older People in Groups

SELF-ASSESSMENT

Because most group leaders do not have personal experience with the issues faced by older adults, the leaders should sensitize themselves to the positive and negative aspects of aging and the developmental issues facing older adults. Leaders need to be aware of their own negative reactions to aging and how this might affect their work.

COHORT EXPERIENCES

There is a wide variation in the experiences and history of older adults. Current 80- to 90-year-old adults grew up in the Great Depression of the 1930s, 65- to 80-year-old adults commonly experienced growing up during World War II, and the Baby Boomers (ages 55–65 years) were teenagers or young adults during the political and sexual revolution of the 1960s.

TYPICAL THEMES IN GROUP MEETINGS

- **Continuity with the past:** Older adults enjoy recalling, reliving, and reminiscing about past accomplishments.
- **Understanding the modern world:** They often use groups to understand and adapt to the modern world.
- **Independence:** They worry about becoming dependent. Physical and cognitive impairments are threats to independence. Loss of family members and friends is also a threat. Leaders should be familiar with the grieving processes.
- **Changes in family relationships:** Family relationships, especially with children and grandchildren, are increasingly important as social roles change.
- **Changes in resources and environment:** Living on a fixed income focuses older people on the importance of their disposable income. They are more vulnerable to community and neighborhood changes because of their physical and financial limitations.

GROUP LEADERSHIP

- The pace of group meetings should be slowed.
- Greater emphasis should be placed on using wisdom and experience rather than learning new information.
- The group should be encouraged to use life review strategies such as autobiography and reminiscence.
- Teaching new coping skills should be placed within the context of previous attempts to resolve issues and problems (Toseland & Rizzo, 2004).

COMMON NURSING INTERVENTION GROUPS

Nurses lead groups of varying types that are geared toward a specific content area such as medication management, symptom management, anger management, and self-care skills. In addition, nurses' groups focus on other issues such as stress management, relaxation, and women's issues. A competent leader integrates group leadership, knowledge, and skills with nursing interventions that fit a selected group. Most groups can be adapted to a virtual environment.

Medication Groups

Nurse-led medication groups are common in psychiatric nursing. Not all medication groups are alike, so the nurse must be clear regarding the purpose of each specific medication group (Box 14.5). A medication group can be used primarily to transmit information about medications, such as action, dosage, and side effects, or it can focus on issues related to medications, such as compliance, management of side effects, and lifestyle adjustments. Many nurses incorporate both perspectives.

Assessing a member's medication knowledge is important before they join the group to determine what the individual would like to learn. People with mental illness may have difficulty remembering new information, so assessment of cognitive abilities is important. Assessing attention span, memory, and problem-solving skills gives valuable information that nurses can use in designing the group. The nurse should determine the members' reading and writing skills to select effective patient education materials.

An ideal group is one in which all members use the same medication. This situation is rare. Usually, the group members are using various medications. The nurse should know which medications each member is taking,

---

BOX 14.5
Medication Group Protocol

PURPOSE: Develop strategies that reinforce a self-medication routine.

DESCRIPTION: The medication group is an open, ongoing group that meets once a week to discuss topics germane to self-administration of medication. Members will not be asked to disclose the names of their medications.

MEMBER SELECTION: The group is open to any person taking medication for a mental illness or emotional problem who would like more information about medication, side effects, and staying on a regimen. Referrals from mental health providers are encouraged. Each person will meet with the group leader before attending the group to determine if the group will meet the individual's learning needs.

STRUCTURE: The format is a small group, with no more than eight members and one psychiatric nurse group leader facilitating a discussion about the issues. Topics are rotated.

TIME AND LOCATION: 2:00 to 3:00 PM, every Wednesday at the Mental Health Center

COST: No charge for attending

TOPICS
- How Do I Know If My Medications Are Working?
- Side Effect Management: Is It Worth It?
- Hints for Taking Medications Without Missing Doses!
- Health Problems That Medications Affect.
- (Other topics will be developed to meet the needs of group members.)

EVALUATION: Short pretest and posttest for instructor's use only

---

but to avoid violating patient confidentiality, the nurse needs to be careful not to divulge that information to other patients. If group members choose, they can share the names of their medications with one another. A small group format works best, and the more interaction, the better. Using a lecture method of teaching is less effective than involving the members in the learning process. The nurse should expose the members to various audio and visual educational materials, including workbooks, videotapes, and handouts. The nurse should ask members to write down information to help them remember and learn through various modes. Evaluation of the learning outcomes begins with the first class. Nurses can develop and give pretests and posttests, which in combination can measure learning outcomes.

Symptom Management Groups

Nurses often lead recovery-oriented groups that focus on helping patients deal with a severe and persistent mental illness. Handling hallucinations, being socially appropriate, and staying motivated to complete activities of daily living are a few common topics. In symptom management groups, members also learn when a symptom indicates that relapse is imminent and what to do about it. Within the context of a symptom management group, patients can learn how to avoid relapse.

Anger Management Groups

Anger management is another common topic for a nurse-led group, often in the inpatient setting. The purposes of an anger management group are to discuss the concept of anger, identify antecedents to aggressive behavior, and develop new strategies to deal with anger other than verbal and physical aggression (see Chapter 20). The treatment team refers individuals with histories of being verbally and physically abusive, usually to family members, to these groups to help them better understand their emotions and behavioral responses. Impulsiveness and emotional lability are problems for many of the group members. Anger management usually includes a discussion of associated stressful situations, events that trigger anger, feelings about the situation, and unmet personal needs.

Self-Care Groups

Another common nurse-led recovery-oriented psychiatric group is a self-care group. People with psychiatric illnesses often have self-care deficits and benefit from the structure that a group provides. These groups are challenging because members usually know how to perform these daily tasks (e.g., bathing, grooming, performing personal hygiene), but their illnesses cause them to lose the motivation to complete them. The leader not only reinforces the basic self-care skills but also, more importantly, helps identify strategies that can motivate the patients and provide structure to their daily lives.

Reminiscence Groups

Reminiscence therapy has been shown to be a valuable intervention for older clients. In this type of group, members are encouraged to remember events from past years. Such a group is easily implemented. Usually, a simple question about an important family event will spark memories. Reminiscence groups are usually associated with patients who have dementia who are having difficulty with recent memory. Reminiscence groups can also be used as an intergenerational intervention with healthy older adults and children. These groups can also reduce symptoms of depression, improve aspects of quality of life, and improve negative attitudes toward old age (Siverová & Bužgová, 2018).

SUMMARY OF KEY POINTS

- The definition of group can vary according to theoretic orientation. A general definition is that a group is two or more people who have at least one common goal or issue. Group dynamics are the interactions within a group that influence the group's development and process.

- Groups can be open, with new members joining at any time, or closed, with members admitted only once. Either small or large groups can be effective, but dynamics change in different size groups.

- Virtual applications are emerging as an important tool in leading groups. The group leader must adapt the technology to the purpose of the group and address issues of confidentiality and privacy when using the internet.

- The process of group development occurs in phases: beginning, middle, and termination. These stages are not fixed but dynamic. The process challenges the leader to guide the group. During the working stage, the group addresses its purpose.

- Leading a group involves many different functions, from obtaining and receiving information to testing and evaluating decisions. The leader should explain the rules of the group at the beginning of the group.

- Verbal communication includes the communication network and group themes. Nonverbal communication is more complex and involves eye contact, body posture, and the mood of the group. Decision-making groups can be victims of groupthink, which can have positive or negative outcomes. Groupthink research is ongoing.

- Seating arrangements can affect group interaction. The fewer physical barriers there are, such as tables, the better the communication. Everyone should be a part of the group, and no one should sit outside of it. In the most interactive groups, members face one another in a circle.

- Leadership skills involve listening; tracking verbal and nonverbal behaviors; and maintaining a neutral, nonjudgmental style.

- Although there are only two formal group roles, leader and member, there are many informal group roles. These roles are usually categorized according to purpose—task functions, maintenance functions, and individual roles. Members who assume task functions encourage the group members to stay focused on the group's task. Those who assume maintenance functions worry more about the group working together than the actual task itself. Individual roles can either enhance or detract from the work of the group.

- The leader should address behaviors that challenge the leadership, group process, or other members to determine whether to intervene. In some instances, the leader redirects a monopolizing member; at other times, the leader lets the group deal with the behavior. Group conflict occurs in most groups.

- There are many different types of groups. Most groups can be adapted to a virtual platform. Psychiatric nurses lead psychoeducation and support groups. Mental health specialists who are trained to provide intensive therapy lead psychotherapy groups. Consumers lead self-help groups, and professionals assist only as requested. Leading age-related groups requires attention to the developmental, physical, social, and intellectual abilities of the participants. Themes of older adult groups include continuity with the past, understanding the modern world, independence, and changes in family and resources. Group leadership for older adult groups builds on participants' previous experiences and coping abilities in developing new coping skills.

- Medication, symptom management, anger management, and self-care groups are common nurse-led groups focused on specific interventions.

Unfolding Patient Stories: Randy Adams

Part 2

Recall from Chapter 7 Randy Adams, a veteran with symptoms of posttraumatic stress disorder (PTSD) and neurocognitive problems, which manifested after a recent car accident. He has resisted getting care from the Veterans Affairs hospital. How can he benefit from group therapy and be encouraged to attend? What group interventions would the nurse consider for a client with PTSD, who is reexperiencing war events? How can the nurse foster communication and group interactions when he has difficulty expressing his feelings and decreased concentration?

CRITICAL THINKING CHALLENGES

1. Group members are very polite to one another and are superficially discussing topics. You would assess the group as being in which phase? Explain your answer.

2. After three sessions of a support group, two members begin to share their frustration with having a mental illness. The group is moving into which phase of group development? Explain your answer.

3. Define the roles of the task and maintenance functions in groups. Observe your clinical group and identify classmates who are assuming task functions and maintenance functions.

4. Observe a patient group for at least five sessions. Discuss the seating pattern that emerges. Identify the communication network and the group themes. Then identify the group's norms and standards.

5. Participate in a virtual support or self-help group. Identify the strengths and limitations of using the virtual technology.

6. Discuss the conditions that lead to groupthink. When is groupthink positive? When is groupthink negative? Explain.

7. List at least six behaviors that are important for a group leader, including one for age-related groups. Justify your answers.

8. During the first meeting, one member seems very anxious and tends to monopolize the conversation. Discuss how you would assess the situation and whether you would intervene.

9. At the end of the fourth meeting, one group member angrily accuses another of asking too many questions. The other members look on quietly. How would you assess the situation? Would you intervene? Explain.

Movie Viewing Guides

12 Angry Men: 1998. In this excellent film, a young man stands accused of fatally stabbing his father. A jury of his "peers" is deciding his fate. This jury is portrayed by an excellent cast, including Jack Lemmon, George C. Scott, Tony Danza, and Ossie Davis. At first, the case appears to be "open and shut." This film depicts an intense struggle to reach a verdict and is an excellent study of group process and group dynamics.

VIEWING POINTS: Identify the leaders in the group. How does leadership change throughout the film? Do you find any evidence of groupthink? How does the group handle conflict?

REFERENCES

Brown, N. W. (2018). *Psychoeducational groups: Process and practice* (4th ed.). Taylor & Francis Group.

Chien, W., Bressington, D., Yip, A., & Karatzias, T. (2017). An international multi-site, randomized controlled trial of a mindfulness-based psychoeducation group programme for people with schizophrenia. *Psychological Medicine*, 47(12), 2018–2096.

Christensen, S. S. (2019). Escape from the diffusion of responsibility: A review and guide for nurses. *Journal of Nursing Management*, 27(2), 264–270. https://doi-org.libproxy.siue.edu/10.1111/jonm.12677

Cleary, M., Lees, D., & Sayers, J. (2019). Leadership, thought diversity, and the influence of groupthink. *Issues in Mental Health Nursing*, 40(8), 731–733. https://doi.org/10.1080/01612840.2019.1604050

Colditz, J. B., Rothenberger, S. D., Liebschutz, J. M., Rollman, B. L., & Kraemer, K. L. (2020). COVID-19 social distancing and online mutual help engagement for alcohol use recovery. *Journal of Addiction Medicine*, 10.1097/ADM.0000000000000797. Advance online publication. https://doi.org/10.1097/ADM.0000000000000797

Corey, M. S., Corey, G., & Corey, C. (2018). *Group process and practice* (10th ed.). Cengage Learning.

Etain, B., Scott, J., Cochet, B., Bellivier, F., Boudebesse, C., Drancourt, N., Lauer, S., Dusser, I., Yon, L., Fouques, D., Richard, J. R., Lajnef, M., Leboyer, M., & Henry, C. (2018). A study of the real-world effectiveness of group psychoeducation for bipolar disorders: Is change in illness perception a key mediator of benefit. *Journal of Affective Disorders*, 227, 714–720. https://doi.org/10.1016/j.jad.2017.11.072

Firth, N., Delgadillo, J., Kellett, S., & Lucock, M. (2020). The influence of socio-demographic similarity and difference on adequate attendance of group psychoeducational cognitive behavioural therapy. *Psychotherapy Research: Journal of the Society for Psychotherapy Research*, 30(3), 362–374. https://doi.org/10.1080/10503307.2019.1589652

Frias, C. E., Garcia-Pascual, M., Montoro, M., Ribas, N., Risco, E., & Zabalegui, A. (2020). Effectiveness of a psychoeducational intervention for caregivers of people with dementia with regard to burden, anxiety and depression: A systematic review. *Journal of Advanced Nursing*, 76(3), 787–802. https://doi.org/10.1111/jan.14286

Janis, I. (1972). *Victims of groupthink*. Houghton Mifflin.

Janis, I. (1982). *Groupthink* (2nd ed.). Houghton Mifflin.

Jansen, W. S., Meeussen, L., Jetten, J., & Ellemers, N. (2020). Negotiating inclusion: Revealing the dynamic interplay between individual and group inclusion goals. *European Journal of Social Psychology*, 50, 520–533. https://doi.org/10.1002/ejsp.2633

Jiao, N., Zhu, L., Chong, Y. S., Chan, W. S., Luo, N., Wang, W., Hu, R., Chan, Y. H., & He, H. G. (2019). Web-based versus home-based postnatal psychoeducational interventions for first-time mothers: A randomised controlled trial. *International Journal of Nursing Studies*, 99, 103385. https://doi.org/10.1016/j.ijnurstu.2019.07.002

Leach, H. J., Potter, K. B., & Hidde, M. C. (2019). A group dynamics-based exercise intervention to improve physical activity maintenance in breast cancer survivors. *Journal of Physical Activity & Health*, 16(9), 785–791. https://doi.org/10.1123/jpah.2018-0667

Lewin, K. (1939). Experiments in social space. *Harvard Educational Review*, 9, 21–32.

Lockhart, N. C. (2017). Social network analysis as an analytic tool for task group research: A case study of an interdisciplinary community of practice. *The Journal for Specialists in Group Work*, 62(3), 152–175.

Moon, S., & Park, K. (2020). The effect of digital reminiscence therapy on people with dementia: A pilot randomized controlled trial. *BMC Geriatrics*, 20(1), 166. https://doi.org/10.1186/s12877-020-01563-2

Pomeroy, A., Rowe, P., Clark, A., Walker, A., Kerr, A., Chandler, E., Barber, M., Baron, J. C., & SWIFT Cast Investigators (2016). Skills, knowledge and attributes of support group leaders: A systematic review. *Patient Education and Counseling*, 96, 672–688.

Richardson, A. E., Broadbent, E., & Morton, R. P. (2019). A systematic review of psychological interventions for patients with head and neck cancer. *Supportive Care in Cancer*, 27(6), 2007–2021. https://doi.org/10.1007/s00520-019-04768-3

Siverová, J., & Bužgová, B. (2018). The effect of reminiscence therapy of quality of life, attitudes to ageing, and depressive symptoms on institutionalized elder adults with cognitive impairment: A quasi-experimental study. *International Journal of Mental health Nursing*, 27(5), 1430–1439.

Toseland, R. W., & Rizzo, V. M. (2004). What's different about working with older people in groups? *Journal of Gerontological Social Work*, 44(1/2), 5–23.

Wu, J., Balliet, D. Peperkoorn, L. S., Romano, A., & Van Lange, P. A. M. (2020). Cooperation in groups of different sizes: The effects of punishment and reputation-based partner choice. *Frontiers in Psychology*, 10, 2956. https://doi.org/10.3389/fpsyg.2019.02956

Yalom, I., & Leszcz, M. (2005). *The theory and practice of group psychotherapy*. Basic Books.

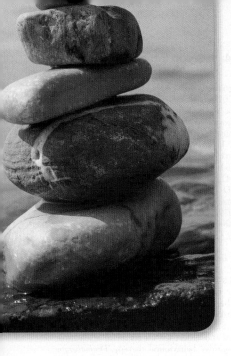

15
Family Assessment and Interventions

Mary Ann Boyd

KEYCONCEPTS

- comprehensive family assessment
- family

LEARNING OBJECTIVES

After studying this chapter, you will be able to:

1. Examine the changing family structure and mental health implications.

2. Discuss the impact of mental disorders on a family system.

3. Complete a genogram that depicts the family history, relationships, and mental disorders across at least three generations.

4. Develop a plan for a comprehensive family assessment.

5. Discuss nursing interventions that are useful in caring for families.

KEY TERMS

- Boundaries • Differentiation of self • Dysfunctional • Emotional cutoff • Extended family • Family development
- Family life cycle • Family projection process • Family structure • Genogram • Multigenerational transmission process • Nuclear family emotional process • Resilience • Sibling position • Subsystems • Transition times • Triangles

INTRODUCTION

A family is a group of people, connected emotionally, or by blood, or in both ways, that has developed patterns of interaction and relationships. Family members have a shared history and a shared future. Family includes the entire emotional system of three, four, or even five generations held by blood, and legal, emotional, and/or historical ties. Relationships with parents, siblings, and other family members go through transitions as they move through life. Families are unique in that, unlike all other groups, they incorporate new members only by birth, adoption, or marriage, and members can leave only by divorce or death (McGoldrick et al., 2016).

> **KEYCONCEPT Family** is a group of people, connected by emotions, blood, or both, that has developed patterns of interaction and relationships. Family members have a shared history and a shared future (McGoldrick et al., 2016).

The psychiatric nurse interacts with families in various ways. Because of the interpersonal and chronic nature of many mental disorders, psychiatric nurses often have frequent and long-term contact with families. Involvement may range from meeting family members only once or twice to treating the whole family as a patient. Unlike a therapeutic group (see Chapter 14), the family system has a history and continues to function when the nurse is not there. The family reacts to past, present, and anticipated future relationships within at least a three-generation family system. This chapter explains how to integrate important family concepts into the nursing process when providing nursing care to families experiencing mental health problems.

CHANGING FAMILY STRUCTURE

Although families may be defined differently within various cultures, they all play an important role in our lives and influence who and what we are. Traditionally, families are considered a source of guidance, security, love, and understanding. This is also true for people experiencing mental illnesses and emotional problems. Often the family assumes primary care for the person with mental illness and supports that individual through recovery. For patients, the family unit may provide their only constant support throughout their lives.

Family structure and size influence the strength of a family system. Family structure and size have changed drastically in recent times and so have the functions and roles of family members.

Family Size

Family size in the United States has decreased. In 1790, about one third of all households, including servants, those individuals enslaved, and other people not related to the head, consisted of seven people or more. By 1960, only 1 household in 20 consisted of 7 people or more. The average family household in 2018 was 2.6 people. Married couples make up 47.8% of the households in the United States; almost half of adults today do not live with a spouse (U.S. Census Bureau, 2018).

Contemporary Roles

Men and women's family roles have changed drastically in the past years. Many women work outside the home and many men are involved in parenting. Today, most women, including those who are mothers, work—both in dual-income families and in single-parent families. Women make up 46.9% of the American civilian work force. More than half of the female work force is married, and only 27% of married mothers and 7% of married fathers with children are stay-at-home parents (Livingston, 2018b).

Mobility and Relocation

Families are more mobile and may change residences frequently. Leaving familiar environments and readjusting to new surroundings and lifestyles stress the family system. These moves impose separation from the **extended family**, which traditionally has been a stabilizing force and a much needed support system.

Family Composition

Unmarried Couples

More unmarried couples are cohabitating before or instead of marrying. In the United States, 53% of adults age 18 and older are married, down from 58% in 1995. During that time, the cohabitation rate increased from 3% to 7%. More than half of cohabiters are raising children, including about a third who are living with a child they share with their partner. There is variation in marriage rates by race and ethnicity. Fifty-seven percent White adults and 63% of Asian adults are married; fewer than half of the Hispanic (48%) and Black adults (33%) are married. The majority of cohabiters have only lived with one partner. Most Americans view cohabitation as acceptable even without marriage plans (Horowitz et al., 2019). (Stepler, 2017)

Single-Parent Families

It is estimated that 50% to 60% of American children will reside at some point in a single-parent home. Almost a quarter of U.S. children live with a singlesolo parent, more than any other nation (Kramer, 2019). Singlesolo parents are overwhelmingly female. Among singlesolo parents, 42% are White and 28% are Black. Single mothers are more than twice as likely to be Black as cohabiting mothers (30% vs. 12%) and approximately four times as likely as married mothers (7% are Black) (Livingston, 2018a).

Stepfamilies

Remarried families or stepfamilies have a unique set of challenges that are not completely understood. More than 50% of U.S. families are remarried or recoupled (U.S. Census Bureau, 2018). Many parents find that step-parenting is much more difficult than parenting a biologic child. The bonding that occurs with biologic children rarely occurs with the stepchildren, whose natural bond is with a parent not living with them. However, the step-parent often assumes a measure of financial and parental responsibility. The care and management of children often become the primary stressor to the marital partners. In addition, the children are faced with multiple sets of parents whose expectations may differ. They may also compete for the children's attention. It is not unusual for second marriages to fail because of the stressors inherent in a remarried family.

Childless Families

Couples can be involuntarily childless because of infertility or voluntarily childless by choice. Approximately 10% to 15% of all couples in the reproductive age are involuntarily childless. As the opportunities for women have increased, many people have chosen not to have children. Research on childlessness is sparse, but it appears lifetime childlessness is associated with long-term illness, poorer midlife physical function for men, and poorer cognition. The studies on depression are mixes in later life (Keenan & Grundy, 2018).

Lesbian, Gay, Bisexual, Transsexual, and Queer or Questioning Families

Among the most stigmatized people are those who are lesbian, gay, bisexual, transsexual, and queer or questioning (LGBTQ). It is estimated that most LGBTQ populations have encountered some form of verbal harassment or violence in their lives. Higher rates of depression, stress, and low self-esteem have been seen in this population than in similar heterosexual groups (Wang et al., 2020). However, these mental health problems may improve as public acceptance increases.

Although, historically, some believed that being LGBTQ was a result of faulty parenting or personal choice, evidence shows that sexual orientation and identity are determined early in life by a combination of factors, including genetic predisposition, biologic development, and environmental events (see Chapter 35). In the past, it was also believed that sexual orientation could be changed through counseling by making a concerted effort to establish new relationships. However, no evidence supports the hypothesis that changes in sexual orientation are possible.

FAMILY MENTAL HEALTH

Families can be viewed as a system often consisting of several generations with multiple health care needs. In a mentally healthy family, members live in harmony among themselves and within society. These families support and nurture their members throughout their lives. However, stress and illnesses can negatively affect a family's overall mental health. Ideally, families can access health care services in an integrated system where primary health services and mental health care are linked.

Family Dysfunction

A family becomes **dysfunctional** when interactions, decisions, or behaviors interfere with the positive development of the family and its individual members. Most families have periods of dysfunction such as during a crisis or stressful situation when the coping skills are not available. Families usually adapt and regain their mentally healthy balance. A family can be mentally healthy and at the same time have a member who has a mental illness. Conversely, a family can be dysfunctional and have no member with a diagnosable mental illness.

Effects of Mental Illness on Family Functioning

Family members with mental disorders have special needs. Many adults with mental disorders live with their parents well into their 30s and beyond. For these adults with persistent mental illness, the family serves several functions that those without mental illness do not need. Such functions include the following:

- *Providing support.* People with mental illness have difficulty maintaining nonfamilial support networks and may rely exclusively on their families.
- *Providing information.* Families often have complete and continuous information about care and treatment over the years.
- *Monitoring services.* Families observe the progress of their relative and report concerns to those in charge of care.
- *Advocating for services.* Family groups advocate for money for residential care services.

The stigma associated with having a family member with a psychiatric disorder underlies much of the burden and stress the caregivers experience. Families can become socially isolated and financially stressed and lose employment opportunities as they struggle to care for their loved one. Frustration, anxiety, and low self-esteem may result (Yin et al., 2020).

Conflicts can occur between parents and mental health workers who place a high value on independence. Members of the mental health care system may criticize families for being overly protective when, in reality, the patient with mental illness may face real barriers to independent living. Housing may be unavailable; when available, quality and conditions may be inadequate. The patient may fear leaving home, may be at risk for relapse if they do leave, or may be too comfortable at home to want to leave. When long-term caregivers, usually the parents, die, their adult children with mental illness experience housing disruptions and potentially traumatic transitions. Siblings who have other responsibilities expect to be less involved than their parents in the care and oversight of the mentally ill brother or sister. Few families actually plan for this difficult eventuality (Fekadu et al., 2019).

Nurses must use an objective and rational approach when discussing independence and dependence of those with mental illness who live with aging parents. Family emotions often obscure the underlying issues, but nurses can diffuse such emotions, so that everyone can explore the alternatives comfortably. Although separation must eventually occur, the timing and process vary according to each family's particular situation. Parents may be highly anxious when their adult children first leave home and need reassurance and support.

COMPREHENSIVE FAMILY ASSESSMENT

A comprehensive family assessment is the collection of all relevant data related to family health, psychological well-being, and social functioning to identify problems for which the nurse can generate nursing diagnoses. The assessment consists of a face-to-face interview with family members and can be conducted during several sessions. Nurses conduct a comprehensive family assessment when they care for patients and their families for an extended period. They also use them when a patient's mental health problems are so complex that family support is important for optimal care (Box 15.1).

> **KEYCONCEPT A comprehensive family assessment** is the collection of all relevant data related to family health, psychological well-being, and social functioning to identify problems for which the nurse can generate nursing diagnoses.

Relationship Building

In preparing for a family assessment, nurses must concentrate on developing a relationship with the family. Although necessary when working with any family, relationship development is particularly important for families from ethnic minority cultures; because of the discrimination that they have experienced, they may be less likely to trust those from outside their family or community. Developing a relationship takes time, so the nurse may need to complete the assessment during several meetings rather than just one.

To develop a positive relationship with a family, nurses must establish credibility with the family and address its immediate intervention needs. To establish credibility, the family must see the nurse as knowledgeable and skillful. Possessing culturally competent nursing skills and projecting a professional image are crucial to establishing credibility. With regard to immediate intervention needs, a family that needs shelter or food is not ready to discuss a member's medication regimen until the first needs are met. The nurse will make considerable progress in establishing a relationship with a family when they help members meet their immediate needs.

Genograms

Families possess various structural configurations (e.g., single-parent, multigenerational, same-gender relationships). The nurse can facilitate taking the family history by completing a **genogram**, which is a multigenerational schematic depiction of biologic, legal, and emotional relationships from generation to generation. The nurse can use a genogram as a framework for exploring relationships and patterns of health and illness.

Creating Genograms

A genogram includes the age, dates of marriage and death, and geographic location of each member. Symbols are used in the genogram and are defined in a legend. Squares represent men, and circles represent women; ages are listed inside the squares and circles. Horizontal lines represent marriages with dates; vertical lines connect parents and children. Genograms can be particularly useful in understanding family history, composition, relationships, and illnesses (Fig. 15.1).

Genograms vary from simple to elaborate. The patient's and family's assessment needs guide the level of detail. In a small family with limited problems, the genogram can be rather general. In a large family with multiple problems, the genogram should reflect these complexities. Thus, depending on the level of detail, nurses collect various data. They can study important events such as marriages, divorces, deaths, and geographic movements. They can include cultural or religious affiliations, education and economic levels, and the nature of the work of each family member. Psychiatric nurses should always include mental disorders and other significant health problems in the genogram.

Analyzing and Using Genograms

For a genogram to be useful in assessment, the nurse needs to analyze the data for family composition, relationship problems, and mental health patterns. Nurses can begin with composition. How large is the family? Where do family members live? A large family whose members live in the same city is more likely to have support than a family in which distance separates members. Of course, this is not always the case. Sometimes even when family members live geographically close, they are emotionally distant from one another.

The nurse should also study the genogram for relationship and illness patterns. For relationship patterns, the nurse may find a history of divorces or family members who do not keep in touch with the rest of the family. The nurse can then explore the significance of these and other relationships. For illness patterns, alcoholism, often seen across several generations, may be prevalent in men on one side of a family. The nurse can then hypothesize that alcoholism is one of the mental health risks for the family and design interventions to reduce the risk. Or the nurse may find via a genogram that members of a family's previous generation were in "state hospitals" or had "nerve problems."

Family Physical and Mental Health

The family assessment includes a thorough picture of physical and mental health status and how the status affects family functioning. The family with multiple

BOX 15.1

Family Mental Health Assessment

I. Family members present

Name	Age	Relationship
_____	_____	_____
_____	_____	_____
_____	_____	_____

II. Health status

Member	Disorder and current treatment
_____	_____
_____	_____

III. Mental health status

Member	Disorder and current treatment
_____	_____
_____	_____

IV. Impact of mental illness on family function
Describe the changes that occur in the family as a result of the family member's disorder. _____
_____
_____

V. Family life cycle
Describe the family life cycle phase and any transitions that are occurring._____
_____

VI. Communication patterns
Describe the family communication patterns in terms of usual times of communication (morning, dinner, etc.), which family members talk to each other, who communicates the family rules, who carries out discipline. Identify triangulated messages. _____
_____
_____

VII. Stress and coping
Identify current family stressful events and family coping mechanisms. _____
_____

VIII. Problem-solving skills
Determine who solves problems in the family. Are the problem-solving skills of the family able to manage most family problems? _____
_____
_____

IX. Family system (from the genogram)
Family composition _____

Health and illness patterns _____

Relationship patterns _____

Social functioning patterns _____

Financial and legal status _____

Formal and informal network _____

X. Nursing diagnoses _____
_____
_____

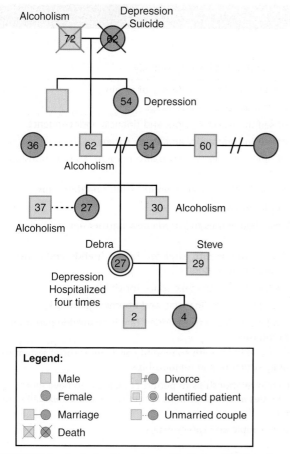

FIGURE 15.1 Analysis of genogram for Debra. Illness patterns are depression (paternal aunt, grandmother [suicide]) and alcoholism (brother, father, grandfather). Relationship patterns show that the parents are divorced and neither sibling is married.

health problems, both physical and mental, must try to manage these problems as well as obtain the many financial and health care resources the family members need.

Physical Health Status

The family health status includes the physical illnesses and disabilities of all members; the nurse can record such information on the genogram and also include the physical illnesses and disabilities of other generations. Illnesses of family members are an indication not only of their physical status but also of the stress currently being placed on the family and its resources. The nurse should pay particular attention to any physical problems that affect family functioning. For example, if a member requires frequent visits to a provider or hospitalizations, the whole family will feel the effects of focusing excessive time and financial resources on that member. The nurse should explore how such situations specifically affect other members.

Mental Health Status

Detecting mental disorders in families may be difficult because these disorders often are hidden or the "family secret." Very calmly, the nurse should ask family members to identify anyone who has experienced mental illness. The nurse should record the information on the genogram as well as in the narrative. If family members do not know if anyone in the family had or has a mental illness, the nurse should ask if anyone was treated for "nerves" or had a "nervous breakdown." A good family history of mental illness across multiple generations helps the nurse understand the significance of mental illness in the current generation. If one family member has a serious mental illness, the whole family will be affected. Usually, siblings of the mentally ill member receive less parental attention than the affected member.

Family's Psychological Domain

Assessment of the family's psychological domain focuses on the family's development and life cycle, communication patterns, stress and coping abilities, and problem-solving skills. One aim of the assessment is to understand the relationships within the family. Although family roles and structures are important, the true value of the family is in its relationships, which are irreplaceable. For example, if a parent leaves or dies, another person (e.g., stepparent, grandparent) can assume some parental functions but can never really replace the emotional relationship with the missing parent.

Family Development

Family development is a broad term that refers to all the processes connected with the growth of a family, including changes associated with work, geographic location, migration, acculturation, and serious illness. In optimal family development, family members are relatively differentiated (capable of autonomous functioning) from one another, anxiety is low, and the parents have good emotional relationships with their own families of origin.

Family Life Cycles

The concept of **family life cycle** refers to a system evolving through phases based on significant events related to the arrival and departure of members, such as birth or adoption, child-rearing, departure of children from home, occupational retirement, and death. Identifying the family life cycle is helpful in assessing family relationships, roles, and stresses. The family life cycle is a process of expansion, contraction, and realignment of relationship systems to support the entry, exit, and development of family members (Table 15.1)

TABLE 15.1   PHASES OF THE FAMILY LIFE CYCLE

Family Life Cycle Phase	Emotional Process of Transition: Key Prerequisite Attitudes	Changes in the System to Proceed Developmentally
Emerging young adults	Accepting emotional and financial responsibility for self	a. Differentiation of self in relation to family of origin b. Development of intimate peer relationships c. Establishment of self in respect to work and financial independence d. Establishment of self in community and larger society e. Establishment of one's worldview, spirituality, religion, and relationship to nature f. Parents shifting to consultative role in young adult's relationships
Couple formation: The joining of families	Commitment to new system	a. Formation of couple systems b. Expansion of family boundaries to include new partner and extended family c. Realignment of relationships with extended family, friends, and larger community to include new partners
Families with young children	Accepting new members into the system	a. Adjustment of couple system to make space for children b. Collaboration in child-rearing, financial, and housekeeping tasks c. Realignment of relationships with extended family to include parenting and grandparenting roles d. Realignment of relationships with community and larger social system to include new family structure and relationships
Families with adolescents	Increasing flexibility of family boundaries to permit children's independence and grandparents' frailties	a. Shift of parent–child relationships to permit adolescent to have more independent activities and relationships and to move more flexibility into and out of system b. Refocus on midlife couple and career issues c. Begin shift toward caring for older generation
Launching children and moving on at midlife	Accepting a multitude of exits from and entries into the system	a. Renegotiation of couple system as a dyad b. Development of adult-to-adult relationships between parents and grown children c. Realignment of relationships to include in-laws and grandchildren d. Realignment of relationships with community and larger social system to include new structure and constellation of family relationships e. Exploration of new interests or career given the freedom from child care responsibilities f. Dealing with care needs, disabilities, and death of parents (grandparents)
Families in late middle age	Accepting the shifting generational roles	a. Maintaining or modifying own and/or couple and social functioning and interests in face of physiologic decline: exploration of new familial and social role options b. Supporting more central role of middle generations c. Making room in the system for the wisdom and experience of elders d. Supporting the older generation without overfunctioning for them
Families nearing the end of life	Accepting the realities of limitations and death and the completion of one cycle of life	a. Dealing with loss of spouse, siblings, and other peer b. Making preparations for death and legacy c. Managing reversed roles in caretaking between middle and older generations d. Realignment of relationships with larger community and social system to acknowledge changing life cycle relationships

McGoldrick, M., Garcia Preto, N., & Carter, B. (2016). Overview: The life cycle in its changing context: Individual, family and social perspectives. In M. McGoldrick, N. Garcia Preto, & B. Carter (Eds.). *The expanding family life cycle: Individual, family, and social perspectives* (5th ed., pp. 24–25). © 2016. Reprinted by permission of Pearson Education, Inc.

(McGoldrick et al., 2016). A family's life cycle is conceptualized in terms of phases throughout the years. To move from one phase to the next, the family system undergoes changes. Structural and potential structural changes within phases can usually be handled by rearranging the family system (first-order changes), but transition from one phase to the next requires changes in the system itself (second-order changes). An example of a first-order change is when all the children are finally in school and the stay-at-home parent returns to work. The system is rearranged, but the structure remains the same. In second-order changes, the family structure does change, such as when a member moves away from the family home to live independently.

> **NCLEXNOTE** Apply family life cycle phases to a specific family with a member who has a psychiatric disorder. Identify the emotional transitions and the required family changes.

The nurse should not view a family model as "the normal" life cycle because a family's system is always evolving. As second marriages, career changes in midlife, and other life events occur with increasing frequency, this traditional model is being modified and redesigned to address contemporary structural and role changes. This model also may not fit many cultural groups. Variations of the family life cycle are presented for the divorced and remarried family (Table 15.2).

Transition times are the addition, subtraction, or change in status of family members. During transitions, family stresses are more likely to cause symptoms or dysfunction. Significant family events, such as the death of a member or the introduction of a new member, also affect the family's ability to function. During transitions, families may seek help from the mental health system.

Cultural Variations

In caring for families from diverse cultures, the nurse should examine whether the underlying assumptions and frameworks of the dominant life cycle models apply. Even the concept of "family" varies among cultures. For example, the dominant White middle-class culture's definition of family refers to the intact nuclear family. Many children grow up with parents from separate cultures where they experience differences in daily living. For Italian Americans, the entire extended network of aunts, uncles, cousins, and grandparents may be involved in family decision-making and share holidays and life cycle transitions. For African Americans, the family may include a broad network of kin and community that includes long-time friends who are considered family members (McGoldrick et al., 2016).

Cultural groups also differ in the importance they give to certain life cycle transitions. For example, Irish

American families may emphasize the wake, viewing death as an important life cycle transition. African American families may emphasize funerals, going to considerable expense and delaying services until all family members arrive. Italian American and Polish American families may place great emphasis on weddings (McGoldrick et al., 2016).

The life cycle of Mexican immigrant families can be examined in the context of *familismo* (a value of close connection between immediate and extended family members), parental authority, and extended family. The impact of living in a different country, learning a different language, and lack of extended family may create family conflict as they adjust to a different cultural environment. Their children are faced with academic expectations that need parental involvement and support. Family emotional climate increases as both parents share parenting responsibilities (Valdez & Martinez, 2019).

Work and Family Conflict

While work can provide the economic security of a family, it can also cause stress. Parents are often torn between responsibilities of work and home. Conflict between two expectations can lead to additional family stress and poorer mental health (see Box 15.2).

Families in Poverty

Prior to the coronavirus disease 2019 pandemic, 10.5% of the U.S. population lived below the poverty rate. During the pandemic, the poverty rate in the United States reached 17.5% (Boghani, 2020). As the impact of the pandemic is beginning to subside, the poverty rate is expected to decrease. A disproportionate number of children from minority groups live in poverty. LGBTQ people have a poverty rate of 21.6%, much higher than others (Badgett et al., 2019).

The family life cycle of those living in poverty may vary from those with adequate financial means. People living in poverty struggle to make ends meet, and family members may face difficulties in meeting their own or other members' basic developmental needs. To experience poverty does not mean that a family is automatically dysfunctional. But poverty is an important factor that can force even the healthiest families to crumble.

Communication Patterns

Family communication patterns develop over a lifetime and are important information during an assessment. Some family members communicate more openly and honestly than others. In addition, family subgroups

TABLE 15.2   FAMILY LIFE CYCLE FOR THE DIVORCING AND REMARRYING FAMILIES

Phase and Task	Emotional Process	Developmental Issues
Divorce		
Decision to divorce	Acceptance of inability to resolve marital problems sufficiently to continue relationship	Acceptance of one's own part in the failure of the marriage
Planning the breakup of the system	Supporting viable arrangements for all parts of the system	a. Working cooperatively on problems of custody, visitation, and finances b. Dealing with extended family about the divorce
Separation	a. Willingness to continue cooperative coparental relationship and joint financial support of children b. Working on resolution of attachment to spouse	a. Mourning loss of intact family b. Restructuring marital and parent–child relationships and finances; adaptation to living apart c. Realignment of relationships with extended family; staying connected with spouse's extended family
Divorce	Working on emotional divorce: overcoming hurt, anger, guilt, and so on	a. Mourning loss of intact family; giving up fantasies of reunion b. Retrieving hopes, dreams, expectations from the marriage c. Staying connected with extended families
Postdivorce Family		
Single parent (custodial household or primary residence)	Willingness to maintain financial responsibilities, continue parental contact with ex-spouse, and support contact of children with ex-spouse and their family	a. Making flexible visitation arrangements with ex-spouse and family b. Rebuilding own financial resources c. Rebuilding own social network
Single parent (noncustodial)	Willingness to maintain financial responsibilities and parental contact with ex-spouse and to support custodial parent's relationship with children	a. Finding ways to continue effective parenting b. Maintaining financial responsibilities to ex-spouse and children c. Rebuilding own social network
Remarriage		
Entering new relationship	Recovery from loss of first marriage (adequate "emotional divorce")	Recommitment to marriage and to forming a family with readiness to deal with the complexity and ambiguity
Conceptualizing and planning new marriage and family	Accepting one's own fears and those of new spouse and children about forming a new family Accepting the need for time and patience for adjustment to complexity and ambiguity of the following: a. Multiple new roles b. Boundaries: space, time, membership, and authority c. Affective issues: guilt, loyalty conflicts, desire for mutuality, unresolvable past hurts	a. Working on openness in the new relationships to avoid pseudomutuality b. Planning for maintenance of cooperative financial and coparental relationships with ex-spouses c. Planning to help children deal with fears, loyalty conflicts, and membership in two systems d. Realignment of relationships with extended family to include new spouse and children e. Plan maintenance of connections for children with extended family of ex-spouses
Remarriage and reconstruction of family	a. Resolution of attachment to previous spouse and ideal of "intact" family b. Acceptance of different models of family with permeable boundaries	a. Restructuring family boundaries to allow for inclusion of new spouse—stepparent b. Realignment of relationships and financial arrangements to permit interweaving of several systems c. Making room for relationships of all children with all parents, grandparents, and other extended family d. Sharing memories and histories to enhance stepfamily integration
Renegotiation of remarried family at all future life cycle transitions	Accepting evolving relationships of transformed remarried family	a. Changes as each child graduates, marries, dies, or becomes ill b. Changes as each spouse forms new couple relationship, remarries, moves, becomes ill, or dies

McGoldrick, M., Garcia Preto, N., & Carter, B. (2016). The remarriage cycle: Divorced, multinuclear and recoupled families. In M. McGoldrick, N. Garcia Preto, & B. Carter (Eds.). *The expanding family life cycle: Individual, family, and social perspectives* (5th ed., pp. 413–414). © 2016. Reprinted by permission of Pearson Education, Inc.

BOX 15.2

Parenting Stress

Cherry, K. E., Gerstein, E. D., & Ciciolla, L. (2019). Parenting stress and children's behavior: Transactional models during Early Head Start. Journal of Family Psychology: JFP : Journal of the Division of Family Psychology of the American Psychological Association (Division 43), 33(8), 916–926. https://doi.org/10.1037/fam0000574

THE QUESTION: Is parental stress linked to childhood behavior?

METHODS: Data were taken from the Early Head Start Family and Child Experiences Study, where 835 parent–child dyads were assessed at 1, 2, and 3 years. Parenting stress and behavior problems were measured at all three time points, while family conflict and observed parental supportiveness were measured at ages 2 and 3.

FINDINGS: Results indicated that parenting stress and children's behavior problems were relatively stable over time and influenced each other. Family conflict escalated children's behavior problems at age 1 and parenting stress at age 3, while parental supportiveness served a protective role in parent–child relationship.

IMPLICATIONS FOR NURSING: Early prevention programs should focus on both children's behavior and parenting stress in the first year and work to reduce family conflict and increase parental supportiveness.

develop from communication patterns. Just as in any assessment interview, the nurse should observe the verbal and nonverbal communication of the family members. Who sits next to each other? Who talks to whom? Who answers most questions? Who volunteers information? Who changes the subject? Which subjects seem acceptable to discuss? Which topics are not discussed? Can spouses be intimate with each other? Are any family secrets revealed? Does the nonverbal communication match the verbal communication? Nurses can use all of this information to help identify family problems and communication issues.

Nurses should also assess the family for its daily communication patterns. Identifying which family members confide in one another is a place to start examining ongoing communication. Other areas include how often children talk with parents, which child talks to the parents most, and who is most likely to discipline the children. Another question considers whether family members can express positive and negative feelings. In determining how open or closed the family is, the nurse explores the type of information the family shares with nonfamily members. For example, whereas one family may tell others about a member's mental illness, another family may not discuss any illnesses with those outside the family.

Stress and Coping Abilities

One of the most important assessment tasks is to determine how family members deal with major and minor stressful events and their available coping skills. Some families seem able to cope with overwhelming stresses, such as the death of a member, major illness, or severe conflict, but other families seem to fall apart over relatively minor events. Some family caregivers of persons with mental illness have **resilience**, the ability to recover or adjust to challenges over time. For some families, they not only survive the day-to-day stresses of caring for a family member with a serious mental health problem but also seem to grow stronger and healthier. It is important for the nurse to listen to which situation a family appraises as stressful and help the family identify usual coping responses. The nurse can then evaluate these responses. On the other hand, if the family's responses are maladaptive (e.g., substance abuse, physical abuse), the nurse will discuss the need to develop coping skills that lead to family well-being (see Chapter 19).

NCLEXNOTE Identifying stressful events and coping mechanisms should be a priority in a family assessment.

Problem-Solving Skills

Nurses assess family's problem-solving skills by focusing on the more recent problems the family has experienced and determining the process that members used to solve them. For example, a child is sick at school and needs to go home. Does the mother, father, grandparent, or babysitter receive the call from the school? Who then cares for the child? Underlying the ability to solve problems is the decision-making process. Who makes and implements decisions? How does the family handle conflict? All of these data provide information regarding the family's problem-solving abilities. After these abilities are identified, the nurse can build on these strengths in helping families deal with additional problems.

Family Social Domain

An assessment of the family's social domain provides important data about the operation of the family as a system and its interaction within its environment. Areas of concern include the system itself, social and financial status, and formal and informal support networks.

Family Systems

Just as any group can be viewed as a system, a family can be understood as a system with interdependent members.

Family system theories view the family as an open system whose members interact with their environment as well as among themselves. One family member's change in thoughts or behavior can cause a ripple effect and change in everyone else's. For example, a mother who decides not to pick up her children's clothing from their bedroom floors anymore forces the children to deal with the cluttered rooms and dirty clothes in a different way than before.

One common scenario in the mental health field is the effect of a patient's improvement on the family. With new medications and treatment, patients are more likely to be able to live independently, and this subsequently changes the responsibilities and activities of family caregivers. Although on the surface members may seem relieved that their caregiving burden is lifted, in reality, they must adjust their time and energies to fill the remaining void. This transition may not be easy because it is often less stressful to maintain familiar activities than to venture into uncharted territory. Families may seem as though they want to keep an ill member dependent, but in reality, they are struggling with the change in their family system.

Several system models are used in caring for families: the Wright Leahey Calgary model (Shajani & Snell, 2019); Bowen family system (1975, 1976); and Minuchin, Lee, and Simon's (1996) structural family system.

Calgary Family Model

Lorraine M. Wright and Maureen Leahey developed the Calgary Family Assessment Model and the Calgary Family Intervention Model. These nursing models are based on systems, cybernetics, and communication and change theories (Shajani & Snell, 2019). Families seek help when they have family health and illness problems, difficulties, and suffering. These two models are multidimensional frameworks that conceptualize the family into structural, developmental, and functional categories. Each assessment category contains several subcategories. Structure is further categorized into internal (e.g., family, gender, sexual orientation), external (i.e., extended family and larger systems), and context (i.e., ethnicity, race, social class, religion, spirituality, environment). Family developmental assessment is organized according to stages, tasks, and attachments. Functional assessment areas include instrumental (e.g., activities of daily living) and expressive (i.e., communication, problem-solving roles, beliefs).

The Calgary Family Assessment Model and Calgary Family Intervention Model are built around four stages: engagement, assessment, intervention, and termination. The *engagement* stage is the initial stage in which the family is greeted and made comfortable. In the *assessment* stage, problems are identified and relationships among family members and health providers develop. During this stage, the nurse opens space for the family members to tell their story. The *intervention* stage is the core of the clinical work and involves providing a context in which the family can make changes (see Intervention section in this chapter). The *termination* phase refers to the process of ending the therapeutic relationship (Shajani & Snell, 2019).

Family Systems Therapy Model

Murray Bowen (1913–1990) recognized the power of a system and believed that there is a balance between the family system and the individual. Bowen developed several concepts that professionals often use today when working with families (Bowen, 1975, 1976; Kerr, 2019).

Differentiation of self involves two processes: intrapsychic and interpersonal. Intrapsychic differentiation means separating thinking from feeling: a differentiated individual can distinguish between thoughts and feelings and can consequently think through behavior. For example, a person who has experienced intrapsychic differentiation, even though angry, will think through the underlying issue before acting. However, the feeling of the moment will drive the behavior of an undifferentiated individual. Interpersonal differentiation is the process of freeing oneself from the family's emotional chaos. That is, the individual can recognize the family turmoil but avoid reentering arguments and issues. For Bowen, the individual must resolve attachment to this chaos before they can differentiate into a mature, healthy personality.

Triangles: According to Bowen, the triangle is a three-person system and the smallest stable unit in human relations. Cycles of closeness and distance characterize a two-person relationship. When anxiety is high during periods of distance, one party "triangulates" a third person or thing into the relationship. For example, two partners may have a stable relationship when anxiety is low. When anxiety and tension rise, one partner may be so uncomfortable they confide in a friend instead of the other partner. In these cases, triangulating reduces the tension but freezes the conflict in place. In families, triangulating occurs when a husband and wife diffuse tension by focusing on the children. To maintain the status quo and avoid the conflict, which tends to produce symptoms in the child (e.g., bed wetting, fear of school), one of the parents develops an overly intense relationship with one of the children.

Family projection process: Through this process, the triangulated member becomes the center of the family conflicts; that is, the family projects its conflicts onto the child or other triangulated person. Projection is an anxious, enmeshed concern. For example, a husband and wife are having difficulty deciding how to spend money. One of their children is having difficulty with interpersonal relationships in school. Instead of the parents resolving their differences over money, one parent focuses on the child's needs and becomes intensely involved in the child's issues. The other parent then relates coolly and distantly to the involved parent.

Nuclear family emotional process: This concept describes patterns of emotional functioning in a family in a single generation. This emotional distance is a patterned reaction in daily interactions with the spouse.

Multigenerational transmission process: Bowen believed that one generation transfers its emotional processes to the next generation. Certain basic patterns among parents and children are replicas of those of past generations, and generations to follow will repeat them. The child who is the most involved with the family is least able to differentiate from their family of origin and passes on conflicts from one generation to another. For example, a spouse may stay emotionally distant from his partner just as his father was with his mother.

Sibling position: Children develop fixed personality characteristics based on their sibling position in their families. For example, a first-born child may have more confidence and be more outgoing than the second-born child, who has grown up in the older child's shadow. Conversely, the second-born child may be more inclined to identify with the oppressed and be more open to other experiences than the first-born child. These attitudinal and behavioral patterns become fixed parts of both children's personalities. Knowledge of these general personality characteristics is helpful in predicting the family's emotional processes and patterns. These theoretical ideas of Bowen have not been supported by research, but the more general principle that a child's position in the family origin affects the child has significant empirical support (Bleske-Rechek & Kelley, 2014; Green & Griffiths, 2014).

Emotional cutoff: If a member cannot differentiate from their family, that member may just flee from the family, either by moving away or avoiding personal subjects of conversation. Yet a brief visit from parents can render these individuals helpless.

In using the family systems therapy model, the nurse can observe family interactions to determine how differentiated family members are from one another. Are members autonomous in thinking and feeling? Do triangulated relationships develop during periods of stress and tension? Are family members interacting in the same manner as their parents or grandparents? How do the personalities of older siblings compare with those of younger siblings? Who lives close to one another? Does any family member live in another city? The Bowen model can provide a way of assessing the system of family relationships (Yektatalab et al., 2017).

Family Structure Model

Salvador Minuchin (1921–2017) emphasizes the importance of family structure. In their model, the family consists of three essential components: structure, subsystems, and boundaries.

Family structure is the organized pattern in which family members interact. As two adult partners come together to form a family, they develop the quantity of their interactions or how much time they spend interacting. For example, a newly married couple may establish their evening interaction pattern by talking to each other during dinner but not while watching television. The quality of the interactions also becomes patterned. Whereas some topics are appropriate for conversation during their evening walk (e.g., reciting daily events), controversial or emotionally provocative topics are relegated to other times and places (Minuchin et al., 1996).

Family rules are important influences on interaction patterns. For example, "family problems stay in the family" is a common rule. Both the number of people in the family and its development also influence the interaction pattern. For instance, the interaction between a single mother and her children changes when she remarries and introduces a stepfather. Over time, families repeat interactions, which develop into enduring patterns. For example, if a mother tells her son to straighten his room and the son refuses until his father yells at him, the family has initiated an interactional pattern. If this pattern continues, the child will come to see the father as the disciplinarian and the mother as incompetent. However, the mother will be more affectionate to her son, and the father will remain the disciplinarian on the "outside."

Subsystems develop when family members join together for various activities or functions. Minuchin et al. (1996) view each member, as well as dyads and other larger groups that form, as a subsystem. Obvious groups are parents and children. Sometimes, there are "boy" and "girl" systems. Such systems become obvious in an assessment when family members talk about "the boys going fishing with dad" and "the girls going shopping with mother." Family members belong to several different subgroups. A mother may also be a wife, sister, and daughter. Sometimes, these roles can conflict. It may be acceptable for a woman to be very firm as a disciplinarian in her role as mother. However, in her sister, wife, or daughter role, similar behavior would provoke anger and resentment.

Boundaries are invisible barriers with varying permeabilities that surround each subsystem. They regulate the amount of contact a person has with others and protect the autonomy of the family and its subsystems. If family members do not take telephone calls at dinner, they are protecting themselves from outside intrusion. When parents do not allow children to interrupt them, they are establishing a boundary between themselves and their children. According to Minuchin et al. (1996), the spouse subsystem must have a boundary that separates it from parents, children, and the outside world. A clear boundary between parent and child enables children to interact with their parents but excludes them from the spouse subsystem.

Boundaries vary from rigid to diffuse. If boundaries are too rigid and permit little contact from outside subsystems, disengagement results, and disengaged individuals are relatively isolated. On the other hand, rigid boundaries permit independence, growth, and mastery within the subsystem, particularly if parents do not hover over their children, telling them what to do or fighting their battles for themselves. Enmeshed subsystems result when boundaries are diffuse. That is, when boundaries are too relaxed, parents may become too involved with their children, and the children learn to rely on the parents to make decisions, resulting in decreased independence. According to Minuchin et al. (1996), if children see their parents as friends and treat them as they would treat their peers, then enmeshment exists.

Autonomy and interdependence are key concepts, important both to individual growth and family system maintenance. Relationship patterns are maintained by universal rules governing family organization (especially power hierarchy) and mutual behavioral expectations. In the well-functioning family, boundaries are clear, and a hierarchy exists with a strong parental subsystem. Problems result when there is a malfunctioning of the hierarchical arrangement or boundaries or a maladaptive reaction to changing developmental or environmental requirements. Minuchin et al. (1996) believe in clear, flexible boundaries by which all family members can live comfortably.

In the family structural theory, what distinguishes normal families is not the absence of problems but a functional family structure to handle them. Husbands and wives must learn to adjust to each other, rear their children, deal with their own parents, cope with their jobs, and fit into their communities. The types of struggles change with developmental stages and situational crises. The psychiatric nurse assesses the family structure and the presence of subsystems or boundaries. The nurse uses these data to determine how the subsystems and boundaries affect the family's functioning. Helping family members change a subsystem, such as including younger and older children together in family activities, may improve family functioning.

Social and Financial Status

Social status is often linked directly to financial status. The nurse should assess the occupations of the family members. Who works? Who is primarily responsible for the family's financial support? Families of low social status are more likely to have limited financial resources, which can place additional stresses on the family. Cultural expectations and beliefs about acceptable behaviors may cause additional stress when in conflict with beliefs of caregivers. Nurses can use information regarding the family's financial status to determine whether to refer the family to social services.

Formal and Informal Support Networks

Both formal and informal networks are important in providing support to individuals and families and should be identified in the assessment. These networks are the link among the individual, families, and the community. Assessing the extent of formal support (e.g., hospitals, agencies) and informal support (e.g., extended family, friends, and neighbors) gives a clearer picture of the availability of support. In assessing formal support, the nurse should ask about the family's involvement with government institutions and self-help groups such as Alcoholics Anonymous. Assessing the informal network is particularly important in cultural groups with extended family networks or close friends because these individuals can be major sources of support to patients. If the nurse does not ask about the informal network, these important people may be missed. Nurses can inquire whether family members volunteer at schools, local hospitals, or nursing homes. They can also ask whether the family attends religious services or activities.

FAMILY INTERVENTIONS

Family interventions focus on supporting the integrity and functioning of the family as defined by its members. Although family therapy is reserved for mental health specialists, the generalist psychiatric mental health nurse can implement several interventions, such as counseling, promotion of self-care activities, supportive therapy, education and health teaching, and the use of genograms.

In implementing any family intervention, flexibility is essential, particularly when working with culturally diverse groups. The nurse creates the context for change by making sure the interventions are possible for the family (Shajani & Snell, 2019). For example, weekly appointments may be ideal but impossible for a busy family. To implement successful, culturally competent family interventions, nurses need to be open to modifying the structure and format of the sessions. Longer sessions are often useful, especially when a translator or interpreter is used. Nurses also need to respect and work with the changing family composition of family and nonfamily participants (e.g., extended family members, intimate partners, friends and neighbors, community helpers) in sessions. Because of the stigma that some cultural groups associate with seeking help, nurses may need to hold intervention sessions in community settings (e.g., churches and schools) or at the family's home. If adequate progress is made, it is time to decrease the frequency of sessions and move toward termination. Families may move toward termination if they recognize that improvement has been made (Shajani & Snell, 2019).

Counseling

Nurses often use counseling when working with families because it is a short-term problem-solving approach that addresses current issues. The nurse should avoid taking sides by forming an alliance with one family member or subgroup (Shajani & Snell, 2019). If the assessment reveals complex, long-standing relationship problems, the nurse needs to refer the family to a family therapist. If the family is struggling with psychiatric problems of one or more family members or the family system is in a life cycle transition, the nurse should use short-term counseling. Instead of giving advice, the counseling sessions should focus on specific issues or problems using sound group process theory. Usually, a problem-solving approach works well after an issue has been identified (see Chapter 19).

Promoting Self-Care Activities

Families often need support in changing behaviors that promote self-care activities. For example, families may inadvertently reinforce a family member's dependency out of fear of the patient being taken advantage of in work or social situations. A nurse can help the family explore how to meet the patient's need for work and social activity and at the same time help alleviate the family's fears.

Caregiver distress or role strain can occur in families that are responsible for the care of members with long-term illness. Family interventions can help families deal with the burden of caring for members with psychiatric disorders. Family intervention may decrease the frequency of relapse (in persons with schizophrenia) and encourage compliance with medication (Okpokoro et al., 2014).

Supporting Family Functioning and Resilience

Supporting family functioning involves various nursing approaches. In meeting with the family, the nurse should identify and acknowledge its values. In developing a trusting relationship with the family, the nurse should confirm that all members have a sense of self and self-worth. Encouraging positive thinking and participating in support groups will contribute to the family's well-being. Supporting family subsystems (e.g., encouraging the children to play while meeting with the spouses) reinforces family boundaries. Based on assessment of the family system's operation and communication patterns, the nurse can reinforce open, honest communication.

In communicating with the family, the nurse needs to observe boundaries constantly and avoid becoming triangulated into family issues. An objective, empathic leadership style can set the tone for the family sessions.

Providing Education and Health Teaching

One of the most important family interventions is education and health teaching, particularly in families with mental illness. Families have a central role in the treatment of mental illnesses. Members need to learn about mental disorders, medications, actions, side effects, and overall treatment approaches and outcomes. For example, families are often reluctant to have members take psychiatric medications because they believe the medications will "drug" the patient or become addictive. The family's beliefs about mental illnesses and treatment can affect whether patients will be able to manage their illness.

Using Genograms

Genograms not only are useful in assessment but also can be used as intervention strategies. Nurses can use genograms to help family members understand current feelings and emotions as well as the family's evolution over several generations. Genograms allow the family to examine relationships from a factual, objective perspective. Often, family members gain new insights and can begin to understand their problems within the context of their family system. For example, families may begin to view depression in an adolescent daughter with new seriousness when they see it as part of a pattern of several generations of women who have struggled with depression. A husband, raised as an only child in a small Midwestern town, may better understand his feelings of being overwhelmed after comparing his family structure with that of his wife, who comes from a large family of several generations living together in the urban Northeast (Box 15.3).

BOX 15.3

John and Judy Jones

John and Judy Jones were married 3 years ago after their graduation from a small liberal arts college in the Midwest. Judy's career choice required that she live on the East Coast where she should be near her large family. John willingly moved with her and quickly found a satisfying position. After about 6 months of marriage, John became extremely irritable and depressed. He kept saying that his life was not his own. Judy was very concerned but could not understand his feelings of being overwhelmed. His job was going well, and they had a very busy social life, mostly revolving around her family, whom John loved. They decided to seek counseling and completed the following genogram:

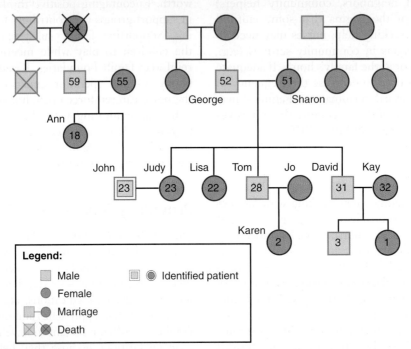

Legend:

⬜ Male   ⬜● Identified patient

🔴 Female

⬜● Marriage

⊠ ⊗ Death

After looking at the genogram, both John and Judy began to realize that part of John's discomfort had to do with the number of family members who were involved in their lives. Judy and John began to redefine their social life, allowing more time with friends and each other.

SUMMARY OF KEY POINTS

- The family is an important societal unit that often is responsible for the care and coordination of treatment of members with mental disorders. The family structure, size, and roles are rapidly changing. Traditional health care services will have to adapt to meet the mental health care needs of these families.

- A family is a group of people who are connected emotionally, by blood, or in both ways that has developed patterns of interactions and relationships. Families come in various compositions, including nuclear, extended, multigenerational, single-parent, and same-gender families. Cultural values and beliefs define family composition and roles.

- Nurses complete a comprehensive family assessment when they care for families for extended periods or if a patient has complex mental health problems.

- In building relationships with families, nurses must establish credibility and competence with the family. Unless the nurse addresses the family's immediate needs first, the family will have difficulty engaging in the challenges of caring for someone with a mental disorder.

- The genogram is an assessment and intervention tool that is useful in understanding health problems, relationship issues, and social functioning across several generations.

- In assessing the family, the nurse determines physical and mental health status and their effects on family functioning.

- Family members are often reluctant to discuss the mental disorders of family members because of the stigma associated with mental illness. In many instances, family members do not know whether mental illnesses were present in other generations.

- The family psychological assessment focuses on family development, the family life cycle, communication patterns, stress and coping abilities, and problem-solving skills. One assessment aim is to begin to understand family interpersonal relationships.

- The family life cycle is a process of expansion, contraction, and realignment of the relationship systems to support the entry, exit, and development of family members in a functional way. The nurse should determine whether a family fits any of the life cycle models. Families living in poverty may have a condensed life cycle.

- In assessing the family social domain, the nurse compiles data about the system itself, social and financial status, and formal and informal support networks.

- The family system model proposes that a balance should exist between the family system and the individual. A person not only needs family connection but also needs to be differentiated as an individual. Important concepts include triangles, family projection process, nuclear family emotional process, multigenerational transmission, sibling position, and emotional cutoff.

- The family structure model explains patterns of family interaction. Subsystems develop that also influence interaction patterns. Boundaries can vary from rigid to relaxed. The rigidity of the boundaries affects family functioning.

- Family interventions focus on supporting the family's integrity and functioning as defined by its members. Family nursing interventions include counseling, promotion of self-care activities, supportive therapy, education and health teaching, and the use of genograms. Mental health specialists, including advanced practice nurses, conduct family therapy.

- Education of the family is one of the most useful interventions. Teaching the family about mental disorders, life cycles, family systems, and family interactions can help the family develop a new understanding of family functioning and the effects of mental disorders on the family.

CRITICAL THINKING CHALLENGES

1. How can a group of people who are unrelated by blood consider themselves a family?

2. Interview a family with a member who has a mental illness and identify who provides support to the individual and family during acute episodes of illness.

3. Interview someone from another culture regarding family beliefs about mental illness. Compare them with your own.

4. Develop a genogram for your family. Analyze the genogram for its pattern of health problems, relationship issues, and social functioning.

5. A female patient, divorced with two small children, reports that she is considering getting married again to a man whom she met 6 months ago. She asks for help in considering the advantages and disadvantages of remarriage. Using the remarried family formulations life cycle model, develop a plan for structuring the counseling session.

6. Define Minuchin et al.'s term *family structure* and use that definition in observing your own family and its interaction.

7. Discuss what happens to a family that has rigid boundaries.

8. A family is finding it difficult to provide transportation to a support group for an adult member with mental illness. The family is committed to his treatment but is also experiencing severe financial stress because of another family illness. Using a problem-solving approach, outline a plan for helping the family explore solutions to the transportation problem.

Movie Viewing Guides

Call Me by Your Name: 2017. In 1983, the Perlmans invite a 24-year-old, American graduate student, Oliver, to spend 6 weeks with them over the summer to help Professor Perlman with his work. The location is northern Italy in a 17th century villa, where the Perlmans spend their summers and Hannukah. Oliver associates with the Perlmans 17-year-old son Elio and Elio's friends. During the course of 6 weeks, Oliver and Elio realize their strong attraction to each other and develop a clandestine relationship.

VIEWING POINTS: Observe your feelings as you watch this movie. Identify the cultural mores that prevent Oliver and Elio from being open about their relationship.

My Big Fat Greek Wedding: 2002. This movie is about Fotoula "Toula" Portokalos, a Greek-American woman who falls in love with a non-Greek protestant fellow, Ian Miller. Toula is the only one in her family who had not met her family expectations of marrying a Greek and having children. Toula is stuck working in the family business, a restaurant, and her sister has the perfect Greek family. Toula's father is adamantly opposed to marriage to a non-Greek. A wedding is eventually planned with multiple problems throughout the year.

VIEWING POINTS: Discuss the stigma that faces Toula and Ian as they plan their life together. How would you intervene if Toula approached you for help with her family? Identify the cultural beliefs that are shaping and interfering with the wishes of the newly engaged couple.

REFERENCES

Badgett, V. B. L., Choi, S. K., & Wilson, B. D. M. (2019). *LGBT poverty in the United States: A study of difference between sexual orientation and gender identity groups.* Research that Matters. Williams Institute, School of Law, UCLA. https://williamsinstitute.law.ucla.edu/wp-content/uploads/National-LGBT-Poverty-Oct-2019.pdf

Bleske-Rechek, A., & Kelley, J. A. (2014). Birth order and personality: A within-family test using independent self-reports from both firstborn and laterborn siblings. *Personality and Individual Differences, 56*(1), 15–18.

Boghani, P. (2020, December 8). How COVID has impacted poverty in America. Frontline. PBS. https://www.pbs.org/wgbh/frontline/article/covid-poverty-america/

Bowen, M. (1975). Family therapy after twenty years. In S. Arieti, D. Freedman, & J. Dyrud (Eds.). *American Handbook of Psychiatry* (2nd ed., Vol. 5, pp. 379–391). Basic Books.

Bowen, M. (1976). Theory in the practice of psychotherapy. In P. Guerin (Ed.), *Family therapy: Theory and practice* (pp. 42–90). Gardner Press.

Fekadu, W., Mihiretu, A., Craig, T., & Fekadu, A. (2019). Multidimensional impact of severe mental illness on family members: Systematic review. *BMJ open, 9*(12), e032391. https://doi.org/10.1136/bmjopen-2019-032391

Green, B., & Griffiths, E. C. (2014). Birth order and post-traumatic stress disorder. *Psychology, Health & Medicine, 19*(1), 24–32.

Horowitz, J. M., Graf, N., & Livingston, G. (2019). The landscape of marriage and cohabitation in the U.S. *Marriage and cohabitation in the U.S.*, Pew Research Center. https://www.pewsocialtrends.org/2019/11/06/the-landscape-of-marriage-and-cohabitation-in-the-u-s/

Keenan, K., & Grundy, E. (2018). Fertility history and physical and mental health changes in European older adults. *European Journal of Population = Revue europeenne de demographie, 35*(3), 459–485. https://doi.org/10.1007/s10680-018-9489-x

Kerr, M. (2019). *Bowen theory's secrets: Revealing the hidden lives of families.* W.W. Norton & Company.

Kramer, S. (2019). U.S. has world's Highest rate of children living in single-parent households. *Fact Tank: News in the numbers.* Pew Research Center.

Livingston, G. (2018a, April 25). The changing profile of unmarried parents. *Social and Demographic Trends.* Pew Research Center. https://www.pewsocialtrends.org/2018/04/25/the-changing-profile-of-unmarried-parents/#:~:text=In%201968%2C%20just%2012%25%20were,as%20were%2088%25%20in%201968

Livingston, G. (2018b, September 24). Stay-at-home moms and dads account for about one-in-five U.S. parents. *Fact tank: News in numbers.* Pew Research Center. https://www.pewresearch.org/fact-tank/2018/09/24/stay-at-home-moms-and-dads-account-for-about-one-in-five-u-s-parents/

McGoldrick, M., Garcia Preto, N., & Carter, B. (2016). The life cycle in its changing context: Individual, family and social perspectives. In M. McGoldrick, N. Garcia Preto, & B. Carter (Eds.). *The expanding family life cycle: Individual, family, and social perspectives* (5th ed.). Pearson.

Minuchin, S., Lee, W., & Simon, G. (1996). *Mastering family therapy: Journey of growth and transformation* (2nd ed.). John Wiley & Sons.

Okpokoro, U., Adams, C. E., & Sampson, S. (2014). Family intervention (brief) for schizophrenia. *Cochrane Database Syst Rev, (3),* CD009802.

Shajani, Z., & Snell, D. (2019). *Wright & Leahey's nurses and families: A guide to family assessment and intervention.* 7e. F. A. Davis: Philadelphia.

Stepler, R. (2017). Number of U.S. adults cohabiting with a partner continues to rise, especially among those 50 and older. *Fact Tank: News in the Numbers.* Pew Research Center. https://www.pewresearch.org/fact-tank/2017/04/06/number-of-u-s-adults-cohabiting-with-a-partner-continues-to-rise-especially-among-those-50-and-older/

U.S. Census Bureau. (2018). Households and families. https://data.census.gov/cedsci/table?q=families&hidePreview=false&tid=ACSST1Y2018.S1101&vintage=2018

Valdez, C. R., & Martinez, E. (2019). Mexican immigrant fathers' recognition of and coping with maternal depression: The influence of meaning-making on marital and co-parenting roles among men participating in a family intervention. *Journal of Latina/o Psychology, 7*(4), 304–321. https://doi.org/10.1037/lat0000132

Wang, K., Burke, S. E., Przedworski, J. M., Wittlin, N. M., Onyeador, I. N., Dovidio, J. F., Dyrbye, L. N., Herrin, J., & van Ryn, M. (2020). A comparison of depression and anxiety symptoms between sexual minority and heterosexual medical residents: A report from the medical trainee CHANGE Study. *LGBT Health,* 10.1089/lgbt.2020.0027. Advance online publication. https://doi.org/10.1089/lgbt.2020.0027

Yektatalab, S., Seddigh Oskouee, F., & Sodani, M. (2017). Efficacy of Bowen Theory on marital conflict in the family nursing practice: A randomized controlled trial. *Issues in Mental Health Nursing, 38*(3), 253–260. https://doi.org/10.1080/01612840.2016.1261210

Yin, M., Li, Z., & Zhou, C. (2020). Experience of stigma among family members of people with severe mental illness: A qualitative systematic review. *International Journal of Mental Health Nursing, 29*(2), 141–160. https://doi.org/10.1111/inm.12668

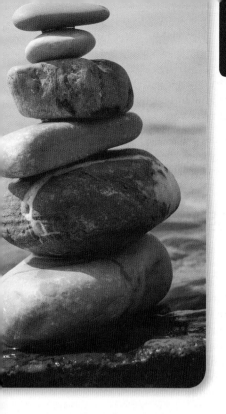

Mental Health Across the Life Span

16

Mental Health Promotion for Children and Adolescents

Catherine Gray Deering

KEYCONCEPTS

- egocentric thinking
- invincibility fable

LEARNING OBJECTIVES

After studying this chapter, you will be able to:

1. Describe common stressors for children and adolescents.

2. Identify risk factors for the development of psychopathology in childhood and adolescence.

3. Describe protective factors in the mental health promotion of children and adolescents.

4. Analyze the role of the nurse in mental health promotion for children and families.

KEY TERMS

- Adverse childhood events • Attachment • Bibliotherapy • Bullying • Child abuse and neglect • Developmental delays • Early intervention programs • Family preservation • Fetal alcohol syndrome • Formal operations • Normalization • Protective factors • Psychoeducational programs • Relational aggression • Resilience • Risk factors • Social skills training • Vulnerable child syndrome

INTRODUCTION

Children and adolescents respond to the stresses of life in different ways according to their developmental levels. **Resilience** is the phenomenon by which some children at risk for psychopathology—because of genetic or experiential circumstances (or both)—attain good mental health, maintain hope, and achieve healthy outcomes (Garcia-Dia et al., 2013). This chapter examines specific determinants of childhood and adolescent mental health, discusses the effects of common childhood stressors, and identifies **risk factors** for psychopathology, or the characteristics that increase the likelihood of developing a disorder. This chapter also considers **protective factors**, or the characteristics that reduce the probability that a child will develop a disorder, and provides guidelines for mental health promotion and risk reduction. Over the past two decades, a large body of research on diverse populations has established a strong connection between **adverse childhood events** (e.g., abuse, neglect, domestic violence, household substance abuse and mental illness, parental separation or divorce, and incarceration of family members) and later physical and mental health problems (Hays-Grudo & Morris, 2020). Nurses are in a key position to identify and intervene with children and adolescents at risk for psychopathology by virtue of their close contact with families in health care settings and their roles as educators. Knowing the difference between typical and atypical child development is crucial in helping parents to view their children's behavior realistically and to respond appropriately.

CHILDHOOD AND ADOLESCENT MENTAL HEALTH

Supportive social networks and positive childhood and adolescent experiences maximize the mental health of children and adolescents. Children are more likely to be mentally healthy if they have good physical health, positive social development, an easy temperament (adaptable, low intensity, and positive mood), and secure **attachment** through the emotional bonds formed between them and their parents at an early age. These areas are considered in the mental health assessment of children (see Chapter 36). **Developmental delays** not only slow the child's progress but also can interfere with the development of positive self-esteem. Children with an easy

temperament can adapt to change without intense emotional reactions. A secure attachment helps the child test the world without fear of rejection.

> **NCLEXNOTE** Attachment and temperament are key concepts in the behavior of children and adolescents in any health care setting. Apply these concepts to any pediatric patient.

COMMON PROBLEMS IN CHILDHOOD

Children and adolescents are faced with many challenges while growing up. Loss is an inevitable part of life. All children experience significant losses, the most common being death of a grandparent, parental divorce, death of a pet, and loss of friends through moving or changing schools. Learning to mourn losses can lead to a renewed appreciation of the precious value of life and close relationships. Sibling rivalry, illness, and common adolescent risk-taking tendencies also may pose challenges for children as they grow and develop.

Death and Grief

Vast research shows that similar to adults, children who experience major losses are at risk for mental health problems, particularly if the natural grieving process is impeded. However, the grieving process differs somewhat between children and adults (Table 16.1).

TABLE 16.1 GRIEVING IN CHILDHOOD, ADOLESCENCE, AND ADULTHOOD		
Children	**Adolescents**	**Adults**
View death as reversible; do not understand that death is permanent until about age 7 years.	Understand that death is permanent but may flirt with death (e.g., reckless driving, unprotected sex) because of omnipotent feelings.	Understand that death is permanent; may struggle with spiritual beliefs about death.
Experiment with ideas about death by killing bugs, staging funerals, acting-out death in play.	May be fascinated by death, enjoy morbid books and movies, listen to rock music about death and suicide.	May try not to think about death, depending on cultural background.
Mourn through activities (e.g., mock funerals, playing with things owned by the loved one); may not cry.	Mourn by talking about the loss, crying, and reflecting on it, sometimes becoming dramatic (e.g., overidentifying with the lost person, developing poetic or romantic ideas about death).	Mourn through talking about the loss, crying, reviewing memories, and thinking privately about it.
May not discuss the loss openly but may instead express grief through regression, somatic complaints, behavior problems, or withdrawal.	Often withdraw when mourning or seek comfort through peer groups; may feel parents do not understand their feelings.	Usually discuss loss openly, depending on level of support available; may feel there is a "time limit" on how long it is socially acceptable to grieve.
Need repeated explanations to fully understand the loss; it may be helpful to read children's books that explain death.	Need permission to grieve openly because they may believe they should act strong or take care of the adults involved; need acceptance of their sometimes extreme reactions.	Need friends, family, and other supportive people to listen and allow them to mourn for however long it takes; need opportunities to review their feelings and memories.

Children's responses to loss reflect their developmental level. As early as age 3 years, children have some concept of death. For example, the death of a goldfish provides an opportunity for the child to grasp the idea that the fish will never swim again. However, not until about age 7 years can most children understand the permanence of death. Before this age, they may verbalize that someone has "died" but in the next sentence ask when the dead person will be "coming back". Some adolescents, age 11 to 18, may believe they are immune to death and engage in risky behaviors, such as driving dangerously. This phenomenon is known as the *invincibility fable* because adolescents view themselves in an egocentric way, as unique and invulnerable to the consequences experienced by others.

> **KEYCONCEPT The invincibility fable** is an aspect of **egocentric thinking** in adolescence that causes teens to view themselves as immune to dangerous situations, such as unprotected sex, fast driving, and drug abuse.

If the concept of death is difficult for adults to grasp, it is particularly important to be sensitive to children's struggle to understand and cope with it. Most children closely watch their parents' response to grief and loss and use fantasy to fill the gaps in their understanding. In many cases, family members take turns grieving, with children sensing that their parents are so overwhelmed by their own emotional pain that they cannot bear the children's grief. They also see adults taking turns being strong for each other.

Loss and Early Childhood

A child, ages 2 to 6, may react more to the parents' distress about a death than to the death itself. Young children who depend totally on their parents may be frightened when they see their parents upset. Anything the parent can do to alleviate their children's anxiety, such as reassuring them that the parent will be okay and continuing the child's routine (e.g., normal bedtimes, snacks, play times), will help the child to feel secure (Worden, 2018). Because preschool-aged children have limited ability to verbalize their feelings, they may need to express them through fantasy play and activities, such as mock funerals. Books that explain death, such as *Charlotte's Web* by E. B. White, may also be helpful. Parents should take care not to use euphemisms that could fuel misconceptions of death, such as "They went to sleep." Young children may interpret these messages literally and fear going to sleep (because they might die) or focus their natural, grief-related anger on the irrational idea that the person deliberately has not returned. The best approach is to explain honestly that the person has died and is not coming back, elicit the child's understanding and questions about what has happened, and

then repeat this process continually as the child gradually begins to grasp the reality of the situation. The decision of whether to take a young child to a funeral may be particularly complex. Figure 16.1 enumerates some factors to consider.

Loss and the Middle Childhood Years

Children, age 6 to 11, understand the permanence of death more clearly than do younger children age 2 to 6, but they may still struggle to articulate their feelings. Children in this age group, age 6 to 11, may express their grief through somatic complaints, regression, behavior problems, withdrawal, and even anger toward their parents. They may think that others expect them to cry and react with immediate emotional intensity to the death; when they do not react this way, they feel guilty.

The death of a sibling can be a particularly difficult loss for both the child and the family. Common reactions to this are for the surviving child to feel guilt because of natural sibling rivalry and for the parents to unconsciously endow the surviving child with qualities of the lost sibling as if to fill the empty space in the family (Worden, 2018). Of course, the death of a parent can be even more devastating. The surviving parent's psychological functioning has a major impact on the child's adjustment to the loss (Bugge et al., 2014). Parents should provide grieving children with support, nurturance, continuity, and the opportunity to remember the lost person in concrete ways through photographs, stories, and family activities that allow the child to memorialize the loved one.

Loss and Adolescents

Adolescents who are in Piaget stage of **formal operations**, characterized by the ability to use abstract reasoning to conceptualize and solve problems, can better understand death as an abstract concept (see Chapter 7). Because adolescents tend to be idealistic and to think in extremes, they may even have poetic or romantic notions about death. Many teenagers become fascinated with morbid rock music, movies, and books. Although they may be able to express their thoughts and feelings about death more clearly than younger children, they often are reluctant to do so for fear of being viewed as childish. Some adolescents assume a parental role in the family after a death, denying their own needs. School settings may be particularly helpful in providing group and individual support for grieving adolescents who may fear being viewed as different from their peers (Lytje, 2017). Structured programs for children and adolescents can prevent complicated (pathologic) bereavement.

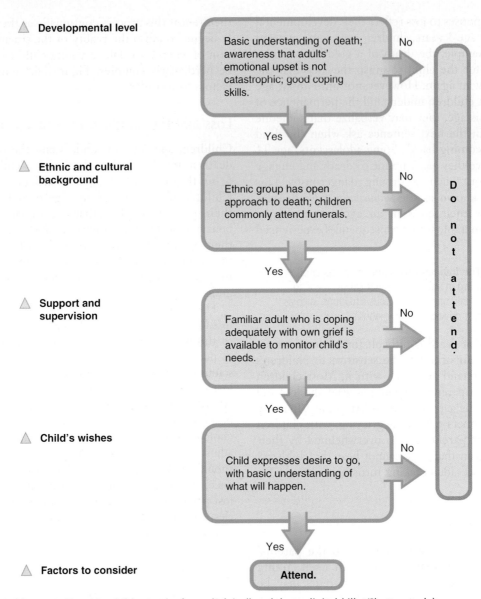

FIGURE 16.1 Decision tree: Should a child attend a funeral? (pixelheadphoto digitalskillet/Shutterstock.)

Separation and Divorce

Although many families adapt to separation and divorce without long-term negative effects for the children, youth often show at least temporary difficulties in dealing with this common stressor (Demir-Dagnas, 2020). Parental separation and divorce change the family structure, usually resulting in a substantial reduction in the contact that children have with one of their parents. The child's response to divorce is similar to the response to death. In some ways, divorce may be harder for the child to understand because the noncustodial parent is gone but still alive, and the parents have made a conscious choice to separate. Children of divorce are at increased risk for emotional, behavioral, and academic problems. However, the response to the loss that divorce imposes

varies depending on the child's temperament; the parents' interventions; and the level of stress, change, and conflict surrounding the divorce (Hetherington & Kelly, 2002). A major change in socioeconomic status, such as moving from dual-earner status to single-parent family status, may account for much of the variation in levels of distress among divorcing families (Ryan & Claessens, 2013).

The first 2 or 3 years after the couple's breakup tend to be the most difficult. Typical childhood reactions include confusion, guilt, depression, regression, somatic symptoms, acting-out behaviors (e.g., stealing, disobedience), fantasies that the parents will reunite, fear of losing the custodial parent, and alignment with one parent against the other. After an initial adjustment period, children usually accept the reality of the situation and begin coping adaptively. Most divorced parents eventually remarry new partners, which often imposes another period of coping difficulties for the children. Children with stepparents and stepsiblings are at renewed risk for emotional and behavioral problems as they struggle to cope with the new relationships (Browning & Artelt, 2014).

Protective factors against emotional problems in children of divorce and remarriage include a structured home and school environment with reasonable and consistent limit setting and a warm, supportive relationship with stepparents (Kelly, 2012). Helpful interventions for children of divorce include education regarding children's reactions; promotion of regular and predictable visitation; reduction of conflict between the parents through counseling, mediation, and clear visitation policies; continuance of usual routines; and family counseling to facilitate adjustment after remarriage (Table 16.2). It is also important to make it clear to children that the divorce was not caused by them. Egocentric thinking, which is normal for children, may cause children to believe that they are at the root of the problem. Some evidence shows that it is not the divorce

TABLE 16.2	PLAY THERAPY WITH A 4-YEAR-OLD CHILD WHOSE PARENTS ARE DIVORCING	
Patient Statement	**Nurse Response**	**Analysis and Rationale**
(Child smashes two cars together and makes loud, crashing sound.)	That's a loud crash. They really hit hard.	Child may be expressing anger and frustration nonverbally through play. Nurse attempts to establish rapport with child by relating at child's level using age-appropriate vocabulary.
Crrrash!	I know a boy who gets so mad sometimes that he feels like smashing something.	Child is engrossed in fantasy play, typical of preschoolers. Children often use toys as symbols of human figures (animism). Nurse uses indirect method of eliciting child's feelings because preschoolers often do not express feelings directly. Reference to another child's anger helps to normalize this child's feelings.
Yeah!	Sounds like you feel that way sometimes, too.	Child is beginning to relate to nurse and sense her empathy. Nurse reflects the child's feelings to facilitate further communication.
Yeah, when my mom and dad fight.	It's hard to listen to parents fighting. Sometimes, it's scary. You wonder what's going to happen.	Child is experiencing frustration and helplessness related to family conflict. Nurse expresses empathy and attempts to articulate child's feelings because preschool children have a limited ability to identify and label feelings.
My mom and dad are getting a divorce.	That's too bad. What's going to happen when they get the divorce?	Child has basic awareness of the reality of parents' divorce but may not understand this concept. Nurse expresses empathy and attempts to assess the child's level of understanding of the divorce.
Dad is not going to live in our house.	Oh, I guess you'll miss having him there all the time. It would be nice if you all could live together, but I guess that's not going to happen.	Preschool child focuses on the effects the divorce will have on him (egocentrism). Child seems to have a clear understanding of the consequences of the divorce. Nurse articulates the child's perspective and reinforces the reality of the divorce to avoid fueling child's possible denial and reconciliation fantasies.
(Silently moves cars across the floor.)	What do you think is the reason your parents decided to get a divorce?	Child expresses sadness nonverbally. Nurse further attempts to assess the child's understanding of the circumstances surrounding the divorce.
Because I did it.	What do you mean—you did it?	Child provides clue that he may be feeling responsible. Nurse uses clarification to fully assess child's understanding.
I made them mad because I left my bike in the driveway and Dad ran over it.	How? Do you think that is why they're getting the divorce?	Child uses egocentric thinking to draw conclusion that his actions caused the divorce. Nurse continues to clarify the child's thinking. The goal is to elicit the child's perceptions, so that misperceptions can be corrected.
Yeah, they had a big fight.	They may have been upset about the bike, but I don't think that is why they're getting a divorce.	The nurse goes on to explain why parents get divorced and to provide opportunities for the child to ask questions.
Why?	Because parents get divorced when they're upset with *each other*—when they can't get along—not when they're upset with their children.	

itself but rather the continuing conflict between the parents that is most damaging to children (Havermans et al., 2014). Parents manage divorce better if they can remember that children naturally idealize and identify with both parents and need to view both of them positively. Therefore, it is helpful for parents to guard against making negative statements about each other and focus on evidence of their former partner's love and respect for the child.

> **KEYCONCEPT In egocentric thinking,** children naturally view themselves as the center of their own universe. Common examples of this are children looking out the car window at night and claiming that "the moon is following me" and children sitting in front of the television set, blocking the view for the parent, but believing that if they can see the television, the parent can, too. This kind of magical, self-focused thinking is charming, but it has a downside when children believe that they have caused a divorce or death in the family because of their own actions.

Sibling Relationships

Until recently, the role of siblings in children's development was underemphasized. A growing body of research shows that sibling relationships significantly influence personality development. Positive sibling relationships can be protective factors against the development of psychopathology (Fig. 16.2), particularly in troubled families in which the parents are emotionally unavailable (Bank & Kahn, 2014). Thus, nurses should emphasize to

parents that minimizing sibling rivalry and maximizing cooperative behavior will benefit their children's social and emotional development throughout life.

Sibling rivalry begins with the birth of the second child. Often, this event is traumatic for the first child who, up until then, was the sole focus of the parents' attention (Nadelman & Begun, 2014). The older sibling usually reacts with anger and may reveal not-so-subtle fantasies of getting rid of the new sibling (e.g., "I dreamed that the new baby died."). Parents should recognize that these reactions are natural and allow the child to express feelings, both positive and negative, about the baby while reassuring the child that they have a very special place in the family. Allowing the older child opportunities to care for the baby and reinforcing any nurturing or affectionate behavior will promote positive bonding (Kramer & Ramsburg, 2002).

Some sibling rivalry is natural and inevitable, even into adulthood. However, intense rivalry and conflict between siblings correlate with behavior problems in children. However, positive temperament and effective, supportive coparenting can buffer against the negative outcomes associated with sibling conflict (Kolak & Volling, 2013). One factor that can exacerbate this sibling rivalry is differential treatment of children. Although it is natural and appropriate for parents to use different methods to manage children with different personalities, parents must be sensitive to their children's perceptions of their behavior

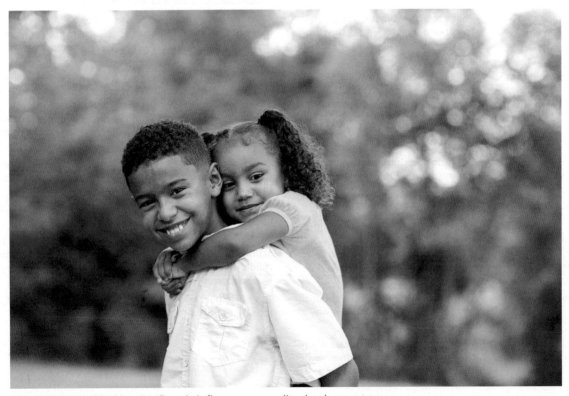

FIGURE 16.2 Sibling relationships significantly influence personality development.

and emphasize each child's strengths. Helping each child to develop a separate identity based on unique talents and interests can minimize rivalry and perceptions of favoritism.

Children with siblings who have psychological disorders are also at increased risk for mental health problems (Ma et al., 2015) (However, recent studies suggest that siblings may be an important source of support for children with mental health problems [Bojanowski et al., 2020]), and they may provide a buffer against parental conflict in families (Davies et al., 2019). Nurses should be alert to behavior problems of other family members and include siblings in family interventions.

Bullying

Children have been victimized by bullies throughout history, but this problem has only recently become a topic of widespread concern for mental health professionals.

Bullying is defined as repeated, deliberate attempts to harm someone, usually unprovoked. An imbalance in strength is a part of the pattern, with most victims having difficulty defending themselves. Boys are more likely to use physical aggression, and bigger boys usually pick on smaller, weaker ones (Hymel & Swearer, 2015). Some studies suggest that girls are more likely to use **relational aggression**, which involves disrupting peer relationships by excluding or manipulating others and spreading rumors. Cyberbullying (spreading pictures, rumors, or smear campaigns via the Internet) has become an increasingly common phenomenon that can have devastating effects because of the speed and scope of its impact (Carpenter & Hubbard, 2014).

Children who have insecure attachments, who have distant or authoritarian parents, and who have been physically, sexually, or verbally abused are at risk for becoming bullies (Rodkin & Hodges, 2003). On the other side, victims of bullies often suffer from low self-esteem and relationship difficulties, even into adulthood.

Nurses who work with children and adolescents should assess for the occurrence of bullying by asking direct questions because this problem is often hidden (Hensley, 2013). Immediate intervention should involve a coordinated effort by the school, parents, bullies, and victims because studies show that bullying does not occur in a vacuum. Rather, numerous "henchmen", supporters, and bystanders participate in the process (Olweus, 2003). The most effective programs involve educating and changing the climate in the whole school (not just working with the bullies) (Nickerson, 2019).

Physical Illness

Many children experience a major physical illness or injury at some point during development. Hospitalization and intrusive medical procedures are acutely traumatic for most children. The likelihood of lasting psychological problems resulting from physical illness depends on the child's developmental level and previous coping mechanisms, the family's level of functioning before and after the illness, and the nature and severity of the illness. As with any major stressor, the perception of the event (i.e., meaning of the illness) will influence the family's ability to cope. One possible outcome of early childhood illness or injury is the phenomenon of **vulnerable child syndrome**, in which the family perceives the child as fragile despite current good health, causing them to be overprotective (Duncan & Caughy, 2009).

Common childhood reactions to physical illness include regression (e.g., loss of previous developmental gains in toilet training, social maturity, autonomous behavior), sleep and feeding difficulties, behavior problems (negativism, withdrawal), somatic complaints that mask attempts at emotional expression (e.g., headaches, stomach aches), and depression. Infants and children younger than school age are particularly vulnerable to separation anxiety during illness and may regress to earlier levels of anxiety about strangers, becoming fearful of health care providers. Young children often have magical thinking about the illness, and their tendency to process information in concrete terms may lead to misperceptions about the illness and treatment procedures (e.g., dye vs. die; stretcher vs. stretch her) (Deering & Cody, 2002). Adolescents may be concerned about body image and maintaining their sense of independence and control.

Nurses must remember that parents are the primary resource to the child and the experts who know the child's needs and reactions. Thus, nurses must maintain a collaborative approach in working with parents of physically ill children. If the child is a sick infant, nurses should take care to allow the normal attachment process between parents and the infant to unfold, despite health care professionals' efforts to assume some parenting functions.

Many parents react with guilt to their child's illness or injury, especially if the illness is genetically based or partially the result of their own behavior (e.g., drug or alcohol abuse during pregnancy). Parents may project their guilt onto each other or health care professionals, lashing out in anger and blame. Nurses should view this behavior as part of the grieving process and help parents to move forward in caring for their children and regaining competence. Teaching parents how to care for their children's medical problems and reinforcing their successes in doing so will help.

Chronic physical illness in childhood presents a unique set of challenges. Although most children with chronic illnesses and their families are remarkably resilient and adjust to the stressors and regimens involved in their care, children with chronic health conditions are significantly more likely to experience psychiatric symptoms than are their healthy peers (Secinti et al., 2017). Conditions that affect the central nervous system (CNS) (e.g., infections, metabolic diseases, CNS malformations, brain and spinal cord trauma) are particularly likely to result in psychiatric difficulties. Nurses who understand pathophysiologic processes are in a unique position to assess the interaction between biologic and psychological factors that contribute to mental health problems in chronically ill children (e.g., lethargy from high blood sugar levels or respiratory problems, mood swings from steroid use). Inactivity and lack of sensory stimulation from hospitalization or bed rest may contribute to neurologic deficits and developmental delays.

The major challenge for a chronically ill child is to remain active despite the limitations of the illness and to become fully integrated into school and social activities. Children who view themselves as different or defective will experience low self-esteem and be more at risk for depression, anxiety, and behavior problems. Studies show that parental perceptions of the child's vulnerability predict greater adjustment problems even after controlling for age and disease severity (Anthony et al., 2003). Educating parents and helping them to foster maximum independence within the limitations of the child's health problem is the key. Nurses in primary care settings are in a good position to promote integrated mental health care to children with physical health problems.

Adolescent Risk-Taking Behaviors

Adolescence is a time of growing independence and, consequently, experimentation. Emotional extremes prevail. To adolescents, the world seems great one day and terrible the next; people are either for them or against them. Adolescents are struggling to consolidate their abilities to control their impulses and react to the many "crises" that may seem trivial to adults but are very important to teens. Biologic changes (e.g., onset of puberty, height and weight changes, hormonal changes), psychological changes (increased ability for abstract thinking), and social changes (dating, driving, increased autonomy) are all significant. Unevenness in adolescent brain development, specifically in the amygdala, may contribute to difficulties with impulse control or the ability to "think twice" before acting (Steinberg, 2019).

Teenagers test different roles and struggle to find a peer group that fits their unfolding self-image. During this process, many adolescents experiment with risk-taking behaviors, such as smoking, using alcohol and drugs, having unprotected sex, engaging in truancy or delinquent behaviors, and running away from home. Although most youths eventually become more responsible, some develop harmful behavior patterns and addictions that endanger their mental and physical health. One recent trend is self-mutilation or cutting by adolescents who use this as a cry for help or a tension release (Askew & Byrne, 2009; Lloyd-Richardson et al., 2020). Adolescents whose psychiatric problems have already developed are particularly vulnerable to engaging in risky behaviors because they have limited coping skills, may attempt to self-medicate their symptoms, and may feel increased pressure to fit in with other teens.

Several approaches to mental health promotion with adolescents are recommended. First, intervening at the peer group level through education programs, alternative recreation activities, and peer counseling is most successful. Second, training in values clarification, problem-solving, social skills, and assertiveness helps give adolescents the skills to cope with situations in which they are pressured by their peers. If just one person can find the strength to express an unpopular viewpoint in a group and decline to participate in a destructive activity, others will quickly follow. It takes enormous courage, as well as concrete knowledge and practice with assertiveness, to speak up in these situations. A third type of intervention is a program that uses team efforts by teachers, parents, community leaders, and teen role models. These programs help at-risk youth by building self-esteem, setting positive examples, and working to involve the youth in community activities.

Approaches that have not proved effective include mere education about dangerous activities without behavior training and programs that provide inadequate training for the professionals implementing them. In any intervention, it is also important to keep in mind that adolescents are skeptical of authority figures and tend to take cues from one another. Nurses working with teenagers find it helpful to use a discussion approach that encourages questioning and argument as opposed to talking down to or "talking at" teenagers (Deering & Cody, 2002).

RISK FACTORS FOR CHILDHOOD PSYCHOPATHOLOGY

Understanding the risk factors for psychopathology is vital in mental health promotion and the prevention of disorders. Any intervention must recognize and work to address these factors if it is to be successful.

Poverty and Homelessness

Children are born into their parents' socioeconomic class, and the effects of intergenerational poverty impact all aspects of their development (Miller-Smith, 2020). Lack of proper nutrition and access to prenatal and infant care places children from poor families at risk for physical and mental health problems. Adolescence may be truncated when children from impoverished families are forced into adult roles as parents work long hours to meet basic needs (Dashiff et al., 2009; see Chapter 15).

Although crime, drug abuse, gang activity, and teenage pregnancy are seen in adolescents from all socioeconomic backgrounds, children living in poverty may be more vulnerable to these problems because they may view their options as limited. Thus, they may have an increased need to maintain a tough image and struggle more for a sense of control over their environment. The obstacles inherent in overcoming the effects of poverty can seem insurmountable to young people.

A major focus of preventive nursing interventions for disadvantaged families involves simply forming an alliance that conveys respect and willingness to work as an advocate to help patients gain access to resources. In terms of Maslow need hierarchy, families living in poverty may be more focused on survival needs (e.g., food, shelter) than self-actualization needs (e.g., insight-oriented psychotherapy for themselves or their children). Unless the nurse can work as a partner with the family and address the issues that are most pressing for the family with an active, problem-solving approach, other types of intervention may be fruitless. At the same time, it is inappropriate to assume that poor families will be resistant to or unable to benefit from psychotherapy or other mental health interventions.

Additional risks arise from homelessness in children and teens, which may result from loss of shelter for the entire family, running away, or being thrown out of their homes (Box 16.1; see also Chapter 41). For youths who are homeless, there is an increased risk for physical health problems (e.g., nutrition deficiencies, infections, chronic illnesses), mental health problems (particularly developmental delays in language, fine or gross motor coordination, and social development; depression; anxiety; disruptive behavior disorders), and educational underachievement. Many homeless youth have been physically and/or sexually abused, leading to elevated rates of mental disorders (Wong et al., 2016). Adolescents who run away from an abusive home can find themselves living on the streets where staying alive and developing self-reliance are a daily struggle.

The living conditions of many shelters place children at risk for lead poisoning and communicable diseases and make the regular sleep, feeding, play, and bathing patterns important for normal development nearly impossible. Nurses working with homeless families need to be aware of the effects of this lifestyle on children because they have a limited ability to speak for themselves and because their needs are often overlooked.

Child Abuse and Neglect

Early recognition and reduction of risk factors are the keys to preventing **child abuse and neglect**, which includes any actions that endanger or impair a child's physical, psychological, or emotional health and development. Risk factors for child abuse and neglect include high levels of family stress, drug or alcohol abuse, a stepparent or parental boyfriend or girlfriend who is unstable or unloving toward the child, and lack of social support for the parents. In addition, young children (particularly

---

BOX 16.1

Attention, Externalizing, and Internalizing Problems of Youth Exposed to Parental Incarceration

Boch, S. J., Warren, B. J. W., & Ford, J. L. (2019). Attention, externalizing, and internalizing problems of youth exposed to parental incarceration. Issues in Mental Health Nursing, 40(6), 466–475.

THE QUESTION: How does parental incarceration affect children's mental health, and how does exposure to additional adverse childhood experiences (ACEs) influence these outcomes?

METHODS: Nurse researchers examined data from a sample of adolescents in a racially, ethnically, and socioeconomically representative area of a Columbus, Ohio (n = 613). Face-to-face interviews were conducted in the home, along with surveys of adolescents and their caregivers. The researchers performed regression analyses to answer to their questions.

FINDINGS: Youth who were exposed to parental incarceration were more likely to have their caregiver-report attention, internalizing (e.g., depression, anxiety), externalizing (e.g., disobedience, anger), and total problem behaviors, after controlling for socioeconomic characteristics. Youth exposed to parental incarceration experienced an average of 15 additional ACEs compared with their unexposed peers, who averaged 4 ACEs.

IMPLICATIONS FOR NURSING: The nurse researchers conclude that the experience of parental incarceration may be viewed as a marker of accumulative risk for mental health problems in youth. The combination of the incarceration and the increased exposure to additional ACEs has an apparent cumulative effect. The ACEs may be part of the pathway toward incarceration (e.g., poverty, parental substance abuse) or a direct consequence of the incarceration (e.g., loss of parent, out-of-home placement). Either way, this vulnerable population needs additional screening, trauma-informed care, and interventions. The article cites other research showing that one in every 14 youth in the United States has experienced parental incarceration. Nurses should screen for ACEs among youth whose parents have been incarcerated and work with community or school organizations to implement evidence-based interventions.

---

those younger than 3 years) and children with a history of prematurity, medical problems, and severe emotional problems are at high risk because they place great demands on their parents. Abuse can have lifelong effects on development. Children who have been maltreated are more likely to enter aggressive relationships, abuse drugs or alcohol to numb emotions, develop eating disorders, become depressed, and engage in self-destructive behavior (Kolko & Berkout, 2017).

Nurses are legally mandated to report any reasonable suspicion of abuse and neglect to the appropriate state authorities. Box 16.2 lists signs of physical and sexual abuse in children. Mandated reporting laws allow the state to investigate the possibility of abuse, provide protection to children, and link families with support and

---

BOX 16.2

Signs of Possible Child Abuse

SEXUAL ABUSE

- Bruises or bleeding on the genitals or in the rectum
- Sexually transmitted infection (e.g., HIV, gonorrhea, syphilis, herpes genitalis)
- Vaginal or penile discharge
- Sore throats
- Enuresis or encopresis
- Foreign bodies in the vagina or rectum
- Pregnancy, especially in a young adolescent
- Difficulty in walking or sitting
- Sexual acting out with siblings or peers
- Sophisticated knowledge of sexual activities
- Preoccupation with sexual ideas
- Somatic complaints, especially abdominal pain and constipation
- Sleep difficulties
- Hyperalertness to the environment
- Withdrawal
- Excessive daydreaming or seeming preoccupied
- Regressed behavior

PHYSICAL ABUSE

- Bruises or lacerations, especially in clusters on back, buttocks, thighs, or large areas of the torso
- Fractures inconsistent with the child's history
- Old and new injuries at the same time
- Unwilling to change clothes in front of others; wears heavy clothes in warm weather
- Identifiable marks from belt buckles, electrical cords, or handprints
- Cigarette burns
- Rope burns on arms, legs, face, neck, or torso from being bound and gagged
- Adult-size bite marks
- Bald spots interspersed with normal hair
- Shrinking at the touch of an adult
- Fear of adults, especially parents
- Apprehensive when other children cry
- Scanning the environment, staying very still, failing to cry when hurt
- Aggression or withdrawal
- Nondiscriminatory seeking of affection
- Defensive reactions when questioned about injuries
- History of being taken to many different clinics and emergency departments for different injuries

*Note. Because many injuries do not represent child abuse, a careful history must be taken.

---

services. Nurses are immune from liability for reporting suspected abuse, but they may be held legally accountable for not reporting it. The decision to report abuse sometimes poses an ethical dilemma for nurses as they try to balance the need to maintain the family's trust against the need to protect the child. This decision is further complicated by the knowledge that if temporary out-of-home placement is necessary, the quality of the placement may not be optimum, and the child and family may suffer in the process of the separation.

To minimize damaging the nurse–family relationship, experts recommend that nurses report abuse in the presence of the parents, preferably with the parent initiating the telephone call. The professional should explain that reporting is necessary to provide safety for the child and to obtain services for the family. If the parents cannot be present when the report is made, the nurse should, at minimum, notify the family that the report was made.

Preventing child abuse and neglect occurs with any intervention that supports the parents with physical, financial, mental health, and medical resources that will reduce stress within the family system. Early intervention and family support programs are considered the cornerstone of preventive efforts. A major protective factor against psychopathology stemming from abuse and neglect is the establishment of a supportive relationship with at least one adult who can provide empathy, consistency, and possibly, a corrective experience (e.g., a foster parent or other family member) for the child (Yoon et al., 2019).

Nurses working with abused children should resist the temptation to view the child as the only victim. Remembering that most abusive parents were abused as children and therefore may have limited coping mechanisms or little access to positive parental role models will help the nurse keep empathy toward the parents. After state agencies intervene to establish the child's safety, a family systems approach that is supportive of the whole family unit is most effective.

Substance-Abusing Families

Children whose parents are substance abusing (see Chapter 31) live in an unpredictable family environment, coping with stress that may disrupt their ability to perform in school and lead to other emotional problems. The codependency movement, which emphasizes the effects of addiction on family members and groups such as Adult Children of Alcoholics and Al-Anon, has brought increasing attention to the effects of parental substance abuse on child development.

Biologic factors affecting children of those who abuse substances include **fetal alcohol syndrome**, nutritional deficits stemming from neglect, and neuropsychiatric dysfunction (Hughes et al., 2019). Genetic factors are at least partly responsible for the well-documented increased risk for substance abuse among children whose parents abuse substances. Recent studies are beginning to link a family history of anxiety disorders and alcoholism with genetically transmitted anxiety disorders, which may be a precursor to alcohol abuse. The precise mechanism of family transmission of alcoholism is still unknown. Recent studies suggest that children of those who abuse substances may inherit a predisposition to a nonspecific form of biologic dysregulation that may be expressed either as alcoholism or some other psychiatric disorder (e.g., hyperactivity, conduct disorder, depression), depending on the individual's developmental history.

Children of those who abuse substances are at high risk for both substance abuse and behavior disorders (Straussner & Fewell, 2011). Moreover, some evidence shows that other factors related to addiction, such as family stress, violence, divorce, dysfunction, and other concurrent parental psychiatric disorders (e.g., depression, anxiety), are as important as the substance abuse itself in increasing this risk (Ritter et al., 2002). The experience of growing up in a substance-abusing family is marked by unpredictability, fear, and helplessness because of the cyclic nature of addictive patterns.

Even for children who do not experience significant psychopathology, the experience of growing up in a substance-abusing family can lead to a poor self-concept when children feel responsible for their parents' behavior, become isolated, and learn to mistrust their own perceptions because the family denies the reality of the addiction. The recent upsurge in opioid abuse has posed particular challenges for families (Sapp & Hooten, 2019). The experience of growing up with an opioid-addicted parents has been characterized as living with ambiguous loss, as the parent may be physically present but psychologically absent due to preoccupation with obtaining and using the drug (Mechling et al., 2018). Despite the well-documented risk for children in substance-abusing families, there is no uniform pattern of outcomes, and many children prove resilience. School-based interventions with children from substance-abusing families can significantly increase resilience (Gance-Cleveland & Mays, 2008).

Out-of-Home Placement

The tendency to blame parents and view out-of-home placement as a refuge for children has sharply declined in recent years. This change in attitudes results from public awareness of the deficiencies in the foster care system, greater support for parents' rights, and increased knowledge of the biologic basis for many of the disorders of parents and children that lead to out-of-home placement. **Family preservation** involves supporting and educating the family to secure the attachment between children and parents and to preserve the family unit and prevent the removal of children from their homes. Today, children are removed from their homes only as a last resort. Family support services are designed to assist families with access to resources and education regarding child-rearing, monitor and facilitate the development of the bond between child and caregiver, and increase the caregiver's confidence in their abilities (Turnbull et al., 2007).

However, despite latest trends toward family preservation, an increasing number of children are placed in foster homes, group homes, or residential treatment centers—in many cases for months to years (Bruskas,

2008). Factors leading to the increased number of children in out-of-home placement include increased willingness of the public and professionals to report child abuse and neglect; the epidemic proportions of substance abuse and cases of acquired immunodeficiency syndrome; and the increasing number of families living in poverty. Those may lead to abuse, neglect, and homelessness. About 50% of children in out-of-home placement are adolescents, but the numbers of infants and young children are growing, particularly those with serious physical and emotional problems, who pose particular challenges for placement (Scribano, 2010). Infants who are abandoned by drug-abusing parents and children with human immunodeficiency virus (HIV) whose parents are sick or deceased need permanent out-of-home placements, which are often difficult to find. When children with mental health needs are placed in foster care, a family support team is required to meet regularly, with the goal of providing holistic care, avoiding overuse of psychotropic medication, and moving toward a permanent placement that will provide stability (Bertram, 2018).

The adjustment to an out-of-home placement can be viewed through the conceptual framework of Bowlby's stages of coping with parental separation. According to Bowlby (1960), the child initially responds to separation from parents with protest (crying, kicking, screaming, pleading, and attempting to elicit the parent's return). The child then moves to a state of despair (listlessness, apathy, and withdrawal, which lead to some acceptance of caregiving by others but a reluctance to reattach fully). Finally, the child experiences detachment if the child and new parent cannot manage to form an emotional bond. Because children often experience multiple placements, the potential for a disrupted attachment may be great by the time the child faces the prospect of a permanent family. After repeatedly undergoing separation and mourning, the child learns that rejection is inevitable and may automatically maintain distance from a new caregiver.

Typical coping styles seen in children exposed to multiple placements include detachment, diffuse rage, chronic depression, antisocial behavior, low self-esteem, and chronic dependency or exaggerated demands for nurturing and support. Sometimes, these symptoms develop into attachment disorders that can be difficult to treat. It takes a very committed and resilient parent to continue caring for a child who does not reinforce attempts at caregiving and who exhibits these kinds of significant emotional and behavior problems.

INTERVENTION APPROACHES

The goal of health promotion and prevention interventions is to maximize the mental health of children and adolescents. The selected interventions should allow maximal autonomy for the child and family; keep the family unit intact, if possible; and provide the appropriate level of care to meet the needs of the child and family. A view of parents as partners is important to effective interventions. Interdisciplinary approaches are ideal in which the nurse acts as coordinator, case manager, and advocate to establish linkages with physicians and nurse practitioners, teachers, speech and language specialists, social workers, and other professionals to develop and implement a comprehensive biopsychosocial plan of intervention (Box 16.3). Support groups are available for every kind of stressor that a family can experience, including substance abuse, death, divorce, and coping with a chronic illness. A continuum of modalities of care is available to children and families (Fig. 16.3).

Early intervention programs offer regular home visits, support, education, and concrete services to those in need. The assumption underlying these programs is that parents are the most consistent and important individuals in children's lives, and they should be afforded the opportunity to define their own needs and priorities. With support and education, parents are empowered to respond more effectively to their children. The effectiveness of these programs may be the key to preventing the placement of children outside the home (Heckman, 2013).

Psychoeducational programs designed to teach parents and children basic coping skills for dealing with various stressors are a particularly effective form of mental health intervention. By focusing on **normalization** (teaching families normal behaviors and expected responses) and providing families with information about typical child development and expected reactions to various stressors, families feel less isolated, know what to expect, and put their reactions into perspective. For example, if families learn that anger is a natural part of grieving, they will be less likely to view it as abnormal and more likely to accept and cope with it constructively.

Social skills training is useful with youth who have low self-esteem or aggressive behavior or who are at high risk for substance abuse (Bloomquist, 2013; Kvarme et al., 2010). Social skills training involves instruction, feedback, support, and practice with learning behaviors that help children to interact more effectively with peers and adults. When combined with assertiveness training, social skills training can be particularly helpful in providing children with coping skills to resist engaging in addictive or antisocial behaviors and to prevent social withdrawal under stress. Social skills training may be particularly helpful for children who are bullies or who are rejected by their peers (Fopma-Loy, 2000).

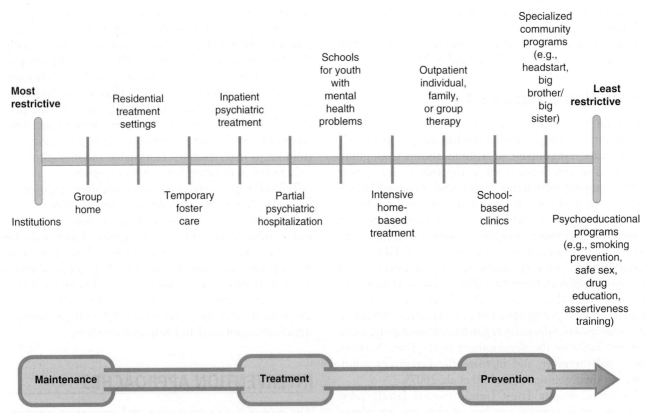

FIGURE 16.3 The continuum of mental health care for children and adolescents.

BOX 16.3

Preventive Interventions with an Adolescent in Crisis

Ben and Rita were just transferred to a second foster home after being removed from their mother's care when she relapsed on cocaine and left them unattended. The plan is for the two children to return to their mother's home after she completes a 30-day drug treatment program. Ben, a high school freshman, is in the school nurse's office asking for aspirin for another headache.

The nurse notices that Ben's nose looks inflamed, he is sniffling, and he seems more "hyper" than usual. In a concerned tone of voice, she asks him if he has been using cocaine, and he snaps back, "Just because my mother's a coke head doesn't give you the right to suspect me!" When the nurse gently says, "Tell me about what's been happening with your mother; I had no idea," Ben responds less defensively and explains the situation about the foster home and his mother's drug problem. He says that if it weren't for Rita, his younger sister, he would have run away by now. His foster parents are "making him" go to school, but he's going to drop out as soon as he returns to live with his mother. The only thing that he likes about school is playing basketball, and the basketball coach, who is his physical education teacher, wants him on the team.

After a lengthy talk with Ben, the nurse finishes the assessment interview and concludes that he is at risk for drug abuse, running away, and dropping out of school. He is also showing symptoms of depression, which he may be attempting to medicate with cocaine. Protective

factors for Ben include his strong attachment to his sister, his ability and willingness to express his thoughts and feelings, his interest in basketball, and a positive relationship with the basketball coach.

The nurse develops a plan with Ben to attend the weekly drug and alcohol discussion group at the school, so he can talk with other teens from substance-abusing families and learn coping skills to prevent addiction. The nurse contacts the basketball coach, who agrees to find a student mentor who can shoot hoops with Ben and help him come up with a plan to stay in school, maybe find a part time job, and join the basketball team. Ben agrees to check in regularly with the nurse to report how the plan is working and revise it if needed. The nurse feels optimistic that with support from his peers, coach, mentor, and herself, Ben can overcome what is probably a genetically based risk for depression and addiction. Ben shows signs of resilience. He is motivated to "keep his act together for Rita", capable of forming positive attachments, and willing to seek help when he knows where to find it.

WHAT DO YOU THINK?

• If Ben "forgets" to check in regularly with the nurse, what would be the next course of action?

• When are the times Ben is most susceptible to change his mind about staying in school and avoiding drugs? What action should be taken to avoid these times?

A wide variety of books are available to help children understand issues such as death, divorce, chronic illness, stepfamilies, adoption, and birth of a sibling. In addition, many mental health organizations and public health agencies have pamphlets designed to educate parents about various physical and psychological problems. By supplying concrete information and advice, these reading materials help to reduce anxiety by pointing out common reactions to the various stressors, so that families do not feel alone.

SUMMARY OF KEY POINTS

■ Children who experience major losses, such as death or divorce, are at risk for developing mental health problems.

■ Sibling relationships have significant effects on personality development. Positive sibling relationships can be protective factors against the development of mental health problems.

■ Bullying is a severe problem that is often hidden yet can cause long-standing psychological harm; it must be addressed on a school-wide level.

■ Medical problems in childhood and adolescence may cause psychological problems when illness leads to

regression or lack of full participation in family, school, and social activities.

■ Striving for identity and independence may lead adolescents to take part in high-risk activities (e.g., drug use, unprotected sex, smoking, delinquent behaviors) that may lead to mental health problems.

■ Poverty, homelessness, abuse, neglect, and parental substance abuse all create conditions that undermine a child's ability to make normal developmental gains and contribute to vulnerability for various emotional and behavioral problems.

■ Children who experience disrupted attachments because of out-of-home placements may have difficulty forming close relationships with their new parents and trusting others.

■ Family support services and early intervention programs are designed to prevent removal of the child from the family because of abuse or neglect and to keep a strong, nurturing family system.

■ Psychoeducational approaches, such as training opportunities, group experiences, and **bibliotherapy**, provide children and families with the information and skills to promote their own mental health.

CRITICAL THINKING CHALLENGES

1. Analyze a case of a family that is grieving a loss and compare the parents' and children's reactions. Include an evaluation of how each child's reactions differ, depending on their developmental level.

2. Watch a movie or read a book that provides a child's view of death, divorce, or some other loss and consider how adults may be insensitive to the child's reactions.

3. Examine your own developmental history and pinpoint periods when stressful life events might have increased the risk for emotional problems for you or other family members. What protective factors in your own personality and coping skills and in the environment around you helped you to maintain your good mental health?

4. What aspects of life are more stressful for children than for adults? (i.e., How is it different to experience life as a child?)

5. Examine how your own social and cultural background may either facilitate or create barriers to your ability to interact with families from other ethnic groups or those who are poor or homeless.

6. Allow yourself to reflect on how your own judgmental attitudes might interfere with your ability to communicate effectively with families who have abused or neglected their children.

7. Why is the process of normalization of feelings such a powerful intervention with children and families? What kinds of mental health issues, developmental processes, or both would benefit from teaching related to normal reactions? How can nurses incorporate this kind of intervention into their practice roles?

8. How can nurses expand their roles to have maximal effects on primary, secondary, and tertiary mental health intervention with children and families?

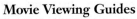

Movie Viewing Guides

Precious: 2009. This powerful and disturbing movie portrays the life of an African American adolescent girl who is physically, sexually, and emotionally abused by her family. It shows the devastating effects of abuse, poverty, substandard schooling, and family dysfunction, at the same time conveying hope through this girl's amazing resilience.

VIEWING POINTS: Give some examples of how Precious uses dissociation to cope with her abuse. What are some of the effective and ineffective interventions illustrated by the professionals interacting with Precious? Explain how Precious illustrates resilience.

Because of Winn Dixie: 2005. This is a heart-rending account of Opal, a 10-year-old girl who overcomes her loneliness after moving to a small town by adopting a dog and reaching out to people in her new community. The movie explores such issues as parental separation, single parenting, substance abuse, and childhood grieving.

VIEWING POINTS: Describe how Opal's grieving process is typical of school-aged children and how it differs from that of her father. What aspects of her coping show resilience? Explain the importance of Opal's dog, Winn Dixie, in the healing process for this family. Discuss how pets may play a key role in the mental health of children. How is the relationship with a pet similar and different from the role of a sibling?

REFERENCES

Anthony, K. K., Gil, K. M., & Schanberg, L. E. (2003). Parental perceptions of child vulnerability in children with chronic illness. *Journal of Pediatric Psychology, 28*(3), 185–190.

Askew, M., & Byrne, M. W. (2009). Biopsychosocial approach to treating self-injurious behaviors: An adolescent case study. *Journal of Child and Adolescent Psychiatric Nursing, 22*(3), 115–119.

Bank, S., & Kahn, M. D. (2014). Intense sibling loyalties. In M. E. Lamb, & B. Sutton-Smith (Eds.), *Sibling relationships: Their nature and significance across the lifespan*. Lawrence.

Bertram, J. (2018). Care planning and decision-making for youth with mental health needs in the foster care system. *Archives of Psychiatric Nursing, 32*, 707–722.

Bloomquist, M. L. (2013). *The practitioner guide to skills training for struggling kids*. Guilford Press.

Bojanowski, S., Gotti, E. G., Wanowski, N., Nisslein, J., & Lemkuhl, U. (2020). Sibling relationships of children and adolescents with mental disorders – Resource or risk factor? *Journal of Family Psychology, 34*(8), 918–926. https://doi.org/10.1037/fam0000721

Bowlby, J. (1960). Grief and mourning in infancy and early childhood. *Psychoanalytic Study of the Child, 15*, 9–52.

Browning, S., & Artelt, E. (2014). "Why are some stepfamilies vulnerable?" In S. Browning & E. Artelt (Eds.), *Stepfamily therapy: A 10-step clinical approach* (pp. 35–68). American Psychological Association.

Bruskas, D. (2008). Children in foster care: A vulnerable population at risk. *Journal of Child and Adolescent Psychiatric Nursing, 21*(2), 70–77.

Bugge, K. E., Darbyshire, P., Rokholt, E. G., Haugstvedt, K. T. S., & Helseth, S. (2014). Young children's grief: Parents' understanding and coping. *Death Studies, 38*(1), 36–43.

Carpenter, L. M., & Hubbard, G. B. (2014). Cyberbullying: Implications for the psychiatric nurse practitioner. *Journal of Child and Adolescent Psychiatric Nursing, 27*(3), 142–148.

Dashiff, C., DiMicco, W., Myers, B., & Sheppard, K. (2009). Poverty and adolescent mental health. *Journal of Child and Adolescent Psychiatric Nursing, 22*(1), 23–32.

Davies, P. T., Parry, L. Q., Bascoe, S. M., Martin, M. J., & Cummings, E. M. (2019). Children's vulnerability to interparental conflict: The protective role of sibling relationship quality. *Child Development, 90*, 2118–2134.

Deering, C. G., & Cody, D. J. (2002). Communicating effectively with children and adolescents. *American Journal of Nursing, 102*(3), 34–42.

Demir-Dagnas, T. (2020). Parental divorce, parent-child ties, and health: Explaining long-term age differences in vulnerability. *Marriage & Family Review*. https://doi.org/10.1080/01494929.2020.1754318

Duncan, A. F., & Caughy, M. O. (2009). Parenting style and the vulnerable child syndrome. *Journal of Child and Adolescent Psychiatric Nursing, 22*(4), 228–234.

Fopma-Loy, J. (2000). Peer rejection and neglect of latency age children: Pathways and group psychotherapy model. *Journal of Child and Adolescent Psychiatric Nursing, 13*(1), 29–38.

Gance-Cleveland, B., & Mays, M. Z. (2008). School-based support groups for adolescents with a substance-abusing parent. *Journal of the American Psychiatric Nurses Association, 14*(4), 297–309.

Garcia-Dia, M. J., DiNapoli, J. M., Garcia-Ona, L., Jakubowski, R., & O'Flaherty, D. (2013). Concept analysis: Resilience. *Archives of Psychiatric Nursing, 27*(6), 264–270.

Havermans, N., Botterman, S., & Matthijs, K. (2014). Family resources as mediators in the relation between divorce and children's school engagement. *The Social Science Journal, 51*(4), 564–579.

Hays-Grudo, J., & Morris, A. S. (2020). *Adverse and protective childhood experiences: A developmental perspective.* American Psychological Association.

Heckman, J. J. (2013). *Giving kids a fair chance.* MIT Press.

Hensley, V. (2013). Childhood bullying: A review and implications for healthcare professionals. *Nursing Clinics of North America, 48*(2), 203–213.

Hetherington, E. M., & Kelly, J. (2002). *For better or for worse: Divorce reconsidered.* W. W. Norton.

Hughes, E., Baca, E., Mahmoud, K. F., Edwards, A., Griffith, K. J., & Matthews, E. (2019). Nurses and fetal alcohol spectrum disorders prevention. *Issues in Mental Health Nursing, 40*(6), 621–625.

Hymel, S., & Swearer, S. M. (2015). Four decades of research on school bullying: An introduction. *American Psychologist, 70*(4), 293–299.

Kelly, J. (2012). Risk and protective factors associated with child and adolescent adjustment following separation and divorce: Social science applications. In K. Kuehnle & L. Drozd (Eds.), *Parenting plan evaluations: Applied research for the family court* (pp. 49–84). Oxford, New York: Oxford University Press.

Kolak, A. M., & Volling, B. L. (2013). Coparenting moderates the association between firstborn children's temperament and problem behavior across the transition to siblinghood. *Journal of Family Psychology, 27*(3), 355–364.

Kolko, D. J., & Berkout, O. V. (2017) Child physical abuse. In S. N. Gold (Ed.), *APA handbook of trauma psychology* (Vol. 1, Chap. 17, pp. 99–115). APA.

Kramer, L., & Ramsburg, D. (2002). Advice given to parents on welcoming a second child: A critical review. *Family Relations: Interdisciplinary Journal of Applied Family Studies, 51*(1), 2–14.

Kvarme, L. G., Helseth, S., Sorum, R., Luth-Hansen, V., Haugland, S., & Natvig, G. K. (2010). The effect of a solution-focused approach to improve self-efficacy in socially withdrawn school children: A non-randomized controlled trial. *International Journal of Nursing Studies, 47*(11), 1389–1396.

Lloyd-Richardson, E., Hasking, P., Lewis, S., Hamza, C., McAllister, M., Baetens, I., & Muehlenkamp, J. (2020). Addressing self-injury in schools, Part 1: Understanding nonsuicidal self-injury and the importance of respectful curiosity in supporting youth who engage in self-injury. *NASN School Nurse, 35*(2), 92–98.

Lytje, M. (2017). Toward a model of loss navigation in adolescence. *Death Studies, 41*(5), 291–302.

Ma, N., Roberts, R., Winefield, H., & Furber, G. (2015). The prevalence of psychopathology in siblings of children with mental health problems: A 20-year systematic review. *Child Psychiatry and Human Development, 46*(1), 130–149.

Mechling, B. M., Ahern, N. R., & Palumbo, R. (2018). Applying ambiguous loss theory to children of parents with an opioid use disorder. *Journal of Child and Adolescent Psychiatric Nursing, 31*(2–3), 53–60.

Miller-Smith, M. (2020). *Families and children living in poverty.* Cognella.

Nadelman, L., & Begun, A. (2014). The effect of the newborn on the older sibling: Mothers' questionnaire. In M. Lamb & B. Sutton-Smith (Eds.), *Sibling relationships: Their nature and significance across the lifespan,* pp. 13–37. Lawrence Erlbaum.

Nickerson, A. B. (2019). Preventing and intervening with bullying in schools: A framework for evidence-based practice. *School Mental Health, 11,* 15–28.

Olweus, D. (2003). A profile of bullying at school. *Educational Leadership, 60*(6), 12–17.

Ritter, J., Stewart, M., Bernet, C., Coe, M., & Brown, S. A. (2002). Effects of childhood exposure to familial alcoholism and family violence on adolescent substance use, conduct problems, and self-esteem. *Journal of Traumatic Stress, 15*(2), 113–122.

Rodkin, P. C., & Hodges, E. V. (2003). Bullies and victims in the peer ecology: Four questions for psychologists and school professionals. *School Psychology Review, 32*(3), 384–400.

Ryan, R. M., & Claessens, A. (2013). Associations between family structure changes and children's behavior problems: The mediating effects of timing and marital birth. *Developmental Psychology, 40*(7), 1219–1231.

Sapp, A. J., & Hooten, P. (2019). Working with families impacted by the opioid crisis: Education, best practices, and hope. *Archives of Psychiatric Nursing, 33*(5), 3–8.

Scribano, P. V. (2010). Prevention strategies in child maltreatment. *Current Opinion in Pediatrics, 22*(5), 616–620.

Secinti, E., Thompson, E. J., Richards, M., & Gaysina, D. (2017). Research review: Childhood chronic physical illness and adult emotional health- A systematic review and mata-analysis. *Journal of Child Psychology and Psychiatry, 58*(7), 753–769.

Steinberg, L. (2019). *Adolescence* (12th ed.). McGraw-Hill.

Straussner, S. L. A., & Fewell, C. F. (2011). *Children of substance-abusing parents: Dynamics and treatment.*

Turnbull, A. P., Summers, J. A., Turnbull, R., Brotherson, M. J., Winton, P., Roberts, R., Snyder, P., McWilliam, R., Chandler, L., Schrandt, S., Stowe, M., Bruder, M. B., Divenere, N., Epley, P., Hornback, M., Huff, B., Miksch, P., Mitchell, L., Sharp, L., & Stroup-Rentier, V. (2007). Family supports and services in early intervention: A bold vision. *Journal of Early Intervention, 29*(3), 187–206.

Wong, C. F., Clark, L. F., & Marlotte, L. (2016). The impact of specific and complex trauma on the mental health of homeless youth. *Journal of Interpersonal Violence, 31*(5), 831.

Worden, J. W. (2018). *Grief counseling and grief therapy: A handbook for the mental health practitioner* (5th ed.). Springer.

Yoon, S., Howell, K., Dillard, R., McCarthy, K. S., Napier, T. R., & Pei, F. (2019). Resilience following child maltreatment: Definitional considerations and developmental variations. *Trauma, Violence & Abuse, 11.* https://doi.org/10.1177/1524838019869094

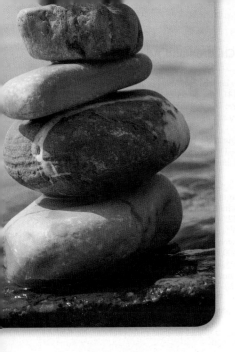

17
Mental Health Promotion for Young and Middle-Aged Adults

Mary Ann Boyd

KEYCONCEPTS

- middle adulthood
- young adulthood

LEARNING OBJECTIVES

After studying this chapter, you will be able to:

1. Describe psychosocial challenges common to young and middle-aged adults.

2. Identify risk factors related to psychopathology in young and middle-aged adults.

3. Describe protective factors in the mental health promotion of young and middle-aged adults.

4. Analyze the role of the nurse in mental health promotion for young and middle-aged adults.

KEY TERMS

- Empty nest • Informal caregivers • Protective factors • Risk factors • Sandwich generation

INTRODUCTION

Young adulthood and middle adulthood are relatively new concepts. In 1900, life expectancy was age 47 (Centers for Diseases Control and Prevention [CDC], 2010). As life expectancy increased, the middle-aged adult emerged. In 2020, life expectancy is averaging 77.8 years ranging from 72 years for Black Americans to 79.9 years for Hispanic Americans (Arias et al., 2021).

Healthy lifestyles, medical advances, and economic success contributed to longevity. U.S. families have achieved unprecedented economic stability that provides for long periods of development. Technologic advances such as economic development, improved nutrition, public health control of infectious diseases, access to health care, and other modern developments have resulted in the lengthening of the life span chronologically in the developed world. This extended adulthood provides for an increased range of life choices, such as education; job selection; and

lifestyle, including relationships, marriage, and family. Such advances do not exist worldwide because of the differences in the chronologic life span in different societies. In many nondeveloped areas, the life span is characterized by a brief childhood followed by a mature adulthood that evolves quickly into old age.

MENTAL HEALTH IN YOUNG AND MIDDLE ADULTHOOD

Psychological changes in adulthood occur slowly and subtly with age and experience, not in a fixed stepwise manner. Until the late 1900s, adult development was viewed as a relatively stationary plateau with the rapid and complex changes of childhood and adolescence forming one steep side and the declining changes of old age the other. Any rigid stage theory of adult life is oversimplifying young and middle adulthood development.

Young and middle adulthood development is viewed as dynamic and multifaceted (Wahl & Kruse, 2005).

The developmental issues reported by young adults, middle-aged adults, and older adults are recurrent, taking new forms as their lives unfold. The developmental concepts of identity, intimacy, and generativity may have their initial blooming during adolescence, young adulthood, and middle age, but they continue to be renegotiated in the face of life stresses such as unemployment and changes in family structure (see Chapter 7).

> **KEYCONCEPT** The generally accepted age range for **young adulthood** is from 18 to 44 years. **Middle adulthood** spans the period from approximately 45 to 65 years.

Chronologic age is also losing its customary social meaning, resulting in a more fluid life cycle. Traditional notions of young adulthood as a time of leaving the parental home and establishing an independent career and family life, of college education taking place during late adolescence, or of the middle adulthood parents facing the **"empty nest"**—a home devoid of children and caregiving responsibilities—are being replaced with fewer age-defined life roles.

The timing of life events such as education, marriage, childrearing, career development, and retirement is becoming less regular, and more alternatives are tolerated by society. Some people never marry, and others retire very early. Many young adults now remain in their parents' homes while they pursue their professional education rather than strike out on their own, as was customary in previous generations. Their middle adulthood parents are often already caring for their own parents, creating the **sandwich generation**, with its responsibilities toward the older generation above and two generations of children below them. Many women choose to marry and establish a family and then return to finish their college education when their children start school. See Table 17.1 for a breakdown of marital status in the U.S. adult population.

TABLE 17.1	MARITAL STATUS OF THE U.S. ADULT POPULATION OVER THE AGE OF 15 YEARS
Marital Status	**Percent of Adult Population**
Married	50.4
Widowed	5.6
Divorced	9.7
Separated	1.9
Never married	32.4

U.S. Census Bureau. (2016). America's families and living arrangements: 2019. https://www.census.gov/search-results.html?q=America%27s+Families+and+Living+Arrangements&page=1&stateGeo=none&searchtype=web&cssp=SERP&_charset_=UTF-8

COMMON CHALLENGES IN ADULTHOOD

Young and middle adulthood are marked by many significant life events. Among them are leaving the primary family home for the first time, getting married (or not), and taking on new caregiving responsibilities. For adults in a breadwinning role, the prospect of unemployment can also present a major life challenge that affects their ability to be effective in other life roles.

Changes in Family Structure

The young adult and middle adulthood years are characterized by changes in family structures. Older adolescents finish school and often leave home, which alters the primary family structure. Marriage establishes new roles for adults who previously lived by themselves or their parents. The arrival of children changes the structure and dynamics of the newly formed family. These are all normal developmental events, but they can also lead to mental distress, physical problems, and social alienation.

Married adults are healthier than those in other non-married groups. Married adults are least likely to experience health problems and least likely to engage in risky health behaviors with one exception: middle adulthood married men have the highest rate of overweight or obesity. Widowed, divorced, or separated adults are more likely to experience serious psychological distress than married adults. In a dysfunctional marriage, problematic eating behaviors increase health problems (Roberson et al., 2018).

The prevalence of physical inactivity in leisure time, current cigarette smoking, and heavier drinking of alcohol is higher in those who are widowed, divorced, separated, never married, or living with a partner (Schoenborn et al., 2018). Rates of separation or divorce are at least twice as high for those with almost any psychiatric disorder as for those without disorder.

Men and women are marrying later than in the 1990s. In 2019, the median age of men who marry for the first time was 30.1 and for women 28.3 years (Statista Research Department, 2021). Men and women who marry in the teen years have the highest probability of divorce, whereas individuals with a higher education are more likely to be married. The percentage of couples who cohabitate decreases as education increases (Lamidi et al., 2019).

There is an emerging trend for fewer women to marry and, at the same time, there is an increase in the percentage of women who cohabitate (Lamidi et al., 2019). There are an increasing number of women who never marry. The proportion of pregnancies occurring in women of at least 35 years of age has increased from 6.2% in 1980 to 22.3% in 2016 (Heazell et al., 2018).

Caring for Others

In 2019, 73.5 million children (younger than the age of 18 years) resided in the United States, up from 64 million in 1990. Most of these children (70%) lived with two parents and approximately 21% lived with only their mother, 4% lived with only their father, and another 3% lived in households with neither parent present. Within these numbers, there are further variations in ethnic groups. Seventy-eight percent of White, non-Hispanic, 70% of Hispanic, and 42% of Black children lived with two parents in 2015 (U.S. Census Bureau, 2019).

Whether functioning in a two-parent or single-parent home, parents who work out of the home must provide for the care and safety of their children during their absence. Childcare outside the home is often disproportionately expensive compared to income and often is not available for parents working evenings, nights, holidays, or weekends and during periods of illness and other crises. Federal support to single-parent families is limited. Working parents could formerly rely on their own parents and other family members to assist with childcare, but today many parents have no family available locally or are also serving as caretakers to family members in addition to their children.

In fact, **informal caregivers**, unpaid individuals who provide care, are the largest source of long-term care services in the United States. It is estimated that more than 47.9 million people provide care to an adult or child, with about 41.8 million of these Americans providing unpaid care to an adult age 50 or older in the last 12 months. Although men are increasingly becoming more involved in caregiving, women comprise the majority and perform the more difficult tasks of caregiving. The duration of caregiving spans from less than a year to more than 40 years, with an average duration of 4.5 years (National Alliance for Caregiving, 2020).

Caregivers are under considerable stress and often neglect their physical and mental health needs. Caregivers also report higher levels of loneliness, anxiety and depressive symptoms, and other mental health problems than non-caregiving peers. In turn, altered physical and mental health reduces the quality, satisfaction, and ability to cope with daily stresses related to caregiving (National Alliance for Caregiving, 2020).

Unemployment

Employment is an important societal value and thus serves as a source of economic, social, and emotional stability and self-esteem. Young and middle-adulthood adults seek and maintain employment that maintains their lifestyle and provides for their children. In a society that is consumer driven, the ability to generate resources becomes critical. Yet shifts in the ownership and organizational structure of companies, downsizing, and the job market's ever-changing demands for workers with particular skills make employment stability questionable, both now and in the future. Career changes and the continuing necessity of training for new positions are now the norm.

In 2020, the United States began facing an economic recession resulting in the coronavirus disease 2019 (COVID-19) pandemic. The unemployment rate jumped to over 14% in spring and by mid 2020, the rate dropped to over 10%, up 3.7% a year earlier. The minority population was especially hit hard, with the unemployment rate of Blacks or African Americans and Hispanics or Latinxs at over 18%. Generally, those with limited education and nonskilled workers remain at special risk for low wages and unemployment (U.S. Bureau of Labor Statistics, 2020).

COVID-19 put single mothers in an impossible situation. Low-income and single mothers often are employed in low-wage jobs, which disappeared. During the national shutdown of businesses, 28% of single mothers lost their jobs. Then as the restrictions on businesses eased with stay-at-home orders, single mothers were faced with returning to work or staying at home with their children who were no longer in school or daycare. Single mothers are another group at high risk for low wages and unemployment.

Within the cohort of unemployed workers, there are twice as many people with mental disorders. Of those with a mental illness who are working, many are underemployed; about 70% who hold college degrees earn less than $10 per hour (NAMI, 2014; SAMSHA, 2014).

MENTAL DISORDERS IN YOUNG AND MIDDLE ADULTHOOD

The great majority of people experience their first diagnostic symptoms of mental illness during late adolescence or early adulthood. By far, the highest rates of mental disorder occur among young adults. Late-life onset of mental disorder (older than age 40 years) is relatively rare, with the exception of cognitive impairment, which typically occurs past the age of 70 years. Recent research suggests that 1 in 5 adults will experience a mental disorder in their lifetime and that within a year, 1 in 25 will experience serious mental illness in the United States (NAMI, 2020).

Changes in the biologic, psychological, and social domains can create a matrix of stress that may foster mental disorder. The vast majority of people with mental disorders do not come to the attention of the mental health system. In fact, fewer than half of those with mental disorders receive any kind of treatment from mental health professionals (Mental Health America, 2020).

RISK FACTORS FOR YOUNG AND MIDDLE ADULTHOOD PSYCHOPATHOLOGY

Mental health promotion and illness prevention are driven by cultivating an awareness of personal risk factors for mental illness and modifying those that can be changed. Specific **risk factors,** or characteristics that increase the likelihood of developing a disorder, can contribute to poor mental health and influence the development of a mental disorder. Risk factors do not cause the disorder or problem and are not symptoms of the illness but are factors that influence the likelihood that the symptoms will appear. The existence of a risk factor does not always mean the person will get the disorder or disease; it just increases the chances. There are many different kinds of risk factors, including genetic, biologic, environmental, cultural, and occupational. Even gender is a risk factor for some disorders (e.g., more women experience depression than men) (see Chapter 25). In general, gender, age, unemployment, and lower education are risk factors associated with mental illness.

Biologic Risk Factors

The biologic functioning of young versus middle-aged adults is a contrast between optimally running physiologic systems and those showing definite signs of wear and inefficiency. Of course, there are wide variations in the health of the various systems within each stage, with some young adults more physiologically and functionally compromised than their middle adulthood counterparts. Most physical and mental systems have completed development by the time an individual reaches young adulthood. In general, the optimal health state of young adults begins to show changes around the age of 30 years. The perception of these physical changes often makes individuals aware of their aging process and may result in threats to bodily integrity and self-esteem. This section reviews the primary changes in the health of physiologic symptoms and possible mental health implications.

Skin

The most obvious change in physical appearance starts with the skin. Although the young adult's skin is smooth and taut, by late young adulthood, the skin begins to lose moisture and tone, and wrinkles develop. Self-esteem issues can erupt as the skin ages, especially for women.

Cardiovascular and Respiratory Systems

Maximum cardiac output is reached between 20 and 30 years of age. Thereafter, blood pressure and cholesterol levels gradually increase. Although men are especially prone to cardiovascular disease in middle age because of testosterone levels, women are not exempt from risk

of heart disease. In a parallel manner, respiratory function also decreases with age. After the age of 30 years, maximum breathing capacity slowly decreases and may be reduced up to 75% compared with during young adulthood. Such changes are compounded if the individual smoked throughout adulthood. Alterations in cardiac and respiratory efficiency may result in limited energy for daily tasks and preference for lower activity levels, which makes exercise less of an enjoyable activity (Hart & Zernicke, 2020).

Sensory Function

Sensory functions are also compromised as an individual moves from young into middle adulthood. Although the visual sense is at its peak in early young adulthood, the lenses of the eyes gradually lose their elasticity around the age of 30 years, and corrective lenses may be necessary. Such changes may result in issues regarding physical appearance that may affect self-esteem. Hearing is optimal in young adulthood, but middle age brings changes in the bones of the inner ear and auditory nerve, resulting in the gradual inability to hear high-pitched tones and detect certain consonants. Such alterations in hearing may also present issues related to body integrity.

Neurologic System

In middle age, brain structural changes are minimal. Although neurons are gradually being lost, changes in cognition are not evident. There may be some slowing of speed of reflexes because of small changes in nerve conduction speed during middle age.

Basal Metabolic Rate

Basal metabolic rate is at maximum functional capacity at the age of 30 years and then gradually decreases at a rate of 2% per decade, related to a gradual loss in highly physiologically active muscle mass. The ratio of fat tissue to lean body mass gradually increases, which may result in weight gain if calories are not restricted. There is currently an epidemic of obesity within the United States because of poor nutrition and low activity levels. Weight gain also raises concerns about changes in physical attractiveness, especially in women. It is also related to decreased cardiac and respiratory efficiency, which makes exercise less of a preferred activity (Patnode et al., 2017).

Sexual and Reproductive Functioning

Concerns about changing physical appearance may also be tied to reactions to changes in sexual functioning. In middle-aged men, testosterone production decreases, resulting in a lower sex drive, more time needed to achieve erection, and production of fewer sperm cells. Men whose sense of self was dependent on the level of sexual functioning typical of young adulthood may experience anxiety over such changes. Diminishing estrogen levels in middle age in women result in the cessation of menses and capacity for pregnancy. The beginning of menopause may bring unpleasant symptoms such as hot flashes, night sweats, fatigue, and nausea. However, most women experience menopause as a relief from menses, fluctuating hormone levels, and the possibility of pregnancy. Women whose view of self was based on sexual characteristics may also be prone to anxiety because of these changes.

Psychosocial Risk Factors

Any of the common challenges of adulthood previously discussed such as unemployment, changing family structure, and caregiving may serve as risks factors for mental disorders. These more general problems reveal underlying risk factors that have shown to be common in the development of mental disorders. Also, risk factors rarely occur in isolation but tend to cluster because one may bring about another, and they influence each other.

Age

The majority of mental disorders occur among young adults and appear to be less common with increasing age. The first symptoms may occur in childhood but are usually evident in late adolescence and early middle adulthood. Such symptoms may be partially tied to the increasing demands for independence and social responsibility that Western society places on developing individuals. As some adults get older, they may experience decreasing stress because of learning to cope more efficiently.

Marital Status

Individuals who are happily married experience higher rates of both physical and mental health compared with those who are single, separated, or divorced. Marriage may serve as a general marker for psychological health and the ability to connect with larger social networks. In contrast, an unhappy marriage can have negative health effects. Unmarried individuals may experience positive physical and mental health especially if they are not isolated from others and have support from a larger social system (Pandey et al., 2019; Robles, 2014).

Unemployment and Other Job Stresses

In this consumer-oriented society, economic stability is a major value. Unemployment is a larger indicator of such socioeconomically related variables such as those experiencing poverty, lack of education, and the ability to obtain economic power within the larger social system. This creates an environment of stress that may contribute to the development of mental disorder or may indicate the negative effect that mental disorder has had on obtaining the education and independence necessary for obtaining job security and advancement. Employment rates for individuals with mental illnesses are notoriously low. Employment declined from 23% in 2003 to 17.8% in 2012. Most adults with a mental disorder want to work and approximately 6 out of 10 can work with the proper supports (NAMI, 2014).

Conversely, employment has its own set of stresses. Many people with low-paying jobs work two jobs, often going directly from one job to another. Shift work causes changes in circadian rhythms and sleep patterns, leading to an increase in stress. Interpersonal problems with coworkers can lead to emotional distress. Challenges even arise related to the different learning styles and career expectations of workers of different ages and backgrounds or who are reentering the workforce.

Gender

Women come to the attention of the mental health system because of their greater awareness of health issues and willingness to seek interventions. However, women also differ in the types of mental disorders that they show. Whereas women are more prone to anxiety and depression, men tend to show problems with impulse control that result in alcohol use disorder and substance use disorder.

History of Child Abuse

Being abused as a child increases the risk of a mental disorder as an adult. Data from a national survey indicated that there are long-term consequences of early childhood abuse. Reported emotional abuse was associated with lower personal control, which in turn leads to lower health ratings (Li et al., 2016).

Prior Mental Disorder

Mental illness tends to be a chronic disorder with symptoms manifesting fairly early in life. Research has shown that mental illness arising in childhood and adolescence predicts further disorder in later years. Because most mental disorders are never cured, the existence of prior symptoms or full-blown disorder is a risk for mental illness at later periods in life. Increased stress provides the ground for the current emergence of symptoms of mental disorders that may have appeared to be in remission (Li et al., 2016).

Coping

Although the quality of coping is important in the reduction of stress, little is known about the continuity and changes in coping styles over the life span. Because past behavior is the best predictor of future behavior, it would appear that coping styles used in the past would be repeated in the present time. The quality of such coping would determine how well stress is handled in the present and sets the stage for continued positive outcomes or more problems in the future.

There is an absence of epidemiologic studies that directly compare adult life stages according to mental health variables such as stress and coping. An exception is the Midlife Development in the United States (MIDUS) Study, which included more than 7,000 subjects between 25 and 74 years of age and those at midlife (defined as 40–60 years). The results of this study that compared young and middle-aged adults suggest that the process of coping improves in quality as life and satisfaction with life. A longitudinal follow-up of MIDUS respondents occurred over 2002 to 2006 and 2011 to 2016. The purposes of the follow-up were to repeat the assessments obtained in the original study and to expand into other areas of biologic and neurologic assessments. There are hundreds of research publications generated from this study. See Box 17.1 for an example.

Well-Being

Mental, physical, and social well-being is an indicator of positive functioning. As part of the Behavioral Risk Factor Surveillance System, a national survey that monitors behaviors that place individuals at risk for health problems and mental, physical, and social well-being was reported in three states. Most adults were satisfied with their work, neighborhood, and education but well-being varied by marital status, health, chronic conditions, and disability. People with disabilities, current smokers, and those who were unemployed or unable to work had low mental well-being (Kobau et al., 2013). In a related study, the prevalence of minor and major depression among pregnant women in the United States was compared. Major depression was not greater among pregnant women than nonpregnant women, but the prevalence of minor depression was greater among pregnant women (Ashley et al., 2015).

Lack of Health Promotion Behaviors

People with mental disorders in young adulthood and middle age appear to lack basic health promotion behaviors. This lack results in high rates of physical illness and premature mortality compared with the general population. This includes low levels of awareness about physical and mental health issues, smoking, poor quality diets, lack of exercise, lack of leisure activities and contact with friends, negative attitudes toward help seeking, and stigma associated with mental health problems (Ashdown-Franks et al., 2020).

> **NCLEXNOTE** People with mental disorders frequently neglect their physical health and have premature mortality. Assessment of physical health and health-promoting activities is important in the care of people with mental disorders because of their high rate of smoking, lack of physical activity, and resistance to seeking help for physical concerns.

Parenting Stress

Young adults often find that the addition of children to the family, particularly the birth of the second child, tends to insulate the nuclear family from larger social networks. The responsibilities and time constraints involved in rearing small children may limit the couple's worldview to the home, and definitions of self may be constricted to the activities of the nuclear family. However, as children grow and create their own lives, the social connectedness of the parents tends to expand. By middle age, couples may anticipate the emancipation of their children and may entertain more options for socializing with other people.

Factors Associated with Suicide

Suicidal ideation and suicide were serious public health problems in the United States before the COVID-19 pandemic (see Chapter 22). The mental health challenges cause the disease, and mitigation activities such as physical distancing and stay-at-home orders made

---

BOX 17.1

Adverse Childhood Experiences and Adult Coping Strategies

Sheffler, J. L., Piazza, J. R., Quinn, J. M., Sachs-Ericsson, N. J., & Stanley, I. H. (2019). Adverse childhood experiences and coping strategies: Identifying pathways to resiliency in adulthood. Anxiety, Stress, and Coping, 32(5), 594–609. https://doi.org/10.1080/10615806.2019.1638699

THE QUESTION: Do coping strategies facilitate the link between adverse childhood experiences (ACEs) and adult psychiatric and physical health outcomes?

METHODS: This study included wave I (n = 7,108), wave II (N = 4,963), and wave III (N = 3,294) of the MIDUS survey. Seven adverse events were related to coping strategies at the 20-year follow-up.

FINDINGS: Wave I adverse ACEs were associated with worse psychiatric and physical health outcomes. At Wave II, the adverse childhood events were associated with greater use of avoidant emotion-focused coping and lower use of problem-focused strategies.

IMPLICATIONS FOR NURSING: Learning coping strategies may be important for promoting mental and physical health in children who have had ACEs.

the problems worse. In a large study during June 2020, 5,412 adults completed a web-based survey related to mental health conditions associated with COVID-19. Approximately twice as many reported serious considerations of suicide during the last 30 days compared with adults answering this same question in the United States in 2018. The percentage of respondents who reported having seriously considered suicide in the 30 days before completing the survey (10.7%) was significantly higher among respondents aged 18 to 24 years (25.5%) and minority racial/ethnic groups (Hispanic respondents [18.6%], non-Hispanic Black respondents [15.1%], self-reported unpaid caregivers for adults [30.7%], and essential workers [21.7%]) (Czeisler et al., 2020).

PROTECTIVE FACTORS

In contrast to risk factors, **protective factors** are characteristics that reduce the probability that a person will develop a mental health disorder or problem or decrease the severity of existing problems. Common protective factors exist in multiple contexts—families, communities, and society. All of these contexts should be considered when promoting mental health. For example, parental involvement can help combat drug abuse in their children, but a strong school policy is also needed. In addition, other community resources must be used to support the drug-free community environment. Targeting only one context is unlikely to make a lasting impact.

INTERVENTION APPROACHES

Many nursing interventions are effective in helping young and middle-aged adults achieve greater mental health. Whereas some are geared toward helping adults cope with the challenges typical of this period of life, others are more specifically designed toward preventing depression and suicide. Another aspect of intervention is helping adults overcome societal pressures that might prevent them from seeking care in the first place.

Mental Health Promotion

The psychiatric mental health nurse supports the young and middle-aged adult through the developmental journey of life. Stresses associated with balancing the psychosocial demands and the adjustment to changes in the biologic, psychological, and social domains can be overwhelming. Validation and education are important interventions in helping these individuals cope with these changes (see Chapter 18).

A person's mental health can be challenged by a variety of factors: Biologic changes or illnesses, psychological

pressures, and interpersonal tensions are only a few. Developing coping strategies to eliminate or reduce the impact of these potentially destructive factors is a part of normal growth and development. In addition, sustaining positive health behaviors such as relaxation, proper nutrition, adequate sleep, regular exercise, and forming a network of trusting relationships can support one's mental health. Mental health promotion focuses on increasing the individual's physical, mental, emotional, and social competencies to increase well-being and actualize potential.

Social Support During Life Transitions

Young and middle-aged adults are prone to many life transitions: entrance into the workforce, job loss, career change, separation, divorce, the birth of children and their eventual leaving home, and changes in health status. Middle-aged adults are also subject to watching their parents' age and possibly lose independence. Both young and middle adults can benefit from education about coping with the stresses involved with such transitions, linking with sources of social support, and anticipating the changes in role and adjustment.

Lifestyle Support

Although health may be at its maximum during the young adult years, changes in bodily appearance and function become evident by the age of 30 years and become more pronounced as middle age begins. Although such changes are inevitable, their magnitude can be tempered by health promotion activities such as attention to regular exercise, good nutrition, adequate sleep, health screening, relaxation, leisure, and other forms of stress management. The young adult years are times of learning positive coping strategies for the stresses inherent to personal, marital, family, and occupational life. Such learning can be enhanced by a social support network consisting of people who are currently undergoing such stresses as well as older people who have the perspective and experience in handling these domains of life. These networks can be informal, such as regular contact with a circle of friends, or more formal, such as support groups sponsored by social, occupational, and religious organizations. A sense of belonging and availability of social support is important for the maintenance of health and recovery from illness of all kinds.

Self-Care Enhancement

The latter part of young adulthood and middle age are times when chronic illnesses such as hypertension, heart disease, and arthritis may become evident. Symptoms of mental disorders may have arisen earlier in life but require continuous care because of their chronic and episodic nature. It is important for both young and middle-aged adults to be educated about the physiologic aspects of such disorders, the advances in medications used in treating them, possible side effects, the importance of medication adherence, lifestyle changes that can be instituted to control such disorders, and the possible use of complementary healing methods (e.g., massage, meditation). Such strategies require a good relationship with a health care provider as well as initiative from individuals to contributing to their own care through seeking and evaluating information available in the media, on the Internet, or from advocacy groups.

Prevention of Depression and Suicide

Suicide is the 10th leading cause of death for all ages in the United States but ranks as the 2nd leading cause of death for people of ages 10 to 34 and the 4th leading cause for people of ages 35 to 54. The suicide rate is consistently higher for males than females. Suicide rates are increasing in most rural counties for both males and females (Hedegaard et al., 2020).

Symptoms of most psychiatric disorders have made their appearance by the time an individual enters young adulthood. In particular, mood disorders may first arise during the young adult years and continue through middle age and older adulthood. Because depression is a significant precipitating factor for suicide, early detection and intervention are critical for managing mood disorders and preventing suicide. Routine screening for depression and associated substance abuse is common in primary care settings.

Reducing the Stigma of Mental Health Treatment

Although mental disorders are common within the community and the rate of treatment has risen over the past 20 years, more than half of people do not receive mental health treatment of any kind. Part of this lack of attention is certainly because of the lack of available treatment in many communities (e.g., rural areas), but another major factor is the stigma that continues to be associated with mental illness and seeking help for mental health problems. Organizations such as the National Alliance on Mental Illness have spearheaded the movement toward viewing mental disorders as biologically based and devoid of moral implications, putting them on par with physical disorders. National Alliance on Mental Illness is an important organization for obtaining information, support, and referrals for treatment for individuals with mental disorders as well as their families.

The Future of Mental Health for Young and Middle-Aged Adults

Young adulthood and middle age can be some of the most productive periods in life. They can also be the most stressful and debilitating because of the rapid rate of social change and economic instability that society is currently experiencing. The division of adulthood into young- and middle-aged stages and the interest in adult development have paved the way for examining the challenges unique to these stages, in which individuals spend the majority of their lives. More needs to be known about the stresses of these stages, the ways that individuals cope, the changes that bring about increased life satisfaction, and the ways in which nurses can support adaptation and ensure health promotion. Such health-promoting interventions may serve as the foundation for future mental health.

Although more is known about childhood and older adults because of the more dramatic and time-dependent aspects of their development, the more subtle changes of adulthood also deserve consideration. Development does not end at childhood, and more needs to be known about the manner in which young adults progress within their lives and achieve the satisfaction reported with middle age.

Research also needs to examine the variables that promote and protect mental health as well as understanding risk factors. Researchers and clinicians often equate promotive or protective factors with the absence of risk factors. This is tantamount to equating health with the absence of illness. Models of thriving and flourishing in response to life's challenges have been proposed by theorists as a more appropriate model for mental health promotion rather than adequate functioning or the lack of criteria for a psychiatric disorder. Those who flourish do not merely lack psychiatric disorders; they also have lower risk for cardiovascular disease and other chronic physical illnesses, fewer health-related limitations, lower health care utilization, fewer missed days of work, and high resilience and intimacy. The adoption of such positive models has implications not only for prevention of mental illness but also for more proactive interventions that ensure continued wellness that progresses into older adulthood.

SUMMARY OF KEY POINTS

■ Western families have achieved unprecedented economic stability that provides for long periods of development and a range of choices in lifestyle.

■ The periods of young and middle adulthood do not exist in less developed countries; a brief childhood progresses quickly into old age.

■ Western society has recently shown greater tolerance for the timing of life events such as education, marriage, and childrearing.

- The periods of young and middle adulthood are characterized by changes in family structure caused by children leaving and returning home, marriage, and divorce.

- Caregiving for both children and older parents is a potential stress faced by both young and middle-aged adults.

- Unemployment is a growing common problem in adulthood, particularly for single mothers and African Americans.

- Mental disorders are most common in young adults, with the first symptoms evident in late adolescence and young adulthood, with the exception of cognitive impairment.

- As individuals progress from young to middle adulthood, they experience changes from optimally running physiologic systems to those showing wear and inefficiency.

- Psychosocial risk factors for mental disorders include age, marital status, unemployment and job stresses, gender, prior mental disorder, coping, lack of health promotion behaviors, parenting stress, and factors associated with suicide.

- Despite decreases in the efficiency of physiologic functioning, young and middle-aged adults often lack health-promoting behaviors, especially if they have mental disorders.

- Suicide is a growing problem in young and middle-aged adulthood, especially in the light of the recent COVID-19 pandemic and economic downturns. It requires early detection and treatment.

- Social support and stress management are important in helping people to cope with the stresses involved in life transitions.

- Fewer than half of individuals receive treatment for their mental health issues, and stigma remains toward those experiencing problems.

- Mental health promotion in adulthood needs to embrace positive models of people who flourish in life rather than those who lack mental illness. Little is known about the factors that promote or protect mental health.

CRITICAL THINKING CHALLENGES

1. What are your assumptions about the psychosocial tasks that should be accomplished by an individual in American society who is young versus middle aged? Describe the challenges that each age group faces in terms of education, marriage, career, children, financial stability, and health and the expected outcomes for each of these challenges.

Then compare your answers with another person's. In which areas do you agree and disagree? Why do the perceptions of the tasks of young and middle-aged adulthood differ from person to person?

2. Describe the modifiable risk factors for mental disorders for young and middle-aged adults and suggest mental health promotion activities that can be used to address these risk factors.

3. What factors do you think are protective or promotive of mental health? How do physical health and mental health overlap? What kinds of interventions may promote both physical and mental health?

Movie Viewing Guides

The Kids Are All Right: 2010. This is a film about a lesbian couple and their adolescent daughter and son who were both conceived from the same anonymous donor via artificial insemination. The daughter, who is preparing to leave home for college, decides to initiate contact with her biologic father. The introduction of the father, although pleasant at first, ultimately reveals the strains in the family's relationships and functioning. This film illustrates the children negotiating the identity tasks of adolescence and ambivalently assuming initial responsibilities of young adulthood. The parents mirror their children's struggles in terms of renegotiating the roles played in their marriage, their lesbian identities, the level of independence given to their children, and acknowledging the imminent "empty nest."

VIEWING POINTS: Identify the life transitions faced by each of the family members in the film. How does each member cope with the stresses they are experiencing? How are the developmental issues the parents are facing similar to their children's? How did the entrance of the father highlight the conflicts and ultimately change the dynamics in this family?

REFERENCES

Arias, E., Tejada-Vera, M. S., & Ahmad, F. (2021). Provisional life expectancy estimates for January through June, 2020. *National Vital Statistics Rapid Release*. Centers for Diseases Control and Prevention Report No. 010. https://www.cdc.gov/nchs/data/vsrr/VSRR10-508.pdf

Ashdown-Franks, G., Firth, J., Carney, R., Carvalho, A. F., Hallgren, M., Koyanagi, A., Rosenbaum, S., Schuch, F. B., Smith, L., Solmi, M., Vancampfort, D., & Stubbs, B. (2020). Exercise as medicine for mental and substance use disorders: A meta-review of the benefits for neuropsychiatric and cognitive outcomes. *Sports Medicine (Auckland, N.Z.)*, 50(1), 151–170. https://doi.org/10.1007/s40279-019-01187-6

Ashley, J. M., Harper, B. D., Arms-Chavez, C. J., & LoBello, S. G. (2015). Estimated prevalence of antenatal depression in the US population. *Archives of Women's Mental Health*, 19(2), 395–400.

Centers for Diseases Control and Prevention. (2010). Table 22. Life expectancy at birth, at 65 years of age, and at 75 years of age, by race and sex: United States, selected years 1900–2007. https://www.cdc.gov/nchs/data/hus/2010/022.pdf

Czeisler, M. É., Lane, R. I., Petrosky, E., Wiley, J. F., Christensen, A., Njai, R., Weaver, M. D., Robbins, R., Facer-Childs, E. R., Barger, L. K., Czeisler, C. A., Howard, M. E., & Rajaratnam, S. M. W. (2020). Mental health, substance use, and suicidal ideation during the COVID-19 pandemic – United States, June 24–30, 2020. *Morbidity and Mortality Weekly Report*, *69*(32), 1049–1057. https://doi.org/10.15585/mmwr.mm6932a1

Hart, D. A., & Zernicke, R. F. (2020). Optimal human functioning requires exercise across the lifespan: Mobility in a 1g environment is intrinsic to the integrity of multiple biological systems. *Frontiers in Physiology*, *11*, 156. https://doi.org/10.3389/fphys.2020.00156

Heazell, A., Newman, L., Lean, S. C., & Jones, R. L. (2018). Pregnancy outcome in mothers over the age of 35. *Current Opinion in Obstetrics & Gynecology*, *30*(6), 337–343. https://doi.org/10.1097/GCO.0000000000000494

Hedegaard, H., Curtin, S. C., & Warner, M. (2020). Increase in suicide mortality in the United States, 1999–2018. *NCHS Data Brief. No. 362.* Nation Center for Health Statistics. Centers for Disease Control and Prevention. U. S. Department of health and Human Services. https://www.cdc.gov/nchs/data/databriefs/db362-h.pdf

Henderson, T. (2020). Single mothers hit hard by job losses. *Demographics, Economy, Health & Labor.* Pew Research Center. https://www.pewtrusts.org/en/research-and-analysis/blogs/stateline/2020/05/26/single-mothers-hit-hard-by-job-losses

Kobau, R., Bann, C., Lewis, M., Zack, M. M., Boardman, A. M., Boyd, R., Lim, K. C., Holder, T., Hoff, A. K., Luncheon, C., Thompson, W., Horner-Johnson, W., & Lucas, R. E. (2013). Mental, social and physical well-being in New Hampshire, Oregon, and Washington, 2010 Behavioral Risk Factor Surveillance System: Implications for public health research and practice related to Healthy People 2020 foundation health measures on well-being. *Population Health Metrics*, *11*(1), 19.

Lamidi, E. O., Manning, W. D., & Brown, S. L. (2019). Change in the stability of first premarital cohabitation among women in the United States, 1983–2013. *Demography*, *56*(2), 427–450. https://doi-org.libproxy.siue.edu/10.1007/s13524-019-00765-7

Li, M., D'Arcy, D., & Meng, X. (2016). Maltreatment in childhood substantially increases the risk of adult depression and anxiety in prospective cohort studies: Systematic review, meta-analysis, and proportional attributable fractions. *Psychological Medicine*, *46*(4), 717–730.

Mental Health America. (2020). The state of mental health in America 2020. https://mhanational.org/sites/default/files/State%20of%20Mental%20Health%20in%20America%20-%202020.pdf

NAMI. (2014). *Road to recovery: Employment and mental illness.* National Alliance on Mental Illness.

NAMI. (2020). You are not alone. National Alliance on Mental Illness. https://www.nami.org/mhstats

National Alliance for Caregiving. (2020). Caregiving in the U.S. 2020: Research report. http://www.caregiving.org

Pandey, K. R., Yang, F., Cagney, K. A., Smieliauskas, F., Meltzer, D. O., & Ruhnke, G. W. (2019). The impact of marital status on health care utilization among Medicare beneficiaries. *Medicine*, *98*(12), e14871. https://doi.org/10.1097/MD.0000000000014871

Patnode, C. D., Evans, C. V., Senger, C. A., Redmond, N., & Lin, J. S. (2017). *Behavioral counseling to promote a healthful diet and physical activity for cardiovascular disease prevention in adults without known cardiovascular disease risk factors: Updated systematic review for the U.S. Preventive Services Task Force.* Agency for Healthcare Research and Quality (US).

Roberson, P., Shorter, R. L., Woods, S., & Priest, J. (2018). How health behaviors link romantic relationship dysfunction and physical health across 20 years for middle-aged and older adults. *Social Science & Medicine (1982)*, *201*, 18–26. https://doi.org/10.1016/j.socscimed.2018.01.037

Robles, T. F. (2014). Marital quality and health: Implications for marriage in the 21st century. *Current Directions in Psychological Science*, *23*(6), 427–432.

SAMSHA. (2014). The NSDUH Report. Center for Behavioral Health. U.S. Department of Health & Human Services.

Schoenborn, C. A., Stommel, M., & Lucas, J. W. (2018). Examining the high rate of cigarette smoking among adults with a GED. *Addictive behaviors*, *77*, 275–286. https://doi.org/10.1016/j.addbeh.2017.04.012

Sheffler, J. L., Piazza, J. R., Quinn, J. M., Sachs-Ericsson, N. J., & Stanley, I. H. (2019). Adverse childhood experiences and coping strategies: Identifying pathways to resiliency in adulthood. *Anxiety, Stress, and Coping*, *32*(5), 594–609. https://doi.org/10.1080/10615806.2019.1638699

Statista Research Department. (2021). Estimated median age of Americans at their first wedding in the United States from 1998 to 2019, by sex. https://www.statista.com/statistics/371933/median-age-of-us-americans-at-their-first-wedding/

U.S. Bureau of Labor Statistics. (2020). State Employment and Unemployment Summary. https://www.bls.gov/news.release/laus.nr0.htm

U.S. Census Bureau. (2019). Living arrangements of children under 18 years and marital status of parents, by age, sex, race, and Hispanic origin and selected characteristics of the child for all children: 2019. https://www.census.gov/data/tables/2019/demo/families/cps-2019.html

Wahl, H., & Kruse, A. (2005). Historical perspective of middle age within the life span. In S. Willis & M. Martin (Eds.), *Middle adulthood: A lifetime perspective* (pp. 3–34). Sage Publishing. https://us.sagepub.com/sites/default/files/upm-assets/5431_book_item_5431.pdf

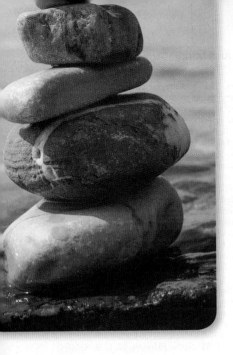

18
Mental Health Promotion for Older Adults

Mary Ann Boyd

KEYCONCEPTS

- late adulthood
- cognitive health

LEARNING OBJECTIVES

After studying this chapter, you will be able to:

1. Describe developmental processes supporting mental health in late adulthood.

2. Describe neurobiologic and psychosocial changes that impact successful aging.

3. Identify risk factors that challenge mental health status.

4. Identify protective factors in the mental health promotion of older adults.

5. Discuss mental health prevention and promotion interventions with older adults.

KEY TERMS

- Bridge employment • Cognitive aging • Cognitive reserve • Crystallized intelligence • Older adult mistreatment
- Fluid intelligence • Functional status • Gerotranscendence • Middle–old • Old–old • Polypharmacy • Resilience
- Social isolation • Working memory • Young–old

INTRODUCTION

The number and proportion of older adults in the United States is rapidly increasing. By 2050, it is expected that Americans aged 65 and older will number nearly 83.7 million, more than double the number of older adults in the United States in 2012. The reason for the rapid growth in the aging population is that Americans are living longer lives (Arias et al., 2021).

More than a quarter of all Americans and two of three older Americans have multiple chronic conditions. Ninety percent of the U.S. health care expenditures are for people with chronic and mental health conditions (CDC, 2020a). Older adults are at somewhat greater risk than younger age groups for the development or recurrence of mental health problems. One in four older adults have a significant mental disorder, with depression, anxiety disorders, and dementia being among the most common (McCombe et al., 2018). There has been a significant increase in use of antianxiety, sedative, and hypnotic medications in community-dwelling older adults as well as an increase in use of antidepressants in this group. Even with a high usage of psychotropic medications, depression often remains untreated in this population.

Yet, despite the high prevalence of psychiatric disorders and mental health problems in later life, older people remain vastly underserved by the current mental health system. This chapter explains the effects of aging on mental health and identifies risks and protective factors related to the mental health problems of older adults.

OLDER ADULT MENTAL HEALTH

Changing needs and personal development characterize older adulthood. This stage of life can be conceptualized in roughly three stages: **young–old** (ages 65 to 74 years), **middle–old** (ages 75 to 84 years), and **old–old** (age 85 years and older). The needs are different in the young–old than in the old–old. Generally, the young–old are challenged to develop new roles after retirement. This group of individuals may need programs and services that help them find meaningful activities. The old–old group tends to need supportive and protective services. However, the aging process is very individualized. Some young–old need supportive services and some in the old–old group are just beginning retirement (Maltais et al., 2019).

> **KEYCONCEPT Late adulthood** can be divided into three chronologic groups: young–old, middle–old, and old–old.

The quality of the journey through older adulthood depends on many factors including biologic changes and psychosocial situations. When older adults retire from their lifelong work, they are challenged to establish a new meaning in life. There are now opportunities to do the things, such as traveling and visiting friends, that were impossible when work and family responsibilities took precedence. If there are health issues, financial limitations, or family problems, the person may not be able to pursue retirement opportunities.

The individual's perception of aging also can impact late adulthood. For example, as once-dependent children grow into adulthood and become parents themselves, they no longer require close attention. No longer having dependent children is viewed positively by some who have more time to pursue personal interests and negatively by others who feel lonely and abandoned. The nurse can be instrumental in helping older adults consider the potential growth opportunities during this time.

COMMON CHALLENGES IN OLDER ADULTHOOD

Changes in vital biologic structures and processes occur gradually over decades and become evident in late adulthood. However, many older adults integrate profound decrements in physical capacity without significantly affecting their ability to function under normal conditions. It is only when functional reserves are needed, such as during an infection, that the absence of these reserves may be observed. Changes in health status, for example, can lead to loss in physical functioning and independence, which in turn can result in an unplanned change in residence. The risk of depression is increased as functional limitation increases and perceived physical health declines (Gouveia et al., 2017).

Physical Changes

Many physical changes occur in older adults. Typically, body fat increases (18% to 36% in men; 33% to 48% in women), total body water decreases (10% to 15%), and muscle mass decreases. In the renal system, there is a predictable decline in glomerular filtration and tubular secretion. Although less efficient, the renal system without disease or injury can function adequately throughout late adulthood (Saxon et al., 2015). Liver function may be reduced because of decreases in blood flow and enzyme activity, resulting in increased blood and tissue concentrations of medications as well as half-life prolongation. Also, fat-soluble drugs may become sequestered in fatty tissue, rather than remaining in the circulating plasma, increasing the risk for drug accumulation and toxicity (see Chapter 11). Age-related changes in the brain are highly individual. For example, cortical thickness and anterior midcingulate cortex in some older adults (60 to 80 years) are indistinguishable from those in younger adults (Sun et al., 2016). For others, there may be a loss of neurons and a general atrophy of the brain (Saxon et al., 2015). Any of these changes over time can compromise the physiologic reserves to manage the everyday stresses of life.

Sensory Changes

All five senses gradually decline in acuity with age, usually beginning in the fourth and fifth decades of life, but these changes do not limit activity until the seventh and eight decades (Saxon et al., 2015). Visual and auditory losses can significantly impact independence and self-mastery. Taste, touch, and smell undergo a uniform dulling although the rate of decline is highly variable among individuals. Sensory decline is important to consider when assessing psychiatrically ill older adults because diminished senses may affect information processing, potentially affecting interpretation of standard mental status examinations. For example, patients who do not reveal hearing difficulty may be evaluated instead for dementia or depression.

Sexuality

Interest in and enjoyment of sexual activities can continue until one's death despite physical changes that affect sexual functioning. Health, a desire to remain sexually active, access to a partner, and a conducive environment contribute to positive sexual experiences. Physiologic changes in women related to sexual functioning include decreasing estrogen levels, alterations in the structural integrity of the vagina (e.g., decreased blood flow, decreased flexibility, diminished lubrication, and diminished response during orgasm), and decreased breast engorgement during arousal (Saxon et al., 2015). Physiologic changes in men include a decline in testosterone production, increased time to achieve erection, less firm erections, decreased urgency for ejaculation, decreased sperm production, and a longer refractory period (i.e., the amount of time before the man can achieve another erection). Problems with sexual performance in aging men are usually centered around erectile dysfunction, which in turn, affects self-esteem (Saxon et al., 2015).

The issue of sexuality in older adults is more complicated than just the physiologic changes. Sexual activity declines with age, with women less likely than men to report being sexually active, but a large number of men and women remain sexually active into their eighth and ninth decades (Macleod et al., 2020). Access to a conducive environment for sexual expression may be hindered if an older adult resides with an adult child or in a nursing home. Stigma associated with sexual activity in later life is also perpetuated by young adults' negative attitudes toward late-life sexuality and further contributes to lack of acceptance that sexual feelings and behaviors are normal at all ages. Lack of acceptance by others, particularly family members, and lack of privacy further contribute to a sense of isolation, loneliness, and poor social support, which are all associated with risks for depression (Srinivasan et al., 2019).

Psychological Changes

Cognitive Health

Cognition includes several mental functions such as attention, thinking, understanding, learning, remembering, solving problems, and making decisions. Cognitive health, the maintenance of optimal cognitive function with age, is multidimensional and relies on a number of interrelated abilities that depend on brain anatomy and physiology. Many cognitive abilities (e.g., knowledge accumulated over a lifetime) are preserved or even enhanced during aging. Additionally, even though there are areas of cognitive decline beginning in middle adulthood, older adults can successfully use compensatory strategies to offset these changes and have a wealth of knowledge, skills, and experiences that younger adults may not have (Lövdén et al., 2020).

KEYCONCEPT Cognitive health is the maintenance of optimal cognitive function with age.

Cognitive aging is a process of gradual, ongoing, yet highly variable changes in cognitive functions that occur as people get older. Cognitive aging is a lifelong process beginning in utero. Normal aging does not impair consciousness, alertness, or attention. Health and environmental factors over a life span influence cognitive aging. Individual factors, including genetics, culture, medical comorbidities, acute illness, customary activity levels, socioeconomic status, education, and personality may modify the development or expression of age-related changes in cognition (IOM, 2015).

Mental Processing Speed and Reaction

Mental processing speed and reaction gradually decline in aging. Generally, it takes longer for older people to process information and give a response, which can lead to problems in reaction times (driving) and interactions with others. These changes may influence other cognitive operations such as working memory, speech processing, and attention. A person's ability to remember spoken word, attend to important information, or perform tasks may also be affected. Decline in processing speed may be offset by experience. For example, if older adults continue to engage in complex activities such as maintaining computer skills, they may not experience a significant decline in processing information. Communication with older adults requires paying special attention to verbal interactions and environmental influences. Hurrying older adults to answer questions may interfere with their ability to provide the correct answer (Saxon et al., 2015). Box 18.1 highlights many of the considerations necessary when interacting with older adults.

BOX 18.1

Communicating with Older Adults

- Focus the person's attention on the exchange of communication; the older adult may need extra time to begin to process information.
- Face the person when speaking to them.
- Minimize distractions in the room, including other people, objects in your hands, noise, and other activities.
- Reduce glare from room lighting by dimming too bright lights. Conversely, avoid sitting in shadows.
- Speak slowly and clearly. Older adults may depend on lip reading, so ensure that the individual can see you. Speak loudly, but do not shout.
- Use short, simple sentences and be prepared to repeat or revise what you have said.
- Limit the number of topics discussed at one time to prevent information overload.
- Ask one question at a time to minimize confusion. Allow plenty of time for the person to answer and express ideas.
- Frequently summarize the important points of the conversation to improve understanding and comprehension.
- Avoid the urge to finish sentences.
- Consider factors such as fatigue and discomfort in structuring the communication.
- If the communication exchange is going poorly, postpone it for another time.

Memory

Older adults often worry about changes in memory as they age. Memory problems in later life are believed to result from encoding or retrieval problems (or both). There are many types of memory (measured by neuropsychologic tests); some remain stable and others decline. **Working memory**, the ability to temporarily hold information in one's mind while it is processed, is central to many functions (see Chapter 8), such as remembering to take medication, processing language, solving problems, making decisions, and learning. Generally, working memory declines with age, especially for complex tasks. Despite these declines, performance of well-learned tasks often shows little declines. For example, there is little evidence that older workers are any less productive than younger workers. In most day-to-day tasks, older adults perform very well (IOM, 2015).

Other factors associated with memory changes include a lack of perceived relevance, sensory problems, not paying attention, a general failure to link the "to be remembered" information to existing knowledge through association, and a lack of using repetition to strengthen memory. The learning abilities of older people may be more selective, requiring motivation ("How important is this information?"), depend on meaningful content ("Why do I need to know this?"), and be related to familiarity with the idea or content. Level of education needs to be considered in evaluating responses on mental status examinations because lack of education may account for poor performance.

Although a decline in memory efficiency may be frustrating for the older individual, it does not necessarily hamper their ability to function daily (IOM, 2015). Threats to memory include medications, depression (impairs concentration and attention), poor nutrition, infection, heart and lung disease (lack of oxygen), thyroid problems (can cause symptoms of depression or confusion that mimic memory loss), alcohol use, and sensory loss (interferes with perception). However, it is important not to confuse memory decline with deficits in memory storage, such as those that are seen in dementias (see Chapter 38).

Intelligence

Intelligence includes both **crystallized intelligence**, knowledge such as language skills or knowledge about a particular topic, and fluid intelligence, that is, processing current or new information. **Fluid intelligence** involves thinking logically and solving problems. Crystallized intelligence remains fairly stable with modest declines in later life. Declines in fluid intelligence begin earlier and are more gradual throughout the life span (IOM, 2015). Similar to other cognitive aspects, intelligence is impacted by other factors, including the environment, social context, knowledge, prior experience, health status, the demands of the task, and support.

Cognitive Reserve

The variability in cognitive aging can partially be explained by the concept of **cognitive reserve**, the resistance to decline in functioning of the brain. Factors that contribute to cognitive reserve include education, occupational attainment, physical activity, and engagement in intellectual and social activities. A deficit in early-life cognitive reserve is often related to socioeconomic status. Staying physically fit and maintaining an active social network can have positive effects in older adults (Bettcher et al., 2019; Lövdén, 2020).

Personality

Personalities and personality traits are generally believed to be stable throughout the life span. Some personality traits are associated with longevity, such as conscientiousness, responsibility, self-control, and traditionalism. Personality traits, such as extroversion, openness to experience, agreeableness, and conscientiousness, are related to successful aging. People who are assessed with low conscientiousness (low self-esteem, acting spontaneously without planning, showing little persistence in pursuing long-term goals, and not being driven by obligations of duty and responsibility) have a higher mortality rate than those with an average sense of conscientiousness. Characteristics of low conscientiousness may lead to unhealthy life choices and risk-taking behavior. Even though we generally believe that personalities are formed by the age of 30 years, evidence shows that personality traits are shaped by the environment and social experiences throughout life. Occupational and romantic experiences and other major life events influence the expression of personality traits in all age groups (Jokela, et al., 2020).

Development

Late-life adult developmental phenomena are not well defined. Early developmental theorists viewed older adults as having the same psychological and social needs as when they were younger. They believed that as the aging person gave up their roles as employee and parent, the individual should replace the role losses with new roles and increase social interaction (Havighurst, 1961). The Disengagement Theory is similar but proposed that the aging individual and society mutually withdraw from each other to prepare the individual for an eventual exit from society (Cumming & Henry, 1960). Later, Erik Erikson identified "integrity versus despair" as a developmental task specific to late adulthood (Erikson & Erikson, 1997). He proposed that the primary task of the older adult is to reflect on their past experiences. If the individual is satisfied with their life, this eighth stage is resolved, and the person attains wisdom and acceptance of death.

Unlike the earlier theories, the Gerotranscendence Theory describes **gerotranscendence** as the continuation or progression toward maturation and shifting from a materialistic and pragmatic view of the world to a more cosmic view. The individual may experience personal growth in dimensions such as spirituality and inner strength with an emphasis on the meaning of life and making positive use of solitude (Tornstam, 2005). The concept of gerotranscendence may be used in establishing health promotion interventions. Gerotranscendence is also congruent with more recent research about mental health in late adulthood, which is more optimistic and addresses successful aging. This approach focuses on generation awareness, awareness of aging, the big picture of life, and a need for solitude (Braam et al., 2016; Lee et al., 2020). See Box 18.2 for one study focusing on enhancing the perception of gerotranscendence.

Emotional Health

Although personality is fairly stable across adulthood, emotional changes are small but generally positive. Aging adults tend to become more emotionally stable, more agreeable, and more conscientious, with a higher level of well-being. These positive changes are thought to be related to the development of better emotional regulation because of life experiences and involvement in meaningful activities, networks, and goals. Threats to emotional and physical well-being include limitations in daily activities, physical impairments, grief following loss of loved ones, caregiving or challenging living situations, or untreated mental illness such as depression and substance abuse.

Perception of Time

Older adults often comment that time seems to go faster than when they were younger. Experts have yet to agree on an explanation for this experience, but there are several factors that contribute to this change in time perception. The lives of older adults tend to be more stable than their younger counterparts as months, weeks, and years unfold with fewer life changes that demarcate periods of time. Life transitions of younger persons are often dramatically different from each other, such as children growing up and leaving home, job changes, and relocation. Aging adults have less time in life than younger people. Younger persons often plan for their future, whereas time for older adults is limited. Thus, the present is the older adult's future, whereas a younger person prepares for a different future than their present life (Löckenhoff & Rutt, 2017; Rutt & Löckenhoff, 2016).

Social Changes
Functional Status

Functional status, the extent to which a person can independently carry out personal care, home management, and social functions in everyday life in a way that has meaning and purpose, often changes during the later years. Estimates of the prevalence of functional dependency vary, but in general, studies show that difficulty in performing activities of daily living and instrumental activities of daily living increases with advancing age and that cognitive impairment significantly predicts functional decline (Cornelis et al., 2019). It is important to remember that most older adults live in the community and perceive that they are aging well despite chronic illnesses and some physical disability. A sense of control and self-efficacy contributes to an older person's sense of self-mastery despite limitations.

Retirement

Research shows an association between successful aging and a happy retirement. The ability to adapt to change and remain engaged and involved in life and social networks contributes to the successful negotiation of the retirement transition. Voluntary retirement is associated with

---

BOX 18.2
Gerotranscendence: Perception and Depression

Shu-Chuan Chen, Moyle, W., & Jones, C. (2019). Feasibility and effect of a multidimensional support program to improve gerotranscendence perception and depression for older adults: A pragmatic cluster-randomized control study. Research in Gerontological Nursing, 12(3), 148–158. https://doi-org.libproxy.siue.edu/10.3928/19404921-20190212-01

THE QUESTION: Is it feasible to improve gerotranscendence and reduce depression in community-dwelling older adults through providing a multidimensional support program (MSP)?

METHODS: Using a cluster-randomized control trial design, four sites (98 participants) were randomly assigned to a MSP or control group.

FINDINGS: The MSP was found to significantly enhance the perception of gerotranscendence in older adults but not their level of depression.

IMPLICATIONS FOR NURSING: This study demonstrated that the MSP is a feasible and effective program to improve perception of gerotranscendence and may potentially lead to positive psychological well-being for older adults.

postretirement well-being. For many, **bridge employment** (paid work for those receiving a pension) alleviates the negative consequences of retirement for those who are forced to retire involuntarily (Carlstedt et al., 2018). On the other hand, changing roles and circumstances can cause stress and contribute to poorer mental health (Voss et al., 2020).

Financial concerns certainly impact one's adjustment to retirement. Social Security Annuity continues to provide the largest single source of income for older adults, but retirement income security now often requires earnings from working in later life (Quinn & Cahill, 2016). The traditional "three-legged stool" on which retirement rests—Social Security, pensions, and savings and investments—disproportionately excludes some groups, such as people of color, LGBTQIA (Lesbian, Gay, Bisexual, Transgender, Questioning, Intersex, Asexual) members, women, and immigrants who have faced barriers to education, health, a stable work history, or financial stability. Many no longer have pensions or savings to sustain them in retirement (Tamborini & Kim, 2020).

Economic downturns have significant implications in terms of personal financial concerns; there is increased competition for jobs as well as a potential delay in retirement. Although mandatory retirement is becoming a thing of the past, older workers may be overlooked for promotions and employment opportunities because of their age and likelihood of retiring. Pensions are no longer the economic mainstay of retirement. The recent pandemic from coronavirus disease 2019 (COVID-19) accelerated unemployment and retirements of older workers who often had health issues, increasing their risks of contracting the deadly disease. Food insecurity became commonplace (Wolfson & Leung, 2020).

Leisure and Social Activities

As with younger populations, lifestyle is crucial in late adulthood. As age increases, participation in leisure and social activities decreases for many people. Health conditions such as depression, lung disease, and diabetes may prevent participation in home maintenance and leisure activities, especially walking, gardening, and active sports. Maintaining a positive mental attitude and participating in cognitively engaging, regularly scheduled leisure activities appear to exert a protective factor and is associated with a reduced risk of dementia even after adjusting for baseline cognitive status. Higher education levels are also associated with increased participation in both formal and informal activities (Gholamnezhad et al., 2020).

Family Relationship Changes

As family relationships change, interpersonal relationship strains can develop. Disappointments with the lifestyles of adult children and changes in caregiving responsibilities

affect the quality of a long-term family relationship. In some instances, the young–old assume caregiving responsibilities for their old–old relatives. It is also common for grandparents to assume some caregiving responsibilities for their grandchildren. Although there are stresses associated with grandparenting, positive benefits appear to outweigh negatives except when combined with other intensive caregiving (Arpino & Gómez-León, 2020). The frequency of grandparents raising grandchildren in co-parenting and custodial households has increased significantly in the past 35 years, occurring most frequently in African American families (Whitley et al., 2016).

Cultural Impact

With our communities increasingly becoming a reflection of multiple ethnic histories and values, the aging population is likewise becoming more diverse. In 2010, 80% of the adults aged 65 years or older were non-Hispanic White. By 2030, older non-Hispanic White adults will make up 71.2% of the population, whereas Hispanics will make up 12%, non-Hispanic Blacks nearly 10.3%, and Asian American 5.4%. By 2050, older non-Hispanic White adults will account for only about 58% of the total population aged 65 or older (CDC, 2020a). Underrepresented groups face disparities in access to and provision of health care. At the same time, they have higher-than-average health care needs (Borson et al., 2019). Cultural variations also exist in family expectations of and responsibilities for older adults. For example, some groups, such as the Chinese, tend to highly value the experience and wisdom of their elders, and family members feel a responsibility for their care (Ma & Saw, 2020).

Community Factors

Although most older adults live in their own homes, they may find themselves living in changing or deteriorating neighborhoods with inadequate social resources, such as place of worship and community, shopping, and health care centers. Relocating to smaller and more protective housing may be welcomed by some and fiercely resisted by others.

Residential Care

Residential care in foster care homes, family homes, personal care homes, residential care facilities, or assisted living arrangements provides the older adult with a protected environment. The quality of services and affordability of the arrangement need to be carefully evaluated to determine whether the older adult's needs and abilities match the care provided in that facility, including staff training and staffing patterns, medication supervision, approaches to behavior management, activities provided, services available (e.g., care management, family support, counseling, day care), safety and security issues, provision of personal care with attention to dignity and privacy, health and nutrition concerns, full disclosure of costs and funding, and payment issues.

RISK FACTORS FOR OLDER ADULT PSYCHOPATHOLOGY

Chronic Illnesses

Although the frequency of acute conditions declines with advancing age, about 80% of older adults have at least one chronic health condition; 50% have at least two. Poor physical health is associated with mental disorders both as a risk factor and as an outcome, with those with severe disabilities reporting lower levels of well-being (Happell et al., 2017). Common chronic conditions that cause activity limitation include arthritis, hypertension, heart disease, and respiratory disorders. Chronic illnesses can reduce physiologic capacity and consequently increase functional dependency. In addition, during acute episodes of illness, many older adults lose functional ability because they have limited reserves or cannot mobilize reserves to regain their premorbid performance levels.

Alcohol Use Disorder and Substance Use Disorder

Alcohol use disorder and substance use disorder are underestimated and undertreated. Substance use disorder is associated with poor health outcomes, higher health care utilization, and increased complexity of the course of the disorder. In addition, older adults with substance use disorder problems have increased disability and impairment, compromised quality of life, increased caregiver stress, increased mortality, and a higher risk of suicide. Excessive alcohol use accounts for more than 21,000 deaths each year among adults 65 years or older (Chhatre et al., 2017). The majority of older adults with substance use disorder do not receive adequate treatment (Rhee & Rosenheck, 2020).

Polypharmacy

More than 87% of older adults use prescription medication. The prevalence of **polypharmacy**, the use of five or more medications, in older adults ages 62 to 85 years is 90% in long-term care facilities (Talebreza & McPherson, 2020). The aging process affects pharmacokinetics and the strength and number of protein-binding sites (see Chapter 11). These changes place older adults at increased risk for adverse drug reactions. Difficulties in managing medications arising from memory impairment further compound the problem of medication misuse. Serious problems result when the treatment regimen and care delivery specific to prescribed medications are not coordinated. These problems are compounded when an older adult uses over-the-counter drugs, herbal remedies, and home or folk remedies without considering their potential interaction with prescribed drugs. Prescribers can follow the principles delineated in Box 18.3 to improve drug therapy in the older adult population.

BOX 18.3

Drug Therapy Interventions

- Minimize the number of drugs that the patient uses, keeping only those drugs that are essential. One third of the residents in one long-term care facility received 8 to 16 drugs daily.
- Always consider alternatives among different drug classifications or dosage forms that are more suitable for older adult patients.
- Implement preventive measures to reduce the need for certain medications. Such prevention includes health promotion through proper nutrition, exercise, and stress reduction.
- Most age-dependent pharmacokinetic changes lead to potential accumulation of the drug; therefore, medication dosages should start low and go slow.
- Exercise caution when administering medication with a long half-life or in an older adult with impaired renal or liver function. Under these conditions, the time may be extended between doses.
- Be knowledgeable of each drug's properties, including such factors as half-life, excretion, and adverse effects

(e.g., venlafaxine HCl [Effexor], a structurally novel antidepressant that inhibits the reuptake of serotonin and norepinephrine, requires regular monitoring of the patient's blood pressure.

- Assess the patient's clinical history for physical problems that may affect excretion of medications.
- Monitor laboratory values (e.g., creatinine clearance) and urinary output in patients receiving medications eliminated by the kidneys.
- Monitor plasma albumin levels in patients receiving drugs that have high binding affinity to protein.
- Regularly monitor the patient's reaction to all medications to ensure a therapeutic response.
- Look for potential drug interactions that may complicate therapy. Antacids lower gastric acidity and may decrease the rate at which other medications are dissolved and absorbed.
- Instruct patients to consult with their providers before taking any over-the-counter medications.

Bereavement and Loss

Older adults experience many losses—friends and family members die, physical health can be compromised, choices and independence may be limited, and social status may diminish. Loss of one's spouse, particularly when the relationship has been long and satisfying, constitutes a major life event. Women are more likely to lose their spouses and tend to be widowed at a younger age than are men. Consequently, women have more time to adjust and develop substitute social relationships to replace the spouse. Conversely, men tend to lose their wives at an older age, have fewer social networks to replace the spouse, and express feelings of loneliness and abandonment. Because of differences in longevity, men and women usually experience life events at different ages. Regardless of gender differences, survivors are at higher risk for depression and face financial issues after the death of a loved one. Health care professionals should work closely with grieving survivors to help them understand that their lives will be displaced for some time. Support sessions on the grief process and financial and employment planning could become a standard part of care.

Older Adults Experiencing Poverty

In the past 50 years, the number of individuals experiencing poverty aged 65 and older has steadily decreased, from 28.5% in 1966 to 9.2% in 2017. In 2018, three million older Whites (7.3%) were poor, compared to 18.9% of older African Americans, 11.7% of Asians, and 19.5% of older Hispanics (Administration for Community Living, 2020). Whereas the proportion of older adults who live in poverty has decreased, the number of aged poor has increased from 3.1 million in 1974 to 44.7 million in 2017. However, certain groups are more vulnerable to poverty than others, including widows, divorced women, and never married men and women. Individuals aged 80 and older have the highest poverty rate, especially women. The poverty rate of women aged 80 and older is 13.5% compared with 8.7% for men. Poverty rates also vary by race in older adults. The poverty rate is lowest among the non-Hispanic White population (5.8% for men and 8.0% for women) and highest among the Black population (16.1% for men and 21.5% for women) (Li & Dalaker, 2019).

The aging of the population has significant implications for healthcare costs associated with Medicare as two million baby boomers were eligible to sign up by the end of 2015.

Social Isolation

Social isolation, the relative absence of social relationships, is recognized as detrimental to quality of life and premature mortality. Meaningful interactions are important to the physical and mental health of older adults. Staying active, continuing to work, caring for others, and/or engaging with family, friends, and community contribute to the well-being of the older person. Since the older adult population was very vulnerable to COVID-19 transmission, social isolation became a strategy to prevent transmission of the illness. While social isolation protected many from physical illness, it led to negative consequences of loneliness and depression (Smith et al., 2020). As a result of the sheltering in place and other social distancing strategies, loneliness is higher than prior to the pandemic and associated with depression and suicidal ideation (Killgore et al., 2020).

Lack of Social Support and Suicide

Closely related to social isolation, a lack of social support is linked to transition into an institutional setting. When older adults can go to movies, dinner, or a casino and visit family and friends, they are more likely to remain in independent living. Dissatisfaction with social life, lack of participation in organizations, and being distant from others are associated with a wish for death (Bernier et al., 2020; Oh, 2019). Safety concerns are always a priority. Any suicidal ideation should be identified and a safety plan developed (see Box 18.4).

BOX 18.4

Risk Factors for Suicide in Late Life (Age Older than 65 Years)

- Depression
- Prior attempts at suicide
- Marked feelings of hopelessness; lack of interest in future plans
- Feelings of loss of independence or sense of purpose
- Medical conditions that significantly limit functioning or life expectancy
- Impulsivity due to cognitive impairment
- Social isolation
- Family discord or losses (i.e., recent death of a loved one)
- Inflexible personality or marked difficulty adapting to change
- Access to lethal means (i.e., firearms, other weapons, etc.)
- Daring or risk-taking behavior
- Sudden personality changes
- Alcohol or medication misuse or abuse
- Verbal suicide threats such as, "You'd be better off without me" or "Maybe I won't be around"
- Giving away prized possessions

Mental Health America. (2021). Preventing suicide in older adults. https://www.mhanational.org/preventing-suicide-older-adults. Reprinted with permission from Mental Health America and National Council on Aging.

Shared Living Arrangements and Older Adult Mistreatment

Older adult mistreatment, intentional actions that cause harm or create a serious risk of harm to a vulnerable older adult by a caregiver or other person who stands in a trust relationship to the individual, has an estimated prevalence of 10%. Actual cases may actually be 14 times the number of reported cases (National Center on Elder Abuse [NCEA], 2017). Clinical and empirical evidence suggests that a shared living arrangement increases the opportunities for contact that can lead to conflict and mistreatment. Abuse of older adults tends to take place where the individuals live: most often in the home where abusers are apt to be adult children, other family members such as grandchildren, or spouses or partners of older adults. Institutional settings, especially long-term care facilities, can also be sources of abuse. The prevalence of mistreatment of the older adult appears to be related to low income, poor health, and lack of social support. Race and ethnic differences have not been shown to play a role (Hernandez-Tejada et al., 2020).

PROTECTIVE FACTORS FOR MENTAL ILLNESS IN OLDER PERSONS

Protective factors for minimizing the occurrence of mental disorders in older adults are similar to those in younger adults. Evidence supports protective factors, which include marriage, education and income level, resilience—and positive outlook, healthy lifestyle, nutrition, and exercise.

The Marriage Effect

It has long been thought that married people have lower mortality rates than unmarried at all ages. Many studies have reported that being part of a couple and the quality of the relationship are positively correlated with longevity and health, including cognitive and emotional function (Karimi et al., 2019). There are several possible explanations for the marriage advantage. For example, married people may be less likely to engage in high-risk and health-damaging behaviors. They may also be more likely to receive care and support when needed. They have shared economic resources and a social network of relatives and friends who can provide vital support at older ages. Negotiating a partner relationship that presents ongoing social and emotional challenges may also contribute to higher functioning (see Fig. 18.1).

Education and Income

Education and income provide older adults with cognitive, economic, and coping reserves that support function

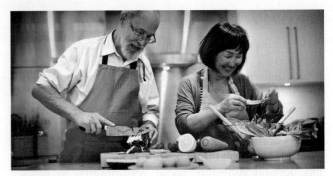

FIGURE 18.1 Lifelong marriage is associated with positive physical and mental health. (Rawpixel/Shutterstock.)

and well-being and are related to physical activity and physical and cognitive function and disability. Those with higher education and income are more likely to engage in physical activity and have the resources to provide care when needed. Higher levels of education are associated with higher levels of cognitive function as well as a lower risk of dementia (Arce Rentería et al., 2019).

Resilience and Positive Outlook

Research has shown that those with a positive attitude toward aging age better and live longer. Although it is not known why a positive attitude increases longevity, it is thought to be linked to the will to live, **resilience** (i.e., the ability to adapt successfully to stress, trauma, or chronic adversity), and a proactive approach to health. It may also be that people with a positive attitude have lower stress. Research has proposed that resilience enables one to adapt positively to adversity, and characteristics associated with resilience include optimism, social engagement, emotional well-being, fewer cognitive complaints, and successful aging (Calderón-Larrañaga et al., 2019).

Healthy Lifestyle

A healthy lifestyle is important in preventing illness and promoting well-being at all ages, including in late adulthood. Such behaviors include not smoking; drinking alcohol in moderation; getting adequate rest and sleep; getting adequate hydration and nutrition, especially fruits and vegetables; exercising; and coping with stress (Perera & Agboola, 2019).

Nutrition

Maintaining a healthy diet can be challenging for older adults. In the United States, the prevalence of obesity is 42.5% of all adults over the age of 60 (CDC, 2020b). The prevalence of undernutrition appears to be high in older adults, especially those living in an institutionalized setting (17%) (Kiesswetter et al., 2020). Factors contributing to undernutrition include living alone, poor appetite, poor intake of fluid and nutritious foods, medications, malignancy, bereavement, and depression. Undernutrition can lead to anemia, inadequate wound healing, increased incidence of pressure sores, impaired elimination, impaired immunologic functions, weakness, fatigue, and mental problems (including depression, dementia, and agitation) (Saxon et al., 2015). Adequate nutrition is an important factor in maintaining mental health.

Physical Activity

Emerging evidence suggests that physical activity is related to positive mental health and may be a protective factor. There is a moderate amount of evidence that exercise can prevent the onset or worsening of depression. Structured exercise programs enhance older persons' overall physical functioning and well-being and reduce anxiety symptoms among sedentary adults with chronic illnesses (Miller et al., 2020).

INTERVENTION APPROACHES

Reducing the Stigma of Mental Health Treatment

The stigma of mental illness continues to interfere with the willingness of older adults to seek treatment. Older adults in America grew up during a time when institutionalization in asylums, electroconvulsive treatments, and other treatment approaches were regarded with fear. This fear can lead to denial of problems. Nurses can help reduce the stigma through educational interventions and facilitation of access to services.

Early Recognition of Depressive Symptoms and Suicide Risk

Depression is one of the most common mental disorders in older adults (see Chapter 23). Even with a high usage of psychotropic medications, depression remains untreated in this population (Blazer & Steffens, 2019). Because depression can be debilitating and can lead to suicide, recognition and early intervention are the keys to avoiding ongoing depressive episodes. Depressive symptoms among older adults are more likely to include vague somatic complaints, cognitive symptoms, hypersomnia, and appetite changes rather than complaints of depressed mood. Early indications of symptomatology can be identified in primary care settings using a screening tool such as the Geriatric Depression Scale (Yesavage et al., 1982). Several preventive interventions are helpful, such as grief counseling for widows and widowers, self-help groups, and physical and social activities.

Monitoring Medications

With the approval of new medications, older adults' health problems can be treated with pharmacologic agents that were not previously available. It is important to make sure that medications are being taken correctly as well as whether they are having the desired effects. Side effects and drug interactions should be carefully monitored to detect untoward symptoms and delirium. Dosages may need to be adjusted slowly. It is important to review all medications, including over-the-counter, natural, and alternative remedies.

Avoiding Premature Institutionalization

Although many people require nursing home care, integrated care in the community is effective and can delay nursing home placement. Home visits that focus on assessment of symptoms and coordination of health care needs can result in older adults receiving their mental health support within the community and, therefore, are able to stay in their current living arrangements. Older adults and those with disabilities prefer to receive community-based care, which to be most effective must include prevention and rehabilitation services as well as acute care.

Promoting Mental Health

Social Support Transitions

Compensating for loss of family by expanding friendship networks and employment may become an important method of establishing a network in late life. Older adults can be prepared for the transition by receiving information about internal developmental processes, sources of social support, and opportunities for personal growth and role supplementation. Interventions to support successful aging promote productive and social engagement, and effective coping groups can be particularly effective in developing a sense of community, decreasing isolation, and strengthening a safety network.

Cognitive Engagement

Frequent engagement in cognitive activities may positively impact cognitive functioning in memory. Successful cognitive aging appears to be supported not only by cognitive reserve but also by the older adult's development and use of compensatory strategies. For example, a nursing intervention would be teaching the patient to write notes to self about upcoming events. Such compensatory strategies support cognitive functioning as well as a sense of personal control.

Lifestyle Support

Lifestyle interventions, such as exercise promotion and nutrition counseling, are particularly important in late life because a tendency to slow down and become more sedentary usually accompanies aging. For many, retirement provides an opportunity to restructure the time that was previously spent working. Developing regular exercise habits can help maintain physical and psychological well-being, especially if done with others. Self-help programs generally include components of exercise, nutrition, health screening, and health habits. Maintaining social support is an integral part of lifestyle support.

Self-Care Enhancement

Enhancing health self-care is a major area for mental health promotion. Education of older adults and their families is crucial to ensuring adherence to agreed-upon care regimens. The nurse must consider the individual's educational level, pace of learning, and visual and hearing deficits. The nurse should provide instructional aids, large-print labeling, and devices such as medication calendars that encourage adherence. Self-care enhancements assist older adults in the use of compensatory strategies and aid in their being as functionally independent as possible for as long as possible. Supporting a sense of control and decisional capacity is critical to self-care.

Spiritual Support

Spirituality can be extremely important to older adults and can positively affect attitude, particularly as health declines. Participation in a community of faith is associated with better health outcomes and mental well-being (Lima et al., 2020). Supporting contact with spiritual leaders important to the patient is an ongoing mental health promotion intervention. The nurse can also support a patient's spiritual growth by exploring the meanings that a particular life change has for the patient. In late life, existential issues such as experiencing losses, redefining meanings in existence, and living in the present become the standard, replacing the performance and future orientation that characterize earlier adulthood.

Community Services

Community care options are needed that provide both sustenance and growth. Examples of supportive services that foster independent community living include information and referral services; transportation and nutrition services; legal and protective services; comprehensive older adult community centers; homemaker and handyman services; matching of older with younger individuals to share housing; and use of the supports available through places of worship, community groups, or mental health

and other community agencies (e.g., area agencies on aging) to maintain older adults in the community for as long as possible. The availability and accessibility of these services vary greatly, and eligibility requirements may exist.

POSITIVE MENTAL AGING

At this time, there are many questions about the course of aging for future cohorts of older adults. It is probable that some of the losses and decrements associated with aging are in fact artifacts of a more sedentary, less healthy lifestyle over a lifetime. Furthermore, we must consider that positive mental aging is more than the absence of mental disorders and impairment but rather is more a reflection of resilience—the capacity to adapt, feel in control, and make decisions about care and life. Most important is to listen to older adults themselves. Research shows that four qualities contribute to successful aging: the capacity to adapt to change, engagement and involvement in life, the importance of stability and security with reliable social support, and, least important, physical health (Jeste et al., 2013). As nurses, it is incumbent upon us to help older adults to recognize and use their strengths to cope with and transcend losses and limitations. Recognizing and tapping into the wisdom accumulated over a lifetime may help older adults to negotiate the many challenges faced in later life.

SUMMARY OF KEY POINTS

- Changes in vital biologic structures and processes occur, but older adults can sustain some structural losses without losing function.
- All five senses (sight, hearing, touch, taste, and smell) decline with age, which may affect information processing.
- Although older adults experience many physical changes, they can and have the desire to remain sexually active.
- Threats to cognitive function in older adults include medication side effects, depression, poor nutrition, infection, heart and lung disease, thyroid problems, alcohol use, and sensory loss.
- Intelligence and personality are stable throughout the life span; however, reaction time slows with age.
- Major changes in social roles with aging include retirement, loss of partner, and changes in residence.
- Polypharmacy is prevalent in older adults, particularly in nursing homes. Ongoing assessment of medications is needed to prevent inappropriate medication administration.
- Older people are at higher risk for poverty and suicide.

- Older adults are vulnerable to COVID-19, which leads to social isolation and increased mortality.

- Mental health protective factors include marriage, education, resilience and positive outlook, and healthy lifestyle (including nutrition and exercise).

- Interventions to prevent mental illness include reducing the stigma of mental health treatment, preventing depression and suicide, monitoring medications, and preventing premature institutionalization.

- Nurses can provide a number of interventions to promote mental health, addressing social support transitions, cognitive engagement, lifestyle support, self-care enhancement, spiritual support, and community-based services.

- Positive mental aging is more than the absence of mental disorders and impairment but rather is more a reflection of resilience, which is the capacity to adapt, feel in control, and be engaged, with a positive outlook.

CRITICAL THINKING CHALLENGES

1. Compare the three late adulthood chronologic groups in terms of age. Using the recommendations in Box 18.1, interview people representing each of the three chronologic groups about their views of mental health.

2. Highlight normal biologic changes that occur during the aging process.

3. Hypothesize why IQ tests and personality do not change with time.

4. Explain the concept of gerotranscendence and use the concept to explain differences between the young–old and the old–old.

5. Identify positive and negative perspectives of retirement.

6. Explain why chronic illnesses, polypharmacy, and poverty are all risk factors for mental health problems in later life.

7. Describe mental health promotion interventions that relate to social support transitions, cognitive engagement, lifestyle support, and self-care.

8. Describe factors that contribute to successful aging.

Movie Viewing Guides
Driving Miss Daisy: 1989. This delightful film stars Jessica Tandy as Daisy Werthan, a cantankerous older woman. Morgan Freeman plays Hoke Colburn, Daisy's chauffeur. This beautiful story examines a relationship between two people who have more in common than just getting old. *Driving Miss Daisy* challenges some of the myths about getting old.

VIEWING POINTS: Identify the normal behaviors in the growth and development of older adults. Observe the verbal and nonverbal communication of Daisy and Hoke. How do they support each other?

REFERENCES

Administration for Community Living. (2020). 2019 Profile of older Americans. Administration on Aging. U.S. Department of health and Human Services. https://acl.gov/sites/default/files/Aging%20and%20Disability%20in%20America/2019ProfileOlderAmericans508.pdf

Arce Rentería, M., Vonk, J., Felix, G., Avila, J. F., Zahodne, L. B., Dalchand, E., Frazer, K. M., Martinez, M. N., Shouel, H. L., & Manly, J. J. (2019). Illiteracy, dementia risk, and cognitive trajectories among older adults with low education. *Neurology, 93*(24), e2247–e2256. https://doi.org/10.1212/WNL.0000000000008587

Arias, E., Tejada-Vera, M. S., & Ahmad, F. (2021). Provisional life expectancy estimates for January through June, 2020. *National Vital Statistics Rapid Release*. Centers for Diseases Control and Prevention Report No.010. https://www.cdc.gov/nchs/data/vsrr/VSRR10-508.pdf

Arpino, B., & Gómez-León, M. (2020). Consequences on depression of combining grandparental childcare with other caregiving roles. *Aging & Mental Health, 24*(8), 1263–1270. https://doi.org/10.1080/13607863.2019.1584788

Bernier, S., Lapierre, S., & Desjardins, S. (2020). Social interactions among older adults who wish for death. *Clinical Gerontologist, 43*(1), 4–16. https://doi.org/10.1080/07317115.2019.1672846

Bettcher, B. M., Gross, A. L., Gavett, B. E., Widaman, K. F., Fletcher, E., Dowling, N. M., Buckley, R. F., Arenaza-Urquijo, E. M., Zahodne, L. B., Hohman, T. J., Vonk, J., Rentz, D. M., & Mungas, D. (2019). Dynamic change of cognitive reserve: Associations with changes in brain, cognition, and diagnosis. *Neurobiology of Aging, 83*, 95–104. https://doi.org/10.1016/j.neurobiolaging.2019.08.016

Blazer, D. G., & Steffens, D. C. (2019). Older adults. In L. W. Roberts (Ed.). *The American psychiatric publishing textbook of geriatric psychiatry* (7th ed., pp. 1213–1241). American Psychiatric Publishing.

Borson, S., Korpak, A., Carbajal-Madrid, P., Likar, D., Brown, G. A., & Batra, R. (2019). Reducing barriers to mental health care: Bringing evidence-based psychotherapy home. *Journal of the American Geriatrics Society, 67*(10), 2174–2179. https://doi.org/10.1111/jgs.16088

Braam, A. W., Galenkamp, H., Derkx, P., Aartsen, M. J., & Deeg, D. J. (2016). Ten-year course of cosmic transcendence in older adults in the Netherlands. *International Journal of Aging & Human Development, 84*(1), 44–65. https://doi.org/10.1177/0091415016668354

Calderón-Larrañaga, A., Vetrano, D. L., Welmer, A. K., Grande, G., Fratiglioni, L., & Dekhtyar, S. (2019). Psychological correlates of multimorbidity and disability accumulation in older adults. *Age and Ageing, 48*(6), 789–796. https://doi.org/10.1093/ageing/afz117

Carlstedt, A. B., Brushammar, G., Bjursell, C., Nystedt, P., & Nilsson, G. (2018). A scoping review of the incentives for a prolonged work life after pensionable age and the importance of "bridge employment". *Work (Reading, Mass.), 60*(2), 175–189. https://doi.org/10.3233/WOR-182728

Centers for Disease Control and Prevention. (2020a). *Health and economic cost of chronic diseases*. National Center for Chronic Disease Prevention and Health Promotion (NCCDPHP). https://www.cdc.gov/chronicdisease/about/costs/index.htm#ref1

Centers for Disease Control and Prevention. (2020b). Prevalence of obesity and severe obesity among adults: United States, 2017–2018. National Center for Health Statistics. https://www.cdc.gov/nchs/products/databriefs/db360.htm

Chhatre, S., Cook, R., Mallik, E., & Jayadevappa, R. (2017). Trends in substance use admissions among older adults. *BMC Health Services Research, 17*(1), 584. https://doi.org/10.1186/s12913-017-2538-z

Cornelis, E., Gorus, E., Van Schelvergem, N., & De Vriendt, P. (2019). The relationship between basic, instrumental, and advanced activities of daily living and executive functioning in geriatric patients with neurocognitive disorders. *International Journal of Geriatric Psychiatry, 34*(6), 889–899. https://doi.org/10.1002/gps.5087

Cumming, E., & Henry, W. E. (1960). *Growing old: The process of disengagement.* Basic Books

Erikson, E. H., & Erikson, J. M. (1997). *The lifecycle completed, extended version.* W.W. Norton & Company.

Gholamnezhad, Z., Boskabady, M. H., & Jahangiri, Z. (2020). Exercise and dementia. *Advances in Experimental Medicine and Biology, 1228*, 303–315. https://doi.org/10.1007/978-981-15-1792-1_20

Gouveia, É. R. Q., Gouveia, B. R., Ihle, A., Kliegel, M., Maia, J. A., Bermudez i Badia, S., & Freitas, D. L. (2017). Correlates of health-related quality of life in young-old and old-old community-dwelling older adults. *Quality of Life Research: An International Journal of Quality of Life Aspects of Treatment, Care & Rehabilitation*, 26(6), 1561–1569. https://doi-org.libproxy.siue.edu/10.1007/s11136-017-1502-z

Happell, B., Wilson, K., Platania-Phung, C., & Stanton, R. (2017). Physical health and mental illness: Listening to the voice of carers. *Journal of Mental Health*, 26(2), 127–133. https://doi-org.libproxy.siue.edu/10.3109/09638237.2016.116785

Havighurst, R. J. (1961). Successful aging. *The Gerontologist*, 1(1), 8–13.

Hernandez-Tejada, M. A., Frook, G., Steedley, M., Watkins, J., & Acierno, R. (2020). Demographic-based risk of reporting psychopathology and poor health among mistreated older adults in the national elder mistreatment study wave II. *Aging & Mental Health*, 24(1), 22–26. https://doi.org/10.1080/13607863.2018.1509296

IOM (Institute of Medicine). (2015). *Cognitive aging: Progress in understanding and opportunities for action*. The National Academies Press.

Jeste, D. V., Savla, G. N., Thompson, W. K., Vahia, I. V., Glorioso, D. K., Martin, A. S., Palmer, B. W., Rock, D., Golshan, S., Kraemer, H. C., & Depp, C. A. (2013). Association between older age and more successful aging: Critical role of resilience and depression. *American Journal of Psychiatry*, 170(2), 188–196.

Jokela, M., Airaksinen, J., Virtanen, M., Batty, G. D., Kivimäki, M., & Hakulinen, C. (2020). Personality, disability-free life years, and life expectancy: Individual participant meta-analysis of 131,195 individuals from 10 cohort studies. *Journal of Personality*, 88(3), 596–605. https://doi.org/10.1111/jopy.12513

Karimi, R., Bakhtiyari, M., & Masjedi Arani, A. (2019). Protective factors of marital stability in long-term marriage globally: A systematic review. *Epidemiology and Health*, 41, e2019023. https://doi.org/10.4178/epih.e2019023

Kiesswetter, E., Colombo, M. G., Meisinger, C., Peters, A., Thorand, B., Holle, R., Ladwig, K. H., Schulz, H., Grill, E., Diekmann, R., Schrader, E., Stehle, P., Sieber, C. C., & Volkert, D. (2020). Malnutrition and related risk factors in older adults from different health-care settings: An *enable* study. *Public Health Nutrition*, 23(3), 446–456. https://doi.org/10.1017/S1368980019002271

Killgore, W., Cloonan, S. A., Taylor, E. C., & Dailey, N. S. (2020). Loneliness: A signature mental health concern in the era of COVID-19. *Psychiatry Research*, 290, 113117. https://doi.org/10.1016/j.psychres.2020.113117

Lee, Y. W., Kim, N. C., Ahn, S. Y., Cho, M. O., Choi, K. S., Kong, E. S., Kim, C. G., Kim, H. K., & Chang, S. O. (2020). Exploring the subjective frame of references in the development of gerotranscendence in Korean older adults: Q Methodology. *Journal of Transcultural Nursing*, 1043659620903775. https://doi.org/10.1177/1043659620903775

Li, Z., & Dalaker, J. (2019). *Poverty among Americans aged 65 and older*. Congressional Research Service https://crsreports.congress.gov. R45791

Lima, S., Teixeira, L., Esteves, R., Ribeiro, F., Pereira, F., Teixeira, A., & Magalhães, C. (2020). Spirituality and quality of life in older adults: A path analysis model. *BMC Geriatrics*, 20(1), 259. https://doi.org/10.1186/s12877-020-01646-0

Löckenhoff, C. E., & Rutt, J. L. (2017). Age differences in self-continuity: Converging evidence and directions for future research. *The Gerontologist*, 57(3), 396–408. https://doi.org/10.1093/geront/gnx010.

Lövdén, M., Fratiglioni, L., Glymour, M. M., Lindenberger, U., & Tucker-Drob, E. M. (2020). Education and cognitive functioning across the life span. *Psychological Science in the Public Interest: A Journal of the American Psychological Society*, 21(1), 6–41. https://doi.org/10.1177/1529100620920576

Ma, K., & Saw, A. (2020). An international systematic review of dementia caregiving interventions for Chinese families. *International Journal of Geriatric Psychiatry*, 35(11), 1263–1284. https://doi.org/10.1002/gps.5400

Macleod, A., Busija, L., & McCabe, M. (2020). Mapping the perceived sexuality of heterosexual men and women in mid- and later life: A mixed-methods study. *Sexual Medicine*, 8(1), 84–99. https://doi.org/10.1016/j.esxm.2019.10.001 64–569

Maltais, M., Boisvert-Vigneault, K., Rolland, Y., Vellas, B., de Souto Barreto, P., & MAPT/DSA Study Group. (2019). Longitudinal associations of physical activity levels with morphological and functional changes related with aging: The MAPT study. *Experimental Gerontology*, 128, 110758. https://doi.org/10.1016/j.exger.2019.110758

McCombe, G., Fogarty, F., Swan, D., Hannigan, A., Fealy, G. M., Kyne, L., Meagher, D., & Cullen, W. (2018). Identified mental disorders in older adults in primary care: A cross-sectional database study. *The European Journal of General Practice*, 24(1), 84–91. https://doi.org/10.1080/13814788.2017.1402884

Miller, K. J., Gonçalves-Bradley, D. C., Areerob, P., Hennessy, D., Mesagno, C., & Grace, F. (2020). Comparative effectiveness of three exercise types to treat clinical depression in older adults: A systematic review and network meta-analysis of randomised controlled trials. *Ageing Research Reviews*, 58, 100999. https://doi.org/10.1016/j.arr.2019.100999

National Center on Elder Abuse (NCEA). (2017). The facts of elder abuse. *Administration on aging*. U.S. Department of Health & Human Services. https://ncea.acl.gov/NCEA/media/Publication/NCEA_TheFactsofEA_2019_5.pdf

Oh, A., (2019). Social support and patterns of institutionalization among older adults: A Longitudinal Study. *Journal of the American Geriatrics Society*, 67(12), 2622–2627. https://doi.org/10.1111/jgs.16184.

Perera, N., & Agboola, S. (2019). Are formal self-care interventions for healthy people effective? A systematic review of the evidence. *BMJ Global Health*, 4(Suppl 10), e001415. https://doi.org/10.1136/bmjgh-2019-001415

Quinn, J. F., & Cahill, K. E. (2016). The new world of retirement income security in America. *American Psychologist*, 71(4), 321–333.

Rhee, T. G., & Rosenheck, R. A. (2020). Alcohol use disorder among adults recovered from substance use disorders. *The American Journal on Addictions*, 29(4), 331–339. https://doi.org/10.1111/ajad.13026

Rutt, J. L., & Lockenhoff, C. E. (2016). From past to future. Temporal self-continuity across the life span. *Psychology and Aging*, 31(6), 631–639.

Saxon, S. V., Perkins, E. A., & Etten, M. J. (2015). *Physical change and aging: A guide for the helping professions* (6th ed.). Springer.

Smith, M. L., Steinman, L. E., & Casey, E. A. (2020). Combatting social isolation among older adults in a time of physical distancing: The COVID-19 Social Connectivity Paradox. *Frontiers in Public Health*, 8, 403. https://doi.org/10.3389/fpubh.2020.00403

Srinivasan, S., Glover, J., Tampi, R. R., Tampi, D. J., & Sewell, D. D. (2019). Sexuality and the older adult. *Current Psychiatry Reports*, 21(10), 97. https://doi.org/10.1007/s11920-019-1090-4

Sun, F. W., Stepanovic, M. R., Andreano, J., Barrett, L. F., Touroutoglou, A., & Dickerson, B. C. (2016). Youthful brains in older adults: Preserved neuroanatomy in the default mode and salience networks contributes to youthful memory in superaging. *Journal of Neuroscience*, 36(37), 9659–9668.

Talebreza, S., & McPherson, M. L. (2020). Recognizing and managing polypharmacy in advanced illness. *The Medical Clinics of North America*, 104(3), 405–413. https://doi.org/10.1016/j.mcna.2019.12.003

Tamborini, C. R., & Kim, C. (2020). Are you saving for retirement? Racial/ethnic differentials in contributory retirement savings plans. *The Journals of Gerontology. Series B, Psychological Sciences and Social Sciences*, 75(4), 837–848. https://doi.org/10.1093/geronb/gbz131

Tornstam, L. (2005). *Gerotranscendence: A developmental theory of positive aging*. Springer Publishing Company.

Voss, M. W., Wadsworth, L. L., Birmingham, W., Merryman, M. B., Crabtree, L., Subasic, K., & Hung, M. (2020). Health effects of late-career unemployment. *Journal of Aging and Health*, 32(1), 106–116. https://doi.org/10.1177/0898264318806792

Whitley, D. M., Kelley, S. J., & Lamis, D. A. (2016). Depression, social support, and mental health: A longitudinal mediation analysis in African American custodial grandmothers. *The International Journal of Aging*, 82(2–3), 166–187.

Wolfson, J. A., & Leung, C. W. (2020). Food insecurity and COVID-19: Disparities in early effects for US adults. *Nutrients*, 12(6), 1648. https://doi.org/10.3390/nu12061648

Yesavage, J. A., Brink, T. L., Rose, T. L., Lum, O., Huang, V., Adey, M., & Leirer, V. O. (1982). Development and validation of a geriatric depression screening scale: A preliminary report. *Journal of Psychiatric Research*, 17(1), 37–49.

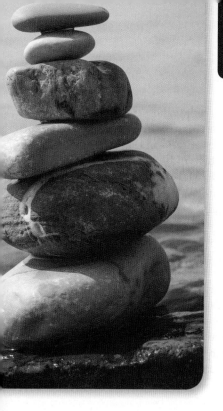

Prevention of Mental Disorders

19

Stress and Mental Health

Kelley McGuire

KEYCONCEPTS

- appraisal
- allostatic load
- adaptation
- coping
- stress

LEARNING OBJECTIVES

After studying this chapter, you will be able to:

1. Discuss the concept of stress as it relates to mental health and mental illness.

2. Differentiate acute stress from chronic stress.

3. Discuss the factors that lead to allostatic load.

4. Discuss psychosocial factors that influence the experience of stress.

5. Discuss the variety of stress responses experienced by individuals.

6. Explain the role of coping and adaptation in maintaining and promoting mental health.

7. Apply critical thinking skills to the nursing process for a person experiencing stress.

KEY TERMS

- Acute stress • Allostasis • Chronic stress • Diathesis • Emotion-focused coping • Emotions • General adaptation syndrome • Homeostasis • Problem-focused coping • Reappraisal • Social functioning • Social network • Social support • Stress response • Transactional stress model

INTRODUCTION

Stress is a natural part of life, yet it is one of the most complex concepts in health and nursing. Although often thought of as negative, depending on the source of the stress, it can be a positive experience. During severe stress, some people draw on resources that they never realized they had and grow from those experiences. However, early childhood stress and trauma, unresolved stress, or chronic stress can have negative mental and physical health consequences.

Stress is also associated with the development or exacerbation of symptoms of mental illness. For example, a stressful event may precipitate a psychosis. Family caregivers can develop depression as they continually monitor their family member, cope with illness-related behaviors, and often witness deterioration of their partner (Crespo et al., 2019).

Stress is approached from several overlapping theoretical perspectives—physiologic, psychological, and social. Consequently, there are many definitions of stress depending upon the theoretical perspective. This chapter provides an overview of the major evidence-based theories of stress and describes the applicability of the models in the practice of nursing.

BIOLOGIC PERSPECTIVES OF STRESS

Physiologic responses to stress are automatic and differ based on the event, duration, and intensity. Homeostasis and allostasis are the foundation of the physiologic responses to stressful events.

Homeostasis versus Allostasis

The concept of **homeostasis**, which is the body's tendency to resist physiologic change and hold bodily functions relatively consistent, well-coordinated, and usually stable, was introduced by Walter Cannon in the 1930s. The body's internal equilibrium is regulated by physiologic processes such as blood glucose, pH, and oxygen; set points (normal reference ranges of physiologic parameters) are maintained (Cannon, 1932).

Allostasis is a term used to describe how the body adapts to maintain physiologic stability. Allostasis is a dynamic regulatory process involving functions of the autonomic nervous system, the hypothalamic–pituitary–adrenal (HPA) axis, and the cardiovascular, metabolic, and immune systems respond to internal and external stimuli (McEwen, 2017).

Acute Stress

Acute stress, an intense biopsychosocial reaction to a threatening event, is time limited (usually less than a month) but can occur repeatedly. It can lead to physiologic allostatic load/overload, which in turn can have a negative impact on a person's health (McEwen, 2017).

Acute stress is associated with the "fight-or-flight" response. When the brain (amygdala and hippocampus) interprets an event as a threat, the hypothalamus and autonomic nervous system are signaled to secrete adrenaline, cortisol, and epinephrine. These hormones activate the sympathetic nervous system and physiologic stability is challenged. A "fight-or-flight" response occurs when the heart rate, blood pressure, and blood sugar increase. Energy is mobilized for survival. As the sympathetic system is activated, the parasympathetic is muted (Table 19.1). After there is no longer a need for more energy and the threat is over, the body returns to a state of homeostasis.

Chronic Stress

Chronic stress is an ongoing physiologic reaction to events resulting in "wear and tear" on the body and negatively impacts health and well-being. The adaptive physiologic changes that occur during acute stress become maladaptive when prolonged and contribute to the risk for illness. The relationship between chronic stress and illness was identified many years ago with the introduction of the general adaptation syndrome (GAS).

TABLE 19.1	FIGHT AND FLIGHT: PHYSIOLOGIC CHANGES	
Sympathetic Nervous System Effect	**Purpose**	**Parasympathetic Nervous System Conservation of Energy**
Increased serum glucose	Increased energy	Decreased sexual and sex hormone activity
Increased cardiac output and blood pressure (increase in renin and angiotensin)	Increased blood flow	Decreased growth, repair, and maturation
Increased oxygen tension and hematocrit	Increased supply of oxygen in blood	Decreased digestion, assimilation, and whole food distribution
Other Physiologic Changes		
Effect	**Purpose**	
Increased immune responses	Reduced risk of infections	
Heightened vigilance in the brain	Increased decision-making attention and memory	
Hyperactivation of the hemostatic and coagulation system	Prevention of excessive bleeding from wounds	

Adapted from Diamond, J. W. (2009). Allostatic medicine: Bringing stress, coping, and chronic disease into focus: Part 1. *Integrative Medicine, 8*(6), 40–44.

General Adaptation Syndrome

Hans Seyle, who is credited with initiation of the study of stress, defined stress as a nonspecific response to an irritant, a perceived danger, or a life threat. He called stress evoked by positive emotions or events *eustress* and stress evoked by negative feelings and events *distress*. He showed that corticosteroid secretion from the pituitary gland increased during stress and contributed to development of illnesses. Seyle described this process as **general adaptation syndrome (GAS)** (Selye, 1956, 1974). This early work set the stage for our understanding of the role of the HPA in chronic stress.

When the HPA axis is activated under conditions of stress, the hypothalamus secretes corticotropin-releasing hormone, because of which the pituitary gland increases secretion of adrenocorticotropic hormone (corticotropin), which in turn stimulates the adrenocortical secretion of cortisol. Over time, excessive exposure to cortisol contributes to the dysregulation of the autonomic nervous system.

Allostatic Load

Allostatic load (AL) is a term used to describe the wear and tear on a person's body and brain resulting from chronic stress. The cumulative changes of the biologic regulatory systems (cardiovascular, metabolic, and immune) is indicated by abnormal laboratory values and may increase the risk of disease and illness. As wear and tear on the brain and body occurs, there is a corresponding increase in the AL (Fig. 19.1). The greater the AL, the greater the state of chronic stress and, ultimately, the more negative changes in health (Guidi et al., 2021; McEwen, 2017).

> **KEYCONCEPT Allostatic load** is the consequence of the wear and tear on the body and brain and leads to ill health.

Paradoxically, the same systems that are protective in acute stress can damage the body when activated by chronic stress. The benefits of the increase in circulating cortisol to the human body are initially adaptive, but if it continues, it can be quite damaging to both mental (depression) and physical (immune, cardiovascular, and metabolic) health (Anisman, 2015; McVicar et al., 2013; Sterling, 2012).

Consequences of Chronic Stress

In chronic stress, the immune system is suppressed. Cortisol is primarily immunosuppressive and contributes to reduction in lymphocyte numbers and function (primarily T-lymphocyte and monocyte subsets) and natural killer activities. The immune cells have receptors for cortisol and catecholamines that can bind with lymphatic cells and suppress the immune system. The continuous sustained activation of the sympathetic nervous system; HPA axis; cardiovascular, metabolic, and immune systems contribute to a hormonal overload, leading to impairment in memory, immunity, cardiovascular, and metabolic function (McEwen, 2017).

Over time, chronic stress compromises health and increases susceptibility to illnesses. For instance, children who have suffered psychological neglect, abuse, or parental loss are more likely to experience elevated AL in adulthood (Guidi et al., 2021). Elevation of white blood cell counts and lower counts of T, B, and natural killer cells are found in those who face academic examinations, job strain, caregiving for a family member experiencing dementia, marital conflict, and daily stress. Altered parameters of immune function are present in those with negative moods (chronic hostility, depression, and anxiety), social isolation, and marital disagreement. Antibody titers to Epstein–Barr and herpes simplex viruses are also

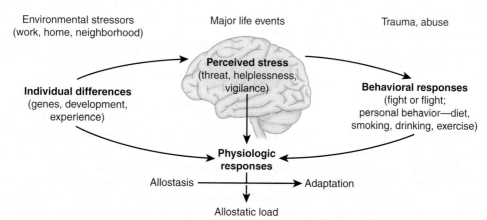

FIGURE 19.1 The development of allostatic load in response to stress. (Redrawn from McEwen, B. S. [1998]. Protective and damaging effects of stress and stress mediators. *New England Journal of Medicine, 3*[38], 171–179. Copyright © 1998 Massachusetts Medical Society. Reprinted with permission from Massachusetts Medical Society.)

BOX 19.1

Research for Best Practice: Allostatic Load

Chyu, L. & Upchurch, D. M. (2018). A longitudinal analysis of allostatic load among a multi-ethnic sample of midlife women: Findings from the study of women's health across the nation. Women's Health Issues, 28(3), 258–266.

THE QUESTION: Does AL increase over time (reflecting health declines and physiological aging) in midlife women (42–52 years old)? Is lower socioeconomic status associated with higher AL?

METHODS: A community-based, multisite, prospective study examined biopsychosocial changes during menopausal transition among a cohort of midlife women (N = 1,932; 13,391 observations). Ten biomarkers were used to represent AL across cardiovascular, inflammatory, metabolic, and neuroendocrine systems. AL scores were calculated at baseline and at annual visits at seven time points. Higher AL scores indicated poorer health.

FINDINGS: Older age at baseline, lower household income, African-American race, and speaking and reading English only were significant predictors of higher AL scores.

IMPLICATIONS FOR NURSING: AL can be used to identify high-risk women and begin early prevention and intervention to reduce disease burden and disparities at the population level.

---

elevated in stressed populations. If the stress is long term, the immune alteration continues (McEwen, 2017).

Health disparities found in lower socioeconomic groups, racial and ethnic minorities, and older adults may be partly explained by the chronic stress they tend to experience. These groups have been found to have elevated AL. AL has been found to differ by race, where Black Americans display greater levels than White Americans. Further, the effects of elevated AL may present differently based on gender, where high AL is more often associated with depression in Black men and White women than their corresponding counterpart (Guidi et al., 2021; McEwen, 2017) (see Box 19.1).

Chronic Stress and Mental Illness

When stress is associated with the development or exacerbation of a mental illness, the diathesis–stress model can be applied. A **diathesis** is a genetic predisposition that increases susceptibility of developing a disorder. This model describes how stress can trigger the development or exacerbation of an illness (Kalamatianos & Canellopoulos, 2019). Exposure to childhood trauma can lead to negative long-term health consequences on mental and physical health throughout life (American Society for the Positive Care of Children, 2021); for example, a

woman whose mother had a long history of depression (indicating a genetic predisposition to mental disorders for the daughter) and who was assaulted as she was leaving work and sustained multiple injuries. Her first manic episode occurred within 2 months (see Chapter 22).

No one lives in a stress-free environment, yet stress reduction leads to positive mental health. Conversely, many patients attribute their first illness episode to a stressful event such as an assault, rape, or family tragedy.

PSYCHOSOCIAL PERSPECTIVES OF STRESS

The **Transactional Stress Model** describes the psychological experience of stress. This model views stress as an interactive process arising from real or perceived internal or external environmental demands that are appraised as threatening or benign (Fig. 19.2) (Lazarus & Folkman, 1984). The external environment includes physical aspects such as air quality, cleanliness of food and water, temperature, and noise and social aspects such as living arrangements and personal contacts.

> **KEYCONCEPT Stress** is a process arising from real or perceived internal or external environmental demands that are appraised as threatening or benign (Lazarus & Folkman, 1984).

Appraisal

Appraisal is the individual perception that an event or situation is a threat. One situation may be perceived as threatening to one person but not to another (Box 19.2). The more important or meaningful the event, the more vulnerable the person is to stress. For example, chest pain is threatening not only because of the immediate pain and incapacitation but also because the pain may mean a heart attack is occurring. The individual is afraid that they may not have the physiologic resources to survive the attack.

> **KEYCONCEPT Appraisal** is the process where potentially stressful events are evaluated for meaning and significance to individual well-being (Lazarus & Folkman, 1984).

Appraisal is a complex process that includes many aspects—the demands, constraints, and resources are balanced with personal goals and beliefs. A critical factor is the risk that the event poses to a person's well-being (Carpenter, 2016; Lazarus, 2001).

The appraisal process has two levels: primary and secondary. In a primary appraisal, a person evaluates the events occurring in their life as a threat, harm, or challenge. During primary appraisal of an event, the person determines whether (1) the event is relevant, (2) the event is consistent with their values and beliefs, and (3) a personal commitment is present. In the vignette, Susan's

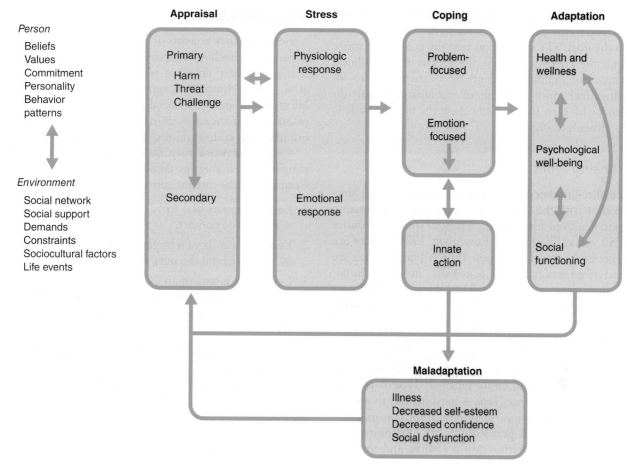

FIGURE 19.2   Stress, coping, and adaptation model.

BOX 19.2 CLINICAL VIGNETTE

Stress Responses to an Examination

Two students are preparing for the same examination. Susan is genuinely interested in the subject, prepares by studying throughout the semester, and reviews the content 2 days before test day. The night before the examination, she goes to bed early, gets a good night's sleep, and wakes refreshed but is slightly nervous about the test. She wants to do well and expects a difficult test but knows that she can retake it at a later date if she does poorly.

In contrast, Joanne is not interested in the subject matter and does not study throughout the semester. She "crams" 2 days before the test date and does an "all-nighters" the night before. This is the last time that Joanne can take the examination, but she believes that she will pass because she has already taken it twice and is familiar with the questions. If she does not pass, she will not be able to return to school. On entering the room, Joanne is physically tired and somewhat fearful of not passing the test. As she looks at the test, she instantly realizes that it is not the examination she expected. The questions are new. She begins hyperventilating and tremoring. After yelling obscenities at the teacher, she storms out of the room. She is very distressed and describes herself as "being in a panic."

What Do You Think?

- How are the students' experiences different? Are there any similarities?
- Are there any nursing diagnoses that apply to Joanne's situation?

commitment to the goal of doing well on the test was consistent with her valuing the content, which in turn motivated her to study regularly and prepare carefully for the examination. She believed that the test would be difficult. Joanne had a commitment to pass the test but did not value the content. Unlike Susan, Joanne believed that the test would be relatively easy because she expected the questions to be the same as those on the previous examination.

In a secondary appraisal, the person determines if they possess the necessary coping mechanisms to overcome the event. In the example, Susan was nervous but took the test. Joanne's secondary appraisal of the test-taking situation began with the realization that she might not pass the test because the questions were different. She acted impulsively by blaming the teacher for giving a different examination and storming out of the room. She clearly did not cope effectively with a difficult situation.

Values and Goals

Cultural, ethnic, family, and religious values shape the significance and importance of the event. For example, one person may value a high-paying salary and another may value the freedom to move around without the boundaries of material things.

If a goal (such as maintaining an important position) is important, a person is more likely to do what it takes to reach the goal. The more important the goal or the more difficult the goal is to obtain, the greater the likelihood of stress. For example, students who earn mostly or all As often feel more stress about examinations than do students who earn Bs and Cs because the higher grade is more difficult to obtain.

Personality Types

Personality influences the appraisal process and the ability to cope with the stress. The association of personality types to health or illness status has been studied for more than 50 years (Friedman & Rosenman, 1974). There are four general personality types. Type A personalities are characterized as competitive, aggressive, ambitious, impatient, alert, tense, and restless. They think, speak, and act at an accelerated pace and reflect an aggressive, hostile, and time-urgent style of living that is often associated with increased psychophysiologic arousal (Bokenberger et al., 2014; Roy, 2018). In contrast, type B personalities do not exhibit these behaviors and generally are more relaxed, easygoing, and easily satisfied. Type B personalities are less likely than Type A personalities to engage in risky health behaviors such as alcohol consumption and smoking. Type B personalities are also more likely to practice preventative care measures and wellness activities (Korotkov et al., 2011). Type B personalities are described as accepting and relaxed. They are unlikely to experience a lack of time for commitments and are able to commit time for relaxation (Iswari, 2020).

Type C personalities are described as having difficulty expressing emotion and are introverted, respectful, conforming, compliant, and eager to please and avoid conflict. They respond to stress with depression and hopelessness. This personality type was initially associated with the development of cancer, specifically breast cancer in women, presumably due to the changes that occur within endocrine and immune function (Lală et al., 2010; Romo-González et al., 2018). It is more likely that this personality type will experience more depression and difficult marital adjustment (Bozo et al., 2017).

Type D (distressed) personalities experience a tendency toward negative emotions and pessimism. These individuals are more likely to be socially inhibited and are unlikely to show their emotions to others. Despite some overlap, the characteristics of type D personalities are different than depression and anxiety (Kim et al., 2020). There is mixed research support for an association between a type D personality and mental health disorders and poor physical health status (Marchesi et al., 2014; Stevenson & Williams, 2014). Emerging data suggest that type D personality is related to outcome severity of acute coronary syndrome and diabetes (Conti et al., 2016; Garcia-Retamero et al., 2016).

Social Networks

A **social network** consists of linkages among a defined set of people with whom an individual has personal contacts. A social identity develops within this network (Azmitia et al., 2008). Emotional support, material aid, services, information, and new social contacts increase personal resources, enhance the ability to cope with change, and influence the course of illnesses (Li & Wu, 2010).

A social network may be small, or it may be large, consisting of numerous family and community contacts. Contacts can be categorized according to three levels:

1. Level I consists of 6 to 12 people with whom the person has close contact.
2. Level II consists of a larger number of contacts, 30 to 40 people whom the person sees regularly.
3. Level III consists of an even larger number of people with whom a person has direct contact, such as the grocer and mail carrier, and can represent several hundred people.

Each person's social network is slightly different. Multiple contacts allow several networks to interact. Generally, the larger the network, the more support is available. An ideal network structure is fairly dense and interconnected; people within the network are in contact with one another. Dense networks are better able to respond in times of stress and crisis and to provide emotional support to those in distress. For example, residents of a small town are more likely to provide food and shelter to fire victims than neighbors in a large urban area who have little contact with each other.

Ideally, a balance between intense and less intense relationships exists in a social network. When relationships are intense and include only one or two people, the opportunity to interact with other network members is limited. However, isolation can occur without at least a few intense relationships.

Social networks provide opportunities for give and take. Network members both provide and receive support, aid, services, and information. Reciprocity is particularly important because most friendships do not last without the give and take of support and services. A person who is always on the receiving end eventually becomes isolated from others.

Distinguishing a social network from social networking and social media is vital. Because social media has grown in popularity throughout the past two decades, there is controversial evidence about the relationship between social media usage and mental health outcomes (Aalbers et al., 2019). While some studies report that social media use increases stress, depression, and experiencing symptoms of loneliness, others report that abstinence from social media decreases life satisfaction for similar reasons (Aalbers et al., 2019; Vally & D'Souza, 2019).

Social Support

One of the important functions of the social network is to provide **social support** in the form of positive interpersonal interactions as part of a dynamic process that is in constant flux and varies with life events and health status (Whatley et al., 2010). Not all interpersonal interactions within a network are supportive. A person can have a large, complex social network but little social support. Some life events, such as marriage, divorce, and bereavement, actually change the level of social support by adding to or subtracting from a person's social network.

Social support serves three functions:

1. Emotional support contributes to a person's feelings of being cared for or loved.

2. Tangible support provides a person with additional resources.

3. Informational support helps a person view situations in a new light (Table 19.2).

Social support enhances health outcomes and reduces mortality by helping members make needed behavior changes and buffering stressful life events. Individuals with strong social support have a lower risk of psychopathology related to an increased likelihood of practicing positive and effective coping strategies to deal with stress (McDonald et al., 2020). In a supportive social environment, members feel helped, valued, and in personal control.

Cultural Factors and Ethnic Identity

Cultural expectations and role strain serve as both demands and constraints in the experience of stress. If a person violates cultural group values to meet role expectations, stress occurs; for example, a person may stay in an abusive relationship to avoid the stress of violating a cultural norm that values lifelong marriage, no matter what the circumstances. The potential guilt associated with norm violation and the anticipated isolation from being ostracized seem worse than the physical and psychological pain caused by the abusive situation. Ethnic identity affirmation describes the recognition of positive attributes of one's ethnic group (McDonald et al., 2020). Evidence suggests ethnic identity can help individuals cope with and manage stressful experiences, including chronic stressors (McDonald et al., 2020).

Employment Factors

Employment is another highly valued cultural norm and provides social, psychological, and financial benefits. In all cultures, work is assigned significance beyond economic compensation. It is often the central focus of adulthood and, for many, a source of personal identity. Even if employment brings little real happiness, being employed implies financial needs are being met. Work offers status, regulates life activities, permits association with others, and provides a meaningful life experience. Although work is demanding, unemployment can be equally or more stressful because of the associated isolation, loss of social status, and potential financial strains.

Gender Influences

Gender expectations often become an additional source of demands and constraints for women, who assume multiple roles. In most cultures, women who work outside the home are expected to assume primary responsibility for care of the children and household duties. Maternal employment offers several benefits; however, increased workplace stress and difficulty finding balance between work and family responsibilities can increase the risk of depression in women (Shepherd-Banigan et al., 2016).

Life Events

In 1967, Holmes and Rahe (1967) presented a psychosocial view of illness by pointing out the complex relationship between life changes and the development of illnesses. They hypothesized that people become ill after they experience major life events, such as marriage, divorce, and bereavement. The more frequent the changes, the greater the possibility of becoming sick. The investigators cited the events that they believed partially accounted for the onset of illnesses and began testing whether these life changes were actual precursors to illness. It soon became clear that not all events have the same effects. For example, the death of a spouse or partner is usually much more devastating and stressful than a change in residence. From their research, the investigators were able to assign relative weights to various life events according to the degree of associated stress. Rahe (1994) devised the Recent Life Changes Questionnaire (Table 19.3) to evaluate the frequency and significance of

TABLE 19.2	EXAMPLES OF FUNCTIONS OF SOCIAL SUPPORT
Function	Example
Emotional support	Attachment, reassurance, being able to rely on and confide in a person
Tangible support	Direct aid such as loans or gifts, services such as taking care of someone who is ill, doing a job or chore
Informational support	Providing information or advice, giving feedback about how a person is doing

Reprinted by permission from Springer: Schaefer, C., Coyne, J., & Lazarus, R. (1982). The health-related functions of social support. *Journal of Behavioral Medicine, 4*(4), 381–406. Copyright © 1981 Springer Nature.

TABLE 19.3   RECENT LIFE CHANGES QUESTIONNAIRE

Directions: Sum the life-change units (LCUs) for your life-changing events during the past 12 months.

250–400 LCUs per year: Minor life crisis

Over 400 LCUs per year: Major life crisis

Life Changes	LCU Values[a]	Life Changes	LCU Values[a]
Family		Begin or end school	32
Death of spouse	105	Change in sleeping habits	31
Marital separation	65	Revision of personal habits	31
Death of close family member	65	Change in eating habits	29
Divorce	62	Change in church activities	29
Pregnancy	60	Vacation	29
Change in health of family member	52	Change in school	28
Marriage	50	Change in recreation	28
Gain of new family member	50	Christmas	26
Marital reconciliation	42	**Work**	
Spouse begins or stops work	37	Fired at work	64
Son or daughter leaves home	29	Retirement from work	49
In-law trouble	29	Trouble with boss	39
Change in number of family get-togethers	26	Business readjustment	38
Personal		Change to different line of work	38
Jail term	56	Change in work responsibilities	33
Sex difficulties	49	Change in work hours or conditions	30
Death of a close friend	46	**Financial**	
Personal injury or illness	42	Foreclosure of mortgage or loan	57
Change in living conditions	39	Change in financial state	43
Outstanding personal achievement	33	Mortgage (e.g., home, car)	39
Change in residence	33	Mortgage or loan less than $10,000 (e.g., stereo)	26
Minor violations of the law	32		

[a]LCU, life-change unit. The number of LCUs reflects the average degree or intensity of the life change.
Reprinted with permission from Rahe, R. H. (2000). Recent Life Changes Questionnaire (RLCQ).

life-changing events. Numerous research studies subsequently demonstrated the relationship between a recent life change and the severity of near-future illness or the development of a new illness (Friborg, 2019; Rahe, 1994; Rahe et al., 2002). Recent studies show that life changes in older adults that resulted in feeling helpless or fearing for their life reported higher body mass index and more chronic illnesses (Seib et al., 2014). If several life changes occur within a short period, the likelihood that an illness will appear is even greater (Tamers et al., 2014).

RESPONSES TO STRESS

A **stress response** includes simultaneous physiologic and emotional responses. The physiologic stress responses were previously discussed. Emotional responses to stress

depend on the significance of the event experience. It is now known that people experience stress differently depending on their gender. Whereas males are more likely to respond to stress with a fight-or-flight response, females have less aggressive responses; they "tend and befriend" (McEwen, 2005).

Emotional Responses

Emotions (psychophysiologic reactions that define a person's mood) are usually ones of excitement or distress marked by strong feelings and usually accompanied by an impulse toward definite action. If the emotions are intense, a disturbance in intellectual functions occurs. When the situation is viewed as a challenge, emotions are more likely to be positive. If the event is evaluated as

TABLE 19.4	CORE RELATIONAL THEMES FOR EACH EMOTION
Emotion	**Relational Meaning**
Anger	A demeaning offense against me and mine
Anxiety	Facing an uncertain, existential threat
Fright	Facing an immediate, concrete, and overwhelming physical danger
Guilt	Having transgressed a moral imperative
Shame	Having failed to live up to an ego ideal
Sadness	Having experienced an irrevocable loss
Envy	Wanting what someone else has
Jealousy	Resenting a third party for the loss of or a threat to another's affection
Disgust	Taking in or being too close to an indigestible object or idea (metaphorically speaking)
Happiness	Making reasonable progress toward the realization of a goal
Pride	Enhancement of one's ego identity by taking credit for a valued object or achievement, either our own or that of someone or a group with whom we identify
Relief	A distressing goal/incongruent condition that has changed for the better or gone away
Hope	Fearing the worst but yearning for better
Love	Desiring or participating in affection, usually but not necessarily reciprocated
Compassion	Being moved by another's suffering and wanting to help

Adapted with permission of Oxford University Press from Lazarus, R. S. (1991). *Emotion and adaptation* (p. 122). Oxford University Press; permission conveyed through Copyright Clearance Center, Inc.

threatening or harmful, negative emotions are elicited. Emotions can be categorized as follows:

- *Negative emotions* occur when there is a threat to, delay in, or thwarting of a goal or a conflict between goals: anger, fright, anxiety, guilt, shame, sadness, envy, jealousy, and disgust.
- *Positive emotions* occur when there is movement toward or attainment of a goal: happiness, pride, relief, and love.

- *Borderline emotions* are somewhat ambiguous: hope, compassion, empathy, sympathy, and contentment.
- *Nonemotions* describe emotional reactions that are too ambiguous to fit into any of the preceding categories: confidence, awe, confusion, and excitement (Lazarus, 2006).

Emotions are expressed as themes that summarize dangers or benefits of each stressful situation. For instance, physical danger provokes fear; a loss leads to feelings of sadness (Table 19.4). Emotions have their own innate responses that are automatic and unique; for example, anger may automatically provoke tremors in one person but both tremors and perspiration in another. Emotions often provoke impulsive behavior. For example, the first impulse of a young musician facing his first performance at Carnegie Hall who experiences stage fright is to run home. As he resists this impulse, he begins coping with his fears in order to perform.

COPING

Coping is a deliberate, planned, and psychological effort to manage stressful demands. The coping process may inhibit or override the innate urge to act. Positive coping leads to adaptation, which is characterized by a balance between health and illness, a sense of well-being, and maximum **social functioning**. When a person does not cope well, maladaptations occur that can shift the balance toward illness, a diminished self-concept, and deterioration in social functioning.

KEYCONCEPT Coping is a deliberate, planned, and psychological effort to manage stressful demands.

There are two types of coping. In **problem-focused coping**, the person addresses the source of stress and solves the problem (eliminating it or changing its effects). In **emotion-focused coping**, the person reduces the stress by reinterpreting the situation to change its meaning (Boxes 19.3 and 19.4).

Different coping strategies will be needed for different situations. Over time, strategies become automatic and develop into patterns for each person. Some situations require a combination of strategies and activities. Ideally, a stressful situation is matched with the needed resources as the events are unfolding. Social support can be critical in helping people cope with difficult situations. Successful coping with life stresses is linked to quality of life and to physical and mental health (Lazarus, 2001).

As a part of the coping process, reappraisal is important because of the changing nature of the stressful situation. **Reappraisal**, which is the same as appraisal

---

BOX 19.3

Ways of Coping: Examples of Problem-Focused Versus Emotion-Focused Coping

PROBLEM-FOCUSED COPING

- When noise from the television interrupts a student's studying and causes the student to be stressed, the student turns off the television and eliminates the noise.
- An abused spouse is finally able to leave her husband because she realizes that the abuse will not stop even though he promises never to hit her again.

EMOTION-FOCUSED COPING

- A husband is adamantly opposed to visiting his wife's relatives because they keep dogs in their house. Even though the dogs are well cared for, their presence in the relative's home violates his need for an orderly, clean house and causes the husband sufficient stress that he copes with by refusing to visit. This becomes a source of marital conflict. One holiday, the husband is given a puppy and immediately becomes attached to the dog, who soon becomes a valued family member. The husband then begins to view his wife's relatives differently and willingly visits their house more often.
- A mother is afraid that her teenage daughter has been in an accident because she did not come home after a party. Then, the woman remembers that she gave her daughter permission to stay at a friend's house. She immediately feels better.

BOX 19.4

Research for Best Practice: Emotion- Versus Problem-Focused Coping for Health Threats

del-Pino-Casado, R., Pérez-Cruz, M., & Frías-Osuna, A. (2014). Coping, subjective burden and anxiety among family caregivers of older dependent. Journal of Clinical Nursing, 23, *3335–3344.*

THE QUESTION: Do stressors, coping, and subjective burden contribute to anxiety in caregivers?

METHODS: Data from 140 family caregivers were analyzed using descriptive statistics, correlation coefficients, and path analysis. Sociodemographic data and several scales were used to collect data.

FINDINGS: Stressors, coping, emotion-focused coping, dysfunctional coping, and subjective burden were related to greater anxiety.

IMPLICATIONS FOR NURSING: Stressors, dysfunctional coping, and subjective burden can be used in clinical practice for early detection of and early intervention for anxiety. Problem solving, positive reappraisal, assertiveness, and control of negative thoughts may not be as effective in reducing anxiety.

---

except that it happens after coping strategies are implemented, provides feedback about the outcomes and allows for continual adjustment and actions to new information.

ADAPTATION

Adaptation can be conceptualized as a person's capacity to survive and flourish (Lazarus, 2006). Adaptation or lack of it affects three important areas: health, psychological well-being, and social functioning. A period of stress may compromise any or all of these areas. If a person copes successfully with stress, they return to a previous level of adaptation. Successful coping results in an improvement in health, well-being, and social functioning. Unfortunately, coping strategies will not always be successful and maladaptation occurs.

> **KEYCONCEPT Adaptation** is a person's capacity to survive and flourish. Adaptation affects three important areas: health, psychological well-being, and social functioning.

It is impossible to separate completely the adaptation areas of health, well-being, and social functioning. A maladaptation in any one area can negatively affect the others. For instance, the appearance of psychiatric symptoms can cause problems in performance in the work environment that in turn elicit a negative self-concept. Although each area will be discussed separately, the reader should realize that when one area is affected, most likely all three areas are affected.

Healthy Coping

Health can be negatively affected by stress when coping is ineffective and the damaging condition or situation is not ameliorated or the emotional distress is not regulated. Examples of ineffective coping include using emotion-focused coping when a problem-focused approach is appropriate, such as if a woman reinterprets an abusive situation as her fault instead of getting help to remove herself from the environment. In addition, if a coping strategy violates cultural norms and lifestyle, stress is often exaggerated. Some coping strategies actually increase the risk for mortality and morbidity, such as the excessive use of alcohol, drugs, or tobacco. Many people use overeating, smoking, or drinking to reduce stress. They may feel better temporarily but are actually increasing their risk for illness. For people whose behaviors exacerbate their illnesses, learning new behaviors becomes important. Healthy coping strategies such as exercising and obtaining adequate sleep and nutrition contribute to stress reduction and the promotion of long-term health.

Psychological Well-Being

An ideal outcome to a stress response is feeling good about how stress is handled. Outcome satisfaction for one person does not necessarily represent outcome satisfaction for another. For example, suppose that two students receive the same passing score on an examination. One may feel a sense of relief, but the other may feel anxious because he appraises the score as too low. Understanding a person's emotional response to an outcome is essential to analyzing its personal meaning. People who consistently have positive outcomes from stressful experiences are more likely to have positive self-esteem and self-confidence. Unsatisfactory outcomes from stressful experiences are associated with negative mood states, such as depression, anger, guilt leading to decreased self-esteem, and feelings of helplessness. Likewise, if the situation was appraised as challenging rather than harmful or threatening, increased self-confidence and a sense of well-being are likely to follow. If the situation was accurately appraised as harmful or threatening but viewed as manageable, the outcome may also be positive.

Social Functioning

Social functioning, the performance of daily activities within the context of interpersonal relations and family and community roles, can be seriously impaired during stressful episodes. For instance, a student who is experiencing the stress of needing to pass an examination to satisfactorily pass a class may not be able to maintain social relationships or keep up with work-related responsibilities satisfactorily. Social functioning continues to be impaired if the person views the outcome as unsuccessful and experiences negative emotions. If successful coping with a stressful encounter leads to a positive outcome, social functioning returns to normal or is improved.

NURSING CARE FOR THE PERSON EXPERIENCING STRESS

The overall goals in the nursing care of the person experiencing stress are to resolve the stressful person–environment situation, reduce the physiologic and psychological stress response, and develop positive coping skills. The goals for those who are at high risk for stress (experiencing recent life changes, vulnerable to stress, or have limited coping mechanisms) are to recognize the potential for stressful situations and strengthen positive coping skills through education and practice.

Stress responses vary from one person to another. Acute stress is easier to recognize than chronic stress. In many instances, living with chronic stress has become a way of life and is no longer recognized. If there are significant emotional or behavioral symptoms in response to an identifiable stressful situation, a diagnosis of adjustment disorder may be made (American Psychiatric Association, 2013). From the assessment data, the nurse can determine any illnesses, the intensity of the stress response, and the effectiveness of coping strategies. Nurses typically identify stress responses in people or family members who are receiving treatment for other health problems.

Telehealth and web-based stress management programs offer promising treatment options for individuals who experience stress. For example, college students are known to experience high levels of stress; however, they rarely seek treatment for a number of reasons such as accessibility and social stigma (Coudray et al., 2019). Web-based programs have been found to be helpful for students experiencing distress (Coudray et al., 2019). Further, the use of telehealth programs have been implemented to assist with mental health care for military personnel experiencing posttraumatic stress disorder with success (Engel et al., 2016). These programs may be instrumental in assisting individuals experiencing to seek guidance from health care professionals.

Mental Health Nursing Assessment

The assessment of a person experiencing stress should include a careful health history, current stressful event, and coping resources. If a psychiatric disorder is present, symptoms may spontaneously reappear even when no alteration has occurred in the patient's treatment regimen.

Physical Assessment

Review of Systems

A systems review can help the nurse identify the person's own unique physiologic response to stress and can also provide important data on the effect of chronic illnesses. These data are useful for understanding the person–environment situation and the person's stress reactions, coping responses, and adaptation.

Physical Functioning

Physical functioning usually changes during a stress response. Typically, sleep is disturbed, appetite either increases or decreases, body weight fluctuates, and sexual activity changes. Physical appearance may be uncharacteristically disheveled—a projection of the person's feelings. Body language expresses muscle tension, which conveys a state of anxiety not usually present. Because exercise is an important strategy in stress reduction, the nurse should assess the amount of physical activity, tolerance for exercise, and usual exercise patterns. Determining the details of the person's exercise pattern and any recent changes can help in formulating reasonable interventions.

Pharmacologic Assessment

In assessing a person's coping strategies, the nurse needs to ask about the use of alcohol, tobacco, marijuana, and any other addictive substances. Many people begin or increase the frequency of using these substances as a way of coping with stress. In turn, substance abuse contributes to the stress behavior. Knowing details about the person's use of these substances (number of times a day or week, amount, circumstances, side effects) helps in determining the role these substances play in overall stress reduction or management. The more important the substances are in the person's handling of stress, the more difficult it will be to change the addictive behavior.

Stress also often prompts people to use antianxiety medication without supervision. Use of over-the-counter and herbal medications is also common. The nurse should carefully assess the use of any drugs or herbal remedies used to manage stress symptoms. If drugs are the primary coping strategy, further evaluation is needed with a possible referral to a mental health specialist. If a psychiatric disorder is present, the nurse should assess medication adherence, especially if the psychiatric symptoms are reappearing.

Psychosocial Assessment

Unlike assessment for other mental health problems, psychological assessment of the person under stress does not ordinarily include a mental status examination. Instead, psychological assessment focuses on the person's emotions and their severity, as well as their coping strategies. The assessment elicits the person's appraisal of risks and benefits, the personal meaning of the situation, and the person's commitment to a particular outcome. The nurse can then understand how vulnerable the person is to stress.

Using therapeutic communication techniques, a person's emotional state is assessed in a nurse–patient interview. By beginning the interview with a statement such as, "Let's talk about what you have been feeling," the nurse can elicit the feelings that the person has been experiencing. Identifying the person's emotions can be helpful in assessing the intensity of the stress being experienced. Negative emotions (anger, fright, anxiety, guilt, shame, sadness, envy, jealousy, and disgust) are usually associated with an inability to cope and severe stress.

After identifying the person's emotions, the nurse determines how the person reacts initially to them. For example, does the person who is angry respond by carrying out the innate urge to attack someone whom the person blames for the situation? Or does that person respond by thinking through the situation and overriding the initial innate urge to act? The person who tends to act impulsively has few real coping skills. For the person who can resist the innate urge to act and has developed coping skills, the focus of the assessment becomes determining their effectiveness.

In an assessment interview, it can be determined whether the person uses problem-focused or emotion-focused coping strategies effectively. Problem-focused coping is effective when the person can accurately assess the situation. In this case, the person sets goals, seeks information, masters new skills, and seeks help as needed. Emotion-focused coping is effective when the person has inaccurately assessed the situation and coping corrects the false interpretation.

Social assessment data are invaluable in determining the person's resources for positive coping. The ability to make healthy lifestyle changes is strongly influenced by the person's health beliefs and family support system. Even the expression of stress is related to social factors, particularly cultural expectations and values.

Assessment could include the use of the Recent Life Changes Questionnaire (refer to Table 19.3) to determine the number and importance of life changes that the patient has experienced within the past year. If several recent life changes have occurred, the person–environment relationship has changed. The person is likely to be either at high risk for or already experiencing stress.

The assessment should include identification of the person's social network. Because employment is the mainstay of adulthood and the source of many personal contacts, assessment of any recent changes in employment status is important. If a person is unemployed, the nurse should determine the significance of the unemployment and its effects on the person's social network. For children and young adults, nurses should note any recent changes in their attendance at school. The nurse should elicit the following data:

- Size and extent of the patient's social network, both relatives and nonrelatives, professional and nonprofessional, and how long known
- Functions that the network serves (e.g., intimacy, social integration, nurturance, reassurance of worth, guidance and advice, access to new contacts)
- Degree of reciprocity between the patient and other network members; that is, who provides support to the patient and who the patient supports
- Degree of interconnectedness; that is, how many of the network members know one another and are in contact

Priorities of Nursing Care

There are several possible priorities of nursing care depending upon the individual's response to stress. For patients with changes in eating, sleeping, or activity, the priorities of care can focus on reestablishing these functional patterns. For other patients, the priorities may focus on psychological issues such as low self-esteem, fear, and hopelessness. Other patients may not have the psychological resources to cope with the situation, which will lead to a focus on coping skills.

Nursing Interventions

People under stress can usually benefit from approaches supporting healthy behaviors. Activities of daily living are usually interrupted, and the affected individuals often feel that they have no time for themselves. The stressed person who is normally well groomed and dressed may appear disheveled and unkempt. Simply reinstating the daily routine of shaving or combing hair can improve the person's outlook on life and ability to cope with the stress.

Stress is commonly manifested in the areas of nutrition and activity. During stressful periods, a person's eating patterns change. To cope with stress, a person may either overeat or become anorexic. Both are ineffective coping behaviors and actually contribute to stress. Educating the patient about the importance of maintaining an adequate diet during the period of stress will highlight its importance. It will also allow the nurse to help the person decide how eating behaviors can be changed.

Exercise can reduce the emotional and behavioral responses to stress. In addition to the physical benefits of exercise, a regular exercise routine can provide structure to a person's life, enhance self-confidence, and increase feelings of well-being. People who are stressed are often not receptive to the idea of exercise, particularly if it has not been a part of their routine. Exploring the patient's personal beliefs about the value of activity will help to determine whether exercise is a reasonable activity for that person.

The person under stress tends to be tense, nervous, and on edge. Simple relaxation techniques help the person relax and may improve coping skills. If these techniques do not help the patient relax, distraction or guided imagery may be taught to the patient (see Chapter 10). In some instances, spiritually oriented interventions can be used. Referral to a mental health specialist for hypnosis or biofeedback should be considered for patients who have severe stress responses.

Psychosocial Nursing Interventions

Numerous interventions help reduce stress and support coping efforts. All of the interventions are best carried out within the framework of a supportive nurse–patient relationship.

Problem Solving

Assisting patients to develop appropriate problem-solving strategies based on personal strengths and previous experiences is important in understanding and coping with stressful situations. Some aspects of any situation cannot be changed, such as a family member's illness or a death of a loved one, but usually there are areas within the patient's control that can be changed. For example, a caregiver cannot reverse the family member's disability, but can arrange for short-term respite.

Encouraging patients to examine times when coping has been successful and examine aspects of that situation can help in identifying strengths and strategies for the current problem. For example, a young mother was completely overwhelmed with feelings of inadequacy after the birth of her third child. Further assessment revealed that the patient's mother had helped during the 6 weeks after the other children had been born. The patient's mother was not available for the third birth. First, the nurse acknowledged and validated that having three children could be overwhelming for anyone. The nurse also explained the postpartum hormonal changes that were occurring, validating that the patient's feelings were typical of many mothers. Finally, together, the nurse and the patient identified resources in her environment that could support her during the postpartum period.

Family Interventions

People who are coping with stressful situations can often benefit from interventions that facilitate family unit functioning and promote the health and welfare of all family members. To intervene with the total family, the stressed person must agree for the family members to be involved. If the data gathered from the assessment of supportive and unsupportive factors indicate that the family members are not supportive, the nurse should assist the patient to consider expanding their social network. If the family is the major source of support, the nurse should design interventions that support the functioning of the family unit. Parent education can also be effective in supporting family unit functioning. If family therapy is needed, the nurse should refer the family to an advanced practice specialist.

Evaluation and Treatment Outcomes

The treatment outcomes established in the initial plan of care guide the evaluation. Individual outcomes relate to improved health, well-being, and social function.

Depending on the level of intervention, there can also be family and network outcomes. Family outcomes may be related to improved communication or social support; for instance, caregiver stress is reduced when other members of the family help in the care of the ill member. Social network outcomes focus on modifying the social network to increase support for the individual.

SUMMARY OF KEY POINTS

- Stress affects everyone. Coping with stress can produce positive and negative outcomes. The person can learn and grow from the experience or maladaptation can occur.

- The concept of homeostasis is the body's tendency to resist physiologic change and hold bodily functions relatively consistent, well-coordinated, and usually stable.

- When the brain interprets an event as a threat, physiologic stability is challenged, and a "fight-or-flight" response occurs.

- Allostasis describes a dynamic regulatory process that maintains homeostasis through a process of adaptation. Physiologic stability is achieved when the autonomic nervous system, the HPA, and the cardiovascular, metabolic, and immune systems respond to internal and external stimuli. As wear and tear on the brain and body occur, there is a corresponding increase in the number of abnormal biologic parameters called the AL. AL is an indication of chronic stress.

- Stress is defined as an environmental pressure or force that puts strain on a person's system. Acute stress can lead to physiologic overload, which in turn can have a negative impact on a person's health, well-being, and social functioning. Chronic stress is associated with AL that can lead to negative health outcomes.

- Stress responses are determined by the interaction with environment and the individual's cognitive appraisal of the risks and benefits of a situation. Stress responses are simultaneously emotional and physiologic, leading to an innate tendency to act.

- Many personal factors, such as personality patterns, beliefs, values, and commitment to an outcome, interact with environmental demands and constraints that produce a person–environment relationship.

- Effective coping can be either problem focused or emotion focused. The outcome of successful coping is adaptation through enhanced health, psychological well-being, and social functioning.

- Within the social network, social support can help a person cope with stress.

- The overall goals in the nursing management of stress are to resolve the stressful person–environment situation, reduce the stress response, and develop positive coping skills.

Unfolding Patient Stories: David Carter

Part 2

Recall from Chapter 12 David Carter, age 28 with schizophrenia who was hospitalized after a violent outburst having paranoid delusions and auditory hallucinations. He lives with his mother and previously worked as a grocery clerk. What can be influencing his increased social isolation? What factors should the nurse consider when developing a plan of care for discharge to promote David's social functioning and lessen his isolation?

CRITICAL THINKING CHALLENGES

1. Compare and contrast the concepts of homeostasis and allostasis.

2. Discuss the impact of acute stress versus chronic stress. Why is chronic stress of more concern than acute stress?

3. Explain why one person may experience the stress of losing a job differently from another.

4. An individual is experiencing being overweight, has hypertension and insomnia, and was recently widowed. The doctor has told them to lose weight and quit smoking. The individual seeks your advice. Would you recommend a problem-focused or an emotion-focused approach?

5. A person at the local shelter announced to the group that they were returning to their partner because it was partly their fault that their partner beat them. Is this an example of problem-focused or emotion-focused coping? Justify your answer.

6. Using the Stress Coping and Adaptation Model (see Fig. 19.2), assess a patient and determine the cognitive appraisal of significant events.

Movie Viewing Guides

Noise: (2007). David Owen (Tim Robbins) copes with the stressful noises of the city, specifically car alarms, by becoming aggressive and destructive. At first, the noise is merely an irritant. Later, he interprets the noise as an assault on everyone. He becomes an activist, protecting others, and gradually becomes very grandiose. As his grandiosity increases, he becomes more and more driven to damage vehicles with active care alarms.

VIEWING POINTS: What is the relationship between the physiologic response to the noise and his eventual grandiose behavior? How would you help him reduce the stressful experience and cope positively? Observe your own feelings throughout the movie. Did you experience stress?

REFERENCES

Aalbers, G., McNally, R. J., Heeren, A., de Wit, S., & Fried, E. I. (2019). Social media and depression symptoms: A network perspective. *Journal of Experimental Psychology: General, 148*(8), 1454–1462.

American Psychiatric Association. (2013). *Diagnostic and statistical manual of mental disorders* (5th ed.). Author.

American Society for the Positive Care of Children. (2021). Get the facts: Adverse childhood experiences (ACES). https://americanspcc.org/get-the-facts-adverse-childhood-experiences/

Anisman, H. (2015). *Stress and your health: From vulnerability to resilience* (1st ed.). John Wiley & Sons, Incorporated.

Azmitia, M., Syed, M., & Radmacher, K. (2008). On the intersection of personal and social identities: Introduction and evidence from a longitudinal study of emerging adults. *New Directions for Child & Adolescent Development, 120*, 1–16.

Bokenberger, K., Pedersen, N. L., Gatz, M., & Dahl, A. K. (2014). The Type A behavior pattern and cardiovascular disease as predictors of dementia. *Health Psychology, 33*(12), 1593.

Bozo, Ö., Yagmur, A., & Eldoğan, D. (2017). Does marital adjustment mediate Type C personality-depressive symptoms relation? A comparison between breast cancer patients and cancer-free women. *Current Psychology*, 1–8. https://doi-org.libproxy.siue.edu/10.1007/s12144-017-9693-6

Cannon, W. B. (1932). *The wisdom of the body*. W. W. Norton & Company.

Carpenter, R. (2016). A review of instruments on cognitive appraisal of stress. *Archives of Psychiatric Nursing, 30*(2), 271–279.

Conti, C., Carrozzino, D., Patierno, C., Vitacolonna, E., & Fulcheri, M. (2016). The clinical link between Type D personality and diabetes. *Frontiers in Psychiatry, 7*, 113.

Coudray, C., Palmer, R., & Frazier, P. (2019). Moderators of the efficacy of a web-based stress management intervention for college students. *Journal of Counseling Psychology, 66*(6), 747–754.

Crespo, M., Guillén, A. I., & Piccini, A. T. (2019). Work experience and emotional state in caregivers of elderly relatives. *The Spanish Journal of Psychology, 22*. E34. https://doi.org/10.1017/sjp.2019.34

Engel, C. C., Jaycox, L. H., Freed, M. C., Bray, R. M., Brambilla, D., Zatzick, D., Litz, B., Tanielian, T., Novak, L. A., Lane, M. E., Belsher, B. E., Olmsted, K. L., Evatt, D. P., Vandermaas-Peeler, R., Unützer, J., & Katon, W. J. (2016). Centrally assisted collaborative telecare for posttraumatic stress disorder and depression among military personnel attending primary care: A randomized clinical trial. *Journal of the American Medical Association: Internal Medicine, 176*(7), 948–956.

Friborg, O. (2019). An improved method for counting stressful life events (SLEs) when predicting mental health and wellness. *Psychology & Health, 34*(1), 64–83.

Friedman, M., & Rosenman, R. (1974). *Type A and your heart*. Knopf.

Garcia-Retamero, R., Petrova, D., Arrebola-Moreno, A., Catena, A., & Ramírez-Hernández, J. A. (2016). Type D personality is related to severity of acute coronary syndrome in patients with recurrent cardiovascular disease. *British Journal of Health Psychology, 21*(3), 694–711.

Guidi, J., Lucente, M., Sonino, N., & Fava, G. A. (2021). Allostatic load and Its impact on health: A systematic review. *Psychotherapy and Psychosomatics, 90*(1), 11–27. https://doi.org/10.1159/000510696

Holmes, T., & Rahe, R. (1967). The social readjustment patient scale. *Journal of Psychosomatic Research, 11*(2), 213–218.

Iswari, T. I. (2020). How does personality type define the choice? A survey to accounting students. *Review of Integrative Business and Economics Research, 9*, 346–360.

Kalamatianos, A., & Canellopoulos, L. (2019). A diathesis-stress model conceptualization of depressive symptomatology. *Psychiatriki, 30*(1), 49–57.

Kim, S. R., Nho, J. H., & Kim, H. Y. (2020). Influence of type D personality on quality of life in university students: The mediating effect of health –

Promoting behavior and subjective health status. *Psychology in the Schools, 57*(5), 768–782.

Korotkov, D., Perunovic, M., Claybourn, M., Fraser, I., Houlihan, M., Macdonald, M., & Korotov, K. A. (2011). The type B behavior pattern as a moderating variable of the relationship between stressor chronicity and health behavior. *Journal of Health Psychology, 16*(3), 397–409.

Lală, A., Bobîrnac, G., & Tipa, R. (2010). Stress levels, alexithymia, type A and type C personality patterns in undergraduate students. *Journal of Medicine and Life, 3*(2), 200.

Lazarus, R. S. (2001). Relational meaning and discrete emotions. In K. R., Scherer, A. Schorr, & T. Johnstone (Eds.), *Appraisal processes in emotion: Theory, methods, research* (pp. 37–67). Oxford University Press.

Lazarus, R. S. (2006). *Stress and emotion: A new synthesis*. Springer.

Lazarus, R. S., & Folkman, S. (1984). *Stress, appraisal and coping*. Springer.

Li, Y., & Wu, S. (2010). Social networks and health among rural-urban migrants in China: A channel or a constraint? *Health Promotion International, 25*(3), 371–380.

Marchesi, C., Ossola, P., Scagnelli, F., Paglia, F., Aprile, S., Monici, A., Tonna, M., Conte, G., Masini, F., De Panfilis, C., & Ardissino, D. (2014). Type D personality in never-depressed patients and the development of major and minor depression after acute coronary syndrome. *Journal of Affective Disorders, 155*, 194–199.

McDonald, A., Thompson, A. J., Perzow, S. E., Joos, C., & Wadsworth, M. E. (2020). The protective roles of ethnic identity, social support, and coping on depression in low-income parents: A test of the adaptation to poverty-related stress model. *Journal of Consulting and Clinical Psychology, 88*(6), 504.

McEwen, B. S. (2005). Stressed or stressed out: What is the difference? *Journal of Psychiatry Neuroscience, 30*(5), 315–318.

McEwen, B. S. (2015). Biomarkers for assessing population and individual health and disease related to stress and adaptation. *Metabolism, 64*(3), S1–S10.

McEwen, B. S. (2017). Neurobiological and systemic effects of chronic stress. *Chronic Stress, 1*(1), 1–171.

McVicar, A., Ravalier, J. M., & Greenwood, C. (2013). Biology of stress revisited: Intracellular mechanisms and the conceptualization of stress. *Stress & Health, 30*(4), 272–279.

Rahe, R. H. (1994). The more things change. *Psychosomatic Medicine, 56*(4), 306–307.

Rahe, R. H., Taylor, C. B., Tolles, R. L., Newhall, L. M., Veach, T. L., & Bryson, S. (2002). A novel stress and coping workplace program reduces illness and healthcare utilization. *Psychosomatic Medicine, 64*(2), 278–286.

Romo-González, T., Martínez, A. J., Hernández-Pozo, M. d. R., Gutiérrez-Ospina, G., & Larralde, C. (2018). Psychological features of breast cancer in Mexican women I: Personality traits and stress symptoms. *Advances in Neuroimmune Biology, 7*(1), 3–15.

Roy, B. (2018). Socio-economic variables: A contributing factor for the development of aggressive behaviour among the students with type A and type B personality. *Indian Journal of community Psychology, 14*(1), 125–132.

Seib, C., Whiteside, E., Lee, K., Humphreys, J., Tran, T. H., Chopin, L., & Anderson, D. (2014). Stress, lifestyle, and quality of life in midlife and older Australian women: Results from the Stress and the Health of Women Study. *Women's Health Issues, 24*(1), e43–e52.

Selye, H. (1956). *The stress of life*. McGraw-Hill.

Selye, H. (1974). *Stress without distress*. J. B. Lippincott.

Shepherd-Banigan, M., Bell, J. F., Basu, A., Booth-LaForce, C., & Harris, J. R. (2016). Workplace stress and working from home influence depressive symptoms among employed women with young children. *International Journal of Behavioral Medicine, 23*(1), 102–111.

Sterling, P. (2012). Allostasis: A model of predictive regulation. *Physiology & Behavior, 106*, 5–15.

Stevenson, C., & Williams, L. (2014). Type D personality, quality of life and physical symptoms in the general population: A dimensional analysis. *Psychology & Health, 29*(3), 365–373.

Tamers, S. L., Okechukwu, C., Bohl, A. A., Guéguen, A., Goldberg, M., & Zins, M. (2014). The impact of stressful life events on excessive alcohol consumption in the French population: Findings from the GAZEL Cohort Study. *PLOS One, 9*(1), e87653.

Vally, Z., & D'Souza, C. G. (2019). Abstinence from social media use, subjective well-being, stress, and loneliness. *Perspectives in Psychiatric Care, 55*(4), 752–759.

Whatley, A. D., DiIorio, C. K., & Yeager, K. (2010). Examining the relationships of depressive symptoms, stigma, social support and regimen-specific support on quality of life in adult patients with epilepsy. *Health Education Research, 25*(4), 575–584.

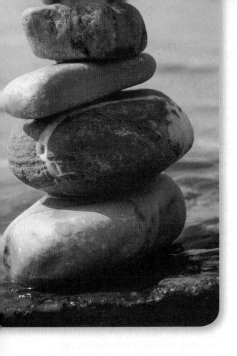

20
Management of Anger, Aggression, and Violence

Sandra P. Thomas

KEYCONCEPTS

- anger
- aggression

- gender, culture, and ethnic differences

- intervention fit
- violence

LEARNING OBJECTIVES

After studying this chapter, you will be able to:

1. Explore the difference between healthy and maladaptive styles of anger.

2. Discuss principles of anger management as a psychoeducational intervention to promote wellness.

3. Discuss the factors that influence aggressive and violent behaviors.

4. Discuss theories used to explain anger, aggression, and violence.

5. Identify behaviors or actions that escalate and de-escalate violent behavior.

6. Recognize the risk for verbal and physical attacks on nurses.

7. Generate options for responding to the expression of anger, aggression, and violent behaviors in clinical nursing practice.

8. Apply the nursing process to the management of anger, aggression, and violence in patients.

KEY TERMS

- Anger management • Catharsis • Instrumental aggression • Inwardly directed anger • Maladaptive anger
- Outwardly directed anger

INTRODUCTION

Maladaptive anger and potentially lethal violent behavior are increasingly evident in contemporary Western society. Temper tantrums of athletes, episodes of road rage, and school shootings often dominate the evening news and social media. Clearly, mismanagement of angry emotion is a serious social problem.

Language pertaining to anger is imprecise and confusing. Some of the words used interchangeably with anger include *annoyance, frustration, temper, resentment, hostility, hatred,* and *rage.* To avoid perpetuating the confusion, three key concepts were selected for use in this chapter: *anger, aggression,* and *violence.* Anger, aggression, and violence should not be viewed as a continuum because one does not necessarily lead to another. That is a myth. Cultural myths about anger abound (Table 20.1).

One goal of this chapter is to dispel confusion between anger as a normal, healthy response to violation of one's integrity and maladaptive anger that is detrimental to one's mental and physical health. Understanding this distinction is an important aspect of emotional intelligence.

TABLE 20.1   CULTURAL MYTHS ABOUT ANGER

Myth

Anger is a knee-jerk reaction to external events.

Anger can be uncontrollable, resulting in crimes of passion such as "involuntary manslaughter."

Anger behavior in adulthood is determined by temperament and childhood experiences.

Men are angrier than women.

People must behave aggressively to get what they want.

A second goal of this chapter is to outline risk factors for aggression and violence and describe preventive interventions, particularly as they pertain to the psychiatric nursing care environment. Verbal and physical aggression and violence also occur across a wide spectrum of other health care settings, including emergency departments, medical–surgical facilities, and primary care. All nurses must develop expertise in prevention and management of aggression. Contrary to a popular misconception, patients who have psychiatric problems are not more violent than other patients, but astute clinicians need to know which patients *might* become aggressive given a combination of known risk factors with specific environmental conditions.

ANGER

Anger is an internal affective state, usually temporary rather than an enduring hostile attitude. If expressed outwardly, anger behavior can be constructive or destructive. Whereas destructive anger alienates other people and invites retaliation, constructive anger can be a powerful force for asserting one's rights and achieving social justice.

Anger is a signal that something is wrong in a situation; thus, the angry individual has the urge to act. The situation is more distressing than a minor annoyance such as a slow grocery line. An interpersonal offense such as unjust or disrespectful treatment (a spouse lying, a coworker taking advantage) often provokes anger. The meaning of an angry episode depends on the relational context. For example, anger is more intense and intermingled with considerable hurt when loved ones violate the implicit relational contract ("If he loved me, how could he lie about that? How can I trust him again?") (Thomas, 2006).

KEYCONCEPT Anger is "a strong, uncomfortable emotional response to a provocation that is unwanted and incongruent with one's values, beliefs, or rights" (Thomas, 2001).

Maladaptive anger: While anger arousal is normal, anger becomes maladaptive when it is too frequent, too

intense, or managed in unhealthy ways: excessive outward expression (e.g., losing temper, yelling) or suppression (i.e., seething inside and ruminating about grievances). Maladaptive anger is linked to psychiatric conditions as well as a plethora of medical conditions. For example, anger and hostility are associated with hospitalizations in patients with heart failure (Endrighi et al., 2019), and *excessive outwardly directed anger* is linked to coronary heart disease (Pimple et al., 2019), metabolic syndrome (Thomas et al., 2020), and myocardial infarction (Buckley et al., 2015; Smeijers et al., 2017). *Suppressed anger* is related to arthritis, breast and colorectal cancer, chronic pain, and hypertension (Kakoo Brioso et al., 2020; Russell et al., 2016; Sommer et al., 2019) and is a risk factor for postpartum depression (Bruno et al., 2017).

In contrast to these maladaptive **anger management** styles, research shows that anger discussed with other people in a constructive way and mindfulness-based stress reduction have a beneficial effect on blood pressure (Lee et al., 2020; Momeni et al., 2016; Thomas, 1997a), as well as statistically significant associations with better general health, a higher sense of self-efficacy, less depression, and a lower likelihood of obesity (Thomas, 1997b). Anger controlled through calming strategies is associated with faster wound healing and other health benefits (Barlow et al., 2019; Gouin et al., 2008). Thus, effective anger management is important in maintenance of emotional wellness and holistic health (Trost et al., 2017).

Skillful anger control is also essential to social and occupational success. People with poor anger control have more conflict at work, change jobs more frequently, take more unwise risks, and have more accidents than people with adaptive anger behavior (Halperin & Reifen Tagar, 2017).

The Experience of Anger

When you are angry, your heart pounds, your blood pressure rises, you breathe faster, your muscles tense, and you clench your jaw or fists as you experience an impulse to do something with this physical energy. Some individuals experience anger arousal as pleasurable, but others find its strong physical manifestations scary and unpleasant. People who were taught that anger is a sin may immediately try to ban it from awareness and deny its existence. However, suppression actually results in greater, more prolonged physiological arousal. A better option is finding a way to safely release the physical energy, either through vigorous physical activity (e.g., jogging) or through a calming activity (e.g., deep breathing). Later, at an opportune time, calmly discussing the incident with the provocateur permits clarification of misunderstandings and resolution of grievances. Box 20.1 invites the reader to explore variations in anger experience.

Self-Awareness Exercise: Personal Experience of Anger

People's reactions differ when they experience anger. Some people report a sense of power, control, and calmness different from their usual experience; others report feeling shaky, tearful, and on the verge of collapse. Still others describe physical sensations of nausea and dizziness.

Think about the last time you felt angry. List the body sensations and other emotions that you experienced. Now ask a friend, colleague, or family member to do the same. Compare lists. What are the similarities and differences between you? How will awareness of these differences help you in your clinical practice?

TABLE 20.2 **STYLES OF ANGER EXPRESSION**

Style	Characteristic Behaviors
Anger suppression	Feeling anxious when anger is aroused Acting as though nothing happened Withdrawing from people when angry Conveying anger nonverbally by body language Sulking, pouting, or ruminating
Unhealthy outward anger expression	Flying off the handle Expressing anger in an attacking or blaming way Yelling, saying nasty things Calling the other person names or using profanity Using fists rather than words to express angry feelings
Constructive anger discussion	Discussing the anger with a friend or family member even if the provocateur cannot be confronted at the time Approaching the person with whom one is angry and discussing the concern directly Using "I" language to describe feelings and request changes in another's behavior

The physiology of anger involves the cerebral cortex, the sympathetic nervous system, the adrenal medulla (which secretes adrenaline and noradrenaline), the adrenal cortex (which secretes cortisol), the cardiovascular system, and even the immune system. From a biologic viewpoint, angry episodes may partially originate from developmental deficits, anoxia, malnutrition, toxins, tumors, neurodegenerative diseases, or trauma affecting the brain.

The Expression of Anger

While the physiological arousal of anger is similar in all people, ways of expressing anger differ. The most common modes, or styles, of anger expression are listed in Table 20.2.

In Western culture, control of anger was the dominant stance from Greco-Roman times to the 20th century. Anger was viewed as sinful, dangerous, and destructive—an irrational emotion to be contained, controlled, and denied. This pejorative view contributed to the development of a powerful taboo against feeling and expressing anger. People who have accepted this persistent taboo may have difficulty even knowing when they are angry. They may use euphemisms such as "a little upset" (Rubin, 1970).

In contrast to the denial or containment of angry emotion, some mental health care providers began to advocate the use of **catharsis** during the early 20th century, based on the animal research of ethologists and on Freud's conceptualization of "strangulated affect"; rather than holding in their anger, people were urged to "vent it," lest there be a dangerous "slush fund" of unexpressed anger building up in the body (Rubin, 1970). The legacy of the ill-advised "ventilationist movement" is still with us, visible in rude, uncivil behavior in the nation's classrooms, offices, roadways, and other public places, as well as in countless homes where loud arguments are a daily occurrence.

More ideally, the clear expression of honest anger may prevent aggression and help to resolve a situation (Thomas, 2009). Suppression of anger, prolonged rumination about the grievance, and malevolent fantasies of revenge do not resolve a problem and may result in negative consequences later. Similarly, antagonistic anger toward an intimate partner or coworker only exacerbates the conflict (Sommer et al., 2016). In contrast, if anger is expressed assertively, beneficial outcomes are possible. In Averill's classic study (1983) of everyday anger, 76% of those who were on the receiving end of someone else's anger reported that they recognized their own faults as a result of the anger incident. Contrary to popular misconception, the relationship with the angry person was strengthened, not weakened.

Special Issues in the Nurse–Patient Relationship

Nurses may withdraw from angry patients and try to hide their own anger because "good nurses" do not get angry at patients. Coldness and distancing on the part of staff are acutely painful to patients (Jalil & Dickens, 2018). What patients want are steady, dependable, confident caregivers who will remain connected with them when they are angry.

Nurses' perceptions and beliefs about themselves as individuals and professionals influence their response to aggressive behaviors. For example, a nurse who considers any expression of anger inappropriate will approach an agitated patient differently from a nurse who considers agitated behavior to be meaningful. Understandably, nurses often shrink from patient anger when their own family backgrounds have been characterized by out-of-control anger or abuse. A nurse who has previously been assaulted by a patient is also more likely to have difficulty dealing with subsequent episodes of aggression (Box 20.2).

Some patients have an uncanny ability to target a nurse's vulnerable characteristics. Although it is normal to become defensive when feeling vulnerable, maintaining personal control is a must. If not, the potential for punitive interventions is greater. Threatening an agitated patient (e.g., "You are going to get an injection if you don't calm down.") will only worsen a volatile situation. Nurses must collaborate with other members of the treatment team when interacting with particularly challenging patients, obtaining consultation from supervisors if necessary.

Assessment of Anger

Both **outwardly directed anger** (particularly the hostile, attacking forms) and **inwardly directed anger**

BOX 20.2

Research for Best Practice: Mental Health Nurses' Emotions and Exposure to Patient Aggression

Jalil, R., Huber, J. W., Sixsmith, J., & Dickens, G. S. (2018). Mental health nurses' emotions, exposure to patient aggression attitudes to and use of coercive measures: Cross-sectional questionnaire survey. International Journal of Nursing Studies, 75, 130–138. https://doi.org/10.1016/j.ijnurstu.2017.07.018

THE QUESTION: What are the relationships between mental health nurses' exposure to patient aggression and their emotions/attitudes toward coercive containment measures and involvement in patient seclusion and restraint?

METHODS: Sixty-eight mental health nurses completed a questionnaire about their exposure to aggression, their attitudes toward seclusion and restraint, and their emotions.

FINDINGS: Verbal aggression that is targeted, demeaning, or humiliating is associated with higher experienced anger provocation and approval of restraints or seclusion, but anger did not predict involvement in the use of restraints or seclusion.

IMPLICATIONS FOR NURSING: Nurses may benefit from interventions that improve their skill and coping strategies for dealing with verbal aggression. Nurses should be sufficiently self-aware to avoid using restraints or seclusion when experiencing anger.

(i.e., anger that is stifled despite strong arousal) produce adverse consequences, indicating a need for anger management intervention. Complicating matters, however, most people's anger styles cannot be neatly categorized as "anger-in" or "anger-out" because they behave differently in different environments (e.g., yelling at assistants in the office, stifling anger at a family member). Therefore, it is necessary to conduct a careful assessment of a patient's behavior pattern across various situations.

The manner of anger expression is not the only important aspect of assessment. The difficulty in regulating the frequency and intensity of anger also must be assessed. Intense anger, evident in clenched fists and readiness to burst when arguing with others, can even trigger a heart attack (Buckley et al., 2015). Having an episode of intense anger caused an 8.5-fold increase in risk of acute coronary occlusion within the next 2 hours. The extent to which anger is creating problems at work or intimate relationships should be evaluated, as well as the use of unhealthy coping techniques such as binge eating, drinking, or medicating their angry distress with over-the-counter or illicit drugs (Feinson & Hornik-Lurie, 2016; Thomas, 2006). Evidence-based practice has been extensively used with thousands of people, permitting comparison of a client with established norms. The Spielberger State-Trait Anger Expression Inventory is one such tool (Spielberger, 1999). This instrument measures the general temperamental proneness to be aroused to anger (trait anger) as well as current feelings (state anger) and several styles of anger expression, including anger-in, anger-out, and control through calming techniques.

Because anger and aggression can be symptomatic of many underlying psychiatric or medical disorders, from posttraumatic stress disorder and bipolar disorder to toxicities and head injuries, first any underlying disorder must be properly evaluated. Only one anger-related disorder, intermittent explosive disorder (IED), appears in the *Diagnostic and Statistical Manual of Mental Disorders* (American Psychiatric Association [APA], 2013). This diagnosis is used when recurring aggressive outbursts cannot be attributed to any other condition. People with IED display aggressive behavior that is disproportionate to the precipitating event, usually a minor provocation by a family member or other close associate (APA, 2013).

Once thought to be rare, more recent research has shown that IED is as common as many other psychiatric disorders (Coccaro, 2019). The disorder usually appears during the teen years and persists over the life course. A national study indicates that the average number of lifetime anger attacks per person is large (43 per person). Because the disorder involves inadequate production or functioning of serotonin, IED is commonly treated with selective serotonin reuptake inhibitors (Cocarro &

Lee, 2019). However, behavior therapy should also be included. Very few people with IED ever choose to be treated for their anger (Rynar & Coccaro, 2018) although the IED population is responsive to treatment (Galbraith et al., 2018).

Culture and Gender Considerations in Assessment

Anger is one of the six universal emotions with identifiable facial features and emotionally inflected speech. People across the globe experience the emotion of anger, along with the impulse to act, but culture is perhaps the most important determinant of what angry individuals actually do. Cultural differences in anger behavior can emanate from the historical trajectories, religions, languages, and customs of a group of people (Thomas, 2006). The same event can provoke very different emotional responses in culturally different persons (e.g., a random act of greeting such as a smile by a stranger could be perceived as insulting by one individual but dismissed with a laugh by someone from another culture).

KEYCONCEPT Gender, culture, and ethnic differences in the experience and expression of anger must be taken into consideration before planning interventions.

Gender role socialization influences beliefs about the appropriateness of "owning" angry emotionality and revealing it to others. In Western cultures, aggressive behavior has traditionally been expected in males and more conciliatory behavior expected in females (see Table 20.2). However, these generalizations may not apply to marginalized underrepresented groups or sexual orientation and gender identification (e.g., individuals who identify as lesbian, gay, bisexual, transgender, and queer or questioning). Some Eastern cultures disapprove of anger for both genders, particularly cultures emphasizing connectedness rather than individualism (e.g., Japanese). Therefore, clients in such cultures may ruminate for lengthy periods about anger episodes rather than verbalizing their feelings. The influence of cultural context was evident in a cross-cultural study showing that greater outward expression of anger actually *reduced* cardiovascular risk in Japanese individuals, while increasing cardiovascular risk in Americans (Kitayama et al., 2015). A more extensive discussion of culture and gender factors can be found in Thomas (2006).

The essential element in a cultural assessment is exploration of what the client learned about anger and its display in their culture and family of origin (the primary bearer of that culture). For example, African Americans may have been taught as children to suppress anger at racist discrimination, but suppression can increase their risk for depression and hypertension; in adulthood, anger at societal racism is one of the main reasons that African Americans seek therapy (Kelly, 2019). Therapy must be tailored in a culturally responsive manner.

Anger Interventions

There are self-regulation and communication techniques that promote the management of anger in nondestructive ways. However, most people lack skill in handling anger constructively. Few people have healthy role models to observe while growing up. Education in anger management can be valuable, both for psychological growth and improved interpersonal relations (Trost et al., 2017).

Anger Management: A Psychoeducational Intervention to Promote Wellness

Anger management is an effective intervention that nurses can deliver to persons whose anger behavior is maladaptive in some way (i.e., interfering with success in work or relationships) but *not violent*. In recent years, there has been an increase in court-mandated "anger management" for persons whose behavior is violent as opposed to angry. When these individuals do not greatly benefit, a conclusion may be drawn that anger management is ineffective. However, psychoeducational anger management courses cannot be expected to modify *violent* behavior. (Interventions designed for aggressive and violent individuals are presented later in the chapter.)

The desired outcomes of any anger management intervention are to teach people to (1) effectively modulate the physiological arousal of anger, (2) alter any irrational thoughts fueling the anger, and (3) modify maladaptive anger behaviors (e.g., blaming, attacking, or suppressing) that prevent problem-solving in daily living. Group work is valuable to anger management clients because they need to practice new behaviors in an interpersonal context that offers feedback and support. The leader of an anger management group functions as a teacher and coach, not as a therapist. Potential participants should be screened and referred to individual counseling or psychotherapy if their anger is chronic. Some individuals have deeper developmental issues that mitigate against their successful participation in anger management groups (Shepherd & Cant, 2020). Exclusion criteria are paranoia, organic disorders, and severe personality disorders (Thomas, 2001). Candidates for psychoeducational anger management classes must have some insight that their behavior is problematic and some desire to enlarge their behavioral repertoire.

Anger management includes both didactic and experiential components. Educational handouts, videos, and workbooks are usually used. Ideally, participants commit to attendance for a series of weekly meetings, ranging from 4 to 10 weeks. Between the group meetings, participants are given homework assignments, such as keeping an anger diary and applying the lessons of the class in their homes and work sites. Fresh anger incidents can be brought to the class for role-plays and group discussion. Feedback from group members assists in reappraisal of situations in less hostile terms and permits practice of new anger behaviors in a supportive atmosphere. It may be useful to conduct gender-specific or culturally specific groups (Thomas, 2001).

Individuals can successfully reduce anger and foster forgiveness for an offender through religious/spiritual anger management strategies such as prayer, meditation, or yoga (Smith-MacDonald et al., 2017).

Effectiveness of anger management has been demonstrated in numerous studies, including college students, angry drivers, angry veterans, various medical and psychiatric outpatients, and parents who have difficulty controlling anger toward their children (Lee & DiGiuseppe, 2018). Family members of patients with alcohol use disorder also can benefit from anger management.

Cognitive-Behavioral Therapy for Anger

Cognitive-behavioral therapy is often recommended for the treatment of uncontrollable anger. The first step is establishing a therapeutic alliance because some angry individuals are not in a stage of readiness to change their behavior. Cognitive-behavioral therapy involves avoidance of provoking stimuli, self-monitoring regarding cues of anger arousal, stimulus control, response disruption, and guided practice of more effective anger behaviors. Relaxation or mindfulness training is often introduced early in the treatment because it strengthens the therapeutic alliance and convinces clients that they can indeed learn to calm themselves when angry. When the body relaxes, there is less physical impetus to act impulsively in a way that one will later regret (Shepherd & Cant, 2020).

AGGRESSION AND VIOLENCE

Aggression and violence command the attention of the criminal justice system as well as the mental health care system. During periods when people are a danger to others, they may be separated from the larger society and confined in prisons or locked psychiatric units. Because nurses frequently practice in these settings, management of aggressive and violent behavior is an essential skill.

Factors That Influence Aggressive and Violent Behavior

The violent individual may feel trapped, frightened, or desperate, perhaps at the end of their rope. The nurse must remember that many violent individuals have experienced childhood abandonment, physical brutality, or sexual abuse. Confinement that replicates earlier experiences of degrading treatment may provoke aggressive response, but humane care may kindle hope of recovery and rehabilitation. The response of the nurse may be critical in determining whether aggression escalates or diminishes. Aggressive or violent behavior does not occur in a vacuum. Both the patient and the context must be considered. Therefore, a multidimensional framework is essential for understanding and responding to these behaviors.

KEYCONCEPT Aggression involves overt behavior intended to hurt, belittle, take revenge, or achieve domination and control. Aggression can be verbal (sarcasm, insults, threats) or physical (property damage, slapping, hitting). Mentally healthy people stop themselves from aggression by realizing the negative consequences to themselves or their relationships.

KEYCONCEPT Impulsive aggression occurs in situations of anger and anxiety when the individual lashes out. **Instrumental aggression** is a goal-directed aggressive behavior that is premeditated and unrelated to immediate feelings of frustration or threat; it is a means to secure a goal or reward.

KEYCONCEPT Violence is extreme aggression and involves the use of strong force or weapons to inflict bodily harm to another person and in some cases to kill. Violence connotes greater intensity and destruction than aggression. All violence is aggressive, but not all aggression is violent.

Theories of Aggression and Violence

This section discusses some of the main theoretical explanations for aggression and violence. A single model or theory cannot fully explain aggression and violence; instead, choose the most useful theories for explaining a patient's experience and for planning interventions.

Biologic Theories

The brain structures most frequently associated with aggressive behavior are the limbic system and the cerebral cortex, particularly the frontal and temporal lobes. Patients with a history of damage to the cerebral cortex are more likely to exhibit increased impulsivity, decreased inhibition, and decreased judgment than are those who have not experienced such damage. The interaction of neurocognitive impairment and social history of abuse or family violence increases the risk for violent behavior, particularly for boys (Golding & Fitzgerald, 2019).

There is increasing evidence that activity of monoamine oxidase A is related to the development of impulsivity and aggression. Inhibition of this enzyme, which affects the activity of norepinephrine, serotonin, and dopamine, may play a significant role in the violence enacted by abused children, especially boys. Low serotonin levels are also associated with irritability, increased pain sensitivity, impulsiveness, and aggression (Burke et al., 2018).

Gender differences in aggressive behavior can partially be explained by neurobiology. Activation of the amygdala is correlated with higher anger scores in men but not in women. When provoked, men also have more activation in the orbitofrontal cortex, rectal gyrus, and anterior cingulate cortex than women. Activation of these areas is associated with aggression (Repple et al., 2018). Sex hormones also play a role in some aggressive behavior, with testosterone associated with aggression (Been et al., 2018). Before reading additional research evidence, try the anger exercise in Box 20.3. What does daily experience suggest about biologically based aspects of the experience and expression of anger?

NCLEXNOTE In caring for a potentially aggressive patient, the nurse should recognize that biochemical imbalance contributes to the person's inability to control aggression.

Psychological Theories

Several psychological explanations exist for aggressive and violent behaviors. This section discusses these theories and their treatment approaches.

BOX 20.3

Self-Awareness Exercise: Intensity of Anger

Imagine this scene:
  You are coming home late at night. You've been at the library studying for midterm examinations and are tired. As you come up the front walk, you trip over a skateboard, probably left by one of the neighborhood children. Before you know it, you are sprawled across the front step.
  What emotions threaten to overwhelm you at that moment? What contributes to the intensity of the anger that you feel?

- The pain where you scraped your leg across the cement?
- Your general state of tiredness?
- The fact that you skipped dinner?
- The five cups of coffee you had today?
- The careless children who left a toy in your way?

  If the same thing had happened when you were well rested and feeling good, would the feeling and the intensity be the same?

Psychoanalytic Theories

Psychoanalytic theorists view emotions as instinctual drives. They view suppression of these drives as unhealthy and possible contributors to the development of psychosomatic or psychological disorders. Some psychoanalysts recommended the use of cathartic approaches to release patients' pent-up anger. Nurses in the mid-20th century often used interventions that directed the patient to "let it out" by pounding a pillow or ripping up telephone books. However, studies did not support the theory that catharsis reduces aggression.

Contemporary psychoanalysts do not adhere to any single explanatory model of aggression, often focusing on patients' tendencies to reenact old childhood conflicts or their defensive attempts to deny vulnerability. In working with angry patients, they focus on issues such as improved control over outbursts, heightened empathy for others, and repair of deficits in the personality structure. During analytic therapy, patients gradually achieve greater insight into unconscious processes (Feindler & Byers, 2006; Fuchshuber & Unterrainer, 2020). Thus, they become aware of the reasons they developed maladaptive anger behaviors.

Behavioral Theories

As behavioral theories came into prominence, anger was viewed as a learned response to a stimulus rather than an instinctual drive. In the 1930s, the frustration–aggression hypothesis was advanced in which a person may experience anger and act violently in response to interference with or blocking of a goal. Laboratory experiments and the reality of everyday experience have proved the limitations of this theory (Thomas, 1990). Not all situations in which one's goal is blocked lead to anger or violence.

Social Learning Theory

In Bandura social learning theory, Bandura focuses on the role of learning and rewards in the expression of aggression and violence (Bandura, 2001). Children's observations of aggressive behaviors among family members and violence in their communities foster a context for learning that aggressive behavior is an acceptable way of getting what they want. According to this view, people develop aggressive and violent behaviors by participating in an environment that rewards aggression, such as violent video games (Teng et al., 2019).

General Aggression Model

The general aggression model is a framework that accounts for the interaction of cognition, affect, and arousal during an aggressive episode (Fig. 20.1) (Allen et al., 2018). In this model, an episode consists of *person*

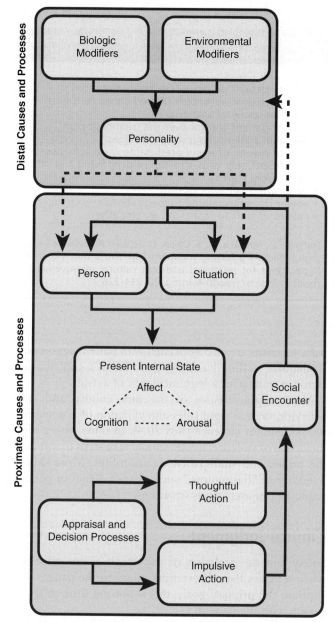

FIGURE 20.1 General aggression model overview. (Redrawn from Anderson, C. A., & Anderson, K. B. [2008]. Men who target women: Specificity of target, generality of aggressive behavior. *Aggressive Behavior, 34*[6], 605–622. Copyright © 2008 Wiley-Liss, Inc. Reprinted by permission of John Wiley & Sons, Inc.)

goals) and cues that trigger memories of similar situations. *Cognition* includes hostile thoughts and scripts (previous behavior patterns and responses to similar episodes). Mood, emotion, and expressive motor responses (automatic reactions to specific emotions) represent the *affect component. Arousal* can be physiologic, psychological, or both.

PROMOTING SAFETY AND PREVENTING VIOLENCE

The paramount aims of psychiatric nurses, particularly those staffing inpatient facilities, are promoting safety and preventing violence. The nurse works toward these goals by establishing therapeutic nurse–patient relationships and creating a therapeutic milieu. Intervening with a potentially violent patient begins with assessment of the history and the predictive factors outlined in the next section.

Assessment for Aggression and Violence

The patient's history is the most important predictor of potential for aggression and violence. Schizophrenia, young age, alcohol use, drug misuse, and hostile–dominant interpersonal styles are also predictors of patient violence (d'Ettorre & Pellicani, 2017). Early life adverse circumstances, such as inadequate maternal nutrition, birth complications, traumatic brain injury, and lead exposure can contribute to risk for aggressive and criminal behaviors in adulthood (Golding & Fitzgerald, 2019). Important markers in the patient's history include previous episodes of rage and violent behavior, escalating irritability, intruding angry thoughts, and fear of losing control.

Characteristics Predictive of Aggression and Violence

The age, gender, and race of patients are *not* good predictors, but several research reports suggest that particular characteristics are predictive of violent behaviors. Usually, but not always, there are some observable precursors to aggression and violence: staring or glaring in an intimating manner, raising voice tone or volume, making sarcastic or demanding comments, and pacing.

Impaired Communication

Impaired communication (including hearing loss and reduced visual acuity), disorientation, and depression have been found to be consistently associated with aggressive behavior among nursing home residents with dementia (Bora et al., 2016).

and situation factors in an ongoing *social interaction*. The episode is mediated through a person's thoughts, feelings, and intensity of arousal. Within this context, the individual appraises the episode and then decides about a follow-up action. The outcome is either thoughtful or impulsive action. The *person factors* include characteristics such as gender, personality traits, beliefs and attitudes, values, goals, and behavior patterns. *Situational factors* include the actual provocation (insults, slights, verbal and physical aggression, interference with achieving

In patients with cognitive impairments, the anticipation of basic needs such as thirst and hunger is important, especially when working with adults and children who cannot readily express their needs. Similarly, the nurse needs to know when the patient last voided and the pattern of bowel movements. The urge to void can be a powerful stimulus to agitated behavior. Regular toileting routines are not just interventions to prevent incontinence. Other discomforts can arise from impaired communication, such as conditions like ingrown toenails and medication side effects.

Physical Condition

The patient's physical condition contributes to the likelihood of aggression. Patients with long-standing poor dietary habits (e.g., indigent patients, patients with alcoholism) often have deficiencies of thiamine and niacin. Increased irritability, disorientation, and paranoia may result. Assessing overall dietary intake is relevant, particularly of good tryptophan sources, such as wheat, flour, corn, milk, and eggs. Intake of caffeine, a potent stimulant, should be assessed and limited as necessary.

Social Factors

The nurse should evaluate social factors, such as crisis conditions in the patient's home, family, or community that could lead to aggression or violent episodes. If assessment reveals stressful actions by family members, such as evicting the patient from the home, attention must be devoted to mobilizing resources for family and community support and alternative housing.

Are financial or legal troubles placing increased stress on the patient? Is the patient experiencing conflict with other patients on the unit or with certain staff? People reenact in new relationships the same behaviors that created problems in old ones. Thus, behavior in a mental health facility provides important clues to a patient's habitual responses to authority figures, opposite-sex peers, and same-sex peers. Assessment data provide direction for interventions such as reassigning roommates or caregivers.

Milieu and Environmental Factors

Angry or out-of-control behavior is highly influenced by contextual factors. Successful psychiatric stabilization and treatment in a hospital often depend on the nature of the unit itself. A busy, noisy hospital unit can quickly provoke an aggressive episode. A rude comment or staff denial of a patient's request can trigger physical assault. Documented times of increased violence include meals, medication, and shift change (Salzmann-Erikson & Yifter, 2020). Crowding and density during times of high

---

BOX 20.4

Characteristics of Unit Culture and Staff Behavior that Predict Patient Violence

- Rigid unit rules
- Lack of patient privacy or boundary violations
- Lack of patient autonomy (locked doors, restraints)
- Strict hierarchy of authority
- Lack of patient control over the treatment plan
- Denial of patient requests or privileges
- Lack of meaningful and predictable ward activities
- Insufficient help with activities of daily living and other needs from staff
- Patronizing behavior of staff
- Power struggles related to medications
- Failure of staff to listen, convey empathy

Hamrin, V., Iennaco, J., & Olsen, D. (2009). A review of ecological factors affecting inpatient psychiatric unit violence: Implications for relational and unit cultural improvements. *Issues in Mental Health Nursing, 30*, 214–226.

---

patient census are also associated with patient aggression. Inadequate staffing has been identified as a contributing factor in units with a high incidence of assault.

Many characteristics of the unit culture and staff behavior, such as rigid rules and violation of boundaries, predict patient violence (Box 20.4). In units with a high incidence of violence, nurses should take steps to improve the milieu and staff–patient relationships. More skilled handling of "flashpoints," such as staff denial of patient requests, can avert crisis situations.

Clinical Judgment

Safety and de-escalation of the situation are priorities when tempers flare. Preventing injury to the patient and staff are the primary goals; this is not the time to try to reason with the patient.

Interventions for Promoting Safety

Both patients and staff have a right to safety in a psychiatric unit. Nursing interventions focus on communication and development of the nurse–patient relationship, cognitive interventions, interventions for the milieu and environment, and violence prevention.

Communication and Development of the Therapeutic Nurse–Patient Relationship

Communicating with a patient who has the potential for aggression or violence follows the same principles discussed in Chapter 10. Aggressive behavior can be a patient's way to communicate a need, especially if there are communication deficits. The patient who behaves aggressively may receive rewards such as more frequent observation and more opportunities to discuss concerns with nurses.

Listening to the Patient's Illness Experience and Concerns

Development of the therapeutic nurse–patient relationship begins with listening. Many patients with persistent mental illness have had traumatic experiences related to previous hospitalizations. Understandably, they may harbor distrust of mental health clinicians and resentment being hospitalized again. Inviting patients and families to talk about their experiences with the health care system may highlight both their concerns and resources. Simply listening to patients' concerns and "being with" them is often as significant as "doing for" them (Box 20.5) (Thomas & Pollio, 2002).

Validating

Patients who experience intense anger and rage can feel isolated and anxious. The nurse can acknowledge these intense feelings by reflecting, "This must be scary for you." Empathic responding can reduce emotional arousal because the patient feels understood and supported (see Chapter 10). By drawing on experience with other patients, the nurse can also reassure the patient that others have felt the same way.

Box 20.5 • THERAPEUTIC DIALOGUE: THE POTENTIALLY AGGRESSIVE PATIENT

P.T. is a 23-year-old patient in the high observation area of an inpatient unit. The patient pacing back and forth, pounding one fist into his other hand. In the past 24 hours, P.T has been more cooperative and less agitated. The behavior the nurse observes now is more like the behavior the patient displayed 2 days ago. Yesterday, the psychiatrist agreed to grant more freedom in the unit if the patient's behavior improved. Even after behavior improvement, the psychiatrist refused to change the restrictions.

INEFFECTIVE APPROACH

Nurse: P.T., I can understand this is frustrating for you.

P.T.: How can you understand? Have you ever been held like a prisoner?

Nurse: I do understand, P.T. Now you must calm down or more privileges will be removed.

P.T. (voice gets louder): But I was told that calm behavior would mean more privileges. Now you are telling me calm behavior only gets me what I have got! Can't you talk to the doctor for me?

Nurse: No, P.T., I can't talk to the doctor. (P.T. appears more frustrated and agitated as the conversation continues.)

EFFECTIVE APPROACH

Nurse: P.T., you look upset (observation). What happened in your conversation with the psychiatrist? (seeking information)

P.T.: Yesterday, the doctor said calmer behavior would mean more freedom in the unit. I have tried to be calmer and not to swear. You said you noticed the difference. But today the doctor says "no" to more freedom.

Nurse: Some people might feel cheated if this happened to them (validation). Is that how you feel?

P.T.: Yeah, I feel real cheated. Nothing I do makes a difference. That's the way it is here, and that's the way it is when I am out of the hospital.

Nurse: Sounds like experiences like this leave you feeling powerless (validation).

P.T.: I don't have any power, anywhere. Sometimes when I have no power, I get mean. At least then people pay attention to me.

Nurse: In this situation with your doctor, what would help you feel that you had some power? (Inviting patient partnership)

P.T.: Well, if the doctor would listen to me or read my chart.

Nurse: I am a bit confused by the psychiatrist's decision. I won't make promises that your privileges will change, but would it be okay with you if I talk with the doctor?

P.T.: That would make me feel like someone is on my side.

CRITICAL THINKING CHALLENGE

- In the first scenario, how did the nurse escalate the situation?
- Compare the first scenario with the second. How are they different?

Providing Choices

When possible, the nurse should provide the patient with choices, particularly patients who have little control over their situation because of their condition. Offering concrete choices is better than offering open-ended options. For example, a patient who is experiencing a manic episode and is confined to their room may have few options in their daily schedule. However, they may be allowed to make choices about food, personal hygiene, and which pajamas to wear.

Cognitive Interventions to Address Aggression

Cognitive interventions are very useful in interacting with a potentially aggressive patient (see Chapter 13). These interventions are useful when the patient is in a nonaggressive state and willing to discuss the irrational thought process underlying aggressive episodes. These periods of interaction allow exploration of the patient's beliefs and provision of reassurance, support, and education.

> **NCLEXNOTE** The best time to teach the patient techniques for managing anger and aggression is when the patient is not experiencing the provoking event. Cognitive therapy approaches are useful and can be prioritized according to responses.

Providing Patient Education

Inpatient hospitalization offers opportunities for education of patients and families about a variety of topics. Nurses can seize "teachable moments" to convey important principles of anger management. For example, after an outburst of loud cursing by J., who mistakenly thought another patient, S., had stolen their cigarettes, the nurse helped them consider what they could have done differently in the situation. J. was more amenable to learning about calming techniques and problem-solving strategies at this time because their behavior had resulted in adverse consequences (estrangement from S., disruption of the dayroom during a popular bingo game, and cancellation of S.'s weekend pass). This incident could also be used for teaching in a subsequent group meeting of inpatients. Many units have daily meetings that permit processing of such conflicts. S. could be invited to express feelings about being falsely accused of stealing. Other patients may reveal how distressed they were when J. was cursing loudly, providing their useful peer feedback about J.'s outburst. Together, group members could generate ideas for more appropriate behavior.

Developing Prevention Strategies

Although patients are not always aware of it, escalation of feelings, thoughts, and behavior from calmness to violence may follow a pattern. Disruption of the pattern can sometimes be a useful means for preventing escalation and helping the patient regain composure. Patients can learn to identify their own personal warning signs of aggression and develop aggression–prevention strategies. Both inpatients and outpatients have benefited from nurse-led group therapy for aggressive behaviors. Group members recognized their underlying feelings of helplessness and loss of control and successfully decreased their aggressive behaviors (Lanza, 2018). Nurses can suggest a variety of strategies to interrupt patterns:

- Counting to 10
- Using a relaxation or breathing technique (see Chapter 11)
- Removing oneself from interactions or stimuli that may contribute to increased distress (voluntarily taking a "cooling-off walk" or "time-out")
- Doing something different (e.g., reading, listening to quiet music, watching television)

Milieu and Environmental Interventions

The inpatient environment can be modified proactively to decrease the potential of aggressive and violent behaviors (Box 20.6).

Reducing Stimulation

For people whose perceptions or thoughts are disordered from brain damage, degeneration, or other thought-processing difficulties, modification of the environment may be one of the main interventions. The patient with a brain injury, progressive dementia, or distorted vision may be experiencing intense and highly confusing stimulation even though the environment, from the nurse's or family's perspective, seems calm and orderly.

Likewise, introducing more structure into a chaotic environment can help decrease the risk for aggressive behavior. It is possible to make stimuli meaningful or to simplify and interpret the environment in many practical ways, such as by identifying people or equipment that may be unfamiliar, providing cues as to what is expected (e.g., posting signs with directions, putting a toothbrush and toothpaste by the sink), and removing or silencing unnecessary stimuli (e.g., turning off paging systems).

BOX 20.6

Environmental Management: Maintaining Patient Safety

DEFINITION

Maintaining patient safety includes identifying and eliminating environmental risks for persons who are at risk of injuring self or others.

ACTIVITIES

- Search the environment routinely to maintain it as hazard free.
- Remove potential weapons (e.g., sharps, ropelike objects) from the environment.
- Search the patient and belongings for weapons or potential weapons
- Monitor the safety of items that visitors bring to the environment.
- Instruct visitors and other caregivers about relevant patient safety issues.
- Limit patient use of potential weapons (e.g., sharps, ropelike objects).
- Monitor patient during use of potential weapons (e.g., razors).
- Place the patient with potential for self-harm with a roommate to decrease isolation and opportunity to act on self-harm thoughts, as appropriate.
- Assign a single room to the patient with potential for violence toward others.
- Place the patient in a bedroom located near a nursing station.
- Limit access to windows unless they are locked and shatterproof, as appropriate.
- Lock utility and storage rooms.
- Provide paper dishes and plastic utensils at meals.
- Place the patient in the least restrictive environment that still allows for the necessary level of observation.
- Provide ongoing surveillance of all patient access areas to maintain patient safety and therapeutically intervene, as needed.
- Remove other individuals from the vicinity of a violent or potentially violent patient.
- Maintain a designated safe area (e.g., seclusion room) for patient to be placed when violent.
- Provide plastic, rather than metal, clothes hangers, as appropriate.

Adapted from the Mental Health Environment of Care Checklist. VHA National Center for Patient Safety, Department of Veterans Affairs. Version 06–01–2015. http://www.patientsafety.va.gov/professionals/onthejob/mental-health.asp

---

Considering the environment from the patient's viewpoint is essential. For instance, if the surroundings are unfamiliar, the patient will need to process more information. Lack of a recognizable pattern or structure further taxes the patient's capacity to encode information. Appropriate interventions include clarifying the meaning and purpose of people and objects in the environment, enhancing the patient's sense of control and the predictability of the environment, and reducing other stimuli as much as possible.

Interventions for Managing Imminent Aggression and Violence

De-Escalation

Authentic engagement with the patient is the core component in a therapeutic de-escalation by the nurse. Creative, patient-centered strategies, not techniques of physical restraint, are of paramount importance. Individualizing interventions is important. In some patients, loudness and pacing can be ignored; in others, these behaviors indicate an escalation of agitation.

De-escalating potential aggression is always preferable to challenging or provoking a patient. De-escalating (commonly known as "talking the person down") is a skill that every nurse can develop. Trying to clarify what has upset the patient is important although not all patients are capable of articulating what provoked them, as in cases where violent acting out has been triggered by delusions or hallucinations (Moylan, 2015). Some analyses will have to take place after a crisis has been diffused. The nurse can use therapeutic communication techniques to prevent a crisis or diffuse a critical situation (see Box 20.5).

The nurse who works with potentially aggressive patients should do so with respect and concern. The goal is to work with patients to find solutions, approaching these patients calmly and empathizing with the patient's perspective. Offering a simple apology to an agitated patient can circumvent a power struggle (Berring et al., 2016). In dealing with aggression, as in other aspects of nursing practice, at times the best intervention is silence. It is easy to equate intervention with activity, the sense that "I must do something." But offering quiet calmness may be enough to help a patient regain control of their behavior.

KEYCONCEPT Intervention fit The nurse who intervenes from within the context of the therapeutic relationship must be cognizant of the fit of a particular intervention.

Interventions that are appropriate in early phases of escalation differ from those used when the patient's agitation is greater. The patient's affective, behavioral, and cognitive response to an intervention provides information about its effects and guides the nurse's next response. The following approaches are important in caring for patients who are aggressive or violent:

- Using nonthreatening body language
- Respecting the patient's personal space and boundaries
- Having immediate access to the door of the room in case you need to leave the room

- Choosing to leave the door open to an office while talking to a patient
- Knowing where colleagues are and making sure those colleagues know where you are
- Removing or not wearing clothing or accessories that could be used to harm you, such as scarves, necklaces, or dangling earrings

Administering and Monitoring PRN Medications

Patients with potential for aggression and violence usually have a PRN (as-needed) medication order for agitation and aggression. Administering a PRN medication is left to the discretion of the nurse, who makes a judgment about the patient after careful assessment. Patients often recognize when a PRN medication is needed.

Avoiding the Use of Seclusion and Restraint

Seclusion and restraint have been used by nurses when patients need to be separated from other patients on the unit. The decision to use seclusion and restraint is a dynamic process involving evaluation of the risks to all who are present, as well as the need to maintain a therapeutic milieu. The decision is usually an interdisciplinary decision that follows ethical and legal standards as well as accrediting guidelines (Moylan, 2015).

The use of seclusion and restraint is now recognized as a traumatic experience for patients. Most patients with a mental disorder have already experienced traumas, usually in childhood. The act of placing an individual in seclusion or restraints retraumatizes the individual (Chieze et al., 2019). Therefore, the trauma-informed care movement has influenced organizational policy making (Moylan, 2015). Many hospitals no longer use restraints as a form of behavioral management. In instances where seclusion and restraint are used, they should be the last resort to protect the patient or the staff. De-escalation interventions should be tried first and clearly documented in the patient's record.

American institutions that receive Medicare or Medicaid reimbursement must adhere to guidelines issued by the Center for Medicare and Medicaid Services. These guidelines specify that a registered nurse must verify the need for restraint or seclusion and then contact the physician or other licensed practitioner; within 1 hour, that practitioner must examine the patient. Individual states have also enacted laws to regulate the use of restraints, and professional organizations released position statements on restraints as the last resort in an emergency (American Psychiatric Nurses Association, 2014).

Restraint-related injuries and deaths have prompted many facilities to ban their use entirely and train staff in alternative techniques. Comfort or sensory rooms are becoming more widespread, providing an appealing alternative to coercive interventions by unit staff. These rooms can provide stimulation for sight, smell, hearing, touch, and taste in a demand-free environment that is controlled by the patient. The rooms may reduce patients' distress and agitation and reduce the need for seclusion and restraint (Björkdahl et al., 2016). Some treatment facilities offer items such as weighted blankets, massage creams, and "squishy" balls to augment other de-escalation measures (Blackburn et al., 2016).

Evaluation and Treatment Outcomes

Treatment outcomes can be considered at both individual and aggregate levels. The desired outcome at the individual level is for the patient to regain or maintain control over aggressive or potentially aggressive thoughts, feelings, and actions. The nurse may observe that the patient shows decreased psychomotor activity (e.g., less pacing), has a more relaxed posture, speaks more directly about feelings of anger and personal needs, requires less sedating medication, shows increased tolerance for frustration and the ability to consider alternatives, and makes effective use of other coping strategies.

If restraints or seclusion have been used, a debriefing occurs with the persons involved in the incident, including the patient. This approach allows for a collaborative, community approach to preventing patient violence and avoids blaming one assailant for incidents provoked by a variety of contextual and interpersonal factors. The practice of prompt debriefing and reflection can ultimately transform a treatment setting to a learning community (Berring et al., 2016).

Evidence of a reduction in risk factors in the treatment setting include decreased noise and confusion in the immediate environment; calmness on the part of nursing staff and others; and a climate of safety, clear expectations, and mutual acceptance and respect. In units, day hospitals, or group home settings, indicators of positive treatment outcomes include a reduction in the number and severity of assaults on staff and other patients, fewer incident reports, and increased staff competency in de-escalating potentially violent situations.

For practice improvement and research purposes, the American Psychiatric Nurses Association Council for Safe Environments recommends measuring violence at a standard rate of incidents per 1,000 days of patient care, using validated tools such as the Overt Aggression Scale and the Modified Version of the Overt Aggression Scale. These tools can be incorporated into nursing assessments and documented in electronic health records. The resultant data can be used to evaluate effectiveness of interventions and adequacy of staffing (Allen et al., 2019).

Responding to Assault on Nurses

Because nurses have extended contact with patients during highly stressful circumstances, there is always the risk that they may be the recipients of patient aggression. Psychiatric nurses are assaulted more often than medical–surgical nurses, but physical violence and mental abuse occur more often in the emergency room than in the mental health unit (Pekurinen et al., 2017).

Assaults on nurses by patients can have both immediate and long-term consequences (see Table 20.3). Reported assaults range from verbal abuse or threats and minor altercations to severe injuries, rape, and murder. Any assault can produce severe consequences for the victim including posttraumatic stress disorder. After a violent incident, the nurse may avoid the patient or watch for any signs of patient remorse; the nurse's response differs depending on the nurse's feelings of safety and comfort with the patient. The nurse's interpretation of the assaultive behavior will depend on many factors such as experience with assault, the type of assault (impulsive or instrumental), and the nurse's injury.

Unfortunately, patient aggression directed toward nurses is often downplayed or tolerated by nurses as "part of the job." Nurses seldom report attacks to the police or prosecute their attackers, but such incidents should be reported to supervisors and possibly to legal authorities, depending on the circumstances. Aggression by patients must be addressed vigorously because it can threaten the other patients, other health care professionals, family members, and visitors, as well as the nursing staff. Reporting violent attacks increases public awareness and increases the likelihood that protective legislation will be enacted. The environment should be modified with the addition of security alarms, video monitors, and de-escalation teams.

All nurses must be provided with training programs in the prevention and management of aggressive behavior. These programs, similar to courses on cardiopulmonary resuscitation, impart both knowledge and skills, lessening the likelihood of emotional freezing in the presence of violent patient behavior. Similar to cardiopulmonary resuscitation training, the courses should be provided to undergraduate students and regularly offered to practicing nurses, so that they have opportunities to reinforce and update what they have learned (Searby et al., 2019). Some states have enacted legislation mandating workplace violence prevention programs, but the curricula vary, and the quality of training lacks systematic evaluation. Commercially marketed training programs have been criticized because they fail to consider the predatory aspect of some patients' violence and fail to cite nursing research.

RESEARCH AND POLICY INITIATIVES

Additional understanding of the phenomena of anger, aggression, and violence as they occur in the clinical setting is needed. Nurses must research the effectiveness of particular anger and aggression management interventions. Although much of this chapter focused on individuals who need to *down*regulate anger, the reader must remember that anger suppressors have a need to *up*regulate their anger and express it more assertively. Learning to express legitimate angry feelings was a significant step in the trajectory of recovery for women who had survived childhood abuse (Thomas et al., 2012). Treatments should be tailored based on assessment data and patients' progress.

There is a moral imperative for nurses to be involved in combating violence in the larger community. Lessening anger and violence in the workplace and the home

TABLE 20.3	NURSES' RESPONSES TO ASSAULT	
Response Type	Personal	Professional
Affective	• Irritability • Depression • Anger • Anxiety • Apathy	• Erosion of feelings of competence, leading to increased anxiety and fear • Feelings of guilt or self-blame • Fear of potentially violent patients
Cognitive	• Suppressed or intrusive thoughts of assault	• Reduced confidence in judgment • Consideration of job change
Behavioral	• Social withdrawal	• Possible hesitation in responding to other violent situations • Possible overcontrolling • Possible hesitation to report future assaults • Possible withdrawal from colleagues • Questioning of capabilities by coworkers
Physiologic	• Disturbed sleep • Headaches • Stomach aches • Tension	• Increased absenteeism because of somatic complaints

demands involvement of all mental health professionals. Nurses can share their expertise with parents, children, teachers, and community agencies. Nurses are well positioned to teach health-promoting anger management classes in diverse practice settings, such as outpatient clinics, schools, and corporate sites. Classes for children and adolescents can be of great benefit because young people are forming the anger habits that will continue into adulthood. Youth who have high levels of anger are at risk for misuse of alcohol and other substances (Serafini et al., 2016) as well as interpersonal conflicts that hamper their educational and occupational success.

SUMMARY OF KEY POINTS

- Anger is an emotional state, usually temporary, that can be expressed constructively or destructively. Destructive anger alienates other people and invites retaliation.

- Anger, aggression, and violence should not be viewed as a continuum. The anger of ordinary people seldom progresses to aggression or violence. Anger does not necessarily lead to aggression or violence.

- Anger management is a useful psychoeducational intervention that is effective with a wide variety of nonviolent individuals. However, anger management is not designed to modify violent behavior.

- Several theories explain anger, aggression, and violence and include neurobiological and psychosocial theories. These theories serve as the basis of assessment and interventions.

- The general aggression model accounts for the interaction of cognition, affect, and arousal during an aggressive episode.

- There is no one factor that predicts aggression or violence. Factors that have been observed to be precursors are staring and eye contact, tone and volume of voice, anxiety, and pacing.

- Nursing interventions can be affective, cognitive, behavioral, or sociocultural. A therapeutic milieu supports a nonviolent culture.

- Nurses who experience assault may experience changes in affective, cognitive, behavioral, and physiological areas.

- Seclusion or restraints should be used only as a last resort.

- Patient aggression and violence are serious concerns for nurses in all areas of clinical practice. Training in policies and procedures for the prevention and management of aggressive episodes should be available in nursing education programs and all work settings.

CRITICAL THINKING CHALLENGES

1. M.J., a 24-year-old, has just been admitted to an inpatient psychiatry unit transferring from the emergency department after being treated for a drug overdose. Patient is sullen when introduced to the roommate and refuses to answer the admission assessment questions. The nurse tells the patient that they will come back in 30 minutes to complete the assessment. A few minutes later, the patient approaches the nursing station and asks in a demanding tone to talk with someone because of being completely ignored.

   a. What frameworks can the nurse use to understand M.J. behavior?

   b. At this point in time, what data are available to develop a plan of care?

   c. What interventions might the nurse choose to use to help M.J. behave in a manner that is consistent with the norms of this inpatient unit?

2. Discuss the influence of gender and cultural norms on the expression of anger. When a nurse is caring for a patient from a culture that the nurse is not familiar with, what could the nurse ask to ensure that their expectations of the patient's behavior are consistent with the gender and cultural norms of the patient?

3. Under what circumstances should people who are aggressive or violent be held accountable for their behavior? Are there any exceptions?

4. When a nurse minimizes verbally abusive behavior by a patient, family member, or health care colleague, what implicit message does they send?

 Movie Viewing Guides
Mandela: Long Walk to Freedom: 2013. South African icon Nelson Mandela displays the gamut of angry behaviors in this biographic epic: (1) righteous anger on behalf of his clients when he was a young lawyer; (2) fiery anger at the cruel persecution of Blacks during apartheid; and (3) violence against the government after the failure of nonviolent protests to achieve freedom from oppression. Bomb throwing at government buildings results in 27 years of imprisonment, which could have created lasting bitterness against his oppressors. Yet after his release, Mandela forgives those who had imprisoned him, becomes the first Black president of his country, and receives the Nobel Peace Prize. This remarkable true story provides many lessons for all.

VIEWING POINTS: Although most of us will never be forced to endure such intolerable conditions, we all experience times of unfair or unkind treatment. How can we learn to use our anger productively or learn to let it go by forgiving those who wronged us?

REFERENCES

Allen, D. E., Mistler, L. A., Ray, R., Batscha, C., Delaney, K., Loucks, J., Nadler-Moodie, M., & Sharp, D. (2019). A call to action from the APNA Council for Safe Environments: Defining violence and aggression for research and practice improvement purposes. *Journal of the American Psychiatric Nurses Association, 25*(1), 7–10.

Allen, J. J., Anderson, C. A., & Bushman, B. J. (2018). The general aggression model. *Current Opinions in Psychology, 19,* 75–80. https://doi.org/10.1016/j.copsyc.2017.03.034

American Psychiatric Association (APA). (2013). *Diagnostic and statistical manual of mental disorders (DSM-5).* Author.

American Psychiatric Nurses Association. (2014). *2014 Position statement on the use of seclusion and restraint.* Author.

Averill, J. R. (1983). Studies on anger and aggression: Implications for theories of emotion. *American Psychologist, 38*(11), 1145–1160.

Bandura, A. (2001). Social cognitive theory: An agentic perspective. *Annual Review of Psychology, 52,* 1–26.

Barlow, M. A., Wrosch, C., Gouin, J. P., & Kunzmann, U. (2019). Is anger, but not sadness, associated with chronic inflammation and illness in older adulthood? *Psychology and aging, 34*(3), 330–340. https://doi.org/10.1037/pag0000348

Been, L. E., Gibbons, A. V., & Meisel, R. L. (2018). Towards a neurobiology of female aggression. *Neuropharmacology.* https://doi.org/10.1016/j.neuropharm.2018.11.039

Berring, L. L., Hummelvoll, J. K., Pedersen, L., & Buus, N. (2016). A co-operative inquiry into generating, describing, and transforming knowledge about de-escalation practices in mental health settings. *Issues in Mental Health Nursing, 37*(7), 451–463.

Björkdahl, A., Perseius, K.-I., Samuelsson, M., & Lindberg, M. H. (2016). Sensory rooms in psychiatric inpatient care: Staff experiences. *International Journal of Mental Health Nursing, 25*(5), 472–479. https://doi.org/10.1111/inm.12205

Blackburn, J., McKenna, B., Jackson, B., Hitch, D., Benitez, J., McLennan, C., & Furness, T. (2016). Educating mental health clinicians about sensory modulation to enhance clinical practice in a youth inpatient mental health unit: A feasibility study. *Issues in Mental Health Nursing, 37*(7), 517–525.

Bora, E., Velakoulis, D., & Walterfang, M. (2016). Meta-analysis of facial emotion recognition in behavioral variant frontotemporal dementia: Comparison with Alzheimer Disease and healthy controls. *Journal of Geriatric Psychiatry and Neurology, 29*(4), 201–211.

Buckley, T., Hoo, S. Y., Fethney, J., Shaw, E., Hanson, P. S., & Tofler, G. H. (2015). Triggering of acute coronary occlusion by episodes of anger. *European Heart Journal: Acute Cardiovascular Care, 4*(6), 493–498.

Bruno, A., Laganà, A. S., Leonardi, V., Greco, D., Merlino, M., Vitale, S. G., Triolo, O., Zoccali, R. A., & Muscatello, M. (2017). Inside-out: the role of anger experience and expression in the development of postpartum mood disorders. The journal of maternal-fetal & neonatal medicine : the official journal of the European Association of Perinatal Medicine, the Federation of Asia and Oceania Perinatal Societies, the International Society of Perinatal Obstetricians, 31(22), 3033–3038. https://doi.org/10.1080/14767058.2017.1362554

Burke, M. W., Fillion, M., Mejia, J., Ervin, F. R., & Palmour, R. M. (2018). Perinatal MAO inhibition produces long-lasting impairment of serotonin function in offspring. *Brain Sciences, 8*(6). pii: E106. https://doi.org/10.3390/brainsci8060106

Chieze, M., Hurst, S., Kaiser, S., & Sentissi, O. (2019). Effects of seclusion and restraint in adult psychiatry: A systematic review. *Frontiers in Psychiatry, 10,* 1–19.

Coccaro, E. F. (2019). Psychiatric comorbidity in Intermittent Explosive Disorder. *Journal of Psychiatric Research, 118,* 38–43. https://doi.org/10.1016/j.jpsychires.2019.08.012

Coccaro, E. F., & Lee, R. J. (2019). 5-HT$_{2c}$ agonist, lorcaserin, reduces aggressive responding in intermittent explosive disorder: A pilot study. *Human Psychopharmacology, 34*(6), e2714. https://doi.org/10.1002/hup.2714

Endrighi, R., Dimond, A. J., Waters, A. J., Dimond, C. C., Harris, K. M., Gottlieb, S. S., & Krantz, D. S. (2019). Associations of perceived stress and state anger with symptom burden and functional status in patients with heart failure. *Psychology & Health, 34*(10), 1250–1266. https://doi.org/10.1080/08870446.2019.1609676

d'Ettorre, G., & Pellicani, V. (2017). Workplace violence toward mental healthcare workers employed in psychiatric wards. *Safety and Health at Work, 8*(4), 337–342.

Feindler, E. L. (2006). *Anger-related disorders: A practitioner's guide to comparative treatments.* Springer.

Feindler, E. L., & Byers, A. (2006). Multiple perspectives on the conceptualization and treatment of anger-related disorders. In E. L. Feindler (Ed.), *Anger-related disorders: A practitioner's guide to comparative treatments* (pp. 303–320). Springer.

Feinson, M. C., & Hornik-Lurie, T. (2016). Binge eating and childhood emotional abuse: The mediating role of anger. *Appetite, 105,* 487–493.

Fuchshuber, J., & Unterrainer, H. F. (2020). Childhood trauma, personality, and substance use disorder: The development of a neuropsychoanalytic addiction model. *Frontiers in Psychiatry, 11,* 531. https://doi.org/10.3389/fpsyt.2020.00531

Galbraith, T., Carliner, H., Keyes, K. M., McLaughlin, K. A., McCloskey, M. S., & Heimberg, R. G. (2018). The co-occurrence and correlates of anxiety disorders among adolescents with intermittent explosive disorder. *Aggressive Behavior, 44*(6), 581–590. https://doi.org/10.1002/ab.21783

Golding, P., & Fitzgerald, J. E. (2019). The early biopsychosocial development of boys and the origins of violence in males. *Infant Mental Health Journal, 40*(1), 5–22.

Gouin, J., Kiecolt-Glaser, J. K., Malarkey, W. B., & Glaser, R. (2008). The influence of anger expression on wound healing. *Brain, Behavior, and Immunity, 22*(5), 699–708.

Halperin, E., & Reifen Tagar, M. (2017). Emotions in conflicts: Understanding emotional processes sheds light on the nature and potential resolution of intractable conflicts. *Current Opinion in Psychology, 17,* 94–98.

Jalil, R., & Dickens, G. L. (2018). Systematic review of studies of mental health nurses' experience of anger and its relationships with their attitudes and practice. *Journal of Psychiatric Mental Health Nursing, 25*(3), 201–213.

Kakoo Brioso, E., Ferreira Cristina, S., Costa, L., & Ouakinin, S. (2020). Correlation between emotional regulation and peripheral lymphocyte counts in colorectal cancer patients. *PeerJ, 8,* e9475. https://doi.org/10.7717/peerj.9475

Kelly, S. (2019). Cognitive behavior therapy with African Americans. In G. Y. Iwamasa & P. A. Hays (Eds.), *Culturally responsive cognitive behavior therapy: Practice and supervision* (2nd ed., pp. 105–128). American Psychological Association.

Kitayama, S., Park, J., Boylan, J., Miyamoto, Y., Levine, C. S., Markus, H., Karasawa, M., Coe, C. L., Kawakami, N., Love, G., & Ryff, C. D. (2015). Expression of anger and ill health in two cultures: An examination of inflammation and cardiovascular risk. *Psychological Science, 26*(2), 211–220. https://doi.org/10.1177710956797614561268

Lanza, M. (2018). Concentric group therapy for aggression: A historical perspective. *Issues in Mental Health Nursing, 39*(10), 883–887. https://doi.org/1080/01612840.2018.1493164

Lee, A., & DiGiuseppe, R. (2018). Anger and aggression treatments: A review of meta-analyses. *Current Opinion in Psychology, 19,* 65–74.

Lee, E., Yeung, N., Xu, Z., Zhang, D., Yu, C. P., & Wong, S. (2020). Effect and acceptability of mindfulness-based stress reduction program on patients with elevated blood pressure or hypertension: A meta-analysis of randomized controlled trials. *Hypertension (Dallas, Tex.: 1979), 76*(6), 1992–2001. https://doi.org/10.1161/HYPERTENSIONAHA.120.16160

Momeni, J., Omidi, A., Raygan, F., & Akbari, H. (2016). The effects of mindfulness-based stress reduction on cardiac patients' blood pressure, perceived stress, and anger: A single-blind randomized controlled trial. *Journal of the American Society of Hypertension: JASH, 10*(10), 763–771. https://doi.org/10.1016/j.jash.2016.07.007

Moylan, L. B. (2015). A conceptual model for nurses' decision-making with the aggressive psychiatric patient. *Issues in Mental Health Nursing, 36*(8), 577–582. https://doi.org/10.3109/01612840.2015.1019019

Pekurinen, V., Willman, L., Virtanen, M., Kivimäki, M., Vahtera, J., & Välimäki, M. (2017). Patient aggression and the wellbeing of nurses: A cross-sectional survey study in psychiatric and non-psychiatric settings. *International Journal of Environmental Research and Public Health, 14*(10), 1245. https://doi.org/10.3390/ijerph14101245

Pimple, P., Lima, B. B., Hammadah, M., Wilmot, K., Ramadan, R., Levantsevych, O., Sullivan, S., Kim, J. H., Kaseer, B., Shah, A. J., Ward, L., Raggi, P., Bremner, J. D., Hanfelt, J., Lewis, T., Quyyumi, A. A., & Vaccarino, V. (2019). Psychological distress and subsequent cardiovascular events in individuals with coronary artery disease. *Journal of the American Heart Association, 8*(9), e011866. https://doi.org/10.1161/JAHA.118.011866

Repple, J., Habel, U., Wagels, L., Pawliczek, C. M., Schneider, F., & Kohn, N. (2018). Sex differences in the neural correlates of aggression. *Brain Structure & Function, 223*(9), 4115–4124. https://doi.org/10.1007/s00429-018-1739-5

Rubin, T. I. (1970). *The angry book.* Collier.

Russell, M. A., Smith, T. W., & Smyth, J. M. (2016). Anger expression, momentary anger, and symptom severity in patients with chronic disease. *Annals of Behavioral, 50*(2), 259–271. https://doi.org/10.1007/s12160-015-9747-7

Rynar, L., & Coccaro, E. F. (2018). Psychosocial impairment in DSM-5 intermittent explosive disorder. *Psychiatry Research, 264,* 91–95. https://doi.org/10.1016/j.psychres.2018.03.077

Salzmann-Erikson, M., & Yifter, L. (2020). Risk factors and triggers that may result in patient-initiated violence on inpatient psychiatric units: An integrative review. *Clinical Nursing Research*, 29(7), 504–520. https://doi.org/10.1177/1054773818823333

Searby, A., Snipe, J., & Maude, P. (2019). Aggression management training in undergraduate nursing students: A scoping review. *Issues in Mental Health Nursing*, 40(6), 503–510. https://doi.org/10.1080/01612840.2019.1565874

Serafini, K., Toohey, M., Kiluk, B., & Carroll, K. (2016). Anger and its association with substance use treatment outcomes in a sample of adolescents. *Journal of Child and Adolescent Substance Abuse*, 25(5), 391–398. https://doi.org/10.1080/1067828x.2015.1049394

Shepherd, G., & Cant, M. (2020). Difficult to change? The differences between successful and not-so-successful participation in anger management groups. *Counseling and Psychotherapy Research*, 20, 214–223. https://doi.org/10.1002/capr.12276

Smeijers, L., Mostofsky, E., Tofler, G. H., Muller, J. E., Kop, W. J., & Mittleman, M. A. (2017). Anxiety and anger immediately prior to myocardial infarction and long-term mortality: Characteristics of high-risk patients. *Journal of Psychosomatic Research*, 93, 19–27. https://doi.org/10.1016/j.jpsychores.2016.12.001

Smith-MacDonald, L., Norris, J. M., Raffin-Bouchal, S., & Sinclair, S. (2017). Spirituality and mental well-being in Combat Veterans: A systematic review. *Military Medicine*, 182(11), e1920–e1940. https://doi.org/10.7205/MILMED-D-17-00099

Sommer, J., Lyican, S., & Babcock, J. (2016). The relation between contempt, anger, and intimate partner violence: A dyadic approach. *Journal of Interpersonal Violence*. https://doi.org/10.1177/0886260516665107

Spielberger, C. D. (1999). *Manual for the State Trait Anger Expression Inventory-2*. Psychological Assessment Resources.

Teng, Z., Nie, Q., Guo, C., Zhang, Q., Liu, Y., & Bushman, B. J. (2019). A longitudinal study of link between exposure to violent video games and aggression in Chinese adolescents: The mediating role of moral disengagement. *Developmental Psychology*, 55(10), 184–195.

Thomas, M. C., Kamarck, T. W., Wright, A., Matthews, K. A., Muldoon, M. F., & Manuck, S. B. (2020). Hostility dimensions and metabolic syndrome in a healthy, midlife sample. *International Journal of Behavioral Medicine*, 27(4), 475–480. https://doi.org/10.1007/s12529-020-09855-y

Thomas, S. P. (1990). Theoretical and empirical perspectives on anger. *Issues in Mental Health Nursing*, 11(3), 203–216.

Thomas, S. P. (1997a). Women's anger: Relationship of suppression to blood pressure. *Nursing Research*, 46(6), 324–330.

Thomas, S. P. (1997b). Angry? Let's talk about it! *Applied Nursing Research*, 10(2), 80–85.

Thomas, S. P. (2001). Teaching healthy anger management. *Perspectives in Psychiatric Care*, 37(2), 41–48.

Thomas, S. P. (2006). Cultural and gender considerations in the assessment and treatment of anger-related disorders. In E. L. Feindler (Ed.), *Anger-related disorders: A practitioner's guide to comparative treatments* (pp. 71–95). Springer.

Thomas, S. P. (2009). *Transforming nurses' stress and anger* (3rd ed.). Springer.

Thomas, S. P., Bannister, S. C., & Hall, J. M. (2012). Anger in the trajectory of healing from childhood maltreatment. *Archives of Psychiatric Nursing*, 26(3), 169–180. https://doi.org/10.1016/j.apnu.2011.09.003

Thomas, S. P., & Pollio, H. R. (2002). *Listening to patients*. Springer.

Thomas, S. P., Shattell, M., & Martin, T. (2002). What's therapeutic about the therapeutic milieu? *Archives of Psychiatric Nursing*, 16(3), 99–107.

Trost, Z., Scott, W., Buelow, M. T., Nowlin, L., Turan, B., Boals, A., & Monden, K. R. (2017). The association between injustice perception and psychological outcomes in an inpatient spinal cord injury sample: The mediating effects of anger. *Spinal Cord*, 55(10), 898–905.

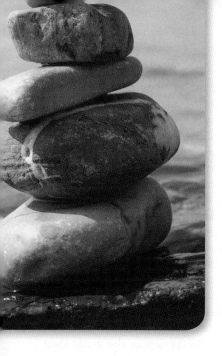

21
Crisis, Loss, Grief, Bereavement, and Disaster Management

Mary Ann Boyd

KEYCONCEPTS

- Bereavement
- Crisis
- Disaster
- Grief
- Loss

LEARNING OBJECTIVES

After studying this chapter, you will be able to:

1. Describe the types of crises and their impact on mental health.

2. Discuss theoretical models explaining grief, uncomplicated bereavement, and complicated bereavement.

3. Discuss the impact of disasters on mental health.

4. Discuss nursing care for persons experiencing crises, loss, grief, bereavement, and disaster.

5. Evaluate the effects of crises, losses, and disasters on lifestyle and survival.

6. Explain the psychological impact of crises, losses, and disasters on survivors of catastrophic events.

KEY TERMS

- ABCs of psychological first aid • Acute grief • Complicated bereavement • Debriefing • Developmental crisis • Dual process model • Loss-oriented coping • Maturational crises • Oscillation • Predeath grief • Restoration-oriented coping • Situational crisis • Traumatic crisis • Uncomplicated bereavement

INTRODUCTION

Successfully surviving crises, loss, and disaster may make a difference between being mentally healthy or mentally ill. This chapter explores the concepts of crisis, loss, grief, bereavement, and disaster management; broadens the scope and understanding of the responses of persons to crisis, loss, and disaster situations; and describes how the nursing process can be used to care for persons experiencing these events.

CRISIS

Adaptation and coping are a natural part of life (see Chapter 19). Crisis occurs when there is a perceived challenge or threat that overwhelms the capacity of the individual to cope effectively with the event at any age. Life is disrupted, and unexpected emotional (e.g., sadness, depression, anxiety) and biologic (e.g., nausea, vomiting, diarrhea, headaches) responses occur (see Box 21.1). Functioning can be severely impaired.

BOX 21.1
Grief

Physical: stunned, weight gain/loss, insomnia, anorexia, exhausted, restless, aching arms, sleep difficulties, headaches, aching arms, feels ill, palpitations, breathlessness, sighing, lack of strength, blurred vision

Emotional: crying, sobbing, sadness, guilt, anger, sense of failure, irritability, resentment, bitterness, denial, frustration, shame, fear of own death, oversensitivity to environment, senses the presence of the deceased

Social: social withdrawal from normal activity, isolation from others

Cognitive: forgetful, difficulty in making decisions, disorganized, concentration is difficult, preoccupation with thoughts of the deceased, time confusion, short attention span, think they are going crazy

---

KEYCONCEPT Crisis is a time-limited event that triggers adaptive or nonadaptive responses to maturational, situational, or traumatic experiences. A crisis results from stressful events for which previous coping mechanisms fail to provide adequate adaptive skills to address the perceived challenge or threat. Adaptation to crisis typically occurs in 6 weeks.

A crisis occurs when an individual is at a breaking point. A crisis can have either positive or negative outcomes. If positive, there is an opportunity for growth and change as new ways of coping are learned. If negative, suicide, homelessness, or depression can result. A crisis generally lasts no more than 4 to 6 weeks. At the end of that time, the person in crisis should have begun to come to grip with the event and begun to harness resources to cope with its long-term consequences. By definition, there is no such thing as a chronic crisis. People who live in constant turmoil are not in crisis but in chaos.

Many events evoke a crisis, such as natural disasters (e.g., floods, tornadoes, earthquakes) and human-made disasters (e.g., wars, bombings, airplane crashes) as well as traumatic experiences (e.g., rape, sexual abuse, assault). In addition, interpersonal events (marriage, birth of a child) create crises in the lives of any person.

Feelings of fear, desperation, and being out of control are common during a crisis, but the precipitating event and circumstances are unusual or rare, perceived as a threat, and specific to the individual. For example, a disagreement with a family member may escalate into a crisis for one person, but not another. If the person is significantly distressed or social functioning is impaired, a diagnosis of acute stress disorder should be considered (American Psychiatric Association [APA], 2013). The person with an acute stress disorder has dissociative symptoms and persistently reexperiences the event (See Chapter 29).

Historical Perspectives of Crisis

The psychiatrist Caplan (1961) defined a crisis as occurring when a person faces a problem that cannot be solved by customary problem-solving methods. When the usual problem-solving methods no longer work, a person's life balance or equilibrium is upset. During the period of disequilibrium, there is a rise in inner tension and anxiety followed by emotional upset and an inability to function. This conceptualization of phases of a crisis is used today (Fig. 21.1). According to Caplan, during a crisis, a person is open to learning new ways of coping to survive. The outcome of a crisis is governed by the kind of interaction that occurs between the person and available key social support systems.

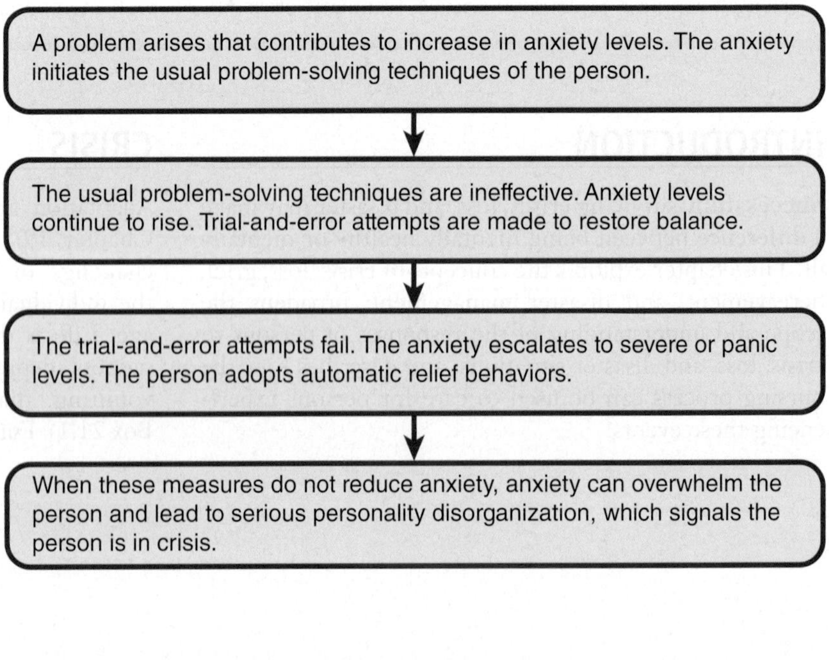

A problem arises that contributes to increase in anxiety levels. The anxiety initiates the usual problem-solving techniques of the person.

↓

The usual problem-solving techniques are ineffective. Anxiety levels continue to rise. Trial-and-error attempts are made to restore balance.

↓

The trial-and-error attempts fail. The anxiety escalates to severe or panic levels. The person adopts automatic relief behaviors.

↓

When these measures do not reduce anxiety, anxiety can overwhelm the person and lead to serious personality disorganization, which signals the person is in crisis.

FIGURE 21.1   Phases of crisis.

Types of Crises

Research has focused on categorizing types of crisis events, understanding responses to a crisis, and developing intervention models that support people through a crisis.

Developmental Crisis

While Caplan was creating his crisis model, Erik Erikson was formulating ideas about crisis and development. He proposed that **maturational crises** are a normal part of growth and development and successfully resolving a crisis at one stage allows one to move to the next. According to this model, the child develops positive characteristics after experiencing a crisis. If they develop fewer desirable traits, the crisis is not resolved (see Chapter 7). The concept of **developmental crisis** continues to be used today to describe significant maturational events, such as leaving home for the first time, completing school, and accepting the responsibility of adulthood.

Situational Crisis

A **situational crisis** occurs whenever a specific stressful event threatens a person's physical and psychosocial integrity and results in some degree of psychological disequilibrium. The event can be an internal one, such as a disease process, or any number of external threats. A move to another city, a job promotion, or graduation from high school can initiate a crisis even though they are positive events. Graduation from high school marks the end of an established routine of going to school, participating in school activities, and doing homework assignments. When starting a new job after graduation, the former student must learn an entirely different routine and acquire new knowledge and skills. If a person enters a new situation without adequate coping skills, a crisis may occur.

Traumatic Crisis

A **traumatic crisis** is initiated by unexpected, unusual events that can affect an individual or a multitude of people. In such situations, people face overwhelmingly hazardous events that entail injury, trauma, destruction, or sacrifice. Examples of events include national disasters (e.g., racial persecutions, riots, war), violent crimes (e.g., rape, murder, kidnappings, and assault and battery), and environmental disasters (e.g., earthquakes, floods, forest fires, hurricanes).

Teamwork and Collaboration: Working Toward Recovery

The goal for people experiencing a crisis is to return to the precrisis level of functioning. The role of the nurse is to provide a framework of support systems that guide the patient through the crisis and facilitate the development and use of positive coping skills.

BOX 21.2

Decision Tree for Determining Referral

Situation: A 35-year-old woman is being seen in a clinic because of minor burns she received during a house fire. Her home was completely destroyed. She is tearful and withdrawn, and she complains of a great deal of pain from her minor burns. Biopsychosocial assessment is completed.

Assessment Result	Nursing Action
Patient has psychological distress but believes that her social support is adequate. She would like to talk to a nurse when she returns for her follow-up visit.	Provide counseling and support for the patient during her visit. Make an appointment for her return visit to the clinic for follow-up.
The patient is severely distressed. She has no social support. She does not know how she will survive.	Refer the patient to a mental health specialist. The patient will need crisis intervention strategies provided by a mental health specialist.

EMERGENCY CARE ALERT ! It is important to be acutely aware that a person in crisis may be at high risk for suicide or homicide. To determine the level of effectiveness of coping capabilities of the person, the nurse should complete a careful assessment for suicidal or homicidal risk. If a person is at high risk for either, the nurse should consider referral for admission to the hospital.

NCLEXNOTE During a crisis, the behaviors and verbalizations of a person may provide data that are indicative of a mental illness. Nursing care should be prioritized according to the severity of responses. After the crisis has been resolved, assess whether the abnormal thoughts or feelings disappear.

During an environmental crisis (e.g., flood, hurricane, forest fire) that affects the well-being of many people, nursing interventions will be a part of the community's efforts to respond to the event. This is covered in more detail in the section of the chapter on disasters. On the other hand, when a personal crisis occurs, the person in crisis may have only the nurse to respond to their needs. After the assessment, the nurse must decide whether to provide the care needed or to refer the person to a mental health specialist. Box 21.2 offers guidance in making this decision.

EVIDENCE-BASED NURSING CARE OF PERSON IN CRISIS

Mental Health Nursing Assessment

Because the response to a crisis is individual and differs from person to person, the nurse should make sure that a very complete assessment is done. The first priority is determining the extent of physical injury or trauma. The person should receive medical care for any injuries. Once medically stable, changes in health practices following the crisis provide clues to the severity of the disruption in functioning.

Physical Health

Maintaining health is important because a crisis can be physically exhausting. Disturbances in sleep and eating patterns and the reappearance of physical or psychiatric symptoms are common. Changes in body function may include tachycardia, tachypnea, profuse perspiration, nausea, vomiting, dilated pupils, and extreme shakiness. Some individuals may exhibit loss of control and have total disregard for their personal safety. If sleep patterns are disturbed or nutrition is inadequate, the individual may not have the physical resources to deal with the crisis.

Emotional and Behavioral Responses

The mental health nursing assessment focuses on the individual's emotions and coping strengths. In the beginning of the crisis, the person may report feelings of numbness and shock. Responses to psychological distress should be differentiated from symptoms of psychiatric illnesses that may be present. Later, as the reality of the crisis sinks in, the person will be able to recognize and describe the felt emotions. The nurse should expect these emotions to be intense and be sure to provide some support during their expression.

Initially, the individual's thoughts and behaviors may be erratic and illogic. The nurse should assess for evidence of depression, confusion, uncontrolled weeping or screaming, disorientation, or aggression. The person may be suffering from a loss of feelings of well-being and safety. In addition, panic responses, anxiety, and fear may be present. The ability to cope by problem-solving may be disrupted. By assessing the person's ability to solve problems, the nurse can evaluate whether they can cognitively cope with the crisis situation and determine the kind and amount of support needed.

Coping Skills

Coping skills should be identified in an assessment of anyone undergoing a crisis. The coping skills of some individuals are sufficient to weather a crisis, but many skills are inadequate for the situation. Unusual behaviors may emerge that are ineffective. There may be evidence of self-mutilation activities or suicide ideation.

Social Functioning and Support

It is critical to assess the person's perception of the problem and the availability of support systems (emotional and financial). The extent of disruption of normal daily activities and routines is assessed to determine the need for additional support. The person may not be shopping, paying bills, or cleaning the house. The nurse should identify the social network of family and friends who are available to provide help and support.

Clinical Judgment

Safety is a priority. Physical consequences of the crisis are the first priority. There may be tachycardia or hyperventilation. Reports of potential self-physical harm such suicide ideation or intention should be the focus of the next intervention. Body systems can change during a crisis. Diarrhea and urinary incontinence can occur. Food and shelter needs should be considered. The emotional and psychological consequences of the crisis such as fear, extreme distress will also be important to address.

THERAPEUTIC RELATIONSHIP

A nurse is often meeting the person in crisis for the first time and will need to skillfully apply therapeutic communication techniques to meet the individual's immediate mental health needs. Patience, listening, and empathy are important tools that along with a calm, nurturing approach can help establish trust. In some instances, the nurse has a relationship with the patient who reaches out during a crisis. In that instance, the nurse will have already established the therapeutic relationship and can quickly provide meaningful support and interventions. Be careful not to give unrealistic or false reassurances of positive outcomes over which you have no control. For example, it is not a good idea to reassure the person that everything with be alright because things may get worse, not better.

> **NCLEXNOTE** Individual responses to a crisis can be best understood by assessing the usual responses of the person to stressful events. The response to the crisis will also depend on the meaning of the event to the person. The use of therapeutic communication principles is a priority when caring for a person who has experienced a crisis or disaster.

MENTAL HEALTH NURSING INTERVENTIONS

Immediate goals during a crisis may be providing first aid, preventing the person from committing suicide or homicide, arranging for food and shelter (if needed), and mobilizing social support. After safety needs are met, the individual can work toward recovery by addressing other goals such as reestablishing self-care routines and using positive coping strategies. Strengths identified in the assessment supporting a healthy lifestyle prior to the crisis should be used to develop a plan of care.

TABLE 21.1	GUIDELINES FOR CRISIS INTERVENTION	
Approach	Rationale	Example
Support the expression (or nonexpression) of feelings according to cultural or ethnic practices.	Emotional support helps the person face reality. The emotional expression by the victim may be culturally driven.	Ask the person to actualize the loss using active and reflective listening. "Where you there when they died?" "Tell me how they died?" "What special remembrances do you have?" If the person is crying, sobbing, or angry; allow for the expression of their emotions. Sit quietly beside. When they are done you can say, "I can tell how terribly sad or angry you are." Try to avoid handing a tissue. Wait for them to look for a tissue before you hand them one.
Help the person think clearly and focus on one implication at a time.	Focusing on all the implications at once can be too overwhelming.	An individual left a partner because of abuse. At first, focus only on living arrangements and safety. "You can say, there are several things we need to focus on now for your safety." At another time, discuss the other implications of the separation.
Avoid giving false reassurances, such as "It will be all right;" "It is for the best."	Giving false reassurances blocks communication. It may not be all right.	Patient: "My doctor told me that I have a terminal illness." Nurse: Restatement: "Your doctor told you that you have a terminal illness. What does that mean to you?"
Clarify fantasies with facts.	Accurate information is needed to solve problems.	A young mother is holding her child who has died. The mother expresses disbelief this has happened. Quietly sit beside her. The longer she holds her child, the realization this has occurred will settle within her. You do not need to point out the obvious.
Link the person and family with community resources, as needed.	Social support can ease the effect of the crisis or loss.	Provide information about a meeting of a support group such as that of the American Cancer Society, Alzheimer Support Groups; Compassionate Friends; resolve through sharing or other local bereavement support groups.

Adapted from Lazarus, R. (1991). *Emotion and adaptation* (p. 122). Oxford University Press; Worden, W. (1991). *Grief counseling and grief therapy: A handbook for the mental health practitioner.* Springer.

The person may have exercised regularly and is ready to use exercise as a way of dealing with the stress. Or the person may have had a healthy diet before the crisis and is now ready to reengage in healthier eating choices. Guidelines for crisis intervention and examples are presented in Table 21.1. Individuals should be encouraged to report any depression, anxiety, or interpersonal difficulties during the recovery period.

Self-Care

A person needs to eat and sleep in order to have the energy to cope with a crisis. Personal hygiene may be suffering. The nurse should encourage the person to reestablish a healthy diet, practice sleep hygiene strategies, and attend to personal grooming. If the person is unable to function, a referral can be made to other health care clinicians. Medication may be needed to help maintain a high level of psychophysical functioning.

Medication Interventions

Medication cannot resolve a crisis, but the judicious use of these agents can help reduce its emotional intensity. For example, the use of an antianxiety medication such as lorazepam may help the person through the initial shock of the crisis (see Box 21.3).

Counseling

Counseling reinforces healthy coping behaviors and interaction patterns. Counseling, which focuses on identifying emotions and positive coping strategies, helps the person integrate the effects of the crisis into a real life experience. Responses to crisis differ with individuals. Some may present with behaviors that indicate transient disruptions in their ability to cope. Others may be totally devastated. At times, virtual counseling may provide the person with enough help that face-to-face counseling is not necessary. If counseling strategies do not work, other stress reduction and coping enhancement interventions can be used (see Chapter 19). The nurse should refer anyone who cannot cope with a crisis to a mental health specialist for an evaluation.

Social Support Strategies

A crisis often disrupts a person's social network, leading to changes in available social support. Development of a new social support network may help the person cope more effectively with the crisis. Supporting the development of new support contacts within the context of available social networks can be done by contacting available local and state agencies for assistance as well as specific private support groups and religious groups.

BOX 21.3

Lorazepam (Ativan)

DRUG CLASS: Benzodiazepine; antianxiety/sedative hypnotic agent

RECEPTOR AFFINITY: Acts mainly at the subcortical levels of the central nervous system (CNS), leaving the cortex relatively unaffected. Main sites of action may be the limbic system and reticular formation. It potentiates the effects of α-aminobutyric acid, an inhibitory neurotransmitter. The exact mechanism of action is unknown.

INDICATIONS: Management of anxiety disorders or for short-term relief of symptoms of anxiety or anxiety associated with depression (oral forms). Also used as preanesthetic medication in adults to produce sedation, relieve anxiety, and decrease recall of events related to surgery (parenteral form). Unlabeled parenteral uses for management of acute alcohol withdrawal.

ROUTE AND DOSAGE: Available in 0.5-, 1-, and 2-mg tablets; 2 mg/mL concentrated oral solution and 2 mg/mL and 4 mg/mL solutions for injection.

Adults: Usually 2–6 mg/day orally, with a range of 1–10 mg/day in divided doses, with the largest dose given at night. 0.05 mg/kg intramuscularly (IM) up to a maximum of 4 mg administered at least 2 h before surgery. Initially 2 mg total or 0.044 mg/kg intravenously (IV) (whichever is smaller). Doses as high as 0.05 mg/kg up to a total of 4 mg may be given 15–20 min before the procedure to those benefiting by a greater lack of recall.

Geriatric patients: Dosage not to exceed adult IV dose. Orally, 1–2 mg/day in divided doses initially, adjusted as needed and tolerated.

Children: Drug should not be used in children younger than 12 years.

HALF-LIFE (PEAK EFFECT): 10–20 h (1–6 h [oral]; 60–90 min IM; 10–15 min IV).

SELECTED ADVERSE REACTIONS: Transient mild drowsiness, sedation, depression, lethargy, apathy, fatigue, light-headedness, disorientation, anger, hostility, restlessness, confusion, crying, headache, mild paradoxical excitatory reactions during first 2 weeks of treatment, constipation, dry mouth, diarrhea, nausea, bradycardia, hypotension, cardiovascular collapse, urinary retention, and drug dependence with withdrawal symptoms.

WARNINGS: Contraindicated in psychoses; acute narrow angle glaucoma; shock; acute alcoholic intoxication with depression of vital signs; and during pregnancy, labor and delivery, and while breastfeeding. Use cautiously in patients with impaired liver or kidney function and those who are debilitated. When given with theophylline, there is a decreased effect of lorazepam. When using the drug IV, it must be diluted immediately before use and administered by direct injection slowly or infused at a maximum rate of 2 mg/min. When giving narcotic analgesics, reduce its dose by at least half in patients who have received lorazepam.

SPECIFIC PATIENT AND FAMILY EDUCATION

- Take the drug exactly as prescribed; do not stop taking the drug abruptly.
- Avoid alcohol and other CNS depressants.
- Avoid driving and other activities that require alertness.
- Notify the prescriber before taking any other prescription or over-the-counter drug.
- Change your position slowly and sit at the edge of the bed for a few minutes before arising.
- Report to the prescriber any severe dizziness, weakness, drowsiness that persists, rash or skin lesions, palpitations, edema of the extremities, visual changes, or difficulty urinating.

Telephone Hotlines

Public and private funding and the efforts of trained volunteers permit most communities to provide crisis services to the public. For example, telephone hotlines for problems ranging from child abuse to suicide are a part of health delivery systems of most communities. Crisis services permit immediate access to the mental health system for people who are experiencing an emergency (such as threatened suicide) or for those who need help with stress or a crisis.

Residential Crisis Services

Many communities provide, as part of the health care network, residential crisis services for people who need short-term housing. The specific residential crisis services available within a community reflect the problems that the community members judge as particularly important. For example, some communities provide shelter for teenage runaways; others offer shelter for abused spouses. Still others provide shelter for people who would otherwise require acute psychiatric hospitalization. These settings provide residents with a place to stay in a supportive, home like atmosphere. The people who use these services are linked to other community services such as financial aid.

Evaluation and Treatment Outcomes

Outcomes developed in cooperation with the person experiencing the crisis guide the evaluation. Once assessment data are clustered and prioritized and the outcomes are determined. Once interventions are developed and implemented in cooperation with the individual in crisis, the person should come through the crisis with improved health, well-being, and social function. If complications occur, the nurse should make appropriate alterations in the entire nursing process or make appropriate referrals.

LOSS, GRIEF, AND BEREAVEMENT

Loss, grief, and bereavement are universal human experiences. The terms bereavement and mourning are used interchangeably to describe the process of healing after a perceived loss. The outcomes of loss, grief and bereavement can range from an increase in psychosocial functioning to maladaptation which can include death, illness, isolation, and/or mental illness. Nurses are important caregivers who are called upon to provide support and guidance during these difficult times. This section focuses on the loss of a loved one.

> **KEYCONCEPT Loss** can evoke minor to complex thoughts, feelings, and behaviors depending on the perceived relationship of the person with the lost loved object or person.

In death, the intensity of the loss is based on perceived relationship to the deceased and the circumstances of the loss. Death can be sudden and unexpected or after a long-term, chronic illness. Stigmatic losses (death associated with a stigmatized event or action such as abortion, AIDS, homicide, and suicide) can also affect coping with and healing after a loss.

The first year after a loss is considered to be the most difficult as holidays, birthdays, anniversaries, and other important life events must be handled by the bereaved. Days surrounding the anniversary date of the death can be difficult for the bereaved.

> **KEYCONCEPT Grief** is a natural, intense, physical, emotional, social, cognitive, or social reaction to the death of a loved one. Spontaneous expressions to loss can include sobbing, crying, anger, and expressions of guilt.

Grief

There are commonalities in grief, but each grief experience is specific to the unique relationship that is lost. While grief is usually associated with death, it can occur without a death and be unrecognized. **Predeath grief** occurs prior to a death such as when a loved one has a terminal illness. The grief symptoms can be severe and are most likely to occur in caregivers of patients at the end of life, particularly dementia patients. Higher predeath grief levels are associated with depressive symptoms, caregiver burden, and less communication within the family about dying. **Acute grief** occurs immediately after the death of a loved one and normally evolves to a permanent state of integrated grief after a process of adaptation. *Integrated grief* is a long-term process where there continues to be mild yearning and other painful emotions, thoughts, and memories, but they are not intrusive. Even though there may be occasional periods of grief intensity, they do not interfere with ongoing life and a sense of well-being. Failure to adapt to the loss can lead to a prolonged grief disorder (PGD) (intense longing for or persistent preoccupation with the deceased that lasts more than 6 months) (Meichsner et al., 2020).

Theories of Bereavement

> **KEYCONCEPT Bereavement** is the process of healing and learning how to cope with the loss. It begins immediately after the loss, and can last months or years. Individual differences, age, religious and cultural practices, and social support influence grief and bereavement.

Stage Theories

There has been wide acceptance that bereavement follows stages (Bowlby & Parkes, 1970; Kubler-Ross, 1969). Although over time, the stage theory of grief and bereavement has been challenged and remains unsupported by empirical evidence, it continues to be used by health care professionals (Corr, 2018; Meichsner et al., 2020).

Dual Process Model

The **dual process model** (DPM) offers a nonlinear explanation of how grieving persons and families come to terms with their loss over time (Stroebe et al., 2010; Stroebe & Schut, 2015). This model can be used to understand how bereaved individuals cope (Fiore, 2019). According to DPM, the person adjusts to the loss by oscillating between **loss-oriented coping** (preoccupation with the deceased) and **restoration-oriented coping** (preoccupation with stressful events as a result of the death including financial issues, new identity as a widow[er]). **Oscillation** is the process of confronting (loss-oriented coping) and avoiding (restoration-oriented coping) the stresses associated with bereavement. At times, the bereaved person is confronted with the loss and memories, and at other times, the person will be distracted and the thoughts and memories will be avoided. The bereaved experiences relief from the intense emotion associated with the loss by focusing on other things. For example, the bereaved person may be recalling a special moment in the relationship such as a wedding or imagining what the person would say about a current event but then switches to thinking about completing tasks that the deceased had previously undertaken (e.g., paying bills, cooking meals). In the loss-oriented coping mode, emotions relate to the relationship with the deceased person; in the restoration-oriented coping, the bereaved person's emotions relate to the stressful events associated with the responsibilities and changes as a result of the loss. Over time, after repeated confrontation with the loss, there is no longer a need to think about certain aspects of the loss (Currie et al., 2019) (see Figure 21.2).

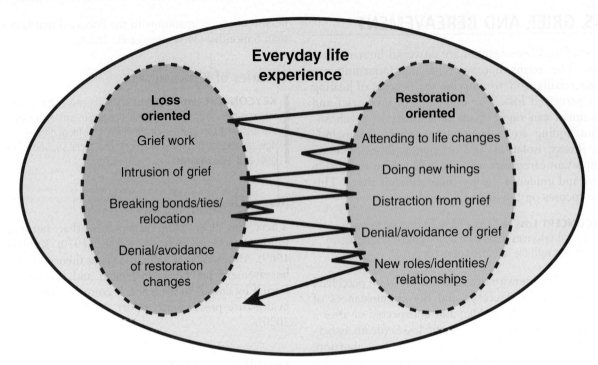

FIGURE 21.2 Dual process model of coping with bereavement. (Redrawn from Stroebe, M., & Schut, H. (1999). The dual process model of coping with bereavement: Rationale and description. *Death Studies, 23*, 213. Used with permission from Taylor & Francis Ltd, https://www.tandfonline.com)

Types of Bereavement

Uncomplicated Bereavement

Most bereaved people experience **uncomplicated bereavement** after the loss of a loved one. Uncomplicated bereavement grief is painful and disruptive, however, there is always movement. Questions surface such as "Why did the death happen?" "Why my loved one?" "Why me?" and, "Why did God allow this to happen?"

The bereavement process is often applied to other situations in which a loss occurs, not necessarily the death of a person. The "empty nest syndrome," divorce, birth of a handicapped child, and death of a pet are other examples of losses were there may be grief and bereavement.

Most bereaved persons do not need clinical interventions and are able to find new meaning and purpose in their lives. Their self-esteem and sense of competency while threatened remain intact. They gradually accept the sense of loss as a reality and are able to move on with their lives. There is little evidence they need or benefit from counseling or therapy. Those who experience suicidal thoughts with a plan and/or suicidal gestures should be evaluated for depression and posttraumatic stress disorder (PTSD) (Hamdan et al., 2020).

Traumatic Grief

Traumatic grief is a term that is used for a more difficult and prolonged grief. In traumatic grieving, external factors influence the reactions and potential long-term outcomes. For example, memories of the traumatic death of the deceased may lead to more traumatic memories including the violent death scene/ The external circumstances of death associated with traumatic grief include (1) suddenness and lack of anticipation; (2) violence, mutilation, and destruction; (3) degree of preventability or randomness of the death; (4) multiple deaths (bereavement overload); and (5) mourner's personal encounter with death involving a significant threat to personal survival or a massive and shocking confrontation with the death (or mutilation) of others (Zetumer et al., 2015).

The deaths of COVID-19 victims are expected to leave several million bereaved families and friends who are high risk for traumatic grief. Funeral ceremonies are suspended. Families are deprived of assisting the dying person because of the contagiousness of the disease. Families are unable to visit loved ones in the hospitals and intensive care units (ICU) which can lead to feelings of guilt. As a result of these factors, an increase in traumatic bereavement and PGD is expected. The multiple deaths of the COVID-19 family members could lead to bereavement overload (Kokou-Kpolou et al., 2020).

Complicated Bereavement

Complicated bereavement or PGD occurs in about 10% to 20% of bereaved persons (Skritskaya et al., 2020). The person is frozen or stuck in a state of chronic mourning which lasts for more than a month to 6 months after a loss. In other words, there is no movement in the thought processes in how the bereaved view and experience their loss. The person may feel bitter over the loss and wish their life could revert to the time they were together.

In complicated grief there is an intense longing and yearning for the person who died that lasts for more than 6 months. Additionally, the person may have trouble accepting the death, an inability to trust others since the death, excessive bitterness related to the death, and feeling that life is meaningless without the deceased person. Individuals who are more vulnerable for developing complicated bereavement are those who have experienced a sudden, unexpected loss, stigmatic loss, or death of a loved one after a long-term chronic illness as these situations have the potential to limit their social support.

Teamwork and Collaboration: Working Toward Recovery

The person with uncomplicated grief may not need mental health team intervention. When grief and bereavement become complicated with ongoing psychological and physical stress, mental health interventions can support an adaptive response to the loss. A priority of concern is always safety. Are there thoughts of suicide? Is depression evident? The individual may need support from a psychiatrist, nurse, psychologist, social worker, counselor or chaplain.

EVIDENCE-BASED NURSING CARE OF PERSON IN GRIEF

Mental Health Nursing Assessment

The initial assessment determines whether the individual is experiencing predeath grief, acute grief, or complicated bereavement. In predeath grief, the terminally ill loved one is alive, but the caregiver has intense sadness, anger, and loneliness over the changes in the relationship with the patient, loss of shared activities, and plans for the future. In acute grief, there are bouts of yearning, sadness and other painful emotions that are frequently intense. There may be intrusive thoughts and memories and heighted reaction to reminders of the loss. In complicated bereavement, the loss occurred at least 6 months prior, daily functioning is impaired with thoughts, yearning and memories of the deceased with evidence of difficulty accepting the loss. Emotional pain exists longer than socially acceptable (Meichsner et al., 2020).

Physical Health

The status of physical health will provide clues to the intensity of the grief. Sleep difficulty, lack of appetite, weight loss can indicate the severity of the grief. Substance use should be determined. One area to determine is how dependent the bereaved was on the deceased for physical care. Who prepared the meals, shopping, or house cleaning?

Cognitions

The thought process should be assessed for negative and maladaptive thoughts. If the person is protesting the death (death should not have happened; it is not fair; could have prevented death) and has a negative view of the world (bad things happen; no one is safe), they are at risk maladaptive thoughts that complicate bereavement. An example of other negative cognitions includes needing the person (i.e., life is unbearable without the person who died) (Skritskaya et al., 2020).

Emotional and Behavioral Responses

Assessing the persons emotional state includes determining current mood and behavior. Poor grooming, disheveled appearance, blank or tearful facial expressions could indicate depression. A suicide risk assessment should be conducted. By asking the question, "Have you wished that you were dead or wished that you could go to sleep and not wake up?", the nurse can determine if further suicide risk assessment should be completed and the patient referred to a therapist (see Chapters 22 and 25).

Social Functioning and Support

Determining the presence of social support is important as well as determining the level of social functioning. Withdrawal from normal social activities or failure to resume previous activities may indicate the onset of depression.

Clinical Judgment

Patient safety is always a priority. If the patient answers "yes" to suicide risk questions, the individual should be referred. If patient is safe, physical health such as eating and sleeping should be addressed. If there are changes in these areas, the nurse should consider depression or an environmental situation such as lack of ability to shop for food as a priority. For an older adult who has lost a spouse or partner, living arrangements could be considered. In many instances, grief may lead to depression because of social isolation and loneliness. Can the bereaved carry out activities of daily living and personal safety without the deceased? Helping the person manage physical health needs could be a priority.

Therapeutic Relationship

A positive therapeutic relationship is critical for the bereaved person who is grieving. The loss of attachment of a loved one leads to pain and emptiness that will take time to heal. A calm, empathic, quiet approach of acceptance of the person's level of pain will promote interaction. Providing an opportunity to share memories about the deceased is not only comforting, but helps to accept the loss. Listening is key. It is important to avoid giving reassurance that everything will be fine. It is appropriate to normalize the grief by reassuring the person that sadness and yearning are normal. Keeping an open, non-judgmental attitude will allow the person to express feelings in a safe environment (Meichsner et al., 2020).

Mental Health Nursing Interventions

The goal of bereavement interventions is to help the person adapt and re-stabilize biopsychosocial systems as the pain and sadness lessens with time. Adaptation involves accepting the reality of the loss and restoring a sense of well-being (Meichsner et al., 2020).

Self-Care

Self-care strategies can range from providing or arranging for physical care for the person to suggesting resources. Adequate nutrition and sleep are critical to support the person through bereavement. Strategies include recommending balanced meals and teaching sleep hygiene techniques.

Medications

Short-term reliance on antidepressants or sleep aids may be useful during acute grief. Careful monitoring of the use of medications is needed to prevent long-term use of these medication.

Counseling

Counseling is very beneficial to individuals experiencing a loss. The counseling goal is to foster adaptive coping and management of painful experiences. The focus of the counseling will be determined by the circumstances of the loss and the relationship of the bereaved to the deceased. If a person is experiencing predeath grief, the nurse identifies the changes associated with the disease and fosters acceptance of the loved one's disease and symptoms. The nurse continues to monitor the health and well-being of the caregiver who may be unaware of the extent of their grief or the toll on their own health. For someone experiencing acute grief, in addition to normalizing the painful, sad feelings, the counseling approaches can encourage engagement with a natural support system or grief support group, and focus on ways to live with the reminders of the loss. If prolonged grief is the primary characteristic with impaired functioning and preoccupation with thoughts of the deceased, the person should be referred to a mental health specialist for further evaluation (Meichsner et al., 2020).

Social Support Strategies

Bereavement can be a highly stressful time with increased physical and psychological demands. This is a time that the bereaved benefit from the support of family, friends, social cultural, and religious communities. Normal life is suspended and a new reality gradually evolves. Social support is especially needed after the busy time of planning a funeral or celebration of life is over and the social community gradually withdraws. Loneliness sets in and the full impact of the loss is realized. During this time, the person is high risk for suicide. Through social support, the individual can begin thinking about their future and focus on their own self-care and well-being.

The COVID-19 pandemic greatly complicates the grieving process for many because of the lack of face-to-face social support for the surviving family members. Not only were they unable to assist their loved one in dying, they do not have access to social support because of restrictions. A priority for family and friends is to find ways to maintain social contacts such as taking advantage of small gatherings or enjoyable activities.

Evaluation and Treatment Outcomes

A positive outcome of bereavement is adaptation to a life without the deceased, but learn to live with the reminders of the deceased. Other positive outcomes include attending to self-care and enjoying social and recreational activities again.

DISASTER AND TERRORISM

A disaster is a sudden ecologic or human-made phenomenon that is of sufficient magnitude to require external help to address the psychosocial needs as well as the physical needs of the victims. Acts of terrorism and pandemics present situations that mimic disasters and are categorized disasters.

> **KEYCONCEPT A disaster** is a sudden overwhelming catastrophic event that causes great damage and destruction that may involve mass casualties and human suffering requiring assistance from all available resources.

Although disasters can affect all members of a society, the most affected are the victims and survivors of the event, as well as nurses and others who are first to respond to the traumatic and life-threatening consequences of the event. The mental health of the survivors of disasters can be severely impacted by the event. Fear, anger, and distress elevate severe anxiety to the panic level, which can result in severe mental illnesses. Unresolved crisis or disastrous events can lead to disorganized thinking. Post-disaster depression is a real risk (North et al., 2018). In addition, the victims may experience the development of acute stress disorder (which has a strong emphasis on dissociative symptoms) and PTSD.

Historical Perspectives of Disasters in the United States

Throughout history, disasters have been portrayed from a fatalistic perspective that humans have little control over catastrophic events. Some cultures contend that natural disasters are acts of God. Other cultures express their belief that natural disaster events can be attributed to gods dwelling within places such as volcanoes, with eruptions being an expression of the gods' anger. Although often caused by nature, disasters can have human origins. Wars and civil disturbances that destroy homelands and displace people are included among the causes of disasters. Other causes include a building collapse, blizzard, drought, earthquake, epidemic, explosion, famine, fire, flood, hazardous material or transportation incident (such as a chemical spill), hurricane, nuclear incident, terrorist attack, and tornado. Often, the unpredictability of such disasters causes fear, confusion, and stress that can have lasting effects on the health of affected communities and their sense of well-being.

Natural Disasters

The busy Atlantic hurricane season of 2020, Hurricane Maria in Puerto Rico in 2018, Hurricane Harvey in Texas in 2017, and the earthquake and tsunami in Japan in 2011 highlight the importance of government preparedness for natural disasters as well as terrorism. In the United States, the lack of government response and breakdown in communication during Maria resulted in thousands of hurricane victims being displaced and injured. Many Puerto Ricans moved to Florida and experienced more emotional and psychological problems than those staying on the island (Scaramutti et al., 2019). The Japan disaster became a cascade of disasters, resulting in the death of thousands of residents and contamination from the damaged nuclear site. Consequences of these disasters will still be occurring months and years after the initial events.

Terrorism

In recent history, we have experienced several attacks of violence and terrorism that are unprecedented in North America. Some examples are the Pittsburgh synagogue in 2019, destruction of the World Trade Center in New York on September 11, 2001, the Sandy Hook school tragedy in 2012, and the Boston Marathon bombing in 2013, all of which shattered North Americans' sense of safety and security.

Since September 11, 2001, the emergency response planning of federal, state, and local agencies has focused on possible terrorist attacks with chemical, biologic, radiologic, nuclear, or high-yield explosive weapons. Before September 11, 2001, government agencies and public health leaders had not incorporated mental health into their overall response plans to bioterrorism. But in the aftermath of the mass destruction of human life and property in 2001, government and health care leaders are recognizing the need for monumental mental health efforts to be implemented during episodes of terrorism and disaster. The psychological and behavioral consequences of a terrorist attack are now included in most disaster plans.

COVID-19 Pandemic

In December 2019, the Wuhan Municipal Health Commission announced an outbreak of severe acute respiratory syndrome coronavirus 2 (SARS-CoV-2). The virus quickly spread globally and in 2020, World Health Organization (WHO) declared COVID-19 a pandemic and the United States declared a National Emergency. In the U.S., an unprepared health care system was quickly overloaded with critically ill patients who needed ICU beds that did not exist. There was a lack of prepared health care workers who were quickly overwhelmed. Mortality rates are high, especially among the older adults and those with comorbidities. Health care and public health care systems are trying to confront this disease around the globe.

While classified as a disaster, COVID-19 is different than a natural disaster that is time-limited. The physical and psychosocial consequences for the affected persons, survivors, health care workers, and community are unprecedented. The effects will be felt for many years and societies will be forever changed.

The mental health of survivors and health care workers is expected to be another "unseen epidemic" (Stawicki et al., 2020). For patients who survive the disease, they may have life-long mental health problems, isolation and stigma. The psychosocial stressors, particularly related to the use of isolation/quarantine, fear and vulnerability are affecting the total community (Torales et al., 2020).

Health care workers are particularly vulnerable to emotional distress because of their risk of exposure to the virus, concern about infecting and caring for their loved ones, shortages of personal protective equipment, longer work hours and involvement in ethical resource allocation (Pfefferbaum & North, 2020). Health care workers are reporting depression, anxiety, insomnia, and PTSD (Lai et al., 2020; Yin et al., 2020).

Phases of Disaster

Long-term mental health consequences are evident in most disasters Natural and human-made disaster can be conceptualized in three phases:

1. *Prewarning of the disaster.* This phase entails preparing the community for possible evacuation of the environment, mobilization of resources, and review of community disaster plans. In some disasters, such as in the 2011 earthquake in Japan, there is very little warning. In other instances, such as the COVID-19 pandemic, there were unheeded warnings more than a decade before the disease appeared.

2. *The disaster event occurs.* In this phase, the rescuers provide resources, assistance, and support as needed to preserve the biopsychosocial functioning and survival of the victims. In large disasters, the rescuers and health care professionals also experience the traumatic event as both residents and health care providers. The victims experience the initial trauma and threats that occur immediately after the disaster such as confusion (communication breakdown), lack of safety (no available law enforcement), and lack of health care services.

3. *Recuperative effort.* In the third phase, the focus is on implementing strategies for healing sick and injured people, preventing complications of health problems, repairing damages, and reconstructing the community. The disruption effects can be traumatic to the community residents. The debris, lack of trust of the government, fragmentation of families, financial problems, lack of adequate housing, inadequate temporary housing, and fear of another disaster contribute to the long-term negative effects of disasters.

Responses to Disaster

Psychiatric nurses encounter three different types of disaster victims. The first category is the victims who may or may not survive. If they survive, the victims often experience severe physical injuries. The more serious the physical injury, the more likely the victim will experience a mental health problem such as PTSD, depression, anxiety, or other mental health problems (Osofsky et al., 2018). Victims and families need ongoing health care to prevent complications related to both their physical and mental health (Sledge & Thomas, 2019).

The second category of victims includes the professional rescuers. These are persons who are less likely to experience physical injury but who often experience psychological stress. The professional rescuers, such as police officers, firefighters, nurses, and so on, have more effective coping skills than do volunteer rescuers who are not prepared for the emotional impact of a disaster. However, many professional responders report experiencing PTSD for many months after the traumatic event in which they were involved (Lewis-Schroeder et al., 2018).

The third category includes everyone else involved in the disaster. Psychological effects may be experienced worldwide by millions of people as they experience terrorism or disaster vicariously or as direct victims of the terrorism/disaster event. After an act of terrorism, most people will experience some psychological stress, including an altered sense of safety, hypervigilance, sadness, anger, fear, decreased concentration, and difficulty sleeping. Others may alter their behavior by traveling less, staying at home, avoiding public events, keeping children out of school, or increasing smoking and alcohol use. After Hurricane Maria, most of Punta Santiago was without electrical power, and more than half of the households sustained severe damage. In the aftermath, schools were closed, jobs were lost. Families were subject to diseases, dependency on aid, and exposure to heat and humidity. Two-thirds of residents surveyed reported an increase in the significant symptoms associated with depression, generalized anxiety, or posttraumatic stress (Ferré et al., 2018) (see Box 21.4).

BOX 21.4

Health Outcomes after Disaster for Older Americans

Bell, S. A., Horowitz, J., & Iwashyna, T. J. (2020). Health outcomes after disaster for older adults with chronic disease: A systematic review. The Gerontologist, 60(7), e535–e547. https://doi.org/10.1093/geront/gnz123

THE QUESTION: Are there associations among disease outcome after weather- and climate-related disasters among older adults?

METHODS: A systematic review of studies on clinical outcomes of four chronic diseases (COPD), end-stage renal disease (ESRD) congestive heart failure (CHJF) and diabetes after disaster exposure.

FINDINGS: Three disasters were the focus of the findings – earthquakes, hurricanes, and wildfires. The outcomes include access to health care and post disaster health care utilization. The review showed that disasters have limited or insignificant effects older adults relative to younger population.

IMPLICATIONS FOR NURSING: Emergency planning and health services for the older adult with multiple chronic conditions remain important to the health of the older adult.

Teamwork and Collaboration: Working Toward Recovery

The role of the behavioral health care worker in disasters, specifically a nuclear detonation in a U.S. city is the support of lifesaving activities and the prevention of additional casualties from fallout. Victims experiencing head injuries or psychic trauma after a disaster may have to be hospitalized. During a disaster, a victim with a mental illness may experience regression to their pretreatment condition. If community mental health facilities are available, they should be directed to seek assistance from mental health care professionals. The victims should receive follow-up care for the disaster response.

EVIDENCE-BASED NURSING CARE OF PERSONS EXPERIENCING DISASTERS

Mental Health Nursing Assessment

The nurse should assess the kind and severity of a natural or human-made disaster or terrorist act to determine the capability of individuals and communities to respond in a supportive way. Assessment includes the ages of the victims, gender, their capability to participate in problem-solving activities related to the devastation left by the disaster, and their level of self-confidence or self-esteem. The nurse should maintain a calm demeanor, obtain and distribute information about the disaster and the victims, and reunite victims and their families. In addition, there is a need to monitor the news media's impact on the mental health of the victims of the crisis. Sometimes the persistence of the news media diminishes the ability of the survivors to achieve closure to the crisis. Constant rehashing of the disaster in the newspapers, television, and online can initiate feelings of anxiety and depression, or increase and prolong the severity of these feelings (van der Velden et al., 2018).

Women exhibit higher levels of distress than men after a disaster, especially pregnant women and older women Children are especially vulnerable to disasters and respond according to their ages and family experiences. Traumatized children and adolescents are high-risk victims of a wide range of behavioral, psychological, and neurologic problems after experiencing various traumatic events (Blake & Fry-Bowers, 2018).

Physical Health

The nurse should assess physical reactions that may involve many changes in body functions, such as tachycardia, tachypnea, profuse perspiration, nausea, vomiting, dilated pupils, and extreme shakiness. Virtually any organ may be involved. Some victims may exhibit panic reactions and loss of control and have a total disregard for their personal safety. The victims may be suicidal or homicidal and are at high risk for injuries that may include infection, trauma, and head injuries. During the rescue, medical care is a priority. Any medical or psychiatric disorders should be assessed and information communicated to the rest of the health care team. Unexplained physical symptoms such as headache, fatigue, pain, chest pain, and gastrointestinal disturbances should be included in the assessment.

Mental Status

During a disaster, fear and hopelessness can immobilize victims. The victims may suffer from loss of feelings of well-being and various psychological problems, including panic responses, anxiety, and fear. Dissociation and fear are predictive of later developing PTSD and depressive symptoms. Victims witnessing others suffer are especially at high risk for future mental health problems and should be assessed for the details of the disaster (Su et al., 2020).

Emotional and Behavioral Responses

The survivors of the disaster may experience traumatic bereavement because of their feelings of guilt that they survived the disaster (Drožđek et al., 2020). Responses to psychological distress need to be differentiated from any psychiatric illness that the person may be experiencing. A response to a disaster may leave the person feeling overwhelmed, incapacitated, and disoriented.

The victims should be assessed for behaviors that indicate a depressed state, presence of confusion, uncontrolled weeping or screaming, disorientation, or aggressive behavior. Ideally, the nurse should assess the coping strategies the victim uses to normally manage stressful situations.

Social Support and Functioning

Cultural values and beliefs help define the significance and meaning of a disaster. In some instances, a disaster can slow development, but usually the customs, beliefs, and value systems remain the same. It is important that first responders and health care teams are sensitive to the cultural and religious beliefs of the community. In many instances, victims' spiritual beliefs and religious faith help them cope with the disaster.

In a disaster, the victims may experience economic distress because of job loss and loss of other resources. This may ultimately lead to psychological distress. In addition, acts of aggression and other mental health problems may emerge (Daks et al., 2020). Again, shelter, money, and food may not be available. The absence of basic human needs such as food, a place to live, or immediate transportation quickly becomes a priority that may precipitate acts of violence.

Clinical Judgment

Because the responses to disaster are so varied, assessment data are critical. What is the disaster -tsunami, terrorism, or pandemic? Priorities for acutely effected persons are maintaining life systems and treating physical. Depending on the long-term impact of the disaster and the type of disaster, nurse will identify coping skills, support systems, and referral sources.

Therapeutic Relationship

Therapeutic communication is key to understanding the extent of the psychological responses to a disaster and to establishing a bridge of trust that communicates respect, commitment, and acceptance. Developing rapport with the victim communicates reassurance and support.

Mental Health Nursing Interventions

The goals of care include helping the victims prioritize and match available resources with their needs, preventing further complications, monitoring the environment, disseminating information, and implementing disease control strategies. People with pre-existing mental health conditions should continue with their treatment plans during an emergency and monitor for any new symptoms (Centers for Disease Control and Prevention [CDC], 2019). The focus of nursing interventions is on the individual, family, and community.

Self-Care

Any physiologic problems or injuries should be treated quickly. During the emergency response, individuals will be triaged to the appropriate level of care. Victims who are primarily distressed and may have somatic symptoms will be treated after those suffering from exposure with critical injuries. The primary public health concern is clean drinking water, food, shelter, and medical care. In natural disasters, contaminated water and food and lack of shelter and medical care may worsen illnesses that already exist. In pandemics, the primary public health concern is stopping the spread of the disease which means isolation of infected person and quarantine of contacts. For communities, a pandemic means mass home-confinement directives – new to Americans.

All patients, families and communities need to be reassured of the caring and commitment of the nurse to their safety, comfort, and well-being throughout the triage process. Ideally, a mental health specialist is an integral member of the triage team. Many of the same interventions used for persons experiencing stress or crisis will be used for these victims. See also Chapter 33 for discussion of somatization. Victims should be encouraged to do necessary chores and participate in decision-making.

Medications

During the treatment process for the psychological consequences of the disaster, it may become necessary to administer an antianxiety medication or sedative, especially in the early phases of recovery.

Counseling

After the initial interventions, the nurse should support the development of resilience, coping, and recovery while providing technical assistance, training, and consultation. A useful model is the **ABCs of psychological first aid** that focuses on A (arousal), B (behavior), and C (cognition). When arousal is present, the intervention goal is to decrease excitement by providing safety, comfort, and consolation. When abnormal or irrational behavior is present, survivors should be assisted to function more effectively in the disaster, and when cognitive disorientation occurs, reality testing and clear information should be provided. In the initial phases, the nurse should assist the victim in focusing on the reality of problems that are immediate, with specific goals that are consistent with available resources as well as the culture and lifestyle of the victim.

Debriefing (the reconstruction of the traumatic events by the victim) may be helpful for some. Long a common practice, debriefing was believed to be necessary in order for the person to develop a healthy perspective of the event and ultimately prevent PTSD. However, debriefing is not useful for everyone. Additionally, cultural groups respond differently to traumatic events. Therefore, compulsory debriefing is not recommended. If the victim has symptoms of PTSD, referral to a mental health clinic for additional evaluation and treatment is important (see Chapter 29).

The nurse should prepare the victim for recovery by teaching about the effects of stress and helping the victim identify personal strengths and coping skills. Positive coping skills should be supported. The victims should be encouraged to report any depression, anxiety, or interpersonal difficulty during the recovery period. After most disasters, support groups are established that help victims and their families deal with the psychological effects of the disaster.

Psychoeducation

When the nurse explains anticipated reactions and behaviors, this helps the victims gain control and improve coping. For example, after a major disaster, they may have excessive worry, preoccupation with the event, and changes in eating and sleeping patterns. With time, counseling, and group work, these symptoms will lessen. Active coping strategies can be presented in multiple media forums, such as television and radio. After the initial shock, victims react by trying to do something to resolve the situation. When victims begin working to remedy the disaster situation, their physical responses become less exaggerated, and they are more able to work with less tension and fear.

Educating the public about the natural recovery process is important. Information gaps and rumors add to the anxiety and stress of the situation. Giving information and direction helps the public and victims to use the coping skills they already possess. Initially, the event may leave individuals and families in a stage of ambiguity with frantic, disorganized behavior. In addition, individuals and family members are concerned about their own physical and psychological responses to the disastrous event.

Community Care

Outreach is especially important because research shows that disaster victims do not access mental health systems. Peer-delivered mental health services are especially effective in identifying and connecting with victims, especially those with predisaster psychiatric problems (Cheng et al., 2020).

Family support systems may need to be reestablished. The health care community should actively reach out to the media and keep the press engaged. Direct attention to stories that inform and help the public respond should be encouraged. Some federal agencies assist victims of disasters. This assistance is available for individual, families, and communities. One of these agencies is the Federal Emergency Management Agency (FEMA). When a disaster occurs, FEMA sends a team of specialists who review the devastation of disaster. They provide counseling and mental health services and arrange for many of the victims to access other services needed for survival, including training programs. In addition, the Substance Abuse and Mental Health Services Administration (SAMHSA) of the Department of Health and Human Services is available to assist both victims of and responders to the disaster. When a disaster disrupts the victim's social network, other resources must be made available for social support.

The social support system provides an environment in which the victims experience respect and caring from the caregivers, the opportunity to ventilate and examine personal feelings regarding the tragedy, and the opportunity to begin the healing and recovery process. Supporting the development of more contacts within the social network can be done by organizing support groups within the area of the disaster that address grief and loss, trauma, psychoeducational needs, and substance abuse. In addition, the nurse may refer the victims to nearby support groups or religious groups that are appropriate to meet their needs.

Evaluation and Treatment Outcomes

To determine the effectiveness of nursing interventions, the nurse should evaluate the outcomes based on the success of resolution of the disaster. The outcomes will depend on the specific disaster and its meaning (appraisal) to the survivors. For example, are the survivors in a safe place? Are the victims able to cope with the disaster? Were the appropriate supports given, so the victims could draw upon their own strengths?

SUMMARY OF KEY POINTS

- A crisis is a time-limited event that occurs when coping mechanisms fail to provide adaptive skills to address a perceived challenge or threat.

- Grief is a natural, intense physical, emotional, social, and cognitive responses to loss, and bereavement is the process of healing after a loss. The variations in grief are influenced by the characteristics of the individual, perceived relationship to the deceased, and the type of loss.

- Stage theories propose that grief and bereavement follow stages/phases. Process models explain bereavement as nonlinear.

- For most persons, bereavement is uncomplicated and there is no need for counseling. Complicated grief occurs in about 10% to 20% of bereaved persons. Interventions such as medication, counseling, and/or a support group may be required for this group.

- Interventions are designed to support people through crises by helping them understand the process of recovery and identify the resources they need and how to get them.

- Disaster is a sudden, overwhelming catastrophic event that causes great damage and may cause mass casualties and human suffering that require assistance from all available resources.

- COVID-19 pandemic is a global disaster that is unprecedented in contemporary times. Psychological consequences effect the individual, family and community.

- Depending on the disaster, interventions are provided to individuals, families, and communities.

CRITICAL THINKING CHALLENGES

1. Compare nursing interventions used for crises, bereavement, and disasters. What are the similarities? What are the differences?

2. After the death of his mother, a 24-year-old single man with bipolar disorder moves into an apartment. He continues to take his medication but feels sad about his mother's death. He is not adjusting well to living alone and tells his nurse that he no longer wants to go to work and feels he would be better off if he joined his mother. The nurse generates the following supporting positive coping related to inadequate support system. Develop a plan of care for this young man.

3. Listen to people who have experienced a loss to determine where they are in the bereavement process. Discuss the role of medication and counseling when used in crisis or bereavement.

4. Compare uncomplicated bereavement to complicated bereavement. How would you recognize the difference? When would it be appropriate to refer a bereaved person to a support group or mental health specialist?

5. There is a terrorist threat in your community. A patient appears in the emergency department convinced he is going to die. How would you proceed with assessing this patient?

6. A patient is recently diagnosed with COVID-19. She refused the vaccine because she does not believe in vaccines. She is showing fear of her treatment and guilt about not taking the vaccine because she is afraid that she has transmitted the disease to her family. What is the first priority in providing her care once she is medically stable?

Unfolding Patient Stories: George Palo

Part 1 (Loss of Wife and Dog)

 George Palo, 90 years old, was diagnosed 6 months ago with minor neurocognitive disorder, Alzheimer's type. He lives independently in an apartment within a retirement community. His wife of 65 years died 3 years ago. He was managing well until the recent loss of his 13-year-old dog. What responses and behaviors associated with bereavement should the nurse consider when assessing him? How can his cognitive disorder complicate the process of grieving? How can the nurse guide his progression through grief and bereavement?

 Movie Viewing Guides
Grace Is Gone (2007): Stanley Phillips (John Cusack) is a manager of a home-supply store and parent of two girls, 12-year-old Heidi (Shelan O'Keefe) and 8-year-old Dawn (Gracie Bednarczyk). His wife is a soldier in Iraq, but the viewers know her by her message left on the family answering machine. When an army captain and chaplain deliver the news that Grace had died bravely in combat, Stanley becomes numb. He impulsively takes his girls to wherever they desire—a theme park in Florida. Most of the movie follows the three on the trip and the father's attempt to delay and deny his wife's death.

VIEWING POINTS: Describe Stanley's reaction when he receives the news of his wife's death. What clues are present that Heidi gradually understands that something terrible has happened?

REFERENCES

American Psychiatric Association. (2013). *Diagnostic and statistical manual of mental disorders (5th ed.)*. Arlington, VA: Author.

Blake, N., & Fry-Bowers, E. K. (2018). Disaster preparedness: Meeting the needs of children. *Journal of Pediatric Health Care, 32*(2), 207–210. https://doi.org/10.1016/j.pedhc.2017.12.003

Bowlby, J., & Parkes, C. M. (1970). Separation and loss within the family. In E. J. Anthony (Ed.), *The child in his family*. New York: Wiley.

Caplan, G. (1961). *An approach to community mental health*. New York: Grune & Stratton.

Centers for Disease Control and Prevention. (2019). Coping with a disaster or traumatic event. https://emergency.cdc.gov/coping/index.asp

Cheng, P., Xia, G., Pang, P., Wu, B., Jiang, W., Li, Y. T., Wang, M., Ling, Q., Chang, X., Wang, J., Dai, X., Lin, X., & Bi, X. (2020). COVID-19 epidemic peer support and crisis intervention via social media. *Community Mental Health Journal, 56*(5), 786–792. https://doi.org/10.1007/s10597-020-00624-5

Corr, C. (2018). Elisabeth Kübler-Ross and the "Five Stages" Model in a sampling of recent American textbooks. *Omega, 82*, 294–322. doi:10.1177/0030222818809766

Currie, E. R., Christian, B. J., Hinds, P. S., Perna, S. J., Robinson, C., Day, S., Bakitas, M., & Meneses, K. (2019). Life after loss: Parent bereavement and coping experiences after infant death in the neonatal intensive care unit. *Death Studies, 43*(5), 333–342. https://doi.org/10.1080/07481187.2018.1474285

Daks, J. S., Peltz, J. S., & Rogge, R. D. (2020). Psychological flexibility and inflexibility as sources of resiliency and risk during a pandemic: Modeling the cascade of COVID-19 stress on family systems with a contextual behavioral science lens. *Journal of Contextual Behavioral Science, 18*, 16–27. https://doi.org/10.1016/j.jcbs.2020.08.003

Drožđek, B., Rodenburg, J., & Moyene-Jansen, A. (2020). "Hidden" and diverse long-term impacts of exposure to war and violence. *Frontiers in Psychiatry, 10*, 975. https://doi.org/10.3389/fpsyt.2019.00975

Ferré, I. M., Negrón, S., Shultz, J. M., Schwartz, S. J., Kossin, J. P., & Pantin, H. (2018). Hurricane Maria's impact on Punta Santiago, Puerto Rico: Community needs and mental health assessment six months postimpact. *Disaster Medicine and Public Health Preparedness, 13*(1), 18–23. https://doi.org/10.1017/dmp.2018.103

Fiore, J. (2019). A systematic review of the dual process model of coping with bereavement (1999–2016). *Omega*. Advance online publication. https://doi.org/10.1177/0030222819893139

Hamdan, S., Berkman, N., Lavi, N., Levy, S., & Brent, D. (2020). The effect of sudden death bereavement on the risk for suicide: The role of suicide bereavement. *Crisis: The Journal of Crisis Intervention and Suicide Prevention, 41*(3), 214–224. https://doi-org.libproxy.siue.edu/10.1027/0227-5910/a000635

Kokou-Kpolou, C. K., Fernández-Alcántara, M., & Cénat, J. M. (2020). Prolonged grief related to COVID-19 deaths: Do we have to fear a steep rise in traumatic and disenfranchised griefs? *Psychological Trauma: Theory, Research, Practice, and Policy*, 12(S1), S94–S95. https://doi-org.libproxy.siue.edu/10.1037/tra0000798

Kubler-Ross, E. (1969). *On death and dying*. Macmillan Publishing Company.

Lewis-Schroeder, N. F., Kieran, K., Murphy, B. L., Wolff, J. D., Robinson, M. A., & Kaufman, M. L. (2018). Conceptualization, assessment, and treatment of traumatic stress in first responders: A review of critical issues. *Harvard Review of Psychiatry*, 26(4), 216–227. https://doi.org/10.1097/HRP.0000000000000176

Lai, J., Ma, S., Wang, Y., Cai, Z., Hu, J., Wei, N., Wu, J., Du, H., Chen, T., Li, R., Tan, H., Kang, L., Yao, L., Huang, M., Wang, H., Wang, G., Liu, Z., & Hu, S. (2020). Factors associated with mental health outcomes among health care workers exposed to coronavirus disease 2019. *JAMA Network Open*, 3(3), e203976. https://doi.org/10.1001/jamanetworkopen.2020.3976

Meichsner, F., O'Connor, M., Skritskaya, N., & Shear, M. K. (2020). Grief before and after bereavement in the elderly: An approach to care. *The American Journal of Geriatric Psychiatry : Official Journal of the American Association for Geriatric Psychiatry*, 28(5), 560–569. https://doi.org/10.1016/j.jagp.2019.12.010

North, C. S., Baron, D., & Chen, A. F. (2018). Prevalence and predictors of postdisaster major depression. Convergence of evidence from 11 disaster studies using consistent methods. *Journal of Psychiatric Research*, 102, 96–101. doi:10.1016/j.jpsychires.2017.12.013

Osofsky, H. J., Weems, C. F., Graham, R. A., Osofsky, J. D., Hansel, T. C., & King, L. S. (2018). Perceptions of resilience and physical health symptom improvement following post disaster integrated health services. *Disaster Medicine and Public Health Preparedness*, 13(2), 223–229. https://doi.org/10.1017/dmp.2018.35

Pfefferbaum, B., & North, C. S. (2020). Mental health and the Covid-19 pandemic. *The New England Journal of Medicine*, 383(6), 510–512. https://doi.org/10.1056/NEJMp2008017

Scaramutti, C., Salas-Wright, C. P., Vos, S. R., & Schwartz, S. J. (2019). The mental health impact of Hurricane Maria on Puerto Ricans in Puerto Rico and Florida. *Disaster Medicine and Public Health Preparedness*, 13(1), 24–27. https://doi.org/10.1017/dmp.2018.151

Sledge, D., & Thomas, H. F. (2019). From disaster response to community recovery: Nongovernmental entities, government, and public health. *American Journal of Public Health*, e1–e8. doi:10.2015/AJPHJ.2018.304895

Skritskaya, N. A., Mauro, C., Garcia de la Garza, A., Meichsner, F., Lebowitz, B., Reynolds, C. F., Simon, N. M., Zisook, S., & Shear, M. K. (2020). Changes in typical beliefs in response to complicated grief treatment. *Depression and Anxiety*, 37(1), 81–89. https://doi.org/10.1002/da.22981

Stawicki, S. P., Jeanmonod, R., Miller, A. C., Paladino, L., Gaieski, D. F., Yaffee, A. Q., De Wulf, A., Grover, J., Papadimos, T. J., Bloem, C., Galwankar, S. C., Chauhan, V., Firstenberg, M. S., Di Somma, S., Jeanmonod, D., Garg, S. M., Tucci, V., Anderson, H. L., Fatimah, L., Worlton, T. J., ... Garg, M. (2020). The 2019–2020 novel coronavirus (Severe Acute Respiratory Syndrome Coronavirus 2) pandemic: A joint American College of Academic International Medicine–World Academic Council of Emergency Medicine Multidisciplinary COVID-19 working group consensus paper. *Journal of Global Infectious Diseases*, 12(2), 47–93. https://doi.org/10.4103/jgid.jgid_86_20

Stroebe, M., & Schut, H. (2015). Family matters in bereavement: Toward an integrative intra-interpersonal coping model. *Perspective on Psychological Science*, 10(6), 873–879.

Stroebe, M., Schut, H., & Boerner, K. (2010). Continuing bonds in adaptation to bereavement: Toward theoretical integration. *Clinical Psychology Review*, 30, 259–268.

Su, S., Frounfelker, R. L., Desrosiers, A., Brennan, R. T., Farrar, J., & Betancourt, T. S. (2020). Classifying childhood war trauma exposure: latent profile analyses of Sierra Leone's former child soldiers. *Journal of Child Psychology and Psychiatry, and Allied Disciplines*. https://doi.org/10.1111/jcpp.13312

Torales, J., O'Higgins, M., Castaldelli-Maia, J. M., & Ventriglio, A. (2020). The outbreak of COVID-19 coronavirus and its impact on global mental health. *The International Journal of Social Psychiatry*, 66(4), 317–320. https://doi.org/10.1177/0020764020915212

van der Velden, P. G., van der Meulen, E., Lenferink, L., & Yzermans, J. C. (2018). Media experiences and associations with mental health among the bereaved of the MH17-disaster: A latent profile analysis. *Scandinavian Journal of Psychology*, 59(3), 281–288. https://doi.org/10.1111/sjop.12426

Yin, Q., Sun, Z., Liu, T., Ni, X., Deng, X., Jia, Y., Shang, Z., Zhou, Y., & Liu, W. (2020). Posttraumatic stress symptoms of health care workers during the corona virus disease 2019. *Clinical Psychology & Psychotherapy*, 27(3), 384–395. https://doi.org/10.1002/cpp.2477

Zetumer, S., Young, I., Shear, M. K., Skritskaya, N., Lebowitz, B., Simon, N., Reynolds, C., Mauro, C., & Zisook, S. (2015). The impact of losing a child on the clinical presentation of complicated grief. *Journal of Affective Disorders*, 170, 15–21.

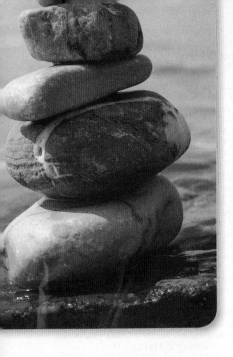

22
Suicide Prevention
Screening, Assessment, and Intervention

Rebecca Luebbert

KEYCONCEPTS

- hopelessness
- lethality
- suicide

LEARNING OBJECTIVES

After studying this chapter, you will be able to:

1. Identify suicide as a major mental health problem in the United States.

2. Define *suicide, suicidality, suicide attempt, parasuicide,* and *suicidal ideation.*

3. Describe population groups that have high rates of suicide.

4. Describe risk factors associated with suicide completion.

5. Identify key factors associated with specific suicide acts.

6. Describe evidence-based interventions used to reduce imminent and ongoing suicide risk.

7. Explain the importance of documentation and reporting when caring for patients who may be at risk of suicide.

KEY TERMS

- Acquired capability for suicide • Case finding • Commitment to treatment statement • Ideation-to-action theories
- Parasuicide • Perceived burdensomeness • Suicidal ideation • Suicidality • Suicide attempt • Suicide contagion
- Thwarted belongingness • Volitional factors

INTRODUCTION

Suicide is one of the major health problems in the United States, accounting for more than 48,000 deaths in 2018 (American Foundation for Suicide Prevention [AFSP], 2020a). Suicide rates have steadily increased in the past 20 years, with a 35% increase in the total suicide rate from 1999 to 2018 (Hedegaard et al., 2020). The public health problem of suicidal behavior is so important that several goals stated in *Healthy People 2020* and retained in *Healthy People 2030* directly target the reduction of deaths by suicide (U.S. Department of Health and Human Services [U.S. DHHS], 2020).

Suicide is so rejected in contemporary society that people with strong suicidal thoughts do not seek treatment for fear of being stigmatized by others. Reports and portrayals of suicide in the popular media and television further stigmatize those who consider or attempt suicide. Society's unwillingness to talk openly about suicide also contributes to the common misperceptions resulting in many myths regarding suicide (Corrigan et al., 2017; Oexle et al., 2020). Box 22.1 presents several myths and facts about suicide.

Suicides are preventable deaths when immediate friends and family and health care providers identify symptoms and use effective interventions. All practicing nurses will come into contact with patients who are thinking about suicide and often can prevent suicides by identifying and intervening with those at risk. Through individual and public education, nurses also can do much to demystify suicide and reduce stigma for those at risk. To reduce the devastating public impact of suicide on those at risk and their families, nurses must be knowledgeable about suicide and be able to implement effective preventive interventions. This chapter contains tools that can be used to reduce the broad effects of suicide and provide appropriate care for patients who are suicidal.

SUICIDE AND SUICIDE ATTEMPT

KEYCONCEPT Suicide is the voluntary act of killing oneself. It is a fatal, self-inflicted destructive act with explicit or inferred intent to die. It is sometimes called suicide completion.

This behavioral definition of suicide is limited and does not consider the complexity of potential underlying mental illness, personal motivations, and situational and family factors that provoke the suicide act. Except for the very young, suicide occurs in all age groups, social classes, and cultures (National Institute of Mental Health [NIMH], 2020).

The term **suicidality** refers to all suicide-related behaviors and thoughts of attempting or completing suicide and suicidal ideation. **Suicidal ideation** is thinking about and planning one's own death. In 2019, 4.8% of adults aged 18 and older had serious thoughts of suicide, with the highest prevalence among young adults aged 18 to 25 (11.8%) (NIMH, 2020). Population studies show that suicidal ideation varies depending on characteristics of the participants and the way suicidal ideation is measured. Although suicidal ideation often does not progress, having recurrent suicidal ideation is associated with poor mental health (Liu et al., 2020).

A **suicide attempt** is a nonfatal, self-inflicted destructive act with explicit or implicit intent to die. In 2018, an estimated 1.4 million Americans attempted suicide, with adult females reporting an attempt 1.4 times more often than males (AFSP, 2020). Suicidal ideation, previous psychiatric hospitalization, and a previous attempt are significant predictors of a completed suicide (Bostwick et al., 2016).

Parasuicide is a voluntary, apparent attempt at suicide, commonly called a suicidal gesture, in which the aim is not death (e.g., taking a sublethal drug). Parasuicidal behavior varies by intent. Some people truly wish to die, but others simply wish to feel nothing for a while. Still others want to send a message about their emotional state. Parasuicide behavior is never normal and should always be taken seriously.

KEYCONCEPT Lethality refers to the probability that a person will successfully complete suicide. Lethality is determined by the seriousness of the person's intent and the likelihood that the planned method of death will succeed. A plan to use an accessible firearm to commit suicide has greater lethality than a suicide plan that involves superficial cuts of the wrist.

Suicide is ranked as the tenth leading cause of death and accounts for 14.2 deaths per 100,000 population. On average, 132 Americans die by suicide each day, with a suicide occurring every 11 minutes in the United States: a rate of 132 completed successful suicides per day. Mountain regions have the highest rate of suicide (Fig. 22.1). Its overall prevalence may be underestimated because suicide can be disguised as vehicular accidents or homicide, especially in young people (AFSP, 2020; Centers for Disease Control and Prevention [CDC], 2020a).

Suicide Across the Life Span
Children, Adolescents, and Young Adults

Suicide is the second leading cause of death among those aged 10 to 34. Mental disorders can lead to poor performance in school, alcohol or other drug abuse, family discord, violence, and suicide. The most recent Youth

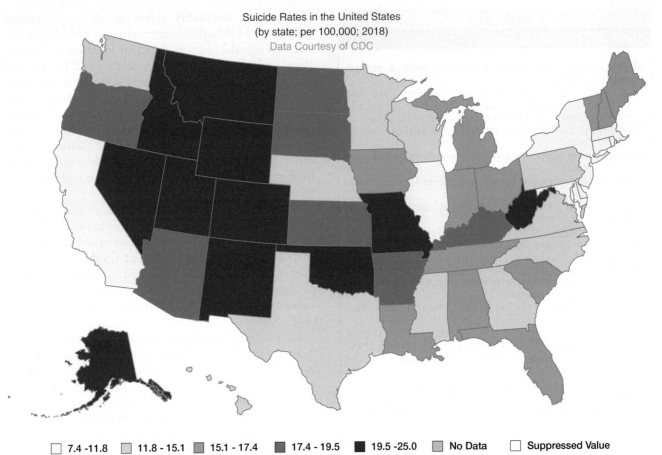

Suicide Rates in the United States
(by state; per 100,000; 2018)
Data Courtesy of CDC

| ☐ 7.4 -11.8 | ☐ 11.8 - 15.1 | ◼ 15.1 - 17.4 | ◼ 17.4 - 19.5 | ◼ 19.5 -25.0 | ◼ No Data | ☐ Suppressed Value |

FIGURE 22.1   Number of deaths attributable to suicide in the United States per 100,000 population, 2018. Data courtesy of CDC. (Retrieved December 2020, from https://www.nimh.nih.gov/health/statistics/suicide.shtml#part_154973)

Risk and Behavior Survey found that in the preceding year among high school students, 18.8% seriously considered attempting suicide, 15.7% made a suicidal plan, 8.9% attempted suicide, and 2.5% were seriously injured in a suicide attempt. Female students were more likely to attempt suicide (11.0%) than male students (6.6%), though males were more likely to die by suicide than females (Ivey-Stephenson et al., 2020).

Adults and Older Adults

Suicide is a major contributor to premature death in adults, ranking the fourth leading cause of death among adults aged 35 to 54. Suicide rates peak during middle age, and a second peak occurs in those aged 75 years and older (Hedegaard et al., 2020; NIMH, 2020). Physical illness, pain, loss, loneliness, social isolation, and disconnectedness are important precipitants to suicide in older adults (Jones & Pastor, 2020; Schmutte & Wilkinson, 2020).

Suicide disproportionally affects those who have served in the military, with suicide rates for Veterans 1.5 times the rate for non-Veterans (U.S. Department of Veterans Affairs, 2019). An estimated 18 veterans die by suicide per day. Depression, Post Traumatic Stress Disorder (PTSD), and combat exposure are some of the leading contributing factors to suicide for both men and women military members (Nichter et al., 2020; Ursano et al., 2020). Other related factors include alcohol or substance dependence, intimate partner problems, legal/administrative stressors, and financial strain (Bryan & Bryan, 2019; Pruitt et al., 2019). For women, military sexual trauma also contributes to suicide ideational and attempts (Griffith, 2019).

Epidemiology and Risk Factors

Suicidal behavior is complex, and there can be many contributing factors. Mental illness is an important factor contributing to suicide in adults. Mood disorders, particularly recurrent depression, are associated with higher risk of suicide. Substance use disorder and personality disorders are also found to influence suicide risk in young adults (Gili et al., 2019). Auditory hallucinations increase the risk for suicide because of the possibility of individuals impulsively responding to "voices" directing them to hurt themselves. Substance abuse increases the likelihood that suicidal ideation will result in both parasuicidal and suicidal behaviors. Box 22.2 identifies risk factors for suicide (CDC, 2020a, 2020b).

BOX 22.2

Suicide Risk Factors

Family history of suicide
Family history of child maltreatment
Previous suicide attempt(s)
History of mental disorders, particularly clinical depression
History of alcohol and substance abuse
Feelings of hopelessness
Impulsive or aggressive tendencies
Cultural and religious beliefs (e.g., belief that suicide is noble resolution of personal dilemma)
Local epidemics of suicide
Isolation, a feeling of being cut off from other people
Barriers to accessing mental health treatment
Loss (relational, social, work, or financial)
Physical illness
Easy access to lethal methods
Unwillingness to seek help because of the stigma attached to mental health and substance abuse disorders or to suicidal thoughts

Centers for Disease Control and Prevention, National Center for Injury Prevention and Control. (2020). Suicide risk and protective factors [Online]. https://www.cdc.gov/violenceprevention/suicide/riskprotectivefactors.html

---

Medical illness contributes to functional disability and also increases the likelihood of chronic depression, which, in turn, contributes to the increased suicide rate of those over the age of 65 (Nelson, 2019). Additionally, symptoms of comorbid illnesses often are similar to depressive disorder, making recognition of depressive disorder by primary care providers difficult. Patients are often reticent to disclose their suicidal thoughts, further complicating detection.

Psychological Risk Factors

Psychological pain, internal distress, low self-esteem, and interpersonal distress have long been associated with suicide (Ducasse et al., 2018). Childhood physical and sexual abuse is linked to suicide, suicide ideation, and parasuicide. Cognitive risk factors include problem-solving deficits, impulsivity, rumination, and hopelessness. Impulsivity, anger, and reduced inhibition increase the risk of suicide. Recent purchase of a handgun increases the risk of self-harm (CDC, 2020b; Crifasi et al., 2015; Wendell et al., 2016).

Social Risk Factors

Social isolation is a primary risk factor for suicide. Social distress leads to despair and can be caused by family discord, parental neglect, abuse, parental suicide, and divorce. Social distress can prevent the patient from accessing the support necessary to prevent suicidal acts. Other social factors associated with suicide risk include economic deprivation, unemployment, poverty, knowing someone who has died by suicide (especially if this person was a family member), and lack of access to behavioral health care (CDC, 2020b; Endo et al., 2017; Suicide Prevention Resource Center [SPRC], 2020a).

Gender

Males have a suicide completion rate nearly four times that of females. White males account for 70% of completed suicides, with middle-aged (ages 45 to 65 years) White men having the highest rate (AFSP, 2020). Men are more likely to use means that have a higher rate of success, with 56% of their suicide deaths by firearms (see Fig. 22.2). Men living in rural areas have a much higher risk of suicide than those in urban areas, and that gap is widening, perhaps attributable to the higher rates of gun ownership in rural areas (Logan et al., 2015). Substance abuse, aggression, hopelessness, emotion-focused coping, social isolation, and feeling little purpose in life have been associated with suicidal behavior in men.

Women across age, racial, and ethnic groups are less likely to die from suicide than are men but are more likely to attempt suicide. Women make three attempts to every attempt by men. Adolescent girls and women aged 10 to 44 years have the highest rate of suicide attempts. Women are less likely to complete a suicide, partly because they are more likely to choose less lethal methods. Women with current or previous exposure to domestic violence are at an increased risk for suicidal behavior (Kavak et al., 2018).

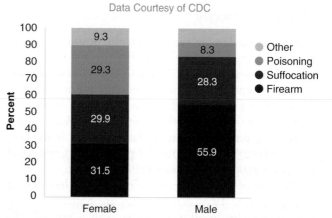

FIGURE 22.2 Suicide deaths by method in the United States (2018). Data courtesy of CDC. (Retrieved December 2020, from https://www.nimh.nih.gov/health/statistics/suicide.shtml#part_154971)

Sexuality

The lesbian, gay, bisexual, transgender, queer, questioning, and intersexed (LGBTQI) community is at increased risk for suicide (National Alliance on Mental Illness [NAMI], 2020). An estimated 1.8 million LGBTQI young people seriously consider suicide each year, with LGBTQI youth nearly five times as likely to attempt suicide compared with heterosexual youth (The Trevor Project, 2020). In lesbian, gay, and bisexual older adults, there are high levels of inadequate general health disability (Fredriksen-Goldsen et al., 2017).

Adolescents in sexual underrepresented groups are often stigmatized and discriminated against. They have more suicidal ideation, more suicide attempts, and are more at risk for completed suicides than their heterosexual peers (Yildiz, 2018). Individuals are more at risk for suicide when they experience conflict with family or friends because of their sexual identity, threat of violence, abuse, bullying, isolation, and other high risk behaviors (American Association of Suicidology, 2019). A nationwide study of youth health behaviors and experiences reported a significantly higher percentage of lesbian, gay, or bisexual students (48%) seriously contemplated suicide, as compared with 13% of heterosexual students, and 23% of lesbian, gay, or bisexual students attempted suicide, as compared to 5% of heterosexual students (Kann et al., 2018).

There are alarming rates of suicide ideation and suicide rates among transgender individuals. In a national study, 40% of transgender adults reported a suicide attempt, with 92% of these individuals making their attempt before the age of 25 (James et al., 2016). Gender-based victimization, discrimination, bullying, violence, rejection by family, friends, and communities are risk factors associated with suicidal behavior (Testa et al., 2017; Virupaksha et al., 2016).

Race and Ethnicity

There is considerable variation in the profile of suicide rates across racial groups, including the age when rates are at their peak and the duration of high rates across several age groups. Rates of suicide among American Indian/Alaska Native people and White people are highest, at 22.1 and 18.0 per 100,000 respectively. Lower suicide rates are found among Asian/Pacific Island individuals (7.0 per 100,000), Hispanics (7.4 per 100,000), and Black (7.2 per 100,000) populations (SPRC, 2020b).

The rate of suicides among White people has steadily increased since 1999. Suicide rates are higher in males than in females in all age groups, with a rate of 22.8 (males) and 6.2 (females) per 100,000. Completed suicides are highest for White individuals between the ages of 35 and 64. Suicide rates among those older than 75 years are also high. The use of firearms is by far the most prominent method of suicide among White people (Hedegaard et al., 2020). Access to firearms contributes to the risk of completed suicides. Firearm ownership is more prevalent in the United States than in any other country, with an estimated 120 firearms per 100 people (Karp, 2018).

Suicide rates among American Indian and Alaska Native (AI/AN) populations are the highest of any racial/ethnic group in the United States. Rates peak during adolescence and young adulthood, then decline (SPRC, 2020a). AI/AN populations engaged in suicidal behavior are more likely to have been exposed to suicide by a family member or friend and more likely to report substance use. For these reasons, community level prevention strategies focusing on survivor support and substance use treatment are critical (Leavitt et al., 2018).

Family cohesion and social support in African American families contribute to the lower rates of suicide in this group. In 2018, the suicide rate among African American females was the lowest among men and women of all ethnicities. Although the overall suicide rate for African American individuals is low, young African American men take their lives at a rate considerably above that of other age groups. Higher rates of suicide in younger men may be associated with disparities in mental health treatment and social factors disproportionally affecting Black adolescents (Lindsey et al., 2019).

Even though the suicide rate for Hispanics is less than half of the overall US rate, in 2017 suicide was the second leading cause of death for Hispanics, aged 15 to 34. Among Hispanic populations, suicide rates remain somewhat consistent across the lifespan, and the death rate for Hispanic men is four times the rate of Hispanic women. Suicide attempts for Hispanic adolescents were 40% greater than non-Hispanic White adolescents (SPRC, 2020a; U.S. DHHS Office of Minority Health [OMH], 2020b).

While the suicide rate for Asian individuals or Pacific Island populations is approximately half of the overall suicide rate in the United States, the scant literature on suicide among Asian populations shows that suicide ideation, plans, and attempts may be more common than popularly believed and vary within Asian ethnic groups. In 2017, suicide was the leading cause of death for Asian American individuals aged 15 to 24. The suicide death rate for men is double that of women. Unlike that of the overall US population, in Asian or Pacific Islander populations, suicide rates peak later in life, in those over the age of 85 (SPRC, 2020a; U.S. DHHS OMH, 2020a). A study of racial/ethnic differences in youth having died by suicide found that Asian American/Pacific Islander youth had significantly lower rates of mental health treatment compared to White youth, consistent with research demonstrating disparities in mental health service utilization (Lee & Wong, 2020).

Pandemic Impact

While the full extent of the impact of coronavirus disease 2019 (COVID-19) on mental health will not be fully realized for quite some time, evidence of mental health challenges related to COVID-19-associated morbidity, mortality, and mitigation activities (including physical distancing and mandated stay-at-home orders) were noted within months of the outbreak in the United States. A national survey of adults in June 2020 found that 41% of respondents reported at least one adverse mental or behavioral health condition related to COVID-19. Symptoms reported included anxiety or depression (31%), trauma/stress (26%), and having started or increased substance use (13%). Nearly 11% of respondents reported having seriously considered suicide in the previous month. In particular, younger adults, members of underrepresented racial/ethnic groups (Hispanic and Black persons), essential workers, and unpaid caregivers for adults were more likely to report disproportionately worse mental health outcomes, increased substance use, and increased suicidal ideation (Czeisler et al., 2020). Distress, anxiety, depression, fear of contagion, uncertainty, chronic stress, isolation, and economic hardship all contribute to a person being more vulnerable to negative impact (Sher, 2020).

Etiology

The convergence of biologic, psychological, and social factors can be directly linked to suicidal behavior. In genetically and physiologically vulnerable individuals, thoughts, feelings, and personality factors can interfere with personal problem-solving, promote impulsivity, and support suicidal behavior. Poverty, unemployment, and social conflict also contribute to suicidal behavior in those at risk for suicide. Figure 22.3 illustrates suicidal thoughts and behaviors among US adults.

Biologic Theories

Depression and severe childhood trauma are linked to suicide. Those who complete suicide often have extremely low levels of the neurotransmitter serotonin. Impairments in the serotonergic system contribute to suicidal behavior. Additionally, dysregulation in the hypothalamic-pituitary-adrenal axis, abnormalities of neurotrophins and neurotrophin receptors, and abnormalities

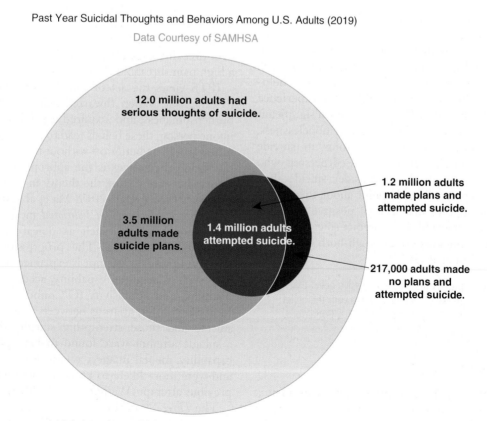

Past Year Suicidal Thoughts and Behaviors Among U.S. Adults (2019)

Data Courtesy of SAMHSA

12.0 million adults had serious thoughts of suicide.

3.5 million adults made suicide plans.

1.4 million adults attempted suicide.

1.2 million adults made plans and attempted suicide.

217,000 adults made no plans and attempted suicide.

FIGURE 22.3 Past year suicidal thoughts and behaviors among U.S. adults (2019). Data courtesy of SAMHSA. (Retrieved December 2020, from https://www.nimh.nih.gov/health/statistics/suicide.shtml#part_154973)

of neuroimmune functions may be associated with suicide risk (Orsolini et al., 2020).

Genetic Factors

Suicide runs in families. First-degree relatives of individuals who have completed suicide have a two to eight times higher risk for suicide than do individuals in the general population. Suicide of a first-degree relative is highly predictive of a serious attempt in another first-degree relative. Children of depressed and suicidal parents have higher rates of suicidal behavior themselves. The genetic link to suicide is evident in twin studies. Suicidal behavior has a 50% concordance for completed suicide (Tidemalm et al., 2011).

There also appears to be a gene/environment connection between early childhood sexual abuse and suicidality. Early childhood adverse experiences appear to lead to genetic changes that modify the expression of the neurologic system, impacting the biologic and psychological development. As a result, there is a propensity to react to stressors, increasing the likelihood of suicidal behavior (Brodsky, 2016).

Psychological Theories

Cognitive Theories

Most evidences on the psychological contributions to suicidal behavior point to cognitive, affective, behavioral, and personality factors that intensify the experience of hopelessness and disconnection from others. Aaron Beck first identified the cognitive triad of hopelessness, helplessness, and worthlessness as integral to the experience of depression (Beck et al., 1979). Since then, a significant evidence base has been established linking hopelessness, loneliness, and other cognitive symptoms to suicide ideation (Klonsky et al., 2017). Depressed persons who are hopeless are more likely to consider suicide than those who are depressed but hopeful about the future. Furthermore, it appears that lack of positive thoughts about the future is more likely to predict suicidal behavior than negative thoughts even though both contribute to hopelessness (Liu et al., 2017).

> **KEYCONCEPT Hopelessness** is the pervasive belief that undesirable events are likely to occur, coupled with the belief that one's situation is unlikely to improve (Ellis & Rutherford, 2008).

Emotional and Personality Factors

Emotional factors and personality traits also play a role in suicidal behavior by enhancing perceptions of helplessness and hopelessness, contributing to poor self-esteem, and interfering with coping efforts. Shame, guilt,

despair, and emotion-focused coping have been linked to suicidal behavior. Loss and grief are also important considerations. Emotional distress often is potentiated by personality traits that contribute to poor self-esteem, impulsivity, and suicidal behavior (Rutter et al., 2020).

Ideation to Action Theories

Suicide ideation does not necessarily lead to suicide attempts. Most people who think of suicide do not act on the idea, but the suicide thoughts of those who do take lethal actions are often indistinguishable from those who do not (see Figure 22.3). Ideation-to-action theories examine factors that identify those who are most likely to attempt suicide. These emerging theories, which are supported by research, provide a basis for discriminating between those who are only thinking about suicide versus those who are likely to engage in suicidal acts.

The *Interpersonal Psychological Theory of Suicidal Behavior (IPTS)*, introduced by Thomas Joiner in 2005, proposes that three interacting factors indicate a high risk of suicide—"thwarted belongingness", perceived burdensomeness, and acquired capability. The term *thwarted belongingness* is used to describe alienation from social relationships or experiences; the human need to belong is not being met. It refers to an individual's feelings of loneliness and isolation, as well as a lack of reciprocal, caring, and meaningful relationships. Perceived burdensomeness is the perception that the individual is a burden to others. Acquired capability for suicide, which develops over time, involves a heightened sense of fearlessness and a high pain threshold (Joiner, 2005).

IPTS views the act of suicide as being very difficult to carry out. When thwarted belongingness, perceived burdensomeness, and acquired capability come together in one person, these beliefs lead to the misperception that others would be better off without them and the idea that sacrificing themselves is the appropriate action to take. Researchers are testing the theory in a variety of clinical situations (Kang et al., 2019; Ma et al., 2016, 2019).

Integrated Motivational Volitional model proposes that motivational factors, such as defeat and entrapment, cause suicide ideation. The progression from suicide ideation to suicide attempt is explained by volitional factors, such as acquired capability, access to lethal means, planning, and impulsivity (O'Connor & Kirtley, 2018). In a study differentiating between those thinking about suicide and those attempting suicide, those reporting a suicide attempt were found to have greater acquired capability, mental imagery about death, and impulsivity, and were more likely to know a friend who had made a previous attempt (Wetherall et al., 2018).

The *Three-Step Theory (3ST)* explains progression from ideation to action in three steps. First, emotional pain and hopelessness cause the suicide ideation. Second, thoughts of suicide become strong as the emotional pain exceeds connectedness. The third step involves the actual attempt when the person has the knowledge and capacity to carry out the suicide (Klonsky et al., 2017). In this model, suicide prevention focuses on reducing pain, increasing hope, improving connections, and reducing capacity to carry out the suicide.

Social Theories

Before the turn of the 20th century, Emile Durkheim (1951[1897]) linked suicide to the social conditions in which people live. Both a lack of social connectedness and social conditions contribute to suicidal behavior. People who are socially connected are less likely to engage in suicidal behavior. When an individual has others they can depend on, suicide can be prevented, even among those at significant risk. Even among people with social bonds, however, lack of community and social resources can interact with physiologic and psychological risk to increase the likelihood of suicide.

Social Distress

A lack of social connection contributes to suicide ideation, attempts, and deaths across the age span. Among adults, those who are single, never married, separated, widowed, living alone, and those reporting loneliness, alienation, and a lack of belongingness, are also more likely to engage in suicidal behavior (Calati et al., 2019). Being socially connected, however, does not in itself reduce risk. Interpersonal conflict, sexual underrepresented groups, and being a victim of bullying can contribute to suicidal behavior, especially in adolescents and young adults (John et al., 2018).

Suicide Contagion

Social exposure to suicide is associated with an increased personal risk for suicidal behavior, particularly among adolescents. Suicidal behavior that occurs after the suicide death of a known other is called suicide contagion or cluster suicide. Suicide contagion seems to work through modeling and is more likely to occur when the individual contemplating suicide is of the same age, gender, and background as the person who died. Contagion can be prompted by the suicide of a friend, an acquaintance, online social networking, or an idolized celebrity. Actions of peer groups, media reports of suicide, and even billboards with content about suicide can trigger suicide behavior among adolescents. In the case of a celebrity suicide, the number of "copycat suicides" is proportional to the amount, duration, and prominence of media coverage (Colman, 2018). Evidence suggests that adolescents can also be influenced by simple individual and community suicide prevention efforts (Zimmerman et al., 2016).

Economic Disadvantage

Poverty and economic disadvantage are associated with depression, suicide ideation, and suicide mortality. Individuals who are not employed, not married, and with low education and low income have a higher risk of suicide. Suicide risk is greater for adults in socially and materially deprived areas (Kerr et al., 2017). Adolescents from impoverished neighborhoods have more suicidal ideation and attempts, and suicides increase as the percentage of boarded-up buildings in a neighborhood increases, particularly if the individuals have a mental disorder (Page et al., 2014).

In impoverished communities, particularly rural America, lack of good schools and employment opportunities leads to unemployment and loss of meaningful social roles. Access to health care is limited in these communities, and there is an increased exposure to others exhibiting suicidal behavior that enhances suicide risk (Carpenter-Song & Snell-Rood, 2017).

Family Response to Suicide

Suicide has devastating effects on everyone it touches, especially family and close friends. One suicide is estimated to leave at least six survivors who are significantly impacted by the loss (Andriessen et al., 2016). In the aftermath of a family member's suicide, survivors experience more grief, anxiety and depression, guilt, shame, self-blame, and dysfunction than families whose loss was because of other reasons and the personal and familial disruption often lasts for years. Although recovery from a loved one's suicide is an ongoing task, survivors who are emotionally healthy before the suicide act and who have social support are able to manage the psychological trauma associated with suicide. Still, the intensity and duration of the postsuicide grief process for many survivors has led to the development of family intervention programs. Although the evidence base for these interventions is still small, strategies that support a positive sense of self, enhance problem-solving, promote the formation of a suicide story, encourage social reintegration, reduce stigma, use journaling, or permit the survivor to debrief may be effective in reducing subjective distress and to resolve grief (Andriessen et al., 2016). These strategies may be most effectively delivered in survivor peer help groups.

Protective Factors

Protective factors buffer individuals from suicidal thoughts and behavior. Although identifying and understanding protective factors is very important, they have not been studied as extensively as risk factors. The Centers for Disease Control and Prevention identifies the following protective factors (CDC, 2020b).

- Effective clinical care for mental, physical, and substance abuse disorders
- Easy access to a variety of clinical interventions and support for help seeking
- Family and community support (connectedness)
- Support from ongoing medical and mental health care relationships
- Skills in problem-solving, conflict resolution, and nonviolent ways of handling disputes
- Cultural and religious beliefs that discourage suicide and support instincts for self-preservation

TREATMENT AND NURSING CARE FOR SUICIDE PREVENTION

Interdisciplinary Treatment and Recovery

The challenges of preventing suicides and promoting healthy coping belong to all disciplines. An interdisciplinary treatment or recovery approach along with peer support is needed for managing the threats of suicide.

Clinical Judgment

 Concept Mastery Alert

A true psychiatric emergency exists when an individual presents with one or more symptoms associated with imminent risk for suicidal behavior. Immediate and focused action is needed to prevent the patient's death.

The first priority is to provide for the patient's safety while initiating the *least* restrictive care possible. In contrast, an example of the *most* restrictive care is an outpatient who is admitted to a locked unit with one staff member who is assigned to observe the person at all times. Hospitalization should be reserved for those whose safety cannot be ensured in an outpatient environment.

Priority Care Issues: Preventing Suicide and Promoting Mental Health

Suicidal ideation, planning, and acts are not easily predicted and, therefore, are difficult to study. As a result, few evidence-based treatments exist that are known to prevent suicide and manage suicidal behavior. There is growing consensus that the suicidal act is part of a continuum of behaviors that extend long before and after a specific suicide behavioral incident. The beginning evidence points to four steps in preventing suicide and promoting long-term mental health: identification of

those thinking about suicide (case finding), assessment to determine an imminent suicidal threat, intervening to change suicidal behavior associated with a specific suicidal threat, and institution of effective interventions to prevent future episodes of suicidal behavior.

Assessment

Case Finding

Case finding refers to identifying people who are at risk for suicide so proper treatment can be initiated. People who are contemplating suicide often do not share their ideation. This lack of disclosure often means that family, friends, and health professionals are unable to intervene until the suicidal ideation and planning have progressed. Yet early identification of suicidal ideation may reduce suicide deaths. Nurses can play important roles in suicide prevention by recognizing the warning signs. See Box 22.3 for the warning signs developed by the American Association of Suicidology (2020); the mnemonic IS PATH WARM can serve as a useful memory aide for these signs. The Columbia Suicide Severity Rating Scale (C-SSRS) is a commonly used evidence-supported suicide risk assessment that measures severity of suicidal ideation, intensity of ideation, suicidal behavior, and lethality (See Chapter 11 for more information about the C-SSRS).

Case finding requires careful and concerned questioning and listening that make the patient feel valued and cared about (Box 22.4). Most standardized health questionnaires

---

BOX 22.3

Warning Signs for Suicide

- **I**—Ideation: Talking or writing about death, dying, or suicide
  - Threatening or talking of wanting to hurt or kill self
  - Looking for ways to kill self: seeking access to firearms, available pills, or other means
- **S**—Substance abuse: Increased substance (alcohol or drug) use
- **P**—Purposelessness: No perceived reason for living; no sense of purpose in life
- **A**—Anxiety: Anxiety, agitation, unable to sleep, or sleeping all the time
- **T**—Trapped: Feeling trapped (like there is no way out)
- **H**—Hopelessness
- **W**—Withdrawal: Withdrawal from friends, family, and society
- **A**—Anger: Rage, uncontrolled anger, seeking revenge
- **R**—Recklessness: Acting reckless or engaging in risky activities, seemingly without thinking
- **M**—Mood change: Dramatic mood changes

Adapted from American Association of Suicidology. (2020). Know the warning signs. https://suicidology.org/resources/warning-signs/

BOX 22.4 • THERAPEUTIC DIALOGUE

SUICIDE

When Caroline sought medical care for a cold from her nurse practitioner, the nurse observed more than a cough and runny nose. Caroline appeared downcast and unusually sad. As the nurse and patient talked, the subject of family life came up, whereupon Caroline began to cry softly. As words tumbled out, she said she had been unhappy at home for a long time. When she was very young, she recalled being happy, but things changed when her brother was born, 4 years after her. Her father began to abuse her sexually, starting when Caroline was 5 years old and continuing until he moved out of the house when she was 12 years old. Caroline suspects her mother knew of the abuse, although she did nothing about it.

Two years ago, Caroline's father committed suicide. Caroline feels relieved about his death but frustrated that she never got a chance to tell him how angry she was with him. Caroline's relationship with her mother has not improved. Caroline says her mother favors her brother and is always telling her she won't amount to anything. Caroline begins to cry harder.

INEFFECTIVE APPROACH

Nurse: Clearly, many things are troubling you. Don't you think that things seem worse now because you have a cold?

Caroline: Well, that could be. What are you going to do to make me feel better?

Nurse: Give you some medicine to help you sleep and clear your nose. I think you should see a psychiatrist, too.

Caroline: I don't need a psychiatrist. I came here for my cold.

Nurse: I know you did, but you seem to be depressed.

Caroline: What are you, some kind of social worker? I am just tired.

Nurse: I am a nurse, and you seem down to me. Are you thinking about suicide?

Caroline: I don't think you know what you're talking about. I want to go now. Could you give me my medicine?

EFFECTIVE APPROACH

Nurse: It seems as though many things have been piling up on you. Does it seem that way to you, too?

Caroline: It sure does. I've just been trying to get through 1 day at a time, but now with this cold and no sleep, I feel like I can't go on.

Nurse: When you say you can't go on, what does that mean to you?

Caroline: Lately, I have been thinking about running away to some place where I can't be found and maybe starting over. But then I think, where would I go? Where would I stay? Who would take care of me?

Nurse: When you think that your plan for escape won't work, what happens?

Caroline: (Starting to cry again.) Then I think that maybe it would be better if I just did what my father did. I really don't think anyone would miss me.

Nurse: So you think you might take your life, like your Dad did?

Caroline: Yeah, and what really scares me is lately I have been thinking about that a lot. I keep saying to myself, "You're just tired," but I am so exhausted now that I can't chase the thoughts away.

Nurse: So, do you think about suicide every day?

Caroline: It seems like I never stop thinking about it.

Nurse: Is there anything you can do to make the thoughts go away?

Caroline: Nothing. (Silence.)

Nurse: What would you do?

CRITICAL THINKING CHALLENGE

In the first interaction, the nurse made two key blunders.

• What were they?
• What effect did they have on the patient?
• How did they interfere with the patient's care?

have questions about suicide thoughts. Many nurses are concerned that asking patients about their suicidal thoughts will provoke a suicide attempt. This belief simply is not true. The patient expressing suicidal ideation often has had these thoughts for some time and may feel more socially connected when another recognizes the seriousness of the situation. Under no circumstances should a patient be promised secrecy about suicidal thoughts, plans, or acts. Instead, tell patients that disclosure of suicidal intent will be shared with other interdisciplinary team members so the safety of the patient can be ensured.

Assessing Risk

After suicidal ideation has been established, the next step is to determine the risk for a suicide attempt. Suicide risk assessment is difficult and whenever possible should proceed only with the assistance of other members of the interdisciplinary treatment team. Assessing for risk includes determining the seriousness of the suicidal ideation, degree of hopelessness, disorders, previous attempt, suicide planning and implementation, and availability and lethality of suicide method. Risk assessment also includes the patient's resources, including coping skills and social supports, that can be used to counter suicidal impulses. Box 22.5 lists some questions that might be asked in assessing the risk for suicide.

The greatest predictor of a future suicide attempt is a previous attempt, partly because the individual already has broken the "taboo" around suicidal behavior. Repeated episodes of self-harm with or without suicidal

intent also increase immediate risk because they increase an individual's capacity to complete suicide. Other important signs of high risk are the presence of suicide planning behaviors (detailed plan, availability of means, opportunity, and capability) and engaging in final acts, such as giving away prized possessions and saying goodbye to loved ones. Although the presence of a specific psychiatric disorder, such as depression, is an important consideration in risk assessment, anxiety, agitation, alcohol use, and impulsivity may be better indicators of immediate risk. However, support from important others, religious prohibitions, responsibility for young children, and employment may provide protection from suicidal impulses.

Ideally, an interdisciplinary team conducts suicide risk assessment in an emergency department or outpatient facility with multiple supports. Nurses practicing in more isolated situations should keep a list of contacts in settings that routinely conduct suicide risk assessments so the contacts may be consulted if a seriously suicidal individual appears in the nurse's setting.

> **NCLEXNOTE** Suicide assessment is always considered a priority. Practice by asking patients about suicidal thoughts and plans. Develop a plan with a suicidal patient that focuses on resisting the suicidal impulse. Apply the assessment process that delineates the (1) intent to die, (2) severity of ideation, (3) availability of means, and (4) degree of planning.

Interventions for Imminent, Intermediate, and Long-Term Suicide Prevention

Interventions for Those at Imminent Risk

There are three urgent priorities for care of a person who is at imminent risk for suicide: reconnecting the patient to other people and instilling hope, restoring emotional stability, and reducing suicidal behavior, and ensuring safety. Reconnecting the patient interpersonally includes listening intently, and without judgment, to the patient's thoughts and feelings and validating their experience and suffering. This intervention directly challenges the patient's belief that no one cares. Using cognitive interventions can help the client regain hope and establish goals for the future (see Chapter 13).

Ensuring Patient Safety

Helping patients develop strategies for making safer choices when distressed is an important goal. Nurses caring for patients who are emerging from the initial hours and days of a suicide attempt can support the patient and focus on managing suicidal urges and developing protective strategies. As the nurse connects with the patient, together they can create a list of personal and professional

---

BOX 22.5

Assessment of Suicidal Episode

INTENT TO DIE

1. Have you been thinking about hurting or killing yourself?
2. How seriously do you want to die?
3. Have you attempted suicide before?
4. Are there people or things in your life who might keep you from killing yourself?

SEVERITY OF IDEATION

1. How often do you have these thoughts?
2. How long do they last?
3. How much do the thoughts distress you?
4. Can you dismiss them or do they tend to return?
5. Are they increasing in intensity and frequency?

DEGREE OF PLANNING

1. Have you made any plans to kill yourself? If yes, what are they?
2. Do you have access to the materials (e.g., gun, poison, pills) that you plan to use to kill yourself?
3. How likely is it that you could actually carry out the plan?
4. Have you done anything to put the plan into action?
5. Could you stop yourself from killing yourself?

resources that can be used when the individual is in crisis. With the nurse's help, the patient can visualize "emotional spaces that are safe places to go" when distressed.

For years, the no-suicide contract was a staple of psychiatric nursing practice and widely used across disciplines as a means of preventing suicide among those at risk. No-suicide contracts are verbal and written "contracts" between the individual at imminent risk for suicide and a health care provider that contain an agreement that the patient will not commit suicide during a specific time period. Careful evaluation of this practice has not established its efficacy in preventing suicidal behavior and suicide deaths. As a consequence, the nurse should avoid engaging in a no-suicide contract with a patient (Matarazzo et al., 2014).

Inpatient Safety Considerations

When hospitalization is considered the best option to ensure the safety of the patient, the nurse has responsibility for providing a safe, therapeutic environment in which human connection, instilling hope, and changing suicidal behavior can occur. There are no evidence-based guidelines for preventing suicides in hospitals. Inpatient suicides do occur. One study reported an average of 50 to 65 hospital inpatient suicides occurring per year in the United States. The vast majority of inpatient suicides take place in psychiatric facilities, and the method used in 70% of these events is hanging (Williams et al., 2018).

Removal of dangerous items and environmental hazards, continuous or intermittent observation of at-risk patients by hospital personnel trained in observation methods, and limitation of outpatient passes are the mainstays of hospital interventions. Observation procedures vary from facility to facility. For patients who require constant supervision, a staff member will be assigned only to the high-risk patient. For less risky patients, observation may entail close or intermittent observations.

Observation is not, in itself, therapeutic. An observation becomes therapeutic when interaction occurs with the patient. Psychiatric intensive care of this kind and restriction of freedom can be very upsetting to the patient who is withdrawn and isolated. Nurses can help patients reestablish personal control by including them in decisions about their care and restricting their behavior only as necessary. Nurses can also reduce the patient's stress while ensuring the patient's safety by intruding as little as possible on the person's exercise of free will. Observational periods can be used to help patients express a broad range of feelings and strengthen their belief in their own abilities to keep themselves safe. During observation, the nurse can help the patient describe feelings and identify ways to manage safety needs (Box 22.6).

BOX 22.6

Suicide Prevention

When teaching the patient and family about suicide and its prevention, be sure to address the following topics:

- Importance of emotional connections to family and friends
- Importance of instilling hope
- Discouraging suicidal ideation, rumination, self-harming behaviors
- Self-validation
- Emotional distress management
- Finding alternatives to suicidal behavior
- Establishing and using a crisis management plan
- Reestablishing the social network of the patient
- Information about treatment of underlying psychiatric disorders

---

Interventions for Intermediate and Long-Term Risk

Patients who are suicidal may need ongoing preventive interventions. The risk varies with the genetic, psychiatric, and psychological profile of the patient and the extent of their social support. Discouragement and hopelessness often persist long past the suicidal episode. Episodes of hopelessness should be anticipated and planned for in the patient's care. Patients should be taught to expect setbacks and times when they are unable to see much of a future for themselves. They should be encouraged to think of times in their lives when they were not so hopeless and consider how they may feel similarly in the future. Helping patients review the goals they already have achieved and at the same time set goals that can be achieved in the immediate future can help them manage periods of discouragement and hopelessness.

Interventions for the Biologic Domain

Patients who have survived a suicide attempt often need physical care of their self-inflicted injury. Overdose, gunshot wounds, and skin wounds are common. There will be biologic interventions for the underlying psychiatric disorder (see Unit VI).

Medication Management

Medication management focuses on treating the underlying psychiatric disorder. Currently, clozapine is the only U.S. Food and Drug Administration–approved medication for suicide risk in individuals with schizophrenia. Studies showing reduced suicide risk in patients with bipolar disorder or major depression taking lithium are not conclusive. For depression, a nonlethal antidepressant, such as a selective serotonin reuptake inhibitor, usually will be prescribed (AFSP, 2020b).

Electroconvulsive Therapy

Electroconvulsive therapy (ECT) has been used in both inpatient and outpatient settings to alleviate severe depression, especially in medically compromised groups, such as older adults, who may not tolerate conventional pharmacotherapy for depression (see Chapter 12). Rapid reduction in depression often leads to a decreased suicide drive. More research is needed to determine the role ECT may play in managing suicidal behavior. At this time, ECT is among several strategies used to decrease suicidal behavior over the long term (AFSP, 2020b; Kellner & Patel, 2018).

Interventions for the Psychological Domain

The goals of treatment in the psychological domain include reducing the capacity for suicidal behavior, increasing tolerance for distress, expanding coping abilities, and developing effective crisis management strategies. During the early part of a hospitalization, the most important way to reduce stress is to help the patient feel more secure and hopeful. As patients become more comfortable in their environment, the nurse can provide education about emotions, help patients explore and link presuicidal beliefs to a positive and hopeful future, support the application of new skills in managing negative thoughts, and help develop effective problem-solving skills.

Challenging the Suicidal Mindset

Teaching patients to distract themselves when thinking about suicide or engaging in negative self-evaluation can help to diminish suicidal ideation, dysfunctional thinking, and emotional reactivity. Simple distracting techniques such as reminding oneself to think of other things or engaging in other activities such as talking on the telephone, reading, or watching a movie are excellent temporary means of distracting the patient from negative cognitive states (see Box 22.6).

Validating the patient and teaching the patient to self-validate are powerful means of reducing suicidal thinking. Patients can learn that everyone experiences emotional distress and can begin to recognize it as a routine event. To manage emotional distress and increase tolerance for it, patients can be taught simple anxiety management strategies such as relaxation and visualization. The patient can be encouraged to write about their emotional experiences.

When negative thoughts and emotions coexist, they reinforce each other and contribute to suicidal ideation. Individuals who are suicidal often believe they are a burden to their family, who would be better off without them and do not feel connected to others. Nurses can challenge negative beliefs, especially the patient's idea that they are a burden to others (see Chapter 13). Ask the patient to describe the events that led to specific suicidal behavior so the patient can be engaged in developing alternative solutions. For each event, work with the patient to identify specific strategies that could be used to manage their distress, sense of disconnection, extreme focus on suicidal ideas, and other experiences that led the person to believe they had no option other than to die.

Developing New Coping Strategies

Preventing suicidal behavior requires that patients develop crisis management strategies, generate solutions to difficult life circumstances other than suicide, engage in effective interpersonal interactions, and maintain hope. The nurse can help the patient develop a written plan that can be used as a blueprint for action when the patient feels that they are losing control. The plan should include strategies that the patient can use to self-soothe; friends and family members that could be called, including multiple phone numbers where they can be reached; self-help groups and services such as suicide hotlines; and professional resources, including emergency departments and outpatient emergency psychiatric services.

Commitment to Treatment

Patients are usually ambivalent about wanting to die. The commitment to treatment statement (CTS) directly addresses ambivalence about treatment by asking the patient to engage in treatment by making a commitment to try new approaches. Different from the no-suicide contract, the CTS does not restrict the patient's rights regarding the option of suicide. Instead, the patient agrees to engage in treatment and access emergency service if needed. Underlying the CTS is the expectation that the patient will communicate openly and honestly about all aspects of treatment, including suicide. This commitment is written and signed by the patient. The efficacy of this approach has yet to be established by systematic research. Whether using the CTS or other means, be observant for lapses in the patient's participation in treatment and discuss them with the patient and other members of the interdisciplinary team.

Interventions for the Social Domain

Poor social skills may interfere with the patient's ability to engage others. The nurse should assess the patient's social capability early in treatment and make necessary provisions for social skills training. The interpersonal relationship with the nurse is an ideal place to begin shaping social behaviors that will help the patient to establish a social network that will sustain them during periods of discouragement or crisis. Participation in support networks, such as recovery groups, clubhouses, drop-in centers, self-help groups, or other therapeutic social engagement, will help the patient become connected to others.

Patients need to anticipate that even some of the people closest to them will feel uncomfortable with their suicidal behavior. Helping the patient to anticipate the stigmatizing behavior of others and how to manage it will go far in reintegrating the patient into a supportive social community. The nurse can also explore the patient's participation in specific social activities such as attending church or community activities.

Evaluation and Treatment Outcomes

The most desirable treatment outcome is the patient's recovery with no future suicide attempts. Short-term outcomes include maintaining the patient's safety, averting suicide, and mobilizing the patient's resources. Whether the patient is hospitalized or cared for in the community, their emotional distress must be reduced. Long-term outcomes must focus on maintaining the patient in psychiatric treatment, enabling the patient and family to identify and manage suicidal crises effectively, and widening the patient's support network.

Continuum of Care

Whether the suicide prevention plan is instituted in the hospital or in an outpatient setting, the patient cannot be released to home until a workable plan of care is in place. The care plan includes scheduling an appointment for outpatient treatment, providing for continuing somatic treatments until the first outpatient treatment visit, ensuring postrelease contact between the patient and significant other, providing for access to emergency psychiatric care, and arranging the patient's environment so it provides both structure and safety.

At the first follow-up visit, the patient and health care provider can establish a plan of care that specifies the intensity of outpatient care. Very unstable patients may need frequent supervision (e.g., telephone or face-to-face meetings or both) in the early days after hospitalization to maintain the patient's safety in the community. These contacts often can be short; their purpose is to convey the ongoing concern and caring of professionals involved in the patient's care. In arranging outpatient care, be certain to refer the patient to a provider who can provide the intensity of care the patient may need.

The patient's outpatient environment should be made as safe as possible before discharge. The nurse must share the care plan with family members so they can remove any objects in the patient's environment that could be used to engage in self-harm. The nurse should explain this measure to the patient to reinforce their sense of self-control. It is important to be reasonable in deciding what to remove from the environment. Patients who are truly determined to kill themselves after discharge will succeed in doing so, using whatever means are available.

Documentation and Reporting

The nurse must thoroughly document encounters with patients who are suicidal. This action is for the patient's ongoing treatment and the nurse's protection. Lawsuits for malpractice in psychiatric settings often involve completed suicides. The medical record must reflect that the nurse took every reasonable action to provide for the patient's safety.

The record should describe the patient's history, assessment, and interventions agreed upon by the patient and nurse. The nurse should document the presence or absence of suicidal thoughts, intent, plan, and available means to illustrate the patient's current and ongoing suicide risk. If the patient denies any suicidal ideation, it is important that the denial is documented. Documentation must include any use of drugs, alcohol, or prescription medications by the patient during 6 hours before the assessment. It should include the use of antidepressants that are especially lethal (e.g., tricyclics), as well as any medication that might impair the patient's judgment (e.g., a sleep medication). Notes should reflect the level of the patient's judgment and ability to be a partner in treatment.

The documentation should reflect if any medications were prescribed, the dosages, and the number of pills dispensed. Notes should reflect the plan for ongoing treatment, including the time of the next appointment with the provider, instructions given to the patient about obtaining emergency care if needed, and the names of family members and friends who will act as supports if the patient needs them.

NURSES' REFLECTION

Caring for suicidal patients is highly stressful and can lead to secondary trauma for the nurse. Nurses who care for suicidal patients must regularly share their experiences and feelings with one another. Talking about how the situations or actions of patients make them feel will help alleviate symptoms of stress. Some nurses find outpatient therapy helpful because it enhances their understanding of what situations are most likely to trigger secondary trauma. By demonstrating how to effectively manage the stressors in their own lives, nurses can be powerful role models for their patients.

SUMMARY OF KEY POINTS

- Suicide is a common and major public health problem.
- Suicide completion is more common in White men, especially older men.
- Parasuicide is more common among women than men.
- People who attempt suicide and fail are likely to try again without treatment.
- Suicidal behavior has genetic, biologic, and psychosocial origins.
- Suicide is associated with feelings of being a burden and not belonging.
- Acquired capability for suicide means that the person is fearless about death and has a high pain threshold.
- A suicide assessment focuses on the intention to die, hopelessness, available means, previous attempts and self-harm behavior, and degree of planning.
- Patients who are in crisis, are depressed, or use substances are at risk for suicide.
- The major objectives of brief hospital care are to maintain the patient's safety, reestablish the patient's biologic equilibrium, help the patient reconnect to others, instill hope, strengthen the patient's cognitive coping skills, and develop an outpatient support system.
- The nurse who cares for suicidal patients is vulnerable to secondary trauma and must take steps to maintain personal mental health.

CRITICAL THINKING CHALLENGES

1. An African American woman who lives with her three children, husband, and mother comes to her primary care provider. She is tearful and very depressed. What factors should be investigated to determine her risk for suicide and need for hospitalization?

2. A woman experiencing poverty with no insurance is hospitalized after her third suicide attempt. Antidepressant medication is prescribed. What kinds of treatment will be most effective in preventing future suicidal behavior?

3. A young man enters his workplace inebriated and carrying a gun. He does not threaten anyone but says that he must end it all. Assuming that he can be disarmed, what civil rights must be considered in taking further action in managing his suicidal risk?

4. You are a nurse in a large outpatient primary care setting responsible for an impoverished population. You want to implement a case-finding program for suicide prevention. Discuss how you would proceed and some potential problems you might face.

Movie Viewing Guides

Daughter of a Suicide: 1996 (Documentary). This personal documentary is the story of a woman whose mother committed suicide when the daughter was 18 years old. The daughter recounts the emotional struggle and depression left as the lifelong legacy of suicide and explores her efforts to heal. Combining digital video, 16-mm, and super-8 film, *Daughter of a Suicide* uses interviews with family and friends to tell the story of both mother and daughter.

VIEWING POINTS: How does this movie show that the effects of suicide do not end with a person's death?

The Virgin Suicides: 1999. After the suicide death of their 13-year-old daughter Cecilia, the Lisbon family becomes recluses. The remaining daughters try to resume their life by defying the withdrawal of their parents. Unsuccessful, the movie climaxes with the suicide deaths of the three remaining teenage girls.

VIEWING POINTS: What conditions in the girls' family led the girls to take their lives?

Paradise Now: 2005. This movie traces the motivations of two suicide bombers in Palestine. It explores how the two young men came to the decision to kill themselves and others and their ambivalence about their impending deaths. Ultimately, one decides to live, and the movie ends with an ambiguous fate of the other. This movie provides insight into the background and troubled thoughts that precede a suicidal act.

VIEWING POINTS: Can suicide be a political act? What other factors in these young men's lives might have contributed to their decision to volunteer as suicide bombers?

REFERENCES

American Association of Suicidology. (2019). Suicidal behavior among lesbian, gay, bisexual, and transgender youth fact sheet [Online]. https://suicidology.org/wp-content/uploads/2019/07/Updated-LGBT-Fact-Sheet.pdf

American Association of Suicidology. (2020). Warning signs [Online]. https://suicidology.org/resources/warning-signs/

American Foundation of Suicide Prevention. (2020a). Suicide facts & figures: United States 2020. https://afsp.org/suicide-statistics

American Foundation of Suicide Prevention. (2020b). Treatment for suicide and suicide attempts. https://afsp.org/treatment

Andriessen, K., Draper, B., Dudley, M., & Mitchell, P. B. (2016). Pre- and postloss features of adolescent suicide bereavement: A systematic review. *Death Studies, 40*(4), 229–246.

Beck, A. T., Rush, A. J., Shaw, B. F., & Emery, G. (1979). *Cognitive therapy of depression.* The Guildford Press.

Bostwick, J. M., Pabatti, C., Geske, J. R., & McKean, A. J. (2016). Suicide attempt as a risk factor for completed suicide: Even more lethal than we know. *American Journal of Psychiatry, 173*(11), 1094–1100.

Brodsky, B. S. (2016). Early childhood environment and genetic interactions: The diathesis for suicidal behavior. *Current Psychiatry Reports, 18,* 86.

Bryan, C. J., & Bryan, A. O. (2019). Financial strain, suicidal thoughts, and suicidal behavior among US military personnel in the National Guard. Crisis: *The Journal of Crisis Intervention & Suicide Prevention, 40*(6), 437–445.

Calati, R., Ferrari, C., Brittner, M., Oasi, O., Olie, E., Carvalho, A. F., & Courtet, P. (2019). Suicidal thoughts and behaviors and social isolation: A narrative review of the literature. *Journal of Affective Disorders, 245,* 653–667.

Carpenter-Song, E., & Snell-Rood, C. (2017). The changing context of rural America: A call to examine the impact of social change on mental health and mental health care. *Psychiatric Services, 68,* 503–506.

Centers for Disease Control and Prevention [CDC]. (2020a). Suicide prevention [Online]. Suicide|Violence Prevention|Injury Center|CDC

Centers for Disease Control and Prevention [CDC]. (2020b). Risk and protective factors [Online]. https://www.cdc.gov/violenceprevention/suicide/riskprotectivefactors.html

Colman, I. (2018). Responsible reporting to prevent suicide contagion. *Canadian Medical Association Journal, 190*(30), E898–E899.

Corrigan, P. W., Sheehan, L., Al-Khouja, M. A., & the Stigma of Suicide Research Team. (2017). Making sense of the public stigma of suicide: Factor analysis of its stereotypes, prejudices, and discriminations. Crisis: *The Journal of Crisis Intervention & Suicide Prevention, 38*(5), 351–359.

Crifasi, C. K., Meyers, J. S., Vernick, J. S., & Webster, D. W. (2015). Effects of changes in permit-to-purchase handgun laws in Connecticut and Missouri on suicide rates. *Preventive Medicine, 79,* 43–49.

Czeisler, M. É., Lane, R. I., Petrosky, E., Wiley, J. F., Christensen, A., Njai, R., Weaver, M. D., Robbins, R., Facer-Childs, E. R., Barger, L. K., Czeisler, C. A., Howard, M. E., & Rajaratnam, S. (2020). Mental health, substance use, and suicidal ideation during the COVID-19 pandemic - United States, June 24-30, 2020. *MMWR. Morbidity and Mortality Weekly Report, 69*(32), 1049–1057. https://doi.org/10.15585/mmwr.mm6932a1

Ducasse, D., Holden, R. R., Boyer, L., Artéro, S., Calati, R., Guillaume, S., Courtet, P., & Olié, E. (2018). Psychological pain in suicidality: A meta-analysis. *The Journal of Clinical Psychiatry, 79*(3), 16r10732. https://doi.org/10.4088/JCP.16r10732

Durkheim, E. (1951 [1897]). *Suicide.* Free Press.

Ellis, T. E., & Rutherford, B. (2008). Cognition and suicide: Two decades of progress. *International Journal of Cognitive Therapy, 1*(1), 47–68.

Endo, K., Ando, S., Shimodera, S., Yamasaki, S., Usami, S., Okazaki, Y., Sasaki, T., Richards, M., Hatch, S., & Nishida, A. (2017). Preference for solitude, social isolation, suicidal ideation, and self-harm in adolescents. *The Journal of Adolescent Health: Official Publication of the Society for Adolescent Medicine, 61*(2), 187–191. https://doi.org/10.1016/j.jadohealth.2017.02.018

Fredriksen-Goldsen, K. I., Kim, H. J., Sui, C., & Bryan, A. E. B. (2017). Chronic health conditions and key health indicators among lesbian, gay, and bisexual older U.S. adults, 2013–2014. *American Journal of Public Health, 107*(8), 1332–1338.

Gili, M., Castellví, P., Vives, M., de la Torre-Luque, A., Almenara, J., Blasco, M. J., Cebrià, A. I., Gabilondo, A., Pérez-Ara, M. A., A, M. M., Lagares, C., Parés-Badell, O., Piqueras, J. A., Rodríguez-Jiménez, T., Rodríguez-Marín, J., Soto-Sanz, V., Alonso, J., & Roca, M. (2019). Mental disorders as risk factors for suicidal behavior in young people: A meta-analysis and systematic review of longitudinal studies. *Journal of Affective Disorders, 245,* 152–162. https://doi.org/10.1016/j.jad.2018.10.115

Griffith, J. (2019). The sexual harassment-suicide connection in the U.S. military: Contextual effects of hostile work environment and trusted unit leaders. *Suicide and Life-Threatening Behavior, 49*(1), 41–53.

Hedegaard, H., Curtin, S. C., & Warner, M. (2020). Increase in suicide mortality in the United States, 1999–2018. NCHS Data Brief, 362. National Center for Health Statistics.

Ivey-Stephenson, A. Z., Demissie, Z., Crosby, A. E., Stone, D. M., Gaylor, E., Wilkins, N., Lowry, R., & Brown, M. (2020). Suicidal ideation and behaviors among high school students - Youth Risk Behavior Survey, United States, 2019. *MMWR Supplements, 69*(1), 47–55. https://doi.org/10.15585/mmwr.su6901a6

James, S. E., Herman, J. L., Ranking, S., Keisling, M., Mottet, L., & Anafi, M. (2016). *The report of the 2015 U.S. Transgender Survey.* National Center for Transgender Equality.

John, A., Glendenning, A. C., Marchant, A., Montgomery, P., Stewart, A., Wood, S., Lloyd, K., & Hawton, K. (2018). Self-harm, suicidal behaviours, and cyberbullying in children and young people: Systematic review. *Journal of Medical Internet Research, 20*(4), e129. https://doi.org/10.2196/jmir.9044

Joiner, T. (2005). *Why people die by suicide.* Harvard University.

Jones, A. L., & Pastor, D. K. (2020). Older adult suicides: What you should know and what you can do. *Home Healthcare Now, 38*(3), 124–130.

Kang, N., You, J., Huang, J., Ren, Y., Lin, M. P., & Xu, S. (2019). Understanding the pathways from depression to suicidal risk from the perspective of the Interpersonal-Psychological Theory of Suicide. *Suicide and Life-Threatening Behavior, 49*(3), 684–694.

Kann, L., McManus, T., Harris, W. A., Shanklin, S. L., Flint, K. H., Queen, B., Lowry, R., Chyen, D., Whittle, L., Thornton, J., Lim, C., Bradford, D., Yamakawa, Y., Leon, M., Brener, N., & Ethier, K. A. (2018). Youth risk behavior surveillance—United States, 2017. *Morbidity and Mortality Weekly Report.* Surveillance Summaries (Washington, D.C.: 2002), *67*(8), 1–114. https://doi.org/10.15585/mmwr.ss6708a1

Karp, A. (2018). Estimating global civilian-held firearms numbers [Online]. http://www.smallarmssurvey.org/fileadmin/docs/T-Briefing-Papers/SAS-BP-Civilian-Firearms-Numbers.pdf

Kavak, F., Akturk, U., Ozdemir, A., & Gultekin, A. (2018). The relationship between domestic violence against women and suicide risk. *Archives of Psychiatric Nursing, 32*(4), 574–579.

Kellner, C. H., & Patel, S. B. (2018). The role of ECT in the suicide epidemic. *Psychiatric Times, 35*(8), 23.

Kerr, W. C., Kaplan, M. S., Huguet, N., Caetano, R., Giesbrecht, N., & McFarland, B. H. (2017). Economic recession, alcohol, and suicide rates: Comparative effects of poverty, foreclosure, and job loss. *American Journal of Preventative Medicine, 52*(4), 469–475.

Klonsky, E. D., Qiu, T., & Saffer, B. Y. (2017). Recent advances in differentiating suicide attempter from suicide ideators. *Current Opinion Psychiatry, 30*(1), 15–20.

Leavitt, R. A., Ertl, A., Sheats, K., Petrosky, E., Ivey-Stephenson, A., & Fowler, K. A. (2018). Suicides among American Indian/Alaska Natives-National Violent Death Reporting System, 18 States, 2003–2014. *Centers for Disease Control and Prevention: Morbidity and Mortality Weekly Report, 67*(8), 237–242.

Lee, C. S., & Wong, Y. J. (2020). Racial/ethnic differences in the antecedents of youth suicide. *Cultural Diversity and Ethnic Minority Psychology, 26*(4), 532–543.

Lindsey, M. A., Sheftall, A. H., & Joe, S. (2019). Trends of suicidal behaviors among high school students in the United States: 1991–2017. *Pediatrids, 144*(5), e20191187.

Liu, R. T., Bettis, A. H., & Burke, T. A. (2020). Characterizing the phenomenology of passive suicidal ideation: A systematic review and meta-analysis of its prevalence, psychiatric comorbidity, correlates, and comparisons with active suicidal ideation. *Psychological Medicine, 50*(3), 367–383.

Liu, Y., Zhang, J., & Sun, L. (2017). Who are more likely to attempt suicide again? A comparative study between the first and multiple timers. *Comprehensive Psychiatry, 78,* 54–60.

Logan, J. E., Skopp, N. A., Reger, M. A., Gladden, M., Smolenski, D. J., Floyd, C. F., & Gahm, G. A. (2015). Precipitating circumstances of suicide among active duty U.S. Army personnel versus U.S. civilians, 2005–2010. *Suicide & Life-threatening Behavior, 45*(1), 65–77. https://doi.org/10.1111/sltb.12111

Ma, J., Batterham, P. J., Calear, A. L., & Han, J. (2016). A systematic review of the predictions of the Interpersonal-Psychological Theory of Suicidal Behavior. *Clinical Psychology Review, 46,* 34–45.

Ma, J. S., Batterham, P. J., Calear, A. L., & Han, J. (2019). Suicide risk across latent class subgroups: A test of the generalizability of the Interpersonal Psychological Theory of Suicide. *Suicide and Life-Threatening Behavior, 49*(1), 137–154.

Matarazzo, B. B., Homaifar, B. Y., & Wortzel, H. S. (2014). Therapeutic risk management of the suicidal patient: Safety planning. *Journal of Psychiatric Practice, 20*(3), 220–224.

National Alliance on Mental Illness (NAMI). (2020). LGBTQI [Online]. https://www.nami.org/Your-Journey/Identity-and-Cultural-Dimensions/LGBTQI

National Institute of Mental Health (NIMH). (2020). Suicide. https://www.nimh.nih.gov/health/statistics/suicide.shtml

Nelson, C. (2019). Management of late-life depression. *Handbook of Experimental pharmacology, 250,* 389–413.

Nichter, B., Hill, M., Norman, S., Haller, M., & Pietrzak, R. H. (2020). Associations of childhood abuse and combat exposure with suicidal ideation and suicide attempt in U.S. military veterans: A nationally representative study. *Journal of Affective Disorders, 276,* 1102–1108.

O'Connor, R. C., & Kirtley, O. J. (2018). The integrated motivational-volitional model of suicidal behaviour. *Philosophical Transactions of the Royal Society of London. Series B, Biological Sciences, 373,* 1754.

Oexle, N., Feigelman, W., & Sheehan, L. (2020). Perceived suicide stigma, secrecy about suicide loss and mental health outcomes. *Death Studies, 44*(4), 248–255.

Orsolini, L., Latini, R., Pompili, M., Serafini, G., Volpe, U., Vellante, F., Fornaro, M., Valchera, A., Tomasetti, C., Fraticelli, S., Alessandrini, M., La Rovere, R., Trotta, S., Martinotti, G., Di Giannantonio, M., & De Berardis, D. (2020). Understanding the complex of suicide in depression: From research to clinics. *Psychiatry Investigation, 17*(3), 207–221. https://doi.org/10.30773/pi.2019.0171

Page, A., Lewis, G., Kidger, J., Heron, J., Chittleborough, C., Evans, J., & Gunnell, D. (2014). Parental socio-economic position during childhood as a determinant of self-harm in adolescence. *Social Psychiatry and Psychiatric Epidemiology, 49*(2), 193–203. https://doi.org/10.1007/s00127-013-0722-y

Pruitt, L. D., Smolenski, D. J., Bush, N. E., Tucker, J., Fuad, I., Hoytt, T. V., & Reger, M. A. (2019). Suicide in the military: Understanding rates and risk factors across the United States' Armed Forces. *Military Medicine, 184*, 432–437.

Rutter, S. B., Cipriani, N., Smith, E. C., Ramjas, E., Vaccaro, D. H., Martin Lopez, M., Calabrese, W. R., Torres, D., Campos-Abraham, P., Llaguno, M., Soto, E., Ghavami, M., & Perez-Rodriguez, M. M. (2020). Neurocognition and the suicidal process. *Current Topics in Behavioral Neurosciences, 46*, 117–153. https://doi.org/10.1007/7854_2020_162

Schmutte, T. J., & Wilkinson, S. T. (2020). Suicide in older adults with and without known mental illness: Reports from the National Violent Death Reporting System, 2002–2016. *American Journal of Preventative Medicine, 58*(4), 584–590.

Sher, L. (2020). The impact of the COVID-19 pandemic on suicide rates. *QJM, 113*(10), 707–712.

Suicide Prevention Resource Center (SPRC). (2020a). Racial and ethnic disparities [Online]. https://www.sprc.org/scope/racial-ethnic-disparities

Suicide Prevention Resource Center (SPRC). (2020b). Risk and protective factors [Online]. https://www.sprc.org/about-suicide/risk-protective-factors

Testa, R. J., Michaels, M. S., Bliss, W., Rogers, M. L., Balsam, K. F., & Joiner, T. (2017). Suicidal ideation in transgender people: Gender minority stress and interpersonal theory factors. *Journal of Abnormal Psychology, 126*(1), 125–136.

Tidemalm, D., Runeson, B., Waern, M., Frisell, T., Carlström, E., Lichtenstein, P., & Långström, N. (2011). Familial clustering of suicide risk: A total population study of 11.4 million individuals. *Psychological Medicine, 41*(12), 2527–2534. https://doi.org/10.1017/S0033291711000833

The Trevor Project. (2020). Preventing suicide: Facts about suicide [Online]. https://www.thetrevorproject.org/resources/preventing-suicide/facts-about-suicide/

United States Department of Health and Human Services. (2020). Healthy people 2030 [Online]. Healthy People 2030 | health.gov. https://health.gov/healthypeople

United States Department of Health and Human Services Office of Minority Health. (2020a). Mental and Behavioral Health: Asian Americans [Online]. https://www.minorityhealth.hhs.gov/omh/browse.aspx?lvl=4&lvlid=54

United States Department of Health and Human Services Office of Minority Health. (2020b). Mental and Behavioral Health: Hispanics [Online]. https://www.minorityhealth.hhs.gov/omh/browse.aspx?lvl=4&lvlid=69

United States Department of Veterans Affairs. (2019). Mental health and suicide data [Online]. https://www.va.gov/PREVENTS/suicide-data.asp

Ursano, R. J., Herberman Mash, H. B., Kessler, R. C., Naifeh, J. A., Fullerton, C. S., Aliaga, P. A., Stokes, C. M., Wynn, G. H., Ng, T., Dinh, H. M., Gonzalez, O. I., Zaslavsky, A. M., Sampson, N. A., Kao, T. C., Heeringa, S. G., Nock, M. K., & Stein, M. B. (2020). Factors associated with suicide ideation in US Army soldiers during deployment in Afghanistan. *JAMA Network Open, 3*(1), e1919935. https://doi.org/10.1001/jamanetworkopen.2019.19935

Virupaksha, H. G., Muralidhar, D., & Ramakrishna, J. (2016). Suicide and suicidal behavior among transgender persons. *Indian Journal of Psychological Medicine, 38*(6), 505–509. https://doi.org/10.4103/0253-7176.194908

Wendell, J., Ratcliff, C. G., Price, E., Petersen, N. J., Dinapoli, E. A., & Cully, J. A. (2016). Factors associated with high frequency of suicidal ideation in medically ill Veterans. *Journal of Psychiatric Practice, 22*(5), 389–397.

Wetherall, K., Cleare, S., Eschle, S., Ferguson, E., O'Connor, D. B., O'Carroll, R. E., & O'Connor, R. C. (2018). From ideation to action: Differentiating between those who thin about suicide and those who attempt suicide in a national study of young adults. *Journal of Affective Disorders, 241*, 475–483.

Williams, S. C., Schmaltz, S. P., Castro, G. M., & Baker, D. W. (2018). Incidence and method of suicide in hospitals in the United States. *Joint Commission Journal on Quality and Patient Safety, 44*(11), 643–650.

Yildiz, E. (2018). Suicide in sexual minority populations: A systematic review of evidence-based studies. *Archives of Psychiatric Nursing, 32*, 650–659.

Zimmerman, G. M., Rees, C., Posick, C., & Zimmerman, L. A. (2016). The power of (Mis) perception: Rethinking suicide contagion in youth friendship networks. *Social Science & Medicine, 157*, 31–38.

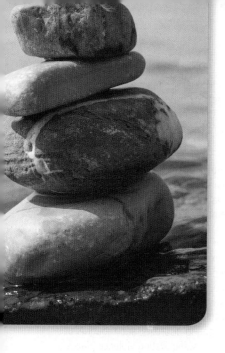

23
Mental Health Care for Survivors of Violence

Beverly Baliko

KEYCONCEPTS

- intimate partner violence
- psychological abuse
- sexual assault

LEARNING OBJECTIVES

After studying this chapter, you will be able to:

1. Describe types of violence and abuse, including intimate partner violence, stalking, rape and sexual assault, child abuse and neglect, and elder abuse.

2. Describe selected theories of violence.

3. Compare the reasons some people become abusive and why some victims remain in violent relationships.

4. Discuss the formation of a therapeutic relationship with a victim of violence.

5. Formulate nursing care plans for survivors of violence and abuse.

6. Describe treatment for perpetrators of abuse.

KEY TERMS

- Child abuse • Child neglect • Cycle of violence • Elder abuse • Intergenerational transmission of violence • Rape
- Revictimization • Stalking

INTRODUCTION

Violence in the form of abuse of intimate partners, children, and older adults is a national health problem. This type of violence permanently changes the survivor's reality and meaning of life. It wounds deeply, endangering core beliefs about the self, others, and the world. It can damage or destroy the survivor's self-esteem.

Nurses encounter survivors of violence and abuse in all health care settings. For this reason, being knowledgeable about abuse risk factors, indicators, causes, assessment techniques, and effective nursing interventions is a must. This chapter presents evidence that can shape contemporary nursing practice in caring for persons and families who survive violence and abuse.

TYPES OF VIOLENCE AND ABUSE

The most common type of abuse occurs as a result of domestic (family) violence; that is, the perpetrator is or formerly was a loved and trusted partner or family member. When this kind of violence occurs, the world and home are no longer safe in the eyes of the survivor. This chapter includes a discussion of intimate partner violence (IPV), **child abuse** and neglect, and **elder abuse** with emphasis on IPV.

Intimate Partner Violence

IPV is a significant public health problem in the United States, and across the globe. Behaviors that constitute

IPV include physical, sexual, and psychological (emotional) abuse or a combination of these perpetrated by a current or former spouse, significant other, or dating partner. The prevalence of IPV can only be estimated, because much abuse goes unreported. The most recent data available suggest that during their lifetimes, 1 in 4 women and nearly 1 in 10 men experience adverse psychological or physical consequences related to physical or sexual violence perpetrated by an intimate partner (Smith et al., 2018). Economic costs associated with acute and chronic medical and mental health services for survivors, lost productivity, and criminal justice activities create a substantial ongoing societal burden (Peterson et al., 2018). Approximately 62% of female murder victims are killed by current or former intimate partners (Violence Policy Center, 2019).

> **KEYCONCEPT Intimate partner violence** involves physical violence, sexual violence, stalking, and psychological aggression (including coercive acts) by a current or former intimate partner. IPV occurs on a continuum from psychological abuse to lethal violence.

Physical Abuse

Physical abuse involves any act of aggression, with or without use of an object or a weapon, that results in injury, pain, or impairment to another. Examples include striking, kicking, shoving, choking, and burning. Frequently, this behavior becomes a pattern that increases in severity over time. Physical abuse not only causes immediate injuries but also contributes to health problems that may persist long after the abuse ends. Although anyone can be a victim or perpetrator of physical abuse, women are far more likely than men to be seriously injured or killed by an intimate partner.

Psychological Abuse

> **KEYCONCEPT Psychological abuse** (also referred to as emotional abuse) involves threats, intimidation, or violence used as a means of asserting dominance and causing fear. Psychological abuse includes behaviors such as criticizing, insulting, humiliating, or ridiculing someone in private or in public. Abusers may destroy property, threaten or harm pets, control or monitor spending and daily activities, or isolate a person from family and friends. Gaslighting is a form of psychological abuse in which the victim is made to question his or her own judgment and perceptions. Perpetrators downplay the consequences of their behavior, deny abusive intent, or argue that actions are somehow justified. They often blame the victim for provoking or otherwise causing the abuse, leaving the victim with feelings of guilt or responsibility. About one third of adults report experiencing psychological abuse by an intimate partner during their lifetime (Smith et al., 2018).

Whereas physical violence may be episodic, psychological abuse is frequently more unrelenting. Over time, psychological abuse is devastating to an individual's self-esteem and self-confidence and can lead to psychiatric and physical disorders resulting from chronic stress. The varieties of abuse used to exert power and control over romantic partners are represented in Figure 23.1.

> **KEYCONCEPT Teen Partner Abuse** Teens and adults are often not aware of the frequency with which teen dating violence occurs. In a recent national survey of adolescents in the United States, 1 in 11 female and 1 in 15 male high school students reported having experienced physical violence by a dating partner in the last year (Centers for Disease Control and Prevention [CDC], 2020a). Sexual violence is also prevalent, reported by 1 in 9 female and 1 in 36 male students. Conflict or relationship problems with parents and peers may be predictors of teen partner abuse. Teens who experience violence in intimate relationships are more likely to develop problems such as depression, substance abuse, eating disorders, and thoughts of suicide. School performance may suffer. Dating violence places youths at higher risk for victimization during college and in subsequent relationships throughout adulthood.

Comorbidities

Besides injuries and death, survivors suffer multiple conditions directly caused by IPV or the chronic stress associated with it. Anxiety disorders, depression, posttraumatic stress disorder, and substance use disorders are all associated with family violence. Examples of health problems associated with IPV include asthma, gastrointestinal conditions, cardiovascular problems, bladder infections, migraines, joint pain, gynecological disorders, and sexually transmitted diseases (STDs) (Office of Women's Health, 2019). Strangulation and blows to the head can cause traumatic brain injuries that have lasting effects on cognition and functioning.

Risk Factors for Intimate Partner Violence

IPV occurs across all demographics and socioeconomic levels. Younger women, women who are divorced or separated, and Native American and Alaska Native women are at highest risk (National Center for Victims of Crime, n.d.). Although women are disproportionately affected, men can also be victims of IPV. Nonheterosexual couples experience IPV at rates similar to heterosexual couples, but victims often receive less support because of social stigma associated with nontraditional relationships. Within any type of relationship, frequent conflicts, jealousy, and possessiveness are associated with an increased risk of violence.

Individual characteristics such as low self-esteem, emotional insecurity, antisocial or borderline personality traits, disorders such as depression and posttraumatic stress disorder or a history of violence increase the likelihood of perpetration of violence (CDC, 2019). There is a strong association of substance use, especially alcohol

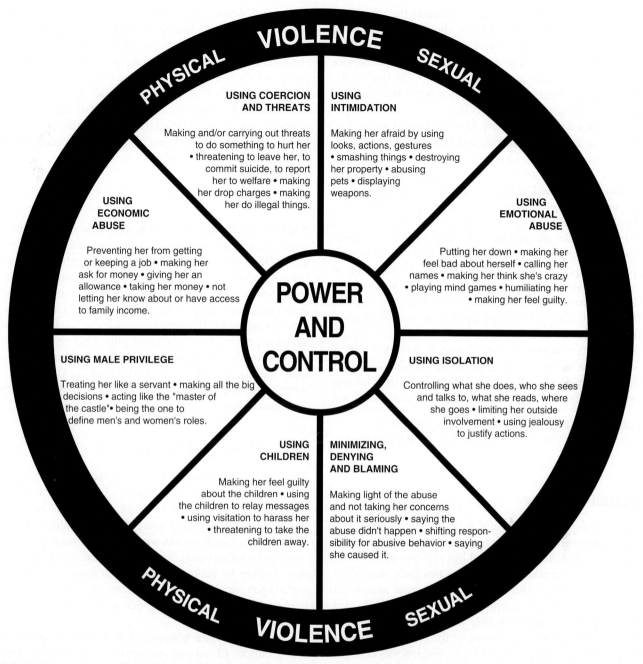

FIGURE 23.1   Power and control wheel. (Courtesy of Domestic Abuse Intervention Programs, 202 East Superior Street, Duluth, MN. 55802 218-722-2781 www.theduluthmodel.org)

abuse, with family violence. The presence of firearms in the home increases the risk of lethal violence.

Personal stressors, such as low income and unemployment, and external stressors, such as natural disasters or economic crises, may challenge individual and family coping, resulting in violence (CDC, 2019). In unstable families, violence sometimes begins or escalates when a pregnancy occurs. Abuse during pregnancy is a significant risk factor for several fetal and maternal complications, including miscarriages, low birth weight, low maternal weight gain, infections, and anemia (Alhusen

et al., 2015). Pregnancy is a window of opportunity for health care providers to screen women for IPV and refer them to the appropriate services.

Impact of the Coronavirus Disease 2019 Pandemic

The coronavirus disease 2019 pandemic resulted in significant psychosocial, health, and economic stressors; decreased contact with social support networks; and disruptions to services. For people in abusive relationships, extended time in contact partners increases the likelihood that violence will occur. Similarly, the absence of school and childcare resources may heighten the risk of child abuse and prevent abuse from being identified. School closures, scarce resources, misinformation in the media, fewer leisure outlets, and changes in job status contribute to family stress and conflict. When stay-at-home orders are in place and agencies are closed, seeking safety and support is more challenging, and travel restrictions can hinder escape plans. There are fewer opportunities to reach out for assistance when the abusive partner is consistently present, often monitoring communications. Abusive partners can withhold access to medications, supplies, or insurance cards to control their victims. Survivors who are at-risk medically might fear leaving their homes to seek assistance. Calls to domestic violence support hotlines have increased nationally, as have domestic violence calls in some police jurisdictions (Ramaswamy et al., 2020). Shelters, which are deemed "essential businesses," remain open. Demand for domestic violence services has historically risen after natural disasters have subsided. Unfortunately, meeting anticipated needs will be challenging, as prior to the pandemic, the capacities of the nearly 1,900 domestic violence programs across the United States were already strained.

> **KEYCONCEPT Sexual violence** includes any form of nonconsenting sexual activity, ranging from verbal threats to penetration.

Sexual Violence

Sexual violence is any type of sexual activity inflicted on a nonconsenting person. Sexual violence can include acts that are not identified as illegal but that are nevertheless traumatic or harmful in that the victim feels objectified, unsafe, or without choice. **Rape** and sexual assault are criminal acts. Rape specifically refers to vaginal, oral, or anal penetration, no matter how slight, with a body part or object, without consent of the victim (Bureau of Justice Statistics, n.d.). In 2013, the rape law was changed to be gender neutral and to state that physical force was not required for a perpetrator to be criminally charged. Rapists sometimes use coercion or threats to gain control over their victims. Rape is a crime of violence and domination, with sexuality used as a weapon. Sexual assault includes a broad range of behavior involving unwanted contact of a sexual nature. Sexual activity that occurs with a person who is unable to consent because of age, mental status, or impairment is considered sexual assault. When the victim is a minor, sexual assault is often referred to as sexual abuse. Most sexual assaults are perpetrated by someone known to the victim. Children are most likely to be sexually abused by family members, caregivers, or others close to them, as are older adults and adults with

disabilities. Adolescents and young adults are especially vulnerable to drug-facilitated assault by acquaintances, which involves the use of "date-rape" drugs, often combined with alcohol, to make a victim incapable of resistance. It is common for sexual assault to occur in conjunction with IPV, as an additional means of intimidation and humiliation. Non-consensual sex within a marriage was exempt from rape laws until the 1970s, and it was not until 1993 that all states had removed that exemption (England, 2020).

Stalking

Stalking is a pattern of repeated unwanted contact, attention, and harassment that often increases in frequency. Stalkers harass and terrorize their victims through behavior that causes fear or substantial emotional distress. Stalking may include such behaviors as following someone, showing up at the person's home or workplace, vandalizing property, using technology to track or harass someone, or sending unwanted gifts. One in 6 women and one in 19 men experience stalking at some point in their lifetime (Smith et al., 2018). Stalking can be prolonged and takes a tremendous toll on victims' health and functioning.

Child Abuse and Neglect

Child abuse includes acts of commission and acts of omission. Acts of commission are intentional harmful behaviors directed toward a child and include physical, sexual, and psychological abuse. **Child neglect** is an act of omission, which occurs when a child's basic physical, emotional, educational, and health care needs are not met. Failure to protect a child from harm, inadequate supervision, or exposure to violence are other forms of neglect (CDC, 2020b). Neglect is the most common form of child abuse.

Children who are younger than 4 years of age, who are products of unwanted pregnancies, or who have developmental or physical disabilities are at highest risk of abuse (CDC, 2020b). Young parents who lack social support, resources, and knowledge of normal childhood development are at increased risk of abusing their children. Multiple stressors, emotional or substance abuse problems, and the use of harsh punishment are additional parental risk factors.

Children who are abused or neglected may develop physical, emotional, and behavioral problems (CDC, 2020b). Their cognitive development may be impaired, and they may exhibit academic difficulties. Abuse leads to problems getting along with or trusting others. Survivors of child abuse are at increased risk for depression, anxiety, low self-esteem, and substance abuse. Adverse experiences in childhood have a negative impact on health and well-being throughout life.

A child who is emotionally or psychologically abused does not have visible injuries to alert others. Nevertheless, psychological abuse severely affects a child's self-esteem and often leaves permanent emotional scars. For many survivors of childhood abuse, emotional abuse is worse than physical abuse. Psychological abuse frequently co-occurs with other types of abuse and can take various forms. Children often believe the abuse is their fault.

Sexual abuse occurs to children of all ages and is frequently perpetrated by someone the child knows and trusts. To maintain their silence, children may be threatened or told that they will not be believed if they disclose the abuse. No child is psychologically prepared to cope with repeated sexual stimulation. A victim of prolonged sexual abuse will develop low self-esteem, a feeling of worthlessness, and a distorted view of sex. The child may become withdrawn, distrustful, or suicidal. Other characteristics of children who have been sexually abused include an unusual interest or avoidance of sexually related content, nightmares, seductiveness, refusal to go to school, conduct problems, secretiveness, and unusual aggressiveness (American Academy of Child & Adolescent Psychiatry, 2020).

Abuse of Older Adults

Older adults and adults who have mental or physical disabilities are vulnerable to abuse. Older individuals may be victims of physical, psychological, or sexual abuse. The most common type of elder abuse is financial abuse, in which older adults may be manipulated by family or caregivers to give up control of their money and are vulnerable to scams and fraud perpetrated by outsiders.

Elder abuse is increasingly recognized as a serious problem in the United States and other countries. As the population continues to age, it is likely that the problem will worsen. The actual prevalence of elder abuse is uncertain, as most abuse is unreported, and relatively little research has focused on this population. An estimated 1 in 10 people over age 60 who live at home suffer some type of abuse, including neglect and exploitation (CDC, 2020c). The abuse usually occurs at the hands of a caregiver or a person the older adult trusts but is a significant problem in nursing homes and assisted living facilities as well.

Individuals who are isolated, have poor support systems, or have mental or physical impairments that foster dependency on others are more vulnerable to harm. Older people may be reluctant to report maltreatment by those they love or on whom they depend, or cognitive deficits may prevent them from being able to articulate their situation. In addition to the obvious physical problems (e.g., injuries, pressure sores, malnutrition) that can result from abuse or neglect, older adults can experience worsening of existing medical conditions and emotional problems such as depression, anxiety, and fearfulness (CDC, 2020c).

Risk factors for those who are more likely to abuse older adults include using drugs or alcohol, high levels of stress, lack of social support, emotional or financial dependence on the older adult, lack of training in taking care of older adults, and depression (CDC, 2020c). Caring for a dependent older adult can be overwhelming. It is important for the nurse to listen to and assess both older adults and their caregivers to help prevent abuse and neglect in this population.

THEORIES OF VIOLENCE

No single cause is sufficient to explain the phenomenon of family violence. The neurobiologic and psychological factors that contribute to anger and poor impulse control (as outlined in Chapter 13) are relevant to the use of aggression in the home. However, the ability of many abusers to refrain from angry outbursts and violence in public settings suggests that their behavior toward family members is not solely attributable to poor self-control. The risk factors discussed in previous sections increase the likelihood of violence occurring but do not cause it. Many people share the same risks but do not engage in violence. Outlined below are a few prominent theories among the many researchers that attempt to explain IPV and other types of violence in the family. Individual characteristics likely intersect with risk factors to produce behavior that is learned and reinforced in families, communities, and society.

Social Learning Theory (Intergenerational Transmission of Violence)

Being a victim of childhood abuse is one of the strongest predictors of violence as an adult. Violent families create an atmosphere of tension, fear, intimidation, and confusion about intimate relationships. Children in violent homes learn that violent behavior is an approved and legitimate way to solve problems and to cope with difficulty. Social learning or **intergenerational transmission of violence** theory posits that children who witness or experience violence in their homes are more likely to perpetuate violent behavior within their own families (Copp et al., 2016). Experiencing harsh physical discipline increases the risk of perpetrating family violence as an adult (Afifi et al., 2017). This learned behavior is reinforced when violence as a means of control or punishment is sanctioned within social systems or when there are inadequate social or legal constraints to discourage such behaviors.

Economic Disadvantage, Community Disorganization, and Attitudes Supportive of Violence

Neighborhoods that are more socially cohesive are more intolerant of deviant behavior. The presence of concentrated economic disadvantage (i.e. neighborhoods with the lowest incomes, high unemployment, and institutional disinvestment); racial or ethnic heterogeneity; and community instability is associated with community disorganization and weak social control, which leads to increased levels of crime and IPV. Within these disadvantaged communities, institutions that normally foster social control, such as churches, schools, and other community organizations, lose their ability to exercise social control over the community. Community disorganization, crime, and weak social control also foster individual acceptance of violence, which, in turn, is associated with increased rates of IPV, child abuse, and elder abuse (Copp et al., 2016).

Imbalances in Relationship Power

Another body of literature suggests that IPV is a manifestation of gender-based imbalances in relationship power. Usually, this perspective explains IPV as violence against women by their male romantic partners related to issues of gender, inequality, power and privilege, patriarchy, and the subordination of women (Namy et al., 2017). Patriarchal systems exist and are supported at the macro level (e.g., government, bureaucracies, religion) and at the micro level (e.g., families), and both levels have gender inequities. Within a patriarchal society, men often hold traditional gender role beliefs. For example, whereas men are heads of households and provide for their families, women are homemakers and mothers. When these beliefs are challenged, such as when women enter the workforce and earn more than their partner, men may feel threatened and respond with violence.

Historically, women and children had few or no rights in most cultures, and in many countries today, women's rights remain limited (Ramsey, 2011). Women and children were considered part of the household over which the male held absolute power and violence was accepted as a permissible way to exercise authority. Even after popular opinion changed and so-called wife-beating became formally illegal in all states in the United States by 1920, IPV was treated differently than other crimes and viewed as a private matter that rarely resulted in arrest or prosecution until the latter part of the 20th century. Until recently, men in the United States were able to use physical violence with relative impunity within the context of intimate relationships. In 1994, *The Violence Against Women Act* (VAWA) (*P.L. 103–122*) became the first U.S. federal policy to combat interpersonal violence and other violence against women. This law declared civil rights for victim-survivors of gender-based violence and created new laws to protect them. The law has been reauthorized several times, with revisions to extend increasingly inclusive protections; however, it expired in early 2019 and as of mid-2020 has not been reauthorized by the current Senate. This is critical because VAWA provides funding for domestic violence services and legal protections for immigrants and other marginalized populations. Despite changes in laws, patriarchal attitudes continue to influence the dynamics of some families, sometimes bolstered by cultural and religious norms (Ogunsiji & Clisdell, 2017).

Cycle of Violence

Many, but not all, cases of IPV reflect a recognized **cycle of violence.** The cycle consists of three recurring phases that often increase in frequency and severity. The cycle is fully described in Figure 23.2.

Factors Influencing Leaving Versus Staying in a Violent Relationship

Many women do not report abuse, fearing retaliation against themselves or their children. Often, they continue to hold strong feelings for their partners despite the abuse. When medical care is required, women may attribute their injuries to other causes; health care providers may be reluctant to inquire about abuse. Provision of assistance to women who are involved in violent intimate relationships can pose unique problems in that seeking support can be dangerous to the women if their activities are discovered by the abusive partner. Therefore, the challenge for health care providers is twofold—ensuring that support is both available and safely accessible, whether or not it is accepted at a given time. Even though it might be difficult to understand why a person would remain in an abusive relationship, it is critical to remain nonjudgmental and to realize that there are valid reasons for deciding to remain in a potentially harmful environment.

Leaving an abusive relationship is a process that can be quite complex. Many women leave and return several times as they learn new coping skills and build support networks before ending the relationship permanently. When abuse is intermittent, and strong emotional and psychological ties to the abusive partner remain, victims continue to hope that the behavior will change. Women who lack job skills, financial resources, and support systems may stay because of economic dependence on their partner. Some are concerned about losing custody of their children if they are unable to provide for them independently.

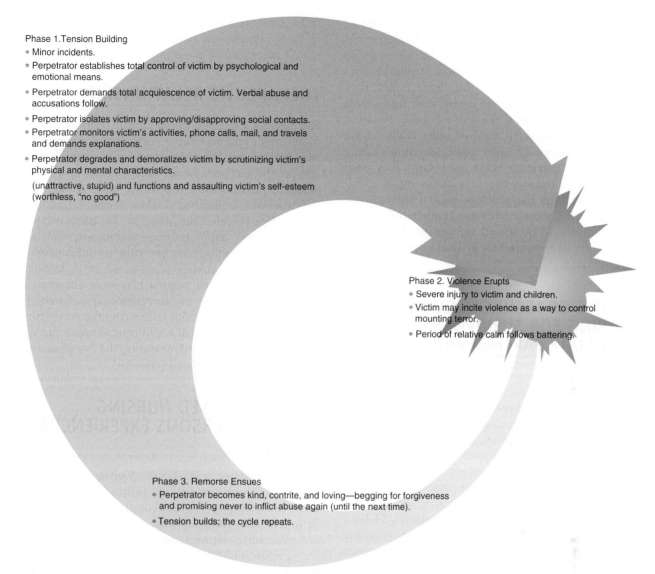

Phase 1.Tension Building

* Minor incidents.

* Perpetrator establishes total control of victim by psychological and emotional means.

* Perpetrator demands total acquiescence of victim. Verbal abuse and accusations follow.

* Perpetrator isolates victim by approving/disapproving social contacts.

* Perpetrator monitors victim's activities, phone calls, mail, and travels and demands explanations.

* Perpetrator degrades and demoralizes victim by scrutinizing victim's physical and mental characteristics.

(unattractive, stupid) and functions and assaulting victim's self-esteem (worthless, "no good")

Phase 2. Violence Erupts

* Severe injury to victim and children.

* Victim may incite violence as a way to control mounting terror.

* Period of relative calm follows battering.

Phase 3. Remorse Ensues

* Perpetrator becomes kind, contrite, and loving—begging for forgiveness and promising never to inflict abuse again (until the next time).

* Tension builds; the cycle repeats.

FIGURE 23.2   The cycle of violence.

Fear is another important factor in deciding whether to leave or stay in a violent relationship. Some women stay because of threats not only against themselves but also against other family members or pets. Women recognize the valid concern that leaving may not stop the violence. If victims attempt to leave or actually do leave the relationship, perpetrators often escalate their violence, stalk their partners, and may even kill them, which makes leaving the time of greatest risk in an abusive relationship (National Coalition against Domestic Violence [NCADV], n.d.).

Safety Issues and Mandatory Reporting

Health care providers, including nurses, are mandated reporters. This means that they must report known or suspected abuse in specific circumstances. Some states require reporting of injuries sustained as a result of abuse. Mandatory reporting for IPV is controversial because it may act as a barrier to disclosure or seeking care (Lippy et al., 2020). Concerns center around triggering involvement with the legal system that can result in removal of children from custody, loss of economic support, or retaliation from the abuser. Black mothers are disproportionally likely to be referred to child protective services for IPV-related concerns. Immigrants, especially those who are undocumented, may fear that discussing IPV will lead to contacts with immigration authorities and deportation or separation from their children.

All states require reporting of known or suspected abuse involving children and vulnerable adults. It is important for nurses to be familiar with the laws of the state in which they practice and with the policies of their organization. Removing children and older adults from their families or caregivers may be necessary to ensure their immediate safety. In most settings, nurses do not have to make this decision alone; rather, they involve other professionals to assist with assessment and alternate placement if the current living situation of an abused or neglected child or older adult cannot be made safe. When an older adult's decision-making is not impaired (*competence* is the legal term), they must be allowed an appropriate degree of autonomy in deciding how to manage the problem even if they choose to remain in the abusive situation (Pomerance, 2015). Forcing someone to do something against their wishes is itself a form of victimization by denying autonomous decision-making.

THE ROLE OF TECHNOLOGY IN CARING FOR SURVIVORS OF INTIMATE PARTNER VIOLENCE

For survivors of violence, technology can be a weapon or a lifeline. Abusers can use technology, to monitor their partner's activities or threaten to post compromising photos or confidential information on a public forum as a means of control. More often, the internet is a valuable source of information and support when using reliable sources such as hotlines, particularly for survivors who are not emotionally ready for in-person meetings or who do not have ready access to nearby services. For those who are in abusive relationships, websites, 24-hour hotlines, and chats provide resources for safety planning (Rempel et al., 2019). Most websites and chats designed for IPV survivors have escape features to disconnect quickly if necessary. Survivors are warned to clear their search histories if there is a risk they are being checked. Technology extends the reach of services for survivors in rural and underserved locations via virtual therapy and consultations, and peer support can come through online groups and texts and messaging apps.

When connecting with a survivor online, confidentiality is crucial. Therapists are careful to use secure platforms that cannot be tracked or monitored. Telemedicine providers should be aware of risks when incorporating screening questions into the visit. Yes or no questions can be used to ensure that the client is alone and it is safe to speak. If a survivor is at risk, messages can be moved to password-protected health portals. When language is a barrier, it is important to utilize certified interpreters who are not family members. Virtual access to services and health care became critical when controlling the spread of the new coronavirus required social distancing and limitation of in-person services. These situations increased safety risks for survivors of IPV and expanded use of technology created opportunities to reduce isolation. In all cases, effective use of technology requires internet or mobile access, which is not universally available.

THERAPEUTIC RELATIONSHIP

Establishing a trusting nurse–patient relationship is one of the most important steps in caring for any person experiencing violence. When interviewing, to establish rapport and put the survivor at ease, start with the least sensitive areas and progress to more sensitive topics (Power, 2017). Survivors are unlikely to disclose sensitive information unless they perceive the nurse to be trustworthy and nonjudgmental. Important considerations in establishing open communication are ensuring confidentiality and providing a quiet, private place in which to interact. A supportive, empathetic approach is most effective. The nurse must continually monitor personal reactions to prevent negative feelings from influencing the nurse–patient relationship in a way that could re-traumatize the survivor. Nurses must make clear during the assessment their responsibility for mandated reporting.

EVIDENCE-BASED NURSING CARE FOR PERSONS EXPERIENCING VIOLENCE

Nurses encounter survivors of violence and abuse in many health care settings, not just in mental health settings. Abuse may be disclosed or discovered by providers in urgent care clinics, primary care settings, obstetrics and gynecology settings, pediatric units, well-child clinics, geriatric units, schools, and nursing homes, among others.

Mental Health Nursing Assessment

Conducting a Safety Assessment First

Once physiologic stability is established, the nurse should determine whether the survivors are in danger for their life, either from homicide or suicide, and, if children are in the home, whether they are in danger. Trauma may trigger suicidal ideation or exacerbate preexisting mental health conditions that place the survivor at risk. Suicide precautions should be initiated if indicated.

Children who are present during abusive episodes are at risk for emotional and developmental harm even if they are not direct recipients of abuse. Exposing a child to violence carries legal consequences in many states (Child Welfare Information Gateway, 2016).

The Danger Assessment Screen is a useful tool for assessing the risk that IPV will end in homicide (Campbell & Humphries, 1993) (Box 23.1). This assessment may

---

BOX 23.1

Danger Assessment

Several risk factors have been associated with homicides (murders) of both batterers and victims in research that has been conducted after the killings have taken place. We cannot predict what will happen in your case, but we would like you to be aware of the danger of homicide in situations of severe battering and to see how many of the risk factors apply to your situation.

1. Has the physical violence increased in frequency during the past year?
2. Has the physical violence increased in severity during the past year or has a weapon or threat with weapon been used?
3. Does your partner ever try to choke you?
4. Is there a gun in the house?
5. Has your partner ever forced you to have sex when you did not wish to do so?
6. Does your partner use drugs? By drugs, I mean "uppers" or amphetamines, speed, angel dust, cocaine, "crack," street drugs, heroin, or mixtures.
7. Does your partner threaten to kill you, or do you believe they are is capable of killing you?
8. Is your partner drunk every day or almost every day? (In terms of quantity of alcohol.)
9. Does your partner control most or all of your daily activities? For instance, does they tell you who you can be friends with, how much money you can take with you for shopping, or when you can take the car?
10. Has your partner ever beaten you while you were pregnant? (If never pregnant by him, check here _____.)
11. Is your partner violently and constantly jealous of you? (For instance, do you? (For instance, say, "If I can't have you, no one can.")
12. Have you ever threatened or tried to commit suicide?
13. Have they ever threatened or tried to commit suicide?
14. Is your partner violent toward the children?
15. Is your partner violent outside the home?

TOTAL YES ANSWERS: _____

Thank you. Please talk to your nurse, advocate, or counselor about what the danger assessment means in terms of your situation.

Adapted from Campbell, J., & Humphreys, J. (Eds.) (1993). *Nursing care of survivors of family violence* (p. 259). St. Louis: Mosby. Copyright © 1993 Elsevier. With permission.

---

help survivors recognize the serious nature of the violence they routinely experience. An abbreviated version of this tool, the Danger Assessment-5 (Messing et al., 2017), can be used for brief screening.

Screening for Violence and Abuse

Because of the prevalence of IPV, the US Preventive Services Task Force recommends universal screening for all women of child-bearing age (2018). However, actual rates of screening in most settings are low. Most survivors do not report violence to health care workers without specifically being asked about it (Power, 2017).

Survivors may be reluctant to report abuse because of shame, embarrassment, fear of not being believed, or fear of retaliation. Survivors who depend on the abuser for care or financial support may be concerned about consequences of disclosure. If the suspected abuser is present, it is important to speak to the survivor alone.

Validated screening tools are readily accessible (Cavner, 2019). Asking specific abuse screening questions substantially increases the detection of abuse. For that reason, nurses must develop a repertoire of age-appropriate, culturally sensitive abuse-related questions. Avoid using terms such as *abuse* and *rape*, because those labels may not be consistent with an individual's perception of their experience. See Boxes 23.2 and 23.3.

Other questions that might be useful in eliciting disclosure are as follows:

- "When there are fights at home, have you ever been hurt or afraid?"
- "It looks like someone has hurt you. Tell me about it."
- "Some women have described problems like yours. If this is happening to you, can we talk about it?"

When survivors are disclosing abuse, they need privacy and time to tell their story. The nurse should listen attentively without offering unsolicited advice or making judgmental remarks about the possible abuse or the perpetrator. Use validating messages to convey that the survivors are believed and that the nurse is concerned for their safety and well-being. Examples of such messages include the following:

- "I'm really sorry this happened to you."
- "I'm glad you told me."
- "It sounds like a frightening experience."
- "It was not your fault."

BOX 23.2

Abuse Assessment Screen

1. Have you ever been emotionally or physically abused by your partner or someone important to you?	YES	NO
2. Within the past year, have you been hit, slapped, kicked, or otherwise physically hurt by someone? If YES, by whom: _____ Number of times: _____ Mark the area of injury on body map.	YES	NO
3. Within the past year, has anyone forced you to have sexual activities? If YES, who: _____ Number of times: _____	YES	NO
4. Are you afraid of your partner or anyone you listed above?	YES	NO

BOX 23.3

Burgess-Partner Abuse Scale for Teens

Directions: During the past 12 months, you and one of your partners may have had a fight. Following is a list of things one of your partners may have done to you. Please circle the number of how often this partner did these things to you. This is not a test and there are no right or wrong answers. Remember, having a partner(s) does not mean you are having sex with the partner(s).

If you have not had a partner in the past 12 months, do not fill this form out.

	Never	Once	A Few Times	More than a Few Times	Routinely or a lot
1. My partner doesn't let me go out with my friends.	0	1	2	3	4
2. My partner tells me what to wear.	0	1	2	3	4
3. My partner says if I don't have sex with them then I don't love them.	0	1	2	3	4
4. My partner says they will hurt me if I talk to another guy/girl.	0	1	2	3	4
5. My partner calls me bad names like bitch.	0	1	2	3	4
6. My partner says they will hurt me with a weapon.	0	1	2	3	4
7. My partner forces me to have sex.	0	1	2	3	4
8. My partner tells me I am stupid or dumb.		1	2	3	4
9. My partner follows me when I do things with my friends or family.	0	1	2	3	4
10. My partner hits or kicks something when they get mad at me.	0	1	2	3	4
11. My partner kicks me.	0	1	2	3	4
12. My partner says they can have sex with other people even though they said I can't.	0	1	2	3	4
13. My partner gives me sexually transmitted infections.	0	1	2	3	4
14. My partner hurts me using a weapon.	0	1	2	3	4
15. My partner forces me to use drugs even though I don't want to.	0	1	2	3	4
16. My partner beats me up so bad.	0	1	2	3	4
17. My partner says they will hurt my family if I don't do what they say.	0	1	2	3	4
18. My partner tells me what school activities I can and can't do.	0	1	2	3	4
19. My partner tells me what friends I can hang out with.	0	1	2	3	4
20. My partner chokes me if they get mad at me.	0	1	2	3	4
21. My partner yells at me if they don't know where I am.	0	1	2	3	4
22. My partner says we can't break up even though I want to.	0	1	2	3	4

How many partners have you had in the past 12 months?_____

Permission is granted for use in research or clinical settings. Burgess, S., & Tavakoli, A. (2005). Psychometric assessment of the Burgess-Partner Abuse Scale for Teens (B-PAST). *Aquichan, 5,* 96–107.

Survivors of IPV may deny the abuse, make excuses for the perpetrator's behavior, or attribute an injury to an unlikely cause. Avoid pressuring or confronting them, but carefully document a description of the survivor's account of how the injury happened, using the survivor's own words.

After assessment is completed in a health care agency and abuse is evident, the nurse should offer the adult survivor use of the telephone. This may be the only time that the survivor can make calls in private to family, who might offer support, or to the police, lawyers, or shelters. Scheduling future appointments may provide the survivor with a legitimate reason to leave the perpetrator and continue to explore options.

Physical Health Assessment

Documentation of abuse or suspected abuse includes a complete history and physical examination. Note vital signs, sleep and appetite disturbances, exaggerated startle responses, flashbacks, and nightmares that may suggest PTSD or depression. Assess for injuries in need of immediate attention. Documentation should include a detailed history of how injuries occurred and a careful description of the injuries. A body map may be used to indicate location, size, and type of injuries. The nurse's documentation may become evidence if there are legal consequences related to the violence, even if the survivor declines to file a report at the time of the incident. Victims of violence experience mild-to-severe physical consequences. Mild injuries may include bruises and abrasions of the head, neck, face, trunk, and limbs. People who are chronically abused may have multiple bruises in various stages of healing. Severe injuries include multiple traumas, major fractures, major lacerations, and internal injuries (including chest and abdominal injuries and subdural hematomas). Loss of vision and hearing can result from blows to the head.

Physical or sexual violence may result in head injuries that can produce changes in cognition, affect, motivation, and behavior. Survivors of sexual abuse may have vaginal and perineal trauma. Anorectal injuries may also be present, including disruption of anal sphincters, retained foreign bodies, and mucosal lacerations. Examination for sexual abuse, acute or chronic events, may require referral to a trained registered nurse in sexual assault, known as a *sexual assault nurse examiner* (SANE). If a SANE nurse is not available, the Emergency Department nurse may take the lead in caring for patients who have experienced sexual assault. Sexual assault examination involves evidence gathering, careful documentation, and attention to psychosocial needs and emotional distress (Delgadillo, 2017). Determine the need for emergency contraception, or prophylactic treatment for human immunodeficiency virus [HIV] or STDs. See Box 23.4 for additional considerations.

BOX 23.4

Special Concerns for Victims of Sexual Assault

ASSESSMENT FOCUS

The history and physical examination of the survivor of sexual assault differ significantly from other assessment routines because the evidence obtained may be used in prosecuting the perpetrator. Therefore, the purpose is twofold:

• To assess the patient for injuries
• To collect evidence for forensic evaluation and proceedings

Usually, someone with appropriate training, such as a nurse practitioner who has taken special courses, examines a victim of rape or sexual assault. Generalist nurses may be involved in treating the injuries that result from the assault, including genital trauma (e.g., vaginal and anal lacerations) and extragenital trauma (e.g., injury to the mouth, throat, wrists, arms, breasts, thighs).

KEY INTERVENTIONS

Nursing intervention to prevent short- or long-term psychopathology after sexual assault is crucial. Psychological trauma after rape and sexual assault includes immediate anxiety and distress and the development of PTSD, depression, panic, and substance abuse.

Key interventions include the following:

• Early treatment because initial levels of distress are strongly related to later levels of posttraumatic stress disorder, panic, and anxiety.
• Supportive, caring, and nonjudgmental nursing interventions during the forensic rape examination are also crucial. This examination often increases survivors' immediate distress because they must recount the assault in detail and submit to an invasive pelvic or anal examination.
• Anxiety-reducing education, counseling, and emotional support, particularly regarding unwanted pregnancies and sexually transmitted infections, including HIV. All survivors should be tested for these possibilities. Treatment may include terminating a pregnancy; administering medications to treat gonorrhea, chlamydia, trichomoniasis, and syphilis; and administering medications that may decrease the likelihood of contracting HIV infection.
• Interventions that are helpful for survivors of domestic violence; these also apply to survivors of sexual assault.

Healthy child development and deviations that may be related to abuse or neglect are critical components of the nursing assessment of children. Assessing developmental milestones, school history, and relationships with siblings and friends is important. Intracranial hemorrhage in an infant in the absence of an obvious cause, such as a motor vehicle accident, may suggest shaken baby syndrome. Infants do not begin to move or ambulate on their own prior to the age of 6 months, when they begin to crawl; therefore, any bruises on an infant before the age of 6 months is cause for suspicion. Any discrepancies between the history and physical examination and implausible explanations for injuries and other symptoms should be an alert to the possibility of abuse (Yaffe, 2010). Children and adolescents who wear clothing that covers parts of the body in a manner inconsistent with the season may be hiding bruises, abrasions, or burns caused by cigarettes or boiling water. Other circumstances that should heighten the suspicion of childhood abuse include multiple fractures or types of fractures (such as spiral fractures) that would only occur in an abusive situation. Other injuries such as bite marks or injuries to the genitals or anus always require further investigation.

For reference when assessing older adults, become familiar with normal aging and signs and symptoms of common illnesses to distinguish those conditions from abuse. Observe for signs of malnutrition or inattention to activities of daily living (ADLs). As with children, bruises, lacerations, and other injuries are suspicious if they are inconsistent with a description of how they occurred. Some older adults are unable to communicate effectively because of dementia or other cognitive impairment. Evidence that excessive medications or physical restraints are being used to control an older adult's behavior should be investigated. Box 23.5 lists indicators of actual or potential abuse that need to be thoroughly assessed for all survivors.

BOX 23.5

History and Physical Findings Suggestive of Abuse

PRESENTING PROBLEM

- Vague information about cause of problem
- Delay between occurrence of injury and seeking of treatment
- Inappropriate reactions of significant other or family
- Denial or minimizing of seriousness of injury
- Discrepancy between history and physical examination findings

FAMILY HISTORY

- Past family violence
- Physical punishment of children
- Children who are fearful of parent(s)
- Father or mother (or both) who demands unquestioning obedience
- Alcohol or drug abuse
- Violence outside the home
- Unemployment or underemployment
- Financial difficulties or poverty
- Use of older adult's finances for other family members
- Finances rigidly controlled by one member

HEALTH AND PSYCHIATRIC HISTORY

- Fractures at various stages of healing
- Spontaneous abortions
- Injuries during pregnancy
- Multiple visits to the emergency department
- Elimination disturbances (e.g., constipation, diarrhea)
- Multiple somatic complaints
- Eating disorders
- Substance abuse
- Depression
- Posttraumatic stress disorder
- Self-mutilation
- Suicide attempts
- Feelings of helplessness or hopelessness
- Low self-esteem
- Chronic fatigue
- Apathy
- Sleep disturbances (e.g., hypersomnia, hyposomnia)
- Psychiatric hospitalizations

PERSONAL AND SOCIAL HISTORY

- Feelings of powerlessness
- Feelings of being trapped
- Lack of trust

- Traditional values about home, partner, and children's behavior
- Major decisions in family controlled by one person
- Few social supports (isolated from family, friends)
- Little activity outside the home
- Unwanted or unplanned pregnancy
- Dependency on caregivers
- Extreme jealousy by partner
- Difficulties at school or work
- Short attention span
- Running away
- Promiscuity
- Child who has knowledge of sexual matters beyond that appropriate for age
- Sexualized play with self, peers, dolls, toys
- Masturbation
- Excessive fears and clinging in children
- Verbal aggression
- Themes of violence in artwork and schoolwork
- Distorted body image
- History of chronic physical or psychological disability
- Inability to perform activities of daily living
- Delayed language development

PHYSICAL EXAMINATION FINDINGS

General Appearance

- Fearful, anxious, hyperactive, hypoactive
- Watching partner, parent, or caregiver for approval of answers to your questions
- Poor grooming or inappropriate dress
- Malnourishment
- Signs of stress or fatigue
- Flinching when approached or touched
- Inappropriate or anxious nonverbal behavior
- Wearing clothing inappropriate to the season or occasion to cover body parts

Vital Statistics

- Elevated pulse or blood pressure
- Other signs of autonomic arousal (e.g., exaggerated startle response, excessive sweating)
- Underweight or overweight

Skin

- Bruises, welts, edema, or scars
- Burns (cigarette, immersion, friction from ropes, pattern like an electric iron or stove)

BOX 23.5 (Continued)

- Subdural hematoma
- Missing hair
- Poor skin integrity: dehydration, decubitus ulcers, untreated wounds, urine burns, or excoriation

Eyes
- Orbital swelling
- Conjunctival hemorrhage
- Retinal hemorrhage
- Black eyes
- No glasses to accommodate poor eyesight

Ears
- Hearing loss
- No prosthetic device to accommodate poor hearing

Mouth
- Bruising
- Lacerations
- Missing or broken teeth
- Untreated dental problems

Abdomen
- Abdominal injuries during pregnancy
- Intraabdominal injuries

Genitourinary System or Rectum
- Bruising, lacerations, bleeding, edema, tenderness
- Untreated infections

Musculoskeletal System
- Recent fractures or old fractures in various stages of healing

- Dislocations
- Limited range of motion in extremities
- Contractures

Neurologic System
- Difficulty with speech or swallowing
- Hyperactive reflexes
- Developmental delays
- Areas of numbness
- Tremors

Mental Status
- Anxiety, fear
- Depression
- Suicidal ideation
- Difficulty concentrating
- Memory loss

Medications
- Medications that are not indicated by physical condition
- Overdose of drugs or medications (prescribed or over the counter)
- Medications not taken as prescribed

Communication Patterns and Relations
- Verbal hostility, arguments
- Negative nonverbal communication, lack of visible affection
- One person answers questions and looks to other person for approval
- Extreme dependency of family members

Psychosocial Assessment

Fear

Living with an abusive partner, parent, or caregiver means living with constant fear and uncertainly. Because victims never know what might precipitate an incident of violence, they are constantly hypervigilant and fearful. The back-and-forth nature of the relationship, that is, alternating between love and violence, is confusing, so the survivor may try to do everything possible to please the abuser in an effort to prevent another violent episode.

Low Self-Esteem

Being the victim of abuse is devastating to healthy self-esteem, or feelings of self-acceptance, self-worth, self-love, and self-nurturing. Emotional abuse may be particularly devastating. Victims are criticized, rejected, devaluated, and ignored. Over time, people begin to internalize the negative messages and may come to believe the abuse is deserved. Low self-esteem has been linked to physical and mental health problems, problems with relationships, may affect survivors' ability to achieve financial independence.

Guilt and Shame

A history of abuse is often associated with guilt and shame. Survivors are ashamed of being manipulated and violated and for having put themselves in such a situation. Abusive partners tell the survivors that the abuse is their fault and many victims believe them. Feelings of humiliation and shame prevent survivors from seeking medical care and other forms of support and reporting abuse to authorities. The experience of being battered is so degrading and humiliating that survivors are often afraid to disclose it to anyone. Many fear that they will not be taken seriously or will be blamed for inciting the abuse or for staying with their abusers. Keeping their circumstances secret and maintaining a front of normality places enormous tension and pressure on survivors.

Problems with Intimacy

Abused children, especially those who have experienced child sexual abuse, experience intrusion, abandonment, devaluation, or pain in the relationship with the abuser instead of the closeness and nurturing that are normal for intimate relationships (American Academy of Child & Adolescent Psychiatry [AACAP], 2020). Consequently, intimacy is associated with shame and fear rather than warmth and caring and with concerns about dominance and submission rather than mutuality. Shame, in turn, is associated with being submissive, feeling devalued, and the desire to retaliate against a person who is seen as the source of humiliation. In adulthood, unresolved feelings of shame, as well as symptoms of PTSD or depression, may disrupt the development of intimacy and interfere with the ability to develop and sustain healthy relationships.

Conversely, some survivors of child abuse and child sexual abuse may engage in risky sexual behavior such as early sexual activity (before age 15 years), promiscuity, and prostitution (AACAP, 2020). These behaviors place survivors at risk for developing STDs and HIV. Survivors who engage in this type of behavior may have learned that sexual activity is a means for securing affection, intimacy, or material rewards such as money or drugs.

Revictimization

Many survivors who experienced childhood trauma are revictimized later in life. Numerous factors are related to **revictimization**, including symptoms of PTSD, dissociation, boundary issues, and feelings of self-blame and shame. Internalized stigma, victim-blaming statements, and past negative social reactions from others affect survivors' self-perception and willingness to disclose subsequent abuse (Kennedy & Prock, 2018). People with abuse histories frequently have difficulty with boundaries. During childhood abuse, they experienced frequent boundary violations and associate those violations with intimate relationships. Excessive use of alcohol and other drugs by survivors makes them more vulnerable and less able to defend themselves. Survivors with substance use problems are more likely to enter a relationship with someone who also uses alcohol or other drugs, placing them at risk for substance-related violence. In a recent study, 82% of female prison inmates with substance use issues reported childhood trauma and revictimization after age 18. Substance use problems typically followed traumatic experiences, contributed to behavioral problems in adolescence, and continued to impair their judgment and functioning in adulthood (Mejia et al., 2015).

Social Networks

An evaluation of social networks provides additional clues of psychological abuse and controlling behavior. Having supportive family or friends is crucial in short-term planning for developing a safety plan and is also important to long-term recovery. A survivor cannot leave an abusive situation with nowhere to go. Supportive family and friends may be willing to provide shelter and

safety, as well as emotional support. As part of safety planning, survivors can set up code words to make contacts aware that help is needed, or ask friends to keep belongings or documents that they may require if they leave home quickly.

Social Isolation

Many perpetrators isolate their family from all social contacts, including other relatives. Some survivors isolate themselves because they are ashamed of the abuse or fear nonsupportive responses. Nurses can assess restrictions on freedom that may suggest abuse and control by asking such questions as "Are you free to go where you want?" "Is staying home your choice?" and "Is there anything you would like to do that you cannot?"

Economic and Emotional Dependency

Women who have young children and depend on the perpetrator financially may believe that they cannot leave the abusive relationship. Those who are emotionally dependent on the perpetrator may experience an intense grief reaction that further complicates their leaving. Older adults and children often depend on the abuser and cannot leave the abusive situation without workable alternatives.

Clinical Judgment

Violence and abuse are critical situations that need to be addressed immediately. The nurse should focus on the individual's personal safety first and any injuries that have occurred.

Mental Health Nursing Interventions

The goals of all nursing interventions in cases of violence are to prevent injury, stop the violence, ensure the survivor's safety, and restore health.

As appropriate concerning age and ability, nursing interventions should empower survivors to act on their own behalf. This must be done in a collaborative partnership. Nurses must be willing to offer support and information and not impose their own values on survivors by encouraging them to leave abusive relationships (Campbell et al., 2009). Strong psychological and economic bonds tie many survivors to their perpetrators. Moreover, adult survivors who are capable of making decisions are the experts about their situations. They are the best judges to determine the appropriate time to leave a relationship.

Intervention strategies for older adults depend on whether the individual accepts or refuses assistance and whether they can make decisions. If the person refuses treatment, it is important to remain nonjudgmental and provide information about available services and emergency contact information. If the older adult appears incapable of making decisions, then guardianship, foster care, or nursing home placement may be needed. The nurse should initiate a referral to a case manager or others who can facilitate further intervention.

Safety Planning

One of the most important interventions when caring for individuals who are in an ongoing abusive relationship is to help survivors develop a safety plan (Domestic Violence Resource Center, 2018). The first step in developing such a plan is helping the survivor recognize the signs of danger. Changes in tone of voice, substance use, and increased criticism may indicate that the perpetrator is losing control. Detecting early warning signs helps survivors to escape before battering begins.

The next step is to devise the escape. For families at risk for violence, this may involve mapping the house for an escape route. The IPV survivor needs to have a bag packed and hidden but readily accessible that includes what is needed to get away. Important things to pack are clothes, a set of car and house keys, bank account numbers, birth certificate, insurance policies and numbers, marriage license, valuable jewelry, important telephone numbers, and money. If children are involved, the adult survivor should make arrangements to get them out safely. That might include arranging a signal to indicate when it is safe for them to leave the house and to meet at a prearranged place.

A safety plan for a child or dependent older adult might include safe places to hide and important telephone numbers, including 911 and those of the police and fire departments and other family members and friends.

Physical Health Interventions

Treatment of trauma symptoms may include cleaning and dressing burns or other wounds and assisting with setting and casting broken bones. Malnourished and dehydrated children and older adults may require nursing interventions such as intravenous therapy or nutritional supplements that alleviate the alteration in nutrition and fluid and electrolyte imbalances. Victims of sexual assault require additional considerations (see Box 23.5).

KEYCONCEPT Individuals who are experiencing IPV need their basic needs met (e.g., safety, housing, food, child care) before their psychological traumas can be addressed.

Promoting Healthy Daily Activity

Teaching sleep hygiene (i.e., practices conducive to healthy sleep patterns) and promoting exercise, leisure

time, and nutrition will help battered survivors regain a healthy physical state and self-care activities. Taking care of themselves may be difficult for survivors who have spent years trying to separate themselves from their bodies (dissociate) to survive years of abuse. Techniques such as going to bed and arising at consistent times, avoiding naps and caffeine, and scheduling periods for relaxation just before retiring may be useful in promoting sleep (Pigeon et al., 2009). Aerobic exercise is a useful technique for relieving anxiety and depression and promoting sleep.

Managing Care of Patients with Mental Health or Substance Abuse Issues

Survivors of abuse and sexual assault, and those in abusive relationships, may experience depression, anxiety, and posttraumatic stress. These disorders interfere with cognitive processes—including judgment, decision-making, and problem-solving—and impede healing even after the survivor is in a safe environment. Trauma-informed cognitive-behavioral therapy and interpersonal therapy specifically targeting psychological consequences of IPV are the most effective treatments for survivors (Arroyo et al., 2017). Refer the survivor to a qualified mental health provider for treatment.

Survivors who have a substance use disorder need referral to a treatment center for such disorders. The treatment center should have programs that address the special needs of survivors. Alcohol- and drug-dependent survivors frequently stop treatment and return to previous dysfunctional use patterns if their violence-related problems are not addressed appropriately (Ullman & Sigurvinsdottir, 2015). Survivors who are impaired by substances are at high risk for HIV infection and other infectious diseases. If survivors do not know their HIV status, they should be encouraged to get tested.

Psychosocial Interventions

Several issues must be addressed for survivors including guilt, shame, and stigmatization. These issues can be approached in several ways. Assisting survivors to verbalize their experience in an accepting nonjudgmental atmosphere is the first step. Directly challenging attributions of self-blame for the abuse and feelings of being dirty and different is another. Helping survivors to identify their strengths and validating thoughts and feelings may help to increase their self-esteem.

Working with Children

Children may need to learn a "violence vocabulary" that allows them to talk about their abuse and assign responsibility for abusive behavior. Children also need to learn that violence is not okay, and it is not their fault. Allowing children to discuss their abuse in the safety of a supportive, caring relationship may alleviate anxiety and fear. Respond to children's disclosures with sensitivity, belief, and a calm demeanor. Avoid pressuring children to talk or share details if they are uncomfortable (Ramamoorthy & Myers-Walls, 2013).

Reenacting the abuse through play is another technique that may be helpful in assisting children to express and work through their anxiety and fear. Play therapy uses dolls, human or animal figures, video games, or puppets to work through anxiety or fears. Other techniques include reading stories about recovery from abusive experiences (literal or metaphoric), using art or music to express feelings, and psychodrama. In addition, teaching strategies to manage fear and anxiety, such as relaxation techniques, coping skills, and imagery, may give the children an added sense of mastering their fear (National Child Traumatic Stress Network, n.d.).

Managing Anger

Anger and rage are part of the healing process for survivors. Expression of intense anger is uncomfortable for many nurses. However, anger expression should be expected from the survivor, so it is necessary to develop comfortable ways to respond. Moreover, an important nursing intervention is teaching and modeling anger expression appropriately. Inappropriate expressions of anger might drive supportive people away. Anger management techniques include appropriately recognizing and labeling anger and expressing it assertively rather than aggressively or passive-aggressively. Assertive ways of expressing anger include owning the feeling by using "I feel" statements and avoiding blaming others. Teaching anger management and conflict resolution may be especially important for children who have seen nothing but violence to resolve problems.

Coping with Anxiety

Anxiety management is a crucial intervention for all survivors. A high comorbidity exists involving trauma, PTSD, and anxiety disorders. During treatment, survivors experience situations and memories that provoke intense anxiety and must know how to soothe themselves when they experience painful feelings. Moreover, most survivors struggle with control issues, especially involving their bodies. Anxiety management skills offer one way to maintain some control over their bodies and choices. See Chapter 16.

Finding Strength and Hope

Providing hope and a sense of control is fundamental for survivors of trauma. Help survivors find hope by assisting them to identify specific strengths and aspects of their lives that are under their control. This type of intervention may empower survivors to find options other than remaining in an abusive relationship. Interventions that focus on empowerment encourage and create opportunities for survivors to make decisions about their lives, thereby restoring a sense of autonomy and competence lost in the abusive environment (Wood, 2015).

Psychoeducation

Other nursing interventions include teaching self-protection skills, healthy relationship skills, and healthy sexuality (Box 23.6). Again, this teaching may be especially important for children who have no role models for healthy relationships. Children also need to know what constitutes controlling and abusive behavior and how to get help for abuse. Survivors also need information about resources, such as shelters for battered women, legal services, government benefits, and support networks. Before giving the survivor any written material, first discuss the possibility that if the perpetrator were to find the information in the survivor's possession, they might use it as an excuse for further battering.

Family Interventions

Family interventions in cases of child abuse focus on behavioral approaches to improve parenting skills. A behavioral approach has multiple components. *Child management skills* help parents manage maladaptive behaviors and reward appropriate behaviors. *Parenting skills* teach parents how to be more effective and nurturing with their children. *Leisure skills* training is important to reduce stress in the household and promote healthy family time. *Household organization* training is another way to reduce stress by teaching effective ways to manage

---

BOX 23.6

Abuse

When caring for the patient who has been abused, be sure to address the following topics in the teaching plan:
• Cycle of violence
• Access to shelters
• Legal services
• Government benefits
• Support network
• Symptoms of anxiety, dissociation, and PTSD
• Safety or escape plan
• Relaxation
• Adequate nutrition and exercise
• Sleep hygiene
• HIV testing and counseling

the multiple tasks that families must perform. Such tasks include meal planning, cooking, shopping, keeping health care providers' appointments (e.g., dental care, health visits, counseling) appointments, and planning family activities (National Center for Parent, Family and Community Engagement, 2015).

Anger control and stress management skills are important parts of behavioral programs for families. Anger control programs teach parents to identify events that increase anger and stress and to replace anger-producing thoughts with more appropriate ones. Parents learn self-control skills to reduce the expression of uncontrolled anger. Stress-reduction techniques include relaxation techniques and methods for coping with stressful interactions with their children.

Community Involvement

Nurses may be involved in interventions to reduce violence at the community level. Many abusive caregivers, parents, and guardians, as well because battered partners, older adults, and children are socially isolated. Developing support networks may help reduce stress and therefore reduce abuse. Community contacts vary for each abuser and survivor but might include crisis hotlines, support groups, and education classes.

Nurses may also make home visits. Home visits provide support to families and provide them with knowledge about stress and management. Abuse of any kind creates a volatile situation, so nurses may be putting themselves or the survivor in danger if they do make home visits. Carefully assess this possibility before proceeding. If necessary, arrange a safe place to meet the survivor instead.

Evaluation and Treatment Outcomes

Evaluation and outcome criteria depend on the setting for interventions. For instance, if a survivor is encountered in the emergency department, successful outcomes might be that injuries are appropriately managed and the patient's immediate safety is ensured. For long-term care, outcome criteria and evaluation might center on ending abusive relationships. Examples of other outcome criteria that would indicate successful nursing interventions are recognizing that one is not to blame for the violence, demonstrating knowledge of strengths and coping skills, and reestablishing social networks.

Evaluation of nursing care for abused children depends on attaining goals mutually set with the parents or guardians. An end to all violence is the optimal outcome criterion; however, attainment of smaller goals indicates progress toward that end. Outcomes such as increased problem-solving and communication skills within the family, increased self-esteem in both children and parents, and increased use of nonphysical forms of discipline may all indicate progress toward the total elimination of child abuse.

Follow-up efforts are important in evaluating the outcomes of elder abuse. The optimal outcome is to end all abuse and keep the older adults in their own living environment, if appropriate. Although the abuse may have been resolved temporarily, it may flare up again. Ongoing support for the caregiver and assistance with caregiving tasks may be necessary if the older adult is to remain at home. Nursing home or assisted living may be the only desirable option if the burden is too great for the family and the likelihood of ongoing abuse or neglect is high.

Another important outcome of nursing intervention with survivors is appropriate treatment of any disorder resulting from abuse (e.g., acute stress disorder, PTSD, anxiety disorders, dissociative identity disorder [DID], major depression, substance abuse). Follow-up nursing assessments should monitor symptom reduction or exacerbation, adherence to any medication regimen, and side effects of medication. The ultimate outcome is to end violence and enable the survivor to return to a more productive, safe, and nurturing life without being continually haunted by memories of the abuse.

Nurses must become accustomed to measuring gains in small steps when working with survivors. Making any changes in significant relationships has serious consequences and can be done only when the adult survivor is ready. It is easy to become angry or discouraged with survivors, so it is important not to communicate such feelings. Discussing such feelings with other staff provides a way of dealing with them appropriately. In such discussions with supervisors or other staff, it is imperative to protect the survivor's confidentiality by discussing feelings around issues, not particular individuals, in order to ensure that survivors cannot be identified.

TREATMENT FOR THE ABUSER

Participants in programs that treat abusers are usually present only because the court has mandated the treatment. Programs are often outpatient groups that meet weekly for an extended period, often 36 to 48 weeks. Some programs advocate longer programs, believing that chronic offenders require from 1 to 5 years of treatment to change abusive behavior. States vary on requiring that treatment programs for abusers contact partners.

Interventions must be culturally sensitive. Many factors can affect violence against others, including socioeconomic status, racial or ethnic identity, country of origin, and sexual orientation; those differences must be addressed. When applicable, intervention programs may require abusers to undergo substance abuse treatment concurrently, so patients are required to remain sober and to submit to random drug testing.

SUMMARY OF KEY POINTS

- The most common type of abuse results from domestic violence.

- IPV is a significant public health problem; it includes physical violence, sexual violence, stalking, and psychological aggression.

- IPV crosses all ethnic, racial, and socioeconomic lines. Women are more likely to be injured or killed by current or former intimate partners than by any other perpetrators.

- Stalking is repeated unwanted contact, attention, and harassment that increase in frequency.

- Child maltreatment includes child abuse (i.e., overt actions that cause harm, potential or threat of harm) and child neglect (i.e., failure to provide needs or to protect from harm or potential harm).

- Older adults may also be physically, emotionally, and sexually abused or neglected. The most common type of elder abuse is economic.

- Among the many theories that have been proposed to explain violence are neurologic problems, psychopathology, alcohol and other drug abuse, intergenerational transmission of violence, and economic and community factors

- A well-documented cycle of violence consists of three phases of increasing frequency and severity.

- Nurses need to be familiar with signs and symptoms of abuse and to be vigilant when assessing patients.

- Nurses need to be nonjudgmental when caring for a victim of abuse. Many reasons a person could cause a person to remain in an abusive situation.

- Nursing interventions include physical health interventions and psychosocial interventions that focus on helping victims identify their strengths and validating thoughts and feelings.

Unfolding Patient Stories: Sandra Littlefield

Part 2

 Recall from Chapter 2 Sandra Littlefield with borderline personality disorder. She has a history of unstable relationships, several divorces, prostitution, poor impulse control, drug and alcohol abuse, anxiety, cutting, and suicide attempts. The nurse ascertains that she was sexually abused as a child. What factors in her history are suggestive of abuse? Describe areas of a psychosocial assessment associated with her behaviors. What nursing interventions and education can help promote her mental health stability?

CRITICAL THINKING CHALLENGES

1. Abuse is a pervasive problem, in which anyone can be a victim (e.g., women, men, children, older adults, gays, lesbians). Why do so few nursing units and nurses make it routine to ask questions about abuse?

2. Abuse is not just a "women's issue". The prevalence of abuse might decrease if men make it a "men's issue" as well. What is preventing this from happening?

3. What are your thoughts and feelings about women who are victims of violence in which both partners (victim and perpetrator) abuse alcohol and other drugs?

4. What are your thoughts and feelings about women who will not leave an abusive relationship?

5. What are some reasons that people remain in abusive relationships?

6. Why do some survivors become involved in more than one abusive relationship?

7. How do you handle your feelings toward abusive parents or relatives who abuse older adults?

8. What are the issues in mandatory reporting of violence toward women, particularly violence?

9. Would your thoughts, feelings, and ability to intervene change if the violent relationship is between same-sex partners?

Movie Viewing Guides

Once Were Warriors: 1994. A mother of 5 children reevaluates her 18-year marriage to her alcoholic, hot-tempered husband when his barroom violence tragically encroaches into their home life. Produced and filmed in New Zealand, this film also presents how urbanization has undermined the culture and strength of the indigenous Maori people.

VIEWING POINTS: What evidence can you find in this film that may reflect intergenerational transmission of violence? In what ways do you think that culture can influence attitudes toward abuse (both positive and negative)? What are positive and negative cultural influences in this film?

Sybil: 1976. Sally Field plays Sybil, a woman who experiences DID after suffering horrible abuse during childhood. Help from a psychiatrist (Joanne Woodward) uncovers the memories that have led to the splitting of Sybil's personality. The movie contains harrowing scenes of the abuse Sybil experienced.

VIEW INTS: What symptoms does Sybil show in the film? How does the psychiatrist work with Sybil's different personalities in this film?

Enough: 2002. Jennifer Lopez stars as a blue-collar beauty (Slim Hiller) who marries the really wrong guy. Eventually, she discovers his philandering and spends the rest of the movie in a nomadic flight from his hot-tempered brutality. Bankrolled by her estranged father, she protects her young daughter. Knowing she must face the inevitable showdown, she turns to self-defense courses for empowerment.

VIEWING POINTS: When did Slim and Mitch's relationship turn destructive? What are the characteristics of an abused partner displayed by Slim? What were Mitch Hiller's primary motives in stalking Slim?

REFERENCES

Afifi, T. O., Mota, N., Sareen, J., & MacMillan, H. L. (2017). The relationships between harsh physical punishment and child maltreatment in childhood and intimate partner violence in adulthood. *BMC public health*, 17(1), 493. https://doi.org/10.1186/s12889-017-4359-8

Alhusen, J. L., Sharps, R. E., & Bullock, L. (2015). Intimate partner violence during pregnancy: Maternal and neonatal outcomes. *Journal of Women's Health*, 24(1), 100–106.

American Academy of Child & Adolescent Psychiatry. (2020). Sexual abuse. https://www.aacap.org/AACAP/Families_and_Youth/Facts_for_Families/FFF-Guide/Child-Sexual-Abuse-009.aspx

Arroyo, K., Lundahl, B., Butters, R., Vanderoo, M., & Wood, D.S. (2017). Short-term interventions for survivors of intimate partner violence: A systematic review and meta-analysis. *Trauma, Violence, & Abuse*, 18(2), 155–171.

Bureau of Justice Statistics. (n.d.). UCR offense definitions. https://www.bjs.gov/ucrdata/offenses.cfm

Burgess, S., & Tavakoli, A. (2005). Psychometric Assessment of the Burgess-Partner Abuse Scale for Teens (B-PAST). *Aquichan*, 5(1), 96–107.

Campbell, J., & Humphreys, J. (Eds.). (1993). *Nursing care of survivors of family violence*. Mosby.

Campbell, J. C., Webster, D. W., & Glass, N. (2009). The danger assessment: Validation of a lethality risk assessment instrument for intimate partner femicide. *Journal of Interpersonal Violence*, 24(4), 653–674.

Cavner, J. (2019). Recommendations for intimate partner violence screening and interventions. *Women's Healthcare: A Clinical Journal for NPs*, 7(1), 44–47.

Centers for Disease Control and Prevention. (2019). Intimate partner violence: Risk and protective factors. National Center for Injury Prevention and Control, Division of Prevention. https://www.cdc.gov/violenceprevention/intimatepartnerviolence/riskprotectivefactors.html

Centers for Disease Control and Prevention. (2020a). Preventing teen dating violence. National Center for Injury Prevention and Control, Division of Prevention. https://www.cdc.gov/violenceprevention/intimatepartnerviolence/teendatingviolence/fastfact.html

Centers for Disease Control and Prevention. (2020b). Child abuse and neglect. National Center for Injury Prevention and Control, Division of Violence Prevention. https://www.cdc.gov/violenceprevention/childabuseandneglect/index.html

Centers for Disease Control and Prevention. (2020c). Preventing elder abuse. National Center for Injury Prevention and Control, Division of Violence Prevention. https://www.cdc.gov/violenceprevention/pdf/elder/EA_Factsheet.pdf

Child Welfare Information Gateway. (2016). *Child witnesses to domestic violence*. U.S. Department of Health and Human Services, Children's Bureau.

Copp, J. C., Giordano, P. C., Longmore, M. A., & Manning, W. D. (2016). The development of attitudes towards intimate partner violence: An examination of key correlates among a sample of young adults. *Journal of Interpersonal Violence*. https://doi.org/10.1177/0886260516651311

Delgadillo, D. (2017). When there is no sexual assault nurse examiner: Emergency nursing care for female adult sexual assault patients. *Journal of Emergency Nursing*, 43(4), 308–315.

Domestic Violence Resource Center. (2018). Safety planning. Retrieved from https://www.dvrc-or.org/safety-planning/

England, D. C. (2020). *The history of marital rape laws*. Criminal Defense Lawyer. https://www.criminaldefenselawyer.com/resources/criminal-defense/crime-penalties/marital-rape.htm

Kennedy, A. C., & Prock, K. A. (2018). "I still feel like I am not normal": A review of the role of stigma and stigmatization among female survivors of child sexual abuse, sexual assault, and intimate partner violence. *Trauma, Violence, and Abuse*, 19(5), 512–527.

Lippy, C., Jumarali, S. N., Nnawulezi, N. A., Williams, E. P., & Burk, C. (2020). The impact of mandatory reporting laws on survivors of intimate partner violence: Intersectionality, help-seeking and the need for change. *Journal of Family Violence* 35, 255–267. https://doi.org/10.1007/s10896-019-00103-w

Mejia, B., Zea, P., Romero, M., & Saldivar, G. (2015). Traumatic experiences and re-victimization of female inmates undergoing treatment for substance abuse. *Substance Abuse Treatment, Prevention, and Policy*, 10(5). https://doi.org/10.1186/1747-597X-10-5

Messing, J. T., Campbell, J. C., & Snider, C. (2017). Validation and adaptation of the Danger Assessment-5: A brief intimate partner violence risk assessment. *Journal of Advanced Nursing*, 73(12), 3220–3230.

Namy, S., Carlson, C., O'Hara, K., Nakuti, J., Bukuluki, P., Lwanyaaga, J., Namakula, S., Nanyunja, B., Wainberg, M. L., Naker, D., & Michau, L. (2017). Towards a feminist understanding of intersecting violence against women and children in the family. *Social Science & Medicine (1982)*, 184, 40–48. https://doi.org/10.1016/j.socscimed.2017.04.042

National Center for Parent, Family and Community Engagement. (2015). *Compendium of parenting interventions*. National Center on Parent, Family, and Community Engagement, Office of Head Start, U.S. Department of Health & Human Services.

National Center for Victims of Crime. (n.d.). *2018 NCVRW Resource Guide: Intimate Partner Violence Fact Sheet*. https://ovc.ojp.gov/sites/g/files/xyckuh226/files/ncvrw2018/info_flyers/fact_sheets/2018NCVRW_IPV_508_QC.pdf

National Child Traumatic Stress Network. (n.d.). *Interventions*. https://www.nctsn.org/what-is-child-trauma/trauma-types/intimate-partner-violence/interventions

National Coalition against Domestic Violence. (n.d.). Why do victims stay? https://ncadv.org/why-do-victims-stay

Office on Women's Health, U.S. Department of Health and Human Services. (2019). Relationships and safety: Effects of violence against women. https://www.womenshealth.gov/relationships-and-safety/effects-violence-against-women

Ogunsiji, O. & Clisdell, E. (2017). Intimate partner violence prevention and reduction: A review of literature. *Health Care for Women International*, 38(5), 439–462.

Peterson, C., Kearns, M. C., McIntosh, W. L., Estefan, L. F., Nicolaidis, C., McCollister, K. E., & Florence, C. (2018). Lifetime economic burden of intimate partner violence among U.S. adults. *American Journal of Preventive Medicine*, 55(4), 433–444.

Pigeon, W., May, P., Perlis, M., Ward, E., Lu, N., & Talbot, N. (2009). The effect of interpersonal psychotherapy for depression on insomnia symptoms in a cohort of women with sexual abuse histories. *Journal of Traumatic Stress*, 22(6), 634–648.

Pomerance, B. (2015). Finding the middle ground on a slippery slope: Balancing autonomy and protection in mandatory reporting of elder abuse. *Marquette Benefits and Social Welfare Law Review*, 16(2), 436–490.

Power, C. (2017). Domestic violence: What can nurses do? *Alabama Nurse*, 44(4), 18–20.

Ramamoorthy, S., & Myers-Walls, J. A. (2013). Talking to a child who has been abused. https://familynurture.org/resources-from-family-nurturing-center/talking-child-abused/

Ramaswamy, A., Ranji, U., & Salganicoff, A. (2020, June 11). *Finding policy responses to rising intimate partner violence during the coronavirus outbreak*. Kaiser Family Foundation.

Ramsey, C. B. (2011). Domestic violence and state intervention in the American West and Australia, 1860–1930. *Indiana Law Journal*, 86(185), 186–255.

Rempel, E., Donelle, L., Hall, J., & Rodger. S. (2019). Intimate partner violence: A review of online interventions. *Informatics for Health and Social Care*, 44, 204–219. https://doi.org/10.1080/17538157.2018.1433675

Smith, S. G., Zhang, X., Basile, K. C., Merrick, M. T., Wang, J., Kresnow, M., & Chen, J. (2018). *National Intimate Partner and Sexual Violence Survey: 2015 Data Brief*. https://www.cdc.gov/violenceprevention/datasources/nisvs/2015NISVSdatabrief.html

Ullman, S. E., & Sigurvinsdottir, R. (2015). Intimate partner violence and drinking among victims of adult sexual assault. *Journal of Aggression, Maltreatment & Trauma*, 24(2), 117–130.

U.S. Preventive Services Task Force. (2018). *Final recommendation statement: Intimate partner violence, elder abuse, and abuse of vulnerable adults: Screening*. https://www.uspreventiveservicestaskforce.org/Page/Document/UpdateSummaryFinal/intimate-partner-violence-and-abuse-of-elderly-and-vulnerable-adults-screening

Violence Policy Center. (2019). When men murder women: An analysis of 2017 homicide data. https://vpc.org/studies/wmmw2019.pdf

Wood, L. (2015). Hoping, empowering, strengthening: Theories used in intimate partner violence advocacy. *Journal of Women and Social Work*, 30(3), 286–301.

Yaffe, M. (2010). Detection and reporting of elder abuse. *Family Medicine*, 42(2), 481–486.

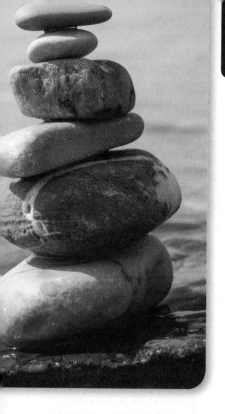

24

Schizophrenia and Related Disorders

Nursing Care of Persons with Thought Disorders

Andrea C. Bostrom

KEYCONCEPTS

- disorganized symptoms
- delusions
- hallucinations
- negative symptoms
- neurocognitive symptoms
- positive symptoms
- psychosis

LEARNING OBJECTIVES

After studying this chapter, you will be able to:

1. Identify key symptoms of schizophrenia.

2. Analyze theories relevant to schizophrenia.

3. Develop strategies to establish a patient-centered, recovery-oriented therapeutic relationship with a person with schizophrenia.

4. Apply a person-centered, recovery-oriented nursing process for patients with schizophrenia.

5. Identify medications used to treat people with schizophrenia and evaluate their effectiveness.

6. Identify and evaluate expected outcomes of nursing care for persons with schizophrenia.

7. Develop wellness strategies for persons with schizophrenia.

8. Differentiate the type of mental health care provided in emergency care, inpatient-focused care, community care, and virtual mental health care.

9. Discuss the importance of integrated health care.

10. Discuss other common schizophrenia spectrum disorders.

KEY TERMS

- Affective lability • Aggression • Agitation • Agranulocytosis • Akathisia • Alogia • Ambivalence • Anhedonia
- Apathy • Autistic thinking • Avolition • Catatonia • Catatonic excitement • Circumstantiality • Clang association
- Command hallucinations • Cholinergic rebound • Concrete thinking • Confused speech and thinking • Delusions
- Echolalia • Echopraxia • Extrapyramidal side effects • Flight of ideas • Gut–brain axis • Hallucinations
- Hypervigilance • Hypofrontality • Illusions • Loose associations • Metonymic speech • Neologisms • Neuroleptic malignant syndrome • Oculogyric crisis • Paranoia • Pressured speech • Prodromal • Psychosis • Referential thinking
- Regressed behavior • Retrocollis • Stereotypy • Stilted language • Tangentiality • Tardive dyskinesia • Torticollis
- Verbigeration • Waxy flexibility • Word salad

Case Study

Arnold, a 53-year-old man who was diagnosed with paranoid schizophrenia at an early age, had been living on the family farm for the last 30 years with his mother. After his mother's death, the farm was to be sold and divided among the siblings, who arranged for Arnold to move to town. Arnold became agitated and threatening and refused to believe that his parents had died and that he would have to leave the farm.

INTRODUCTION

These fascinating schizophrenia spectrum disorders have confounded scientists and philosophers for centuries. Schizophrenia spectrum disorders are among the most severe mental illnesses; they are found in all cultures, races, and socioeconomic groups. Their symptoms have been attributed to possession by demons, considered punishment by gods for evils done, or accepted as evidence of the inhumanity of its sufferers. These explanations have resulted in enduring stigma for people diagnosed with these disorders. Today, the stigma persists, although it has less to do with demonic possession than with society's unwillingness to shoulder the costs associated with housing, treatment, and rehabilitation. All nurses need to understand these disorders.

SCHIZOPHRENIA SPECTRUM DISORDERS OVERVIEW

The schizophrenia spectrum disorders include schizophrenia, schizoaffective, delusional and schizotypal disorders, brief psychotic disorder, schizophreniform disorder, and substance-medication-induced psychotic disorder (American Psychiatric Association [APA], 2013). Schizophrenia is the highlighted disorder in this chapter because it has a broad range of symptoms that are found in other schizophrenia spectrum disorders. A discussion of other disorders follows the content on schizophrenia. Schizotypal disorders will be discussed in Chapter 30.

Central to understanding the problems of persons with schizophrenia spectrum disorders is the concept of **psychosis**, a term used to describe a state in which an individual experiences positive symptoms of schizophrenia, also known as psychotic symptoms (e.g., **hallucinations**; **delusions**; disorganized thoughts, speech, or behavior).

> **KEYCONCEPT Psychosis,** a state in which a person experiences hallucinations, delusions, or disorganized thoughts, speech, or behavior, is the key diagnostic factor in schizophrenia spectrum disorders.

SCHIZOPHRENIA

In the late 1800s, Emil Kraepelin first described the course of the disorder he called *dementia praecox* because of its early onset and notable changes in an individual's cognitive functioning. In the early 1900s, Eugen Bleuler renamed the disorder *schizophrenia*, meaning *split minds*, and began to determine that there was not just one type of schizophrenia but rather a group of schizophrenias. More recently, Kurt Schneider differentiated behaviors associated with schizophrenia as "first rank" symptoms (e.g., psychotic delusions, hallucinations) and "second rank" symptoms (i.e., all other experiences and behaviors associated with the disorder). These pioneering physicians had a great influence on the current diagnostic conceptualizations of schizophrenia that emphasize the heterogeneity of the disorder in terms of symptoms, course of illness, and positive and negative symptoms.

Clinical Course

Schizophrenia robs people of mental health and imposes social stigma. People with schizophrenia struggle to maintain control of their symptoms, which affect every aspect of their lives. The person with schizophrenia displays various interrelated symptoms and experiences and cognitive deficits in several areas.

Because schizophrenia is a disorder of thoughts, perceptions, and behavior, it is sometimes not recognized as an illness by the person experiencing the symptoms. Many people with thought disorders do not believe that they have a mental illness. Their denial of mental illness and the need for treatment poses problems for the family and clinicians. Ideally, in lucid moments, patients recognize that their thoughts are really delusions, that their perceptions are hallucinations, and that their behavior is disorganized. In reality, many patients do not believe that they have a mental illness but agree to treatment to please family and clinicians.

The natural progression of schizophrenia is usually described as a chronic illness that deteriorates over time and with an eventual plateau in the symptoms. Only for older adults with schizophrenia has it been suggested that improvement might occur. In reality, no one really knows what the course of schizophrenia would be if patients were able to adhere to a treatment regimen throughout their lives. Only recently have medications become relatively effective, with manageable side effects. The clinical picture of schizophrenia is complex; individuals differ from one another, and the experience for a single individual may vary from episode to episode.

Prodromal Period

A **prodromal period** (stage of early changes that are a precursor to the disorder) may begin in early childhood. More than half of patients report the following **prodromal** symptoms: tension and nervousness, lack of interest in eating, difficulty concentrating, disturbed sleep, decreased enjoyment and loss of interest, restlessness, forgetfulness, depression, social withdrawal from friends, feeling laughed at, more thinking about religion, feeling bad for no reason, feeling too excited, and hearing voices or seeing things (Jaaro-Peled & Sawa, 2020; Liu et al., 2019a). The benefit of discovering the presence of symptoms early, before they have solidified into a major disorder, is that treatment might be initiated earlier.

Acute Illness

Initially, the behaviors of this illness may be both confusing and frightening to the individual and the family. The symptoms of acute illness usually occur in late adolescence or early adulthood. The behaviors may be subtle; however, at some point they become so disruptive or bizarre that they can no longer be overlooked. These might include episodes of staying up all night for several nights, incoherent conversations, or aggressive acts against oneself or others. For example, one patient's parents reported their son walking around the apartment for several days holding his arms and hands as if they were a machine gun, pointing them at his parents and siblings, and saying "rat-a-tat-tat, you're dead." Another father described his son's first delusional–hallucinatory episode as so convincing that it was frightening. His son began visiting cemeteries and making "mind contact" with the deceased. He saw his deceased grandmother walking around in the home and was certain that pipe bombs were hidden in objects in his home.

As symptoms worsen, patients are less and less able to care for their basic needs (e.g., eating, sleeping, bathing). Substance use is common. Functioning at school or work deteriorates. Dependence on family and friends increases, so those individuals recognize the patients' need for treatment. In the acute phase, individuals afflicted by schizophrenia are at high risk for suicide. Patients may be hospitalized to protect themselves or others.

Initial treatment focuses on alleviation of symptoms through beginning therapy with medications, decreasing the risk of suicide through safety measures, normalizing sleep, and reducing substance use. Functional deficits persist during this period, so the patient and family must begin to learn to cope with these deficits. Emotional blunting diminishes the ability and desire to engage in hobbies, vocational activities, and relationships. Limited participation in social activities spirals into numerous skill deficits, such as difficulty engaging others interpersonally. Cognitive deficits lead to problems recognizing patterns in situations and transferring learning and behaviors from one circumstance to a similar one.

Stabilization

After the initial diagnosis of schizophrenia and initiation of treatment, stabilization of symptoms becomes the focus. Symptoms become less acute but may still be present. Treatment is intense during this period as medication regimens are established, and patients and their families begin to adjust to the idea of a family member having a long-term severe mental illness. Ideally, the use of substances is eliminated. Socialization with others begins to increase, so that rehabilitation begins.

Recovery

The ultimate goal is recovery. For individuals with a severe mental illness like schizophrenia, this will entail learning to live as well as possible with the illness and its symptoms (Cripps & Hood, 2020). Medication generally diminishes the symptoms and allows the person to work toward recovery. However, no medication will cure schizophrenia. As with any chronic illness, following a therapeutic regime will help the individual to live as well as possible with the illness. Living well with schizophrenia requires the patient, family, and providers to work toward acceptance of the illness while offering hope for the best possible outcomes, encouraging autonomy with personal and reasonable goal setting, decreasing self-stigma while creating a positive self-image, finding ways to extract pleasure from life, and creating and maintaining social connections with families and peers (Cripps & Hood, 2020). This can be partially obtained by maintaining a healthy lifestyle, managing the stresses of life, and developing meaningful interpersonal relationships. Family support and involvement are extremely important at this time. After the initial diagnosis has been made, patients and families must be educated to anticipate and expect relapse and know how to cope with it.

Relapses

Relapses can occur at any time during treatment and recovery. They are very detrimental to the successful management of this disorder. Relapse is not inevitable; however, it occurs with sufficient regularity to be a major concern in the treatment of schizophrenia. With each relapse, a longer period of time is needed to recover. Combining medications and psychosocial treatment greatly diminishes the severity and frequency of recurrent relapses (Ceraso et al., 2020; Lauriello & Perkins, 2019).

One major reason for relapse is failure to take medication consistently. Even with newer medications, adherence continues to be a challenge (Chang et al., 2019). Discontinuing medications will almost certainly lead to a relapse (Dufort & Zipursky, 2019). Lower relapse rates are found, for the most part, among groups who carefully follow a treatment regimen.

Many other factors trigger relapse. Impairment in cognition and coping leaves patients vulnerable to stressors. Limited accessibility of community resources, such as public transportation, housing, entry-level and low-stress employment, and limited social services, leaves individuals without access to social support. Income supports that can buffer the day-to-day stressors of living may be inadequate. The degree of stigmatization that the community holds for mental illness attacks the self-concept of patients. Social isolation and the level of responsiveness from family members, friends, and supportive others (e.g., peers and professionals) when patients need assistance also have an impact.

Consider Arnold

Recall that Arnold's relapse was triggered by his mother's death and being forced to leave the family farm.

Diagnostic Criteria

Schizophrenia is characterized by positive and negative symptoms that are present for a significant portion of a 1-month period but with continuous signs of disturbance persisting for at least 6 months (APA, 2013). We define **positive symptoms** as hallucinations and delusions and **negative symptoms** as diminished emotional expression and **avolition** (lack of interest or motivation in goal-directed behavior, such as getting dressed and going to work or school). See Key Diagnostic Characteristics 24.1.

Positive Symptoms of Schizophrenia

Positive symptoms can be thought of as excessive or distorted thoughts and perceptions that occur within the individual but are not experienced by others. Hallucinations and delusions are positive symptoms of schizophrenia. An easy way to remember the difference between hallucinations and delusions is that hallucinations involve one or more of the five senses. Delusions involve only thoughts.

A fairly common hallucination is a command hallucination, that is, an auditory hallucination instructing the patient to act in a certain way, because voices are telling the person to do something. **Command hallucinations** range from innocuous (eat all of your dinner) to very serious (hurt someone or jump in front of a bus).

> **KEYCONCEPT Positive symptoms** reflect an excess or distortion of normal functions, including delusions and hallucinations (APA, 2013).

> **KEYCONCEPT Hallucinations** are perceptual experiences that occur without actual external sensory stimuli. They can involve any of the five senses, but they are usually *visual* or *auditory*. Auditory hallucinations are more common than visual ones. For example, the patient may hear voices carrying on a discussion about their own thoughts or behaviors.

> **KEYCONCEPT Delusions** are erroneous, fixed, false beliefs that cannot be changed by reasonable argument. They usually involve a misinterpretation of experience. For example, the patient believes someone is reading their thoughts or plotting against them. Various types of delusions include the following:
>
> - *Grandiose:* the belief that one has exceptional powers, wealth, skill, influence, or destiny
> - *Nihilistic:* the belief that one is dead or a calamity is impending
> - *Persecutory:* the belief that one is being watched, ridiculed, harmed, or plotted against
> - *Somatic:* beliefs about abnormalities in bodily functions or structures

Negative Symptoms of Schizophrenia

The term *negative symptoms* is used to describe emotions and behaviors that should be present but are diminished in persons with schizophrenia. Negative symptoms are not as dramatic as positive symptoms, but they can interfere greatly with the patient's ability to function day to day. Because expressing emotion is difficult for them, people with schizophrenia laugh, cry, and get angry less often. Their affect is flat; they show little or no emotion when personal loss occurs. They also experience **ambivalence**, which is the concurrent experience of equally strong opposing feelings so that it is impossible to make a decision. Avolition may be so profound that simple activities of daily living (ADLs), such as dressing or combing hair, may not get done. **Anhedonia** prevents the person with schizophrenia from enjoying activities. People with schizophrenia may have limited speech and difficulty

KEY CHARACTERISTICS 24.1 • SCHIZOPHRENIA

Diagnostic Criteria

A. Two (or more) of the following, each present for a significant portion of time during a 1-month period (or less if successfully treated). At least one of these must be (1), (2), or (3):
  1. Delusions
  2. Hallucinations
  3. Disorganized speech (e.g., frequent derailment or incoherence)
  4. Grossly disorganized or catatonic behavior
  5. Negative symptoms (i.e., diminished emotional expression or avolition)

B. For a significant portion of the time since the onset of the disturbance, level of functioning in one or more major areas, such as work, interpersonal relations, or self-care, is markedly below the level achieved prior to the onset (or when the onset is in childhood or adolescence, there is failure to achieve expected level of interpersonal, academic, or occupational functioning).

C. Continuous signs of the disturbance persist for at least 6 months. This 6-month period must include at least 1 month of symptoms (or less if successfully treated) that meet Criterion A (i.e., active-phase symptoms) and may include periods of prodromal or residual symptoms. During these prodromal or residual periods, the signs of the disturbance may be manifested by only negative symptoms or by two or more symptoms listed in Criterion A present in an attenuated form (e.g., odd beliefs and unusual perceptual experiences).

D. SAD and depressive or bipolar disorder with psychotic features have been ruled out because either (1) no major depressive or manic episodes have occurred concurrently with the active-phase symptoms or (2) if mood episodes have occurred during active-phase symptoms, they have been present for a minority of the total duration of the active and residual periods of the illness.

E. The disturbance is not attributable to the physiological effects of a substance (e.g., a drug of abuse, a medication) or another medical condition.

F. If there is a history of autism spectrum disorder or a communication disorder of childhood onset, the additional diagnosis of schizophrenia is made only if prominent delusions or hallucinations, in addition to the other required symptoms of schizophrenia, are also present for at least 1 month (or less if successfully treated).

Target Symptoms and Associated Findings
- Inappropriate affect
- Loss of interest or pleasure
- Dysphoric mood (anger, anxiety, or depression)
- Disturbed sleep patterns
- Lack of interest in eating or refusal of food
- Difficulty concentrating
- Some cognitive dysfunctions, such as confusion, disorientation, or memory impairment
- Lack of insight
- Depersonalization, derealization, and somatic concerns
- Motor abnormalities

Associated Physical Examination Findings
- Physically awkward
- Poor coordination or mirroring
- Motor abnormalities
- Cigarette-related pathologies, such as emphysema and other pulmonary and cardiac problems

Associated Laboratory Findings
- Enlarged ventricular system and prominent sulci in the brain cortex
- Decreased temporal and hippocampal size
- Increased size of basal ganglia
- Decreased cerebral size
- Slowed reaction times
- Abnormalities in eye tracking

Reprinted with permission from the Diagnostic and Statistical Manual of Mental Disorders, Fifth Edition (Copyright ©2013). American Psychiatric Association. All Rights Reserved.

---

saying anything new or carrying on a conversation. These negative symptoms cause the person with schizophrenia to withdraw and experience feelings of severe isolation.

> **KEYCONCEPT Negative symptoms** reflect a lessening or loss of normal functions, such as restriction or flattening in the range and intensity of emotion (diminished emotional expression), reduced fluency and productivity of thought and speech (**alogia**), withdrawal and inability to initiate and persist in goal-directed activity (avolition), and inability to experience pleasure (anhedonia).

Neurocognitive Impairment

Neurocognitive impairment exists in people with schizophrenia and may be independent of positive and negative symptoms. Neurocognition includes memory (short- and long-term); vigilance or sustained attention; verbal fluency or the ability to generate new words; and executive functioning, which includes volition, planning, purposeful action, and self-monitoring behavior. Working memory is a concept that includes short-term memory and the ability to store and process information.

> **KEYCONCEPT Neurocognitive impairment** in memory, vigilance, and executive functioning is related to poor functional outcomes in schizophrenia.

This impairment is independent of the positive symptoms. That is, cognitive dysfunction can exist even if the positive symptoms are in remission. Not all areas of cognitive functioning are impaired. Long-term memory and intellectual functioning are not necessarily affected. However, low intellectual functioning is common and may be related to a lack of educational experiences and opportunities due to the age of illness onset. Neurocognitive dysfunction is often manifested in disorganized symptoms (Vignapiano et al., 2019).

KEYCONCEPT Disorganized symptoms of schizophrenia are findings that make it difficult for the person to understand and respond to the ordinary sights and sounds of daily living. These include **confused speech and thinking**, and disorganized behavior.

Disorganized Thinking

The following are examples of confused speech and thinking patterns:

- **Echolalia**—repetition of another's words that is parrot-like and inappropriate
- **Circumstantiality**—extremely detailed and lengthy discourse about a topic
- **Loose associations**—absence of the normal connectedness of thoughts, ideas, and topics; sudden shifts without apparent relationship to preceding topics
- **Tangentiality**—the topic of conversation is changed to an entirely different topic that is a logical progression but causes a permanent detour from the original focus
- **Flight of ideas**—the topic of conversation changes repeatedly and rapidly, generally after just one sentence or phrase
- **Word salad**—stringing together words that are not connected in any way
- **Neologisms**—words that are made up that have no common meaning and are not recognizable
- **Paranoia**—suspiciousness and guardedness that are unrealistic and often accompanied by grandiosity
- **Referential thinking**—a belief that neutral stimuli have special meaning to the individual, such as a television commentator who is speaking directly to the individual
- **Autistic thinking**—restricts thinking to the literal and immediate so that the individual has private rules of logic and reasoning that make no sense to anyone else
- **Concrete thinking**—lack of abstraction in thinking; inability to understand punch lines, metaphors, and analogies
- **Verbigeration**—purposeless repetition of words or phrases
- **Metonymic speech**—use of words with similar meanings interchangeably
- **Clang association**—repetition of words or phrases that are similar in sound but in no other way, for example, "right, light, sight, might"
- **Stilted language**—overly and inappropriately artificial formal language
- **Pressured speech**—speaking as if the words are being forced out

Disorganized perceptions often create oversensitivity to colors, shapes, and background activities. **Illusions** occur when the person misperceives or exaggerates stimuli that actually exist in the external environment. This is in contrast to hallucinations, which are perceptions in the absence of environmental stimuli. Ancillary symptoms that may accompany schizophrenia include anxiety, depression, and hostility.

Disorganized Behavior

Disorganized behavior (which may manifest as very slow, rhythmic, or ritualistic movement), coupled with disorganized speech, makes it difficult for the person to partake in daily activities. Examples of disorganized behavior include the following:

- **Aggression**—behaviors or attitudes that reflect rage, hostility, and the potential for physical or verbal destructiveness (usually comes about if the person believes someone is going to do them harm)
- **Agitation**—inability to sit still or attend to others, accompanied by heightened emotions and tension
- **Catatonia**—psychomotor disturbances, such as stupor, mutism, posturing, or repetitive behavior
- **Catatonic excitement**—a hyperactivity characterized by purposeless activity and abnormal movements, such as grimacing and posturing
- **Echopraxia**—involuntary imitation of another person's movements and gestures
- **Regressed behavior**—behaving in a manner of a less mature life stage; childlike and immature behavior
- **Stereotypy**—repetitive purposeless movements that are idiosyncratic to the individual and to some degree outside of the individual's control
- **Hypervigilance**—sustained attention to external stimuli as if expecting something important or frightening to happen
- **Waxy flexibility**—posture held in an odd or unusual fixed position for extended periods of time

Disruption in Sense of Self

Many of the symptoms observed in schizophrenia may be attributable to brain deficiencies that affect the individual's experience of "self". The self is difficult to define but is often used to describe who we are: self-concept, self-consciousness, self-awareness, and, for people with schizophrenia, self-disturbance. This self-disturbance leads to significant difficulty determining what thoughts and experiences are internal versus external to the individual. Delusions and hallucinations can be explained by this, as can the person's failures of insight, self-awareness, and self-monitoring (Klaunig et al., 2019). Self-disturbance also suggests ways that adolescents and young adults may be identified during the prodromal period of the illness by their difficulties in integrating self-experiences. Treatment that focuses on self-disturbance aims to help clients to become active agents in their own care. This can be done by helping them to develop concepts of themselves in the world and creating narratives of how their experiences have developed and can be managed in the future in their own unique way (Lysaker & Roe, 2016). Treatment that helps to develop a sense of "self" is possible and integral to recovery (Davidson, 2019).

Schizophrenia Across the Life-Span

Children

The diagnosis of schizophrenia is rare in children before adolescence. When it does occur in children aged 5 or 6 years, the symptoms are essentially the same as in adults. In this age group, hallucinations tend to be visual, and delusions less developed. Because disorganized speech and behavior may be explained better by other disorders that are more common in childhood, those disorders should be considered before applying the diagnosis of schizophrenia to a child.

However, new studies suggest that the likelihood of children later experiencing schizophrenia can be predicted. Developmental abnormalities in childhood, including delays in attainment of speech and motor development, problems in social adjustment, and poorer academic and cognitive performance, have been found to be present in individuals who experience schizophrenia in adulthood. Adults who had childhood cognitive, social, behavioral, and emotional impairments may be at higher risk of developing schizophrenia (Jaaro-Peled & Sawa, 2020).

Older Adults

People with schizophrenia usually get older, and some people develop schizophrenia in late life. For older patients who have had schizophrenia since young adulthood, this may be a time in which they experience some improvement in symptoms or decrease in relapse fluctuations. There is some evidence that suggests that older adults with schizophrenia may be more likely to develop cognitive impairment than those without mental disorders (Shahab et al., 2019). However, their lifestyle is probably dependent on the effectiveness of earlier treatment, the support systems that are in place (including relationships with family members and professionals), and the interaction between environmental stressors and the patient's functional impairments. The cost of caring for older patients with schizophrenia remains high because many are no longer cared for in institutions and because community-based treatment has developed more slowly for this age group than for younger adults.

Epidemiology and Risk Factors

Schizophrenia is found in all cultures and countries. It is prevalent in about 0.48% of the worldwide population (ranging from 0.34% to 0.85%) and is listed within the top 20 illnesses for life lost resulting from premature death and years lived in less than full health (Lin et al., 2018). Its economic costs are enormous. Direct costs include treatment expenses; indirect costs include lost wages, premature death, and involuntary commitment. In addition, employment among people with schizophrenia is one of the lowest of any group with disabilities. The costs of schizophrenia in terms of individual and family suffering are probably inestimable.

People with schizophrenia tend to cluster in the lowest social classes in industrialized countries and urban communities. The symptoms of the illness are so pervasive that it is difficult for these individuals to maintain any type of gainful employment. Homelessness is a problem for people with severe mental illness (e.g., schizophrenia or bipolar illness). People with schizophrenia are more likely to remain homeless with few opportunities for employment (Glick & Olfson, 2018; Wu et al., 2018).

Internal and External Risk Factors

Genetic factors related to cognitive and brain function and brain structure are known risks for schizophrenia. Early neurologic problems, stressful life events, and nonhereditary genetic factors also contribute to the likelihood of developing the disorder. Environmental factors related to schizophrenia include migrant status, having an older father, *Toxoplasma gondii* antibodies, prenatal famine, lifetime cannabis use, obstetric complications, urban rearing, and winter or spring birth (Abrahamyan Empson et al., 2020; Hollander et al., 2020).

Age of Onset

Schizophrenia is usually diagnosed in late adolescence and early adulthood. Men tend to be diagnosed between the ages of 18 and 25 years and women between the ages of 25 and 35 years. The earlier the diagnosis and the longer the psychosis remains untreated, the more severe the disorder becomes (Shahab et al., 2019). Conversely, the earlier the psychosis is recognized and treated within an evidence-based comprehensive program, the better the outcomes (Dixon et al., 2018).

Gender Differences

Men tend to be diagnosed earlier and have a poorer prognosis than women. This may be a sex-linked outcome, but it may also reflect the poorer prognosis for any individual who develops the disorder at an early age (Lewine et al., 2017). When women are diagnosed early, they are at higher risk for physical comorbidities than men (Šimunović Filipčić et al., 2020).

Ethnicity and Culture

Increasingly, efforts are being made to consider culture and ethnic origin when diagnosing and treating individuals with schizophrenia. Racial groups may have varying diagnostic rates of schizophrenia. However, it is not clear whether these findings represent correct diagnosis or misdiagnosis of the disorder based on the cultural bias of the clinician. For instance, schizophrenia has been consistently overdiagnosed among African Americans. African American and Latinx individuals with bipolar disorder are more likely to have misdiagnoses of schizophrenia than are White individuals. Serious mental disorders may remain unrecognized in Asian Americans because of stereotypical beliefs that they are "problem free" (Maura et al., 2017).

Familial Differences

First-degree biologic relatives (e.g., children, siblings, parents) of an individual with schizophrenia have a 10 times estimated greater risk for schizophrenia than the general population. Other relatives may have an increased risk for related disorders, such as schizoaffective disorder (SAD) and schizotypal personality disorder (Hilker et al., 2018).

Comorbidity

Several somatic and psychological disorders coexist with schizophrenia. This results in significant morbidity and mortality for people with schizophrenia, with individuals who have this diagnosis dying up to 20 years earlier than the general population. Physical health conditions and illnesses to which people with schizophrenia are particularly susceptible include tuberculosis, human immunodeficiency disease, hepatitis B and C, osteoporosis, poor dentition, impaired lung function, altered (reduced) pain sensitivity, sexual dysfunction, obstetric complications, cardiovascular problems, hyperpigmentation, obesity, diabetes mellitus (DM), metabolic syndrome with hyperlipidemia, polydipsia, thyroid dysfunction, and hyperprolactinemia (Kessler & Lev-Ran, 2019; Postolache et al., 2019). Early mortality may be from natural causes (cardiovascular, cancer, chronic obstructive pulmonary

disease, DM, and influenza and pneumonia) or unnatural causes (suicide, substance and alcohol abuse, and legal interventions) (Lin et al., 2018). Several health system factors contribute to this, including barriers to obtaining primary care and the primary care providers' lack of preparation and discomfort addressing mental health issues and conditions, the insufficient preparation of mental health practitioners in managing physical illness, the tendency for mental health providers to fail to ask about physical health, and the absence of standards of care that include screening and monitoring medical issues.

The coronavirus disease 2019 pandemic is significantly impacting persons with schizophrenia. Their symptoms, such as delusions, hallucinations, disorganized behavior, cognitive impairment, and poor insight, make it harder for adequate infection control. Many people with schizophrenia live in congregate housing, which compounds the likelihood of infection. Treatment options are less accessible because of the pandemic restrictions related to inpatient and outpatient care (Kozloff et al., 2020).

Substance Abuse and Depression

Among the behavioral comorbidities, substance use is common. Depression may also be observed in patients with schizophrenia. This is an important symptom for several reasons. First, depression may be evidence that the diagnosis of a mood disorder is more appropriate. Second, depression is not unusual in chronic stages of schizophrenia and deserves attention. Third, 50% of people with schizophrenia attempt suicide, and 10% to 15% die by suicide. Risk factors for suicide are untreated psychosis, history of suicide attempt, age younger than 28 years, severity of depression, and substance abuse (Kim et al., 2019; Naguy & Al-Rabaie, 2017).

Diabetes Mellitus and Obesity

Interest has been renewed in the relationship between DM and schizophrenia. Years ago, an association was established between glucose regulation and psychiatric disorders, suggesting that people with schizophrenia may be more prone to type II DM than the general public (Franzen, 1970; Schimmelbusch et al., 1971). Evidence that supports this view includes a higher rate of type II diabetes in first-degree relatives of people with schizophrenia and higher rates of impaired glucose tolerance and insulin resistance among people with schizophrenia. However, obesity, which is associated with type II diabetes, is a growing problem in the United States, in general, and is complicated in schizophrenia treatment by the tendency of individuals to gain weight after their disease is managed with medications. Weight gain in some individuals may be attributed to a return to a healthier living situation, in which regular meals are available and symptoms that interfere with obtaining food regularly (e.g., delusions) are decreased. For others, weight gain may be a medication side effect (Kowalchuk et al., 2019).

Etiology

Schizophrenia is believed to be caused by the interaction of a biologic predisposition or vulnerability and environmental stressors (see the diathesis-stress model discussed in Chapter 13). See Box 24.1 for deficits related to vulnerability in schizophrenia. Environmental stressors include pregnancy or obstetric complications and social adversity, such as migration, unemployment, urban living, childhood abuse, and social isolation or absence of close friends (Hollander et al., 2020).

Biologic Theories

Neuroanatomic Findings

The lateral and third ventricles are somewhat larger, and total brain volume is somewhat less in persons with schizophrenia compared with those without schizophrenia. The thalamus and the medial temporal lobe

---

BOX 24.1

Deficits that Cause Vulnerability in Schizophrenia

COGNITIVE DEFICITS
- Deficits in processing complex information
- Deficits in maintaining a steady focus of attention
- Inability to distinguish between relevant and irrelevant stimuli
- Difficulty forming consistent abstractions
- Impaired memory

PSYCHOPHYSIOLOGIC DEFICITS
- Deficits in sensory inhibition
- Poor control of autonomic responsiveness

SOCIAL SKILLS DEFICITS
- Impairments in processing interpersonal stimuli, such as eye contact or assertiveness
- Deficits in conversational capacity
- Deficits in initiating activities
- Deficits in experiencing pleasure

COPING SKILLS DEFICITS
- Overassessment of threat
- Underassessment of personal resources
- Overuse of denial

Source: McGlashan, T. H. (1994). Psychosocial treatments of schizophrenia: The potential relationships. In N. C. Andreasen (Ed.), *Schizophrenia: From mind to molecule* (pp. 189–215). American Psychiatric Press.

---

structures, including the hippocampus, and superior temporal and prefrontal cortices, tend to be smaller also (Dietsche et al., 2017; Wang et al., 2019).

Genetic Associations

Genetic associations have been identified in a number of regions of the brain, and some have already been tied to neuropathways related to cognitive deficits. The future of treatment of schizophrenia will rely heavily on the outcome of ongoing research (Toulopoulou et al., 2019).

Neurodevelopment

The neurodevelopmental hypothesis explains the etiology of schizophrenia as pathologic processes caused by genetic and environmental factors that begin before the brain reaches its adult state. Evidence suggests that in utero during the first or second trimester, genes involved with cell migration, cell proliferation, axonal outgrowth, and myelination may be affected by neurologic insults, such as viral infections. That is, early neurodevelopmental insults may lead to dysfunction of specific networks that become obvious at adolescence during the normal loss of some plasticity and synapse development (La Barbera et al., 2019).

Neurotransmitters, Pathways, and Receptors

Positron emission tomography (PET) scan findings suggest that in schizophrenia, brain metabolism is generally reduced, with a relative hypermetabolism in the left side of the brain and in the left temporal lobe. Abnormalities exist in specific areas of the brain in the frontal, temporal, and cingulate regions. These findings support further exploration of differential brain hemisphere function in people with schizophrenia (Fig. 24.1). Other PET studies show **hypofrontality**, or a reduced cerebral blood flow and glucose metabolism in the prefrontal cortex of people with schizophrenia and hyperactivity in the limbic area (Buchsbaum, 1990; Hazlett et al., 2019) (Figs. 24.2 and 24.3).

Dopamine Dysregulation

A longstanding explanation of the neurobiological symptoms of schizophrenia is the dopamine hypothesis. Because conventional antipsychotics blocked dopamine and treated the positive symptoms of schizophrenia—specifically, hallucinations and delusions—it was reasoned that *hyperactivity* in the mesolimbic tract at the D2 receptor site in the striatal area (where memory and emotion are regulated) was responsible for these symptoms. Conversely, chronic low levels of dopamine in the

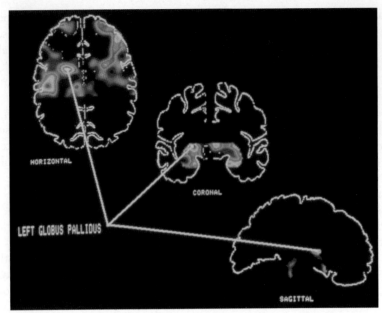

FIGURE 24.1 Area of abnormal functioning in a person with schizophrenia. These three views show the excessive neuronal activity in the left globus pallidus (portion of the basal ganglia next to the putamen). (Courtesy of John W. Haller, PhD, Departments of Psychiatry and Radiology, Washington University, St. Louis.)

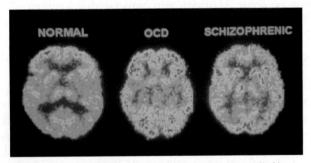

FIGURE 24.2 Metabolic activity in a control subject (*left*), a subject with obsessive-compulsive disorder (*center*), and a subject with schizophrenia (*right*). (Courtesy of Monte S. Buchsbaum, MD, The Mount Sinai Medical Center and School of Medicine, New York.)

prefrontal cortex were thought to underlie cognitive dysfunction in schizophrenia.

Today, research focuses on several of the molecular links to dopamine synthesis and increased release of dopamine. Dopamine has a role in the pathogenesis of schizophrenia, but it is more complicated than previously thought. Dopamine activity is related to other disorders, cortical functioning, and stress (Abi-Dargham, 2020).

Role of Other Receptors

Other receptors are also involved in dopamine neurotransmission, especially serotonergic receptors. It is becoming clear that schizophrenia does not result from dysregulation of a single neurotransmitter or biogenic amine (e.g., norepinephrine, dopamine, or serotonin). Investigators are also hypothesizing a role for glutamate and gamma-aminobutyric acid (GABA) because of the complex interconnections of neuronal transmission and the complexity and heterogeneity of schizophrenia symptoms. The *N*-methyl-D-aspartate class of glutamate receptors is being studied because of the actions of phencyclidine (PCP) at these sites and because of the similarity of the psychotic behaviors that are produced when someone takes PCP (see Figs. 24.1–24.3).

Gut Microbiota

Intestinal flora are necessary for brain development and overall health. Gut bacteria are involved in immune regulation and protect the body through the development of mucosal lymphoid tissue. The **gut–brain axis** (the two-way communication system that connects the gut with the brain) is involved with the intestinal microbiome, neuroendocrine (hypothalamus-pituitary-adrenal axis), immune, and nervous systems. The gut microbiota communicates with the central nervous system (CNS) through the vagus nerve. Emerging research is linking the gut microbiota to the development of mental disorders through the gut–brain axis. It is hypothesized that abnormalities in the gut microbiota increase

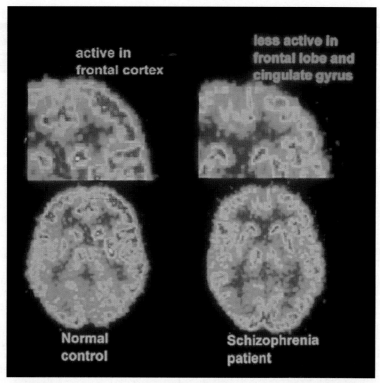

FIGURE 24.3   Positron emission tomography scan with 18F-deoxyglucose shows metabolic activity in a horizontal section of the brain in a control subject (*left*) and in an unmedicated patient with schizophrenia (*right*). *Red* and *yellow* indicate areas of high metabolic activity in the cortex; *green* and *blue* indicate lower activity in the white matter areas of the brain. The frontal lobe is magnified to show reduced frontal activity in the prefrontal cortex of the patient with schizophrenia. (Courtesy of Monte S. Buchsbaum, MD, The Mount Sinai Medical Center and School of Medicine, New York.)

inflammatory cytokines that may cause neuronal damage, cell death, and abnormal brain development (Yuan et al., 2019).

Psychosocial Theories

Social factors can contribute to the changes in brain function that result in schizophrenia and add to the day-to-day challenges of living with a mental illness. Childhood trauma, living in an urban environment, and being a member of a minority are all associated with psychotic syndromes. They can also create barriers to obtaining necessary treatment and recovery (Hollander et al., 2020; Mohammadzadeh et al., 2019). One of the major social stressors is the social stigma that surrounds all mental illnesses (see Chapter 2). The clinical vignette in Box 24.2 describes the impact of living with a stigmatizing illness. Another is the absence of good, affordable, and supportive housing in many communities. With 2010's enactment of insurance parity for mental illness in the Affordable Care Act, it is hoped that quality and continuity of care will be enhanced. Finally, the mental health service delivery system is fragmented; its quality and types of services vary from community to community, based in part on state legislative and mental health department funding differences.

Family Response to Disorder

Initially, families usually experience disbelief, shock, and fear, along with concern for the family member. Families may attribute the episode to taking illicit drugs or to extraordinary stress or fatigue and hope that this is an isolated or transient event. They may be fearful of the behaviors and respond to patient's anger and hostility with fear, confusion, and anxiety. They may deny the severity and chronicity of the illness and only partially engage in treatment. As families begin to acknowledge the disorder and the long-term care nature of recovery, they themselves may feel overwhelmed, angry, and depressed. In many instances, parents become caregivers as the person transitions into adulthood. As caregivers for their adult children, the parents face many challenges accessing health care and resources (Young et al., 2019).

BOX 24.2 CLINICAL VIGNETTE

Graduate Student in Peril

B.G.W. born in 1993, spent most of his teenage years using drugs and alcohol, behavior that started when he was 11 years old. He and his small group of friends spent their teenage years outside of school riding around on bicycles. He failed 8th grade, repeated it, and made it to 10th grade. He was removed permanently from school at the age of 16 years. His dress included a dirty denim jacket or Army fatigues, torn tee shirts with rock band logos, and tight-fitting jeans. At age 16, he was hospitalized for a psychotic episode initiated by lysergic acid diethylamide (LSD); it was the scariest moment of his life. His mind had been getting fuzzier every day; he had dabbled with black magic and Satanism. Later, he admitted that for years he had been trapped in a fantasy land, only partially explained by his drug use.

Years of treatment followed; even with abstinence from drugs, his mental status fluctuated. After antipsychotic agents were prescribed, he began to feel like himself. He was motivated to complete his General Education Diploma (GED) and entered college. He kept his mental illness a secret. While in graduate school, his thoughts, feelings, and behaviors began to change. His thinking became delusional, his moods unpredictable, and his behaviors illogical. Finally, he was hospitalized again, and his condition was stabilized with medication. Currently, he is reapplying to graduate school, and this time he vows to keep people close to him aware of his mental status.

What Do You Think?

- What role did stigma play in the treatment process?
- What information should BGW share with his social network about his mental illness and treatment?

Adapted from Graduate student in peril: A first person account of schizophrenia. (2002). *Schizophrenia Bulletin, 28*(4), 745–755.

BOX 24.3

Research for Evidence-Based Practice—Family-Focused Recovery: Perspectives from Individuals with a Mental Illness

Waller, S., Reupert, A., Ward, B., McCormick, F., & Kidd, S. (2019). Family-focused recovery: Perspectives from individuals with a mental illness. International Journal of Mental Health Nursing, *28(1), 247–255.*

THE QUESTION: How do those with mental illness define *family* and the role of family in their recovery?

METHODS: Purposive sampling and snowballing were used to recruit and conduct semi-structured interviews with 12 people diagnosed with a severe mental illness.

FINDINGS: Participants defined *family* in various ways, with some being very inclusive and others more selective. There was acknowledgment that family contributed to the individual's recovery in myriad ways, although the need for boundaries was stressed.

IMPLICATIONS FOR NURSING: Nurses should recognize that there is not one definition of *family* and that it is important for the patient to define their family.

See Box 24.3 for discussion of recovery-oriented family interventions.

RECOVERY-ORIENTED CARE FOR PERSONS WITH SCHIZOPHRENIA

Teamwork and Collaboration: Working Toward Recovery

The most effective approach to treatment for individuals with schizophrenia involves various disciplines, including nursing (both generalist and advanced practice psychiatric nurses), psychiatry, psychology, social work, occupational and recreational therapy, and pastoral counseling. Individuals with general education in psychology, sociology, and social work often serve as case managers, nursing aides, technicians, and other support personnel in hospitals and community treatment agencies. Peer counselors are sometimes used in community agencies and offer support and hope for a better future.

Patients need help in accepting and understanding their illness, setting goals, and developing a support system that encourages their recovery. Recovery-oriented strategies can address hopelessness associated with suicide attempts or withdrawal from relationships with others and encourage an independent lifestyle. Medication management is central to the treatment of schizophrenia and is the responsibility of the patient, physicians, nurses, and pharmacists. Psychosocial interventions can be implemented by all members of the mental health team and may include cognitive-behavioral, music, vocational, mindfulness, and support therapies. These varied professionals and paraprofessionals are important because of the complex nature of the symptoms, the long-term nature of the disorder, and the need for health promotion support. Complementary and alternative therapies, such as yoga, breathing exercises, relaxation, meditation and mindfulness, and aerobic exercise, may be helpful as adjunctive to the usual care.

Safety Issues

Several special concerns exist when working with people with schizophrenia. A suicide assessment should always be completed when a person is experiencing a psychotic episode. In an inpatient unit, patient safety concerns extend to potentially aggressive actions toward staff and other patients during episodes of psychosis. During times of acute illness, a priority of care is treatment with antipsychotic medications and, in some instances, hospitalization.

Nurses should assess the person's risk for suicide because of the high suicide and attempted suicide rates among persons with schizophrenia (see Chapter 22). One challenge is to distinguish among the displayed behaviors to determine if the person is displaying negative symptoms, side effects of antipsychotic medications, or actual depression and demoralization as a result of this illness. Does the patient speak of suicide, or have delusional thinking that could lead to dangerous behavior, or have command hallucinations telling them to harm self or others? Does the patient have homicidal ideations? Does the patient lack social support and the skills to be meaningfully engaged with other people or a vocation? Does the patient express feelings of not belonging to a social group or being a burden to loved ones? Substance-related disorders are also common among patients with schizophrenia, so that nurses should assess for substance use.

EVIDENCE-BASED NURSING CARE OF PERSONS WITH SCHIZOPHRENIA

Recovery is a long-term journey requiring various nursing interventions at different times. During exacerbation of symptoms, many patients are hospitalized for safety and medication adjustment. During periods of relative stability, the nurse and patient collaborate in developing recovery-oriented strategies that include maintaining a healthy lifestyle, developing positive coping skills, and seeking meaningful relationships. Schizophrenia research is ongoing, and the results are leading to new treatment approaches. It is critical that nurses continually seek out evidence-based strategies through accessing the best possible sources of evidence and formulating clinical questions See Nursing Care Plan 24.1

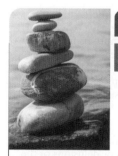

NURSING CARE PLAN 24.1

The Person with Schizophrenia

Arnold is a 53-year-old male with a history of schizophrenia with multiple hospitalizations. He was admitted per mental health court order to the inpatient mental health unit accompanied by the county sheriff. Arnold was given antipsychotic and antianxiety medication in the emergency room for the safety of himself and others after he attempted to strike an emergency room nurse. Arnold had become agitated and threatening while being removed from his family's farm, where he lived with his elderly mother for the past 30 years. Arnold refused to acknowledge that his parents had died.

Setting: Psychiatric Intensive Care Unit

Baseline Assessment: Arnold is dressed in a suit and dress shirt. On admission, he was also wearing a tie, which is his habit whenever he leaves his home. His tie, shoes, and belt were removed after arriving on the unit from the emergency room for safety reasons. Arnold wears his hair short, and he has been completing ADL. Arnold is watchful with a worried and anxious expression. He has a small stack of slightly used paper napkins stored between his shirt and suit jacket and holds a small stack of flattened single-serving milk cartons in his hand. Arnold does not believe that he has schizophrenia and that his previous hospitalizations were attempts by multinational corporations to keep him from following his false beliefs regarding his parent's wishes. Arnold is 5 ft 11 in., weighs 180 lb, BMI 25, BP 140/80, P 78, R 16. Denies suicidal thoughts. Denies using alcohol or illegal drugs. Even though he attended both parents' funerals, he continues to say they are merely away for a while. He has been taking his prescribed medications sporadically. Laboratory values are normal.

Associated Psychiatric Diagnosis	Medications
Schizophrenia, multiple episode, currently in acute episode	Risperidone (Risperdal), 2 mg BID Lorazepam (Ativan), 2 mg PO for agitation PRN

Priority of Care: Alterations in Thought Process

Important Characteristics

- Delusional thinking (believes there is conspiracy against family by multinational corporations, and parents not really deceased)
- Auditory hallucinations (parents talking to him)
- Suspiciousness (refuses to use telephone or other technology)

Associated Considerations

- Uncompensated alterations in brain activity

Nursing Care Plan 24.1 Continued

Outcomes

Initial

- Decreased delusional thinking through accurate interpretation of environment
- Expresses less suspiciousness about family
- Decreased frequency of hearing voices
- Able to participate in activities of increasing length and complexity (e.g., sitting through group and group activities, able to make projects that require increased concentration and contain more steps)

Long-Term

- Able to identify, monitor, and recognize delusional thinking and hallucinations
- Able to use coping mechanisms that will help to minimize or control symptoms of delusions and hallucinations
- Able to develop a reasonable medication routine
- Reestablish self-care activities

Interventions

Interventions	Rationale	Ongoing Assessment
• Initiate a nurse–patient relationship by using an accepting, nonjudgmental approach. • Be patient.	• A therapeutic relationship will provide support as Arnold begins to deal with his life change. • Be patient because his brain is not processing information normally.	• Determine the extent to which Arnold is willing to trust and engage in a relationship. • Determine the length of time Arnold can attend to conversation or activity with others.
• Administer risperidone as prescribed. Observe for affect, side effects, and adverse effects. Begin teaching about the medication and its importance after symptoms subside.	• Risperidone is a D2 and 5-HT2A antagonist and is indicated for the treatment of schizophrenia.	• Make sure Arnold swallows pills. Monitor for relief of positive symptoms using a standardized measure such as the SAPS. Assess side effects, especially extrapyramidal. Monitor blood pressure for orthostatic hypotension and body temperature increase (NMS).
• During hallucinations and delusional thinking, assess significance (what feelings is Arnold experiencing; what actions do the voices or his thoughts suggest he accomplish?). Reassure Arnold that you will keep him safe and that you are aware that his experiences are very real to him even though you may not be having the same experiences (Do not try to convince Arnold that his delusions are not true.) Redirect Arnold to here-and-now activities and experiences.	• It is important to understand the experience and context of the hallucinations and delusions to be able to provide appropriate interventions and redirect the patient to more reality-based activities. By avoiding arguments about the content of the patient's delusional beliefs or the experiences of patient's hallucinations, the nurse will enhance communication. Arguing about delusional thoughts or hallucinatory experiences just places the patient in a position to defend his beliefs.	• Assess the meaning of the hallucinations or delusions of the patient. Monitor whether he is a danger to himself or others. Determine whether patient can be directed to a more reality-based activity.
• Assess ability for self-care activities.	• Disturbed thinking may interfere with Arnold's ability to carry out ADLs.	• Continue to assess: Determine whether Arnold can manage his own self-care.

Priority of Care: Lack of Recognition of Illness and Consequences

Important Characteristics

- Displaces fear of impact of losing parents and home
- Does not perceive personal relevance to behavior
- Unable to admit impact of schizophrenia on life pattern

Associated Considerations

- Anxiety about leaving home
- Lack of control of life situation
- Threat of unpleasant reality

Continued

Nursing Care Plan 24.1 Continued

Outcomes

Initial	Long term
• Avoid hurting self or assaulting other patients or staff. • Decreased anxiety.	• Recognize that parents have died. • Develop coping skills to address moving to a new house.

Interventions

Interventions	Rationale	Ongoing Assessment
• Acknowledge patient's anxiety about parents' absence and loss of family home.	• Beginning with the facts that Arnold accepts as true helps establish a supportive, communication alliance.	• Assess the patient's ability to hear you and respond appropriately to your comments and requests; assess the patient's ability to concentrate on what is being said and happening around him.
• Be genuine and empathic.	• Arnold will benefit from your ability to understand his experience and express that understanding while presenting reality.	• Assess for evidence that the client is less frightened with less potential for striking out.
• Prioritize goals by including maintaining safety, learning about prescribed medication, and participation in treatment activities.	• By having choices, he will begin to develop a sense of control over his behavior.	• Observe the patient's nonverbal communication for evidence of increased agitation.
• Use medications to help the patient relax and maintain more calm: administer lorazepam, 2 mg, for agitation. The PO route is preferable to injection, so offer the patient this choice long before he has lost control.	• Exact mechanisms of action are not understood, but medication is believed to potentiate the inhibitory neurotransmitter GABA, relieving anxiety and producing sedation.	• Observe for a decrease in agitated behavior. • Offering this to the patient early, as fear and agitation are beginning to become evident, prevents the potential for the patient to lose control.

Evaluation

Outcomes	Revised Outcomes	Interventions
• Arnold gradually decreased agitated behavior. • Lorazepam was given regularly for first 2 days.	• Demonstrate control of behavior when discussing realistic discharge plans.	• Problem-solve possible scenarios for discharge.

ADL, activity of daily living; BID, twice a day; GABA, gamma-aminobutyric acid; NMS, neuroleptic malignant syndrome; PO, oral; SAPS, Scale for the Assessment of Positive Symptoms.

Mental Health Nursing Assessment

The nursing assessment should include the biologic, psychological, and social aspects because schizophrenia affects all aspects of the person's life. Not only are symptoms assessed, but strengths are also important in the assessment process.

Physical Health

The nurse should first determine whether any underlying medical disorders are present, particularly those associated with schizophrenia, such as DM, hypertension, and cardiac disease, or a family history of such disorders. Usually, a medical examination is conducted by primary care providers prior to initiation of mental health care. People with schizophrenia have a higher mortality rate from physical illness and often have smoking-related illnesses, such as emphysema as well as other pulmonary and cardiac problems (Seeman, 2019).

Physical Functioning

Physical abilities can be a strength; the potential to maintain optimal physical health should be assessed. Self-care often deteriorates in schizophrenia; sleep may be nonexistent during acute phases. Information regarding physical functioning may best be collected from family members.

Nutrition

A nutritional history should be completed to determine baseline eating habits and preferences. Taking baseline measures for metabolic syndrome is highly recommended and should include weight, waist circumference, cholesterol, and blood sugar (Hammoudeh et al., 2020). A healthy diet is important in managing the illness. Medications can alter normal nutrition, leading to excessive consumption of calories.

Medication

The nurse should obtain a complete list of medications that the patient is taking, including over-the-counter (OTC) agents and herbal supplements. Before initiation of psychiatric medications, standardized assessment of abnormal motor movements should be conducted using one of several assessment tools designed for that purpose, such as the Abnormal Involuntary Movement Scale (AIMS) (see Appendix B), the Dyskinesia Identification System (DISCUS) (Sprague & Kalachnik, 1991), or the Simpson-Angus Rating Scale (Simpson & Angus, 1970), which is designed for Parkinson symptoms.

Substance Use (Alcohol, Illicit Drugs, Tobacco)

The nurse should ask specific questions about alcohol, drug, and tobacco use. The use of these substances is quite common with people with schizophrenia and will significantly influence the treatment approach.

Psychosocial Assessment

The individual who is in an acute phase may be unable to provide an accurate history of early psychosocial issues. Family members' reports help in detailing occurrences of psychotic symptoms of delusions and hallucinations; however, onset of negative symptoms may be more difficult to date. In fact, negative symptoms vary from a slight deviation from normal to a clear impairment. Negative symptoms probably occur earlier than positive symptoms but are less easily recognized. Several assessment scales have been developed to help evaluate clusters of positive and negative symptoms (see Box 24.4).

Mental Status and Appearance

The patient may look eccentric or disheveled or have poor hygiene and bizarre dress. The patient's posture may suggest lethargy or stupor.

BOX 24.4

Rating Scales for Use with Schizophrenia

SCALE FOR THE ASSESSMENT OF NEGATIVE SYMPTOMS (SANS)

Available from Nancy C. Andreasen, MD, PhD, Department of Psychiatry, College of Medicine, The University of Iowa, Iowa City, IA 52242. Copyright 1984.

SCALE FOR THE ASSESSMENT OF POSITIVE SYMPTOMS (SAPS)

Available from Nancy C. Andreasen (see above).

POSITIVE AND NEGATIVE SYNDROME SCALE (PANSS)

Kay, S. R., Fiszbein, A., & Opler, L. A. (1987). The Positive and Negative Syndrome Scale (PANSS) for Schizophrenia. *Schizophrenia Bulletin, 13*, 261–276. Available from first author.

ABNORMAL INVOLUNTARY MOVEMENT SCALE (AIMS)

Guy, W. (1976). *ECDEU: Assessment manual for psychopharmacology* (DHEW Publication No. 76–338). Department of Health, Education, and Welfare, Psychopharmacology Branch.

BRIEF PSYCHIATRIC RATING SCALE (BPRS)

Overall, J. E., & Gorham, D. R. (1988). The Brief Psychiatric Rating Scale (BPRS): Recent developments in ascertainment and scaling. *Psychopharmacology Bulletin, 24*, 97–99.

DYSKINESIA IDENTIFICATION SYSTEM: CONDENSED USER SCALE (DISCUS)

Sprague, R. L., & Kalachnik, J. E. (1991). Reliability, validity, and a total score cutoff for the Dyskinesia Identification Scale System: Condensed User Scale (DISCUS) with mentally ill and mentally retarded populations. *Psychopharmacology Bulletin, 27*(1), 51–58.

SIMPSON-ANGUS RATING SCALE

Simpson, G. M., & Angus, J. W. S. L. (1970). A rating scale for extrapyramidal side effects. *Acta Psychiatrica Scandinavica, 212*(suppl), 11–19. Copyright 1970 Munksgaard International Publishers, Ltd.

Mood and Affect

Patients with schizophrenia often display altered mood states. In some cases, they may show heightened emotional activity; others may display severely limited emotional responses. Affect, the outward expression of mood, is categorized on a continuum: flat (i.e., emotional expression entirely absent), blunted (i.e., expression of emotions present but greatly diminished), and full range of expression. Inappropriate affect is marked by incongruence between the emotional expression and the thoughts expressed (e.g., laughing when telling a sad story). Other common emotional symptoms include the following:

- **Affective lability**—abrupt, dramatic, unprovoked changes in type of emotions expressed
- **Ambivalence**—the presence and expression of two opposing feelings, leading to inaction
- **Apathy**—little emotional expression, diminished interest and desire

Speech

Thought content and other mental processes are expressed in speech. Both content and speech patterns should be assessed by the nurse. Speech content may include obvious obsessions or delusions, loose associations, or flight of ideas. In some instances, as already noted, patients make up their own words (neologisms). Speech may be pressured (words seem to rapidly jump out without pauses) or slow. The nurse should note any difficulty in articulating words (dysarthria) or difficulty in swallowing (dysphagia) as indicators of medication-related side effects.

Thought Process Assessment

Thought process assessment includes determining if any hallucinations, delusions, disorganized communication, or cognitive impairments are present. Because thought process assessment is critical in the nursing assessment, each area is discussed separately in the following sections.

Hallucinations

Hallucinations are the most common example of disturbed sensory perception observed in patients with schizophrenia. Hallucinations are experienced in the sensory modalities (visual, auditory, gustatory, tactile, olfactory); however, auditory hallucinations are the most common type in schizophrenia. Some specific hallucinations may be sufficient to diagnose schizophrenia, such as hearing voices, conversing with each other, or carrying on a discussion with someone who is not there. Because most individuals will not spontaneously share their hallucinatory experiences with an interviewer, the nurse may need to rely on indirect evidence in the patient's behavior, such as (1) pauses during conversations in which the individual seems preoccupied or appears to be listening to someone other than the interviewer, (2) looking toward the perceived source of a voice, or (3) responding to the voices in some manner. Although patients may not spontaneously share their hallucinations, many validate observations of the examiner or admit to a history of hallucinations when asked (see Box 24.5). If a patient has command hallucinations, it is important for the safety of the person and others to know what the voices are telling the patient to do.

Delusions

Delusions are different from strongly held beliefs. Delusions do not change even though strong evidence contradicts the belief. The person continues to hold the belief despite contradictory evidence (APA, 2013). The person's culture must be considered when evaluating delusions. Delusional beliefs are those not sanctioned or held by a cultural or religious subgroup.

Bizarre delusions alone are sufficient to diagnose schizophrenia (APA, 2013). Bizarre delusions are those beliefs that are impossible, illogical, and not derived from ordinary life experiences. Bizarre delusions often include delusions of control (that some outside force controls thoughts and actions), thought broadcasting (that others can read or hear one's thoughts), thought insertion (that someone has placed thoughts into one's mind), and thought withdrawal (that someone is removing thoughts from one's mind). For example, a patient who has been seeing a hypnotist for 2 months reports that the hypnotist continued to read his mind and was "picking his brain away piece by piece." Another patient was convinced that a computer chip was placed in her vagina during a gynecologic examination and that this somehow directly influenced her physical movements and her thoughts.

Remember Arnold?
He believes that his parents are still alive and that they will return. He refuses to leave the farm and insists that everything is left as it is.

Nonbizarre delusions generally have themes of jealousy and persecution and are derived from plausible life experiences. For example, a woman believes that her husband, from whom she has recently separated, is trying to poison her, or a man who believes that members of the Mafia are trying to kill him because, when he was in high school, he reported to the principal that several of his classmates were selling drugs at school (APA, 2013).

Assessing and judging the content of the delusion and exploring other aspects of the delusional experience are helpful in understanding the significance of these false beliefs. The underlying feeling that accompanies the delusion (i.e., fear or inflated self-esteem) should be explored. Other aspects to consider include the conviction with which the delusion is held; the extent to which other aspects of the individual's life are incorporated or affected by the delusion; the degree of internal consistency, organization, and logic evidenced in the delusion; and evaluating the amount of pressure (in terms of preoccupation and concern) individuals feel in their lives as a result of the delusion (Box 24.6).

BOX 24.5 • THERAPEUTIC DIALOGUE: THE PATIENT WITH HALLUCINATIONS

The following conversation took place in Arnold's room during the night checks. The nurse observed that Arnold was talking with someone, but no one else was in the room.

INEFFECTIVE APPROACH

Nurse: Arnold?

Arnold: Yeah?

Nurse: Whom are you talking to?

Arnold: My mother visits me at night. I am telling her about my day.

Nurse: You know, Arnold, you are having a hallucination. Your mother died a few weeks ago.

Arnold: She did not. She is away for a while, but she will be back soon.

Nurse: Arnold. (Looks at nurse.) You are going to have to accept that your mother is gone.

Arnold: Oh yeah? What do you know?

Nurse: Well, we can talk about it in the morning.

Arnold: You don't know what you are talking about.

EFFECTIVE APPROACH

Nurse: Arnold?

Arnold: Yeah?

Nurse: Are you talking to someone?

Arnold: Yes, she visits me at night?

Nurse: Oh, does she talk to you?

Arnold: Yes, she asks me about my day. She visits in the evening.

Nurse: Is there anything else you talk about?

Arnold: No, she leaves after I tell her.

Nurse: OK, how do you feel when she visits you?

Arnold: A little sad, but I like to tell her about my day.

Nurse: A little sad?

Arnold: Yeah, I wish I could see her more.

Nurse: Sounds like you are lonely?

Arnold: Yea, it's nice when you talk with me.

Nurse: I can do that. If you are not asleep when I finish rounds, we can talk more.

CRITICAL THINKING CHALLENGE

• How did the nurse's impatience translate into Arnold's response in the first scenario?

• What effective communicating techniques did the nurse use in the second scenario?

Disorganized Communication

Abrupt shifts in the focus of conversation, which are often altered in schizophrenia, are typically symptomatic of disorganized thinking. Impaired verbal fluency (i.e., ability to produce spontaneous speech) is commonly present. The most severe shifts in focus may occur after only one or two words (i.e., word salad), after one or two phrases or sentences (i.e., flight of ideas or loose associations), or somewhat less severely as a shift that occurs when a new topic is repeatedly suggested and pursued from the current topic (i.e., tangentiality).

Cognitive Impairments

Mental status assessment focuses on eliciting indications of cognitive impairments associated with schizophrenia. Although these impairments vary widely from patient to patient, several primary problems have been identified:

• Attention may be increased and sustained on external stimuli over a period of time (hypervigilance).

• The ability to distinguish and focus on relevant stimuli may be diminished.

BOX 24.6 • THERAPEUTIC DIALOGUE: THE PATIENT WITH DELUSIONS

John joined the nurse in a game of pool. The following conversation occurred as they played.

INEFFECTIVE APPROACH

John: The CIA put a transmitter in my molar, here (points to his right cheek).

Nurse: No one would put a transmitter in your tooth; come on, the CIA isn't looking for you.

John: Yeah, they want to monitor me while I'm here. I know that they have the real Osama bin Laden here in the hospital. They are trying to get the President to intervene with the Michigan Militia. Mark from Michigan told me that.

Nurse: Osama bin Laden can't possibly be here; he died years ago.

John: Maybe—but that was an imposter. They're just trying to keep people from knowing what they're doing.

Nurse: John, Osama bin Laden isn't in the hospital; if he were, I would know it because I work here.

John: (With anger) You don't know anything! You are probably working for the CIA too. I have nothing else to say to you.

EFFECTIVE APPROACH

John: The CIA put a transmitter in my molar, here (points to his right cheek).

Nurse: Oh. Which balls are mine?

John: You get the striped ones. Yeah, they want to monitor me while I'm here. I know that they have the real Osama bin Laden here in the hospital. They are trying to get the President to intervene with the Michigan Militia. Mark from Michigan told me that.

Nurse: Well, I don't know anything about that, but I want you to know that we will keep you safe.

John: Maybe…

Nurse: You sound a little overwhelmed with all the information you have.

John: No, no. I can handle it. The CIA can't do anything to me. I'll never talk.

Nurse: I thought they could hear you when you talk to me.

John: Huh? Oh, that transmitter is so that they can send me misinformation. They send a tower of babble to my brain. They are trying to confuse me so that I stay away from Osama Bin Laden. They all think they can keep me from my mission.

Nurse: Who are they?

John: Everyone in the government. The CIA, FBI, ATF, IRS—all those alphabets.

Nurse: So, everyone in the government is trying to get to you?

John: Well, maybe not everybody. Just the ones that care about money and the militia. I don't think they care about me much in Commerce or Health and Human Services. Although they'd care too if they knew.

Nurse: I would think that's pretty frightening to have all these people out looking for you. You must be scared a lot.

John: It's scary, but I can handle it. I've handled it all my life.

Nurse: You've been in scary situations all your life?

John: Yeah. I don't know. Maybe not scary, just hard. I never seemed to be able to do as well as my parents wanted—or as I wanted.

CRITICAL THINKING CHALLENGE

- How did the nurse's argumentative responses cause the patient to react in the first scenario?
- What effective communication techniques did the nurse use in the second scenario?

- Familiar cues may go unrecognized or be improperly interpreted.
- Information processing may be diminished, leading to inappropriate or illogical conclusions from available observations and information (Dondé et al., 2018; John et al., 2018).

Cognitive impairments are not easy to recognize. By relying only on clinical assessment, the nurse can miss the extent of the impairment. Using a standardized instrument can provide a screening measurement of cognitive function (see Chapter 11). If impairment exists, neuropsychological testing by a qualified psychologist may be necessary.

Memory and Orientation

Impairment in orientation, memory, and abstract thinking is often present. Orientation to time, place, and person may remain relatively intact unless the patient is particularly preoccupied with delusions and hallucinations. Although all aspects of memory may be affected in schizophrenia, registration or the ability to recall within seconds of newly learned information may be particularly diminished. This affects the individual's short- and long-term memory. The ability to engage in abstract thinking may be impaired (see Box 24.7).

Insight and Judgment

Insight and judgment are closely related to each other. Individuals display insight when they recognize that their hallucinations or delusions are symptoms of a mental disorder. Judgment is the ability to decide or act about a situation. If judgment is poor, the person may not recognize personal vulnerabilities and consequently engages in detrimental behavior. For example, the individual may be taken advantage of by others or fail to realize a potentially dangerous situation.

Behavioral Responses

During periods of psychosis, unusual or bizarre behavior often occurs. These behaviors can usually be understood within the context of the patient's disturbed thinking. The nurse needs to understand the significance of the behavior to the individual. For example, one patient moved the family furniture into the yard because he thought that evil spirits were hiding in the furniture. His bizarre behavior was an attempt to protect his family. Another patient painted a sequence of numbers on his bedroom walls. He said that the numbers were the language of the angels. His delusional thoughts were the basis of his behavior.

Because of the negative symptoms, specifically avolition, patients may not seem interested or organized enough to complete normal daily activities. They may stay in bed most of the day or refuse to take a shower. Many times, they agree to get up in the morning and go to work, but they never get around to it. Several specific behaviors are associated with schizophrenia, including stereotypy (i.e., idiosyncratic, repetitive, purposeless movements); echopraxia (i.e., involuntary imitation of others' movements); and waxy flexibility (i.e., posture held in odd or unusual fixed positions for extended periods). In some cases, certain behaviors need to be evaluated carefully to distinguish them from movements that are associated with medication-related side effects, such as grimacing, stereotypical behavior, or agitation.

Self-Concept

In schizophrenia, self-concept is usually poor. Patients often are aware that they are hearing voices that others do not hear. They recognize that they are different from others and are often scared of "going crazy." Many are aware of the loss of expectations for their future achievements. The pervasive stigma associated with having a mental illness contributes to the poor self-concept. Body image can be disturbed, especially during periods of hallucinations or delusions. For example, one patient believed that her body was infected with germs, and she could feel them eating away her insides.

Stress and Coping Patterns

Stressful events are often linked to psychiatric symptoms. It is important to determine stresses from the patient's perspective because a stressful event for one may not be stressful for another. It is also important to determine typical coping patterns, especially negative coping strategies, such as the use of substances or showing aggressive behavior.

BOX 24.7

Arnold's Cognitive Symptoms

Arnold's symptoms of schizophrenia began long before he was actually diagnosed. Throughout school, he had difficulty learning new material. His teachers would describe him as being "slow" or "inattentive." Because he appeared to be functioning normally, his teachers and family attributed his poor academic behavior to lack of interest. His father would often get frustrated with him because he would spend many hours in his bedroom and would not help out on the farm. When prodded to complete schoolwork or a household task, he would often get distracted before finishing the tasks. Family members and teachers quickly learned to provide several prompts for Arnold to complete a task. As he progressed to high school, he was labeled as a "slow learner" and assigned to less demanding classes.

The reality was that Arnold was experiencing unrecognized prodromal cognitive symptoms of schizophrenia. He was having difficulty remembering his assignments. He was having difficulty grasping concepts that other students seemed to easily understand. He was becoming frustrated with his difficulty and retreated to his room. He waited for specific directions that he could easily process. His thinking was concrete, and he had difficulty expressing himself. When he was bombarded with several directions at once, he could not process any of the directions. In his frustration, he would throw objects, frightening others. His family was very concerned with the changes that were occurring with their once easy-going son.

Consider This:

Recall Arnold's symptoms? They appeared after the stress of his parents' death.

Social Network

Several difficulties involving social functioning occur in schizophrenia. As the disorder progresses, individuals can become increasingly socially isolated. On a one-to-one basis, this occurs as the individual seems unable to connect with people in their environment. Several aspects of symptoms already discussed can contribute to this. For example, emotional blunting and anhedonia (the inability to experience pleasure) result in an experience of not being engaged in activities and relationships.

Interpretation of facial expressions and affect displayed by others is often problematic for people with schizophrenia. Cognitive deficits affect social relationships when individuals are unable to recall past interactions and have problems with decision-making and judgment. Other behaviors that affect social relationships are poverty of speech and language and the inability to complete ADLs, which results in poor hygiene, malnutrition, and social isolation.

Functional Status

Functional status of patients with schizophrenia should be assessed initially and at regular intervals. Level of independence, ability to work, ability to maintain an independent living environment, and self-care should be evaluated.

Support Systems

In schizophrenia, support systems become very important in maintaining the patient in the community. The individual may become socially isolated if the treatment and management occur in long-term care facilities and group homes, away from family and friends. One challenge is to identify and maintain the patient's links with family and significant others. Assessment of the formal support (e.g., family, health care providers) and informal support (e.g., neighbors, friends) should be conducted.

Quality of Life

People with schizophrenia often have a poor quality of life, especially older people, who may have spent many years in long-term hospitals. The nurse should assess the patient's quality of life and how it could be improved. Simple changes, such as arranging for a different roommate or improving access to social activities by meeting transportation needs, can greatly improve a patient's quality of life.

Strength Assessment

An important part of recovery is identification of personal and family strengths. Because schizophrenia is usually diagnosed at a young age, the person may be physically fit with little evidence of chronic illness. As the assessment is completed, strengths will emerge. Family support is critical for a person with schizophrenia. Intellectual ability and coping with stress are areas that can be strengths. The following questions are examples that can be used in assessing strengths.

• What do you do for relaxation, fun?
• How do you manage stressful events?
• How do you cope with the voices, thoughts, or impulses?
• Who do you talk with when you are upset?
• Are you hopeful about the future, and if so, what gives you hope for the future?

CLINICAL JUDGMENT

People with schizophrenia have a variety of nursing care needs because of the complexity of this chronic and difficult-to-treat illness. These needs emerge at different times and in different manifestations of the illness. Nurses need to consider the point in time during the progression of schizophrenia, the acceptability of its treatment to the individual, and the availability of community resources in order to best plan care. In many ways, treatment needs should be considered through a matrix of factors including (1) the stage of the illness (prodromal, acute, stable, and recovering); (2) the type, mixture, and intensity of symptoms; (3) the medication effects and side effects; (4) the method and availability of treatment; and (5) sources of social support and recovery-based care. For example, during an episode of psychosis, a nurse needs to be aware of the **symptoms** that affect the patient's **safety**. **Hallucinatory voices** may be telling the individual to self-injure or injure others. **Delusional thinking** may result in **suspicion** or **isolation**. **General functioning and basic care** may be compromised: **sleep** patterns may be severely disrupted, the person may be **undernourished** due to inability to obtain food or fear of eating. There may be **hygiene** issues that interfere with the person's ability to engage in social activities. An acute psychotic episode early in the disease may be accompanied by **grief and loss** due to changes in the expectations of the individual and their family. **Mood disturbances**, specifically depression, may be a priority later in the course of the disorder and may require a significant plan to avoid suicide. **Motivation** may be an issue during the course of the illness: early on as the individual and family wrestle with the implications of the illness and later as the chronicity of the symptoms continues. **Medication management** requires different assessments over the course of the illness. Early on, patients need considerable encouragement to continue taking medications that do not always make them feel comfortable and are not always believed to be necessary. In order to help patients take medications to control symptoms, dosage regimens need to be convenient and easy to follow; medications need to be sufficient to control symptoms without burdening the patient with unpleasant side effects. Long-acting injectable antipsychotic medications may be an answer to the issues of convenience and help to avoid relapse. Late in the illness, medication management needs to be **a mutual process**, particularly for patients who have managed their illness well. **Community resources** differ based on funding and location: rural versus urban; state priorities versus county and city policies. For many individuals with schizophrenia, the course of their illness is not just dependent on their symptoms but also on the availability of resources to help them manage their illness. A very careful and ongoing assessment of needs and issues is important throughout recovery.

NCLEXNOTE When assessing a patient with schizophrenia, the nurse should prioritize the severity of the current responses to the disorder. If hallucinations are impairing function, then managing hallucinations is a priority, and medications are needed immediately. If hallucinations are not a problem, however, coping with negative symptoms becomes a priority.

THERAPEUTIC RELATIONSHIP

Development of the therapeutic nurse-patient relationship centers on developing trust, accepting the person as a worthy human being, and infusing the relationship with hope. People with schizophrenia are often reluctant to engage in any relationship because of previous rejection and, in some instances, an underlying suspiciousness, which is a part of the illness. They are often trying to trust their own thoughts and perceptions, so interactions with another human being may prove to be too overwhelming. If they are hallucinating, their images of other people may be distorted and frightening as well.

The nurse should approach the patient in a calm and caring manner. Engaging the patient in a relationship may take time, but it begins with the first encounter. Short time-limited interactions are best for a patient who is experiencing psychosis. Being consistent in interactions and following through on promises will help establish trust within the relationship.

Establishing a therapeutic relationship is crucial, especially with patients who deny that they are ill. Patients are more likely to agree to and continue treatment if these recommendations are made within the context of a safe, trusting relationship. Even if some patients deny having

mental illness, they may take medication and attend treatment activities because they trust the nurse (Jaeger et al., 2014).

Furthermore, for long-term care and outcomes, recovery-oriented relationships are important. Using the recovery model, all efforts should be made to individualize treatment. Care should be person-centered through partnering with the patient in all aspects of care and encouraging self-direction. Treatment should be focused on strengths and the empowerment of the individual. Patients need encouragement to see that although their diagnosis may seem devastating, recovery is possible (Lean et al., 2019).

MENTAL HEALTH NURSING INTERVENTIONS

Establishing Recovery and Wellness goals

Nurses should aim to help their patients with schizophrenia to maximize their health, given this chronic illness. Goals need to take into consideration the symptoms that accompany schizophrenia, as well as the side effects of the medications used to treat schizophrenia. Helping people to recover and feel the best they can physically with this chronic illness includes the development of healthy day-to-day habits around hygiene, exercise, and nutrition. Nurses also need to be aware of specific issues that can arise for people who have schizophrenia around temperature regulation and fluid and electrolyte balance.

Physical Care

For many people with schizophrenia, the plan of care will include specific interventions to enhance self-care, nutrition, and overall health knowledge. Negative symptoms commonly leave patients unable to initiate these seemingly simple activities. Developing a daily schedule of routine activities (e.g., showering, shaving) can help the patient structure the day. Most patients actually know how to perform self-care activities (e.g., hygiene, grooming) but lack motivation (avolition) to carry them out consistently. Interventions include developing a schedule with the patient for various hygiene-related activities and emphasizing the importance of maintaining appropriate self-care activities. Given the problems related to attention and memory in people with schizophrenia, education about these areas requires careful planning.

Activity, Exercise, and Nutritional Interventions

Encouraging activity and exercise is necessary, not only to maintain a healthy lifestyle but also to counteract the side effects of psychiatric medications that cause weight gain. Because the diagnosis is usually made in late adolescence or early adulthood, it is possible to establish solid exercise patterns early.

During episodes of acute psychosis, patients are sometimes unable to focus on eating. Often when patients begin antipsychotic medication, normal satiety and hunger responses change, and overeating or weight gain can become a problem. Patients report that their appetites increase and cravings for food develop when some medications are initiated. Promoting and maintaining healthy nutrition is a key intervention. Monitoring calorie intake is also important because of the effect many medications have on eating habits.

Weight gain is one of the reasons some patients stop taking their medications. Increased weight places patients at greater risk for several health problems, such as type II DM and early death. Monitoring for DM and managing weight are important activities for all health care providers. Patients should be screened for risk factors of DM, such as family history, obesity as indicated by a body mass index (BMI) exceeding or equal to 27, and age older than 45 years. Patients' weight should be measured at regular intervals and the BMI calculated. Blood pressure readings should be taken regularly. Laboratory findings for triglycerides, high-density lipoprotein cholesterol, and glucose level should be monitored and reviewed regularly. All health care providers should be alert to the development of hyperglycemia, particularly in patients known to have DM who begin taking second-generation antipsychotic agents. A program to address weight gain should be initiated at the earliest sign of weight gain (probably between 5 and 10 pounds over desired body weight). Reduced caloric intake may be accomplished by increasing the patient's access to affordable, healthful, and easy-to-prepare foods. Behavioral management of weight gain includes keeping a food diary, diet teaching, and support groups. Setting small goals and offering a lot of encouragement can lead to some success. (Daumit et al., 2020).

Thermoregulation Interventions

Patients with schizophrenia may have disturbed body temperature regulation. In winter, they may seem to be oblivious to cold weather. In the heat of summer, they may dress for winter. Observing patients' responses to environmental temperatures helps in identifying problems in this area. In patients who are taking psychiatric medications, body temperature needs to be monitored, and the patient needs to be protected from extremes in temperature.

Fluid Balance

Some persons with schizophrenia develop disturbed fluid and electrolyte balance. Nurses should observe for polydipsia (frequently drinking an excessive amount of fluids) or frequent incontinence. These individuals are obsessed with drinking water and compulsively consume fluids. For persons with schizophrenia who demonstrate polydipsia, regulation of their fluid intake is disturbed, resulting in an abnormally low serum sodium level, which can lead to severe water intoxication, a medical emergency.

Nursing interventions include teaching and assisting the patient to develop self-monitoring skills. Fluid intake and weight gain should be monitored to control fluid intake and reduce the likelihood of developing water intoxication. Patients with mild polydipsia are easily treated in outpatient settings and benefit from educational programs that teach them to monitor their own urine's specific gravity and daily weight gains. Patients with moderate polydipsia may respond well to education but still have a more difficult time controlling their own fluid intake, which requires more careful monitoring of intake and weight throughout the day. Patients with severe polydipsia require considerable assistance, probably in an inpatient unit, to restrict their continual water-seeking behavior. These patients may create disruption on the unit, so they are best managed by one-on-one observation to redirect their behavior.

Wellness Challenges

The challenges to the overall wellness of people with schizophrenia include the symptoms of schizophrenia, the effects of medication treatment, and the circumstances around where they live, and their social connections. One example could be addressing a goal related to a healthy diet and exercise. Symptoms of schizophrenia that must be considered are ambivalence, avolition, and lack of motivation. Effects and side effects of medication treatment may include weight gain and sleepiness. Living and social circumstances may include living in group homes with limited access to consistently healthy food, limited funds to purchase healthy food, or living in food deserts in cities or at great distances from food markets in rural towns and communities. These living and social circumstances may limit exercise interventions because housing locations may not be in the safest areas of a city or town.

Wellness goals need to be manageable and specific. Creating goals that focus on small steps is less overwhelming. For instance, selecting a goal to lose 25 pounds may be overwhelming. More manageable goals could be to eat French fries only twice a week and to walk 10 minutes twice a day around the yard of the adult foster care home. Supporting these goals would include conversations around the accomplishment of these activities, as well as measuring outcomes like weight, blood pressure, and hemoglobin A1c, if indicated. Goals can be revised based on levels of success.

Medication Interventions: Antipsychotics

Antipsychotic medications are the treatment of choice for patients with psychosis. Antipsychotic drugs are used because they have the general effect of blocking dopamine transmission, leading to a decrease in psychotic symptoms (see Chapter 12). Some medications also block other receptors of other neurotransmitters to varying degrees (see Table 24.1).

The prescription of first-generation antipsychotics (e.g., haloperidol, chlorpromazine) decreased dramatically with the introduction of second-generation antipsychotics. However, it is important that medication choice be individualized based on each patient's experience and preference, as well as the side effect profiles of selected drugs rather than to limit drug selection to one type or class of antipsychotic medication. This is particularly true during the acute phase of the illness for people with schizophrenia who are known to respond to treatment.

TABLE 24.1	SELECTED ANTIPSYCHOTIC DRUGS	
Generic Name	**Trade Name**	**Dosage Range for Adults (mg/d)**
Second-Generation Antipsychotics		
Aripiprazole	Abilify	10–15
Asenapine	Saphris	10–20
Cariprazine	Vraylar	1.5–6
Clozapine	Clozaril	200–600
Lumateperone	Caplyta	42
Risperidone	Risperdal	4–16
Olanzapine	Zyprexa	10–20
Paliperidone	Invega	3–12
Quetiapine	Seroquel	300–400
Ziprasidone	Geodon	40–160
Lurasidone	Latuda	40–80
Selected First-Generation Antipsychotic Drugs Used to Treat Psychosis in the United States		
Chlorpromazine	NA*	30–800
Fluphenazine	NA	0.5–20
Haloperidol	Haldol	1–15
Loxapine	Loxitane	20–250
Perphenazine	NA	4–32
Pimozide	NA	1–10
Thiothixene	Navane	5–25
Trifluoperazine	NA	5–25

*Not Applicable. No longer available as proprietary formulations.

Second-generation antipsychotic drugs including risperidone (Risperdal), olanzapine (Zyprexa), quetiapine (Seroquel), paliperidone (Invega), ziprasidone (Geodon), aripiprazole (Abilify), iloperidone (Fanapt), asenapine (Saphris), lurasidone (Latuda), cariprazine (Vraylar), and lumateperone (Caplyta) are available in a variety of formulations. See Box 24.8 for more information about risperidone. They are effective in treating both negative and positive symptoms. These drugs also target other neurotransmitter systems, such as serotonin and glutamate. This is believed to contribute to their antipsychotic effectiveness.

Administering Medications

Nursing interventions during the initial acute phase of schizophrenia include prompt, safe, and informed administration of antipsychotic medications. Generally, it takes about 1 to 2 weeks for antipsychotic drugs to effect a change in symptoms. During the stabilization period, the selected drug should be given an adequate trial, generally 6 to 12 weeks, before considering a change in the drug prescription. For maximum absorption, ziprasidone and lurasidone should be given with food. Ziprasidone should be taken with a high-fat meal of 500 calories. For lurasidone, 350 calories should be eaten when administering this (Pfizer, 2020). If treatment effects are not seen, a different antipsychotic agent may be tried. Clozapine is used when no other second-generation antipsychotic is effective; see Box 24.9 for more information about clozapine.

Adherence to a prescribed medication regimen is the best approach to prevent relapse. Unfortunately, adherence to the second-generation antipsychotic agents is not improved from the first-generation antipsychotic. The use of long-acting injectables has improved compliance outcomes (Kane et al., 2020). Box 24.10 provides evidence related to interventions that promote medication adherence for patients with schizophrenia.

Patients with schizophrenia generally face a lifetime of taking antipsychotic medications. Rarely is discontinuation of medications prescribed; however, many patients stop taking medications on their own. Some conditions do require the cessation of medication use, such as **neuroleptic malignant syndrome** (see later discussion), **agranulocytosis** (i.e., dangerously low level of circulating neutrophils), or drug reaction with eosinophilia and systemic symptoms (DRESS) (i.e., fever with a rash and/or swollen lymph glands). Discontinuation is also an option when **tardive dyskinesia** develops. Discontinuation of medications, other than in the circumstances of a medical emergency, should be achieved by gradually lowering the dose over time. This diminishes the likelihood of withdrawal symptoms.

BOX 24.8

Drug Profile: Risperidone (Risperdal)

DRUG CLASS: Atypical antipsychotic

RECEPTOR AFFINITY: Antagonist with high affinity for dopamine D2 and serotonin 5-HT$_2$, also histamine (H1) and α_1-, α_2-adrenergic receptors, weak affinity for D1 and other serotonin receptor subtypes; no affinity for acetylcholine or β-adrenergic receptors

INDICATIONS: Treatment of schizophrenia; short-term treatment of acute manic or mixed episodes associated with bipolar I disorder; and irritability associated with autistic disorder in children and adolescents, including symptoms of aggression toward others, deliberate self-injuriousness, temper tantrums, and quickly changing moods

ROUTES AND DOSAGE: 0.25-, 0.5-, 1-, 2-, 3-, and 4-mg tablets and liquid concentrate (1 mg/mL); orally disintegrating tablets, 0.5, 1, 2, 3, and 4 mg

Adult: Schizophrenia: Initial dose: typically, 1 mg BID. Maximal effect at 6 mg/day. Safety not established above 16 mg/day. Use lowest possible dose to alleviate symptoms.
Bipolar mania: 2 to 3 mg/day
Geriatric: Initial dose, 0.5 mg/day; increase slowly as tolerated
Children: 0.25 mg/day for patients <20 kg and 0.5 mg/day for patients >20 kg

HALF-LIFE (PEAK EFFECT): Mean, 20 h (1 h; peak active metabolite = 3 17 h)

SELECT SIDE EFFECTS: Insomnia, agitation, anxiety, extrapyramidal symptoms, headache, rhinitis, somnolence, dizziness, headache, constipation, nausea, dyspepsia, vomiting, abdominal pain, hypersalivation, tachycardia, orthostatic hypotension, fever, chest pain, coughing, photosensitivity, weight gain

BOXED WARNING: Increased mortality in older patients with dementia-related psychosis

WARNING: Rare development of NMS. Observe frequently for early signs of tardive dyskinesia. Use caution with individuals who have cardiovascular disease; risperidone can cause electrocardiographic changes. Avoid use during pregnancy or while breast feeding. Hepatic or renal impairments increase plasma concentration.

SPECIFIC PATIENT/FAMILY EDUCATION

- Notify your prescriber if tremor, motor restlessness, abnormal movements, chest pain, or other unusual symptoms develop.
- Avoid alcohol and other CNS depressant drugs.
- Notify your prescriber if pregnancy is possible or if planning to become pregnant. Do not breastfeed while taking this medication.
- Notify your prescriber before taking any other prescription or OTC medication.
- May impair judgment, thinking, or motor skills; avoid driving or potentially other hazardous tasks.
- During titration, the individual may experience orthostatic hypotension and should change positions slowly.
- Do not abruptly discontinue.

BID, twice a day; CNS, central nervous system; OTC, over the counter.

BOX 24.9

Drug Profile: Clozapine (Clozaril)

DRUG CLASS: Atypical antipsychotic

RECEPTOR AFFINITY: D1 and D2 blockade, antagonist for 5-HT$_2$, histamine (H1), α-adrenergic, and acetylcholine. These additional antagonist effects may contribute to some of its therapeutic effects. Produces fewer extrapyramidal effects than standard antipsychotics with lower risk for tardive dyskinesia.

INDICATIONS: Severely ill individuals who have schizophrenia and have not responded to standard antipsychotic treatment; reduction in risk of recurrent suicidal behavior in schizophrenia or SADs.

ROUTES AND DOSAGE: Available only in tablet form, 25- and 100-mg doses.

Adult Dosage: Initial dose 25 mg PO twice or four times daily, may gradually increase in 25 to 50 mg/day increments, if tolerated, to a dose of 300 to 450 mg/day by the end of the second week. Additional increases should occur no more than once or twice weekly. Do not exceed 900 mg/day. For maintenance, reduce dosage to lowest effective level.

Children: Safety and efficacy with children younger than age 16 years have not been established.

HALF-LIFE (PEAK EFFECT): 12 h (1 to 6 h)

SELECT ADVERSE REACTIONS: Drowsiness, dizziness, headache, hypersalivation, tachycardia, hypo- or hypertension, constipation, dry mouth, heartburn, nausea or vomiting, blurred vision, diaphoresis, fever, weight gain, hematologic changes, seizures, tremor, akathisia

BOXED WARNING: Agranulocytosis, defined as a granulocyte count of <500 mm^3, occurs at about a cumulative 1-year incidence of 1.3%, most often within 4 to 10 weeks of exposure, but may occur at any time; WBC count before initiation, and weekly WBC counts while taking the drug and for 4 weeks after discontinuation.

BOX 24.9 (*Continued*)

Seizures, myocarditis, and other adverse cardiovascular and respiratory side effects (i.e., orthostatic hypotension).

WARNING: Increased mortality in older patients with dementia-related psychosis; rare development of NMS; *hyperglycemia and DM, tardive dyskinesia,* cases of sudden, unexplained death have been reported; avoid use during pregnancy and while breast feeding.

PRECAUTIONS: Fever, pulmonary embolism, hepatitis, anticholinergic toxicity, and interference with cognitive and motor functions.

SPECIFIC PATIENT/FAMILY EDUCATION

• Need informed consent regarding risk for agranulocytosis. Weekly or biweekly blood draws are required. Notify your prescriber immediately if lethargy, weakness, sore throat, malaise, or other flu-like symptoms develop.
• You should not take clozapine if you are taking other medicines that may cause the same serious bone marrow side effects.

• Inform the patient of risk of seizures, hyperglycemia and diabetes, and orthostatic hypotension. It may potentiate the hypotensive effects of antihypertensive drugs and anticholinergic effects of atropine-like drugs.
• Administration of epinephrine should be avoided in the treatment of drug-induced hypotension.
• Notify your prescriber if pregnancy is possible or if you are planning to become pregnant. Do not breastfeed while taking this medication.
• Notify your prescriber before taking any other prescription or OTC medication. Avoid alcohol or other CNS depressant drugs.
• May cause drowsiness and seizures; avoid driving or other hazardous tasks.
• During titration, the individual may experience orthostatic hypotension and so should change positions slowly.
• Do not abruptly discontinue.

CNS, central nervous system; NMS, neuroleptic malignant syndrome; OTC, over-the-counter; WBC, white blood cell.

BOX 24.10

Research for Evidence-Based Practice: Families and Medication Use and Adherence among Latinos

Hernandez, M. & Barrio, C. (2017). Families and medication use and adherence among Latinos with schizophrenia. Journal of Mental Health, *26(1), 14–20.*

THE QUESTION: What are the perceptions of treatment related to medication use among Latinos with schizophrenia and key family members?

METHODS: Purposive sampling was used to collect data from a total of 34 participants: 14 dyads (made up of 14 patients and 14 key family members) plus 6 key family members of other patients. These six family members, who were interviewed although the patient was not available, were included to provide additional information about family context. Semistructured interviews were conducted with participants in their preferred language.

FINDINGS: Concerns primarily centered on medication side effects. Patients expressed difficulty with low energy, lack of interest in desired activities, and weight gain, among other issues. Family members also noticed changes in patients' affect and behavior. Moreover, families worried about long-term medication use and its effect on patients' health.

IMPLICATIONS FOR NURSING: Family involvement in medication use is important and contributes to patient choices regarding treatment.

Monitoring Extrapyramidal Side Effects

Parkinsonism caused by antipsychotic drugs is identical in appearance to Parkinson disease and tends to occur in older patients. The symptoms are believed to be caused by the blockade of dopamine D_2 receptors in the basal ganglia, which throws off the normal balance between acetylcholine and dopamine in this area of the brain and effectively increases acetylcholine transmission. The symptoms are managed by reducing dosage and thereby increasing dopamine activity or adding an anticholinergic drug, thus decreasing acetylcholine activity, such as benztropine or trihexyphenidyl.

Dystonic reactions are also believed to result from the imbalance of dopamine and acetylcholine, with the latter dominant. Young men seem to be more vulnerable to this particular extrapyramidal side effect. This side effect, which develops rapidly and dramatically, can be very frightening for patients as their muscles tense and their body contorts. The experience often starts with **oculogyric crisis**, in which the muscles that control eye movements tense and pull the eyeball so that the patient is looking toward the ceiling. This may be followed rapidly by **torticollis**, in which the neck muscles pull the head to the side, or **retrocollis**, in which the head is pulled back, or orolaryngeal–pharyngeal hypertonus, in which the patient has extreme difficulty in swallowing. The patient may also experience contorted limbs. These symptoms occur early in antipsychotic drug treatment, when the patient may still be enduring psychotic symptoms, which compounds the patient's fear and anxiety and requires a quick response. The immediate treatment is to administer benztropine 1 to 2 mg, or diphenhydramine (Benadryl), 25 to 50 mg, intramuscularly or intravenously. This is followed by daily administration of anticholinergic drugs and, possibly, by a decrease in dosage antipsychotic medication. See Box 24.11 for more information about benztropine.

Akathisia appears to be caused by the same biologic mechanism as other **extrapyramidal side effects**. Patients are restless and report they feel driven to keep moving. They are extremely uncomfortable. Frequently, this response is misinterpreted as anxiety or increased psychotic symptoms, so that the patient may inappropriately be given increased dosages of an antipsychotic drug, which only perpetuates the side effect. If possible, the dose of antipsychotic drug should be reduced. A beta-adrenergic blocker such as propranolol (Inderal), 20 to 120 mg, may be required. An anticholinergic medication may not be helpful. Failure to manage this side effect is a leading cause of patients ceasing to take antipsychotic medications (see Chapter 12).

Tardive dyskinesia, *tardive dystonia*, and *tardive akathisia* are less likely but still possible to appear in individuals taking second-generation, rather than first-generation, antipsychotics. Table 24.2 describes these and associated motor abnormalities. The term *tardive* means late-appearing, thus all of these movements appear after a person has taken these drugs for a period of time. Thus, tardive dyskinesia is late-appearing abnormal involuntary movements. It can be viewed as the opposite of

---

BOX 24.11

Drug Profile: Benztropine Mesylate

DRUG CLASS: Antiparkinsonism agent

RECEPTOR AFFINITY: Blocks cholinergic (acetylcholine) activity, which is believed to restore the balance of acetylcholine and dopamine in the basal ganglia.

INDICATIONS: Used in psychiatry to reduce extrapyramidal symptoms (acute medication-related movement disorders), including pseudoparkinsonism, dystonia, and akathisia (but not tardive syndromes) caused by neuroleptic drugs such as haloperidol. Most effective with acute dystonia.

ROUTES AND DOSAGE: Available in tablet form, 0.5-, 1-, and 2-mg doses, also injectable 1 mg/mL

Adult Dosage: For acute dystonia, 1 to 2 mg IM or IV usually provides rapid relief. No significant difference in onset of action after IM or IV injection. Treatment of emergent symptoms may be relieved in 1 or 2 days, with 1 to 2 mg PO two to three times a day. Maximum daily dose is 6 mg/day. After 1–2 weeks, withdraw drug to see if continued treatment is needed. Medication-related movement disorders that develop slowly may not respond to this treatment.

Geriatric: Older adults and very thin patients cannot tolerate large doses.

Children: Do not use in children younger than 3 years of age. Use with caution in older children.

HALF-LIFE: 12 to 24 hours; very little pharmacokinetic information is available.

SELECT SIDE EFFECTS: Dry mouth, blurred vision, tachycardia, nausea, constipation, flushing or elevated temperature, decreased sweating, muscular weakness or cramping, urinary retention, urinary hesitancy, dizziness, headache, disorientation, confusion, memory loss, hallucinations, psychoses, and agitation in toxic reactions, which are more pronounced in older adults and occur at smaller doses

WARNING: Avoid use during pregnancy and while breastfeeding. Give with caution in hot weather because of possible heatstroke. Contraindicated with angle-closure glaucoma, pyloric or duodenal obstruction, stenosing peptic ulcers, prostatic hypertrophy or bladder neck obstructions, myasthenia gravis, megacolon, and megaesophagus. May aggravate the symptoms of tardive dyskinesia and other chronic forms of medication-related movement disorder. Concomitant use of other anticholinergic drugs may increase side effects and risk for toxicity. Coadministration of haloperidol or phenothiazines may reduce serum levels of these drugs.

SPECIFIC PATIENT/FAMILY EDUCATION

- Take with meals to reduce dry mouth and gastric irritation.
- Dry mouth may also be alleviated by sucking sugarless candies, maintaining adequate fluid intake, and good oral hygiene; increase fiber and fluids in diet to avoid constipation; stool softeners may be required. Notify your prescriber if urinary hesitancy or constipation persists.
- Notify your prescriber if rapid or pounding heartbeat, confusion, eye pain, rash, or other side effects develop.
- May cause drowsiness, dizziness, or blurred vision; use caution driving or performing other hazardous tasks requiring alertness. Avoid alcohol and other CNS depressants.
- Do not abruptly stop this medication because a flu-like syndrome may develop.
- Use with caution in hot weather. Ensure adequate hydration. May increase susceptibility to heat stroke.

CNS, central nervous system; IM, intramuscular; IV, intravenous; PO, oral.

TABLE 24.2	EXTRAPYRAMIDAL SIDE EFFECTS OF ANTIPSYCHOTIC DRUGS	
Side Effect	Period of Onset	Symptoms
Acute Motor Abnormalities		
Parkinsonism or pseudoparkinsonism	5–30 d	Resting tremor, rigidity, bradykinesia or akinesia, masklike face, shuffling gait, decreased arm swing
Acute dystonia	1–5 d	Intermittent or fixed abnormal postures of the eyes, face, tongue, neck, trunk, and limbs
Akathisia	1–30 d	Obvious motor restlessness evidenced by pacing, rocking, shifting from foot to foot; subjective sense of not being able to sit or be still; these symptoms may occur together or separately
Late-Appearing Motor Abnormalities		
Tardive dyskinesia	Months to years	Abnormal dyskinetic movements of the face, mouth, and jaw; choreoathetoid movements of the legs, arms, and trunk
Tardive dystonia	Months to years	Persistent sustained abnormal postures in the face, eyes, tongue, neck, trunk, and limbs
Tardive akathisia	Months to years	Persistent unabating sense of subjective and objective restlessness

Adapted from Levenson, J.L., Crouse, E.L., & Bozymski, K.M. (2019). Psychopharmacology. In L.W. Roberts, (Eds.), *The American psychiatric publishing textbook of psychiatry* (7th ed.). American Psychiatric Association.

parkinsonism, both in observable movements and in etiology. Whereas muscle rigidity and absence of movement characterize parkinsonism, constant movement characterizes tardive dyskinesia. Typical movements involve the mouth, tongue, and jaw and include lip smacking, sucking, puckering, tongue protrusion, the "bonbon sign" (where the tongue rolls around in the mouth and protrudes into the cheek as if the patient is sucking on a piece of hard candy), athetoid (worm-like) movements of the tongue and chewing. Other facial movements, such as grimacing and eye blinking, may also be present.

Movements in the trunk and limbs are frequently observable with tardive dyskinesia. These include rocking from the hips, athetoid movements of the fingers and toes, jerking movements of the fingers and toes, guitar-strumming movements of the fingers, and foot tapping. The long-term health problems for people with tardive dyskinesia are choking, associated with loss of control of muscles used for swallowing, and compromised respiratory function, leading to infections and possibly respiratory alkalosis.

Because the movements resemble the dyskinetic movements of some patients who have idiopathic Parkinson disease and who have received long-term treatment with l-DOPA (a direct-acting dopamine agonist that crosses the blood–brain barrier), the suggested hypothesis for tardive dyskinesia includes the supersensitivity of the dopamine receptors in the basal ganglia.

An effective treatment for tardive dyskinesia has been elusive. However, antipsychotic drugs mask the movements of tardive dyskinesia and have periodically been suggested as a treatment. This is counterintuitive because these drugs cause the disorder. Second-generation antipsychotic drugs, such as clozapine, may be less likely to cause it; however, recent interest suggests that the tardive dyskinesia is still prevalent but at a lesser rate (Misdrahi et al., 2019). Recently the medications deutetrabenazine and valbenazine have been approved by the U.S. Food and Drug Administration (FDA) and appear to ameliorate the movements of tardive dyskinesia by decreasing the transport of dopamine into storage vesicles (via inhibition of vesicular monoamine transporter 2—VMAT2) and therefore reducing the overall availability of dopamine (Ricciardi et al., 2019). However, the best management remains prevention through using the lowest possible dose of an antipsychotic drug over time that minimizes the symptoms of schizophrenia as well as regular evaluation of movements using tools like the DISCUS (see Box 24.4).

Monitoring Other Side Effects

Orthostatic hypotension is a common side effect of antipsychotic drugs. Primarily an antiadrenergic effect, decreased blood pressure may be generalized or orthostatic. Patients may be protected from falls by teaching them to rise slowly and by monitoring blood pressure before giving the medication. The nurse should monitor and document lying, sitting, and standing blood pressures when any antipsychotic drug therapy begins.

Hyperprolactinemia can occur. When dopamine is blocked in the tuberoinfundibular tract, it can no longer repress prolactin, the neurohormone that regulates lactation and mammary function. The prolactin level increases and, in some individuals, side effects appear. Gynecomastia (i.e., enlarged breasts) can occur in people of both sexes and is understandably distressing to individuals who may be experiencing delusional or hallucinatory body image disturbances. Galactorrhea (i.e., lactation) may also occur. Menstrual irregularities and sexual dysfunction are possible. If these symptoms appear, the medication should be reduced or changed to another antipsychotic agent. Hyperprolactinemia is associated with the use of haloperidol and risperidone.

Sedation is another possible side effect of antipsychotic medication and a frequent reason that patients discontinue medications. Patients should be monitored for the sedating effects of antipsychotic agents. In older patients, sedation can be associated with falls.

Weight gain is related to antipsychotic agents, especially olanzapine and clozapine. Patients may gain as much as 20 or 30 pounds within 1 year. Such increased appetite and weight gain are distressing to patients. Diet teaching and monitoring may have some effect. Another solution is to increase the accessibility of healthful easy-to-prepare food. Simple exercise routines may be helpful.

New-onset DM should be assessed in patients taking antipsychotic drugs. An association has been found between new-onset DM and the administration of second-generation antipsychotic agents, especially after weight gain. Patients should be monitored for clinical symptoms of diabetes. Fasting blood glucose tests and Hemoglobin A1C monitoring are commonly ordered for these individuals.

Cardiac arrhythmias may also occur. Prolongation of the QTc interval is associated with torsade de pointe (polymorphic ventricular tachycardia) or ventricular fibrillation. The potential for drug-induced prolonged QT interval is associated with many drugs. Ziprasidone (Geodon) is more likely than other second-generation antipsychotics to prolong the QT interval and thus change the heart rhythm. For these patients, baseline electrocardiograms may be ordered. Nurses should observe these patients for cardiac arrhythmias.

Agranulocytosis is a reduction in the number of circulating granulocytes and decreased production of granulocytes in the bone marrow, which limits one's ability to fight infection. Agranulocytosis can develop with the use of all antipsychotic drugs, but it is most likely to develop with clozapine use. Although laboratory values below 500 cells/mm^3 are indicative of agranulocytosis, often granulocyte counts drop to below 200 cells/mm^3 with this syndrome.

Patients taking clozapine should have regular blood tests. White blood cell and granulocyte counts should be measured before treatment is initiated and at least weekly or twice weekly after treatment begins. Initial white blood cell counts should be above 3,500 cells/mm^3 before treatment initiation; in patients with counts of 3,500 and 5,000 cells/mm^3, cell counts should be monitored three times a week if clozapine is prescribed. Any time the white blood cell count drops below 3,500 cells/mm^3 or granulocytes drop below 1,500 cells/mm^3, use of clozapine should be stopped, and the patient should be monitored for infection.

However, a faithfully implemented program of blood monitoring should not replace careful observation of the patient. It is not unusual for blood cell counts to drop precipitously over a period of 2 to 3 days. This may not be discovered when the patient is on a strict weekly blood monitoring schedule. Any reported symptoms that suggest a bacterial infection (e.g., fever, pharyngitis, weakness) should be cause for concern, so immediate evaluation of blood count status should be undertaken. Because patients are frequently discharged before the critical period of risk for agranulocytosis, patient education about these symptoms is also essential so that they will report these symptoms, obtain blood monitoring, and reduce their potential exposure to infections. In general, granulocyte levels return to normal within 2 to 4 weeks after discontinuation of use of the medication.

DRESS is a very rare, potentially life-threatening, drug-induced hypersensitivity reaction recently associated with ziprasidone therapy (Geodon). The FDA published a safety announcement related to ziprasidone's association to DRESS. Symptoms include skin eruption, hematologic abnormalities (e.g., eosinophilia, atypical lymphocytosis), lymphadenopathy, and internal organ involvement (e.g., liver, kidney, lung). DRESS has a mortality rate of 10% (U.S. Food and Drug Administration, 2015).

Preventing Drug–Drug Interactions

Antipsychotic medications have the potential to interact with other medications, nicotine, and grapefruit juice. For example, olanzapine and clozapine have the potential to interact with some antidepressants. Some antipsychotics are metabolized faster in smokers than nonsmokers (Chui et al., 2019). Conversely, problems with increased side effects from slower drug metabolism can occur when smoking cessation programs are initiated. Before giving medication, the nurse should check all medications for potential interactions.

Teaching Points

Nonadherence to the medication regimen is an important factor in relapse; the family must be made aware of the importance of the patient's taking medications consistently. Medication education should cover the association between medications and the amelioration of symptoms, side effects, and their management, and interpersonal skills that help the patient and family report medication effects.

Management of Complications

Neuroleptic Malignant Syndrome

Neuroleptic malignant syndrome (NMS) is a life-threatening condition that can develop in reaction to antipsychotic medications. The primary symptoms of NMS are *mental status changes*, *severe muscle rigidity*, and *autonomic changes*, including elevated temperature (usually between 101°F and 103°F), tachycardia, and blood pressure lability. Mental status changes and severe muscle rigidity occur usually within the first week of initiation of antipsychotic therapy and can include two or more of the following: hypertension, tachycardia, tachypnea, prominent diaphoresis, incontinence, mutism, leukocytosis, and laboratory evidence of muscle injury (e.g., elevated creatinine phosphokinase). The incidence of NMS has decreased from 3% to 0.16%, probably because of increased awareness of symptoms, use of atypical antipsychotics, and earlier interventions, such as stopping the offending medication (Schneider et al., 2018). As many as 5% to 15% of affected patients may die as a result of the syndrome. In the past, NMS was probably underreported and may have accounted for unexplained emergency department deaths of patients taking these drugs because their symptoms did not seem serious.

The most important aspects of nursing care for patients with NMS relate to recognizing symptoms early, withholding any antipsychotic or any other dopamine antagonist (e.g., gastric reflux medications), and initiating supportive nursing care (Fig. 24.4). In any patient with muscle rigidity, fluctuating vital signs, abrupt changes in levels of consciousness, or any of the symptoms presented in Box 24.12, NMS should be suspected. The nurse should be especially alert for early signs and symptoms of NMS in high-risk patients, such as those who are

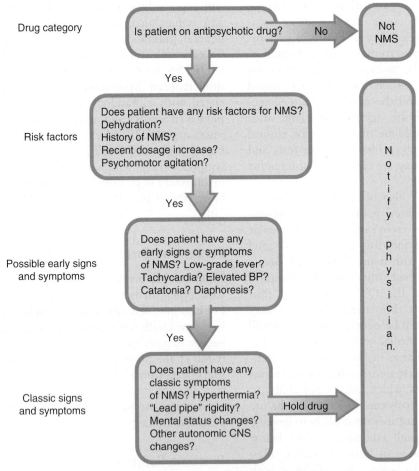

FIGURE 24.4 Action tree for "holding" an antipsychotic drug because of suspected neuroleptic malignant syndrome.

BP, blood pressure; CNS, central nervous system; NMS, neuroleptic malignant syndrome.

BOX 24.12
Recognizing Neuroleptic Malignant Syndrome

Onset: 2 weeks after initiation of antipsychotic treatment or change in dosage
Risk factors: Male gender, preexisting medical or neurologic disorders, depot injection administration, and high ambient temperature

IMMINENT INDICATORS
- Mental status changes
- Muscle rigidity
- Hyperthermia
- Tachycardia
- Hypertension or hypotension
- Tachypnea or hypoxia
- Diaphoresis or sialorrhea
- Tremor
- Incontinence
- Creatinine phosphokinase elevation or myoglobinuria
- Leukocytosis
- Metabolic acidosis

Source: Neuroleptic malignant syndrome. Retrieved on February 20, 2021 from https://rarediseases.org/rare-diseases/neuroleptic-malignant-syndrome/

agitated, physically exhausted, or dehydrated or who have an existing medical or neurologic illness. Patients receiving parenteral or higher doses of neuroleptic drugs or lithium concurrently must also be carefully assessed. The nurse should carefully monitor fluid intake, and fluid and electrolyte status.

NCLEXNOTE Recognition of side effects, including movement disorders, tardive dyskinesia, and weight gain, should lead to interventions. NMS is a medical emergency.

Medical treatment focuses on symptom management and includes administering dopamine agonist drugs, such as bromocriptine (modest success), and muscle relaxants, such as dantrolene or benzodiazepine. Antiparkinsonism drugs are not particularly useful. Some patients experience improvement with electroconvulsive therapy (ECT).

The nurse must frequently monitor vital signs of the patient with symptoms of NMS. In addition, it is important to check the results of the patient's laboratory tests for increased creatine phosphokinase, an elevated white blood cell count, elevated liver enzymes, or myoglobinuria. The nurse must be prepared to initiate supportive measures or anticipate emergency transfer of the patient to a medical-surgical or an intensive care unit.

Treating fever (which frequently exceeds 103°F) is an important priority for these patients. High body temperature may be reduced with a cooling blanket

and acetaminophen therapy. Because many of these patients experience diaphoresis, temperature elevation, or dysphagia, it is important to monitor hydration. Another important aspect of care for patients with NMS is safety. Joints and extremities that are rigid or spastic must be protected from injury. The treatment of these patients depends on the facility and availability of medical support services. In general, patients in psychiatric inpatient units that are separated from general hospitals are transferred to medical-surgical settings for treatment.

Cholinergic Rebound

If patients are prescribed an anticholinergic agent, such as benztropine, for movement disorders and they abruptly stop taking it, they could experience **cholinergic rebound** symptoms including vomiting, excessive sweating, and altered dreams and nightmares. Cholinergic rebound can be especially problematic if patients discontinue other medications with anticholinergic properties (e.g., antipsychotics, antidepressants, antibiotics) at the same time. Medications with anticholinergic properties should be reduced gradually (tapered) over several days. Table 24.3 lists anticholinergic side effects and several antipsychotic medications and interventions to manage them.

TABLE 24.3 NURSING INTERVENTIONS FOR ANTICHOLINERGIC SIDE EFFECTS

Effect	Intervention
Dry mouth	Provide sips of water, hard candies, and chewing gum (preferably sugar free).
Blurred vision	Avoid dangerous tasks; teach patient that this side effect will diminish in a few weeks.
Decreased lacrimation	Use artificial tears if necessary.
Mydriasis	May aggravate glaucoma; teach patient to report eye pain.
Photophobia	Wear sunglasses.
Constipation	High-fiber diet; increased fluid intake; take laxatives as prescribed.
Urinary hesitancy	Privacy; run water in sink; warm water over perineum
Urinary retention	Regular voiding (at least every 2–3 h) and whenever urge is present; catheterize for residual urine; record intake and output; evaluate for benign prostatic hypertrophy.
Tachycardia	Evaluate for preexisting cardiovascular disease.

Anticholinergic Medication Effects and Abuse

The potential exists for abuse of anticholinergic drugs. Some patients may find the anticholinergic effects of these drugs on mood, memory, and perception pleasurable. Although at toxic dosages, patients may experience a mild delirium with disorientation and hallucinations, lesser doses may cause patients to experience greater sociability and euphoria.

Anticholinergic Crisis

An **anticholinergic crisis** is a potentially life-threatening medical emergency caused by an overdose of or sensitivity to drugs with anticholinergic properties. This syndrome (also called anticholinergic delirium) may result from an accidental or intentional overdose of anticholinergic drugs, including atropine, scopolamine, or belladonna alkaloids, which are present in numerous prescription drugs and OTC medicines. The syndrome may also occur in psychiatric patients who are not only receiving therapeutic doses of anticholinergic drugs but also taking other drugs with anticholinergic properties. As a result of either drug overdose or sensitivity, these anticholinergic substances may produce acute delirium or a psychotic reaction resembling schizophrenia. Severe anticholinergic effects may occur in older patients, even at therapeutic levels (Pasina et al., 2019).

The signs and symptoms of anticholinergic crisis are dramatic and physically uncomfortable (Box 24.13). This disorder is characterized by fever, parched mouth, burning thirst, hot dry skin, decreased salivation, decreased bronchial and nasal secretions, widely dilated eyes (bright light becomes painful), decreased ability to accommodate visually, increased heart rate, constipation, difficulty urinating, and hypertension or hypotension. The face, neck, and upper arms may become flushed because of reflexive blood vessel dilation. In addition to peripheral symptoms, patients with anticholinergic psychosis may experience neuropsychiatric symptoms of anxiety, agitation, delirium, hyperactivity, confusion, hallucinations (especially visual), speech difficulties, psychotic symptoms, or seizures. The acute psychotic reaction that is produced resembles schizophrenia. The classic description of anticholinergic crisis is summarized in the following mnemonic: "Hot as a hare, blind as a bat, mad as a hatter, dry as a bone."

In general, episodes of anticholinergic crisis are self-limiting, usually subsiding in 3 days. However, if left untreated, the associated fever and delirium may progress to coma or cardiac and respiratory depression. Although rare, death is generally caused by hyperpyrexia and brain stem depression. After use of the offending drug is discontinued, improvement usually occurs within 24 to 36 hours.

BOX 24.13

Signs and Symptoms of Anticholinergic Crisis

- **Neuropsychiatric signs:** confusion; recent memory loss; agitation; dysarthria; incoherent speech; pressured speech; delusions; ataxia; periods of hyperactivity alternating with somnolence, paranoia, anxiety, or coma
- **Hallucinations:** accompanied by "picking," plucking, or grasping motions; delusions; or disorientation
- **Physical signs:** nonreactive dilated pupils; blurred vision; hot, dry, flushed skin; facial flushing; dry mucous membranes; difficulty swallowing; fever; tachycardia; hypertension; decreased bowel sounds; urinary retention; nausea; vomiting; seizures; or coma

---

A specific and effective antidote, physostigmine, a reversible inhibitor of cholinesterase, is frequently used to treat and diagnose anticholinergic crisis. Administration of this drug rapidly reduces both behavioral and physiologic symptoms. However, the usual adult dose of physostigmine is 1 to 2 mg, intravenously given slowly during a period of 5 minutes because rapid injection of physostigmine may cause seizures, profound bradycardia, or heart block. Physostigmine is relatively short acting, so it may need to be given several times during the course of treatment. This drug provides relief from symptoms for a period of 2 to 3 hours. In addition to receiving physostigmine, patients who intentionally overdose on large amounts of anticholinergic drugs are treated by gastric lavage, administration of charcoal, and catharsis. The dose may be given again after 20 or 30 minutes.

It is important for the nurse to be alert for signs and symptoms of anticholinergic crisis, especially in older and pediatric patients, who are much more sensitive to the anticholinergic effects of drugs, and in patients who are receiving multiple medications with anticholinergic effects. If signs and symptoms of the syndrome occur, the nurse should discontinue use of the offending drug and notify the physician immediately.

Electroconvulsive Therapy

ECT is suggested as a possible alternative when the patient's schizophrenia is not being successfully treated by medication alone. For the most part, this modality is not indicated unless the patient is catatonic or has depression that is not treatable by other means. In general, ECT is not used often for the treatment of schizophrenia, but it may be useful for those persons who are medication resistant, assaultive, and psychotic (Kellner et al., 2020).

Psychosocial Interventions

Psychosocial interventions, such as counseling, conflict resolution, behavior therapy, and cognitive interventions, are appropriate for patients with schizophrenia. The following discussion focuses on applying these interventions.

Therapeutic Interactions

Although antipsychotic medications may relieve positive symptoms, they do not always eliminate hallucinations and delusions. The nurse must continue helping the patient develop creative strategies for dealing with these sensory and thought disturbances. Information about the content of the hallucinations and delusions is necessary, not only to determine whether the medications are effective but also to assess safety and the meaning of these thoughts and perceptions to the patient. In caring for a patient who is experiencing hallucinations or delusions, nursing actions should be guided by three general patient outcomes:

- Decrease the frequency and intensity of hallucinations and delusions.
- Recognize that hallucinations and delusions are symptoms of a brain disorder.
- Develop strategies to manage the recurrence of hallucinations or delusions.

When interacting with a patient who is experiencing hallucinations or delusions, the nurse must remember that these experiences are real to the patient. It is important for the nurse to understand the content and meaning of the hallucinations, particularly those involving command hallucinations.

On the one hand, the nurse should never tell a patient that these experiences are not real. Discounting the experiences blocks communication. On the other hand, it is also dishonest for the nurse to tell the patient that the nurse is having the same hallucinatory experience. It is best to validate the patient's experiences and identify the meaning of these thoughts and feelings to the patient. For example, a patient who believes that they are under surveillance by the Federal Bureau of Investigation probably feels frightened and suspicious of everyone. By acknowledging how frightening it must be to always feel like you are being watched, the nurse focuses on the feelings that are generated by the delusion, not the delusion itself. The nurse can then offer to help the patient feel safe within this environment. The patient, in turn, begins to feel that someone understands them.

Enhancing Cognitive Functioning

After identifying deficits in cognitive functioning, the nurse and patient can develop interventions that target specific deficits. The most effective interventions usually involve the whole treatment team. If the ability to focus or maintain attention is an issue, patients can be encouraged to select activities that improve attention, such as computer games. For memory problems, patients can be encouraged to make lists and to write down important information.

Executive functioning problems are the most challenging for these patients. Patients who cannot manage daily problems may have planning and problem-solving impairments. For these patients, developing interventions that closely simulate real-world problems may help. Through coaching, the nurse can teach and support the development of problem-solving skills. For example, during hospitalizations, patients are given medications and reminded to take them on time. They are often instructed in a classroom setting but rarely have an opportunity to practice self-medication and figure out what to do if their prescription expires, the medications are lost, or they forget to take their medications. Even so, when discharged, patients are expected to take medication at the prescribed dose at the prescribed time. Interventions designed to have patients actively engage in problem-solving behavior with real problems are needed.

Other approaches to helping patients solve problems and learn new strategies for dealing with problems include solution-focused therapy, which focuses on the strengths and positive attributes that exist within each person, and cognitive-behavioral therapy (Jones et al., 2019), which focuses directly on collaboratively determined symptoms and strategies to address them. These therapies involve years of training to master, but certain techniques can be used. For example, the nurse can ask patients to identify the most important problem from their perspective. This focuses the patient on an important issue for them.

Using Behavioral Interventions

Behavioral interventions can be very effective in helping patients improve motivation and organize routine, daily activities, such as maintaining a regular schedule and completing activities. Reinforcement of positive behaviors (getting up on time, completing hygiene, going to treatment activities) can easily be included in a treatment plan. In the hospital, patients gain unit privileges by following an agreed-on treatment plan. In the community, a behavioral intervention is more likely to be combined with other approaches or used for a specific behavior such as smoking (Wilson et al., 2019).

Psychoeducation
Teaching Strategies

Cognitive deficits (e.g., difficulty in processing complex information, maintaining steady focus of attention, distinguishing between relevant and irrelevant stimuli, and forming abstractions) may challenge the nurse planning educational activities. Evidence indicates that people with schizophrenia may learn best in an errorless learning environment (Kern et al., 2018). That is, they are directly given correct information and then encouraged to write it down. Errorless learning is an educational intervention based on the principle of operant conditioning that learning is stronger and more likely to last if it occurs in the absence of errors. Asking questions that encourage guessing is not as effective in helping patients retain information. Trial-and-error learning is avoided.

Teaching and explaining should occur in an environment with minimal distractions. Terminology should be clear and unambiguous. Visual aids can supplement verbal information, but these materials should have simple information stated in simple language. The nurse takes care not to overcrowd the visual material or incorporate images that draw attention away from important content. Teaching should occur in small segments with frequent reinforcement. Most importantly, teaching should occur when the patient is ready. Regular assessments of cognitive abilities with standardized instruments can help determine this readiness. These suggestions can be adapted for teaching during any phase of the illness.

Teaching About Symptoms

Teaching patients that hallucinations and delusions are part of the disorder becomes easier after the medication begins working. When patients believe and acknowledge that they have a mental illness and that some of their thoughts are delusions and some of their perceptions are hallucinations, they can develop strategies to manage their symptoms.

Patients benefit greatly by learning recovery strategies of self-regulation, symptom monitoring, and relapse prevention. By monitoring events, time, place, and stimuli surrounding the appearance of symptoms, the patient can begin to predict high-risk times for symptom recurrence. Cognitive-behavioral therapy is often used in helping patients monitor and identify their emerging symptoms to prevent relapse (Liu et al., 2019b).

Another important nursing intervention is to help the patient identify to whom and where to talk about delusional or hallucinatory material. Because self-disclosure of these symptoms immediately labels someone as having a mental illness, patients should be encouraged to evaluate the environment for negative consequences of disclosing these symptoms. For example, it may be fine to talk about it at home but not at the grocery store.

Teaching How to Cope With Stress

Developing skills to cope with personal, social, and environmental stresses is important to everyone but particularly to those with a severe mental illness. Stresses can easily trigger symptoms that patients are trying to avoid. Establishing regular counseling sessions to support the development of positive coping skills is helpful for both hospitalized patients and those living in the community.

Wellness Strategies

Wellness strategies require providers to consider multiple aspects of what is considered a well-lived life. As with recovery, it is important to establish what "living well with mental illness" means to the individual with schizophrenia. Within the limitations of the illness and its treatment, providers need to work with the person to define wellness. Wellness should be defined beyond just the best physical health possible and includes positive social relationships, engaging leisure and work activities, and spiritual connections, to name a few. To varying degrees, evidence supports interventions such as (1) cognitive training and remediation that focus on cognitive impairments and social functioning (Miley et al., 2020) and could incorporate new methodologies that use virtual reality (Souto et al., 2020); (2) support that provides information about the illness, addresses emotional needs, acknowledges the challenges of the illness, encourages the person, and provides guidance (Beentjes et al., 2020); and (3) goal setting with the individual that uses methodologies like the "Choose-Get-Keep" model that supports client goals over the imposition of provider goals (Anthony et al., 2014).

Social Skills Training

Social skills training, provided either individually or in groups, is also useful when working with patients who have schizophrenia (Vogel et al., 2019). This training teaches patients specific behaviors needed for social interactions. The skills are taught by lecture, demonstration, role-playing, and homework assignments. Nurses may be team members and be involved in case management or provision of services. Furthermore, efforts to offer supportive employment experiences (Carmona et al., 2019) that incorporate patient preferences, rapid job search and employment, and ongoing job supports have shown effectiveness. Although long-term self-sufficiency has not necessarily been achieved, supportive employment has been the most effective vocational rehabilitation method.

Skill-training interventions should be designed to compensate for cognitive deficits. To help patients learn to process complex activities, such as catching a bus, preparing a meal, or shopping for food or clothing, nurses should break the activity into small parts or steps and list them for the patient's reference, for example:

- Leave your apartment with your keys in hand.
- Make sure you have correct bus fare in your pocket.
- Close the door.
- Walk to the corner.
- Turn right and walk three blocks to the bus stop.

 Concept Mastery Alert

If the patient has active psychosis, with symptoms such as hallucinations and social withdrawal, wait until a lucid period to begin social skills training. When a patient is in active psychosis, it is not a good time to introduce additional stressors.

Providing Family Education

Because having a family member with schizophrenia is a life-changing event for the family and friends who provide care and support, educating patients and their families is crucial. It is a primary concern for the psychiatric–mental health nurse. Family support is crucial to help patients maintain treatment. Education should include information about the disease course, treatment regimens, support systems, and life management skills (Box 24.14). The most important factor to stress during patient and family education is the consistent taking of medication.

Promoting Safety

Although violence is not a consistent behavior of people with schizophrenia, it is always a concern during the initial phase when hallucinations or delusions may put patients at risk for harming themselves or others. Nonviolent patients who are experiencing hallucinations

---

BOX 24.14

Psychoeducation Checklist: Schizophrenia

When caring for the patient with schizophrenia, be sure to include the caregiver during planning as appropriate and address the following topic areas in the teaching plan:

- Psychopharmacologic agents, including drug action, dosage, frequency, and possible side effects; stress the importance of adherence to the prescribed regimen
- Management of hallucinations
- Recovery strategies
- Coping strategies (e.g., self-talk, getting busy with something)
- Management of the environment
- Community resources

---

and delusions can also be at risk for victimization by more aggressive patients. The patient who is hallucinating needs to be protected; this may include increased staff monitoring and, if necessary, a safer environment in a secluded area.

Identifying patient risk factors for violence, such as a history of violence can alert the nursing staff of a potential for engaging in aggressive behavior, but careful assessment and management of the immediate environment and treating the psychiatric symptoms are more important in avoiding aggression. The nurse's best approach to avoiding violence or aggression is to demonstrate respect for the patient and the patient's personal space, assess and monitor for signs of fear and agitation, and use preventive interventions before the patient loses control. Patients should be encouraged to discuss their anger and to be involved in their treatment decisions. Medications should be administered as ordered. Because most antipsychotic and antidepressant medications take 1 to 2 weeks to begin moderating behavior, the nurse must be vigilant during the acute illness.

If the patient loses control and is a danger to self or others, restraints and seclusion may be used as a last resort. Health Care Financing Administration guidelines and hospital policy must be followed (see Chapter 4), and staff should be trained in the proper use of seclusion and restraints. In addition, staff need to have planned sessions after all incidents of violence or physical management to analyze the event. These sessions allow clinicians to learn how better to manage these situations and evaluate patients' cues. With sensitive leadership, these sessions can help health care workers to learn more about the interaction of patient and staff characteristics that can contribute to these incidents.

Convening Support Groups

People with mental illness benefit from support groups that focus on daily problems and the stress of dealing with a mental illness. These groups are useful throughout the continuum of care and help reduce the risk of suicide. In the hospital setting, the focus of the group can be simply sharing the experience of living with a mental illness. In the community, a regular support group can provide interaction with people with similar problems and issues. Friendships often develop from these groups. Using peer counseling and support groups is a component of recovery-oriented care, but research is needed to understand these groups' impact on care (Chien et al., 2019).

Implementing Milieu Therapy

Individuals with schizophrenia may be hospitalized or may live in group homes for a long period of time. The challenge is helping people who are unable to live with family members to live harmoniously with strangers who have similar interpersonal difficulties. Arranging the treatment environment to maximize therapy is crucial to the rehabilitation of the patient.

Developing Recovery-Oriented Rehabilitation Strategies

Rehabilitation strategies are used to support the individual's recovery and integration into the community (see Box 24.15). Factors that have been shown to promote recovery include the following:

- Adjustment, coping, and reappraisal
- Responding to the illness
- Social support, close relationships, and belonging

Factors that have a negative impact on the process of recovery include (1) negative interactions and isolation, (2) internal barriers, and (3) uncertainty and hopelessness (Soundy et al., 2015). Community-based psychosocial rehabilitation programs usually offer long-term intensive case management services to adults with schizophrenia. Programs provide a continuum of services to meet the changing needs of people with psychiatric disabilities. Patients set rehabilitation goals, and services are then provided to help "clients" (most programs do not use the term *patients*) reach their goals. Services range from daily home visits to providing transportation, occupational training and supported employment, and group support. Assertive community treatment (ACT) is one example of these types of services and has a solid base of evidence to support its use (Thorning & Dixon, 2020).

Evaluation and Treatment Outcomes

Outcome research related to schizophrenia has redefined previous ways of thinking about the course of the disorder. Schizophrenia was formerly considered to have a progressively long-term and downward course, but it is now known that schizophrenia can be successfully treated and recovery is possible (Vita & Barlati, 2018). In one older but significant study, the researchers interviewed patients 20 to 25 years after diagnosis and found that 50% to 66% experienced significant improvement or recovery (Harding et al., 1987). This study is important because it occurred before the development of second-generation antipsychotic agents. Today, we can be hopeful that even more people can experience improvement or recover from schizophrenia.

Continuum of Care

Continuity of care has been identified as a primary strategy for recovery because individuals with

---

BOX 24.15
A Brother's Perspective

A sibling describes his brother with schizophrenia and the importance of both medications and relationships.

In 1998, at the age of 40 years, Robert was admitted to a psychiatric hospital. His brother was told at the time that he would never be able to live independently, and even if discharged, would only be repeatedly hospitalized. Robert had a long history of treatment and in 1998 he had received various types of antipsychotic medications, but he had not received any of the "new atypical variety." He was prescribed one of these drugs, and within months, the staff who had predicted the most discouraging of outcomes told Robert's brother that he was in the midst of a miraculous recovery—his thinking was clear and free from delusions and they were preparing Robert's discharge.

A few weeks into the discharge planning, Robert called his brother; Robert was distressed because his social worker, whom Robert had known for years from a prior hospitalization, was leaving. The social worker had been abruptly transferred to another hospital. Robert deteriorated rapidly into tantrums, hallucinations, and dangerous behaviors. His discharge was put on hold. Robert's brother's rhetorical question was, "What was the difference between Robert on the same medication on Monday, when he was all right, and Tuesday, when he no longer was?" His answer to Robert's condition was the loss of an important relationship.

Robert is now living in a community-based home where the dedicated staff members have shown that they can maintain rehospitalization rates below 3%.

Robert's brother has interviewed many former psychiatric patients for a book. He found that every one of his interviewees, while attributing their recovery to medications or finding God, or a particular program, also identified an important relationship with one human being who believed in their ability to recover. Most of the time, this person was a professional, such as a social worker, a nurse, or a doctor. Sometimes, however, it was a member of the clergy or family member. A believing relationship....

Robert's brother concluded, "Let's provide a range of medications, and let's study their effectiveness, but let's remember that the pill is the ultimate downsizing. Let's find resources to give people afflicted with mental illness what all of us need: fellow human beings upon whom we can depend on to help us through our dark times and, once through, to emerge into gloriously imperfect lives."

For nurses, it is important to remember that it is not what we do *to* people, but rather, what we do *with* people: give hope, listen to their dreams, help them find ways to get as close as they can.

Adapted from Neugeboren, J. (2006). Meds alone couldn't bring Robert back. *Newsweek*. National Empowerment Center. Retrieved February 20, 2021 from http://power2u.org/meds-alone-couldnt-bring-robert-back/

---

schizophrenia are at risk for becoming "lost" to services if left alone after discharge. Discharge planning encourages follow-up care in the community. In fact, many state mental health systems require an outpatient appointment before discharge. Treatment of people with schizophrenia occurs across a variety of settings. Not only inpatient hospitalization but also partial hospitalization, day treatment, and crisis stabilization can be used effectively.

Emergency Care

Emergency care ideally takes place in a hospital emergency department, but often the crisis occurs in the home. Patients are usually relapsing and do not recognize their bizarre or aggressive behaviors as symptoms. A specially trained crisis team is sent to assess the emergency and recommend further treatment. In the emergency department, patients are brought not only because of relapse but also because of medication side effects or water intoxication. Nurses should refer to the previous discussion for nursing management.

Inpatient-Focused Care

Inpatient hospitalizations are brief and focus on stabilization. Many times, patients are involuntarily admitted for a short period (see Chapter 4). During the stabilization period, the status is changed to voluntary admission, whereby the patient agrees to treatment.

Community Care

Most of the care of persons with schizophrenia is provided in the community through publicly supported recovery-oriented mental health delivery systems. The recovery journey can be long and require a variety of services such as ACT, outpatient therapy, case management, and psychosocial rehabilitation, including clubhouse programs. While the patient is in the community, their health care should be integrated with physical health care. Nurses should be especially vigilant that patients with mental illnesses receive proper primary and medical health care.

> **NCLEXNOTE** Priorities in the patient with acute symptoms of schizophrenia include managing psychosis and keeping the patient safe and free from harming themselves or others. In the community, the priorities are preventing relapse, maintaining psychosocial functioning, engaging in psychoeducation, improving quality of life, and instilling hope.

In some cases, it is not the disorder itself that threatens the mental health of the person with schizophrenia but the stresses of trying to receive care and services. Health care systems are complex and are often at the mercy of outdated policies. Development of assertiveness and conflict resolution skills can help the person in negotiating access to systems that will provide services. Developing a positive support system for stressful periods helps promote a positive outcome.

Virtual Mental Health Care

Telehealth is being used more broadly for many conditions. It is helpful for circumstances where physical distance in rural communities is common or physical distance during pandemics is required. People with schizophrenia who require supportive regular contacts with provider services for counseling, medication and side effect reviews, and assertive community engagement can benefit from telephone or computer-based conferencing. Mobile telephone applications are being developed at a rapid pace as well. These applications can help people to monitor health-related activities like exercise and diet. They can provide education and interventions such as cognitive-behavioral treatment or mindfulness activities. However, the effectiveness of providing care to people with schizophrenia over distances and with mobile applications needs ongoing evaluation to determine to whom these services accrue the most value.

Integration with Primary Care

Traditionally, mental health problems were treated separately from medical needs. It was not uncommon for there to be little connection between the treatment of mental disorders and medical disorders. We now know that a person cannot successfully recover unless physical and mental health care are integrated. The medical needs of persons with schizophrenia are significant and require treatment. There should be a systematic coordination of general and behavior health. Ideally, the patient would have one record where all care would be documented.

Treatment interventions for mental disorders impact the general health status of the person. Frequent communication with primary care providers allows monitoring and adjustment of medical treatment. Medication interactions are a concern when patients are receiving medications from several different clinicians.

SCHIZOAFFECTIVE DISORDER

SAD, a complex and persistent psychiatric illness, is one of the schizophrenia spectrum disorders. SAD is characterized by periods of intense symptom exacerbation alternating with periods of adequate psychosocial functioning. This disorder is at times marked by psychosis, at other times, by mood disturbance. When psychosis and mood disturbance occur at the same time, a diagnosis of SAD is made (APA, 2013). Patients with SAD are more likely to exhibit persistent psychosis than are patients with a mood disorder. They feel that they are on a "chronic roller coaster ride" of symptoms that are often difficult to manage.

The long-term outcome of SAD is generally better than that of schizophrenia but worse than that of mood disorder. These patients resemble the mood disorder group in work function (see Chapter 25) and the schizophrenia group in social function. Persons with SAD usually have higher functioning than those with schizophrenia with severe negative symptoms and early onset of illness (Vardaxi et al., 2018).

Patients with SAD are at risk for suicide. The risk for suicide in patients with psychosis is increased by the presence of depression. Risk factors for suicide increase with the use of alcohol or substances, cigarette smoking, previous suicide attempts, and hospitalizations. Lack of regular social contact may be a factor that confers a long-term risk for suicidal behavior. This risk may be reduced by treatments designed to enhance social networks and contacts, and those focused on helping patients protect themselves against environmental stressors (Simon et al., 2019).

DELUSIONAL DISORDER

Delusional disorder is another schizophrenia spectrum disorder that is characterized by stable and well-systematized delusions that occur in the absence of other psychiatric disorders. A diagnosis of delusional disorder is based on the presence of one or more delusions for at least 1 month (APA, 2013). Delusions are the primary symptom of this disorder. Apart from the direct impact of the delusion, psychosocial functioning is not markedly impaired. Examples of delusions include being followed, poisoned, infected, loved at a distance, or deceived by a spouse or lover.

The course of delusional disorder varies. The onset can be acute, or the disorder can occur gradually and become chronic. Patients usually live with delusions for years, rarely receiving psychiatric treatment unless their delusion relates to their health (somatic delusion), or they act on the basis of their delusion and violate legal or social rules. Full remissions can be followed by relapses. Behavior is remarkably normal except when the patient focuses on the delusion. At that time, thinking, attitudes, and mood may change abruptly. Personality does not usually change, but the patient is gradually and progressively involved with the delusional concern (APA, 2013). Delusional disorder is relatively uncommon in clinical settings.

OTHER PSYCHOTIC DISORDERS

Schizophreniform Disorder

The essential features of schizophreniform disorder are identical to those of schizophrenia, with the exception of the duration of the illness, which can be less than 6 months. Symptoms must be present for at least 1 month to be classified as a schizophreniform disorder. About one-third of the individuals recover, with the other two-thirds developing schizophrenia (APA, 2013).

Brief Psychotic Disorder

In brief psychotic disorder, the length of the episode is at least 1 day but less than 1 month. The onset is sudden and includes at least one of the positive symptoms of schizophrenia. The person generally experiences emotional turmoil or overwhelming confusion and rapid, intense shifts of affect (APA, 2013). Although episodes are brief, impairment can be severe, and supervision may be required to protect the person. Suicide is a risk, especially in younger patients.

Psychotic Disorders Attributable to a Substance

Patients with a psychotic disorder attributable to a substance present with prominent hallucinations or delusions that are the direct physiologic effects of a substance (e.g., drug use, toxin exposure) (APA, 2013). During intoxication, symptoms continue as long as the use of the substance continues. Withdrawal symptoms can last for as long as 4 weeks. Differential diagnosis is recommended.

SUMMARY OF KEY POINTS

- The schizophrenia spectrum disorders include schizophrenia, schizoaffective, delusional, and schizotypal disorders, brief psychotic disorder, schizophreniform disorder, and substance-medication-induced psychotic disorder (APA, 2013). Schizophrenia displays a complex of symptoms typically categorized as positive symptoms (i.e., those that exist but should not), such as delusions or hallucinations and disorganized thinking and behavior, and negative symptoms (characteristics that should be there but are lacking), such as alogia, avolition, anhedonia, and diminished emotional expression.

- The clinical course of schizophrenia begins with a prodromal period in childhood but is usually not recognized as a precursor to schizophrenia. An acute illness usually occurs in late adolescence and may require hospitalization when medication and recovery-oriented care are initiated. In recovery-oriented care, the nurse instills hope and partners with the person with schizophrenia to develop strategies to recover and lead a meaningful life.

- The cause of schizophrenia is thought to be related to genetic, neurodevelopmental, and neurotransmission dysfunction. Environmental stress can trigger acute episodes.

- Nursing assessment begins with the development of the therapeutic relationship and includes biologic, psychological, and social areas.

- Risk for self-injury or injury to others should always be included in the assessment. Establishment of baseline health information should be done before any medications are administered. Several standardized assessment tools are available to help assess characteristic abnormal motor movements.

- In general, the antipsychotic drugs used to treat patients with schizophrenia not only block dopamine transmission in the brain but also cause some troublesome and sometimes serious side effects, primarily anticholinergic side effects and extrapyramidal side effects (i.e., motor abnormalities). Newer second-generation antipsychotic agents block serotonin, as well as dopamine. The nurse should be familiar with these drugs, their possible side effects, and the interventions required to manage or control side effects.

- Extrapyramidal side effects of antipsychotic drugs may appear early in drug treatment and include acute parkinsonism or pseudoparkinsonism, acute dystonia, and akathisia, but they may also appear later after months or years of treatment. The primary example of late-appearing extrapyramidal side effects is tardive dyskinesia, which is a severe syndrome involving abnormal motor movements of the mouth, tongue, jaw, trunk, fingers, and toes.

- Health promotion and wellness interventions are important for overall well-being. People with schizophrenia spectrum disorders have special challenges because their medications can produce a negative impact on their physical health. Nurses can provide education and guidance for positive activity, exercise, and nutrition strategies that can counteract the effect of the medications and symptoms.

- Because schizophrenia is a lifetime disorder and patients require the continued support and care of mental health professionals and family or friends, one of the primary nursing interventions is ensuring that patients and families are properly educated regarding the course of the disorder, importance of drug maintenance, and need for consistent care and support. Positive interaction between patients and their families is key to the success of long-term treatments and outcomes.

- Other schizophrenia spectrum disorders (e.g., schizoaffective, delusional, and schizotypal disorders, brief psychotic disorder, schizophreniform disorder, and substance-medication-induced psychotic disorder) have symptoms similar to those of schizophrenia. Nursing care should be individualized based on a nursing assessment and current evidence related to care.

DEVELOPING CLINICAL JUDGEMENT

1. Describe steps that a nurse should use to make sure an assessment considers the cultural basis of a patient's hallucination and delusions.

2. A patient asks you to explain the difference between "positive" and "negative" symptoms. Develop an answer in "lay" terms for the question.

3. What steps might the nurse take to develop trust in a patient who has hallucinations and delusions and is frightened of other people?

4. Given that a patient with mental illness requires extra efforts at confidentiality and that patients with schizophrenia are often suspicious of their family members, explain ways you can help families and patients develop positive interactions.

5. A patient tells you that she has nothing to live for and everyone would be better off without her. You recognize that she may be having suicidal thoughts. What assessment questions would you ask? How would you help her develop a safety plan?

6. Discuss how therapeutic communication might have to change when working with a person with schizophrenia who is displaying primarily negative symptoms. How will you deal with the person's diminished response to you (both verbally and emotionally) when you are teaching or giving instructions for activities? How will you help the person compensate for some of their cognitive deficits?

7. A person with schizophrenia is admitted during a relapse. He said that he did not want to take his haloperidol anymore because it made him shake. The physician prescribes olanzapine. Develop a medication education plan that includes a comparison between olanzapine and haloperidol.

8. Mr. J. has just received a diagnosis of schizophrenia. During a recent outpatient visit, he confides to a nurse that he just has stress and does not think that he really has any psychiatric problems. Identify assessment areas that should be pursued before the patient leaves his appointment. How would you confront the denial?

9. A patient says his medication is not working. He is taking ziprasidone (Geodon) 40 mg twice a day. He tells you that he takes 40 mg before breakfast

and 40 mg before bed. What interventions are needed to increase the effectiveness of the drug?

10. Ms. J. was prescribed olanzapine (Zyprexa) for schizophrenia 1 month ago. Since her last monthly visit, she has gained 15 pounds. She is considering discontinuing her medication regimen because of the weight gain. Develop a plan to address her weight gain and her intention to discontinue her medication regimen.

11. An older adult in a nursing home has a delusion that her husband is having an affair with her sister. Discuss nonpharmacologic nursing interventions that should be implemented with this patient. How would you explain her delusion to her husband? Develop a plan for clinical management, focusing on psychiatric nursing care, for a patient experiencing this condition.

Identify health promotion activities for a person with schizophrenia who is gaining weight while taking antipsychotics might pursue.

Movie Viewing Guides

A Beautiful Mind: 2001. This Academy Award-winning movie starring Russell Crowe is based on the biography by Sylvia Naasar of the mathematician and Nobel Laureate John Nash. It presents the life and experiences of this man as he dealt with schizophrenia. It shows how his life and work were altered and the effects on his relationships with family and colleagues. The movie depicts how this man came to terms with his illness.

VIEWING POINTS: How does the treatment John Nash received in the 1950s differ from treatment today? How would you classify his symptoms according to the *DSM-5*? What is typical or problematic about Mr. Nash's relationship with the medications prescribed for him?

The Soloist: 2009. Based on a true story, this movie portrays the experience of a reporter/novelist named Steve Lopez (played by Robert Downey, Jr.) when he befriends Nathaniel Anthony Ayers, "the soloist" (played by Jamie Fox), who has severe, persistent, and untreated schizophrenia—and more importantly, exceptional musical talent. Formerly, a student at the prestigious Julliard School of Music in New York City, Ayers now lives on the streets of Los Angeles playing his two-string violin. See also the book by the same title.

VIEWING POINTS: What are the risks and rewards of taking on such a personal relationship? How best can nurses advocate for individuals with severe mental illness (and their family and friends) when community resources are inadequate?

A related Psychiatric-Mental Health Nursing video on the topic of Schizophrenia is available at http://thepoint.lww.com/Boyd7e.

A Practice and Learn Activity related to the video on the topic of Schizophrenia is available at http://thepoint.lww.com/Boyd7e.

Unfolding Patient Stories: Linda Waterfall

Part 2

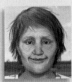

Recall from Chapter 6 Linda Waterfall, a 48-year-old Native American diagnosed with an aggressive form of breast cancer. The recommended treatment is a mastectomy followed by chemotherapy, which she refused. What is the association between her illness and episodes of severe anxiety since diagnosis? How can a secondary mental health disorder contribute to her physical decline from cancer? What psychosocial assessments and interventions should the nurse incorporate into the plan of care to manage her anxiety?

REFERENCES

Abi-Dargham, A. (2020). From "bedside" to "bench" and back: A translational approach to studying dopamine dysfunction in schizophrenia. *Neuroscience and Biobehavioral Reviews, 110,* 174–179. https://doi.org/10.1016/j.neubiorev.2018.12.003

Abrahamyan Empson, L., Baumann, P. S., Söderström, O., Codeluppi, Z., Söderström, D., & Conus, P. (2020). Urbanicity: The need for new avenues to explore the link between urban living and psychosis. *Early Intervention in Psychiatry,14*(4), 398–409. https://doi.org/10.1111/eip.12861

American Psychiatric Association. (2013). *Diagnostic and statistical manual of mental disorders* (5th ed.). Author.

Anthony, W. A., Ellison, M. L., Rogers, E. S., Mizock, L., & Lyass, A. (2014). Implementing and evaluating goal setting in a statewide psychiatric rehabilitation program. *Rehabilitation Counseling Bulletin, 57*(4), 228–237. https://doi.org/10.1177/0034355213505226

Beentjes, T. A. A., van Gaal, B. G. I., van Achterberg, T., & Goossens, P. J. J (2020). Self-management support needs from the perspective of persons with severe mental illness: A systematic review and thematic synthesis of qualitative research. *Journal of the American Psychiatric Nurses Association, 26*(5), 464–482. https://doi.org/10.1177/1078390319877953

Buchsbaum, M. (1990). The frontal lobes, basal ganglia, and temporal lobes as a site for schizophrenia. *Schizophrenia Bulletin, 16,* 377–387.

Carmona, V. R., Gómez-Benito, J., & Rojo-Rodes, J. (2019). Employment support needs of people with schizophrenia: A scoping study. *Journal of Occupational Rehabilitation, 29*(1), 1–10. https://doi.org/10.1007/s10926-018-9771-0

Ceraso, A., Lin, J. J., Schneider-Thoma, J., Siafis, S., Tardy, M., Komossa, K., Heres, S., Kissling, W., Davis, J. M., & Leucht, S. (2020). Maintenance treatment with antipsychotic drugs for schizophrenia. *The Cochrane Database of Systematic Reviews, 8,* CD008016. https://doi.org/10.1002/14651858.CD008016.pub3

Chang, J. G., Roh, D., & Kim, C. H. (2019). Association between therapeutic alliance and adherence in outpatient schizophrenia patients. *Clinical Psychopharmacology and Neuroscience, 17*(2), 273–278. https://doi.org/10.9758/cpn.2019.17.2.273

Chien, W. T., Clifton, A. V., Zhao, S., & Lui, S. (2019). Peer support for people with schizophrenia or other serious mental illness. *Cochrane Database of Systematic Reviews, 4,* CD010880. https://doi.org/10.1002/14651858.CD010880.pub2

Chui, C. Y., Taylor, S. E., Thomas, D., & George, J. (2019). Prevalence and recognition of highly significant medication-smoking cessation interactions in a smoke-free hospital. *Drug and Alcohol Dependence, 200,* 78–81. https://doi.org/10.1016/j.drugalcdep.2019.03.006

Cripps, L., & Hood, C. D. (2020). Recovery and mental health: Exploring the basic characteristics of living well with mental illness. *Therapeutic*

Recreation Journal, *54*(2), 108–127. https://doi.org/10.18666/TRJ-2020-V54-12-9948

Daumit, G. L., Dalcin, A. T., Miller, E. R., Jerome, G. J., Charleston, J. B., Gennusa, J. V., Goldsholl, S., Cook, C., Heller, A., Appel, L. J., Wang, N.-Y.,Daumit, G. L., Dalcin, A. T., Miller, E. R., Charleston, J. B., Crum, R. M., Appel, L. J., Wang, N.-Y., Daumit, G. L. … Wang, N.-Y. (2020). Effect of a comprehensive cardiovascular risk reduction intervention in persons with serious mental illness: A randomized clinical trial. *JAMA Network Open,3*(6), e207247. https://doi.org/10.1001/jamanetworkopen.2020.7247

Davidson, L. (2019). Recovering a sense of self in schizophrenia. *Journal of Personality*, *23*. https://doi.org/10.1111/jopy.12471

Dietsche, B., Kircher, T., & Falkenberg, I. (2017). Structural brain changes in schizophrenia at different stages of the illness: A selective review of longitudinal magnetic resonance imaging studies. *Australian and New Zealand Journal of Psychiatry*, *51*(5), 500–508. https://doi.org/10.1177/0004867417699473

Dixon, L. B., Goldman, H. H., Srihari, V. H., & Kane, J. M. (2018). Transforming the treatment of schizophrenia in the United States: The RAISE initiative. *Annual Review of Clinical Psychology*, *14*, 237–258.

Dondé, C., Silipo, G., Dias, E. C., & Javitt, D. C. (2018). Hierarchical deficits in auditory information processing in schizophrenia. *Schizophrenia Research*, *12*. Pii, S0920-9964(18)30692-3. https://doi.org/10.1016/j.schres.2018.12.001

Dufort, A., & Zipursky, R. B. (2019). Understanding and managing treatment adherence in schizophrenia. *Clinical Schizophrenia & Related Psychoses*. https://doi.org/10.3371/CSRP.ADRZ.121218

Franzen, G. (1970). Plasma free fatty acids before and after an intravenous insulin injection in acute schizophrenic men. *British Journal of Psychiatry*, *116* (531), 173–177.

Glick, I. D., & Olfson, M. (2018). Psychiatric services and "the Homeless": Changing the paradigm. *Journal of Nervous and Mental Disorders*, *206*(5), 378–379. https://doi.org/10.1097/NMD.0000000000000813

Hammoudeh, S., Al Lawati, H., Ghuloum, S., Iram, H., Yehya, A., Becetti, I., Al-Fakhri, N., Ghabrash, H., Shehata, M., Ajmal, N., Amro, I., Safdar, H., Eltorki, Y., & Al-Amin, H. (2020). Risk factors of metabolic syndrome among patients receiving antipsychotics: A retrospective study. *Community Mental Health Journal*, *56*(4), 760–770. https://doi.org/10.1007/s10597-019-00537-y

Harding, C., Zubin, J., & Strauss, J. (1987). Chronicity in schizophrenia: Fact, partial fact or artifact? *Hospital and Community Psychiatry*, *38*(5), 477–486.

Hazlett, E. A., Vaccaro, D. H., Haznedar, M. M., & Goldstein, K. E. (2019). F-18Fluorodeoxyglucose positron emission tomography studies of the schizophrenia spectrum: The legacy of Monte S. Buchsbaum, M. D. *Psychiatry Research*, *271*, 535–540. https://doi.org/10.1016/j.psychres.2018.12.030

Hernandez, M. & Barrio, C. (2017). Families and medication use and adherence among Latinos with schizophrenia. *Journal of Mental Health*, *26*(1), 14–20.

Hilker, R., Helenius, D., Fagerlund, B., Skytthe, A., Christensen, K., Werge, T. M., Nordentoft, M., & Glenthøj, B. (2018). Heritability of Schizophrenia and schizophrenia spectrum based on the nationwide Danish twin register. *Biological Psychiatry*, *83*(6), 492–498. https://doi.org/10.1016/j.biopsych.2017.08.017

Hollander, J. A., Cory-Slechta, D. A., Jacka, F. N., Szabo, S. T., Guilarte, T. R., Bilbo, S. D., Mattingly, C. J., Moy, S. S., Haroon, E., Hornig, M., Levin, E. D., Pletnikov, M. V., Zehr, J. L., McAllister, K. A., Dzierlenga, A. L., Garton, A. E., Lawler, C. P., & Ladd-Acosta, C. (2020). Beyond the looking glass: Recent advances in understanding the impact of environmental exposures on neuropsychiatric disease. *Neuropsychopharmacology: Official Publication of the American College of Neuropsychopharmacology*, *45*(7), 1086–1096. https://doi.org/10.1038/s41386-020-0648-5

Jaaro-Peled, H., & Sawa, A. (2020). Neurodevelopmental factors in schizophrenia. *The Psychiatric Clinics of North America*, *43*(2), 263–274. https://doi.org/10.1016/j.psc.2020.02.010

Jaeger, S., Seißhaupt, S., Flammer, E., & Steinert, T. (2014). Control beliefs, therapeutic relationship, and adherence in schizophrenia outpatients: A cross-sectional study. *American Journal of Health Behavior*, *38*(6), 914–923.

John, Y. J., Zikopoulos, B., Bullock, D., & Barbas, H. (2018). Visual attention deficits in schizophrenia can arise from inhibitory dysfunction in thalamus or cortex. *Computational Psychiatry*, *2*, 223–257. https://doi.org/10.1162/cpsy_a_00023

Jones, C., Hacker, D., Cormac, I., Meaden, A., Irving, C. B., Xia, J., Zhao, S., Shi, C., & Chen, J. (2019). Cognitive behavioral therapy plus standard care versus standard care plus other psychosocial treatments for people with schizophrenia. *Schizophrenia Bulletin*, *45*(2), 284–286. https://doi.org/10.1093/schbul/sby188

Kane, J. M., Schooler, N. R., Marcy, P., Correll, C. U., Achtyes, E. D., Gibbons, R. D., & Robinson, D. G. (2020). Effect of long-acting injectable antipsychotics vs usual care on time to first hospitalization in early-phase schizophrenia: A randomized clinical trial. *JAMA Psychiatry*, *77*(12), 1–8. Advance online publication. https://doi.org/10.1001/jamapsychiatry.2020.2076

Kay, S. R., Fiszbein, A., & Opler, L. A. (1987). The Positive and Negative Syndrome Scale (PANSS) for schizophrenia. *Schizophrenia Bulletin*, *13*, 261–276.

Kellner, C. H., Obbels, J., & Sienaert, P. (2020). When to consider electroconvulsive therapy (ECT). *Acta psychiatrica Scandinavica*, *141*(4), 304–315. https://doi.org/10.1111/acps.13134

Kern, R. S., Zarate, R., Glynn, S. M., Turner, L. R., Smith, K. M., Mitchell, S. S., Sugar, C. A., Bell, M. D., Liberman, R. P., Kopelowicz, A., & Green, M. F. (2018). Improving work outcome in supported employment for serious mental illness: Results from 2 independent studies of errorless learning. *Schizophrenia Bulletin*, *44*(1), 38–45. https://doi.org/10.1093/schbul/sbx100

Kessler, T., & Lev-Ran, S. (2019). The association between comorbid psychiatric diagnoses and hospitalization-related factors among individuals with schizophrenia. *Comprehensive Psychiatry*, *89*, 7–15. https://doi.org/10.1016/j.comppsych.2018.12.004

Kim, S. W., Kim, J. J., Lee, B. J., Yu, J. C., Lee, K. Y., Won, S. H., Lee, S. H., Kim, S. H., Kang, S. H., Kim, E., Lee, J. Y., Kim, J. M., & Chung, Y. C (2019). Clinical and psychosocial factors associated with depression in patients with psychosis according to stage of illness. *Early Intervention in Psychiatry*, *14*(1), 44–52.https://di.org/10.1111/eip.12806

Klaunig, M. J., Trask, C. L., Neis, A. M., Cohn, J. R., Chen, X., Berglund, A. M., & Cicero, D. C. (2019). Associations among domains of self-disturbance in schizophrenia. *Psychiatry Research*, *267*, 187–194. https://doi.org/10.1016/j.psychres.2018.05.082

Kowalchuk, C., Castellani, L. N., Chintoh, A., Remington, G., Giacca, A., & Hahn, M. K. (2019). Antipsychotics and glucose metabolism: How brain and body collide. *American Journal of Physiology, Endocrinology and Metabolism*, *316*(1), E1–E15. https://doi.org/10.1152/ajpendo.00164.2018

Kozloff, N., Mulsant, B. H., Stergiopoulos, V., & Voineskos, A. N. (2020). The COVID-19 global pandemic: Implications for people with schizophrenia and related disorders. *Schizophrenia Bulletin*, *46*(4), 752–757. https://doi.org/10.1093/schbul/sbaa051

La Barbera, L., Vedele, F., Nobili, A., D'Amelio, M., & Krashia, P. (2019). Neurodevelopmental disorders: Functional role of Ambra1 in autism and schizophrenia. *Molecular Neurobiology*, *56*(10), 6716–6724. https://doi.org/10.1007/s12035-019-1557-7

Lauriello, J., & Perkins, D. O. (2019). Enhancing the treatment of patients with schizophrenia through continuous care. *Journal of Clinical Psychiatry*, *80*(1), pii: al18010ah2c. https://doi.org/10.4088/JCP.al18010ah2c

Lean, M., Fornells-Ambrojo, M., Milton, A., Lloyd-Evans, B., Harrison-Stewart, B., Yesufu-Udechuku, A., Kendall, T., & Johnson, S. (2019). Self-management interventions for people with severe mental illness: Systematic review and meta-analysis. *British Journal of Psychiatry*, *214*(5), 260–268. https://doi.org/10.1192/bjp.2019.54

Lewine, R., Martin, M., & Hart, M. (2017). Sex versus gender differences in schizophrenia: The case for normal personality differences. *Schizophrenia Research*, *189*, 57–60. https://doi.org/10.1016/j.schres.2017.02.015

Lin, J., Liang, F., Li, C., & Lu, T. (2018). Leading causes of death among decedents with mention of schizophrenia on the death certificates in the United States. *Schizophrenia Research*, *197*, 116–123. https://doi.org/10.1016/j.schres.2018.01.011.

Liu, Y., Wang, G., Jin, H., Lyu, H., Liu, Y., Guo, W., Shi, C., Meyers, J., Wang, J., Zhao, J., Wu, R., Smith, R. C., & Davis, J. M. (2019a). Cognitive deficits in subjects at risk for psychosis, first-episode and chronic schizophrenia patients. *Psychiatry Research*, *274*, 235–242. https://doi.org/10.1016/j.psychres.2019.01.089

Liu, Y., Yang, X., Gillespie, A., Guo, Z., Ma, Y., Chen, R., & Li, Z. (2019b). Targeting relapse prevention and positive symptom in first-episode schizophrenia using brief cognitive behavioral therapy: A pilot randomized controlled study. *Psychiatry Research*, *272*, 275–283. https://doi.org/10.1016/j.psychres.2018.12.130

Lysaker, P.H., & Roe, D. (2016). Integrative psychotherapy for schizophrenia: Its potential for a central role in recovery oriented treatment. *Journal of Clinical Psychology: In session*, *72*(2), 117–122.

Maura, J., & Weisman de Mamani, A. (2017). Mental health disparities, treatment engagement, and attrition among racial/ethnic minorities with severe mental illness: A review. *Journal of Clinical Psychology in Medical Settings*, *24*(3–4), 187–210. https://doi.org/10.1007/s10880-017-9510-2

Miley, K., Hadidi, N., Kaas, M., & Yu, F. (2020). Cognitive training and remediation in first-episode psychosis: A literature review. *Journal of the American Psychiatric Nurses Association*, *26*(6), 542–554. https://doi.org/10.1177/1078390319877952

Misdrahi, D., Tessier, A., Daubigney, A., Meissner, W. G., Schurhoff, F., Boyer, L., Godin, O., Bulzacka, E., Aouizerate, B., Andrianarisoa, M., Berna, F., Capdevielle, D., Chereau-Boudet, I., D'Amato, T., Dubertret, C., Dubreucq, J., Faget-Agius, C., Lançon, C., Mallet, J., Passerieux, C., ... FACE-SZ (FondaMental Academic Centers of Expertise for Schizophrenia) Group. (2019). Prevalence of and risk factors for extrapyramidal side effects of antipsychotics: Results from the national FACE-SZ cohort. *Journal of Clinical Psychiatry, 80*(1), pii: 18m12246. https://doi.org/10.4088/JCP.18m12246

Mohammadzadeh, A., Azadi, S., King, S., Khosravani, V., & Sharifi Bastan, F. (2019). Childhood trauma and the likelihood of increased suicidal risk in schizophrenia. *Psychiatry Research, 275,* 100–107. https://doi.org/10.1016/j.psychres.2019.03.023

Naguy, A., & Al-Rabaie, A. (2017). Suicidality and survivability in schizophrenia. *Journal of Nervous and Mental Disorders, 205*(7), 585. https://doi.org/10.1097/NMD.0000000000000691

Neugeboren, J. (2006). Meds alone couldn't bring Robert back. *Newsweek.* National Empowerment Center. http://www.power2u.org/articles/recovery/meds.html

Pasina, L., Colzani, L., Cortesi, L., Tettamanti, M., Zambon, A., Nobili, A., Mazzone, A., Mazzola, P., Annoni, G., & Bellelli, G. (2019). Relation between delirium and anticholinergic drug burden in a cohort of hospitalized older patients: An observational study. *Drugs & Aging, 36*(1), 85–91. https://doi.org/10.1007/s40266-018-0612-9

Postolache, T. T., Del Bosque-Plata, L., Jabbour, S., Vergare, M., Wu, R., & Gragnoli, C. (2019). Co-shared genetics and possible risk gene pathway partially explain the comorbidity of schizophrenia, major depressive disorder, type 2 diabetes, and metabolic syndrome. *American Journal of Medical Genetics B Neuropsychiatric Genetics, 180*(3), 186–203. https://doi.org/10.1002/ajmg.b.32712

Pfizer. (2020). GEODON U.S. Physician prescribing information including patient summary of information. http://www.pfizer.com/products/product-detail/geodon

Ricciardi, L., Pringsheim, T., Barnes, T., Martino, D., Gardner, D., Remington, G., Addington, D., Morgante, F., Poole, N., Carson, A., & Edwards, M. (2019). Treatment recommendations for tardive dyskinesia. *Canadian Journal of Psychiatry, 64*(6), 388–399. https://doi.org/10.1177/0706743719828968

Schimmelbusch, W. H., Mueller, P. S., & Sheps, J. (1971). The positive correlation between insulin resistance and duration of hospitalization in untreated schizophrenia. *British Journal of Psychiatry, 118*(545), 429–436.

Schneider, M., Regente, J., Greiner, T., Lensky, S., Bleich, S., Toto, S., Grohmann, R., Stübner, S., & Heinze, M. (2018). Neuroleptic malignant syndrome: Evaluation of drug safety data from the AMSP program during 1993–2015. *European Archives of Psychiatry and Clinical Neuroscience, 270*(1), 23–33. https://doi.org/10.1007/s00406-018-0959-2

Seeman, M. V. (2019). Schizophrenia mortality: Barriers to progress. *Psychiatric Quarterly, 90.* https://doi.org/10.1007/s11126-019-09645-0

Shahab, S., Mulsant, B. H., Levesque, M. L., Calarco, N., Nazeri, A., Wheeler, A. L., Foussias, G., Rajji, T. K., & Voineskos, A. N. (2019). Brain structure, cognition, and brain age in schizophrenia, bipolar disorder, and healthy controls. *Neuropsychopharmacology, 44*(5), 898–906. https://doi.org/10.1038/s41386-018-0298-z

Simon, G. E., Yarborough, B. J., Rossom, R. C., Lawrence, J. M., Lynch, F. L., Waitzfelder, B. E., Ahmedani, B. K., & Shortreed, S. M. (2019). Self-reported suicidal ideation as a predictor of suicidal behavior among outpatients with diagnoses of psychotic disorders. *Psychiatric Services, 70*(3), 176–183. https://doi.org/10.1176/appi.ps.201800381

Simpson, G. M., & Angus, J. W. S. L. (1970). A rating scale for extrapyramidal side effects. *Acta Psychiatrica Scandinavica, 212,* 11–19.

Šimunović Filipčić, I., Ivezić, E., Jakšić, N., Mayer, N., Grah, M., Rojnić Kuzman, M., Bajić, Z., Svab, V., Herceg, M., & Filipčić, I. (2020). Gender differences in early onset of chronic physical multimorbidities in schizophrenia spectrum disorder: Do women suffer more? *Early Intervention in Psychiatry, 14*(4), 418–427. https://doi.org/10.1111/eip.12867

Soundy, A., Stubbs, B., Roskell, C., Williams, S. E., Fox, A., & Vancampfort, D. (2015). Identifying the facilitators and processes which influence recovery in individuals with schizophrenia: A systematic review and thematic synthesis. *Journal of Mental Health, 24*(2), 103–110.

Souto, T., Silva, H., Leite, A., Baptista, A., Queirós, C., & Marques, A. (2020). Facial emotion recognition: Virtual reality program for facial emotion recognition—A trial program targeted at individuals with schizophrenia. *Rehabilitation Counseling Bulletin, 63*(2), 79–90. https://doi.org/10.1177/0034355219847284

Sprague, R. L., & Kalachnik, J. E. (1991). Reliability, validity, and a total score cutoff for the Dyskinesia Identification Scale System: Condensed User Scale (DISCUS) with mentally ill and mentally retarded populations. *Psychopharmacology Bulletin, 27,* 51–58.

Thorning, H., & Dixon, L. (2020). Forty-five years later: The challenge of optimizing assertive community treatment. *Current Opinion in Psychiatry, 33*(4), 397–406. https://doi.org/10.1097/YCO.0000000000000615

Touloupoulou, T., Zhang, X., Cherny, S., Dickinson, D., Berman, K. F., Straub, R. E., Sham, P., & Weinberger, D. R. (2019). Polygenic risk score increases schizophrenia liability through cognition-relevant pathways. *Brain, 142*(2), 471–485. https://doi.org/10.1093/brain/awy279

U.S. Food and Drug Administration. (2015). Ziprasidone. (Geodon). Prescribing Information. www.fda.gov/Drugs/DrugSafety/ucm426391.htm?source=govdelivery&utm_medium=email&utm_source=govdelivery

Vardaxi, C. C., Gonda, X., & Fountoulakis, K. N. (2018). Life events in schizoaffective disorder: A systematic review. *Journal of Affective Disorders, 227,* 563–570. https://doi.org/10.1016/j.jad.2017.11.076

Vignapiano, A., Koenig, T., Mucci, A., Giordano, G. M., Amodio, A., Altamura, M., Bellomo, A., Brugnoli, R., Corrivetti, G., Di Lorenzo, G., Girardi, P., Monteleone, P., Niolu, C., Galderisi, S., Maj, M., & Italian Network for Research on Psychoses. (2019). Disorganization and cognitive impairment in schizophrenia: New insights from electrophysiological findings. *International Journal of Psychophysiology, 145,* 99–108. https://doi.org/10.1016/j.ijpsycho.2019.03.008

Vita, A., & Barlati, S. (2018). Recovery from schizophrenia: Is it possible? *Current Opinion in Psychiatry, 31*(3), 246–255. https://doi.org/10.1097/YCO.0000000000000407

Vogel, J. S., Swart, M., Slade, M., Bruins, J., van der Gaag, M., & Castelein, S. (2019). Peer support and skills training through an eating club for people with psychotic disorders: A feasibility study. *Journal of Behavior Therapy and Experimental Psychiatry, 64,* 80–86. https://doi.org/10.1016/j.jbtep.2019.02.007

Waller, S., Reupert, A., Ward, B., McCormick, F., & Kidd, S. (2019). Family-focused recovery: Perspectives from individuals with a mental illness. *International Journal of Mental Health Nursing, 28*(1), 247–255.

Wang, X., Zhao, N., Shi, J., Wu, Y., Liu, J., Xiao, Q., & Hu, J. (2019). Discussion on the application of multi-modal magnetic resonance imaging fusion in schizophrenia. *Journal of Medical Systems, 43*(5), 131. https://doi.org/10.1007/s10916-019-1215-7

Wilson, S. M., Thompson, A. C., Currence, E. D., Thomas, S. P., Dedert, E. A., Kirby, A. C., Elbogen, E. B., Moore, S. D., Calhoun, P. S., & Beckham, J. C. (2019). Patient-informed treatment development of behavioral smoking cessation for people with schizophrenia. *Behavior Therapy, 50*(2), 395–409. https://doi.org/10.1016/j.beth.2018.07.004

Wu, Y., Kang, R., Yan, Y., Gao, K., Li, Z., Jiang, J., Chi, X., & Xia, L. (2018). Epidemiology of schizophrenia and risk factors of schizophrenia-associated aggression from 2011 to 2015. *Journal of International Medical Research, 46*(10), 4039–4049. https://doi.org/10.1177/0300060518786634

Young, L., Digel Vandyk, A., Daniel Jacob, J., McPherson, C., & Murata, L. (2019). Being parent caregivers for adult children with schizophrenia. *Issues in Mental Health Nursing, 40*(4), 297–303. https://doi-org.libproxy.siue.edu/10.1080/01612840.2018.1524531

Yuan, X., Kang, Y., Zhuo, C., Huang, X. F., & Song, X. (2019). The gut microbiota promotes the pathogenesis of schizophrenia via multiple pathways. *Biochemical Biophysical Research Communication, 512*(2), 373–380. https://doi.org/10.1016/j.bbrc.2019.02.152

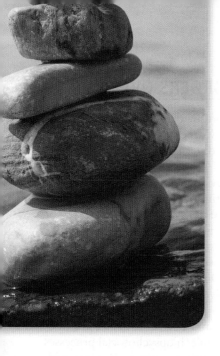

25
Depression
Nursing Care of Persons with Depressive Moods and Suicidal Behavior

Barbara Jones Warren

KEYCONCEPTS

- depression
- mood
- suicidal behavior

LEARNING OBJECTIVES

After studying this chapter, you will be able to:

1. Discuss the role of mood and depression in mental disorders.

2. Delineate the clinical symptoms and course of major depressive disorder, including suicidal behavior.

3. Analyze the primary theories of major depressive disorder and their relationship to suicidal behavior.

4. Develop strategies to establish a patient-centered, recovery-oriented therapeutic relationship with a person with depression.

5. Apply a person-centered, recovery-oriented nursing process for persons with major depressive disorder, including those with suicidal behavior.

6. Identify medications used to treat people with depression and evaluate their effectiveness.

7. Develop wellness strategies for persons with depression.

8. Differentiate the type of mental health care provided in emergency care, inpatient-focused care, community care, and virtual mental health care.

9. Discuss the importance of integrated health care for persons with depression.

10. Describe other depressive disorders.

KEY TERMS

- Affect • Anhedonia • Cytokines • Depression • Depressive disorders • Disruptive mood dysregulation disorder
- Major depressive disorder • Persistent depressive disorder • Premenstrual dysphoric disorder • Serotonin syndrome
- Suicidality

Case Study

Louise is a 31-year-old woman who was admitted voluntarily to an inpatient mental health unit with depression with suicidal ideation. Louise and her husband Brian have three children aged 9, 5, and 3 years.

INTRODUCTION

Most people have bad days or times of feeling sad and overwhelmed. When depressed feelings interfere with daily activities and relationships, however, this mood can impair judgment and contribute to negative views of the world. In some instances, depression is a symptom of a depressive disorder. This chapter discusses mood and depression, depressive disorders, and the related serious issue of suicidal behavior. Major depressive disorder is highlighted.

MOOD AND DEPRESSION

Normal variations in mood occur in response to life events. Normal mood variations (e.g., sadness, euphoria, and anxiety) are time limited and are not usually associated with significant functional impairment. Normal range of mood or affect, the expression of mood, varies considerably both within and among different cultures (Lin & Dmitrieva, 2019).

> **KEYCONCEPTS Mood** is a pervasive and sustained emotion that influences one's perception of the world and how one functions.

Affect, or outward emotional expression, is related to the concept of mood. Affect provides clues to the person's mood. For example, in depression, people often have limited facial expression. Several terms are used to describe affect, including the following:

- *Blunted:* significantly reduced intensity of emotional expression
- *Bright:* smiling, projection of a positive attitude
- *Flat:* absent or nearly absent affective expression
- *Inappropriate:* discordant affective expression accompanying the content of speech or ideation
- *Labile:* varied, rapid, and abrupt shifts in affective expression
- *Restricted or constricted:* mildly reduced in the range and intensity of emotional expression

Depression is the primary mood of depressive disorders. Depression can be overwhelming. Unless appropriately treated, depression persists over time, has a significant negative effect on quality of life, and increases the risk of suicide (Lotfaliany et al., 2018; Tuithof et al., 2018).

> **KEYCONCEPT Depression** is a common mental state characterized by sadness, loss of interest or pleasure, feelings of guilt or low self-worth, disturbed sleep or appetite, low energy, and poor concentration (American Psychiatric Association [APA], 2013; World Health Organization [WHO], 2019).

DEPRESSIVE DISORDERS OVERVIEW

When a sad mood interferes with daily life, a **depressive disorder** may exist that will benefit from treatment. In depressive disorders, a sad, irritable, or empty mood is present with somatic and cognitive changes that interfere with functioning. Several depressive disorders vary according to duration, timing, or cause (APA, 2013). These include disruptive mood dysregulation, major depressive disorder, persistent depressive (dysthymia), premenstrual dysphoric, substance-medication-induced, and other specified depressive and unspecified depressive disorders (APA, 2013). Disruptive mood dysregulation disorder is a new depressive disorder diagnostic category in the *DSM-5*.

The clinical symptoms and course of depressive phenomena are complex, dynamic, biopsychosocial processes involving life span and cultural aspects. Persons with depressive disorders experience a lower quality of life and are at greater risk for development of physical health problems than those who are not depressed. Depressive disorders are so widespread that they are generally diagnosed and treated in the primary care setting. Every nurse will have an opportunity to impact this pandemic health concern (WHO, 2019).

Depressive disorders are characterized by severe and debilitating depressive episodes and are associated with high levels of impairment in occupational, social, and physical functioning. They cause as much disability and distress to patients as chronic medical disorders. Frequently, they are undetected and untreated. Because suicide is a significant risk, these disorders are associated with premature death, especially in those individuals who have been hospitalized for depression (Bachman, 2018).

Depressive Disorders Across the Life Span

Children and Adolescents

Children with depressive disorders have symptoms similar to those seen in adults, with a few exceptions. They are more likely to have anxiety symptoms, such as fear of separation, and somatic symptoms, such as stomach aches and headaches. They may have less interaction with their peers and avoid play and recreational activities that they previously enjoyed. Mood may be irritable, rather than sad, especially in adolescents. See Chapter 37 for discussion of mental health disorders in children.

The risk of suicide, which peaks during the midadolescent years, is very real in children and adolescents. Mortality from suicide, which increases steadily through the teens, is the third leading cause of death for that age group. Findings from research indicate that chronic

TABLE 25.1	INTERVENTIONS TO RELIEVE SIDE EFFECTS OF ANTIDEPRESSANTS	
Side Effect	Pharmacologic Intervention	Nonpharmacologic Intervention
Dry mouth, caries, inflammation of the mouth	Bethanechol 10–30 mg TID Pilocarpine drops	Sugarless gum Sugarless lozenges 6–8 cups of water per day Toothpaste for dry mouth
Nausea, vomiting	Change medication	Take medication with food Soda crackers, toast, tea
Weight gain	Change medication	Nutritionally balanced diet Daily exercise
Urinary hesitation Constipation	Bethanechol 10–30 mg TID Stool softener	6–8 cups of water per day Bulk laxative Daily exercise 6–8 cups of water per day Diet rich in fresh fruits, vegetables, and whole grains
Diarrhea	OTC antidiarrheal	Maintain fluid intake
Orthostatic hypotension		Increase hydration Sit or stand up slowly
Drowsiness	Shift dosing time Lower medication dose Change medication	One caffeinated beverage at strategic time Do not drive when drowsy No alcohol or other recreational drugs Plan for rest time
Fatigue	Lower medication dose> Change medication	Daily exercise
Blurred vision	Bethanechol 10–30 mg TID Pilocarpine eye drops	Temporary use of magnifying lenses until body adjusts to medication
Flushing, sweating	Terazosin 1 mg once daily Lower medication dose Change medication	Frequent bathing Lightweight clothing
Tremor	β-blockers Lower medication dose	Reassure the patient that tremor may decrease as the patient adjusts to medication. Notify the caregiver if tremor interferes with daily functioning

OTC, over-the-counter; TID, three times a day.

victimization increases the risk for depression and suicide ideation and attempts (Brunstein et al., 2019). The use of substances intensifies depressive symptomatology and the risk of suicide (Johns et al., 2018). See Chapter 22 for further discussion of suicide in children and adolescents.

Older Adults

Depression in older adults is often undetected or inadequately treated (Kok & Reynolds, 2017). However, it is estimated that 8% to 20% of older adults in the community and as many as 37% in primary care settings experience depressive symptoms (Blazer & Steffens, 2015). Treatment is successful in 60% to 80%,

but response to treatment is slower than in younger adults. Depression in older adults is often associated with chronic illnesses, such as heart disease, stroke, and cancer; symptoms may have a more somatic focus. Depressive symptomatology in this group may be confused with symptoms of bipolar, dementia, or cerebrovascular accidents. Hence, differential diagnosis may be required to ascertain the root and cause of symptoms. See Chapter 38 for further discussion of mental health disorders in older adults.

Suicide is a very serious risk for older adults, especially for men. Suicide rates peak during middle age, but a second peak occurs in those aged 75 years and older (Ivey-Stephenson et al., 2017) (see Box 25.1 and Chapter 22).

MAJOR DEPRESSIVE DISORDER

Clinical Course

Major depressive disorder is commonly a progressively recurrent illness. With time, episodes tend to occur more frequently, become more severe, and are of a longer duration. Onset of depression may occur at any age. However, the initial onset may occur in puberty; the highest onset occurs within persons in their 20s (APA, 2013). Recurrences of depression are related to age of onset, increased intensity and severity of symptoms, and presence of psychosis, anxiety, and/or personality features. The risk for relapse is higher in persons who have experienced initial symptoms at a younger age and incur other mental disorders (Hoertel et al., 2017).

Diagnostic Criteria

The primary diagnostic criterion for major depressive disorder is one or more moods, which is either a depressed mood or a loss of interest or pleasure in nearly all activities for at least 2 weeks. Four of seven additional symptoms must be present: disruption in sleep, appetite (or weight), concentration, or energy; psychomotor agitation or retardation; excessive guilt or feelings of worthlessness; and suicidal ideation (Key Diagnostic Characteristics 25.1).

The incidence of misdiagnosis is often greater for persons who are treated by someone from culturally and ethnically different populations. Their explanation of their symptomatology may be expressed using different terminology, or the underrepresented group may feel uncomfortable with a clinician from a different culture (Hornberger et al., 2016; Warren, 2020).

Epidemiology and Risk Factors

The prevalence of major depressive disorder within the U.S. population is approximately 10.4% within a 12-month time period, with a lifetime prevalence of 20.6%. Individuals between the ages of 18 and 29 years have a higher prevalence rate than those persons aged 65 and older. Episodes typically last more than 6 months. Females have a higher prevalence rate than males (13.4% vs. 7.2%). Depression is more prevalent in younger adults, White adults, and Native American adults than among African American, Asian American, and Hispanic adults (Hasin et al., 2018).

Data from the WHO indicate that depression is the leading cause of years lost because of disability. More than 50% of persons who recover from an initial episode of depression experience another episode within 5 to 10 years (WHO, 2019).

Risk factors for the development of depression include the following:

• Prior episode of depression
• Family history of depressive disorder
• Lack of social support
• Lack of coping abilities
• Presence of life and environmental stressors
• Current substance use or abuse
• Medical and/or mental illness comorbidity

Consider Louise

Her sister died as a result of drowning 2 months ago. She has been telling her husband that she just wants to go to sleep and not wake up. What risk factors do you recognize?

Ethnicity and Culture

Culture can influence the experience and communication of symptoms of depression. Persons from culturally and ethnically diverse populations may formulate and describe their depressive symptomatology differently than in the clinical language used for diagnosis. For example, expressions such as "heartbrokenness" (Native American and Middle Eastern), "brain fog" (persons from the West Indies), "zar", and "running amok" may be used in place of such terms as *depressed, sad, hopeless,* and *discouraged.*

In some cultures, somatic symptoms, rather than sadness or guilt, may predominate. Individuals from various Asian cultural groups may have complaints of weakness, tiredness, or imbalance. "Problems of the heart" (in Middle Eastern cultures) or of being "heartbroken" (among Native Americans of the Hopi tribe) may be the way that persons from these cultural groups express their depressive experiences. Culturally distinctive experiences need to be assessed to ascertain any presence of depressive disorder from a "normal" cultural emotional response (Pedersen et al., 2016).

KEY CHARACTERISTICS 25.1 • MAJOR DEPRESSIVE DISORDER 296.XX

296.2X MAJOR DEPRESSIVE DISORDER, SINGLE EPISODE
296.3X MAJOR DEPRESSIVE DISORDER, RECURRENT

Diagnostic Criteria

A. Five (or more) of the following symptoms have been present during the same 2-week period and represent a change from previous functioning; at least one of the symptoms is either (1) depressed mood or (2) loss of interest or pleasure.

Note: Do not include symptoms that are clearly attributable to another medical condition.

1. Depressed mood most of the day, nearly every day, as indicated by either subjective report (e.g., feels sad, empty, hopeless) or observation made by others (e.g., appears tearful). (**Note:** In children and adolescents, can be irritable mood.)
2. Markedly diminished interest or pleasure in all, or almost all, activities most of the day, nearly every day (as indicated by either subjective account or observation).
3. Significant weight loss when not dieting or weight gain (e.g., a change of more than 5% of body weight in a month), or decrease or increase in appetite nearly every day. (**Note:** In children, consider failure to make expected weight gain.)
4. Insomnia or hypersomnia nearly every day.
5. Psychomotor agitation or retardation nearly every day (observable by others, not merely subjective feelings of restlessness or being slowed down).
6. Fatigue or loss of energy nearly every day.
7. Feelings of worthlessness or excessive or inappropriate guilt (which may be delusional) nearly every day (not merely self-reproach or guilt about being sick).
8. Diminished ability to think or concentrate, or indecisiveness, nearly every day (either by subjective account or as observed by others).
9. Recurrent thoughts of death (not just fear of dying), recurrent suicidal ideation without a specific plan, or a suicide attempt or a specific plan for committing suicide.

The symptoms cause clinically significant distress or impairment in social, occupational, or other important areas of functioning.

The episode is not attributable to the physiologic effects of a substance or to another medical condition.

B. The symptoms cause clinically significant distress or impairment in social, occupational, or other important areas of functioning.

C. The episode is not attributable to the physiologic effects of a substance or to another medical condition.

Note: Criteria A to C represent a major depressive episode.

Note: Responses to a significant loss (e.g., bereavement, financial ruin, losses from a natural disaster, a serious medical illness, or disability) may include the feelings of intense sadness, rumination about the loss, insomnia, poor appetite, and weight loss noted in Criterion A, which may resemble a depressive episode. Although such symptoms may be understandable or considered appropriate to the loss, the presence of a major depressive episode in addition to the normal response to a significant loss should also be carefully considered. This decision inevitably requires the exercise of clinical judgment based on the individual's history and the cultural norms for the expression of distress in the context of loss.

The occurrence of the major depressive episode is not better explained by schizoaffective disorder, schizophrenia, schizophreniform disorder, delusional disorder, or other specified and unspecified schizophrenia spectrum and other psychotic disorders.

There has never been a manic episode or a hypomanic episode.

Note: This exclusion does not apply if all of the manic-like or hypomanic-like episodes are substance induced or are attributable to the physiologic effects of another medical condition.

Comorbidity

Major depressive disorders often co-occur with other psychiatric disorders, including those that are substance related. Depression often is associated with a variety of chronic medical conditions, particularly endocrine disorders, cardiovascular disease, and neurologic disorders (Lotfaliany et al., 2018).

Etiology

Biologic Theories

Genetic

Family, twin, and adoption studies demonstrate that genetic influences undoubtedly play a substantial role in the etiology of mood disorders. Major depressive disorder tends to run in families and has a heritable component. Currently, a major research effort is focusing on developing a more accurate paradigm regarding the contribution of genetic factors to the development of mood disorders (Howard et al., 2019).

Neurobiologic Hypotheses

Neurobiologic theories of the etiology of depression emerged in the 1950s. These theories posit that major depression is caused by a deficiency or dysregulation in central nervous system (CNS) concentrations of the neurotransmitters norepinephrine, dopamine, and serotonin or in their receptor functions. These hypotheses arose in part from observations that some pharmacologic agents elevated mood; subsequent studies identified their mechanisms of action. All antidepressants currently available have their therapeutic effects on these neurotransmitters or receptors. Current research continues to focus on the role of neurotransmitters and the neurobiology of depression (Joca et al., 2015).

Neuroendocrine and Neuropeptide Hypotheses

Major depressive disorder is associated with multiple endocrine alterations, specifically of the hypothalamic–pituitary–adrenal axis, the hypothalamic–pituitary–thyroid axis, the hypothalamic–growth hormone axis, and the hypothalamic–pituitary–gonadal axis. In addition, mounting evidence indicates that components of neuroendocrine axes (e.g., neuromodulatory peptides, such as corticotropin-releasing factor) may themselves contribute to depressive symptoms. Evidence also suggests that the secretion of these hypothalamic and growth hormones is controlled by many of the neurotransmitters implicated in the pathophysiology of depression (Gong et al., 2019).

Psychoneuroimmunology

Psychoneuroimmunology is a recent area of research into a diverse group of proteins known as *chemical messengers* between immune cells. These messengers, called cytokines, signal the brain and serve as mediators between immune and nerve cells. The brain is capable of influencing immune processes, and conversely, immunologic response can result in changes in brain activity. Increased cytokine levels are associated with depression and cognitive impairment indicating that inflammatory reactions are involved in the development of some mental health disorders (Himmerich et al., 2019).

Psychological Theories

Psychological theories that serve as a basis for nursing practice for persons with a mental health disorder are explained in Chapter 7. Depression is one of the disorders treated from a psychological perspective. The following discussion identifies theoretical models often used in nursing care.

Psychodynamic Factors

Most psychodynamic theorists acknowledge some debt to Freud's original conceptualization of the psychodynamics of depression, which ascribes the cause to an early lack of love, care, warmth, and protection and resultant anger, guilt, helplessness, and fear regarding the loss of love. The ensuing conflict between wanting to be loved and fear of rejection engenders pathologic self-punishment (also conceptualized as aggression turned inward), self-rejection, low self-esteem, and depressive symptoms (see Chapter 7).

Behavioral Factors

The behavioral psychologists hold that depression primarily results from a severe reduction in rewarding activities or an increase in unpleasant events in one's life. The subsequent depression then leads to further restriction of activity, thereby decreasing the likelihood of experiencing pleasurable activities, which, in turn, intensifies the mood disturbance. Affected individuals often self-criticize and believe that they do not have the coping skills to deal with life's stresses. If family members believe that the person is "sick" and so lacks the necessary coping skills, they inadvertently reinforce the hopeless self-view of the depressed person.

Cognitive Factors

The cognitive approach maintains that irrational beliefs and negative distortions of thought about the self, the environment, and the future engender and perpetuate depressive effects (see Chapter 7). These depressive cognitions can be learned socially from family members or lack of experience in developing coping skills. These individuals think differently than nondepressed individuals and view their environment and themselves in negative ways. They blame themselves for any misfortunes that occur and see situations as being much worse than they are.

Developmental Factors

Developmental theorists posit that depression may result from the loss of a parent through death or separation or lack of emotionally adequate parenting. These factors may delay or prohibit the realization of appropriate developmental milestones.

Social Theories

Family Factors

Family theorists ascribe maladaptive patterns in family interactions as contributing to the onset of depression, particularly in the onset and occurrence of depression in younger individuals. A family becomes dysfunctional when interactions, decisions, or behaviors interfere with the positive development of the family and its individual members. Most families have periods of dysfunction, such as during a crisis or stressful situation when coping skills are not available. Unhealthy interactions within a family system can have a negative impact on one or more family members who do not have the coping skills to deal with the situation.

Environmental Factors

Depression has long been understood as a multifactorial disorder that occurs when environmental factors (e.g., death of family member) interact with the biologic and psychological makeup of the individual. Major depression may follow adverse or traumatic life events, especially those that involve the loss of an important human relationship or role in life. Social isolation, deprivation, and financial deprivation are associated with depression (Ge et al., 2017).

Family Response to Disorder

Depression in one family member affects the whole family. Spouses, children, parents, siblings, and friends experience frustration, guilt, and anger when a family member is immobilized and cannot function. It is often hard for others to understand the depth of the mood and how disabling it can be. Financial hardship can occur when the affected family member cannot work and instead spends days in bed. The lack of understanding and difficulty of living with a depressed person can lead to abuse. Women between the ages of 18 and 45 years constitute the majority of those experiencing depression. This incidence may affect women's ability to not only have productive lives and take care of themselves but to also take care of their children or other family members for whom they may have responsibility. Moreover, research indicates that the incidence of depression may be higher in children whose mothers experience depression (Drury et al., 2016).

Remember Louise?

According to her husband, Louise has neglected her self-care and that of her children since her sister's death. Brian is very understanding and supportive of Louise's need to grieve, but he is concerned that this is more than grief. Brian says that he is afraid to leave her alone and the children are suffering. What recommendations would you suggest to Louise's husband? Are there indications that Louise's grief is developing into depression?

RECOVERY-ORIENTED CARE FOR PERSONS WITH DEPRESSIVE DISORDERS

Teamwork and Collaboration: Working Toward Recovery

Depressive disorders are the most commonly occurring mental disorders, but they are usually treated within the primary care setting, rather than psychiatric setting. Nursing practice requires a coordinated ongoing interaction among patients, families, and health care providers to deliver comprehensive services. This includes using the complementary skills of both psychiatric and medical care colleagues for forming overall goals, plans, and decisions and for providing continuity of care as needed. Collaborative care between the primary care provider and mental health specialist is also key to achieving remission of symptoms and physical well-being, restoring baseline occupational and psychosocial functioning, and reducing the likelihood of relapse or recurrence.

Individuals with depression enter mental health settings when their symptoms become so severe that hospitalization is needed, usually after suicide attempts, or if they self-refer because of incapacitation. Antidepressants are indicated for depression and are discussed later in this chapter. Interdisciplinary treatment of these disorders, which is often lifelong, needs to include a wide array of health professionals in all areas. The specific goals of treatment are as follows:

- Reduce or control symptoms and, if possible, eliminate signs and symptoms of the depressive syndrome.
- Improve occupational and psychosocial function as much as possible.
- Reduce the likelihood of relapse and recurrence through recovery-oriented strategies.

Cognitive and Interpersonal Therapies

Recent studies suggest that short-term cognitive and interpersonal therapies may be as effective as pharmacotherapy in milder depressions. In many instances, cognitive-behavioral therapy (CBT) is an effective strategy for preventing relapse in patients who have had only a partial response to pharmacotherapy alone (APA, 2013). CBT is implemented in individual or group therapy by a trained clinician.

- Interpersonal therapy seeks to recognize, explore, and resolve the interpersonal losses, role confusion and transitions, social isolation, and deficits in social skills that may precipitate depressive states. It maintains that losses must be mourned and related affects appreciated, role confusion and transitions must be recognized and resolved, and social skills deficits must be overcome to acquire social supports.

Combination Therapies

For patients with severe or recurrent major depressive disorder, the combination of psychotherapy (including interpersonal, cognitive-behavioral, behavior, brief dynamic, or dialectical behavioral therapies) and pharmacotherapy has been found to be superior to treatment using a single modality. Clinical practice guidelines suggest that the combination of medication and psychotherapy is particularly useful in more complex situations (e.g., depression in the context of concurrent, chronic general-medical, or other psychiatric disorders, or in patients who fail to experience complete response to either treatment alone). Psychotherapy, in combination with medication, is also used to address collateral issues, such as medication adherence or secondary psychosocial problems (Dunlop et al., 2019). If medications and psychotherapy are not effective, other options are available: electroconvulsive therapy (ECT), light therapy, and repetitive transcranial magnetic stimulation (rTMS), discussed later in the chapter.

Alternative Therapies

Alternative or complementary therapies are often used in the treatment of depression. Acupuncture, yoga or tai chi, meditation, guided imagery, and massage therapy are a few therapies that may be helpful to palliate depression. Music or art therapy is also used often in conjunction with medication or psychotherapy.

Safety Issues

The overriding concern for people with mood disorders is safety because these individuals may experience self-destructive thoughts and suicidal ideation. Hence, the assessment of possible suicide risk should be routinely conducted in any person who is depressed (see Chapter 22).

EVIDENCE-BASED NURSING CARE OF PERSONS WITH DEPRESSIVE DISORDER

An awareness of the risk factors for depression, a comprehensive and culturally competent mental health nursing assessment, history of illness, and past treatment are key to formulating a treatment or recovery plan and to evaluating outcomes. Interviewing a family member or close friend about the patient's day-to-day functioning and specific symptoms may help determine the course of the illness, current symptoms, and level of functioning. The family's level of support and understanding of the disorder also need to be assessed. See Nursing Care Plan 25.1.

Mental Health Nursing Assessment

The mental health nursing assessment focuses on the physical consequences of the depression, as well as the psychosocial aspects. The symptoms of depression are similar to those of some medical problems or medication

side effects. Often, the mental health nurse is the only clinician who provides holistic care to a person with depression who is often treated by other disciplines.

Physical Health

The nursing assessment should include a physical systems review and thorough history of medical problems, with special attention to CNS function, endocrine function, anemia, chronic pain, autoimmune illness, diabetes mellitus, or menopause. Additional medical history includes surgeries, medical hospitalizations, head injuries, episodes of loss of consciousness, pregnancies, childbirths, miscarriages, and abortions. A complete list of prescribed and over-the-counter (OTC) medications and herbal supplements should be compiled, including the reason a medication was prescribed or its use discontinued. A physical examination is recommended with baseline vital signs and baseline laboratory tests, including a comprehensive blood chemistry panel, complete blood counts, liver function tests, thyroid function tests, urinalysis, and electrocardiograms (see Chapter 11).

The following symptoms are characteristics of depression and should be assessed:

- *Appetite and weight changes:* In major depression, changes from baseline include a decrease or increase in appetite with or without significant weight loss or gain (i.e., a change of more than 5% of body weight in 1 month). Weight loss occurs when the person is not dieting. Older adults with moderate-to-severe depression need to be assessed for dehydration as well as weight changes.

- *Sleep disturbance:* The most common sleep disturbance associated with major depression is insomnia, which is broken into three categories: initial insomnia (difficulty falling asleep), middle insomnia (waking up during the night and having difficulty returning to sleep), and terminal insomnia (waking too early and being unable to return to sleep). Less frequently, the sleep disturbance is hypersomnia (i.e., prolonged sleep episodes at night or increased daytime sleep). The individual with either insomnia or hypersomnia complains of not feeling rested on awakening.

- *Tiredness, decreased energy, and fatigue:* Fatigue associated with depression is a subjective experience of feeling tired regardless of how much sleep or physical activity a person has had. Even the smallest tasks require substantial effort.

NCLEXNOTE In determining severity of depressive symptoms, nursing assessment should explore physical changes in appetite and sleep patterns and decreased energy. Remember these three major assessment categories. A question in the test may state several patient symptoms and expect the student to recognize that the patient being described is depressed.

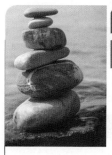

NURSING CARE PLAN 25.1

The Person with Depressive Disorder

Louise is a 31-year-old woman with a diagnosis of major depressive disorder with suicidal ideation. She feels hopeless, helpless, and worthless. She is grieving the loss of her sister and also feels that she has failed her. She believes her family would be better off without her. She has lost interest and pleasure in everything that she used to enjoy. She lacks energy to get out of bed or do basic self-care. Her thoughts are negative and distorted. Her facial expression is sad and restricted. She has difficulty smiling or seeing humor in a situation.

Setting: Intensive Care Psychiatric Unit in a General Hospital

Baseline Assessment: Louise is oriented to time, place, and person. She is dressed in a sweatshirt and sweatpants. Her appearance is disheveled, she has a slight body odor, and her hair is not combed. Her physical care plan reveals a recent 15 lb weight loss, insomnia, and loss of appetite. Her vital signs and laboratory values are within normal limits. She denies having a suicidal plan but says she wants to go to sleep and not wake up. Her husband said he is very worried about her because "she is physically there but not available to any of us."

Associated Psychiatric Diagnosis	Medications
Major depressive disorder	Initiated escitalopram (Lexapro) 20 mg/day

Priority of Care: Safety and Suicide Prevention

Important Characteristics	Associated Considerations
Feelings of hopelessness Expresses desire to die Lethal means available	Recently lost sister Believes she is a burden to family

Outcomes

Initial	Discharge
1. Remain free from self-harm. 2. Identify factors that led to suicidal intent and methods for managing suicidal impulses if they return. 3. Accept treatment of depression by trying the SSRI antidepressants and psychotherapy.	1. Agrees to continue with outpatient therapy. 2. Agrees to take antidepressant. 3. Agrees that family can remove gun(s) from home.

Interventions

Interventions	Rationale	Ongoing Assessment
Initiate a nurse–patient relationship by demonstrating an acceptance of Louise as a worthwhile human being through the use of nonjudgmental statements and behavior.	A sense of worthlessness often underlies suicide ideation. The positive therapeutic relationship can support hopefulness.	Assess the stages of the relationship and determine whether a therapeutic relationship is actually being formed. Identify indicators of trust.
Initiate suicide precautions per hospital policy.	Safety of the individual is a priority with people who have suicide ideation.	Determine intent to harm self—plan and means.
Discuss with family members removal of lethal weapons from home.	Suicidal behavior is often impulsive. Removing means of suicide may prevent persons from acting on impulsive thoughts.	Follow-up with the patient and family member about removing lethal weapons.

Continued

Nursing Care Plan 25.1 Continued

Evaluation

Outcomes	Revised Outcomes	Interventions
Has not harmed herself.	Identify strategies to resist suicide attempts in the future.	Discuss antecedents that led to the suicide attempt. Discuss initiation of an antidepressant.

Priority of Care: Hopelessness

Important Characteristics	Associated Considerations
Decreased affect	Loss of sister
Decreased appetite	
Insomnia	
Lack of initiative	
States she has no reason to live	

Outcomes

Initial	Discharge
Accept support through the nurse–patient relationship. Identify hopelessness as a pervasive feeling.	Express feelings of being hopeful for the future.

Interventions

Interventions	Rationale	Ongoing Assessment
Establish a trusting therapeutic relationship.	Therapeutic relationships are effective in instilling hope.	Observe verbal and nonverbal cues that increase communications.
Enhance Louise's sense of hope by being attentive, validating your interpretation of what is being said or experienced, and helping him verbalize what she is expressing nonverbally.	By showing respect for the patient as a human being who is worth listening to, the nurse can support and help build the patient's sense of self.	Determine whether the patient confirms interpretation of situation and if she can verbalize what she is expressing nonverbally.
Assist to reframe and redefine negative statements ("not a burden but missing your sister").	Reframing an event positively rather than negatively can help the patient view the situation in an alternative way.	Assess whether Louise is feeling more hopeful.
Participate in a recovery group focusing on hope.	Group support can be very effective in discussing hope and identifying strategies to establish hopefulness.	Determine if the patient is attending group sessions and participating in discussions.

Evaluation

Outcomes	Revised Outcomes	Interventions
Able to discuss future events in a positive manner.	Discuss specific plans for future events.	Continue with cognitive approaches when discussing future events.
Attending recovery group regularly.	None.	

SSRI, selective serotonin reuptake inhibitor.

Consider This:

Recall that Louise has not been eating because she is not hungry and has lost 15 lb over the last 6 weeks. She is also not sleeping well. She wakes up during the middle of the night and cannot go back to sleep. What symptoms of depression is Louise experiencing?

Physical Functioning

Physical functioning is an integrated component of a person's biopsychosocial existence. It is really the manner in which a person matches their age-appropriate developmental stage and is able to successfully enact daily tasks of living. It focuses on how healthy a person is and how well they take care of themselves (Warren, 2020).

Medication

In addition to a physical assessment, an assessment of current medications should be completed. The frequency and dosage of prescribed medications, OTC medications, and use of herbal or culturally related medication treatments should be explored. In depression, the nurse must always assess the possible lethality of the medication the patient is taking. For example, if a patient has sleeping medications at home, the individual should be further queried about the number of pills in the bottle. Patients also need to be assessed for their use of alcohol, marijuana, and other mood-altering medications, as well as herbal substances because of the potential for drug–drug interactions. For example, patients taking antidepressants that affect serotonin regulation could also be taking St. John wort (*Hypericum perforatum*) to fight depression. The combined drug and herb could interact to cause serotonin syndrome (altered mental status, autonomic dysfunction, and neuromuscular abnormalities). SAMe (S-adenosyl-L-methionine) is another herbal preparation that patients may be taking. Patients need to be advised of possible adverse side effects of SAMe taken with any prescribed antidepressant because the exact action of this herb remains unclear.

Substance Use Assessment

A significant proportion of persons (40%–60%) with a depressive disorder have a substance use disorder also. Conversely, alcohol use disorder increases the risk of a depressive disorder more than fourfold (Tolliver & Anton, 2015). These co-occurring disorders have an adverse impact on both mood and substance use outcomes. It is important that the nurse assesses the use of substances and consider the impact of co-occurring disorders (see Chapter 42).

Psychosocial Assessment

The psychosocial assessment for persons who have major depressive disorder includes the mental status (mood and affect, thought processes and content, cognition, memory, and attention), coping skills, developmental history, psychiatric family history, patterns of relationships, quality of support system, education, work history, and impact of physical or sexual abuse on interpersonal function. See Chapter 11. The nurse should identify the individual's strengths, as well as problem areas, by asking the patient to describe their thoughts, feelings and behaviors before the current depressive episode. Including a family member or close friend in the assessment process can be helpful. The following discussion identifies key assessment areas for a person who is depressed.

Mental Status and Appearance

Mood and Affect

The person with major depressive disorder has a sustained period of feeling depressed, sad, or hopeless and may experience anhedonia (loss of interest or pleasure). The patient may report "not caring any more" or not feeling any enjoyment in activities that were previously considered pleasurable. In some individuals, this may include a decrease in or loss of libido (i.e., sexual interest or desire) and sexual function. In others, irritability and anger are signs of depression, especially in those who deny being depressed. Individuals often describe themselves as depressed, sad, hopeless, discouraged, or "down in the dumps". If individuals complain of feeling "blah", having no feelings, constantly tired, or feeling anxious, a depressed mood can sometimes be inferred from their facial expression and demeanor (APA, 2013).

Numerous assessment scales are available for assessing depression. Easily administered self-report questionnaires can be valuable detection tools. These questionnaires cannot be the sole basis for making a diagnosis of major depressive episode, but they are sensitive to depressive symptoms. The following are five commonly used self-report scales:

- General Health Questionnaire (GHQ)
- Center for Epidemiological Studies Depression Scale (CES-D)
- Beck Depression Inventory (BDI)
- Zung Self-Rating Depression Scale (SDS)
- PRIME-MD

Clinician-completed rating scales may be more sensitive to improvement in the course of treatment, can assess symptoms in relationship to the depressive diagnostic criteria, and may have a slightly greater specificity than do self-report questionnaires in detecting depression. These include the following:

- Hamilton Rating Scale for Depression (HAM-D)
- Montgomery-Asberg Depression Rating Scale (MADRS)
- National Institute of Mental Health Diagnostic Interview Schedule (DIS)

Thought Content

Depressed individuals often have an unrealistic negative evaluation of their worth or have guilty preoccupations or ruminations about minor past failings. Such individuals often misinterpret neutral or trivial day-to-day events as evidence of personal defects. They may also have an exaggerated sense of responsibility for untoward events. As a result, they feel hopeless, helpless, worthless, and powerless. The possibility of disorganized thought processes (e.g., tangential or circumstantial thinking) and perceptual disturbances (e.g., hallucinations, delusions) should also be included in the assessment.

Cognition and Memory

Many individuals with depression report an impaired ability to think, concentrate, or make decisions. They may appear easily distracted or complain of memory difficulties. In older adults with major depression, memory difficulties may be the chief complaint and may be mistaken for early signs of dementia (pseudodementia) (APA, 2013). When the depression is fully treated, the memory problem often improves or fully resolves.

Behavioral Responses

Changes in patterns of relating (especially social withdrawal) and changes in level of occupational functioning are commonly reported and may represent a significant deterioration from baseline behavior. Increased use of "sick days" may occur. For people who are depressed, special attention should be given to the individual's spiritual dimension and religious background.

Self-Concept

A positive self-esteem can be protective for the development of severe depression. A low self-esteem is associated with several health problems such as obesity, cardiovascular events, and depression (Alghawrien et al., 2020; Ngo et al., 2020). Assessing self-esteem helps in establishing goals and direction for treatment.

Stress and Coping Patterns

The individual should be assessed for coping patterns. How does the person cope with the everyday stresses of life? How does the person cope with the depression and how does the depression impact the person's ability to cope with daily stressors? The nurse helps the patient identify positive coping patterns such as meditating, talking to a loved one and negative coping patterns such as overeating and using alcohol or nonprescribed drugs.

Suicidal Behavior

Patients with major depressive disorder are at increased risk for suicide. The development of suicide behavior is a complex phenomenon because symptoms are often hidden or veiled by somatic symptoms.

KEYCONCEPT Suicidal behavior is the occurrence of persistent thought patterns and actions that indicate a person is thinking about, planning, or enacting suicide.

Suicidal ideation includes thoughts that range from a belief that others would be better off if the person were dead or thoughts of death (passive suicidal ideation) to actual specific plans for committing suicide (active suicidal ideation). See Chapter 22. The frequency, intensity, and lethality of these thoughts can vary and can help to determine the seriousness of intent. The more specific the plan and the more accessible the means, the more serious becomes the intent. The risk for suicide needs to be initially assessed in patients who incur depressive disorders as well as reassessed throughout the course of treatment.

Suicidal ideation is not a normal reaction to stress. Persons who express any suicidal ideation need immediate mental health assessment regarding the depth of their thoughts and intentions. Risk factors for suicide ideation include lack of availability and inadequacy of social supports; family violence, including physical or sexual abuse; past history of suicidal ideation or behavior; presence of psychosis or substance use or abuse; and decreased ability to control suicidal impulses. See Chapter 22.

Ethnic and cultural differences exist regarding suicidal behavior. Men often use firearms. Women often use pills or other poisonous substances to commit suicide. Children often use suffocation. Data on suicide completion rates are reported highest in persons from Native Americans, Alaskan Natives, and those of non-Hispanic White descent. These rates are lowest for persons from Hispanic, non-Hispanic Black, and Asian and Pacific Islander descent. Ongoing research regarding suicide in veterans indicates that they have a higher risk than persons in the general population (Smigelsky et al., 2020). Psychological stress and previously diagnosed psychiatric disorders are major risk factors for veterans. Counseling and supportive services need to be provided to family and friends of persons who attempt or die by suicide because family and friends may experience feelings of grief, guilt, anger, and confusion (Link et al., 2020).

> **NCLEXNOTE** The possibility of suicide should always be a priority with patients who are depressed. Assessment and documentation of suicide risk should always be included in patient care.

Strength Assessment

Throughout the assessment, the nurse should be observing for strengths such as positive physical health status, coping skills, and social support. The following questions may be used to determine a person's strength:

- When you have been depressed before, how did you cope with the feelings?
- What do you do to relax?
- Do you reach out to anyone when you are feeling down?
- When you are not depressed, what makes you feel good?

CLINICAL JUDGMENT

There are several symptoms and effects of depression that could potentially require nursing care. In collaboration with the individual, the nurse can establish priorities of care. Suicidal thoughts and behaviors are always the first priority. If a patient does not have suicidal thoughts, the nurse can focus on the physical impact of the depression, such as lack of sleep, loss of appetite, and lack of energy, to carry out daily routines. Feelings of hopelessness and low self-esteem are usually present and need attention. Many people who are depressed have difficulty making decisions. As the priorities are established, the results of the strength assessment should be identified. These strengths will help the person recover from the depressed state.

THERAPEUTIC RELATIONSHIP

One of the most effective tools for caring for any person with a mental disorder is the therapeutic relationship. For a person who is depressed, there are a number of effective approaches:

- Establishment and maintenance of a supportive relationship based on the incorporation of culturally competent interventions and strategies
- Availability in times of crisis
- Vigilance regarding danger to self and others
- Education about the illness and treatment goals
- Encouragement and feedback concerning progress

- Guidance regarding the patient's interactions with the personal and work environment
- Realistic goal setting and monitoring
- Support of individual strengths in treatment choices.

Interacting with individuals who are depressed is challenging because they tend to be withdrawn and have difficulty expressing feelings and engaging in interpersonal interactions. The therapeutic relationship can be strengthened through the use of cognitive interventions as well as the nurse's ability to win the patient's trust through the use of culturally competent strategies in the context of empathy (Box 25.2).

Cheerleading, or being overly cheerful to a person who is depressed, blocks communication and can be quite irritating to depressed patients. Nurses should avoid approaching patients with depression with an overly cheerful attitude. Instead, a calm, supportive empathic approach helps keep communication open.

> **NCLEXNOTE** Establishing the patient–nurse relationship with a person who is depressed requires an empathic quiet approach that is grounded in the nurse's understanding of the cultural needs of the patient.

MENTAL HEALTH NURSING INTERVENTIONS

Establishing Recovery and Wellness Goals

Nursing intervention selection is a collaborative process between the patient and the nurse. As goals and interventions are agreed by both the nurse and the patient, the person's strengths (e.g., motivation to get better, resources, family support) should be emphasized in making treatment choices.

Physical Care

Because weeks or months of disturbed sleep patterns and nutritional imbalance only worsen depression, one of the first nursing interventions is helping the person re-establish normal sleep patterns and healthy nutrition. Supporting self-care management by encouraging patients to practice positive sleep hygiene and eat well-balanced meals regularly helps the patient move toward remission or recovery.

Deep-breathing exercises three times a day have been shown to reduce self-reported depressive symptoms within 4 weeks in patients with coronary heart disease (Box 25.3). Activity and exercise are also important for improving depressed mood state. Most people find that regular exercise is hard to maintain. People who are depressed may find it impossible. When teaching about

BOX 25.2 • THERAPEUTIC DIALOGUE: APPROACHING THE DEPRESSED PATIENT

Louise is severely depressed and has not left her hospital room since admission to the mental health unit. She has missed breakfast and is not interested in taking a shower or getting dressed.

INEFFECTIVE APPROACH

Nurse: Hello, Louise. My name is Sally. How are you feeling today?

Louise: I didn't sleep last night and need to rest. Please go away.

Nurse: Sorry, but it is time to get up. You have already missed breakfast. You have to take a quick shower now to get to group on time.

Louise: I have no interest in taking a shower or going to group.

Nurse: Why are you here if you don't want to be treated?

Louise: Go away. I don't want you in this room.

EFFECTIVE APPROACH

Nurse: Good morning. My name is Sally. I am your nurse today.

Louise: I didn't sleep last night and need to rest. Please go away.

Nurse: You didn't sleep well last night?

Louise: No, I can't remember when I was able to sleep through the night?

Nurse: Oh, I see. Is that why you missed breakfast?

Louise: I'm just not hungry. I have no energy.

Nurse: Lack of appetite and lack of energy are very common when people are depressed.

Louise: Really?

Nurse: Yes, so let's take one step at time. I'd like to help you get up.

Louise: Ok, I might be able to sit up.

Nurse: (Helps her sit up). Now, let's walk to the bathroom.

Louise: (Walks to the bathroom). Now what?

Nurse: Let's work on your AM care.

CRITICAL THINKING CHALLENGE

• What ineffective techniques did the nurse use in the first scenario and how did they impair communication?

• What effective techniques did the nurse use in the second scenario and how did they facilitate communication?

BOX 25.3

Research for Evidence-Based Practice: Breathing Exercise and Cognitive-Behavioral Interventions

Chien, H., Chung, Y., Yeh, M., & Lee, J. F. (2015). Breathing exercise combined with cognitive behavioural intervention improves sleep quality and heart rate variability in major depression. Journal of Clinical Nursing, 24(21–22), 3206–3214.

QUESTION: Do CBT and breathing exercises improve sleep quality and heart rate variability in major depression?

METHODS: Eighty-nine participants completed this study. One group ($n = 43$) received CBT combined with a breathing relaxation exercise for 4 weeks and the other group ($n = 43$) did not. Sleep quality and heart rate variability were measured at baseline, posttest 1 and 2, and follow-up.

FINDINGS: The group using the cognitive-behavioral intervention with the breathing exercise improved sleep quality and variability of heart rate significantly more than the control group.

IMPLICATIONS FOR NURSING: Nurses should consider using cognitive-behavioral interventions with breathing exercises for those who are depressed to improve their mood and reduce their depressive symptoms.

---

exercise, it is important to start with the current level of patient activity and increase it slowly. For example, if the patient is spending most of the time in bed, encouraging the patient to get dressed every day and walk for 5 or 10 minutes may be all that patient can tolerate. Gradually, patients should be encouraged to have a regular exercise program and to slowly increase their food intake. These activities are consistent with wellness goals.

Wellness Challenges

Depression robs the individual of energy to carry out simple activities. Previous wellness activities from physical activities, nutrition, and stress management often disappear during depression. The side effects of the antidepressants may actually interfere with normal wellness activities. The nurse should work with the individual to re-establish these activities. The individual may not feel like doing anything, but through the nurse–patient relationship, the nurse should seek commitment to gradually incorporate wellness activities. See Chapter 1 and Box 25.4.

Medication Interventions

Antidepressant medications have proved effective in all forms of major depression. To date, controlled trials have shown no single antidepressant drug to have greater efficacy in the treatment of major depressive disorder. See 12 for a list of antidepressant medications, usual dosage range, half-life, and therapeutic blood levels.

An antidepressant is selected based primarily on an individual patient's target symptoms; genetic factors; responses related to cultural, racial, and ethnic influences; and a pharmacologic agent's side-effect profile. Other factors that may influence choice include prior medication response, drug interactions and contraindications, concurrent medical and psychiatric disorders, patient age, and cost of medication. Selecting medications on the basis of pharmacogenetic properties improves symptom remission (Bousman et al., 2019).

BOX 25.4

Wellness Challenges

- Coping effectively with lack of energy and sadness
  - Strategies: Start with the easiest—take a walk after dinner; talk to a friend.
- Stress management.
  - Strategies: Say "no" to being a perfectionist; consider a massage; meditation.
- Decreasing feelings of worthlessness.
  - Strategies: Keep a list of accomplishments, help others; keep busy.
- Understanding the stigma of depression.
  - Strategies: Educate yourself and others about depression; join a support group.
- Recognizing the need for physical activity, healthy foods, and sleep.
  - Strategies: Track physical activity, diet, and sleep in a journal.
- Developing a sense of connection, belonging, and a support system.
  - Strategies: Contact at least one friend, attend religious service.
- Expanding a sense of purpose and meaning in life
  - Strategies: Pray, meditate, help others, volunteer.

The newer antidepressants, selective serotonin reuptake inhibitors (SSRIs), serotonin-norepinephrine reuptake inhibitors (SNRIs), and the norepinephrine dopamine reuptake inhibitor (NDRI) are used most often because these drugs selectively target the neurotransmitters and receptors thought to be associated with depression and minimize side effects. See Box 25.5. Individualizing dosages is usually done by fine-tuning medication dosage based on patient feedback. The tricyclic antidepressants (TCAs) and monoamine oxidase inhibitors (MAOIs) are being used less often than the other agents. See Box 25.6. Given their dietary restrictions, MAOIs usually are reserved for patients whose depression fails to respond to other antidepressants or patients who cannot tolerate typical antidepressants.

NCLEXNOTE Patients may be reluctant to take prescribed antidepressant medications or may self-treat depression based on their cultural beliefs and values (Jung et al., 2020). A culturally competent nursing care and teaching plan needs to address the importance for adherence to a medication regimen and emphasize any potential drug–drug interactions.

Administering Medications

Antidepressants are available in oral form and should be taken as prescribed (see Box 25.7). Even after the first episode of major depression, medication should be continued for at least 6 months to 1 year after the patient achieves complete remission of symptoms. If the patient experiences a recurrence after tapering the first course of treatment, the regimen should be reinstituted for at least another year, and if the illness reoccurs, medication should be continued indefinitely (Schatzberg & DeBattista, 2019).

Monitoring Medications

Patients should be carefully observed for therapeutic and side effects of the antidepressants. In the depths of depression, saving medication for a later suicide attempt is quite common. During antidepressant treatment, the nurse should monitor and document vital signs, plasma drug levels (as appropriate), liver and thyroid function tests, complete blood counts, and blood chemistry to make sure that patients are receiving a therapeutic dosage and are adherent to the prescribed regimen. Results of these tests also help evaluate for toxicity (see Chapter 11 for therapeutic blood levels).

Baseline orthostatic vital signs should be obtained before initiation of any medication, and in the case of medications known to have an impact on vital signs, such as TCAs, MAOIs, or SNRIs, they should be monitored on a regular basis. If these medications are administered to children or older adults, the dosage should be lowered to accommodate the physiologic state of the individual.

BOX 25.5

Drug Profile: Escitalopram Oxalate (LEXAPRO)

DRUG CLASS: Antidepressant

RECEPTOR AFFINITY: A highly SSRI with low affinity for 5-HT 1–7 or α- and β-adrenergic, dopamine D_{1-5}, histamine H_{1-3}, muscarinic M_{1-5}, and benzodiazepine receptors or for Na^+, K^+, Cl^-, and Ca^{++} ion channels that have been associated with various anticholinergic, sedative, and cardiovascular side effects.

INDICATIONS: Treatment of major depressive disorder, generalized anxiety disorder

ROUTES AND DOSAGES: Available as 5-, 10-, and 20-mg oral tablets

Adults: Initially 10 mg once a day. May increase to 20 mg after a minimum of 1 week. Trials have not shown greater benefit at the 20-mg dose.

Geriatric: 10-mg dose is recommended. Adjust dosage related to the drug's longer half-life and the slower liver metabolism of older adult patients.

Renal Impairment: No dosage adjustment is necessary for mild-to-moderate renal impairment.

Children: Safety and efficacy have not been established in this population.

HALF LIFE (PEAK EFFECT): 27 to 32 hours (4–7 hours)

SELECTED ADVERSE REACTIONS: Most common adverse events include insomnia, ejaculation disorder, diarrhea, nausea, fatigue, increased sweating, dry mouth, somnolence, dizziness, and constipation. Most serious adverse events include ejaculation disorder in men; fetal abnormalities and decreased fetal weight in pregnant patients; and serotonin syndrome if coadministered with MAOIs, St. John wort, or SSRIs, including citalopram (Celexa), of which escitalopram (Lexapro) is the active isomer.

BOXED WARNING: Suicidality in children, adolescents, and young adults

WARNING: There is potential for interaction with MAOIs. Lexapro should not be used in combination with an MAOI or within 14 days of discontinuing an MAOI.

SPECIFIC PATIENT AND FAMILY EDUCATION

- Do not take in combination with citalopram (Celexa) or other SSRIs or MAOIs. A 2-week washout period between escitalopram and SSRIs or MAOIs is recommended to avoid serotonin syndrome.
- Families and caregivers should be advised of the need for close observation and communication with the prescriber.
- Notify your prescriber if pregnancy is possible or being planned. Do not breast-feed while taking this medication.
- Use caution driving or operating machinery until you are certain that escitalopram does not alter your physical abilities or mental alertness.
- Notify your prescriber of any OTC medications, herbal supplements, and home remedies being used in combination with escitalopram.
- Ingestion of alcohol in combination with escitalopram is not recommended, although escitalopram does not seem to potentiate mental and motor impairments associated with alcohol.
- MAOI, monoamine oxidase inhibitor; OTC, over-the-counter; SSRI, selective serotonin reuptake inhibitor. http://www.accessdata.fda.gov/drugsatfda_docs/label/2014/021323s044,021365s032lbl.pdf

Managing Side Effects

Many people stop taking the prescribed antidepressants because of the side effects. (See Box 25.8.) Ideally, side effects are minimal and can be alleviated by nonpharmacologic interventions. For example, if patient is having difficulty going to sleep, avoiding caffeinated products may help (Table 25.1). SSRIs tend to be safer and have fewer side effects than the older medications. The most common reason individuals stop taking their SSRIs are gastrointestinal side effects, including diarrhea, cramping, and heartburn. The most common side effects associated with TCAs are the antihistaminic side effects (e.g., sedation weight gain) and anticholinergic side effects (potentiation of CNS drugs, blurred vision, dry mouth, constipation, urinary retention, sinus tachycardia, and decreased memory).

For the MAOIs, the most common side effects are headache, drowsiness, dry mouth and throat, constipation, blurred vision, and orthostatic hypotension. Additional selected adverse effects of MAOIs include insomnia, nausea, agitation, dizziness, asthenia, weight loss, and postural hypotension. Although priapism was not reported during clinical trials, the MAOIs are structurally similar to trazodone, which has been associated with priapism (prolonged painful erection). For those taking, MAOIs, close attention to dietary restrictions should be given. See Chapter 12 for tyramine-restricted diets.

EMERGENCY CARE ALERT ! If coadministered with food or other substances containing tyramine (e.g., aged cheese, beer, red wine), MAOIs can trigger a hypertensive crisis that may be life threatening. Symptoms include a sudden, severe pounding, or explosive headache in the back of the head or temples, racing pulse, flushing, stiff neck, chest pain, nausea and vomiting, and profuse sweating.

BOX 25.6

Drug Profile: Mirtazapine (Remeron)

DRUG CLASS: Antidepressant

RECEPTOR AFFINITY: Believed to enhance central noradrenergic and serotonergic activity antagonizing central presynaptic α_2-adrenergic receptors. Mechanism of action is unknown.

INDICATIONS: Treatment of depression

ROUTES AND DOSAGE: Available as 15- and 30-mg tablets

Adults: Initially, 15 mg/day as a single dose preferably in the evening before sleeping. Maximum dosage is 45 mg/day.

Geriatric: Use with caution; reduced dosage may be needed.

Children: Safety and efficacy have not been established.

HALF-LIFE (PEAK EFFECT): 20 to 40 hours (2 hours)

SELECTED ADVERSE REACTIONS: Somnolence, increased appetite, dizziness, weight gain, elevated cholesterol or triglyceride and transaminase levels, malaise, abdominal pain, hypertension, vasodilation, vomiting, anorexia, thirst, myasthenia, arthralgia, hypoesthesia, apathy, depression, vertigo, twitching, agitation, anxiety, amnesia, increased cough, sinusitis, pruritus, rash, urinary tract infection, mania (rare), agranulocytosis (rare)

BOXED WARNING: Suicidality in children, adolescents, and young adults

WARNING: Contraindicated in patients with known hypersensitivity. Use with caution in older adults, patients who are breast-feeding, and patients with impaired hepatic function. Avoid concomitant use with alcohol or diazepam, which can cause additive impairment of cognitive and motor skills.

SPECIFIC PATIENT AND FAMILY EDUCATION
- Take the dose once a day in the evening before sleep.
- Families and caregivers should be advised of the need for dose observation and communication with the prescriber.
- Avoid driving and performing other tasks requiring alertness.
- Notify your prescriber before taking any OTC or other prescription drugs.
- Avoid alcohol and other CNS depressants.
- Notify your prescriber if pregnancy is possible or planned.
- Monitor temperature and report any fever, lethargy, weakness, sore throat, malaise, or other "flulike" symptoms.
- Maintain medical follow-up, including any appointments for blood counts and liver studies.

CNS, central nervous system; OTC, over-the-counter.

BOX 25.7

Guidelines for Administering and Monitoring Antidepressant Medications

Nurses should do the following in administering and monitoring antidepressant medications:
- Observe the patient for cheeking or saving medications for a later suicide attempt.
- Monitor vital signs (such as orthostatic vital signs and temperature): obtain baseline data before the initiation of medications.
- Monitor periodically results of liver and thyroid function tests, blood chemistry, and complete blood count as appropriate and compare with baseline values.
- Monitor the patient symptoms for therapeutic response and report inadequate response to prescriber.
- Monitor the patient for side effects and report to the prescriber serious side effects or those that are chronic and problematic for the patient. (Table 25.1 indicates pharmacologic and nonpharmacologic interventions for common side effects.)
- Monitor drug levels as appropriate. (Therapeutic drug levels for antidepressants are listed in Chapter 12.)
- Monitor dietary intake as appropriate, especially with regard to MAOI antidepressants.
- Inquire about patient use of other medications, alcohol, "street" drugs, OTC medications, and herbal supplements that might alter the desired effects of prescribed antidepressants.

MAOI, monoamine oxidase inhibitor; OTC, over-the-counter.

Management of Complications

Suicidality

Suicidality is mentioned in a "black box" warning on all antidepressants, indicating an increased risk of suicide exists in children, adolescents, and young adults with major depressive or other psychiatric disorders. After the age of 24 years, the suicidality risk does not increase and after 65, the risk of suicide actually decreases when taking an antidepressant. The SSRIs are the least lethal of the antidepressants, but fatalities have been reported (Schatzberg & DeBattisa, 2019).

EMERGENCY CARE ALERT ! If possible, TCAs should not be prescribed for patients at risk for suicide. Lethal doses of TCAs are only three to five times the therapeutic dose, and more than 1 g of a TCA is often toxic and may be fatal. Death may result from cardiac arrhythmia, hypotension, or uncontrollable seizures.

Serum TCA levels should be evaluated when overdose is suspected. In acute overdose, almost all symptoms develop within 12 hours. Anticholinergic effects are prominent and include dry mucous membranes, warm and dry skin, blurred vision, decreased bowel motility, and urinary retention. CNS suppression (ranging from drowsiness to coma) or an agitated delirium may occur.

BOX 25.8

Antidepressants and Common Side Effects in Treating Depression

MEDICATIONS	COMMON SIDE EFFECTS	MEDICATIONS	COMMON SIDE EFFECTS
Selective Serotonin Reuptake Inhibitors (SSRIs)		**Tricyclic Antidepressants**	
Fluoxetine (Prozac) Sertraline (Zoloft) Paroxetine (Paxil) Fluvoxamine (Luvox) Citalopram (Celexa) Escitalopram (Lexapro)	Gastrointestinal distress Sedation Anticholinergic effects Weight gain or loss in some people Sexual dysfunction Dizziness Diaphoresis	Amitriptyline Amoxapine Clomipramine (Anafranil) Imipramine (Torfanil) Desipramine (Norpramin) Doxepin Nortriptyline (Aventyl, Pamelor) Protriptyline (Vivactil)	Drowsiness Anticholinergic effects Orthostatic hypotension Palpitations Tachycardia Impaired coordination Increased appetite Diaphoresis Weakness Disorientation Sexual side effects (impotence, changes in libido)
Serotonin Norepinephrine Reuptake Inhibitors (SNRIs)			
Desvenlafaxine (Pristiq extended release) Duloxetine (Cymbalta) Levomilnacipran (Fetzima) Venlafaxine (Effexor XR)	Gastrointestinal distress Anticholinergic effects Insomnia or sedation Decreased appetite Sexual dysfunction Abnormal dreams Dizziness Jitteriness Hypertension Irritability Photosensitivity	**Tetracyclic Antidepressants**	
		Maprotiline	Blurred vision Dizziness Lightheadedness Sedation Dry mouth Libido changes Impotence Weight changes
Norepinephrine Dopamine Reuptake Inhibitor (NDRI)		**Monoamine Oxidase Inhibitors**	
Bupropion (Wellbutrin)	Anticholinergic effects Headache Agitation Gastrointestinal distress Insomnia Anorexia Anxiety Weight loss Diarrhea and flatulence	Isocarboxazid (Marplan)	Dizziness Headache Nausea Dry mouth Constipation Drowsiness Sleep disturbance Orthostatic hypotension
Alpha$_2$ Antagonist		Phenelzine (Nardil)	Orthostatic hypotension Edema Dizziness Headache Drowsiness Sleep disturbance
Mirtazapine (Remeron)	Sedation Anticholinergic effects Appetite increase Weight gain Hypercholesterolemia Weakness and lack of energy Dizziness Hypertriglyceridemia	Tranylcypromine (Parnate)	Orthostatic hypotension Dizziness Headache Drowsiness Sleep disturbance Restlessness Central nervous system stimulation
Other Antidepressants			
Trazadone (Oleptro)	Sedation Anticholinergic effects Headache Dizziness Nausea/vomiting	Selegiline (Emsam)	Application site reaction Headache Insomnia Diarrhea Dry mouth Orthostatic hypotension Dyspepsia
Vilazodone (Viibryd)	Diarrhea Nausea Dizziness Dry mouth Insomnia Abnormal dreams		
Vortioxetine (Brintellix)	Nausea Diarrhea Dizziness Dry mouth Constipation Vomiting		

Basic overdose treatment includes induction of emesis, gastric lavage, and cardiorespiratory supportive care.

MAOIs are more lethal in overdose than are the newer antidepressants and thus should be prescribed with caution if the patient's suicide potential is elevated (see Chapter 12). An MAOI generally is given in divided doses to minimize side effects.

Serotonin Syndrome

Serotonin syndrome is a potentially serious side effect caused by drug-induced excess of intrasynaptic serotonin, 5-hydroxytryptamine (5-HT) (see Box 25.9). First reported in the 1950s, it was relatively rare until the introduction of the SSRIs. Serotonin syndrome is most often reported in patients taking two or more medications that increase CNS serotonin levels by different mechanisms (Duignan et al., 2020). The most common drug combinations associated with serotonin syndrome involve the MAOIs, the SSRIs, and the TCAs.

Although serotonin syndrome can cause death, it is mild in most patients, who usually recover with supportive care alone. Unlike neuroleptic malignant syndrome, which develops within 3 to 9 days after the introduction of neuroleptic medications (see Chapter 24), serotonin syndrome tends to develop within hours or days after starting or increasing the dose of serotonergic medication. Symptoms include altered mental status, autonomic dysfunction, and neuromuscular abnormalities. At least three of the following findings must be present for a diagnosis: mental status changes, agitation, myoclonus, hyperreflexia, fever, shivering, diaphoresis, ataxia, and diarrhea. In patients who also have peripheral vascular disease or atherosclerosis, severe vasospasm and hypertension may occur in the presence of elevated serotonin levels. In addition, in a patient who is a slow metabolizer of SSRIs, higher-than-normal levels of these antidepressants may circulate in the blood. Medications that are not usually considered serotonergic, such as dextromethorphan and meperidine have been associated with the syndrome (Dy et al., 2017).

EMERGENCY CARE ALERT ! The most important emergency interventions are stopping use of the offending drug, notifying the prescriber, and providing necessary supportive care (e.g., intravenous fluids, antipyretics, cooling blanket). Severe symptoms have been successfully treated with antiserotonergic agents, such as cyproheptadine (Frye et al., 2020).

BOX 25.9

Serotonin Syndrome

CAUSE: Excessive intrasynaptic serotonin

HOW IT HAPPENS: Combining medications that increase CNS serotonin levels, such as SSRIs + MAOIs; SSRIs + St. John wort; or SSRIs + diet pills; dextromethorphan or alcohol, especially red wine; or SSRI + street drugs, such as LSD, MMDA, or ecstasy

SYMPTOMS: Mental status changes, agitation, ataxia, myoclonus, hyperreflexia, fever, shivering, diaphoresis, diarrhea

TREATMENT
- Assess all medications, supplements, foods, and recreational drugs ingested to determine the offending substances.
- Discontinue any substances that may be causative factors. If symptoms are mild, treat supportively on an outpatient basis with propranolol and lorazepam and follow-up with the prescriber.
- If symptoms are moderate to severe, hospitalization may be needed with monitoring of vital signs and treatment with intravenous fluids, antipyretics, and cooling blankets.

FURTHER USE: Assess on a case-by-case basis and minimize risk factors for further medication therapy.
- CNS, central nervous system; LSD, lysergic acid diethylamide; MAOI, monoamine oxidase inhibitor; MMDA, 3-methoxy-4,5-methylenedioxyamphetamine; SSRI, selective serotonin reuptake inhibitor.

Monitoring for Drug Interactions

Several potential drug interactions are associated with antidepressants. Alcohol consumption should be avoided when taking any antidepressant because SSRIs are metabolized in the liver; other medications that are also metabolized by the same enzyme can cause an increase in drug levels leading to toxicity and serotonin syndrome. For example, if migraine medications known as "triptans" are given with the SSRIs, serotonin syndrome can occur. Bupropion cannot be given at the same time as an MAOI. Grapefruit should not be consumed while taking trazodone. It is beyond the scope of this text to review drug–drug interactions in detail. Nurses should check with pharmacy resources for any drug–drug interactions when administering medications.

Teaching Points

If depression goes untreated or is inadequately treated, episodes can become more frequent, more severe, longer in duration, and can lead to suicide. Patient education involves explaining this pattern and the importance of continuing medication use after the acute phase of treatment to decrease the risk for future episodes. Patient concerns regarding long-term antidepressant therapy need to be assessed and addressed. All teaching points need to be developed and delivered using a culturally competent approach to enhance patient adherence.

Patients should also be advised not to take herbal substances such as St. John wort or SAMe if they are also taking prescribed antidepressants. St. John wort should also not be taken if the patient is taking nasal decongestants, hay fever, and asthma medications containing monoamines, amino acid supplements containing phenylalanine, or tyrosine. The combination may cause hypertension.

Other Somatic Therapies

Electroconvulsive Therapy

Although its therapeutic mechanism of action is unknown, ECT is an effective treatment for patients with severe depression. It is generally reserved for patients whose disorder is refractory or intolerant to initial drug treatments and who are so severely ill that rapid treatment is required (e.g., patients with malnutrition, catatonia, or suicidality).

ECT is contraindicated for patients with increased intracranial pressure. Other high-risk patients include those with recent myocardial infarction, recent cerebrovascular accident, retinal detachment, or pheochromocytoma (a tumor in the cells of the adrenal gland) and those at risk for complications of anesthesia. Older age has been associated with a favorable response to ECT, but the effectiveness and safety in this group have not been shown. Because depression can increase the mortality risk for older adults, in particular, and some older adults do not respond well to medication, effective treatment is especially important for this age group (Hermida et al., 2020).

The role of the nurse in the care of the patient undergoing ECT is to provide educational and emotional support for the patient and family, assess baseline or pretreatment levels of function, prepare the patient for the ECT process, monitor and evaluate the patient's response to ECT, provide assessment data with the ECT team, and modify treatment as needed (see Chapter 12 for more information). The actual procedure, possible therapeutic mechanisms of action, potential adverse effects, contraindications, and nursing interventions are described in detail in Chapter 12.

Light Therapy (Phototherapy)

Light therapy is described in Chapter 12. Given current research, light therapy is an option for well-documented mild-to-moderate seasonal, nonpsychotic, winter depressive episodes in patients with recurrent major depressive disorders, including children and adolescents. Evidence also indicates that light therapy can be as effective as antidepressants (Geoffroy et al., 2019).

Repetitive Transcranial Magnetic Stimulation

In 2008, the U.S. Food and Drug Administration approved rTMS for the treatment of patients with mild treatment-resistant depression. In rTMS, a magnetic coil placed on the scalp at the site of the left motor cortex releases small electrical pulses that stimulate the site of the left dorsolateral prefrontal cortex in the superficial cortex. This rapidly changing magnetic field stimulates the brain sufficiently to depolarize neurons and exert effects across synapses. These pulses (similar in type and strength as a magnetic resonance imaging machine) easily pass through the hair, skin, and skull, requiring much less electricity than ECT. The patient is awake, reclining in an rTMS chair during the procedure, and can resume normal activities immediately after the procedure. Because anesthesia is not required, no risks are associated with sedation. Treatment of depression typically consists of 20 to 30 sessions, lasting 37 minutes each over 4 to 6 weeks. Depending on the level of practice and training, the nurse's role in the use of the rTMS varies from patient education, pre- and postprocedure care to performing the procedure (Sehatzadeh et al., 2019).

Psychosocial Interventions

Therapeutic Interactions

Individuals experiencing depression have often withdrawn from daily activities, such as engaging in family activities, attending work, and participating in community functions. During hospitalization, patients often withdraw to their rooms and refuse to participate in unit activity. Nurses help the patient balance the need for privacy with the need to return to normal social functioning. Even though depressed patients should not be approached in an overly enthusiastic manner, they should be encouraged to set realistic goals to reconnect with their families and communities. Explain to patients that attending social activities, even though they do not feel like it, will promote the recovery process and help them achieve their goals.

Enhancing Cognitive Functioning

Cognitive interventions such as thought stopping and positive self-talk can dispel irrational beliefs and distorted attitudes and, in turn, reduce depressive symptoms during the acute phase of major depression (see Chapter 13). Nurses should consider using cognitive approaches when caring for persons who are depressed. The use of cognitive interventions in the acute phase of treatment combined with medication is now considered first-line treatment for mildly to moderately depressed outpatients.

NCLEXNOTE A cognitive therapy approach is recommended for helping persons restructure the negative thinking processes related to a person's concept of self, others, and the future. This approach should be included in most nursing care plans for patients with depression.

Using Behavioral Interventions

Behavioral interventions are effective in the acute treatment of patients with mildly to moderately severe depression, especially when combined with pharmacotherapy. Therapeutic techniques include activity scheduling, social skills training, and problem solving. Behavioral therapy techniques are described in Chapter 7.

Psychoeducation

Teaching about Symptoms

Patients with depression and their significant others often incorrectly believe that their illness is their own fault and that they should be able to "pull themselves up by their bootstraps and snap out of it." Persons from some cultural groups believe that the symptoms of depression may be a result of someone placing a hex on the affected person because the person has done something evil. It is vital to be culturally competent to be effective in teaching patients and their families about the treatment modalities for depression.

Patients need to know the full range of suitable treatment options before consenting to participate in treatment. Information empowers patients to ask questions, weigh risks and benefits, and make the best treatment choices. The nurse can provide opportunities for patients to question, discuss, and explore their feelings about past, current, and planned use of medications and other treatments. Developing strategies to enhance adherence and to raise awareness of early signs of relapse can be important aids to increasing treatment efficacy and promoting recovery (Box 25.10).

Wellness Strategies

Teaching persons how to develop wellness goals and strategies is an evidence-based approach that psychiatric

---

BOX 25.10

Psychoeducation Checklist: Major Depressive Disorder

When caring for the patient with a major depressive disorder, be sure to include the following topic areas in the teaching plan:
- Psychopharmacologic agents, including drug action, dosing frequency, and possible side effects
- Risk factors for recurrence; signs of recurrence
- Adherence to therapy and treatment program
- Recovery strategies
- Nutrition
- Sleep measures
- Self-care management
- Goal setting and problem solving
- Social interaction skills
- Follow-up appointments
- Community support services

---

nurses can implement to build patients' recovery process (Anthony, 1993; Jacob, 2015). This teaching combines approaches that strengthen a person's clinical and emotional (i.e.,biopsychosocial) functioning (Ohrnberger et al., 2017). The client and the psychiatric nurse set mutual goals that may focus on healthy eating, exercise, and cognitive-behavioral change (Roosenschoon et al., 2019). The psychiatric nurse can engage patients in role-playing in order to learn and practice social skills that can be used in their everyday interactions with other individuals.

Providing Family Education

The family needs education and support during and after the treatment of family members. Because major depressive disorder is a recurring disorder, the family needs information about specific antecedents to a family member's depression and what therapeutic steps to take. For example, one patient may routinely become depressed during the fall of each year, with one of the first symptoms being excessive sleepiness. For another patient, a major loss, such as a child going to college or the death of a pet, may precipitate a depressive episode. Families of older adults need to be aware of the possibility of depression and related symptoms, which often occur after the deaths of friends and relatives. Families of children who are depressed often misinterpret depression as behavioral problems.

Promoting Safety

In many cases, patients are admitted to the psychiatric hospital because of a suicide attempt. Suicidality should continually be evaluated, and the patient should be protected from self-harm (see Chapter 22). During the depths of depression, patients may not have the energy to complete a suicide. As patients begin to feel better and have increased energy, they therefore may be at a greater risk for suicide. If a previously depressed patient appears to have become energized overnight, they may have decided to commit suicide and thus may be relieved that the decision is finally made. The nurse may misinterpret the mood improvement as a positive move toward recovery; however, this patient may be very intent on suicide. These individuals should be carefully monitored to maintain their safety.

Convening Support Groups

Individuals who are depressed can receive emotional support in groups and learn how others deal with similar problems and issues. As group members serve as role models for new group members, they also benefit as their self-esteem increases, which strengthens their ability to address their issues (see Chapter 14). Group interventions are often used to help an individual cope with depression associated with bereavement or chronic medical illness. Group interventions are also commonly used to educate patients and families about their disorder and medications.

Nurses are exceptionally well positioned to engage patients and their families in the active process of improving daily functioning, increasing knowledge and skill acquisition, and increasing independent living. Consumer-oriented support groups can help to enhance the self-esteem and the support network of participating patients and their families. Advice, encouragement, and the sense of group camaraderie may make an important contribution to recovery (APA, 2013). Organizations providing support and information include the Depression and Bipolar Support Network (DBSA), National Alliance on Mental Illness (NAMI), and the Mental Health Association and Recovery, Inc. (a self-help group).

Implementing Milieu Therapy

While hospitalized, milieu therapy (see Chapter 11) helps depressed patients maintain socialization skills and continue to interact with others. When depressed, people are often unaware of the environment and withdraw into themselves. On a psychiatric unit, depressed patients should be encouraged to attend and participate in unit activities. These individuals have decreased energy levels and thus may be moving more slowly than others; however, their efforts should be praised.

Family Interventions

Patients who perceive high family stress are at risk for greater future severity of illness, higher use of health services, and higher health care expense. Marital and family problems are common among patients with mood disorders; comprehensive treatment requires that these problems be assessed and addressed. They may be a consequence of the major depression but may also predispose persons to develop depressive symptoms or inhibit recovery and resilience processes. Marital and family therapy may reduce depressive symptoms and the risk for relapse in patients with marital and family problems. The depressed spouse's depression has marked impact on the marital adjustment of the nondepressed spouse. Treatment approaches should be designed to help couples be supportive of each other, to adapt, and to cope with the depressive symptoms within the framework of their ongoing marital relations. Many family nursing interventions may be used by the psychiatric nurse in providing targeted family-centered care. These include the following:

- Monitoring patient and family for indicators of stress
- Teaching stress management techniques
- Counseling family members on coping skills for their own use
- Providing necessary knowledge of options and support services
- Facilitating family routines and rituals
- Assisting the family to resolve feelings of guilt
- Assisting the family with conflict resolution
- Identifying family strengths and resources with family members
- Facilitating communication among family members

Developing Recovery-Oriented Rehabilitation Strategies

William Anthony (1993) developed a model on recovery from mental illness. The model resonates with patients, families, friends, and psychiatric nurses. The evidenced-based practice model stresses the concept of hope that persons with mental illness develop and enact in their everyday lives (Anthony, 1993). Recovery is not just the emphasis on clinical symptoms. Persons develop new techniques that enhance their strengths in the areas of knowledge regarding their personalities and abilities to develop social support systems (Ohrnberger et al., 2017). In addition, persons learn other evidence-based approaches that help them to increase and maintain their physical and emotional health (Jacob, 2015; Khoury, 2019). Community organizations such as WRAP (Wellness Recovery Action Planning), NAMI, and Mental health boards have recovery evidence-based programs for persons, their families, and mental health providers (Jacob, 2015). Recovery represents a community extended and focused patient-driven approach that puts them in charge: some define it as person-centered but persons who incur mental illness define it as their evidence-based approach to life.

Evaluation and Treatment Outcomes

The major goals of treatment are to help the patient to be as independent as possible and to achieve stability, remission, and recovery from major depression. It is often a lifelong struggle for the individual. Ongoing evaluation of the patient's symptoms, functioning, and quality of life should be carefully documented in the patient's record in order to monitor outcomes of treatment.

Continuum of Care

Mild-to-moderate depression is often first recognized in primary care settings. Primary care nurses should be able to recognize depression in these patients and make appropriate interventions or referrals

Emergency Care

Those with more severe depressive symptoms may be directly admitted to inpatient and outpatient mental health settings or emergency departments

Inpatient-focused Care

Although most patients with major depression are treated in outpatient settings, brief hospitalization may be required if the patient is suicidal or psychotic (Mitchell et al., 2017). Nurses working on inpatient units provide a wide range of direct services, including administering and monitoring medications and target symptoms; conducting psychoeducational groups; and more generally, structuring and maintaining a therapeutic environment.

Community Care

The continuum of care beyond these settings may include partial hospitalization or day treatment programs; individual, family, or group psychotherapy; and home visits. Nurses providing home care have an excellent opportunity to detect undiagnosed depressive disorders and make appropriate referrals.

Virtual Mental Health Care

Commonly known as Telehealth, virtual mental health care emerged in response to client and psychiatric-mental health educator and practitioner needs (Tyson et al., 2019). *Telehealth* is defined as the use of electronic approaches and communications that support clinical and professional health care that facilitate biobehavioral health needs (Tyson et al., 2019). Telehealth extends psychiatric nurses ability to assess, diagnose, and treat clients, as well as collaborate with other health care providers. Video and phone conferencing technologies facilitate the process. The use of virtual mental health helps psychiatric nurses to assess quality education and provide evidenced-based psychiatric care to persons from underserved populations and those living in rural areas (Tyson et al., 2019).

Integration with Primary Care

Depression is often treated in the primary care setting with readily available antidepressants. Unfortunately, the primary treatment for depression in this setting is medication. Many individuals need more than medication but do not access mental health services for a variety of reasons such as stigma, fear of being labeled as mentally ill, and lack of resources. There are also several medical problems associated with depression, such as hypothyroidism (Uhlenbusch et al., 2019). Pain is a common problem for individuals who are depressed (Zis et al., 2017). It is important to communicate with the primary care provider to coordinate care.

The medical home delivery model is becoming widely accepted in the United States. If a patient is cared within a medical home model, all of their health and mental health needs are coordinated by one health provider. Meaningful long-term relationships can be developed. The advantage of a medical home is a recognition and coordination of all health care needs. This model is helpful when many of the health disorders, associated with depression, occur. For example, substance abuse, obesity, are cardiovascular disorders are associated with depression and mood disorders (Berg et al., 2018).

OTHER DEPRESSIVE DISORDERS

Other depressive disorders with similar symptoms are treated similarly to the major depressive disorders. Nursing care should be individualized and based on their patients' mental health needs and strengths. A diagnosis of persistent depressive disorder (*dysthymia*) is made if major depressive disorder symptoms last for 2 years for an adult and 1 year for children and adolescents. These individuals are depressed for most of each day (APA, 2013). A major depressive disorder may precede the persistent depressive disorder or co-occur with it.

Premenstrual dysphoric disorder is characterized by recurring mood swings, feelings of sadness, or sensitivity to rejection in the final week before the onset of menses. The mood begins to improve a few days after menses begins. Stress, history of interpersonal trauma, seasonal changes are associated with this disorder (APA, 2013).

Disruptive mood dysregulation disorder is characterized by severe irritability and outbursts of temper. The onset of disruptive mood dysregulation disorder begins before the age of 10 when children have verbal rages and/or are physically aggressive toward others or property. These outbursts are outside of the normal temper tantrums children display. They are more severe than what would be expected developmentally and occur frequently (i.e., two or three times a week). The behavior disrupts family functioning as well as the child's ability to succeed in school and social activities. This disorder can co-occur with attention-deficit/hyperactivity disorder. See Chapter 37.

Disruptive mood dysregulation disorder is similar to pediatric bipolar disorder, but the *DSM-5* differentiates it from bipolar disorder. Children with this disorder have similar deficits in recognition of emotion through facial expression, decision-making, and control as those with bipolar disorder. More research is needed in understanding this disorder.

SUMMARY OF KEY POINTS

- Moods influence perception of life events and functioning. Depressive disorders are characterized by persistent or recurring disturbances in mood that cause significant psychological distress and functional impairment (typified by feelings of sadness, hopelessness, loss of interest, and fatigue).

- Depressive disorders include major depressive disorder, persistent depressive disorder (dysthymia), premenstrual dysphoric disorder, disruptive mood dysregulation disorder, and others related to medical conditions, medications, or substance use.

- Risk factors include a family history of depressive disorders, prior depressive episodes; lack of social support; stressful life events; substance use; and medical problems, particularly chronic or terminal illnesses.

- Treatment of major depressive disorder primarily includes antidepressant medication, psychotherapy, or a combination of both. ECT, light therapy, and rTMS are also used.

- Nurses must be knowledgeable regarding culturally competent strategies related to the use of antidepressant medications, pharmacologic therapeutic effects and associated side effects, toxicity, dosage ranges, and contraindications. Nurses must also be familiar with ECT protocols and associated interventions. Patient education and the provision of emotional support during the course of treatment are also nursing responsibilities.

- Many symptoms of depression (e.g., weight and appetite changes, sleep disturbance, decreased energy, fatigue) are similar to those of medical illnesses. Assessment includes a thorough medical history and physical examination to detect or rule out medical or psychiatric comorbidity.

- Mental health nursing assessment includes assessing mood; speech patterns; thought processes and content; suicidal or homicidal thoughts; cognition and memory; and social factors, such as patterns of relationships, quality of support systems, and changes in occupational functioning. Several self-report scales are helpful in evaluating depressive symptoms.

- Establishing and maintaining a therapeutic culturally competent nurse–patient relationship is key to successful outcomes. Nursing interventions that foster the therapeutic relationship include being available in times of crisis, providing understanding and education to patients and their families regarding goals of treatment, providing encouragement and feedback concerning the patient's progress, providing guidance in the patient's interpersonal interactions with others and work environment, and helping to set and monitor realistic goals.

- Psychosocial interventions for depressive disorders include self-care management, cognitive therapy, behavior therapy, interpersonal therapy, patient and family education regarding the nature of the disorder and treatment goals, marital and family interventions, and group interventions that include medication maintenance support groups and other consumer-oriented support groups.

CRITICAL THINKING CHALLENGES

1. Describe how you would do a suicide assessment on the patients who come into a primary care office and are distraught and expressing concerns about their ability to cope with their current situation.

2. Describe how you would approach the patient who does not want to talk with you.

3. Describe how you would approach the patients who are expressing concern that the diagnosis of depressive disorder will negatively affect their social and work relationships.

4. Your depressed patients do not seem inclined to talk about their depression. Describe the measures you would take to initiate a therapeutic relationship with them.

5. Compare the side effects of the SSRIs, TCAs, and MAOIs.

6. Think about all the above situations and relate them to persons from culturally and ethnically diverse populations (e.g., African, Latinx, or Asian descent; Jewish or Jehovah Witness religions; across the life span of individuals from children to older adult populations).

Unfolding Patient Stories: Li Na Chen

Part 2

Recall from Chapter 3 Li Na Chen with major depressive disorder who was hospitalized following her third suicide attempt with an overdose. She is transitioning to a partial hospitalization program before formal transition to home. Her husband is concerned about their two children, ages 12 and 14, and his ability to handle her once she is home. What questions can the nurse ask to clarify the husband's concerns? How can Li Na's depression and attempted suicide affect her husband and children? What psychosocial interventions can the nurse consider to support Li Na and her family once she is home?

Movie Viewing Guides
About Schmidt: (2002). This movie is about a 67-year-old man, Warren Schmidt, played by Jack Nicholson, who retires from his job as

an insurance company executive. He experiences work withdrawal and a lack of direction for his retirement. His wife, Helen, irritates him, and he has no idea what to do to fill his days. While watching television one day, he is moved to sponsor a child in Africa with whom he begins a long, one-sided correspondence. When his wife dies unexpectedly, he is initially numb, then sad, and finally angry when he discovers that she had an affair with his best friend many years ago. He is estranged from his only daughter, Jeanie, whose wedding to Randall, a man he thinks is beneath her, is imminent. The movie follows Warren as he searches for connection and meaning in his life.

SIGNIFICANCE: Warren Schmidt demonstrates a common phenomenon among older adults when they retire. He also shows the impact of grief superimposed on initial dysthymia or depression.

VIEWING POINTS: Look for the changes in Schmidt's manifestations of depression in different situations. Note how he experiences the various stages of grieving. What do you think about Schmidt's search for significance and meaning in his life?

Dead Poet's Society: (1989). This film portrays John Keating, played by Robin Williams, as a charismatic English teacher in a conservative New England prep school for boys in 1959. John brings his love of poetry to the students and encourages them to follow their dreams and talents and make the most of every day. His efforts put him at odds with the administration of the school, particularly the headmaster, played by Norman Lloyd, as well as Tom Perry, the father of one of his students, played by Kurtwood Smith. Tom's son, Neil, played by Robert Sean Leonard, chooses to act in a school play despite the objection of his father to any extracurricular activities. When Neil cannot reconcile his love of theater and his father's expectations that he pursues a career in medicine, he kills himself. John Keating blames himself for the death, as does the school administration. He is fired by the administration but has a moment of pride when his students demonstrate their ability to think and act for themselves.

SIGNIFICANCE: This film accurately portrays the sensitivity of adolescents and their longing for worthwhile role models. It also shows adolescent growth and development in a realistic manner. It demonstrates the combination of factors that accompany a decision to commit suicide. We can see how Neil feels caught between his desires and the demands of his father. In the cultural context of the late 1950s, few children or adolescents dared to challenge or defy their parents, especially such a domineering man as Tom Perry.

VIEWING POINTS: Look for the differences in Neil's behavior with his peers and his father or other adults besides Mr. Keating. What, if any, clues do you get that Neil might attempt suicide? What actions by any of the main characters might have prevented his suicide?

A related Psychiatric-Mental Health Nursing video on the topic of Depression is available at http://thepoint.lww.com/Boyd7e.

A Practice and Learn Activity related to the video on the topic of Depression is available at http://thepoint.lww.com/Boyd7e.

REFERENCES

Alghawrien, D., Al-Hussami, M., & Ayaad, O. (2020). The impact of obesity on self-esteem and academic achievement among university students. *International Journal of Adolescent Medicine and Health.* https://doi.org/10.1515/ijamh-2019-0137

American Psychiatric Association (APA). (2013). *Diagnostic and statistical manual of mental disorders DSM-5* (5th ed.). Author.

Anthony, W. A. (1993). Recovery from mental illness: The guiding vision of the mental health service system in the 1990s. *Psychosocial Rehabilitation Journal, 16*(4), 11–23.

Bachman, S. (2018). Epidemiology of suicide and the psychiatric perspective. *International Journal of Environmental Research and Public Health, 15*(7). pii: E1425. https://doi.org/10.3390/ijerph15071425

Berg, S. K., Rasmussen, T. B., Thrysoee, L., Thorup, C. B., Borregaard, B., Christensen, A. V., Mols, R. E., Juel, K., & Ekholm, O. (2018). Mental health is a risk factor for poor outcomes in cardiac patients: Findings from the national DenHeart survey. *Journal of Psychosomatic Research, 112,* 66–72. https://doi.org/doi:10.1016/j.jpsychores.2018.07.002

Blazer, D. G., & Steffens, D. C. (2015). Depressive disorders. In D. G. Blazer, D. C. Steffens, & M. Thakur (Eds.), *The American Psychiatric Publishing Textbook of Geriatric Psychiatry* (5th ed.). American Psychiatric Association.

Bousman, C. A., Arandjelovic, K., Mancuso, S. G., Eyre, H. A., & Dunlop, B. W. (2019). Pharmacogenetic tests and depressive symptom remission: A meta-analysis of randomized controlled trials. *Pharmacogenomics, 20*(1), 37–47. https://doi.org/10.2217/pgs-2018-0142

Brunstein, K. A. (2019). Bi-directional longitudinal associations between different types of bullying victimization, suicide ideation/attempts, and depression among a large sample of European adolescents. *Journal of Psychology and Psychiatry and Allied Disciplines, 60*(2), 209–215. https://doi.org/10.1111/jcpp.12951

Chien, H., Chung, Y., Yeh, M., & Lee, J. F. (2015). Breathing exercise combined with cognitive behavioural intervention improves sleep quality and heart rate variability in major depression. *Journal of Clinical Nursing, 24*(21–22), 3206–3214.

Drury, S. S., Scaramella, L., & Zeanah, C. H. (2016). The neurobiological impact of postpartum maternal depression: Prevention and intervention approaches. *Child Adolescent Psychiatric Clinics of North America, 25,* 179–200.

Duignan, K. M., Quinn, A. M., & Matson, A. M. (2020). Serotonin syndrome from sertraline monotherapy. *The American Journal of Emergency Medicine, 38*(8), 1695.e5–1695.e6. https://doi.org/10.1016/j.ajem.2019.158487

Dunlop, B.W., LoParo, D., Kinkead, B., Mletzko-Crowe, T., Cole, S. P., Nemeroff, C. B., Mayberg, H. S., & Craighead, W. E. (2019). Benefits of sequentially adding cognitive-behavioral therapy or antidepressant medication for adults with nonremitting depression. *American Journal of Psychiatry, 176*(4), 275–286. https://doi.org/10.1176/appi.ajp.2018.18091075

Dy, P., Arcega, V., Ghali, W., & Wolfe, W. (2017). Serotonin syndrome caused by drug to drug interaction between escitalopram and dextromethorphan. *BMJ Case Reports.* https://doi.org/10.1136/bcr-2017-221486

Frye, J. R., Poggemiller, A. M., McGonagill, P. W., Pape, K. O., Galet, C., & Liu, Y. M. (2020). Use of cyproheptadine for the treatment of serotonin syndrome: A case series. *Journal of Clinical Psychopharmacology, 40*(1), 95–99. https://doi.org/10.1097/JCP.0000000000001159

Ge, L., Yap, C. W., Ong, R., & Heng, B. H. (2017). Social isolation, loneliness and their relationships with depressive symptoms: A population-based study. *PLoS One, 12*(8), e0182145. doi: 10.1371/journal.pone.0182145

Geoffroy, P. A., Schroder, C. M., Reynaud, E., & Bourgin, P. (2019). Efficacy of light therapy versus antidepressant drugs, and of the combination versus monotherapy, in major depressive episodes: A systematic review and meta-analysis. *Sleep Medicine Reviews, 48*, 101213. https://doi.org/10.1016/j.smrv.2019.101213

Gong, C., Duan, X., Su, P., Wan, Y., Xu, Y., Tao, F., & Sun, Y. (2019). Heightened HPA-axis stress reactivity and accelerated pubertal progression predicts depressive symptoms over 4-year follow up. *Psychoneuroendocrinology, 103*, 259–265. https://doi.org/10.1016/j.psyneuen.2019.02.001

Hasin, D. S., Sarvet, A. L., Meyers, J. L., Saha, T. D., Ruan, W. J., Stohl, M., & Grant, B. F. (2018). Epidemiology of adult DSM-5 major depressive disorder and its specifiers in the United States. *JAMA Psychiatry, 75*(4), 336–346. https://doi.org/10.1001/jamapsychiatry.2017.4602

Hermida, A. P., Tang, Y. L., Glass, O., Janjua, A. U., & McDonald, W. M. (2020). Efficacy and safety of ECT for behavioral and psychological symptoms of dementia (BPSD): A retrospective chart review. *The American Journal of Geriatric Psychiatry, 28*(2), 157–163. https://doi.org/10.1016/j.jagp.2019.09.008

Himmerich, H., Patsalos, O., Lichtblau, N., Ibrahim, M., & Dalton, B. (2019). Cytokine research in depression: Principles, challenges, and open questions. *Frontiers in Psychiatry, 10*, 30. https://doi.org/10.3389/fpsyt.2019.00030

Hoertel, N., Blanco, C., Oquendo, M. A., et al., Blanco, C., Oquendo, M. A., Wall, M. M., Olfson, M., Falissard, B., Franco, S., Peyre, H., Lemogne, C., & Limosin, F. (2017). A comprehensive model of predictors of persistence and recurrence in adults with major depression: Results from a national 3-year prospective study. *Journal of Psychiatric Research, 95*, 19–27. https://doi.org/10.1016/j.jpsychires.2017.07.022

Hornberger, A. P., Medley-Proctor, K., Nettles, C. D., Cimporescu, M. A., & Howe, G. W. (2016). The influence of the racial/ethnic match of interviewer and respondent on the measurement of couple's relationship quality and emotional functioning. *Couple and Family Psychology: Research and Practice, 5*(1), 12–26.

Howard, D. M., Adams, M. J., Clarke, T. K., Hafferty, J. D., Gibson, J., Shirali, M., Coleman, J., Hagenaars, S. P., Ward, J., Wigmore, E. M., Alloza, C., Shen, X., Barbu, M. C., Xu, E. Y., Whalley, H. C., Marioni, R. E., Porteous, D. J., Davies, G., Deary, I. J., Hemani, G., … McIntosh, A. M. (2019). Genome-wide meta-analysis of depression identifies 102 independent variants and highlights the importance of the prefrontal brain regions. *Nature Neuroscience, 22*(3), 343–352. https://doi.org/10.1038/s41593-018-0326-7

Ivey-Stephenson, A. Z., Crosby, A. E., Jack, S., Haileyesus, T., & Kresnow-Sedacca, M. J.(2017). Suicide trends among and within urbanization levels by sex, race/ethnicity, age group, and mechanism of death—United States, 2001–2015. *MMWR Surveillance Summaries, 66*(No. SS-18), 1–16. http://dx.doi.org/10.15585/mmwr.ss6618a1

Jacob, K. S. (2015). Recovery model of mental illness: A complementary approach to psychiatric care. *Indian Journal of Psychological Medicine, 37*(2), 117–119. https://doi.org/10.4103/0253-7176.155605

Joca, S. R., Moreira, F. A., Wegener, G. (2015). Atypical neurotransmitters and the neurobiology of depression. *CNS & Neurological Disorders Drug Targets, 14*(8), 1001–1011.

Johns, M. M., Lowry, R., Rasberry, C. N., Dunville, R., Robin, L., Pampati, S., Stone, D. M., & Mercer Kollar, L. M. (2018). Violence victimization, substance use, and suicide risk among sexual minority high school students—United States, 2015–2017. *MMWR Morbidity Mortality Weekly Report, 67*(43), 1211–1215. https://doi.org/10.15585/mmwr.mm6743a4

Jung, H., Cho, Y. J., Rhee, M. K., & Jang, Y. (2020). Stigmatizing beliefs about depression in diverse ethnic groups of Asian Americans. *Community Mental Health Journal, 56*(1), 79–87. https://doi.org/10.1007/s10597-019-00481-x

Khoury, E. (2019). Recovery attitudes and recovery practices have an impact on psychosocial outreach interventions in community mental health care. *Frontiers in Psychiatry, 10*. https://doi.org/10.3389/fpsyt.2019.00560

Kok, R. M., & Reynolds, C.F. (2017). Management of depression in older adults: A review. *JAMA, 317*(20), 2114–2122.

Lin, J., & Dmitrieva, J. (2019). Cultural orientation moderates the association between desired affect and depressed mood among Chinese international students living in the United States. *Emotion, 19*(2), 371–375. https://doi.org/10.1037/emo0000415

Link, K. A., Garrett-Wright, D., & Jones, M. S. (2020). The burden of farmer suicide on surviving family members: A qualitative study. *Issues in Mental Health Nursing, 41*(1), 66–72. https://doi.org/10.1080/01612840.2019.1661048

Lotfaliany, M., Bowe, S. J., Kowal, P., Orellana, L., Berk, M., & Mohebbi, M. (2018). Depression and chronic diseases: Co-occurrence and communality of risk factors. *Journal of Affective Disorders, 241*, 461–468. https://doi.org/10.1016/j.jad.2018.08.011

Mitchell, A. M., Kane, I., Kameg, K. M., Stark, K. H., & Kameg, B. (2017). Integrated management of self-directed injury. In K. R. Tusaie & J. J. Fitzpatrick (Eds.), *Advanced practice psychiatric nursing: Integrating psychotherapy, psychopharmacology, and complementary and alternative approaches* (2nd ed., pp. 443–471). Springer Publishing Company.

Ngo, H., VanderLaan, D. P., & Aitken, M. (2020). Self-esteem, symptom severity, and treatment response in adolescents with internalizing problems. *Journal of Affective Disorders, 273*, 183–191. https://doi.org/10.1016/j.jad.2020.04.045

Ohrnberger, J., Fichera, E., & Sutton, M. (2017). The relationship between physical and mental health: A mediation analysis. *Social Sciences & Medicine, 195*, 42–49.

Pedersen, C. A., Lonner, W. J., Draguus, J. G., Trimble, J. E., Scharrón-del Río, M.R. (Eds.) (2016). *Counseling across cultures* (7th ed.). Sage Publishing.

Roosenschoon, B. J., Kamperman, A. M., Deen, M. L., Weeghel, J. V., & Mulder, C. L. (2019). Determinants of clinical, functional and personal recovery for people with schizophrenia and other severe mental illnesses: A cross-sectional analysis. *PLoS One, 14*(9), e0222378. https://doi.org/10.1371/journal.pone.0222378

Schatzberg, A. F., & DeBattista, C. (2019). *Manual of clinical psychopharmacology* (9th ed.). American Psychiatric Publishing.

Sehatzadeh, S., Daskalakis, Z. J., Yap, B., Tu, H. A., Palimaka, S., Bowen, J. M., & O'Reilly, D. J. (2019). Unilateral and bilateral repetitive transcranial magnetic stimulation for treatment-resistant depression: A meta-analysis of randomized controlled trials over 2 decades. *Journal of Psychiatry & Neuroscience, 44*(2), 1–13.

Smigelsky, M. A., Jardin, C., Nieuwsma, J. A., Brancu, M., Meador, K. G., Molloy, K. G., VA Mid-Atlantic MIRECC Workgroup, & Elbogen, E. B. (2020). Religion, spirituality, and suicide risk in Iraq and Afghanistan era veterans. *Depression and Anxiety, 37*(8), 728–737. https://doi.org/10.1002/da.23013

Tolliver, B. K., & Anton, R. F. (2015). Assessment and treatment of mood disorders in the context of substance abuse. *Dialogues in Clinical Neuroscience, 17*(2), 181–190.

Tuithof, M., Ten Have, M., van Dorsselaer, S., Kleinjan, M., Beekman, A., & de Graaf, R. (2018). Course of subthreshold depression into a depressive disorder and its risk factors. *Journal of Affective Disorders, 241*, 206–215. https://doi.org/10.1016/j.jad.2018.08.010

Tyson, R. L., Brammer, S., & McIntosh, D. (2019). Telehealth in psychiatric educations: Lessons from the field. *Journal of the American Psychiatric Nurses Association, 25*(4), 266–271.

Uhlenbusch, N., Löwe, B., Härter, M., Schramm, C., Weiler-Normann, C., & Depping, M. K. (2019). Depression and anxiety in patients with different rare chronic diseases: A cross-sectional study. *PLoS One, 14*(2), e0211343. https://doi.org/10.1371/journal.pone.0211343

Warren, B. J. (2020). The synergistic influence of life experiences and cultural nuances on development of depression: A cognitive behavioral perspective. *Issues in Mental Health Nursing, 41*(1), 3–6.

World Health Organization (WHO). (2019). Evidence-based recommendations for management of depression in non-specialized health settings. Retrieved February 20, 2019, from http://www.who.int/mental_health/mhgap/evidence/depression/en/index.html

Zis, P., Daskalaki, A., Bountouni, I., Sykioti, P., Varrassi, G., & Paladini, A. (2017). Depression and chronic pain in the elderly: Links and management challenges. *Clinical Interventions in Aging, 12*, 709–720. https://doi.org/10.2147/CIA.S113576

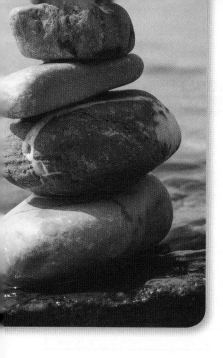

26
Bipolar Disorders
Nursing Care of Persons with Mood Lability

Mary Ann Boyd

KEYCONCEPTS

- mania
- mood lability

LEARNING OBJECTIVES

After studying this chapter, you will be able to:

1. Discuss the role of mania and mood lability in mental disorders.

2. Delineate the clinical symptoms and course of bipolar disorder.

3. Analyze the theories of bipolar disorder and their relationship to mood lability.

4. Develop strategies to establish a patient-centered, recovery-oriented therapeutic relationship with a person with bipolar disorder.

5. Apply a person-centered, recovery-oriented nursing process for persons with bipolar disorder.

6. Identify medications used to treat people with bipolar disorder and evaluate their effectiveness.

7. Develop wellness strategies for persons with bipolar disorder.

8. Differentiate the type of mental health care provided in emergency care, inpatient-focused care, community care, and virtual mental health care.

9. Discuss the importance of integrated health care for persons with bipolar disorder.

10. Describe other other bipolar and related disorders.

KEY TERMS

- Bipolar I disorder • Bipolar II disorder • Cyclothymic disorder • Elation • Elevated mood • Euphoria • Expansive mood • Grandiosity • Hypomania • Mania • Mood lability • Rapid cycling • Social rhythms

Case Study

Christine is a 34-year-old female who has a history of bipolar I disorder. She is brought to the emergency room by the police from the airport, where she was demanding a plane ticket to Hawaii. She became very belligerent when she did not get her ticket. She is wearing an evening dress with several pieces of expensive jewelry. How would you document Christine's behavior and appearance? Was her belligerent behavior at the airport excessive considering the circumstances? How would you support her?

INTRODUCTION

Everyone has ups and downs. Mood changes are a part of everyday life; expression of feeling is integral to communication. But when moods are so pervasive that they cloud reasoning and judgment, they become problematic and interfere with interpersonal relationships. In some instances, extreme moods such as mania are symptoms of mental disorders. This chapter discusses bipolar disorders that are characterized by severe mood changes, with bipolar I disorder highlighted.

MANIA

Mania is one of the primary symptoms of bipolar disorders. It is recognized by an elevated, expansive, or irritable mood. Mania is easily recognized by the cognitive changes that occur. Elevated self-esteem is expressed as **grandiosity** (exaggerating personal importance) and may range from unusual self-confidence to grandiose delusions. Speech is pressured (push of speech); the person is more talkative than usual and at times is difficult to interrupt. There is often a flight of ideas (illogical connections between thoughts) or racing thoughts. Distractibility increases.

> **KEYCONCEPT Mania** is primarily characterized by an abnormally and persistently elevated, expansive, or irritable mood.

In mania, the need for sleep is decreased and energy is increased. The individual often remains awake for long periods or wakes up several times at night full of energy. Initially, there is an increase in goal-directed activity that is purposeful (e.g., cleaning the house), but it deteriorates into hyperactivity, agitation, and disorganized behavior. Social activities, occupational functioning, and interpersonal relationships are eventually impaired. There can be excessive involvement in pleasurable activities with little regard for painful consequences (e.g., excessive spending, risky sexual behavior, drug or alcohol abuse) (Box 26.1). Persons with mania are often hospitalized to prevent self-harm.

Even though mania is primarily associated with bipolar disorders, other psychiatric disorders, including schizophrenia, schizoaffective disorder, anxiety disorders, some personality disorders (borderline personality disorder and histrionic personality disorder), substance abuse involving stimulants, and adolescent conduct disorders, may have symptoms that mimic a manic episode. Mania can also be caused by medical disorders or their treatments, certain metabolic abnormalities, neurologic disorders, central nervous system (CNS) tumors, and medications.

BOX 26.1 CLINICAL VIGNETTE

The Patient With Mania

George was a day trader on the stock market. Initially, he was quite successful and, as a result, upgraded his lifestyle with a more expensive car; a larger, more luxurious house; and a boat. When the stock market declined dramatically, George continued to trade, saying that if he could just find the "right" stock he could earn back all of the money he had lost. He spent his days and nights in front of his computer screen, taking little or no time to eat or sleep. He defaulted on his mortgage and car and boat payments and was talking nonstop to his wife. She brought him to the hospital for evaluation.

What Do You Think?
- What behavioral symptoms of mania does George exhibit?
- What cognitive symptoms of mania does George exhibit?

Mood lability is the term used for the rapid shifts in moods that often occur in bipolar disorder. One month a person is happy, and the next month they are in the depths of depression. These mood shifts leave everyone around the person confused and interfere with social interaction.

> **KEYCONCEPT Mood lability** is alterations in moods with little or no change in external events.

Rapid cycling is an extreme form of mood lability that can occur in bipolar disorders. In its most severe form, rapid cycling includes continuous cycling between subthreshold mania and depression or **hypomania** and depression.

BIPOLAR DISORDERS OVERVIEW

Bipolar and related disorders are characterized by periods of mania or hypomania that alternate with depression. These disorders are further classified as bipolar I, bipolar II, and cyclothymic disorders, depending on the severity of the manic and depressive symptoms. Bipolar disorder may also be related to substance abuse, prescription use, or a medical condition.

BIPOLAR I DISORDER

Bipolar I disorder is the classic manic-depressive disorder with mood swings alternating from depressed to manic. Although the depression component is similar to that experienced in a major depressive disorder, in this disorder there is also a distinct period (of at least 1 week or less if hospitalized) of abnormally and persistently elevated, expansive, or irritable mood with abnormally increased goal-directed behavior or energy (American

Psychiatric Association [APA], 2013). An **elevated mood** can be expressed as **euphoria** (exaggerated feelings of well-being) or **elation** (feeling "high," "ecstatic," "on top of the world," or "up in the clouds"). An **expansive mood** is characterized by lack of restraint in expressing feelings; an overvalued sense of self-importance; and a constant and indiscriminate enthusiasm for interpersonal, sexual, or occupational interactions.

For some people, an irritable mood instead of an elevated mood is pervasive during mania. Such individuals are easily annoyed and provoked to anger, particularly when their wishes are challenged or thwarted. Maintaining social relationships during these episodes is difficult.

> ### Consider Christine
> When Christine is brought to the hospital, she is experiencing grandiose delusions. She believes that she is starting a business. She has spent a large amount of money over a short period of time on clothes and jewelry. Her neighbors reported that she was selling household goods in her yard. Her mood is labile. She is loud and condescending toward staff members. She has push of speech and flight of ideas. What behaviors are characteristic of bipolar disorder?

Clinical Course

Bipolar I disorder is a chronic multisystemic cyclic disorder. Those with an earlier onset have more frequent episodes than persons who develop the illness later in life. Bipolar disorder is a progressive condition with prodromal, symptomatic, and residual states. The progressive nature of this disorder can be arrested with an early diagnosis, proper treatment, and individually tailored management (Muneer & Mazommil, 2018). An early onset and a family history of illness are associated with multiple episodes or continuous symptoms. Symptoms of the illness can be unpredictable and variable. Bipolar I disorder can lead to severe functional impairment, such as alienation from family, friends, and coworkers; indebtedness; job loss; divorce; and other problems of living (Dell'Osso et al., 2020).

Diagnostic Criteria

To be diagnosed with bipolar I disorder, at least one manic episode or mixed episode and a depressive episode have to occur. See Key Diagnostic Characteristics 26.1. The term *mixed episode* is used when mania and depression occur at the same time, which leads to extreme

anxiety, agitation, and irritability. These individuals are clearly miserable and are at high risk for suicide.

Bipolar I Disorder Across the Life Span

Children and Adolescents

Only recently has bipolar disorder been recognized in children. Although it has not been well studied, depression usually appears first. Somewhat different than in adults, the hallmark of childhood bipolar disorder is intense rage. Children may display seemingly unprovoked rage episodes for as long as 2 to 3 hours. The symptoms of bipolar disorder reflect the developmental level of the child. Children younger than 9 years exhibit more irritability and emotional lability; older children exhibit more classic symptoms, such as euphoria and grandiosity. The first contact with the mental health system often occurs when the behavior becomes disruptive, possibly 5 to 10 years after its onset. These children often have other psychiatric disorders, such as attention-deficit hyperactivity disorder or conduct disorder (Arnold et al., 2020). See Chapter 36.

Older Adults

The onset of bipolar disorder can also occur in older adults. Symptoms are similar to the earlier onset bipolar disorder, but the incidence of mania decreases with age. Older adults with bipolar disorder have more neurologic abnormalities and cognitive disturbances (confusion and disorientation) than younger patients (Dols & Beekman, 2020). See Chapter 39.

Epidemiology and Risk Factors

Risk factors for bipolar disorders include a family history of mood disorders, prior mood episodes, lack of social support, stressful life events, substance use, and medical problems, particularly chronic or terminal illnesses (Faedda et al., 2019).

Age of Onset

Bipolar disorders have an estimated prevalence of 1% to 4% (Loftus, et al., 2020). The onset of the majority of cases occurs in early life, from the ages of 14 to 21 years, with fewer cases occurring after 40 years of age (Bolton et al., 2020).

Gender

Although no significant gender differences have been found in the incidence of bipolar I and bipolar II

KEY CHARACTERISTICS 26.1 • BIPOLAR I DISORDER 296.XX

296.4X—BIPOLAR I, CURRENT OR MOST RECENT EPISODE MANIC
296.4X—BIPOLAR I, CURRENT OR MOST RECENT EPISODE HYPOMANIC
296.4X—BIPOLAR I, CURRENT OR MOST RECENT EPISODE DEPRESSED

Diagnostic Criteria

The essential feature of a manic episode is a distinct period during which there is an abnormally, persistently elevated, expansive, or irritable mood and persistently increased activity or energy that is present for most of the day, nearly every day, for a period of at least 1 week (or any duration if hospitalization is necessary), accompanied by at least three additional symptoms from Criterion B. If the mood is irritable rather than elevated or expansive, at least four Criterion B symptoms must be present.

Manic Episode

A. A distinct period of abnormally and persistently elevated, expansive, or irritable mood and abnormally and persistently increased goal-directed activity or energy, lasting at least 1 week and present most of the day, nearly every day (or any duration if hospitalization is necessary).
B. During the period of mood disturbance and increased energy or activity, three (or more) of the following symptoms (four if the mood is only irritable) are pres-

ent to a significant degree and represent a noticeable change from usual behavior:
1. Inflated self-esteem or grandiosity
2. Decreased need for sleep (e.g., feels rested after only 3 hours of sleep)
3. More talkative than usual or pressure to keep talking
4. Flight of ideas or subjective experience that thoughts are racing
5. Distractibility (i.e., attention too easily drawn to unimportant or irrelevant external stimuli), as reported or observed
6. Increase in goal-directed activity (either socially, at work or school, or sexually) or psychomotor agitation (i.e., purposeless non–goal-directed activity)
7. Excessive involvement in activities that have a high potential for painful consequences (e.g., engaging in unrestrained buying sprees, sexual indiscretions, or foolish business investments)

Reprinted with permission from the *Diagnostic and Statistical Manual of Mental Disorders*, Fifth Edition (Copyright © 2013). American Psychiatric Association. All Rights Reserved.

---

disorder diagnoses, gender differences have been reported in phenomenology, course, and treatment response. In addition, some data show that female patients with bipolar disorder are at greater risk for depression and mixed episodes than are male patients, but male patients may be at greater risk for manic episodes (Fellinger et al., 2019).

Ethnicity and Culture

Although there is a general belief that no significant racial and ethnic differences related to bipolar disorder exist, most of the research is based on White individuals who have not experienced a disparity in access to health care. A lack of representation from ethnic/racial groups makes it difficult to determine the impact of race and ethnicity on the morbidity of people with bipolar disorder. Also, African American individuals with bipolar disorder are more likely to be misdiagnosed as having schizophrenia, schizoaffective, or major depressive disorders, and older African American individuals are more likely to use general medical services for treatment than mental health services (Akinhanmi et al., 2018, 2020).

Comorbidity

The two most common comorbid mental health conditions are anxiety disorders (panic disorder and social

phobia are the most prevalent) and substance use (most commonly alcohol and marijuana). Individuals with a comorbid anxiety disorder are more likely to experience a more severe course. A history of substance use further complicates the course of illness and results in less chance for remission and poorer treatment compliance (Loftus et al., 2020; Spoorthy et al., 2019). Bipolar disorder is associated with several medical conditions, such as irritable bowel syndrome, asthma, migraine, multiple sclerosis, and cerebellar diseases (Flowers et al., 2020; Sinha, et al., 2018).

Etiology

The etiology of mood disorders is unknown, but the current thinking is that bipolar disorder results when an interaction exists between the genetic predisposition and psychosocial stress, such as abuse or trauma (Carvalho et al., 2020).

Biologic Theories

Chronobiologic Theories

Sleep disturbance is common in individuals with bipolar disorder, especially mania. Sleep patterns appear to be regulated by an internal biologic clock center in the hypothalamus. Artificially induced sleep deprivation is known to precipitate mania in some patients with bipolar disorder. It is possible that circadian dysregulation underlies the sleep–wake disturbances of bipolar disorder. Seasonal changes in light exposure also trigger affective episodes in some patients, typically depression in winter and hypomania in the summer in the northern hemisphere (Rosenthal et al., 2020).

Genetic Factors

Results from family, adoption, and twin studies indicate that bipolar disorder is highly heritable. Studies of monozygotic twins show risks from 40% to 70% of acquiring the illness if their identical twin has the disorder (Johansson et al., 2019). No one gene or sequence of genes is responsible for the pathology of bipolar disorder. Evidence suggests that the genetic etiologies of schizophrenia and bipolar disorders overlap (Smeland et al., 2020).

Chronic Stress, Inflammation, and Kindling

The role of an allostatic load or wear and tear on the body (see Chapter 19) is thought to contribute to cognitive impairment, comorbidity, and eventual mortality of those with bipolar disorder. As the allostatic load increases, the number of mood episodes increases, which, in turn, increases physical and mental health problems. An interaction between stress and brain development is viewed as dynamic; individuals have different kinds of stress adaptation depending on their neurobiologic responses (Dargél et al., 2020).

The characteristic mood dysregulation of bipolar I disorder is associated with a decrease in serum brain-derived neurotrophic factor, oxidative stress resulting in DNA damage, and inflammation. Pro-inflammatory cytokines bind to neuronal death receptors, leading to cell death. In some patients with repeated episodes, there is a decrease in hippocampal volume and reduction in prefrontal grey matter (Muneer, 2020).

A closely related concept is the kindling theory that posits that as genetically predisposed individuals experience repetitive subthreshold stressors at vulnerable times, mood symptoms of increasing intensity and duration occur. Eventually, a full-blown depressive or manic episode erupts. Each episode leaves a trace and increases the person's vulnerability or sensitizes the person to have another episode with less stimulation. In later episodes, there may be little or no stress occurring before the depression or mania. The disorder takes on a life of its own, and over time, the time between episodes decreases (Carvalho et al., 2020).

Psychosocial Theories

Psychosocial theories are useful in planning recovery-oriented interventions that focus on reducing

environmental stress and trauma in genetically vulnerable individuals. It is now generally accepted that psychosocial and environmental events contribute to the severity of the disorder and the frequency of the mood episodes. Two promising theories are currently receiving research support.

The *behavioral approach system dysregulation* theory proposes that individuals with bipolar disorder are overly sensitive and overreact to relevant cues when approaching a reward. That is, the intensity of the goal-motivated behavior leads to manic symptoms such as euphoria, decreased need for sleep, and excessive self-confidence. Conversely, the system is deactivated and leads to depressive symptoms such as decreased energy, hopelessness, and sadness (Arfaie et al., 2018).

The *social rhythm disruption theory* is consistent with the research on circadian rhythm dysregulation previously discussed. According to this theory, there are environmental factors that set the circadian clock, such as the rising and setting of the sun. There are also social cues or **social rhythms** that can set the circadian clock, such as the time we get out of bed, our first contact in the morning (person), when we start our day, have dinner, and go to bed. These are patterned social events. Individuals with bipolar disorder have fewer regular social rhythms than those without bipolar disorder. This theory suggests that when patterned social events are disrupted, mood swings are more likely to appear (Crowe & Inder, 2018).

Family Response to Disorder

Bipolar disorder can devastate families, who often feel that they are on an emotional merry-go-round, particularly if they have difficulty understanding the mood shifts. A major problem for family members is dealing with the consequences of impulsive behavior during manic episodes, such as taking on excessive debt, assault charges, and sexual infidelities.

Remember Christine?

She has been married for 2 years to Karl, who was unaware of her bipolar disorder. He believed that she used to take antidepressants but that she no longer needed them. Her episode at the airport occurred when he was out of town. He is concerned about her health and their new financial obligations. How do you explain that Karl was unaware of Christine's illness? How would you explain Christine's illness to her husband?

RECOVERY-ORIENTED CARE FOR PERSONS WITH BIPOLAR DISORDER

Teamwork and Collaboration: Working Toward Recovery

An important recovery goal is to minimize or prevent both manic and depressive episodes, which tend to accelerate over time. The fewer the episodes, the more likely the person can live a fully productive life. Three interconnected pathways can lead to relapse: stressful life events, medication nonadherence, and disruption in social rhythms (Crowe et al., 2016). Patients with bipolar disorder have a complex set of issues and have the best chance of recovery by working with an interdisciplinary team. Nurses, physicians, social workers, psychologists, and activity therapists all have valuable expertise. For children with bipolar disorder, schoolteachers and counselors are included in the team. For older adult patients, the primary care physician becomes part of the team. Helping the patient and family learn about the disorder and manage it throughout a lifetime is critical for recovery.

The primary treatment modalities are medications, psychotherapy, education, and support. Mood stabilizers and antipsychotics are the mainstay medications in the treatment of bipolar disorders. Mood stabilizers are discussed later in this chapter. Antipsychotics are discussed in Chapter 24. Long-term psychotherapy may help prevent symptoms by reducing the stresses that trigger episodes and increasing the patient's acceptance of the need for medication. Patients should be encouraged to keep their appointments with the therapist, be honest and open, do the assigned homework, and give the therapist feedback on whether the treatment is effective.

Safety Issues

Risk of suicide is always present for those having a depressive or manic episode (Ballard et al., 2020). During a depressive episode, the patient may believe that life is not worth living. During a manic episode, the patient may believe that they have supernatural powers, such as the ability to fly.

During a manic episode, poor judgment and impulsivity lead to risk-taking behaviors that can have dire consequences for the patient and family. For example, when one patient gambled all of his family's money away, he blamed his partner for letting him have access to the money. A physical confrontation with the partner resulted.

As patients recover from a manic episode, they may be so devastated by the consequences of their impulsive behavior and poor judgment that suicide seems like the only option.

Consider This:

Consider Christine's history of poor judgment during a manic episode. She left her first husband and their two children during her third manic episode. At that time, Christine went to Hawaii and stayed there for several months without informing her family of her whereabouts. She was homeless most of the time. Once Christine is stable, what interventions will support long-term remission of bipolar disorder?

EVIDENCE-BASED NURSING CARE OF PERSONS WITH BIPOLAR DISORDER

The nursing care of patients with a bipolar disorder is one of the most interesting yet greatest challenges in psychiatric nursing. In general, the behavior of patients with bipolar disorder is normal between mood episodes. The nurse's first contact with the patient is usually during a manic or depressive episode. See Nursing Care Plan 26.1.

Mental Health Nursing Assessment

Recovery-oriented nursing care begins with the initial assessment through engaging the patient in a partnership and empowering the person to make decisions in setting overall goals of care (Box 26.2). During acute episodes, the patient's judgment may be impaired, but as the manic or depressive symptoms subside, the person will be able to participate in care decisions.

Physical Health

The physical health assessment should follow the process explained in Chapter 11. Target assessment symptoms include the changes and severity of activity, eating, and sleep patterns. The patient may not sleep, resulting in irritability and physical exhaustion. Diet and body weight usually change during a manic or depressive episode. Laboratory studies, such as thyroid function and electrolytes, should be completed to detect evidence of malnutrition and fluid imbalance. Abnormal thyroid functioning can be responsible for the mood and behavioral disturbances. In mania, patients often become hypersexual and engage in risky sexual practices. Changes in sexual practices should be included in the assessment.

A careful assessment of current medications is important in determining physical status. Many times,

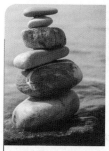

NURSING CARE PLAN 26.1

The Patient with Bipolar I Disorder

Christine, a 34-year-old woman, is admitted involuntarily to the inpatient unit, following an altercation at the airport when she became loud and belligerent and caused a ruckus. She believes that she has special powers over others and has a direct connection to God. She stated she needed to leave town because of the "three men" in her house, who are chasing her. She is accompanied by her mother and husband, Karl. She believes that she is being taken to a safe place, which can protect her from the men who were chasing her.

Her mother stated that Christine was first diagnosed with bipolar disorder at age 22 after her first child was born. She received treatment for 2 years. After her second pregnancy, she refused to take her medication. During her third manic episode, she left her husband and children. She was reunited with her parents 4 years later and reinitiated treatment. After her marriage to Karl, she stopped her medication. Karl believed that Christine had a history of depression but did not realize that she has bipolar disorder. He wants to be supportive and help her.

Setting: Intensive Care Psychiatric Unit in a General Hospital

Baseline Assessment: A 34-year-old woman who is flamboyantly dressed in a cocktail dress with several pieces of expensive jewelry. She is oriented to time, place, and person, but she believes she has special powers. She states that she is "not suicidal—I have a mission." She is displaying push of speech and flight of ideas. She is hyperverbal and hyperactive. It is difficult to interrupt her thoughts. She states she has not slept for several days and does not need to sleep because she is gifted. She is not taking any medications and denies substance use except for an occasional marijuana joint. She admits to taking mood stabilizers in the past but states that they made her gain weight. She does not want to take that medication again. BP 130/70, P 70, R 18, Ht. 5'5', Wt 125 (BMI 20.8).

Associated Psychiatric Diagnosis	Medications
Bipolar I disorder	Ziprasidone (Geodon) 40 mg PO BID (Give with a full meal) Lorazepam 1 mg PO q4h as needed for anxiety or agitation

Priority of Care: Lack of Problem-Solving Ability

Important Characteristics	Associated Considerations
Denial of problems obvious to others Projection of blame or responsibility for problems	Biochemical/neurophysiologic imbalance

Outcomes

Initial	Discharge
1. Increase problem-solving ability	4. Agree to continue medication and follow-up
2. Identify factors that led to current manic episode	5. Attend support group
3. Accept treatment of bipolar disorder	

Interventions

Interventions	Rationale	Ongoing Assessment
Initiate a nurse–patient relationship by demonstrating an acceptance of Christine as a worthwhile human being through the use of nonjudgmental statements and behavior Administer ziprasidone 40 mg BID per health care provider order	The positive therapeutic relationship can maintain the patient's dignity and open communication	Assess the stages of the relationship, and determine whether a therapeutic relationship is actually being formed. Identify indicators of trust

Continued

Nursing Care Plan 26.1 Continued

(Christine refused mood stabilizers because of side effects.) Teach Christine the therapeutic and side effects of medication Instruct her to take medication with a full meal	Most new antipsychotics are indicated for mood disorders. Best absorption of ziprasidone occurs when taken with a full meal	Determine effectiveness of medication. Observe for side effects

Evaluation

Outcomes	Revised Outcomes	Interventions
Increased ability to problemsolve Is dressing appropriately for situation Taking medication as prescribed after discharge Considering attending support groups	Take medication as prescribed	Continue to encourage Christine to attend support groups

Priority of Care: Unable to Cope with Life Stressors

Important Characteristics	Associated Considerations
Asking for help Reported difficulty with life stressors Inability to problem solve Insufficient access to social support Destructive behavior toward self Frequent illnesses Substance abuse	Altered mood (mania) caused by changes secondary to body chemistry (bipolar disorder) Sensory overload secondary to excessive activity

Outcomes

Initial	Discharge
1. Accept support through the nurse–patient relationship 2. Identify areas of ineffective coping 3. Examine the current efforts at coping 4. Identify areas of strength 5. Learn new coping skills	6. Practice new coping skills 7. Focus on strengths

Interventions

Interventions	Rationale	Ongoing Assessment
Identify the current stresses in Christine's life, including bipolar disorder	When areas of concern are verbalized by the patient, she will be able to focus on one issue at a time. If she identifies the mental disorder as a stressor, she will more likely be able to develop strategies to deal with it	Determine whether Christine is able to identify problem areas realistically. Continue to assess for suicidality
Identify Christine's strengths in dealing with past stressors	By focusing on past successes, she can identify strengths and build on them in the future	Assess whether Christine can identify any previous successes in her life
Assist Christine in discussing, selecting, and practicing positive coping skills (e.g., jogging, yoga, thought stopping)	New coping skills take a conscious effort to learn and will at first seem strange and unnatural. Practicing these skills will help the patient incorporate them into her coping strategy repertoire	Assess whether Christine follows through on learning new skills

Continued

Nursing Care Plan 26.1 Continued

Assist patient in coping with bipolar disorder, beginning with education about it	A mood disorder is a major stressor in a patient's life. To manage the stress, the patient needs a knowledge base	Determine Christine's knowledge about bipolar disorder
Administer lorazepam as needed for anxiety or agitation	Benzodiazepine helps decrease anxiety and calm the patient	Assess for target action, side effects, and toxicity

Evaluation

Outcomes	Revised Outcomes	Interventions
Christine is easily engaged in a therapeutic relationship. She examined the areas in her life where she coped ineffectively	Establish a therapeutic relationship with a therapist at the mental health clinic	Refer to mental health clinic
She identified her strengths and how she coped with stressors and especially her illness in the past. She is willing to try medications again, in hopes of not gaining weight	Continue to view illness as a potential stressor that can disrupt life	Seek advice immediately if there are any problems with medications
She learned new problem-solving skills and reported that she learned a lot about her medication. She is committed to complying with her medication regimen. She identified new coping skills that she could realistically do. She will focus on strengths	Continue to practice new coping skills as stressful situations arise	Discuss with therapist the outcomes of using new coping skills. Attend bipolar support group

---

BOX 26.2

Research for Evidence-Based Practice: Promoting Personal Recovery

Crowe, M & Inder, M. (2018). Staying well with bipolar disorder: A qualitative analysis of five-year follow-up interviews with young people. Journal of Psychiatric and Mental Health Nursing, 25(4), 236–244. https://doi.org/10.1111/jpm.12455

THE QUESTION: How do participants in psychotherapy for young people with bipolar disorder describe their experiences of the intervention and its impact on living with the disorder?

METHODS: A qualitative study was conducted 5 years after participants had completed a psychotherapy intervention in a randomized controlled trial for young people with bipolar disorder. Thirty people were recruited and interviewed regarding their experiences.

FINDINGS: Three themes were identified: self-awareness in the context of bipolar disorder, understanding bipolar disorder, and learning to stay well with bipolar disorder.

IMPLICATIONS FOR NURSING: Nurses can promote factors recognized by their patients as being helpful in learning to stay well, including self-awareness, understanding the unique characteristics of their disorder, learning to take care of the self, and stabilization of social rhythms.

manic or depressive episodes occur after patients stop taking their medication. Exploring reasons for discontinuing the medication will help in planning adherence strategies in the future. Some stop taking their medications because of side effects; others do not believe they have a mental disorder. The use of alcohol and other substances should be carefully assessed. Usually, a drug screen is ordered. In some instances, patients have been taking an antidepressant as prescribed for depression without realizing that a bipolar disorder existed.

Psychosocial Assessment

The psychosocial assessment should follow the process explained in Chapter 11. Individuals with bipolar disorder can usually participate fully in this part of the assessment.

Mental Status and Appearance

Mood

By definition, bipolar disorder is a disturbance of mood. If the patient is depressed, using an assessment tool for depression may help determine the severity of depression. If mania predominates, evaluating the quality of the mood (e.g., elated, grandiose, irritated, or agitated) becomes important. Usually, mania is diagnosed by clinical observation.

Cognition

In a depressive episode, an individual may not be able to concentrate enough to complete cognitive tasks,

BOX 26.3 CLINICAL VIGNETTE

The Personal Experience of Mania

Sam is a 35-year-old man who was diagnosed with bipolar disorder 10 years ago. He is now being successfully treated and has insight into his disorder. In a recent discussion with his close friend, he describes his personal experience of mania.

At first, I started having more energy and felt happy most of the time. I decided to date a couple of women because I thought my girlfriend Jill was rather boring. Within a couple of weeks, I started sleeping less, but I thought that meant I could do more things. I decided to go back to school to be a scientist—thought I could save the world. I started to apply to graduate school and became very upset when I was told that I did not have the prerequisites for biochemistry. I was so mad that I started threatening the admissions counselor, who, in turn, called the police. My family was called. They convinced the police that I would not bother the school again. After that, I started drinking and smoking pot. I had periods of confusion, and my family said I became disoriented. There is a lot I don't remember. Eventually, I was hospitalized and started on medication.

What Do You Think?

• At what point could have an early intervention prevented Sam from progressing to a major manic episode?
• Why does Sam not remember the complete manic episode?

such as those called for in a mental status assessment. During the acute phase of a manic or depressive episode, mental status may be abnormal, and in a manic phase, judgment is impaired by extremely rapid, disjointed, and distorted thinking. Moreover, feelings such as grandiosity can interfere with executive functioning. See Box 26.3.

Thought Disturbances

Psychosis commonly occurs in patients with bipolar disorder, especially during acute episodes of mania. Auditory hallucinations and delusional thinking are part of the clinical picture. In children and adolescents, however, psychosis is not so easily disclosed.

Behavioral Responses

Behavior varies according to mood. In periods of mania and poor judgment, there may be episodes of uncharacteristic behaviors such as excessive spending, impulsive gambling, or sexual activities. Behaviors during a manic episode can lead to life-long relationships or legal problems. During periods of depression, remorse for the consequences of poor judgment and behavior contributes to the negative mood state. See Chapter 25.

Self-Concept

The self-concept of an individual with bipolar disorder is generally consistent with others who have stigmatized mental disorders. Even though bipolar disorder is less stigmatized than schizophrenia, the behaviors that are characteristic of persons with these disorders are often not recognized as symptoms of a disorder, but as a character flaw. Consequently, even in periods of mania, self-esteem is severely impaired.

Stress and Coping Patterns

Stress and coping are critical assessment areas for a person with bipolar disorder. A stressful event often triggers a manic or depressive episode. In some instances, no particular stressors preceded the episode, although it is important to discuss the possibility. Determining the patient's usual coping skills for stresses lays the groundwork for developing interventional strategies. Negative coping skills, such as substance use or aggression, should be identified because these skills should be replaced with positive coping skills.

Social Network

Cultural views of mental illness influence the patient's acceptance of the disorder. During illness episodes, patients often behave in ways that jeopardize their social relationships. Losing a job and going through a divorce are common events. When performing an assessment of social function, the nurse should identify changes resulting from a manic or depressive episode.

Functional Status

Symptoms of bipolar disorder can interfere with daily functioning. Sleep, nutrition, and hygiene often suffer during manic or depressive episodes. The individuals are often unable to maintain normal functioning and activities of daily living.

Support Systems

The nurse should assess the available support systems. Individuals who have had been symptomatic may have destroyed their support networks as a result of the depressive or manic behavior. The nurse should determine if there are any positive support systems that can help the person toward recovery.

Risk Assessment

Persons with bipolar disorder are at high risk for injury to themselves and others, with 23% to 26% attempting suicide. People with bipolar disorder account for 3.4% to 14% of all suicide deaths, with self-poisoning and hanging being the most common methods (Schaffer et al., 2015). Child abuse, spouse abuse, or other violent behaviors may occur during severe manic or depressive episodes; thus, patients should be assessed for suicidal or homicidal risk. In addition, they are at high risk for comorbid mental disorders, such as substance abuse and anxiety disorders. Significant risks for cardiovascular and metabolic diseases are found in this group (Grover et al. 2020). Smoking is also a major health hazard (Smith et al., 2020).

Several risk factors associated with bipolar disorders make patients more vulnerable to relapses and resistant to recovery. Among these are high rates of nonadherence to medication therapy, obesity, marital conflict, separation, divorce, unemployment, and underemployment. Even those who take their medication regularly are likely to experience recurrences and may have difficulty keeping jobs and maintaining significant relationships

Social and Occupational Functioning

One of the tragedies of bipolar disorder is its effect on social and occupational functioning. Individuals with this disorder are often employed, but when unrecognized symptoms erupt, their job is often jeopardized. Manifestations of their symptoms often result in being excluded from social and occupational groups.

Quality of Life

The quality of life for someone with bipolar disorder depends upon their ability to manage their symptoms, maintain meaningful employment, and engage in relationships. Some individuals are able to manage their symptoms, adhere to a treatment plan, and live productive lives. Others struggle with symptoms that interfere with their ability to work and maintain meaningful, supportive relationships.

Strength Assessment

The nurse should always be listening for thoughts, feelings, or behaviors that could be identified as strengths. For example, one patient recognized an increase in drinking alcohol as a sign that he was beginning a manic episode and made an appointment with a health care provider. The following questions may be used to determine a person's strength.

- What healthy behaviors do you routinely practice?
- Are there any cues that a manic or depressive episode will occur?
- Who provides emotional support to you?
- What do you do to relax? Manage stress?

- What makes you feel good when you are on medication?
- How do you remember to take your medications?

CLINICAL JUDGMENT

The priority of nursing care is always patient safety. Is the patient likely to self-injure or hurt another person? See Chapter 20. After the patient's safety is established, the nurse analyzes the assessment data for other priorities. For example, sleep deprivation, inadequate nutrition, and dehydration may be imminent needs. The person may be depressed or manic and unable to function socially. The person's coping skills may not be effective, and the person's job may be in jeopardy.

THERAPEUTIC RELATIONSHIP

Interacting with a person with mania is interesting and, at times, exhausting. The individual often quickly jumps from subject to subject and is usually unable to sit still. When in a manic state, the individual can be very engaging and intense. Their stories may be very grandiose. The nurse should acknowledge the verbal content but recognize that many of the thoughts, feelings, and behaviors are symptomatic of mania and then try to re-focus the patient. If a person is in a depressive state, the nurse should use the same approach as when caring for a person with a depressed disorder as discussed in Chapter 25.

People with mania are typically impatient with others and may express irritability at someone's perceived incompetence and lack of understanding of their special powers. When interacting with a person with bipolar disorder, the nurse should remain calm and avoid any arguments. This is not the time to confront the person about their unrealistic perceptions of their status. For example, one agitated person was convinced that he owned a hotel. The nurse acknowledged how difficult it must be to have such responsibilities. He agreed with her and subsequently became less agitated. See Box 26.4.

BOX 26.4

Interacting with a Person with Mania

- Use a calm, nonthreatening approach.
- Be direct and use simple commands (e.g., time for lunch, let's go to group).
- Avoid open-ended sentences; redirect conversation if flight of ideas occurs; avoid confrontation and arguments.
- Limit interaction time and recognize the patient's need for space and movement.
- Do not place demands on patients that may be interpreted as excessive.

In some instances, a person who has mania cannot sit still long enough to have a meaningful interaction. The nurse can initiate a conversation while walking with the patient, but there will be times when the nurse needs to give the patient space to avoid increasing agitation.

A therapeutic relationship can actually be instrumental in preventing a relapse. When a person is in the depths of a depression or the height of mania, therapeutic interaction is critical in helping the person take steps in recovery from either the depression or mania. However, often long periods of time pass when the affected person is living comfortably with bipolar disorder and attending to other issues.

MENTAL HEALTH NURSING INTERVENTIONS

Establishing Recovery and Wellness Goals

The person with a bipolar disorder has emotional ups and downs with periods of poor judgment and erratic behavior. However, there are many periods (months to years) where there are few symptoms. The periods of stable mental health are perfect times to focus on stress reduction, illness management, and relapse prevention. During these relatively quiet periods, it is possible to establish recovery and wellness goals. Goals focus on managing the long-term illness and supporting well-being. Recovery and wellness goals are interrelated. For example, preventing relapse includes managing stress (wellness dimension) that can trigger erratic behavior (mental health goals).

Physical Care

In a state of mania, the patient's physical needs are rest, adequate hydration and nutrition, and reestablishment of physical well-being. Self-care has usually deteriorated. For a patient unable to sit long enough to eat, snacks and high-energy foods that can be eaten while moving should be provided. Consumption of alcohol should be avoided. Sleep hygiene is a priority but may not be realistic until medications have taken effect. Limiting stimuli can be helpful in decreasing agitation and promoting sleep.

NCLEXNOTE Protection of patients with mania is always a priority. Ongoing assessment should focus on irritability, fatigue, and the potential for harming self or others.

After the patient's mood stabilizes, the nurse should focus on monitoring changes in physical functioning in sleep or eating behavior and teaching patients to identify antecedents to mood episodes such as a family argument or a financial problem. Strategies for dealing with future events can then be identified. The patient can begin to problem solve the best approach for future episodes.

A regular sleep routine should be maintained if possible. High-risk times for manic episodes, such as changes in work schedule (day to night), should be avoided if possible. Patients should be encouraged to monitor the amount of their sleep each night and report decreases in sleep of longer than 1 hour per night because this may be a precursor to a manic episode.

Highlighting the recovery concept of hope will support the person who has had multiple episodes and is frustrated with the impact of several episodes (Box 26.5). In educating persons with bipolar disorder, the nonlongitudinal nature of the disorder should be emphasized.

Wellness Challenges

Many self-care interventions that prevent or delay symptoms are also wellness strategies. For example, individuals with bipolar disorder who relapse often describe a stressful life event that led to the manic episode. These individuals appear to be more sensitive to life events than people without the disorder. The emotional dimension of wellness focuses on developing skills for coping with stress. If the individuals can strengthen their coping skills, they may be able to be less sensitive to stressful life events. See Box 26.6.

Medication Interventions

Medications are essential in bipolar disorder to achieve two goals: rapid control of symptoms and prevention of future episodes or, at least, reduction in their severity and frequency.

Mood-Stabilizing Drugs

The mainstays of pharmacotherapy are the mood-stabilizing drugs, including lithium carbonate (Lithium), divalproex sodium (Depakote), carbamazepine (Tegretol), and lamotrigine (Lamictal). Antidepressant therapy is not recommended in persons with bipolar depression because of a risk of switching from depression to mania.

Lithium Carbonate

Lithium is the most widely used mood stabilizer (Box 26.7). Combined response rates from five studies demonstrate that 70% of patients experienced at least partial improvement with lithium therapy. However, for many patients, lithium is not a fully adequate treatment for all phases of the illness, and particularly during the

BOX 26.5 • THERAPEUTIC DIALOGUE: INSTILLING HOPE

 Christine is sitting in the dayroom of an inpatient unit with tears in her eyes. She acknowledges that she has bipolar disorder and wishes that she had been taking her medication and told her husband about her previous relapses.

INEFFECTIVE APPROACH

Nurse: Christine, I am glad that you realize that you have bipolar disorder and want to take your medication. You must commit to staying on your medicine, or you will lose your second husband.

Christine: No one understands what it is like to have this problem. I don't quite understand how this little pill and seeing a shrink will help.

Nurse: Well, medication and therapy will help.

Christine: You don't know what I am talking about.

EFFECTIVE APPROACH

Nurse: Christine, I hope that you are feeling better.

Christine: No one understands what it is like to have this problem. I don't quite understand how this little pill and seeing a shrink will help.

Nurse: Let's talk about it. What does it feel like to have bipolar disorder?

Christine: Sometimes it is wonderful—on top of the world, but after the mood goes away, having this problem is terrible. The bad times outweigh the good feelings.

Nurse: Other people have said the same thing. Many people decide to take their medication and "check in" with a mental health provider in order to stay on track and avoid the bad times that can happen after a manic period.

Christine: Really?

Nurse: There are many successful people with bipolar disorder who find that taking medication helps keep order in their life. I can give you information about a support group.

Christine: Ok, I'm willing to try.

Nurse: Now, what about this medication. Are you willing to try it also? This medication is an effective treatment for bipolar disorder and has helped others to control moods.

Christine: Okay, but I want to know more about this medication.

Nurse: It's a deal. We can spend some time talking about your medications after dinner.

CRITICAL THINKING CHALLENGE

• How did the nurse block communication with Christine in the first scenario? Did she seem hopeful after the interaction?

• How did the nurse instill hope in Christine in the second scenario?

BOX 26.6

Wellness Challenges

• Reducing emotional responses to daily stresses
  • Strategies: Re-frame experiences, use problem-focused coping techniques, relaxation
• Supporting positive circadian rhythms consistent with relapse prevention needs
  • Establish sleep hygiene, eating routines
• Establishing a healthy diet with reducing substance use
  • Eat at regular times, maintain a healthy diet
• Seeking pleasant environments that support well-being
  • Strategies: Seek comfortable, relaxing living arrangements, explore community resources that support people with bipolar disorder
• Satisfying current and future financial situations
  • Strategies: Seek financial counseling, protect resources during periods of relapses

• Satisfying and enriching work
  • Strategies: Select job opportunities that are consistent with health promotion activities
• Recognizing the need for physical activity, healthy foods, and sleep
  • Strategies: Encourage regular physical activity, discuss healthy diets, encourage establishing healthy sleep hygiene routines
• Developing a sense of connection, belonging, and a support system
  • Strategies: Explore expanding a positive support system
• Expanding a sense of purpose and meaning in life
  • Strategies: Focus on goals, values, and beliefs; read inspiring stories or essays

BOX 26.7

Drug Profile: Lithium Carbonate

DRUG CLASS: Mood stabilizer

RECEPTOR AFFINITY: Alters sodium transport in nerve and muscle cells, increases norepinephrine uptake and serotonin receptor sensitivity, slightly increases intraneuronal stores of catecholamines, and delays some second messenger systems. Mechanism of action is unknown.

INDICATIONS: Treatment and prevention of manic episodes in bipolar affective disorder.

ROUTES AND DOSAGE: 150-, 300-, and 600-mg capsules. Lithobid, 300-mg slow-release tablets; Eskalith CR, 450-mg controlled-release tablets; lithium citrate, 300-mg/5 mL liquid form.

Adults: In acute mania, optimal response is usually 600 mg TID or 900 mg BID. Obtain serum levels twice weekly in acute phase. Do not rely on serum levels alone. Maintenance: Use lowest possible dose to alleviate symptoms and maintain serum level of 0.6 to 1.2 mEq/L. In uncomplicated maintenance, obtain serum levels every 2 to 3 months. Monitor patient's side effects.

Geriatric: Increased risk for toxic effects; use lower doses; monitor frequently.

Children: **6 to 12 years:** 15 to 60 mg/kg/day in 3 to 4 divided doses.

HALF-LIFE (PEAK EFFECT): Mean, 24 hours (peak serum levels in 1 to 4 hours). Steady state reached in 5 to 7 days.

SELECTED ADVERSE REACTIONS: Weight gain.

WARNING: Avoid use during pregnancy or while breast-feeding. Hepatic or renal impairments increase plasma concentration.

SPECIFIC PATIENT/FAMILY EDUCATION
- Avoid alcohol and other CNS depressant drugs.
- Notify your prescriber if pregnancy is possible or planned. Do not breastfeed while taking this medication.
- Notify your prescriber before taking any other prescriptions, OTC medications, or herbal supplements.
- May impair judgment, thinking, or motor skills; avoid driving or other hazardous tasks.
- Do not abruptly discontinue use.
- BID, twice a day; CNS, central nervous system; OTC, over-the-counter; TID, three times a day.

TABLE 26.1 LITHIUM BLOOD LEVELS AND ASSOCIATED SIDE EFFECTS

Plasma Level	Side Effects or Symptoms of Toxicity
<1.5 mEq/L Mild side effects	Metallic taste in mouth
	Fine hand tremor (resting)
	Nausea
	Polyuria
	Polydipsia
	Diarrhea or loose stools
	Muscular weakness or fatigue
	Weight gain
	Edema
	Memory impairments
1.5–2.5 mEq/L Moderate toxicity	Severe diarrhea
	Dry mouth
	Nausea and vomiting
	Mild to moderate ataxia
	Incoordination
	Dizziness, sluggishness, giddiness, vertigo
	Slurred speech
	Tinnitus
	Blurred vision
	Increasing tremor
	Muscle irritability or twitching
	Asymmetric deep tendon reflexes
	Increased muscle tone
>2.5 mEq/L Severe toxicity	Cardiac arrhythmias
	Blackouts
	Nystagmus
	Coarse tremor
	Fasciculations
	Visual or tactile hallucinations
	Oliguria, renal failure
	Peripheral vascular collapse
	Confusion
	Seizures
	Coma and death

acute phase, supplemental use of antipsychotics and benzodiazepines is often beneficial (Table 26.1).

NCLEXNOTE Monitoring blood levels of lithium carbonate and divalproex sodium is an ongoing nursing assessment for patients receiving these medications. Side effects of mood stabilizers vary.

Lithium is a salt; the interaction between lithium levels and sodium levels in the body and the relationship between lithium levels and fluid volume in the body remain crucial issues in its safe, effective use. The higher the sodium levels, the lower the lithium level will be and vice versa. Thus, changes in dietary sodium intake can affect lithium blood levels that, in turn, may affect therapeutic results or increase the incidence and severity of side effects. The same principle applies to fluid volume. If body fluid decreases significantly because of hot weather, strenuous exercise, vomiting, diarrhea, or drastic reduction in fluid intake for any reason, then lithium levels can rise sharply, causing an increase in

TABLE 26.2	LITHIUM INTERACTIONS WITH MEDICATIONS AND OTHER SUBSTANCES
Substance	**Effect of Interaction**
ACE inhibitors, such as: • Captopril • Lisinopril • Quinapril	Increase serum lithium; may cause toxicity and impaired kidney function
Acetazolamide	Increases renal excretion of lithium; decreases lithium levels
Alcohol	May increase serum lithium level
Caffeine	Increases lithium excretion; increases lithium tremor
Carbamazepine	Increases neurotoxicity despite normal serum levels and dosage
Fluoxetine	Increases serum lithium levels
Haloperidol	Increases neurotoxicity despite normal serum levels and dosage
Loop diuretics, such as furosemide	Increase lithium serum levels but may be safer than thiazide diuretics; potassium-sparing diuretics (e.g., amiloride, spironolactone) are safest
Methyldopa	Increases neurotoxicity without increasing serum lithium levels
NSAIDs, such as • Diclofenac • Ibuprofen • Indomethacin • Piroxicam	Decrease renal clearance of lithium Increase serum lithium levels by 30%–60% in 3–10 days Aspirin and sulindac do not appear to have the same effect
Osmotic diuretics, such as: • Urea • Mannitol • Isosorbide	Increase renal excretion of lithium and decreases lithium levels
Sodium chloride	High sodium intake decreases lithium levels; low sodium diets may increase lithium levels and lead to toxicity
Thiazide diuretics, such as • Chlorothiazide • Hydrochlorothiazide	Promote sodium and potassium excretion; increase lithium serum levels; may produce cardiotoxicity and neurotoxicity
TCAs	Increases tremor; potentiates pharmacologic effects of tricyclic antidepressants

Note. ACE, angiotensin-converting enzyme; NSAID, nonsteroidal anti-inflammatory drug; TCA, tricyclic antidepressant.

side effects, progressing to lethal lithium toxicity. The key is to start with a lower dose and then increase it slowly to maximize the therapeutic response and avoid overshooting the therapeutic window. See Table 26.2 for lithium interactions with other drugs. See Chapter 12 for further discussion of lithium's possible mechanisms of action, pharmacokinetics, side effects, and toxicity.

Lithium toxicity can range from mild to severe, requiring immediate medical attention and prompt intervention. *Mild toxicity* symptoms include lethargy, drowsiness, coarse hand tremor, muscle weakness, nausea, vomiting, and diarrhea. *Moderate toxicity* is associated with confusion, dysarthria, nystagmus, myoclonic twitches, and ECG changes. *Severe toxicity* is life-threatening and associated with grossly impaired consciousness, increased deep tendon reflexes, seizures, syncope, renal insufficiency, coma, and death.

Lithium toxicity can be caused by an overdose (ingesting a large amount at one time) or by other effects of concomitant medications that increase blood concentrations of lithium, such as loop diuretics, ACE inhibitors, or NSAIDs. Chronic kidney disease increases the risk of toxicity, and use of lithium increases the risk of chronic kidney disease. Renal function generally declines with long-term use of lithium. Treatment includes maintaining airway, managing changes in consciousness, inserting a nasogastric tube, and performing gastric lavage. Hemodialysis may be necessary (Tobita et al, 2020).

> **EMERGENCY CARE ALERT !** If symptoms of moderate or severe toxicity (e.g., cardiac arrhythmias, blackouts, tremors, seizures) are noted, withhold additional doses of lithium, immediately obtain a blood sample to analyze the lithium level, and push fluids if the patient can take fluids. Contact the physician for further direction about relieving the symptoms.

Mild side effects tend to subside or can be managed by nursing measures (Table 26.3).

 Concept Mastery Alert

Fine tremors are mild side effects of lithium. They are made worse by stress, so the nurse should assist the client in minimizing exposure to stressors. Lithium therapy can continue unless the tremors interfere with the client's quality of life.

TABLE 26.3 INTERVENTIONS FOR LITHIUM SIDE EFFECTS

Side Effect	Intervention
Edema of feet or hands	Monitor intake and output of water; check for possible decreased urinary output
	Monitor sodium intake
	Patient should elevate legs when sitting or lying
	Monitor weight
Fine hand tremor	Provide support and reassurance if it does not interfere with daily activities
	Tremor worsens with anxiety and intentional movements; minimize stressors
	Notify prescriber if tremor interferes with patient's work so that compliance may be an issue
	More frequent smaller doses of lithium may also help
Mild diarrhea	Take lithium with meals
	Provide for fluid replacement
	Notify prescriber if it worsens; may need a change in medication preparation or may be early sign of toxicity
Muscle weakness, fatigue, or memory and concentration difficulties	Provide support and reassurance; this side effect will usually pass after a few weeks of treatment.
	Short-term memory aids such as lists or reminder calls may be helpful
	Notify prescriber if side effect becomes severe or interferes with the patient's desire to continue treatment
Metallic taste	Suggest sugarless candies or throat lozenges
	Encourage frequent oral hygiene
Nausea or abdominal discomfort	Consider dividing the medication into smaller doses or giving it at more frequent intervals
	Give medication with meals
Polydipsia	Reassure patient that this is a normal mechanism to cope with polyuria
Polyuria	Monitor intake and output
	Provide reassurance and explain the nature of this side effect
	Explain that this side effect causes no physical damage to the kidneys
Toxicity	Withhold medication
	Notify prescriber
	Use symptomatic treatments

Divalproex Sodium

Divalproex sodium (Depakote), an anticonvulsant, has a broader spectrum of efficacy and has about equal benefit for patients with pure mania as for those with other forms of bipolar disorder (i.e., mixed mania, rapid cycling, comorbid substance abuse, and secondary mania) (Box 26.8). The recommended initial dose is 750 mg daily, increase as rapidly as possible to achieve therapeutic response or desired plasma level. The maximum recommended dosage is 60 mg/kg/day (Depakote Prescribing Information, 2019). Divalproex is usually initiated at 250 mg twice a day or lower. In the inpatient setting, it can be initiated in baseline liver function tests and a complete blood count with platelets should be obtained before starting therapy, and patients with known liver disease should not be given divalproex sodium. The black box warns of hepatotoxicity. Optimal blood levels appear to be in the range of 50 to 150 ng/mL. Levels should be obtained weekly until the patient is stable and then every 6 months. Divalproex sodium is associated with increased risk for birth defects.

Cases of life-threatening pancreatitis have been reported in adults and children receiving valproate, both initially and after several years of use. Some cases were described as hemorrhagic, with a rapid progression from onset to death. If pancreatitis is diagnosed, valproate use should be discontinued (Depakote Prescribing Information, 2019).

Carbamazepine

Carbamazepine, an anticonvulsant, also has mood-stabilizing effects. Data from various studies suggest that it may be effective in patients who experience no response to lithium. The most common side effects of carbamazepine are dizziness, drowsiness, nausea, and vomiting, which may be avoided with slow incremental dosing. Carbamazepine has a boxed warning for aplastic anemia and agranulocytosis, but frequent clinically unimportant decreases in white blood cell counts also occur. Estimates of the rate of severe blood dyscrasias vary from 1 in 10,000 patients treated to a more recent estimate of 1 in 125,000 (Schatzberg &

BOX 26.8

Drug Profile: Divalproex Sodium (Depakote)

DRUG CLASS: Antimanic agent.

RECEPTOR AFFINITY: Thought to increase level of inhibitory neurotransmitter, GABA, to brain neurons. Mechanism of action is unknown.

INDICATIONS: Mania, epilepsy, migraine.

ROUTES AND DOSAGE: Available in 125-mg delayed-release capsules, and 125-, 250-, and 500-mg enteric-coated tablets.

Adult Dosage: Dosage depends on symptoms and clinical picture presented; initially, the dosage is low and gradually increased, depending on the clinical presentation.

HALF-LIFE (PEAK EFFECT): 6 to 16 hours (1–4 hours).

SELECTED ADVERSE REACTIONS: Sedation, tremor (may be dose related), nausea, vomiting, indigestion, abdominal cramps, anorexia with weight loss, slight elevations in liver enzymes, hepatic failure, thrombocytopenia, transient increases in hair loss.

BOXED WARNING: Hepatotoxicity, teratogenicity, pancreatitis.

WARNING: Use cautiously during pregnancy and lactation. Contraindicated in patients with hepatic disease or significant hepatic dysfunction. Administer cautiously with salicylates; may increase serum levels and result in toxicity.

SPECIFIC PATIENT AND FAMILY EDUCATION
- Take with food if gastrointestinal upset occurs.
- Swallow tablets or capsules whole to prevent local irritation of mouth and throat.
- Notify your prescriber before taking any other prescription or OTC medications or herbal supplements.
- Avoid alcohol and sleep-inducing OTC products.
- Avoid driving or performing activities that require alertness.
- Do not abruptly discontinue use.
- Keep appointments for follow-up, including blood tests to monitor response.
- GABA, gamma-aminobutyric acid; OTC, over-the-counter.

DeBattista, 2019). Mild, nonprogressive elevations of liver function test results are relatively common. Carbamazepine is associated with increased risk for birth defects.

In patients older than 12 years, carbamazepine is begun at 200 mg once or twice a day. The dosage is increased by no more than 200 mg every 2 to 4 days, to 800 to 1,000 mg a day or until therapeutic levels or effects are achieved. It is important to monitor for blood dyscrasias and liver damage. Liver function tests and complete blood counts with differential are the minimal pretreatment laboratory tests, and they should be repeated about 1 month after initiating treatment and at 3 months, 6 months, and yearly. Other yearly tests assessments should include electrolytes, blood urea nitrogen, thyroid function tests, urinalysis, and eye examinations. Carbamazepine levels are measured monthly until the patient is on a stable dosage. Studies suggest that blood levels in the range of 8 to 12 ng/mL correspond to therapeutic efficacy. See Table 26.4 for carbamazepine's interactions with other drugs. See Chapter 12 for further discussion of carbamazepine's possible mechanisms of action, pharmacokinetics, side effects, and toxicity.

EMERGENCY CARE ALERT ! Both valproate and carbamazepine may be lethal if high doses are ingested. Toxic symptoms appear in 1 to 3 hours and include neuromuscular disturbances, dizziness, stupor, agitation, disorientation, nystagmus, urinary retention, nausea and vomiting, tachycardia, hypotension or hypertension, cardiovascular shock, coma, and respiratory depression.

TABLE 26.4	SELECTED MEDICATION INTERACTIONS WITH CARBAMAZEPINE
Interaction	**Drug Interacting with Carbamazepine**
Increased carbamazepine levels	Erythromycin
	Cimetidine
	Propoxyphene
	Isoniazid
	Calcium channel blockers (verapamil)
	Fluoxetine
	Danazol
	Diltiazem
	Nicotinamide
Decreased carbamazepine levels	Phenobarbital
	Primidone
	Phenytoin
Drugs whose levels are decreased by carbamazepine	Oral contraceptives
	Warfarin, oral anticoagulants
	Doxycycline
	Theophylline
	Haloperidol
	Divalproex sodium
	Tricyclic antidepressants
	Acetaminophen: increased metabolism but also increased risk for hepatotoxicity

Lamotrigine

For a depressive episode, mood stabilizers such as lamotrigine (Lamictal), which requires a dose titration are frequently prescribed (Box 26.9). Lamotrigine is approved by the U.S. Food and Drug Administration (FDA) for the maintenance treatment of bipolar disorder. It may be particularly effective for rapid cycling and in the depressed phase of bipolar illness. If lamotrigine is given with valproic acid (Depakote), the dose should be reduced. Valproic acid decreases the clearance of lamotrigine. Lamotrigine does have an FDA black box warning for rash. Nurses should be especially vigilant for the appearance of any rash. If a rash does appear, it is most likely benign. However, it is not possible to predict whether the rash is benign or serious (Stevens–Johnson syndrome).

BOX 26.9

Drug Profile: Lamotrigine (Lamictal)

DRUG CLASS: Antiepileptic

RECEPTOR AFFINITY: Lamotrigine has a weak inhibitory effect on the serotonin 5-HT$_3$ receptor. It does not exhibit high-affinity binding: adenosine A$_1$ and A$_2$; adrenergic α_1, α_2, and β; dopamine D$_1$ and D$_2$; GABA-A and -B; histamine H$_1$; kappa opioid; muscarinic acetylcholine; and serotonin 5-HT$_2$.

INDICATIONS: Epilepsy, bipolar disorder (acute mood with standard therapy).

ROUTES AND DOSAGE: Available in tablets: 25, 100, 150, and 200 mg scored.

CHEWABLE DISPERSIBLE TABLETS: 2, 5, and 25 mg.

HALF-LIFE (PEAK EFFECT): 32 hours, but can be increased if taking valproate.

SELECTED ADVERSE REACTIONS: Dizziness, somnolence, and other symptoms and signs of CNS depression.

BOXED WARNING: Lamotrigine can cause serious rashes requiring hospitalization and discontinuation of treatment. The incidence of these rashes, which have included Stevens–Johnson syndrome, is approximately 0.3% to 0.8% in pediatric patients (aged 2–17 years) and 0.08% to 0.3% in adults receiving LAMICTAL.

WARNING: Hypersensitivity reaction, multiorgan failure, blood dyscrasias, and suicidal behavior and ideation have occurred.

SPECIFIC PATIENT AND FAMILY EDUCATION

- Do not drive a car or operate other complex machinery until you have gained sufficient experience taking lamotrigine.
- Lamotrigine may cause a serious rash that may cause you to be hospitalized or to stop taking lamotrigine; it may rarely cause death.
- CNS, central nervous system; GABA, gamma-aminobutyric acid.

Antipsychotics

Several atypical antipsychotics that were primarily developed for the treatment of schizophrenia are also FDA approved for treatment of various symptoms of bipolar disorder. See Table 26.5. The dosages for the treatment of patients with bipolar disorder are generally lower than for those for schizophrenia. Recently, these agents have become a mainstay of treatment because they provide some of the broadest efficacy and are more likely used as the only medication to treat bipolar disorder than the mood stabilizers. Complications such as neuroleptic malignant syndrome can occur if antipsychotics are used in treating the mood disorder. An overview of antipsychotics is presented in Chapter 12, and they are discussed in detail in Chapter 25.

Administering and Monitoring Medications

During acute mania, patients may not believe that they have a psychiatric disorder and may refuse to take medication. Because their energy level is still high, they can be very creative in avoiding medication. Through patience and the development of a trusting relationship, patients will more likely begin to participate in a shared decision-making process. It is important for patients to have a sense of empowerment and participation in treatment even during the most acute episodes. After patients begin to take medications, symptom improvement should be evident. If a patient is very agitated, a benzodiazepine may be given for a short period.

Monitoring Side Effects

Patients with bipolar disorder order are usually treated with several medications. In addition, patients may be taking other "nonpsychiatric" medications. In some instances, one agent is used to augment the effects of another, such as supplemental thyroid hormone to boost antidepressant response in depression. Possible side effects for each medication should be listed and cross-referenced. When a side effect appears, the nurse should document the side effect and notify the prescriber so that further evaluation can be made. In some instances, medications should be changed.

Management of Complications

It is a well-established practice to combine mood stabilizers with antidepressants or antipsychotics. The previously discussed drug interactions should be considered when caring for a person with bipolar disorder. One big challenge is monitoring alcohol, drugs, over-the-counter (OTC) medications, and herbal supplements. A complete list of all medications should be maintained and evaluated for any potential interaction.

TABLE 26.5	FOOD AND DRUG ADMINISTRATION-APPROVED ANTIPSYCHOTICS FOR THE TREATMENT OF SYMPTOMS OF BIPOLAR DISORDER	
Antipsychotic Agent	**FDA Indication for Bipolar Disorder**	**Adult Dosage**
Aripiprazole (Abilify)	Acute treatment of manic and mixed episodes associated with bipolar disorder	10–30 mg/day
Aripiprazole (Abilify Maintena)	Maintenance monotherapy for treatment for bipolar I disorder in adults	300 mg monthly (extended-release, injectable suspension)
Asenapine (Saphris)	Acute treatment of manic or mixed episodes associated with bipolar I disorder as monotherapy or adjunctive treatment to lithium or valproate	5–10 mg BID
Cariprazine Vraylar	Acute treatment of manic or mixed episodes associated with bipolar I disorder in adults	3–6 mg/day
Lurasidone (Latuda)	Depressive episodes associated with bipolar I disorder as monotherapy or as adjunctive treatment to lithium or valproate	20–120 mg daily with food (comprising 350 calories)
Olanzapine (Zyprexa)	Acute treatment of manic or mixed episodes associated with bipolar I disorder (monotherapy and in combination with lithium or valproate) and maintenance treatment of bipolar I disorder	10–15 mg daily
Quetiapine (Seroquel)	Bipolar I disorder, manic or mixed episodes; bipolar disorder, depressive episodes	300–800 mg daily
Risperidone (Risperdal)	Bipolar mania, combination of risperidone with lithium or valproate for short-term treatment of acute manic or mixed episodes associated with bipolar I disorder	2–6 mg daily
Risperidone (Risperdal Consta)	Monotherapy or adjunctive to lithium or valproate for maintenance treatment of bipolar I disorder	25–50 mg every 2 weeks (extended-release, injectable suspension)
Ziprasidone (Geodon)	Acute manic or mixed episodes associated with bipolar disorder, with or without psychotic features	40–80 mg with food (comprising 500 calories)

Note. FDA, U.S. Food and Drug Administration.

Promoting Adherence

Adherence to a complex medication regimen over months to years is difficult. Yet one of the primary reasons that acute symptoms reappear is because of discontinuation of medications. It is important to recognize that taking medication as prescribed over time is difficult. Nurses can help patients and families incorporate taking medications into their lifestyles by developing realistic plans. The use of pillboxes, reminders, and other cues will increase the likelihood of adherence.

Teaching Points

For patients who are taking lithium, it is important to explain that a change in dietary salt intake can affect the therapeutic blood level. If salt intake is reduced, the body will naturally retain lithium to maintain homeostasis. This increase in lithium retention can lead to toxicity. After the patient has been stabilized on a lithium dose, salt intake should remain constant. This is fairly easy to do except during the summer, when excessive perspiration can occur. Patients should increase salt intake during periods of perspiration, increased exercise, and dehydration. Most

mood stabilizers and antidepressants can cause weight gain. Patients should be alerted to this potential side effect and should be instructed to monitor any changes in eating, appetite, or weight. Weight reduction techniques may need to be instituted. Patients should also be clearly instructed to check with the nurse or physician before taking any OTC medications, herbal supplements, or other complementary and alternative treatment approaches.

Other Somatic Therapies

Electroconvulsive therapy (ECT) may be a treatment alternative for patients with severe mania who exhibit unremitting, frenzied physical activity. Other indications for ECT are acute mania that is unresponsive to antimanic agents or high suicide risk. ECT is safe and effective in patients receiving antipsychotic drugs. Use of valproate or carbamazepine will elevate the seizure threshold, requiring some adjustments in treatment.

Transcranial magnetic stimulation is another option for bipolar depression. Most of the research has focused on depressive phase rather than the mania episode. There may be cognitive benefits, such as improvement in verbal fluency, memory, and executive functioning. The research is ongoing (Gold et al., 2019).

Psychosocial Interventions

Medications are necessary for treatment of bipolar disorder, but it is only one aspect of recovery. Psychosocial strategies are critical in successful treatment and prevention of relapse.

Therapeutic Interactions

Through therapeutic interaction, treatment and recovery strategies are developed. It is also important to help the patient understand the disorder and manage the mood lability and dysfunctional thoughts that are often precursors to a manic or depressive episode. The nurse partners with the patient in developing strategies to remember to take medications, identify therapeutic and side effects, and know when and how to contact a clinician. Particularly important are enhancing social and occupational functioning, improving quality of life, increasing the patient and family's acceptance of the disorder, and reducing suicide (Crowe et al., 2016).

Enhancing Cognitive and Behavioral Functioning

Individual cognitive-behavioral therapy, individual interpersonal therapy, and adjunctive therapies (such as those for substance use) are all recommended psychotherapeutic approaches.

There is emerging evidence supporting the use of interpersonal and social rhythm therapy and sleep/light manipulation targeting social rhythms to promote mood stability. The goals of this approach are to stabilize daily social rhythms that impact circadian rhythms, understand the link between mood and regularity of social rhythms, and develop self-awareness of bipolar disorder, chrono-disruptors, early warning signs, and effective actions to take (Crowe et al., 2016, 2020).

Psychoeducation

Teaching Strategies

Psychoeducation is designed to provide information on bipolar disorder and its successful treatment and recovery. The nurse provides information about the illness and obstacles to recovery. In the interest of improved medication adherence, listening carefully to the patient's concerns about the medication, dosing schedules and dose changes, and side effects helps individualize teaching approaches. Resistance to accepting the illness and taking medication, the symbolic meaning of medication taking, and worries about the future are discussed openly. See Box 26.10.

BOX 26.10

Psychoeducation Checklist: Bipolar I Disorder

When caring for the patient with a bipolar I disorder, be sure to include the following topic areas in the teaching plan:
- Psychopharmacologic agents, including drug action, dosage, frequency, and possible side effects
- Medication regimen adherence
- Recovery plan
- Relapse prevention plan
- Strategies to decrease agitation and restlessness
- Safety measures
- Self-care management
- Follow-up laboratory testing
- Support services

Teaching About Symptoms

Helping the patient recognize warning signs and symptoms of relapse, cope with residual symptoms, and improve functional impairments are important interventions. Watching for early warning signs and triggers can mean early treatment. Family members should be included in developing an emergency plan for recognizing and intervening if relapse symptoms occur. See Box 26.11.

BOX 26.11

Relapse Prevention and Emergency Plan

COMMON INDICATORS FOR RELAPSE

Mania

Reading several books or newspapers at once
Cannot concentrate on one topic
Talking faster than usual
Feeling irritable
Hungry all the time
Friends remark on changes in mood
More energy than usual

Depression

Quit cooking, cleaning, daily chores
Avoid people
Crave foods (e.g., chocolate)

Headaches
Do not care about other people
Sleeping more or restless sleep
People are irritating to be around

EMERGENCY PLAN

Keep a list of emergency contacts (primary health care provider, close family members)
Keep a current list of all medications, including their dosages
Information about other health problems
Symptoms that indicate others need to take responsibility for care
Treatment preferences (who, where, medications, advanced directive location)

Wellness Strategies

Mental health promotion activities should be the focus during remissions. During this period, patients have an opportunity to learn new coping skills that promote positive mental health. Stress management and relaxation techniques can be practiced for use when needed. A plan for managing emerging symptoms can also be developed during this period.

Social Skills Training

Social skills training may or may not be needed for the person with a bipolar disorder. Even though their social skills will be impaired during periods of mania or depression, once symptoms are controlled, the individual should return to previous level of functioning. There are instances when an individual does need help with social skills, such as learning to listen to others, taking time to finish projects, and organizing daily living demands of cooking, cleaning, and shopping. For these individuals, a social skills group is useful.

Providing Family Education

Family psychoeducation strategies are particularly useful in decreasing the risk of relapse and hospitalization. The sooner the education is begun, the more effective this approach is (Sampogna et al., 2018). Marital and family interventions are often needed at different periods in the life of a person with bipolar disorder. For the family with a child with this disorder, additional parenting skills are needed to manage the behaviors. The goals of family interventions are to help the family understand and cope with the disorder. Interventions may range from occasional counseling sessions to intensive family therapy.

Promoting Safety

The safety issues previously discussed should be addressed with the individual and family before a manic or depressive episode emerges. The nurse can help the individual and family identify specific thoughts and behaviors associated with unsafe situations. For example, during manic episodes, one patient would often threaten airlines and government officials. Within a therapeutic relationship, the nurse and patient agreed that the first call would be to the nurse or another family member who, in turn, would seek more intensive treatment, such as a medication adjustment.

The individual should keep a safety plan for suicidal ideations close at hand to be used when thoughts occur. Firearms, weapons, and unused lethal medication should be removed from the environment.

Convening Support Groups

Support groups are helpful for people with this disorder. Participating in groups allows the person to meet others with the same disorder and to learn management and preventive strategies. Support groups also are helpful in dealing with the stigma associated with mental illness.

Implementing Milieu Therapy

In the hospital or treatment setting, a calm, therapeutic milieu is usually the responsibility of the nurse. An overly stimulating environment can result in behavior escalation for persons with mania. A noisy unit, frequent demands for group and individual participation and lack of privacy cause an escalation in behavior.

Developing Recovery-Oriented Rehabilitation Strategies

The recovery plan should be developed with the patient and should include treatment for the disorder, mental health promotion strategies, and wellness activities. Building on the person's strengths and resilience will foster a healthy lifestyle and well-being.

Evaluation and Treatment Outcomes

Desired treatment outcomes are stabilization of mood and enhanced quality of life. Primary tools for evaluating outcomes are nursing observation and patient self-report. (Nursing Care Plan 26.1—which sets forth a plan of care for Christine, the case study patient in this chapter—is available at http://thepoint.lww.com/Boyd7e.)

Continuum of Care

In today's health care climate, with efforts to reduce hospitalization, most patients with bipolar disorder are treated in a community setting. Hospitalizations are usually brief; recovery is emphasized, and medication regimen promotes adherence. Psychoeducation helps in understanding and managing the disorder, and supportive psychotherapy helps these individuals move toward recovery. Patients need extended and continued follow-up to monitor medication trials and side effects, reinforce self-care management, and provide continued psychosocial support.

Emergency Care

Emergency care is necessary during periods of depression or mania, when there are safety issues such as suicidal or homicidal ideation. Agitation and aggression in an emergency department are not unusual, and staff are usually well prepared to de-escalate the situation. another critical situation when a person is unwillingly brought to the hospital for treatment. Assaults in the emergency departments can lead to patient and staff injuries (Lawrence et al., 2020).

Inpatient-Focused Care

Inpatient hospitalization is necessary for patients who are severely psychotic or who are an immediate threat to themselves or others. In acute mania, nursing interventions focus on patient safety because patients are prone to injury because of hyperactivity and are often unaware of injuries they sustain. Distraction may also be effective when a patient is talking or acting inappropriately. Removal to a quieter environment may be necessary if other interventions have not been successful, but the patient should be carefully monitored. During acute mania, patients are often impulsive, disinhibited, and interpersonally inappropriate, so the nurse should avoid direct confrontations or challenges.

During manic phases, patients usually violate others' boundaries. For example, roommate selection for patients requiring hospital admittance needs to be carefully considered. If possible, a private room is ideal because patients with bipolar disorder tend to irritate others, who quickly tire of the intrusiveness. These patients may miss the cues indicating anger and aggression from others. The nurse should protect the patient who is manic from self-harm, as well as harm from other patients.

The length of stay in an inpatient unit will be relatively short, 3 to 5 days. The plan of care will focus on medication management, including control of side effects, initiation or revision of a recovery plan, psychoeducation, and promotion of self-care. Nurses should be familiar with drug–drug interactions and with interventions to help control side effects.

Intensive Outpatient Programs

Intensive outpatient programs for several weeks of acute-phase care during a manic or depressive episode are used when hospitalization is not necessary or to prevent or shorten hospitalization. These programs are usually called partial hospitalization. Close medication monitoring and milieu therapies that foster restoration of a patient's previous adaptive abilities are the major nursing responsibilities in these settings.

Setting up frequent office visits and crisis telephone calls are additional nursing interventions that can help shorten or prevent hospitalization during the acute phase of a manic episode. Family sessions or psychoeducation that includes the patient are alternatives. Severely and persistently ill patients may need ongoing intensive treatment, but the frequency of visits can be decreased for patients whose conditions stabilize and who enter the continuation or the maintenance phase of treatment.

Community Care

Persons with bipolar disorder are treated throughout the continuum of care. When symptoms are acute, hospitalization may be necessary. Other times, minimal interaction with the mental health providers is needed. The individual will need to be seen regularly to monitor symptoms and medications.

Virtual Mental Health Care

The use of telemedicine can be very effective for persons with bipolar disorder during periods of remission. Telephone contacts are a useful strategy for monitoring medication adherence (Basit et al., 2020). The use of telephones is relatively inexpensive and widespread. The use of smartphones allows frequent reminders of medication dosage and is unobtrusive. They can also be used for texting and voice-based mobile interventions.

Integration With Primary Care

There are several reasons that coordination of care is very important for persons with bipolar disorder. A large proportion of persons with bipolar disorder are treated in the primary care setting. There may be an average of 6 to 8 years between onset of symptoms and diagnosis. Because there may be several episodes of depression before there is a manic episode, bipolar disorder is often misdiagnosed as depression in primary care, leading to a delay in treatment. If antidepressants are prescribed for someone with a bipolar disorder, these medications may precipitate a manic episode. The need exists to improve the health of this population. Collaborative care of mental health with primary care increases the likelihood that a person would be screened for bipolar disorder, resulting in an early diagnosis and effective treatment (Cerimele et al., 2019). Patients with bipolar disorder frequently require primary care management for comorbidities, such as cardiovascular and metabolic disorders.

OTHER BIPOLAR AND RELATED DISORDERS

In **bipolar II disorder**, the individual is mostly depressed, which can severely affect their social and occupational life. Even though there are brief periods of elevated, expansive, or irritable moods, bipolar II disorder is not as easily recognized as bipolar I disorder because the symptoms are less dramatic. Hypomania, a mild form of mania, is characteristic of bipolar II disorder. Judgment remains fundamentally intact.

In a **cyclothymic disorder**, hypomanic symptoms occur alternating with numerous periods of depressive symptoms. However, these symptoms are less severe than the bipolar disorders. To be diagnosed with this disorder, the symptoms have to be present for at least 2 years of numerous periods of hypomanic symptoms.

Illicit drugs, prescription medications, and some medical conditions such as changes in thyroid functioning can be responsible for manic like behavior. These symptoms cause significant distress and impairment in social functioning.

SUMMARY OF KEY POINTS

- Bipolar and related disorders are characterized by one or more manic episodes or mixed mania (co-occurrence of manic and depressive states) that cause marked impairment in social activities, occupational functioning, and interpersonal relationships and may require hospitalization to prevent self-harm.

- In bipolar and related disorders, there are periods of mania or hypomania that alternate with depression. These disorders are classified as bipolar I disorder, bipolar II disorder, or cyclothymic disorder, depending on the severity of the manic and depressive symptoms. Bipolar disorder may also be related to substance abuse, prescription drug use, or a medical condition.

- Manic episodes are periods in which the individual experiences abnormally and persistently elevated, expansive, or irritable mood characterized by inflated self-esteem, decreased need to sleep, excessive energy or hyperactivity, racing thoughts, easy distractibility, and an inability to stay focused. Other symptoms can include hypersexuality and impulsivity.

- Bipolar disorders are underreported and are often misdiagnosed. Bipolar I disorder is more dramatic than bipolar II disorder, so it is easier to diagnose.

- Genetics plays a role in the etiology of bipolar disorders. Risk factors include a family history of mood disorders, prior mood episodes, lack of social support, stressful life events, substance use, and medical problems, particularly chronic or terminal illnesses.

- Mental health nursing assessment includes assessing mood; speech patterns; thought processes and thought content; suicidal or homicidal thoughts; cognition and memory; and social factors, such as patterns of relationships, quality of support systems, and changes in occupational functioning. Several self-report scales are helpful in evaluating depressive symptoms.

- Many symptoms of bipolar depression, such as weight gain and appetite changes, sleep disturbance, decreased energy, and fatigue, are similar to those of medical illnesses. Assessment includes a thorough medical history and physical examination to detect or rule out medical or psychiatric comorbidity.

- Establishing and maintaining a therapeutic nurse–patient relationship is key to successful outcomes. Shared decision-making with the patient leads to positive outcomes. Recovery-oriented nursing interventions that foster the therapeutic relationship include being available in times of crisis, providing understanding and education to patients and their families regarding goals of treatment and recovery, providing encouragement and feedback concerning the patient's progress, providing guidance in the patient's interpersonal interactions with others and work environment, and helping to set and monitor realistic goals.

- Pharmacotherapy includes mood stabilizers used alone or in combination with antipsychotics or benzodiazepines to treat psychosis, agitation, or insomnia. Electroconvulsive therapy is a valuable alternative for patients with severe mania that does not respond to other treatments.

- Recent major advances in bipolar disorder treatment research validate the efficacy of integrated psychosocial and pharmacologic treatment involving family or couple therapies, psychoeducational programs, and individual cognitive-behavioral or interpersonal therapies.

- Psychosocial interventions for bipolar disorders include self-care management, cognitive therapy, behavior therapy, interpersonal therapy, patient and family education regarding the nature of the disorder and treatment goals, marital and family therapy, and group therapy that includes medication maintenance support groups and other consumer-oriented support groups.

- The use virtual health care strategies can be very effective in monitoring medication adherence and providing virtual therapy and psychoeducation.

CRITICAL THINKING CHALLENGES

1. A patient tells you that he no longer needs medication because he has special powers that protect him from evil forces. He no longer needs sleep and can see things that others do not see. What approaches would you use to help the patient decide to take his medication?

2. Describe how you would approach a patient who is expressing concern that the diagnosis of bipolar disorder will negatively affect her social and work relationships.

3. Your patient with mania is experiencing physical hyperactivity that is interfering with his sleep and nutrition. Describe the actions you would take to meet the patient's needs for rest and nutrition.

4. Prepare a hypothetical discussion with a patient with potential bipolar disorder concerning the advantages and disadvantages of lithium versus divalproex sodium for treatment of bipolar disorder.

5. Think about all of the aforementioned situations and relate them to persons from culturally and ethnically diverse populations (e.g., African American, Latinx, or Asian descent; Jewish or Jehovah Witness religions; across the life-span of individuals from children to older adult populations).

Unfolding Patient Stories: Sharon Cole

Part 2

Recall from Chapter 10 Sharon Cole diagnosed with bipolar disorder who is admitted to the orthopedic unit following surgery for a fractured ankle from a fall during a manic episode. She is exhibiting manic behavior postoperatively with grandiose thoughts, irritability, and wanting to leave the hospital. What are the benefits of having a sitter at her bedside? What education would the nurse provide to a sitter without prior experience caring for a client with bipolar disorder and manic behavior? What instructions would promote safety for the patient and the sitter and deter a potentially volatile situation?

Movie Viewing Guides

Silver Linings Playbook (2012). Pat Solatano (Bradley Cooper), a former teacher and recent divorcee, suffers from bipolar disorder and was recently released from a mental health facility. He moves in with his parents and is determined to win his ex-wife back. This highly acclaimed, romantic comedy depicts the impact of a mental disorder on a person's life and shows that recovery is possible.

SIGNIFICANCE: This movie is a realistic portrayal of the life of someone with bipolar disorder who is struggling to live a happy, healthy, and meaningful life. The viewers can see a day-to-day experience of recovery.

VIEWING POINTS: Identify the role of the courts in the initial treatment of Pat's illness. Discuss the role of nonadherence to medication. How does the illness shape Pat's views of the world? What behaviors are characteristic of persons with bipolar disorder?

Michael Clayton (2007). Arthur Edens (Tom Wilkinson), a successful corporate lawyer, is experiencing the stress of a high-profile legal case and stops taking his medication. Consequently, he has a manic episode with delusions about one of the jurors, whom he eventually contacts. The story traces the attempts by his colleague and friend Michael Clayton (George Clooney) to repair the damage Arthur's behavior has caused to the lawsuit and to get his friend treated before his mania further damages his life.

SIGNIFICANCE: Viewers can gain insight into the devastating impact of mental illness on the successful career of a well-respected attorney. This film depicts the poor judgment, impulsivity, and consequences of a full-blown mania episode.

VIEWING POINTS: Identify the mania symptoms that Arthur displays. What feelings are evoked when you see the strange behavior that he exhibits? If Arthur were your patient, how would you approach him, and what medication would you expect him to be prescribed?

A related Psychiatric-Mental Health Nursing video on the topic of Bipolar Disorders is available at http://thepoint.lww.com/Boyd7e.

A Practice and Learn Activity related to the video on the topic of Bipolar Disorders is available at http://thepoint.lww.com/Boyd7e.

REFERENCES

Akinhanmi, M. O., Biernacka, J. M., Strakowski, S. M., McElroy, S. L., Balls Berry, J. E., Merikangas, K. R., Assari, S., McInnis, M. G., Schulze, T. G., LeBoyer, M., Tamminga, C., Patten, C., & Frye, M. A. (2018). Racial disparities in bipolar disorder treatment and research: A call to action. *Bipolar Disorders, 20*(6), 506–514. https://doi.org/10.1111/bdi.12638

Akinhanmi, M., El-Amin, S., Balls-Berry, J. E., Vallender, E. J., Ladner, M., Geske, J., Coombes, B., Biernacka, J., Kelsoe, J., Bipolar Genome Study (BiGS), & Frye, M. A (2020). Decreased core symptoms of mania and utilization of lithium/mood stabilizing anticonvulsants in U.S. bipolar I patients of African vs European ancestry. *Journal of Affective Disorders, 260*, 361–365. https://doi.org/10.1016/j.jad.2019.09.022

American Psychiatric Association. (2013). *Diagnostic and statistical manual of mental disorders* (5th ed.). Author.

Arfaie, A., Safikhanlou, S., Bakhshipour Roodsari, A., Farnam, A., & Shafiee-Kandjani, A. R. (2018). Assessment of behavioral approach and behavioral inhibition systems in mood disorders. *Basic and Clinical Neuroscience, 9*(4), 261–268. https://doi.org/10.32598/bcn.9.4.261

Arnold, L. E., Van Meter, A. R., Fristad, M. A., Youngstrom, E. A., Birmaher, B. B., Findling, R. L., Horwitz, S., & Black, S. R. (2020). Development of bipolar disorder and other comorbidity among youth with attention-deficit/hyperactivity disorder. *Journal of Child Psychology and Psychiatry, and Allied Disciplines, 61*(2), 175–181. https://doi.org/10.1111/jcpp.13122

Ballard, E. D., Farmer, C. A., Shovestul, B., Vande Voort, J., Machado-Vieira, R., Park, L., Merikangas, K. R., & Zarate, C. A. Jr., (2020). Symptom trajectories in the months before and after a suicide attempt in individuals with bipolar disorder: A STEP-BD study. *Bipolar Disorders, 22*(3), 245–254. https://doi.org/10.1111/bdi.12873

Basit, S. A., Mathews, N., & Kunik, M. E. (2020). Telemedicine interventions for medication adherence in mental illness: A systematic review. *General Hospital Psychiatry*, *62*, 28–36. https://doi.org/10.1016/j.genhosppsych.2019.11.004

Bolton, S., Warner, J., Harriss, E., Geddes, J., & Saunders, K. E. (2020). Bipolar disorder: Trimodal age at onset distribution. *Bipolar Disorders*, .10.1111/bdi.13016. Advance online publication. https://doi.org/10.1111/bdi.13016.

Carvalho, A. F., Firth, J., & Vieta, E. (2020). Bipolar disorder. *The New England Journal of Medicine*, *383*(1), 58–66. https://doi.org/10.1056/NEJMra1906193

Cerimele, J. M., et al. (2019). Bipolar disorder in primary care: A qualitative study of clinician and patient experiences with diagnosis and treatment. *Family Practice*, *36*(1), 32–37. https://doi.org/10.1093/fampra/cmy019

Crowe, M., Beaglehole, B., & Inder, M. (2016). Social rhythm interventions for bipolar disorder: A systematic review and rationale for practice. *Journal of Psychiatric and Mental Health Nursing*, *23*(1), 3–11.

Crowe, M., & Inder, M. (2018). Staying well with bipolar disorder: A qualitative analysis of five-year follow-up interviews with young people. *Journal of Psychiatric and Mental Health Nursing*, *25*(4), 236–244. https://doi.org/10.1111/jpm.12455

Crowe, M., Inder, M., Swartz, H. A., Murray, G., & Porter, R. (2020). Social rhythm therapy: A potentially translatable psychosocial intervention for bipolar disorder. *Bipolar Disorders*, *22*(2), 121–127. https://doi.org/10.1111/bdi.12840

Dargél, A. A., Volant, S., Brietzke, E., Etain, B., Olié, E., Azorin, J. M., Gard, S., Bellivier, F., Bougerol, T., Kahn, J. P., Roux, P., Aubin, V., Courtet, P., Leboyer, M., Henry, C., & FACE-BD collaborators. (2020). Allostatic load, emotional hyper-reactivity, and functioning in individuals with bipolar disorder. *Bipolar Disorders*, 10.1111/bdi.12927. Advance online publication. https://doi.org/10.1111/bdi.12927

Dell'Osso, B., Vismara, M., Benatti, B., Cirnigliaro, G., Grancini, B., Fineberg, N. A., Van Ameringen, M., Hollander, E., Stein, D. J., Menchon, J. M., Rodriguez, C. I., Nicolini, H., Lanzagorta, N., Pallanti, S., Grassi, G., Lochner, C., Marazziti, D., Hranov, G., Karamustafalioglu, O., Hranov, L., ... Zohar, J. (2020). Lifetime bipolar disorder comorbidity and related clinical characteristics in patients with primary obsessive compulsive disorder: A report from the International College of Obsessive-Compulsive Spectrum Disorders (ICOCS). *CNS Spectrums*, *25*(3), 419–425. https://doi.org/10.1017/S1092852919001068

Depakote Prescribing Information. (February 2019). [Online]. Accessed November 1, 2020. Available at: https://www.accessdata.fda.gov/drugsatfda_docs/label/2019/018723s061lbl.pdf.

Dols, A., & Beekman, A. (2020). Older age bipolar disorder. *Clinics in Geriatric Medicine*, *36*(2), 281–296. https://doi.org/10.1016/j.cger.2019.11.008

Faedda, G. L., Baldessarini, R. J., Marangoni, C., Bechdolf, A., Berk, M., Birmaher, B., Conus, P., DelBello, M. P., Duffy, A. C., Hillegers, M., Pfennig, A., Post, R. M., Preisig, M., Ratheesh, A., Salvatore, P., Tohen, M., Vázquez, G. H., Vieta, E., Yatham, L. N., Youngstrom, E. A., ... Correll, C. U.. (2019). An International Society of Bipolar Disorders task force report: Precursors and prodromes of bipolar disorder. *Bipolar Disorders*, *21*(8), 720–740. https://doi.org/10.1111/bdi.12831

Fellinger, M., Waldhoer, T., König, D., Hinterbuchinger, B., Pruckner, N., Baumgartner, J., Vyssoki, S., & Vyssoki, B. (2019). Seasonality in bipolar disorder: Effect of sex and age. *Journal of Affective Disorders*, *243*, 322–326. https://doi.org/10.1016/j.jad.2018.09.073

Flowers, S. A., Ward, K. M., & Clark, C. T. (2020). The gut microbiome in bipolar disorder and pharmacotherapy management. *Neuropsychobiology*, *79*(1), 43–49. https://doi.org/10.1159/000504496

Gold, A. K., Ornelas, A. C., Cirillo, P., Caldieraro, M. A., Nardi, A. E., Nierenberg, A. A., & Kinrys, G. (2019). Clinical applications of transcranial magnetic stimulation in bipolar disorder. Brain and Behavior, *9*(10), e01419. https://doi.org/10.1002/brb3.1419

Grover, S., Mehra, A., Chakravarty, R., Jagota, G., & Sahoo, S. (2020). Change in prevalence of metabolic syndrome in patients with bipolar disorder. *Asian Journal of Psychiatry*, *47*, 101876. https://doi.org/10.1016/j.ajp.2019.101876

Johansson, V., Kuja-Halkola, R., Cannon, T. D., Hultman, C. M., & Hedman, A. M. (2019). A population-based heritability estimate of bipolar disorder: In a Swedish twin sample. *Psychiatry Research*, *278*, 180–187. https://doi.org/10.1016/j.psychres.2019.06.010

Lawrence, R. E., Rolin, S. A., Looney, D. V., Birt, A. R., Stevenson, E. M., Dragatsi, D., Appelbaum, P. S., & Dixon, L. B. (2020). Physical Assault in the Psychiatry Emergency Room. *The Journal of the American Academy of Psychiatry and the Law*, 10.29158/JAAPL.200022-20. Advance online publication. https://doi.org/10.29158/JAAPL.200022-20

Loftus, J., Scott, J., Vorspan, F., Icick, R., Henry, C., Gard, S., Kahn, J. P., Leboyer, M., Bellivier, F., & Etain, B. (2020). Psychiatric comorbidities in bipolar disorders: An examination of the prevalence and chronology of onset according to sex and bipolar subtype. *Journal of Affective Disorders*, *267*, 258–263. https://doi.org/10.1016/j.jad.2020.02.035

Muneer, A. (2020). The discovery of clinically applicable biomarkers for bipolar disorder: A review of candidate and proteomic approaches. *Chonnam Medical Journal*, *56*(3), 166–179. https://doi.org/10.4068/cmj.2020.56.3.166

Muneer, A., & Mazommil, R. (2018). The staging of major mood disorders: Clinical and neurobiological correlates. *Psychiatry Investigation*, *15*(8), 747–758. https://doi.org/10.30773/pi.2018.05.26

Rosenthal, S. J., Josephs, T., Kovtun, O., & McCarty, R. (2020). Seasonal effects on bipolar disorder: A closer look. *Neuroscience and Biobehavioral Reviews*, *115*, 199–219. https://doi.org/10.1016/j.neubiorev.2020.05.017

Sampogna, G., Luciano, M., Del Vecchio, V., Malangone, C., De Rosa, C., Giallonardo, V., Borriello, G., Pocai, B., Savorani, M., Steardo, L. Jr, Lampis, D., Veltro, F., Bartoli, F., Bardicchia, F., Moroni, A. M., Ciampini, G., Orlandi, E., Ferrari, S., Biondi, S., Iapichino, S., ... Fiorillo, A. (2018). The effects of psychoeducational family intervention on coping strategies of relatives of patients with bipolar I disorder: results from a controlled, real-world, multicentric study. *Neuropsychiatric Disease and Treatment*, *14*, 977–989. https://doi.org/10.2147/NDT.S159277

Schaffer, A., Isometsä, E. T., Tondo, L., Moreno, D. H., Sinyor, M., Kessing, L. V., et al. (2015). Epidemiology, neurobiology and pharmacological interventions related to suicide deaths and suicide attempts in bipolar disorder: Part I of a report of the International Society for Bipolar Disorders Tasks Force on Suicide in Bipolar Disorder. *Australian & New Zealand Journal of Psychiatry*, *49*(9), 785–802.

Schatzberg, A. F., & DeBattista, C. (2019). *Manual of clinical psychopharmacology* (9th ed.). American Psychiatric Publishing.

Sinha, A., Shariq, A., Said, K., Sharma, A., Jeffrey Newport, D., & Salloum, I. M. (2018). Medical comorbidities in bipolar disorder. *Current Psychiatry Reports*, *20*(5), 36. https://doi.org/10.1007/s11920-018-0897-8

Smeland, O. B., Bahrami, S., Frei, O., Shadrin, A., O'Connell, K., Savage, J., Watanabe, K., Krull, F., Bettella, F., Steen, N. E., Ueland, T., Posthuma, D., Djurovic, S., Dale, A. M., & Andreassen, O. A. (2020). Genome-wide analysis reveals extensive genetic overlap between schizophrenia, bipolar disorder, and intelligence. *Molecular Psychiatry*, *25*(4), 844–853. https://doi.org/10.1038/s41380-018-0332-x

Smith, P. H., Chhipa, M., Bystrik, J., Roy, J., Goodwin, R. D., & McKee, S. A. (2020). Cigarette smoking among those with mental disorders in the US population: 2012–2013 update. *Tobacco Control*, *29*(1), 29–35. https://doi.org/10.1136/tobaccocontrol-2018-054268

Spoorthy, M. S., Chakrabarti, S., & Grover, S. (2019). Comorbidity of bipolar and anxiety disorders: An overview of trends in research. *World Journal of Psychiatry*, *9*(1):7–29. https://doi.org/10.5498/wjp.v9.i1.7

Tobita, S., Sogawa, R., Murakawa, T., Kimura, S., Tasaki, M., Sakamoto, Y., Monji, A., & Irie, H. (2020). The importance of monitoring renal function and concomitant medication to avoid toxicity in patients taking lithium. *International Clinical Psychopharmacology*, 10.1097/YIC.0000000000000320. Advance online publication. https://doi.org/10.1097/YIC.0000000000000320

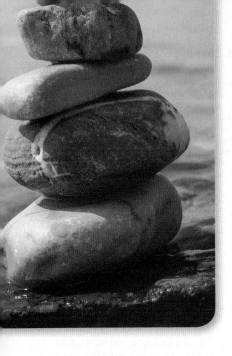

27
Anxiety Disorders
Nursing Care of Patients with Anxiety, Phobia, and Panic

Mary Ann Boyd

KEYCONCEPTS

- anxiety
- panic
- phobia

LEARNING OBJECTIVES

After studying this chapter, you will be able to:

1. Discuss the role of anxiety and panic in mental disorders.

2. Delineate the clinical symptoms and course of panic disorder, including phobias.

3. Analyze the primary theories explaining panic disorder and their relationship to anxiety.

4. Develop strategies to establish a patient-centered, recovery-oriented therapeutic relationship with a person with a panic disorder.

5. Apply a person-centered, recovery-oriented nursing process for persons with a panic disorder.

6. Identify medications used to treat people with a panic disorder and evaluate their effectiveness.

7. Develop wellness strategies for persons with a panic disorder.

8. Differentiate the type of mental health care provided in emergency care, inpatient-focused care, community care, and virtual mental health care.

9. Discuss the importance of integrated health care for persons with panic disorder.

10. Describe other anxiety disorders.

KEY TERMS

- Agoraphobia • Depersonalization • Exposure therapy • Flooding • Implosive therapy • Interoceptive conditioning • Panic attacks • Panic control treatment • Positive self-talk • Reframing • Specific phobia disorder • Social anxiety disorder • Systematic desensitization

Case Study

Doug is a 50-year-old man who lives with his wife Norma and two sons; Greg, a sophomore in college, and Leon, a high school student. Norma was recently laid off from her job and has been unable to find employment. The family is now experiencing financial and marital problems. Leon was recently expelled from school for drug and alcohol use. Doug had an argument with his boss and is afraid that he will lose his job. He appears at the emergency department for chest pain and is convinced he is having a heart attack. All lab test results are normal. Consider how the nurse can help Doug deal with his health issues.

INTRODUCTION

Anxiety is part of many emotional problems and mental disorders. At one time, most mental conditions with anxiety aspects were categorized as "anxiety disorders," but today anxiety disorders have been redefined. Trauma–stressor-related disorder and obsessive–compulsive disorder, both previously identified as anxiety disorders, are now categorized as separate disorders (American Psychiatric Association [APA], 2013). Trauma- and stressor-related disorders, as well as dissociative disorders, are discussed in Chapter 29. Obsessive–compulsive disorders are discussed in Chapter 28. In this chapter, panic disorder is highlighted.

NORMAL VERSUS ABNORMAL ANXIETY RESPONSE

Anxiety is an unavoidable human condition that takes many forms and serves different purposes. Anxiety can be positive and can motivate one to act, or it can produce paralyzing fear, causing inaction. *Normal anxiety* is described as being of realistic intensity and duration for the situation and is followed by relief behaviors intended to reduce or prevent more anxiety (Peplau, 1989). A "normal anxiety response" is appropriate to the situation and can be used to help the individual identify which underlying problem has caused the anxiety.

> **KEYCONCEPT Anxiety** is an uncomfortable feeling of apprehension or dread that occurs in response to internal or external stimuli; it can result in physical, emotional, cognitive, and behavioral symptoms.

During a perceived threat, rising anxiety levels cause physical and emotional changes in all individuals. A normal emotional response to anxiety consists of three parts: physiologic arousal, cognitive processes, and coping strategies. Physiologic arousal, or the fight-or-flight response, is the signal that an individual is facing a threat. Cognitive processes decipher the situation and decide whether the perceived threat should be approached or avoided. Coping strategies are used to resolve the threat. Box 27.1 summarizes many physical, affective, cognitive, and behavioral symptoms associated with anxiety. The factors that determine whether anxiety is a symptom of a mental disorder include the intensity of anxiety relative to the situation, the trigger for the anxiety, and the particular symptom clusters that manifest the anxiety. Table 27.1 describes the four degrees of anxiety and associated perceptual changes and patterns of behavior. Anxiety is a component of all the disorders discussed in this chapter.

PHOBIAS

> **KEYCONCEPT Phobia** is an irrational fear of an object, person, or situation that leads to a compelling avoidance.

The development of a phobia may be the outcome of extreme anxiety. Phobias are often present in anxiety disorders but may also develop into a specific phobia disorder (discussed later).

Defense Mechanisms and Anxiety

Defense mechanisms are used to reduce anxiety by preventing or diminishing unwanted thoughts and feelings. See Chapter 10 for definitions. Defense mechanisms can be helpful in coping with everyday problems, but they become problematic when overused. The first step is identifying a person's use of defense mechanisms. The next step is determining whether the reasons the defense mechanisms are being used support healthy coping or are detrimental to a person's health. What may be healthy for one person may be unhealthy for another. See Box 27.2.

ANXIETY DISORDERS OVERVIEW

The primary symptoms of anxiety disorders are fear and anxiety. Even though symptoms of anxiety disorders can be found in healthy individuals, an anxiety disorder is diagnosed when the fear or anxiety is excessive or out of proportion to the situation. An individual's ability to work and interpersonal relationships may be impaired. Anxiety disorders are differentiated by the situation or objects that provoke fear, anxiety, or avoidance behavior and related cognitive thoughts (APA, 2013).

Anxiety disorders are the most common of the psychiatric illnesses treated by health care providers. Approximately 40 million American adults (older than 18 years old) or about 18.1% of this age group within a given year have an anxiety disorder. Direct and indirect costs of treating anxiety disorders amount to tens of billions of dollars. Women experience anxiety disorders more often than men by a 2:1 ratio. Anxiety disorders may also be associated with other mental or physical comorbidities, such as heart disease, respiratory disease, and mood disorders (Stein et al., 2018). The relationship between depression and anxiety disorders is particularly strong. A single patient may concurrently have more than one anxiety disorder or other psychiatric disorders as well.

Anxiety disorders tend to be chronic and persistent, with full recovery more likely among those who do not

BOX 27.1

Symptoms of Anxiety

PHYSICAL SYMPTOMS

Cardiovascular

Sympathetic
Palpitations
Heart racing
Increased blood
  pressure

Parasympathetic
Actual fainting
Decreased blood
  pressure
Decreased pulse rate

Respiratory
Rapid breathing
Difficulty getting air
Shortness of breath
Pressure of chest
Shallow breathing
Lump in throat
Choking sensations
Gasping
Spasm of bronchi

Neuromuscular
Increased reflexes
Startle reaction
Eyelid twitching
Insomnia
Tremors
Rigidity
Spasm
Fidgeting

Pacing
Strained face
Unsteadiness
Generalized weakness
Wobbly legs
Clumsy motions

Skin
Flushed face
Pale face
Localized sweating
  (palm region)
Generalized sweating
Hot and cold spells
Itching

Gastrointestinal
Loss of appetite
Revulsion about food
Abdominal discomfort
Diarrhea
Abdominal pain
Nausea
Heartburn
Vomiting

Eyes
Dilated pupils

Urinary Tract Parasympathetic
Pressure to urinate
Increased frequency of
  urination

AFFECTIVE SYMPTOMS
Edgy
Impatient
Uneasy
Nervous
Tense
Wound-up
Anxious
Fearful
Apprehensive
Scared
Frightened
Alarmed
Terrified
Jittery
Jumpy

COGNITIVE SYMPTOMS

Sensory-Perceptual
Mind is hazy, cloudy,
  foggy, dazed
Objects seem blurred or
  distant
Environment seems
  different or unreal
Feelings of unreality
Self-consciousness
Hypervigilance

Thinking Difficulties
Cannot recall important
  things
Confused
Unable to control
  thinking

Difficulty concentrating
Difficulty focusing
  attention
Distractibility
Blocking
Difficulty reasoning
Loss of objectivity and
  perspective
Tunnel vision

Conceptual
Cognitive distortion
Fear of losing control
Fear of not being able
  to cope
Fear of physical injury
  or death
Fear of mental disorder
Fear of negative
  evaluations
Frightening visual
  images
Repetitive fearful
  ideation

BEHAVIORAL SYMPTOMS
Inhibited
Tonic immobility
Flight
Avoidance
Speech dysfluency
Impaired coordination
Restlessness
Postural collapse
Hyperventilation

Adapted from Beck, A. T., & Emery, C. (1985). *Anxiety disorders and phobias: A cognitive perspective* (pp. 23–27). Basic Books.

TABLE 27.1 DEGREES OF ANXIETY

Degree of Anxiety	Effects on Perceptual Field and on Ability to Focus Attention	Observable Behavior
Mild	Perceptual field widens slightly. Able to observe more than before and to see relationships (make connection among data). Learning is possible.	Is aware, alert, sees, hears, and grasps more than before. Usually able to recognize and identify anxiety easily.
Moderate	Perceptual field narrows slightly. Selective inattention: does not notice what goes on peripheral to the immediate focus but can do so if attention is directed there by another observer.	Sees, hears, and grasps less than previously. Can attend to more if directed to do so. Able to sustain attention on a particular focus; selectively inattentive to contents outside the focal area. Usually able to state, "I am anxious now."
Severe	Perceptual field is greatly reduced. Tendency toward dissociation: to not notice what is going on outside the current reduced focus of attention; largely unable to do so when another observer suggests it.	Sees, hears, and grasps far less than previously. Attention is focused on a small area of a given event. Inferences drawn may be distorted because of inadequacy of observed data. May be unaware of and unable to name anxiety. Relief behaviors generally used.

(continued)

TABLE 27.1	DEGREES OF ANXIETY (*Continued*)	
Degree of Anxiety	**Effects on Perceptual Field and on Ability to Focus Attention**	**Observable Behavior**
Panic (e.g., terror, horror, dread, uncanniness, awe)	Perceptual field is reduced to a detail, which is usually "blown up," that is, elaborated by distortion (exaggeration), or the focus is on scattered details; the speed of the scattering tends to increase. Massive dissociation, especially of contents of self-system. Felt as an enormous threat to survival. Learning is impossible.	Says, "I'm in a million pieces," "I'm gone," or "What is happening to me?" Perplexity, self-absorption. Feelings of unreality. Flights of ideas or confusion. Fear. Repeats a detail. Many relief behaviors used automatically (without thought). The enormous energy produced by panic must be used and may be mobilized as rage. May pace, run, or fight violently. With dissociation of contents of self-system, there may be a very rapid reorganization of the self, usually going along pathologic lines (e.g., a "psychotic break" is usually preceded by panic).

Adapted with permission from Peplau, H. (1989). Theoretical constructs: Anxiety, self, and hallucinations. In A. O'Toole & S. Welt (Eds.), *Interpersonal theory in nursing practice: Selected works of Hildegarde E. Peplau.* Springer.

BOX 27.2		
Consequences of Decreasing Anxiety Using Defense Mechanisms		
Defense Mechanism	**Positive Consequences**	**Negative Consequences**
Altruism	Satisfies internal needs through helping others	Prevents examination of underlying fears or concerns
Denial	Avoids feelings associated with recognizing a problem	Avoidance of major problem that should be addressed
Displacement	By taking out frustrations on an unsuspecting or vulnerable person, animal, or object, anxiety is reduced and the individual is protected from anticipated retaliation from the source of the frustration	Does not deal with problem and inappropriately expresses feelings towards a more vulnerable person or object
Intellectualization	Able to analyze events in a distant, objective, analytical way	Inability to acknowledge feelings that may be interfering with relationships
Projection	By assigning unwanted thoughts, feelings or behaviors to another person or object, the individual does not have to acknowledge undesirable or unacceptable thoughts or feelings	Does not acknowledge undesirable or unwanted feelings or thoughts and can act on inaccurate interpretation of the other person's thoughts and behaviors
Rationalization	Avoids anxiety by explaining an unacceptable or disappointing behavior or feeling in a logical, rationale way. May protect self-esteem and self-concept	Avoids the reality of a situation, which may be detrimental to the individual
Reaction Formation	Reduces anxiety by taking the opposite feeling. Hides true feelings, which may be appropriate in many situations	Unable to acknowledge personal feelings about others, which leads to negative consequences
Regression	When stressed, abandons effective coping strategies and reverts to behaviors used earlier in development. These strategies are comfortable and may be effective	May reengage in detrimental behaviors such as smoking, drinking, or inappropriate interpersonal responses leading to ineffective coping
Repression	Avoids unwanted thoughts and anxiety by blocking thoughts, experiences from conscious awareness	Cannot recall traumatic events that should be addressed to be healthy (i.e., rape)
Sublimation	Avoids anxiety and channels maladaptive feelings or impulses into socially acceptable behaviors. Maintains socially acceptable behavior	By not recognizing maladaptive feelings, the individual cannot address underlying feelings
Suppression	Reduces anxiety by intentionally avoiding thinking about disturbing problems, wishes, feelings, or experiences. Useful in many situations such as test-taking situations	Avoiding problem situation prevents finding a solution to the problem

have other mental or physical disorders (Andreescu & Lee, 2020). Anxiety disorders tend to first episode in late adolescence or young adult.

Anxiety Disorders Across the Life Span

Prompt identification, diagnosis, and treatment of individuals with anxiety disorders may be difficult for special populations such as children and older adult patients. Often, the symptoms suggestive of anxiety disorders may go unnoticed by caregivers or are misdiagnosed because they mimic cardiac or pulmonary pathology rather than a psychological disturbance. Children and adolescents are discussed in Chapter 37; older adults are discussed in Chapter 38.

Children and Adolescents

Anxiety disorders are among the most common conditions of children and adolescents. If left untreated, symptoms persist and gradually worsen and sometimes lead to suicidal ideation and suicide attempts, early parenthood, drug and alcohol dependence, and educational underachievement later in life (Carballo et al., 2020).

Separation anxiety disorder (i.e., excessive fear or anxiety concerning separation from home or attachment figures) usually first occurs in childhood. Affected children experience extreme distress when separated from home or attachment figures, worry about them when separated from them, and worry about untoward events (i.e., getting lost) and what will happen to them. This disorder is discussed in Chapter 37.

A rare disorder typically seen in childhood is selective mutism, in which children do not initiate speech or respond when spoken to by others (APA, 2013). Children with this disorder are often very anxious when asked to speak in school or read aloud. They may suffer academic impairment because of their inability to communicate with others.

Older Adults

Generally speaking, the prevalence of anxiety disorders declines with age. However, in the older adult population, rates of anxiety disorders are as high as mood disorders, which commonly co-occur. This combination of depressive and anxiety symptoms has been shown to decrease social functioning, increase somatic (physical) symptoms, and increase depressive symptoms (Meuret et al., 2020). In one study, nearly half of primary care patients with chronic pain had at least one attendant anxiety disorder. Detecting and treating anxiety is an important component of pain management (Kroenke et al., 2019). Because the older adult population is at risk for suicide, special assessment of anxiety symptoms is essential.

PANIC DISORDER

Panic is an extreme, overwhelming form of anxiety often experienced when an individual is placed in a real or perceived life-threatening situation. Panic is normal during periods of threat but is abnormal when it is continuously experienced in situations that pose no real physical or psychological threat. Some people experience heightened anxiety because they fear experiencing another panic attack. This type of panic interferes with the individual's ability to function in everyday life and is characteristic of panic disorder.

| **KEYCONCEPT Panic** is a normal but extremely overwhelming form of anxiety, often experienced when an individual is placed in a real or perceived life-threatening situation.

Clinical Course

The onset of panic disorder is typically between 20 and 24 years of age. The disorder usually surfaces in childhood but may not be diagnosed until later. Panic disorder is treatable, but studies have shown that even after years of treatment, many people remain symptomatic. In some cases, symptoms may even worsen (APA, 2013).

Panic Attacks

Panic attacks are characteristic of panic disorder. A panic attack is a sudden, discrete period of intense fear or discomfort that reaches its peak within a few minutes and is accompanied by significant physical discomfort and cognitive distress (APA, 2013). Panic attacks usually peak in about 10 minutes but can last as long as 30 minutes before returning to normal functioning. The physical symptoms include palpitations, chest discomfort, rapid pulse, nausea, dizziness, sweating, paresthesias (burning, tickling, pricking of skin with no apparent reason), trembling or shaking, and a feeling of suffocation or shortness of breath. Cognitive symptoms include disorganized thinking, irrational fears, **depersonalization** (being detached from oneself), and a decreased ability to communicate. Usually, feelings of impending doom or death, fear of going crazy or losing control, and desperation ensue.

The physical symptoms can mimic those of a heart attack. Individuals often seek emergency medical care because they feel as if they are dying, but most have negative cardiac workup results. People experiencing panic attacks may also believe that the attacks stem from an underlying major medical illness (APA, 2013). Even with medical testing and assurance of no underlying disease, they often remain unconvinced.

Remember Doug?

He had chest pains and believed he was having a heart attack. How can you help Doug recognize that even though he is not having a heart attack, his symptoms are serious and that his panic attack could indicate an underlying anxiety disorder? Why wouldn't you tell him that everything is normal?

KEYCONCEPT Physical symptoms of panic attack are similar to cardiac emergencies. These symptoms are physically taxing and psychologically frightening to patients. Recognition of the seriousness of panic attacks should be communicated to the patient.

In a panic disorder, recurrent unexpected panic attacks are followed by persistent concern about experiencing subsequent panic attacks. Because of fear of future attacks, these affected individuals modify normal behaviors to avoid future attacks (APA, 2013). Panic attacks are either expected with an obvious cue or trigger or unexpected with no such obvious cue. The first panic attack is usually associated with an identifiable cue (e.g., anxiety-provoking medical conditions, such as asthma, or in initial trials of illicit substance use), but subsequent attacks are often unexpected without any obvious cue (Box 27.3). Panic attacks not only occur in panic disorder but can also occur in other mental disorders such as depression, bipolar disease, eating disorders, and some medical conditions such as cardiac or respiratory disorders (APA, 2013).

Diagnostic Criteria

Panic disorder is a chronic condition that has several exacerbations and remissions during the course of the disease. The disabling panic attacks often lead to other symptoms, such as phobias.

Other diagnostic symptoms include palpitations, sweating, shaking, shortness of breath or smothering, sensations of choking, chest pain, nausea or abdominal distress, dizziness, derealization or depersonalization, fear of going crazy, fear of dying, paresthesias, and chills or hot flashes (APA, 2013) (see Key Diagnostic Characteristics 27.1).

Disorder Across the Life Span

Children

Panic disorder is more likely to occur in adolescents than in younger children. It is estimated that panic disorder is experienced by 1% of adolescents aged 15 to 19.

BOX 27.3 CLINICAL VIGNETTE

Panic Disorder

Susan, a 22-year-old female, has experienced several life changes, including a recent engagement, loss of her father to cancer and heart disease, graduation from college, and entrance to the workforce as a computer programmer in a large inner-city company. Because of her active lifestyle, her sleep habits have been poor. She frequently uses sleeping aids at night and now drinks a full pot of coffee to start each day. She continues to smoke to "relieve the stress." While sitting in heavy traffic on the way to work, she suddenly experienced chest tightness, sweating, shortness of breath, feelings of being "trapped," and foreboding that she was going to die. Fearing a heart attack, she went to an emergency department, where her discomfort subsided within a half hour. After several hours of testing, the doctor informed her that her heart was healthy. During the next few weeks, she experienced several episodes of feeling trapped and slight chest discomfort on her drive to work. She fears future "attacks" while sitting in traffic and while in her crowded office cubicle.

What Do You Think?
• What risk factors does Susan have that might contribute to the development of panic attacks?
• What lifestyle changes do you think would help Susan reduce stress?

Children and adolescents with panic disorder are most likely experiencing another anxiety or mood disorder. Panic disorder has a significant impact on social and academic functioning and normal development (Baker & Waite, 2020).

Older Adults

Panic disorder occurs in the older adult, but it is an understudied disorder. It is unclear whether the disorder was present, but undiagnosed in early or middle adulthood or had its onset in the later years. In the older adult, panic disorder is associated with significant functional impairment, which compounds any functional issues associated with other comorbid disorders such as dementia (Pace et al., 2020).

Epidemiology and Risk Factors

Panic disorder has a moderately high lifetime prevalence in the general population with 1% to 2% 1-year prevalence rate and 4.8% lifetime rate (Olaya et al., 2018). Increased risk is associated with being female, middle aged, of low socioeconomic status, and widowed, separated, or divorced. The estimates of isolated panic attacks may affect 22.7% of the population. Panic disorders occur in several cultures, but the panic symptoms may be experienced differently across racial/ethnic groups (Assari, 2017).

KEY CHARACTERISTICS 27.1 • PANIC DISORDER

Diagnostic Criteria

A. Recurrent unexpected panic attacks. A panic attack is an abrupt surge of intense fear or intense discomfort that reaches a peak within minutes, and during which time four (or more) of the following symptoms occur:
Note: The abrupt surge can occur from a calm state or an anxious state.
  1. Palpitations, pounding heart, or accelerated heart rate
  2. Sweating
  3. Trembling or shaking
  4. Sensations of shortness of breath or smothering
  5. Feelings of choking
  6. Chest pain or discomfort
  7. Nausea or abdominal distress
  8. Feeling dizzy, unsteady, light-headed, or faint
  9. Chills or heat sensations
  10. Paresthesias (numbness or tingling sensations)
  11. Derealization (feelings of unreality) or depersonalization (being detached from oneself)
  12. Fear of losing control or "going crazy"
  13. Fear of dying
Note: Culture-specific symptoms (e.g., tinnitus, neck soreness, headache, uncontrollable screaming, or crying) may be seen. Such symptoms should not count as one of the four required symptoms.

B. At least one of the attacks has been followed by 1 month (or more) of one or both of the following:
  1. Persistent concern or worry about additional panic attacks or their consequences (e.g., losing control, having a heart attack, "going crazy")
  2. A significant maladaptive change in behavior related to the attacks (e.g., behaviors designed to avoid having panic attacks, such as avoidance of exercise or unfamiliar situations)
C. The disturbance is not attributable to the physiologic effects of a substance (e.g., a drug or substance use disorder, a medication) or another medical condition (e.g., hyperthyroidism, cardiopulmonary disorders)
D. The disturbance is not better explained by another mental disorder (e.g., the panic attacks do not occur only in response to feared social situations, as in social anxiety disorder; in response to circumscribed phobic objects or situations, as in specific phobia; in response to obsessions, as in obsessive–compulsive disorder; in response to reminders of traumatic events, as in post-traumatic stress disorder; or in response to separation from attachment figures, as in separation anxiety disorder).

Target Symptoms

Discrete period of intense fear or discomfort with four (or more) of the following symptoms that develop abruptly and reach a peak within 10 minutes:

- Palpitations, pounding heart, or accelerated heart rate
- Sweating
- Trembling or shaking
- Sensations of shortness of breath or smothering
- Feelings of choking
- Chest pain or discomfort
- Nausea or vomiting
- Feeling dizzy, unsteady, light-headed, or faint
- Derealization (feeling of unreality) or depersonalization (being detached from oneself)
- Fear of losing control or going crazy
- Fear of dying
- Paresthesias (numbness or tingling sensations)
- Chills or hot flushes
- Great apprehension about the outcome of routine activities and experiences
- Loss or disruption of important interpersonal relationships
- Demoralization
- Possible major depressive episode

Associated Findings

- Nocturnal panic attack (waking from sleep in a state of panic)
- Constant or intermittent feelings of anxiety related to physical and mental health
- Pervasive concerns about abilities to complete daily tasks or withstand daily stressors
- Excessive use of drugs or other means to control panic attacks

Associated Physical Examination Findings

- Transient tachycardia
- Moderate elevation of systolic blood pressure

Associated Laboratory Findings

- Compensated respiratory alkalosis (decreased carbon dioxide, decreased bicarbonate levels, almost normal pH)

Other Targets for Treatment

- Loss or disruption of important interpersonal or occupational activities
- Demoralization
- Possible major depressive episode

Reprinted with permission from the *Diagnostic and statistical manual of mental disorders* (5th ed.). (Copyright ©2013). American Psychiatric Association. All Rights Reserved.

Family history, alcohol use disorder and substance and stimulant use disorder, smoking tobacco, and severe stressors are risk factors for panic disorder. People who have several anxiety symptoms and those who experience separation anxiety during childhood often develop panic disorder later in life. Early life traumas and adverse events, self-stigma, a history of physical or sexual abuse, socioeconomic or personal disadvantages, and behavioral inhibition have also been associated with an increased risk for anxiety disorders in children (Bourdon et al., 2019; Kolek et al, 2019).

Comorbidity

Patients may experience other anxiety disorders, depression, eating disorder, substance use disorder, or schizophrenia (Meuret et al., 2020). Although people with panic disorder are thought to have more somatic complaints than the general population, panic disorder does correlate with some medical conditions, including vertigo, cardiac disease, gastrointestinal disorders, asthma, and those related to cigarette smoking.

Etiology

Biologic Theories

There appears to be a substantial familial predisposition to panic disorder with an estimated heritability of 48% (Forstner et al., 2019). Studies show brain abnormalities in the "fear network" (amygdala, hippocampus, thalamus, midbrain, pons, medulla, and cerebellum) and changes in volume in different brain areas (Asok et al., 2019).

Serotonin and Norepinephrine

Serotonin and norepinephrine are both implicated in panic disorders. Norepinephrine effects act on those systems most affected by a panic attack—the cardiovascular, respiratory, and gastrointestinal systems. Serotonergic neurons are distributed in central autonomic and emotional motor control systems regulating anxiety states and anxiety-related physiologic and behavioral responses (Hornboll et al., 2018).

Gamma-Aminobutyric Acid

Gamma-aminobutyric acid (GABA) is the most abundant inhibitory neurotransmitter in the brain. GABA receptor stimulation causes several effects, including neurocognitive effects, reduction of anxiety, and sedation. GABA stimulation also results in increased seizure threshold. Abnormalities in the benzodiazepine–GABA–chloride ion channel complex have been implicated in panic disorder (Asok et al., 2019).

Hypothalamic–Pituitary–Adrenal Axis

Research implicates a role of the hypothalamic–pituitary–adrenal axis in panic disorders (Quagliato & Nardi, 2018). A current explanation is that as stress hormones are activated, anxiety increases, which can lead to a panic attack. See Chapter 19.

Psychosocial Theories

Psychoanalytic and Psychodynamic Theories

Psychodynamic theories examine anxiety that develops after separation and loss. Many patients link their initial panic attacks with recent personal losses. However, the empirical evidence remains inadequate for a psychodynamic explanation. It remains unclear why some patients develop panic disorder, whereas others with similar experiences develop other disorders (Cackovic et al., 2020).

Cognitive-Behavioral Theories

Learning theory underlies most cognitive-behavioral explanations of panic disorder. Classic conditioning theory suggests that one learns a fear response by linking an adverse or fear-provoking event, such as a car accident, with a previously neutral event, such as crossing a bridge. One becomes conditioned to associate fear with crossing a bridge. Applying this theory to people with panic disorder has limitations. Phobic avoidance is not always developed secondary to an adverse event.

Further development of this theory led to an understanding of **interoceptive conditioning**, an association between physical discomforts, such as dizziness or palpitations, and an impending panic attack. For example, during a car accident, the individual may experience rapid heartbeat, dizziness, shortness of breath, and panic. Subsequent experiences of dizziness or palpitations, unrelated to an anxiety-provoking situation, incite anxiety and panic. Furthermore, people with panic disorder may misinterpret mild physical sensations (e.g., sweating, dizziness) as being catastrophic, causing panic as a result of learned fear (catastrophic interpretation). Some researchers hypothesize that individuals with a low sense of control over their environment or with a particular sensitivity to anxiety are vulnerable to misinterpreting normal stress. Controlled exposure to anxiety-provoking situations and cognitive countering techniques has proven successful in reducing the symptoms of panic.

Family Response to Disorder

Persons with a panic disorder may inadvertently cause excessive fears, phobias, or excessive worry in other family members. Families may limit social functions to prevent a panic attack. Those affected need a tremendous amount of support and encouragement from significant others.

RECOVERY-ORIENTED CARE FOR PERSONS WITH PANIC DISORDER

Teamwork and Collaboration: Working Toward Recovery

Nurses are pivotal in providing a safe and therapeutic inpatient environment and teaching patients strategies for managing anxiety and fears. The nurse also administers prescribed medication, monitors its effects, and provides medication education. Advanced practice nurses, licensed clinical social workers, or licensed counselors provide individual psychotherapy sessions as needed. Often, a clinical psychologist gives psychological tests and interprets the results to assist in diagnosing and treating the panic disorder.

Panic Control Treatment

Panic control treatment involves intentional exposure (through exercise) to panic-invoking sensations such as dizziness, hyperventilation, tightness in the chest, and sweating. Identified patterns become targets for treatment. Patients are taught to use breathing training and cognitive restructuring to manage their responses and are instructed to practice these techniques between therapy sessions to adapt the skills to other situations.

Systematic Desensitization

Systematic desensitization, another exposure method used to desensitize patients, exposes the patient to a hierarchy of feared situations that the patient has rated from least to most feared. The patient is taught to use muscle relaxation as levels of anxiety increase through multisituational exposure. Planning and implementing exposure therapy require special training. Because of the multitude of outpatients in the treatment for panic disorder and agoraphobia (discussed later in chapter), exposure therapy is a useful tool for home health psychiatric nurses. Outcomes of home-based exposure treatment are similar to clinic-based treatment outcomes.

Implosive Therapy

Implosive therapy is a provocative technique useful in treating panic disorder and agoraphobia in which the therapist identifies phobic stimuli for the patient and then presents highly anxiety-provoking imagery to the patient, describing the feared scene as dramatically and vividly as possible. **Flooding** is a technique used to desensitize the patient to the fear associated with a particular anxiety-provoking stimulus. Desensitizing is done by presenting feared objects or situations repeatedly without session breaks until the anxiety dissipates. For example, a patient with ophidiophobia (i.e., a morbid fear of snakes) might be presented with a real snake repeatedly until the patient's anxiety decreases.

Exposure Therapy

Many of the treatment approaches used for panic disorder are effective for phobias (discussed in later chapters). **Exposure therapy** is the treatment of choice for phobias. The patient is repeatedly exposed to real or simulated anxiety-provoking situations until they become desensitized and anxiety subsides.

Cognitive-Behavioral Therapy

Cognitive-behavioral therapy (CBT) is a highly effective tool for treating individuals with panic disorder. It is considered a first-line treatment for those with panic and other anxiety disorders and is often used in conjunction with medications, including selective serotonin reuptake inhibitors (SSRIs) (Bilet et al., 2020). The goals of CBT include helping the patient to manage their anxiety and correcting anxiety-provoking thoughts through interventions, including cognitive restructuring, breathing training, and psychoeducation.

Safety Issues

Panic attack symptoms mimic a heart attack—chest pain, palpitations, dyspnea. It is important to rule out any cardiac problems prior to diagnosing and treating a panic attack. Research shows that persons with panic disorder have higher oxidative stress due to impaired serotonin metabolism, which is related to heart disease (Aghayan et al., 2020).

Panic disorder is associated with an increased risk of suicide. A 3-year prevalence of suicide attempt in a sample of adults with panic disorder is 4.6%. Factors that independently predicted suicide attempts include psychopathology, prior history of suicide attempts, lower physical health-related quality of life, and greater number of stressful life events in the past year (Scheer et al., 2020).

EVIDENCE-BASED NURSING CARE OF PERSONS WITH PANIC DISORDER

Individuals often first seek help in the emergency department for their physical symptoms, but they are told that there are no life-threatening cardiac or neurologic causes for the severe physical symptoms. Although no laboratory tests exist to confirm anxiety disorders, a careful clinical assessment will reveal the presence of an anxiety disorder. See Nursing Care Plan 27.1.

Mental Health Nursing Assessment

A comprehensive nursing assessment includes overall physical and mental status, suicidal tendencies and thoughts, cognitive thought patterns, avoidance behavior patterns, and family and cultural factors. Patients can be encouraged to keep a daily log of the severity of anxiety and the frequency, duration, and severity of panic episodes. This log will be a basic tool for monitoring progress as symptoms decrease.

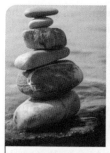

NURSING CARE PLAN 27.1

The Patient with Panic Disorder

Douglas is a 50-year-old man who is being evaluated in the emergency department by a nurse from the mental health crisis team. Doug was brought into the emergency department by his wife after experiencing chest pain early in the evening. He arrived in a state of severe level of anxiety and believed that he was having a heart attack. An ECG and laboratory values were normal.

Setting: Day Treatment Program, Adult Psychiatric Services

Baseline Assessment: Doug arrived at the ED trembling, dizzy, pale, experiencing tachycardia, nausea, and feelings of dread. He could not follow directions and responded poorly to redirection. His attention and thoughts are scattered.

Associated Psychiatric Diagnosis	Medications
Panic disorder	Paroxetine CR (Paxil) 12.5 mg every day
History of hypertension	Lisinopril (Zestril) 20 mg daily
	Lorazepam (Ativan) 1 mg q6h PRN for extreme anxiety

Priority of Nursing Care: Anxiety

Important Characteristics	Associated Considerations
Trembling, increased pulse	Impending panic attacks
Fearful, irritable, scared, worried	Panic attacks
Apprehensive	

Outcomes

Initial	Long-term
Develop skills to decrease impact of panic attack	Carry out normal daily living and social activities outside of the house

Interventions

Interventions	Rationale	Ongoing Assessment
Meet daily with Doug to assess whether he has had a panic attack within the last 24 hours.	Asking Doug to monitor panic attacks will provide data regarding potential antecedents to attacks.	Determine whether Doug has had a panic attack.
Using a calm reassuring approach, encourage verbalization of feelings, perceptions, and fears. Identify periods of time when anxiety level is at its highest.	Discussing the experience of anxiety will help the patient notice when his anxiety increases.	Explore the antecedents and determine whether he was able to practice techniques from education programs.
Teach Doug how to perform relaxation techniques.	Having strategies to deal with impending panic attack will decrease the intensity of the experience.	Observe effectiveness of his technique and changes in anxiety/panic episodes.
Teach Doug about the actions and side effects of paroxetine. Explain the purposes of the medication. Track the number of PRN medications that are used for anxiety. Also, monitor for use of alcohol and herbal supplements.	Panic attacks are neurobiologic occurrences that respond to medications.	Determine whether panic attacks decrease over time and whether there are side effects.
		Determine his commitment to living a more normal life.

Evaluation

Outcomes	Revised Outcomes	Interventions
Doug's panic attacks decreased to once a week. Attended day treatment program every day. Able to go to grocery store.	Increase social activity outside of house.	Meet with Doug twice a week to monitor progress. Continue to reinforce the use of strategies in managing anticipatory anxiety.

Panic Attack Assessment

The assessment of the person with a panic disorder focuses on identifying the characteristics of the panic attack and the individual's strengths and problems. If the panic attack occurs in the presence of the nurse, direct assessment of the symptoms should be made and documented. Questions to ask the patient might include the following:

- What were you doing when the panic attack occurred?
- What did you experience before and during the panic episode, including physical symptoms, feelings, and thoughts?
- When did you begin to feel that way? How long did it last?
- Do you have an explanation for what caused you to feel and think that way?
- Have you experienced these symptoms in the past? If so, under what circumstances?
- Has anyone in your family ever had similar experiences?
- What do you do when you have these experiences to help you to feel safe?
- Have the feelings and sensations ever gone away on their own?

Physical Health

Key assessment areas of physical health that could have precipitated the panic attack include sleep patterns, activity levels, and health conditions.

Sleep Patterns and Physical Activity

Sleep is often disturbed in patients with panic disorder. In fact, panic attacks can occur during sleep, so the patient may fear sleep for this reason. Nurses should closely assess the impact of sleep disturbance because fatigue may increase anxiety and susceptibility to panic attacks. Panic disorder can be improved through active participation in a routine exercise program. If the patient does not exercise routinely, define the barriers to it. If exercise is avoided because of chronic muscle tension, poor muscle tone, muscle cramps, general fatigue, exhaustion, or shortness of breath, the symptoms may indicate poor physical health.

Nutrition

A nutritional assessment is important because people with panic disorder have increased rates of eating disorder behavior when compared to individuals without panic disorder (Garcia et al., 2020). The assessment is especially in women who are more likely to have a comorbid eating disorder than men. The nurse should inquire about the food and drink intake on a typical day and also include questions about binge or fasting behavior.

Medication

Several medications can cause anxiety. Bronchodilators, oral contraceptives, amphetamines (i.e., methylphenidate), steroids, thyroid medication, and several other medications can increase anxiety. Additionally, medicines that contain caffeine, such as some pain and anti-inflammatory agents, decongestants (i.e., phenylephrine), and some illegal drugs (cocaine), also increase anxiety.

Substance Use

Caffeine, pseudoephedrine, amphetamines, cocaine, or other stimulants are associated with panic disorder and may stimulate a panic attack. Tobacco use can also contribute to the risk for panic symptoms. Many individuals with panic disorder use alcohol or central nervous system (CNS) depressants in an effort to self-medicate anxiety symptoms; withdrawal from CNS depressants may produce symptoms of panic.

Other Physical Assessment Areas

Recent changes in physical status should be assessed. For example, pregnant patients should be assessed carefully for an underlying panic disorder. Although pregnancy may actually protect the mother from developing panic symptoms, postpartum onset of panic disorder requires particular attention. During a time that tremendous effort is spent on family, postpartum onset of panic disorder negatively affects lifestyle and decreases self-esteem in affected women, leading to feelings of overwhelming personal disappointment.

Psychosocial Assessment

A psychosocial assessment includes the patient's report of the symptoms and a careful cognitive, behavioral, and social assessment. The assessment should include the following behavioral responses, self-concept, stress and coping patterns, social network, functional status, and support systems. See Chapter 11.

Self-Report Scales

Self-evaluation is difficult in panic disorder. Often the memories of the attack and its triggers are irretrievable. Several tools are available to characterize and rate the patient's state of anxiety. Examples of these symptom and behavioral rating scales are provided in Box 27.4. All of these tools are self-report measures and as such are

---

BOX 27.4

Rating Scales for Assessment of Panic Disorder and Anxiety Disorders

PANIC SYMPTOMS

Panic-Associated Symptom Scale (PASS)

Argyle, N., Delito, J., Allerup, P., Maier, W., Albus, M., Nutzinger, D., et al. (1991). The Panic-Associated Symptom Scale: Measuring the severity of panic disorder. *Acta Psychiatrica Scandinavica, 83,* 20–26.

Acute Panic Inventory

Dillon, D. J., Gorman, J. M., Liebowitz, M. R., Fyer, A. J., & Klein, D. F. (1987). Measurement of lactate-induced panic and anxiety. *Psychiatry Research, 20,* 97–105.

National Institute of Mental Health Panic Questionnaire (NIMH PQ)

Scupi, B. S., Maser, J. D., & Uhde, T. W. (1992). The National Institute of Mental Health Panic Questionnaire: An instrument for assessing clinical characteristics of panic disorder. *Journal of Nervous and Mental Disease, 180,* 566–572.

COGNITIONS

Anxiety Sensitivity Index

Reiss, S., Peterson, R. A., & Gursky, D. M. (1986). Anxiety sensitivity, anxiety frequency, and the prediction of fearfulness. *Behaviour Research and Therapy, 24,* 1–8.

Agoraphobia Cognitions Questionnaire

Chambless, D. L., Caputo, G. C., Bright, P., & Gallagher, R. (1984). Assessment of fear in agoraphobics: The Body Sensations Questionnaire and the Agoraphobic Cognitions Questionnaire. *Journal of Consulting and Clinical Psychology, 52,* 1090–1097.

Body Sensations Questionnaire

Chambless, D. L., Caputo, G. C., Bright, P., & Gallagher, R. (1984). Assessment of fear in agoraphobics: The Body Sensations Questionnaire and the Agoraphobic Cognitions Questionnaire. *Journal of Consulting and Clinical Psychology, 52,* 1090–1097.

PHOBIAS

Mobility Inventory for Agoraphobia

Chambless, D. L., Caputo, G. C., Jasin, S. E., Gracely, E., & Williams, C. (1985). The mobility inventory for agoraphobia. *Behavior Research and Therapy, 23,* 35–44.

Fear Questionnaire

Marks, I. M., & Matthews, A. M. (1979). Brief standard self-rating for phobic patients. *Behaviour Research and Therapy, 17,* 263–267.

ANXIETY

State-Trait Anxiety Inventory (STAI)

Spielberger, C. D., Gorsuch, R. L., & Luchene, R. E. (1976). *Manual for the State-Trait Anxiety Inventory.* Consulting Psychologists Press.

Penn State Worry Questionnaire (PSWQ)

16 items developed to assess the trait of worry.

Meyer, T., Miller, M., Metzger, R., & Borkovec, T. (1990). Development and validation of the Penn State Worry Questionnaire. *Behaviour Research and Therapy, 28*(6), 487–495.

Beck Anxiety Inventory

21 items rating the severity of symptoms on a 4-point scale.

Beck, A., Epstein, N., Brown, G., & Steer, R. (1988). An inventory for measuring clinical anxiety: The Beck Anxiety Inventory. *Journal of Consulting and Clinical Psychology, 56,* 893–897.

---

limited by the individual's self-awareness and openness. However, the Hamilton Rating Scale for Anxiety, provided in Table 27.2, is an example of a scale rated by the clinician (Hamilton, 1959). This 14-item scale reflects both psychological and somatic aspects of anxiety.

Mental Status Examination

During a mental status examination, individuals with panic disorder may exhibit anxiety symptoms, including restlessness, irritability, poor concentration, and apprehensive behavior. Disorganized thinking, irrational fears, and a decreased ability to communicate often occur during a panic attack. Assess by direct questioning whether the patient is experiencing suicidal thoughts, especially if they are abusing substances or taking antidepressant medications.

Cognitive Thought Patterns

Catastrophic misinterpretations of trivial physical symptoms can trigger panic symptoms. After they have been identified, these thoughts should serve as a basis for individualizing patient education to counter such false beliefs. Table 27.3 presents a scale to assess catastrophic misinterpretations of the symptoms of panic.

Several studies have found that individuals who feel a sense of control have less severe panic attacks. Individuals who fear loss of control during a panic attack often make the following type of statements:

- "I feel trapped."
- "I'm afraid others will know or that I'll hurt someone."
- "I feel alone. I can't help myself."
- "I'm losing control."

These individuals also tend to show low self-esteem, feelings of helplessness, demoralization, and overwhelming fears of experiencing panic attacks. They may have difficulty with assertiveness or expressing their feelings.

Social Network

Marital and parental functioning can be adversely affected by panic disorder. During the assessment, the nurse

TABLE 27.2	HAMILTON RATING SCALE FOR ANXIETY

Max Hamilton designed this scale to help clinicians gather information about anxiety states. The symptom inventory provides scaled information that classifies anxiety behavior and assists the clinician in targeting behaviors and achieving outcome measures. Provide a rating for each indicator based on the following scale:

0 = None

1 = Mild

2 = Moderate

3 = Severe

4 = Severe, grossly disabling

Item	Symptoms	Rating
Anxious mood	Worries, anticipation of the worst, fearful anticipation, irritability	
Tension	Feelings of tension, fatigability, startle response, moved to tears easily, trembling, feelings of restlessness, inability to relax	
Fear	Of dark, strangers, being left alone, animals, traffic, crowds	
Insomnia	Difficulty in falling asleep, broken sleep, unsatisfying sleep, and fatigue on waking; dreams, nightmares, night terrors	
Intellectual (cognitive)	Difficulty concentrating, poor memory	
Depressed mood	Loss of interest, lack of pleasure in hobbies, depression, early waking, diurnal swings	
Somatic (sensory)	Tinnitus, blurring of vision, hot and cold flushes, feelings of weakness, prickly sensation	
Somatic (muscular)	Pains and aches, twitching, stiffness, myoclonic jerks, grinding of teeth, unsteady voice, increased muscular tone	
Cardiovascular symptoms	Tachycardia, palpitations, pain in chest, throbbing of vessels, fainting feelings, missing beat	
Respiratory symptoms	Pressure or constriction in chest, choking feelings, sighing, dyspnea	
Gastrointestinal symptoms	Difficulty in swallowing, gas, abdominal pain, burning sensation, abdominal fullness, nausea, vomiting, looseness of bowels, loss of weight, constipation	
Genitourinary symptoms	Frequency of micturition, urgency of micturition, amenorrhea, menorrhagia, development of frigidity, premature ejaculation, loss of libido, impotence	
Autonomic symptoms	Dry mouth, flushing, pallor, tendency to sweat, giddiness, tension headache, raising of hair	
Behavior at interview	Fidgeting, restlessness or pacing, tremor of hands, furrowed brow, strained face, sighing or rapid respiration, facial pallor, swallowing, belching, brisk tendon jerks, dilated pupils, exophthalmos	

Reprinted from Hamilton, M. (1959). The assessment of anxiety states by rating. *British Journal of Medical Psychology, 32*, 54.

should try to grasp the patient's understanding of how panic disorder with or without severe avoidance behavior has affected their life, along with that of the family. Pertinent questions include the following:

- How has the disorder affected your family's social life?
- What limitations related to travel has the disorder placed on you or your family?
- What coping strategies have you used to manage symptoms?
- How has the disorder affected your family members or others?

Cultural Factors

Cultural competence calls for the understanding of cultural knowledge, cultural awareness, cultural assessment skills, and cultural practice. Therefore, cultural differences must be considered in the assessment of panic disorder. Different cultures interpret sensations, feelings, or understandings differently. For example, symptoms of anxiety might be seen as witchcraft or magic (APA, 2013). Several cultures do not have a word to describe *anxiety* or *anxious* and instead may use words or meanings to suggest physical complaints. (Moitra, 2018). Many over-the-counter (OTC) herbal remedies contain

TABLE 27.3	PANIC ATTACK COGNITIONS QUESTIONNAIRE			

Rate each of the following thoughts according to the degree to which you believe each thought contributes to your panic attack.

1 = Not at all   3 = Quite a lot

2 = Somewhat   4 = Very much

1. I'm going to die.	1	2	3	4
2. I'm going insane.	1	2	3	4
3. I'm losing control.	1	2	3	4
4. This will never end.	1	2	3	4
5. I'm really scared.	1	2	3	4
6. I'm having a heart attack.	1	2	3	4
7. I'm going to pass out.	1	2	3	4
8. I don't know what people will think.	1	2	3	4
9. I won't be able to get out of here.	1	2	3	4
10. I don't understand what is happening to me.	1	2	3	4
11. People will think I am crazy.	1	2	3	4
12. I'll always be this way.	1	2	3	4
13. I am going to throw up.	1	2	3	4
14. I must have a brain tumor.	1	2	3	4
15. I'll choke to death.	1	2	3	4
16. I'm going to act foolish.	1	2	3	4
17. I'm going blind.	1	2	3	4
18. I'll hurt someone.	1	2	3	4
19. I'm going to have a stroke.	1	2	3	4
20. I'm going to scream.	1	2	3	4
21. I'm going to babble or talk funny.	1	2	3	4
22. I'll be paralyzed by fear.	1	2	3	4
23. Something is physically wrong with me.	1	2	3	4
24. I won't be able to breathe.	1	2	3	4
25. Something terrible will happen.	1	2	3	4
26. I'm going to make a scene.	1	2	3	4

Adapted from Clum, G. A. (1990). *Panic attack cognitions questionnaire. Coping with panic: A drug-free approach to dealing with anxiety attacks.* Pacific Grove, CA: Brooks/Cole. Reprinted with permission from Dr. George A. Clum.

substances that may induce panic by increasing the heart rate, basal metabolic rate, blood pressure, and sweating (see Chapter 11).

Strength Assessment

During the assessment, the patient's strengths will emerge. For example, a patient may tell you that he does not drink alcohol or use tobacco. Another may relate that he would like to exercise. Still another patient has a supportive partner or family member. The nurse can support these positive behaviors.

CLINICAL JUDGMENT

Suicide prevention is the first priority when caring for a person with a panic disorder. People with panic disorder are often depressed and consequently are at high risk for suicide. Adolescents with panic disorder are at higher risk for suicidal thoughts or may attempt suicide more often than other adolescents. Panic symptoms in early adolescence predict high risk for late adolescent depression and suicide ideation (Barzilay et al., 2020).

Once the nurse establishes that there is no indication of a risk for suicide, the nurse assesses whether the individual may be depressed, lonely, and socially isolated. Panic attacks may be unpredictable, leading the person to be fearful of another attack. Self-esteem may be low as feelings of powerlessness emerge. The patient may be experiencing physical panic symptoms, such as dizziness and hyperventilation. Because the whole family is affected by one member's symptoms, the family's needs may need to be considered.

The patient's strengths should be considered in planning care. For example, the person may be motivated to gain more control through making lifestyle changes. There may be evidence of family support. Outcomes will depend upon the particular health care issue and the interventions that are agreed upon by the patient and nurse.

THERAPEUTIC RELATIONSHIP

The therapeutic relationship is a critical aspect of helping the person work toward recovery. These individuals may appear to be very nervous or anxious throughout the interaction. The nurse should help the patient relax and be comfortable with discussing fears and anxiety. A calm, understanding approach in a comfortable environment will help the person relax and be willing to engage in a therapeutic relationship.

MENTAL HEALTH NURSING INTERVENTIONS

Establishing Mental Health and Wellness Goals

The course of panic disorder culminates in phobic avoidance as the affected person attempts to avoid situations that increase panic. Even though identifying and avoiding anxiety-provoking situations are important during therapy, drastically changing lifestyle to avoid situations does not aid recovery. Goals and interventions that focus on developing a healthy lifestyle, supporting a sense of accomplishment and control, and reducing anxiety and panic are particularly helpful in reducing the number and severity of the attacks.

Physical Care

COVID-19 causes additional fear and anxiety in persons with panic disorder. Physical distancing may exacerbate feeling of seclusion and lead to detrimental prolonged health effects. Quarantine and social isolation can easily prevent an individual with panic disorder from following up with medical issues, such as changes in cardiac functioning. Fears of being infected may prevent the person from picking up regular medications from the local pharmacy or grocery shopping (Pera, 2020).

Psychiatric mental health nurses who make home visits often provide the person with both medical and mental health care. Nurses should consider providing care that is usually given by other nurses.

Teaching Breathing Control

Hyperventilation is common. Often, people are unaware that they take rapid shallow breaths when they become anxious.

Teaching patients breathing control can be helpful. Focus on the breathing and help them to identify the rate, pattern, and depth. If the breathing is rapid and shallow, reassure the patient that exercise and breathing practice can help change this breathing pattern. Then, assist the patient in practicing abdominal breathing by performing the following exercises:

- Instruct the patient to breathe deeply by inhaling slowly through the nose. Have them place a hand on the abdomen just beneath the rib cage.
- Instruct the patient to observe that when one is breathing deeply, the hand on the abdomen will actually rise.
- After the patient understands this process, ask them to inhale slowly through the nose while counting to five, pause, and then exhale slowly through pursed lips.
- While the patient exhales, direct attention to feeling the muscles relax, focusing on "letting go."

- Have the patient repeat the deep abdominal breathing for 10 breaths, pausing between each inhalation and exhalation. Count slowly. If the patient complains of light-headedness, reassure them that this is a normal feeling while deep breathing. Instruct the patient to stop for 30 seconds, breathe normally, and then start again.
- The patient should stop between each cycle of 10 breaths and monitor normal breathing for 30 seconds.
- This series of 10 slow abdominal breaths followed by 30 seconds of normal breathing should be repeated for 3 to 5 minutes.
- Help the patient to establish a time for daily practice of abdominal breathing.

Abdominal breathing may also be used to interrupt an episode of panic as it begins. After patients have learned to identify their own early signs of panic, they can learn the four-square method of breathing, which helps divert or decrease the severity of the attack. Patients should be instructed as follows:

- Advise the patient to practice during calm periods and to begin by inhaling slowly through the nose, count to four, and then hold the breath for a count of four.
- Direct the patient to exhale slowly through pursed lips to a count of four and then rest for a count of four (no breath).
- Finally, the patient may take two normal breaths and repeat the sequence.

After patients practice the skill, the nurse should assist them in identifying the physical cues that will alert them to use this calming technique.

Teaching Nutritional Planning

Maintaining regular and balanced eating habits reduces the likelihood of hypoglycemic episodes, light-headedness, and fatigue. To help teach the patient about healthful eating and ways to minimize physical factors contributing to anxiety:

- Advise the patient to reduce or eliminate substances in the diet that promote anxiety and panic, such as food coloring, monosodium glutamate, and caffeine (withdrawal from which may stimulate panic). Patients need to plan to reduce caffeine consumption and then eliminate it from their diet. Many OTC remedies are now used to boost energy or increase mental performance; some of these contain caffeine. A thorough assessment should be made of all OTC products used to assess the potential of anxiety-provoking ingredients.
- Instruct the patient to check each substance consumed and note whether symptoms of anxiety occur and whether the symptoms are relieved by not consuming the product.

Teaching Relaxation Techniques

Teaching the patient relaxation techniques is another way to help individuals with panic and anxiety disorders. Some are unaware of the tension in their bodies and first need to learn to monitor their own tension. Isometric exercises and progressive muscle relaxation are helpful methods to learn to differentiate muscle tension from muscle relaxation. This method of relaxation is also useful when patients have difficulty clearing the mind, focusing, or visualizing a scene, which are often required in other forms of relaxation, such as meditation. Box 27.5 provides one method of progressive muscle relaxation.

BOX 27.5

Teaching Progressive Muscle Relaxation

Choose a quiet, comfortable location where you will not be disturbed for 20 to 30 minutes. Your position may be lying or sitting, but all parts of your body should be supported, including your head. Wear loose clothing, taking off restrictive items, such as glasses and shoes.

Begin by closing your eyes and clearing your mind. Moving from head to toe, focus on each part of your body and assess the level of tension. Visualize each group of muscles as heavy and relaxed.

Take two or three slow abdominal breaths, pausing briefly between each breath. Imagine the tension flowing from your body.

Each muscle group listed subsequently should be tightened (or tensed isometrically) for 5 to 10 seconds and then abruptly released; visualize this group of muscles as heavy, limp, and relaxed for 15 to 20 seconds before tightening the next group of muscles. There are several methods to tighten each muscle group, and suggestions are provided subsequently. Each muscle group may be tightened two to three times until relaxed. Do not overtighten or strain. You should not experience pain.

- Hands: tighten by making fists
- Biceps: tighten by drawing forearms up and "making a muscle"
- Triceps: extend forearms straight, locking elbows
- Face: grimace, tightly shutting mouth and eyes
- Face: open mouth wide and raise eyebrows
- Neck: pull head forward to chest and tighten neck muscles
- Shoulders: raise shoulders toward ears
- Shoulders: push shoulders back as if touching them together
- Chest: take a deep breath and hold for 10 seconds
- Stomach: suck in your abdominal muscles
- Buttocks: pull buttocks together
- Thighs: straighten legs and squeeze muscles in thighs and hips
- Calves: pull toes carefully toward you, avoid cramps
- Feet: curl toes downward and point toes away from your body

Finally, repeat several deep abdominal breaths and mentally check your body for tension. Rest comfortably for several minutes, breathing normally, and visualize your body as warm and relaxed. Get up slowly when you are finished.

Promoting Increased Physical Activity

Physical exercise can effectively decrease the occurrence of panic attacks by reducing muscle tension, increasing metabolism, increasing serotonin levels, and relieving stress. Exercise programs reduce many of the precipitants of anxiety by improving circulation, digestion, endorphin stimulation, and tissue oxygenation. In addition, exercise lowers cholesterol levels, blood pressure, and weight. After assessing for contraindications to physical exercise, assist the patient in establishing a routine exercise program. Engaging in 10- to 20-minute sessions on treadmills or stationary bicycles two to three times weekly is ideal during the winter months. Casual walking or bike riding during warmer weather promotes health. Help the patient to identify community resources that promote exercise.

Wellness Challenges

Many of the strategies that promote wellness are the same as those used to treat anxiety. For the person who is anxious or fearful, the individual may be more comfortable with a gradual incorporation of the strategies. Many wellness strategies for the person who is anxious should focus on physical health. See Box 27.6.

Medication Interventions

Some antidepressants (e.g., SSRIs and serotonin–norepinephrine reuptake inhibitors [SNRIs]) and

---

BOX 27.6

Wellness Challenges for the Person with Anxiety

WELLNESS CHALLENGES

- Coping effectively with daily stresses without excessive worry
  - Strategies: Develop a daily schedule, allow time to relax, avoid trying to multitask, deep breathing, mindfulness
- Satisfying and enriching work
  - Strategies: Choose activities that are consistent with your skills and knowledge, consider other possibilities if job is too stressful.
- Incorporate physical activity, healthy foods, and adequate sleep into daily life
  - Strategies: Schedule regular physical activity, make a weekly menu of healthy meals, establish healthy sleep hygiene routines
- Developing a sense of connection, belong, and a support system
  - Strategies: Join a support group, seek out recreational activities with friends and families
- Expanding a sense of purpose and meaning in life
  - Strategies: Focus on goals, values, and beliefs, read inspiring stories or essays

antianxiety medication (e.g., benzodiazepines) are U.S. Food and Drug Administration, approved for treating people with panic disorders (see Table 27.4).

Selective Serotonin Reuptake Inhibitors

The SSRIs are recommended as the first drug option in the treatment of patients with panic disorder. They have the best safety profile, and if side effects occur, they tend to be present early in treatment before the therapeutic effect takes place. Hence, the SSRIs should be started at low doses and titrated every 5 to 7 days. Antidepressant therapy is recommended for long-term treatment of the disorder and antianxiety as adjunctive treatment (Zugliani et al., 2019). The SSRIs produce anxiolytic effects by increasing the transmission of serotonin by blocking serotonin reuptake at the presynaptic cleft. The initial increase in serotonergic activity with SSRIs may cause temporary increases in panic symptoms and even panic attacks. After 4 to 6 weeks of treatment, anxiety subsides, and the antianxiety effect of the medications begins (see Chapter 12). Increased serotonin activity in the brain is believed to decrease norepinephrine activity. This decrease lessens cardiovascular symptoms of tachycardia and increased blood pressure, which are associated with panic attacks. See Chapter 25 for administration and monitoring side effects.

NCLEXNOTE Psychopharmacologic treatment is almost always needed. Antidepressants are the medications of choice. Antianxiety medication is used only for short periods of time.

Serotonin–Norepinephrine Reuptake Inhibitors

The SNRIs increase levels of both serotonin and norepinephrine by blocking their reuptake presynaptically. Classified as antidepressants, the SNRIs are also used in anxiety disorders. Venlafaxine is the most commonly used SNRI (see Table 27.4). These medications have been shown to reduce the severity of panic and anticipatory anxiety. Similar to the SSRIs, they should not be abruptly discontinued (see Chapter 12).

Benzodiazepine Therapy

The high-potency benzodiazepines have produced antipanic effects; their therapeutic onset is much faster than that of antidepressants (see Table 27.4). Therefore, benzodiazepines are tremendously useful in treating intensely distressed patients. Alprazolam (Xanax), lorazepam (Ativan), and clonazepam (Klonopin) are widely used for panic disorder. They are well tolerated but carry the risk for withdrawal symptoms upon discontinuation of use (see Box 27.7). The benzodiazepines are still commonly used for panic disorder even though the SSRIs are recommended for first-line treatment of panic disorder (Quagliato et al., 2018).

Administering and Monitoring Benzodiazepines

Treatment may include administering benzodiazepines concurrently with antidepressants for the first 4 weeks and then tapering the benzodiazepine to a maintenance

TABLE 27.4	MEDICATION FOR PANIC DISORDER			
Medication	**Starting Dose (mg/day)**	**Therapeutic Dose**	**Side Effects**	
SSRIs			Class effects: nausea, anorexia, tremors, anxiety, sexual dysfunction, jitteriness, insomnia, suicidality	
Fluoxetine (Prozac)	10	20–60	Class effects	
Sertraline (Zoloft)	25	50–200	Class effects, loose stools	
Paroxetine (Paxil)	10	10–60	Class effects, drowsiness, fatigue	
Paroxetine (controlled release) (Paxil CR)	12.5	12.5–75	Class effects	
SNRIs			Class effects: nausea, sweating, dry mouth, dizziness, insomnia, somnolence, sexual dysfunction, hypertension	
Venlafaxine (extended release)	37.5	75–300	Class effects	
Benzodiazepines			Class effects: sedation, cognitive slowing, physical dependence	
Clonazepam (Klonopin)	0.25 TID	0.5–2.0 BID	Class effects	
Alprazolam (Xanax)	0.25 TID	0.5–1.5 TID	Class effects	

BID, two times a day; SNRIs, serotonin–norepinephrine reuptake inhibitors; SSRIs, selective serotonin reuptake inhibitors; TID, three times a day.

BOX 27.7

Alprazolam (Xanax)

DRUG CLASS: Antianxiety agent

RECEPTOR AFFINITY: Exact mechanism of action is unknown; believed to increase the effects of γ-aminobutyrate.

INDICATIONS: Management of anxiety disorders, short-term relief of anxiety symptoms or depression-related anxiety, panic attacks with or without agoraphobia.

ROUTES AND DOSAGES: Available in 0.25-, 0.5-, 1-, and 2-mg scored tablets.
Adults: For anxiety: Initially, 0.25 to 0.5 mg PO TID titrated to a maximum daily dose of 4 mg in divided doses. For panic disorder: Initially, 0.5 mg PO TID increased at 3- to 4-day intervals in increments of no more than 1 mg/day.
Geriatric Patients: Initially, 0.25 mg BID to TID, increased gradually as needed and tolerated.

HALF-LIFE (PEAK EFFECT): 12 to 15 hours (1 to 2 hours).

SELECTED ADVERSE REACTIONS: Transient mild drowsiness, initially; sedation, depression, lethargy, apathy, fatigue, light-headedness, disorientation, anger, hostility, restlessness, headache, confusion, crying, constipation, diarrhea, dry mouth, nausea, and possible drug dependence.

WARNINGS: Contraindicated in patients with psychosis, acute narrow-angle glaucoma, shock, acute alcoholic intoxication with depressed vital signs, pregnancy, labor and delivery, and breastfeeding. Use cautiously in patients with impaired hepatic or renal function and severe debilitating conditions. Risk for digitalis toxicity if given concurrently with digoxin. Increased CNS depression if taken with alcohol, other CNS depressants, and propoxyphene (Darvon).

SPECIFIC PATIENT AND FAMILY EDUCATION

- Avoid using alcohol, sleep-inducing drugs, and other OTC drugs.
- Take the drug exactly as prescribed, and do not stop taking the drug without consulting your primary health care provider.
- Take the drug with food if gastrointestinal upset occurs.
- Avoid driving a car or performing tasks that require alertness if drowsiness or dizziness occurs.
- Report any signs and symptoms of adverse reactions.
- Notify your primary health care provider if severe dizziness, weakness, or drowsiness persists or if rash or skin lesions, difficulty voiding, palpitations, or swelling of the extremities occurs.
- BID, two times a day; CNS, central nervous system; OTC, over-the-counter; PO, oral; TID, three times a day.

---

dose. This strategy provides rapid symptom relief but avoids the complications of long-term benzodiazepine use. Benzodiazepines with short half-lives do not accumulate in the body, but benzodiazepines with half-lives of longer than 24 hours tend to accumulate with long-term treatment, are removed more slowly, and produce less intense symptoms on discontinuation of use (see Chapter 12).

Short-acting benzodiazepines, such as alprazolam, are associated with rebound anxiety, or anxiety that increases after the peak effects of the medication have decreased. Medications with short half-lives (alprazolam, lorazepam) should be given in three or four doses spaced throughout the day, with a higher dose at bedtime to allay anxiety-related insomnia. Clonazepam, a longer-acting benzodiazepine, requires less frequent dosing and has a lower risk for rebound anxiety.

Because of their depressive CNS effects, benzodiazepines should not be used to treat patients with comorbid sleep apnea. In fact, these drugs may actually decrease the rate and depth of respirations. Exercise caution in older adult patients for these reasons. Discontinuing medication use requires a slow taper during a period of several weeks to avoid rebound anxiety and serious withdrawal symptoms. Benzodiazepines are not indicated in the chronic treatment of patients with substance use disorder but can be useful in quickly treating anxiety symptoms until other medications take effect.

Symptoms associated with withdrawal of benzodiazepine therapy are more likely to occur after high doses and long-term therapy. They can also occur after short-term therapy. Withdrawal symptoms manifest in several ways, including psychological (e.g., apprehension, irritability, agitation).

Monitoring Side Effects

SSRIs should not be given with monoamine oxidase inhibitors (MAOIs) because of potential drug interaction. Drugs that interact with benzodiazepines include the tricyclic antidepressants (TCAs) and digoxin; interaction may result in increased serum TCA or digoxin levels. Alcohol and other CNS depressants, when used with benzodiazepines, increase CNS depression. Their concomitant use is contraindicated. Histamine-2 blockers (e.g., cimetidine) used with benzodiazepines may potentiate sedative effects. Monitor closely for effectiveness in patients who smoke; cigarette smoking may increase the clearance of benzodiazepines.

Management of Complications

The side effects of benzodiazepine medications generally include headache, confusion, dizziness, disorientation, sedation, and visual disturbances. Sedation should be monitored after beginning medication use or increasing the dose. The patient should avoid operating heavy machinery until the sedative effects are known.

Concurrent use of SSRIs and the MAOIs is contraindicated. These antidepressants should not be given together.

Teaching Points

Warn patients to avoid alcohol because of the chance of CNS depression. In addition, warn them not to operate heavy machinery until the sedative effects of the medication are known.

Psychosocial Interventions

Therapeutic Interactions

Peplau (1989) devised general guidelines for nursing interventions that might be successful in treating patients with anxiety. These interventions help the patient attend to and react to input other than the subjective experience of anxiety. They are designed to help the patient focus on other stimuli and cope with anxiety in any form (Table 27.5). These general interventions apply to all anxiety disorders and therefore are not reiterated in subsequent sections.

Enhancing Cognitive Functioning

Distraction

After patients can identify the early symptoms of panic, they may learn to implement distraction behaviors that take the focus off the physical sensations. Some activities include initiating conversation with a nearby person or engaging in physical activity (e.g., walking, gardening, or housecleaning). Performing simple repetitive activities such as snapping a rubber band against the wrist, counting backward from 100 by 3s, or counting objects along the roadway might also deter an attack.

Reframing

Reframing is a cognitive technique that can change the way a situation, event, or person is viewed and reduce the impact of anxiety-provoking thoughts. People with anxiety disorders often view themselves negatively and use "should statements" and "negative labels." Should statements lead to rigid rules and unrealistic expectations? By encouraging patients to avoid the use of should statements and reframe their views, they can change their beliefs to be more realistic. For example, if a patient says, "I should be a better parent" or "I'm a useless failure," the nurse could ask the person to identify the positive aspects of parenting and other successes.

TABLE 27.5	NURSING INTERVENTIONS BASED ON DEGREES OF ANXIETY
Degree of Anxiety	**Nursing Interventions**
Mild	Assist patient to use the energy anxiety provides to encourage learning.
Moderate	Encourage patient to talk: to focus on one experience, to describe it fully, and then to formulate the patient's generalizations about that experience.
Severe	Allow relief behaviors to be used but do not ask about them. Encourage the patient to talk: ventilation of random ideas is likely to reduce anxiety to a moderate level.
Panic	Stay with the patient. Allow pacing and walk with the patient. No content inputs to the patient's thinking should be made by the nurse. (They burden the patient, who will distort them.) Be direct with the fewest number of words: e.g., "Drink this" (give liquids to replace lost fluids and to relieve dry mouth); "Say what's happening to you," "Talk about yourself," or "Tell what you feel now" (to encourage ventilation and externalization of inner, frightening experience). Pick up on what the patient says, for example, Patient: "What's happening to me—how did I get here?" Nurse: "Say what you notice." Use short phrases to the point of the patient's comment. Do not touch the patient; patients experiencing panic are very concerned about survival, are experiencing a grave threat to self, and usually distort intentions of all invasions of their personal space.

Adapted from Peplau, H. (1989). Theoretical constructs: Anxiety, self, and hallucinations. In A. O'Toole & S. Welt (Eds.), *Interpersonal theory in nursing practice: Selected works of Hildegarde E. Peplau*. Springer.

Consider This:
Could distraction and reframing help Doug reduce his anxiety and frequency of his panic attacks? What interventions would you recommend and why?

Positive Self-Talk

During states of increased anxiety and panic, individuals can learn to counter fearful or negative thoughts by using another cognitive approach. **Positive self-talk** involves planning and rehearsing positive coping statements "This is only anxiety, and it will pass," "I can handle these symptoms," and "I'll get through this" are examples of positive self-talk. These types of positive statements can give the individual a focal point and reduce fear when panic symptoms begin. Handheld cards that offer positive statements can be carried in a purse or wallet so the person can retrieve them quickly when panic symptoms are felt (Box 27.8).

BOX 27.8 • THERAPEUTIC DIALOGUE PANIC DISORDER

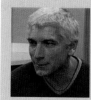

Doug is admitted to an inpatient unit following another severe panic attack. He had an argument with his high school son, who continues to use alcohol and marijuana. Financial problems are also escalating.

INEFFECTIVE APPROACH

Nurse: Oh.... Why are you crying?

Doug: (Looks up, gives a nervous chuckle.) Obviously, because I'm upset. I am tired of living this way. I just want to be normal again. I can't even remember what that feels like.

Nurse: You look normal to me. Everyone has bad days. It'll pass.

Doug: I've felt this way longer than you've been alive. I've tried everything, and nothing works.

Nurse: You're not the first depressed person that I've taken care of. You just need to go to groups and stay out of your room more. You'll start feeling better.

Doug: (Angrily) Oh, it's just that easy. You have no idea what I'm going through! You don't know me! You're just a kid.

Nurse: I can help you if you help yourself. A group starts in 5 minutes, and I'd like to see you there.

Doug: I'm not going to no damn group! I want to be alone so I can think!

Nurse: (Looks about anxiously.) Maybe I should come back after you've calmed down a little.

EFFECTIVE APPROACH

Nurse: Doug, I noticed that you are staying in your room more today. What's troubling you?

Doug: (Looks up) I feel like I've lost complete control of my life. I'm so anxious, and nothing helps. I'm tired of it.

Nurse: I see. That must be difficult. Can you tell me more about what you are feeling right now?

Doug: I feel like I'm going crazy. I worry all the time about having panic attacks. They make me scared I'm going to die. Sometimes I think I'd be better off dead.

Nurse: (Remains silent, continues to give eye contact.)

Doug: Do you know what it's like to be a prisoner to your emotions? I can't even go to work sometimes, and when I do, it's terrifying. I don't know what to think anymore.

Nurse: Doug, you have lived with this disorder for a long time. You say that the medications do not work to your liking, but what has helped you in the past?

Doug: Well, I learned in relaxation group that panic symptoms are probably caused by chemicals in my brain that are not working correctly. I learned that medications can help, but they don't work well for me. I tried an exposure plan and relaxation techniques to deal with my fears of leaving the house and my chronic anxiety. That did help some, but it's scary to do.

Nurse: It sounds like you have learned a lot about your illness, one that can be treated, so that you don't always have to feel this way.

Doug: This is easier to say right now when I'm here and can get help if I need it. It's hard to remember this when I'm in the middle of a panic attack and think I'm dying.

Nurse: It's harder when you're alone?

Doug: Much harder! And I'm alone so much of the time.

Nurse: Let's talk about some ways you can manage your panics when you're alone. Tell me some of the techniques you've learned.

CRITICAL THINKING CHALLENGE

• What tone is established by the nurse's opening question in the first scenario?

• Which therapeutic communication techniques did the nurse use in the second scenario to avoid the pitfalls encountered in the first scenario?

• What information was uncovered in the second scenario that was not touched on in the first?

• What predictions can you make about the interpersonal relationship likely to develop between the nurse and the patient in each scenario?

NCLEXNOTE Cognitive interventions give patients with anxiety a sense of control over the recurring threats of panic and obsessions.

Psychoeducation

Psychoeducation programs help to teach patients and families about the symptoms of panic. Individuals with panic disorder legitimately fear going crazy, losing control, or dying because of their physical symptoms. Attempting to convince a patient that such fears are groundless only heightens anxiety and impedes communication. Information and physical evidence (e.g., electrocardiogram results, laboratory test results) should be presented in a caring and open manner that demonstrates acceptance and understanding of their situation.

Box 27.9 suggests topics for individual or small-group discussion. It is especially important to cover such topics as the differences between panic attacks and heart attacks, the difference between panic disorder and other psychiatric disorders, and the effectiveness of various treatment methods.

Wellness Strategies

Individuals with panic disorder, especially those with significant anxiety sensitivity, may need assistance in reevaluating their lifestyle. Time management can be a useful tool. In the workplace or at home, underestimating the time needed to complete a chore or being overly involved in several activities at once increases stress and anxiety. Procrastination, lack of assertiveness, and difficulties with prioritizing or delegating tasks intensify these problems.

Writing a list of chores to be completed and estimating time to complete them provide concrete feedback to the individual. Crossing out each activity as it is completed helps the patient to regain a sense of control and accomplishment. Large tasks should be broken into a series of smaller tasks to minimize stress and maximize sense of achievement. Rest, relaxation, and family time—frequently omitted from the daily schedule—must be included.

Providing Family Education

In addition to learning the symptoms of panic disorder, nurses should have information sheets or pamphlets available concerning the disorder and any medications prescribed. Parents, especially single parents, will need assistance in child-rearing and may benefit from services designed to provide some respite. Moreover, the entire family will need support in adjusting to the disorder. A referral for family therapy is indicated, because involving the entire family in the therapy process is imperative. Families experience the symptoms, treatments, clinical setbacks, and recovery from chronic mental illnesses as a unit. Misunderstandings, misconceptions, false information, and the stigma of mental illness, singly or collectively, impede recovery efforts.

Convening Support Groups

Participation in supportive groups is helpful in managing anxiety and fears (Barkowski et al., 2020). Persons with panic disorders are usually comfortable in groups with individuals who have other mental disorders and issues. As they participate in a group, they are able to share their fears of an impending panic attack and identify strategies to deal with their fears.

Developing Recovery-Oriented Rehabilitation Strategies

Recovery begins with an understanding of the components of recovery discussed in Chapters 2 and 9. As the components of recovery are explained, the nurse should continue to engage the person in a collaborative decision-making process. The nurse's role in developing recovery-oriented strategies is to negotiate the most effective, evidence-based strategies. The nurse should encourage healthy behaviors supporting wellness as well as strategies directed toward illness management. Empowering the person to make choices that best match the individual's lifestyle increases the likelihood of treatment adherence and recovery. It will also foster a feeling of hopefulness. Some treatment recommendations will not be followed. For example, some persons will attend support groups, but others only want individual psychotherapy. The nurse should encourage the patient to commit to as many recovery strategies that are realistic.

BOX 27.9

Panic Disorder

When caring for a patient with panic disorder, be sure to include the following topic areas in the teaching plan:
- Psychopharmacologic agents (anxiolytics or antidepressants) if ordered, including drug action, dosage, frequency, and possible adverse effects
- Breathing control measures
- Nutrition
- Exercise
- Progressive muscle relaxation
- Distraction behaviors
- Exposure therapy
- Time management
- Positive coping strategies

Evaluation and Treatment Outcomes

Although many researchers consider panic disorder a chronic, long-term condition, the positive results from outcome studies should be shared with patients to provide encouragement and optimism that patients can learn to manage these symptoms. Outcome studies have demonstrated success with panic control treatment, CBT therapy, exposure therapy, and various medications specific to certain symptoms.

Continuum of Care

Emergency Care

Because individuals with panic disorder are likely to first present for treatment in an emergency department or primary care setting, nurses working in these settings should be involved in early recognition and referral. Consultation with a psychiatrist or mental health professional by the primary care physician can decrease both costs and overall patient symptoms. Several interventions may be useful in reducing the number of emergency department visits related to panic symptoms. Psychiatric consultation and nursing education can be provided in the emergency department to explore other avenues of treatment. Remembering that the patient experiencing a panic attack is in crisis, nurses can take several measures to help alleviate symptoms, including the following:

- Stay with the patient and maintain a calm demeanor. (Anxiety often produces more anxiety, and a calm presence will help calm the patient.)

- Reassure the patient that you will not leave, that this episode will pass, and that they are in a safe place. (The patient often fears dying and cannot see beyond the panic attack.)

- Give clear concise directions using short sentences. Do not use medical jargon.

- Walk or pace with the patient to an environment with minimal stimulation. (The patient in panic has excessive energy.)

- Administer PRN (i.e., as-needed) anxiolytic medications as ordered and appropriate. (Pharmacotherapy is effective in treating those patients with acute panic attack.)

After the panic attack has resolved, allow the patient to vent their feelings. This often helps the patient in clarifying their feelings.

Inpatient-Focused Care

Inpatient settings provide control for the stabilization of the acute panic symptoms and initiation of recovery-oriented strategies. Medication use often is initiated here because patients who show initial panic symptoms require in-depth assessment to determine the cause. As recovery begins, crisis stabilization, medication management, milieu therapy, and psychotherapies are introduced, and outpatient discharge linkage appointments are set.

Community Care

Most individuals with panic disorder are treated on an outpatient basis. Referral lists of community resources and support groups are useful in this setting. A discussion about the recovery and the importance of the 10 components helps healing begin (see Chapters 2 and 9). Nurses are more directly involved in treatment, conducting psychoeducation groups on relaxation and breathing techniques, symptom management, and anger management. Advanced practice nurses conduct CBT and individual and family psychotherapy. In addition, medication monitoring groups reemphasize the role of medications, monitor for side effects, and enhance treatment compliance overall.

As with any disorder, a continuum of patient care across multiple settings is crucial. Patients are treated in the least restrictive environment that will meet their safety needs. As the patient progresses through treatment, the environment of care changes from an emergency or inpatient setting to outpatient clinics or individual therapy sessions.

Virtual Mental Health Care

Virtual mental health services are more important now because of the impact of the coronavirus pandemic. The pandemic increased anxieties, depression, and grief. Face-to-face therapies increase anxiety about the risk of infection in individuals who already have significant anxieties. Virtual treatment is ideal. Most therapies discussed in this chapter are available in a virtual format. The patient needs to be cautioned about selecting services that are credible. Support groups such as the National Alliance on Mental Illness and the Anxiety and Depression Association of America are easily accessed online and provide resources for clinicians and patients.

Integration With Primary Care

Coordination of care between mental health and primary care leads to safer management of anxiety disorders. Some groups are more likely to seek out care in primary care rather than in mental health clinics. People with anxiety disorders are often treated in the primary care environment, particularly those who experience panic disorder.

Because panic attacks mimic cardiac difficulties, it is important that the patient continues to seek health care monitoring with medical clinicians. Primary care providers are often asked to treat the physical consequences of anxiety, such as hypertension and obesity (Penninx & Lange, 2018). Anxiety can be caused by physical health issues, such as immune, metabolic, and cardiovascular problems. Many prescription and non-prescription drugs can cause anxiety such as asthma, blood pressure, steroid, and thyroid medications. Without coordination of care, the clinicians will not be able to make a meaningful assessment, which could lead to the wrong treatment (Love & Love, 2019).

GENERALIZED ANXIETY DISORDER

Generally speaking, patients with generalized anxiety disorder (GAD) feel frustrated, disgusted with life, demoralized, and hopeless. They may state that they cannot remember a time that they did not feel anxious. They experience a sense of ill-being and uneasiness and a fear of imminent disaster. Over time, they may recognize that their chronic tension and anxiety are unreasonable.

Clinical Course

The onset of GAD is insidious. Many patients complain of being chronic worriers. GAD affects individuals of all ages. About half of individuals with GAD report an onset in childhood or adolescence, although onset after 20 years of age is also common. Adults with GAD often worry about matters such as their job, household finances, health of family members, or simple matters (e.g., household chores or being late for appointments). The intensity of the worry fluctuates and stress tends to intensify the worry and anxiety symptoms (APA, 2013).

Patients with GAD may exhibit mild depressive symptoms, such as dysphoria. They are also highly somatic, with complaints of multiple clusters of physical symptoms, including muscle aches, soreness, and gastrointestinal ailments. In addition to physical complaints, patients with GAD often experience poor sleep habits, irritability, trembling, twitching, poor concentration, and an exaggerated startle response. People with this disorder often are seen in a primary care setting with somatic symptoms (DeMartini et al., 2019).

Diagnostic Criteria

GAD is characterized by excessive worry and anxiety (apprehensive expectation) for at least 6 months. The anxiety does not usually pertain to a specific situation; rather, it concerns several real-life activities or events. Ultimately, excessive worry and anxiety cause great distress and interfere with the patient's daily personal or social life.

BOX 27.10

Generalized Anxiety Disorder

When caring for the patient with GAD, be sure to include the following topic areas in the teaching plan:
- Psychopharmacologic agents (benzodiazepines, antidepressants, nonbenzodiazepine anxiolytics, β-blockers) if ordered, including drug action, dosage, frequency, and possible adverse effects
- Breathing control
- Nutrition and diet restriction
- Sleep measures
- Progressive muscle relaxation
- Time management
- Positive coping strategies

Nursing Care

Nursing care for the person with GAD is similar to the care of the individual with a panic disorder. In many instances, antidepressants and an antianxiety agent will be prescribed. Nursing interventions should focus on helping the person target specific areas of anxiety and reducing the impact of the anxiety. See Box 27.10.

OTHER ANXIETY DISORDERS

Other disorders exist that have anxiety as their defining feature. These include generalized phobia, agoraphobia, specific phobias, and social anxiety disorder.

Agoraphobia

Agoraphobia is fear or anxiety triggered by about two or more situations such as using public transportation, being in open spaces, being in enclosed places, standing in line, being in a crowd, or being outside of the home alone (APA, 2013). When these situations occur, the individual believes that something terrible might happen and that escape may be difficult. The individual may experience panic like symptoms or other embarrassing symptoms (e.g., vomiting, diarrhea) (APA, 2013). Agoraphobia leads to avoidance behaviors. Such avoidance interferes with routine functioning and eventually renders the person afraid to leave the safety of home. Some affected individuals continue to face feared situations but with significant trepidation (i.e., going in public only to pay bills or to take children to school). Agoraphobia may occur with panic disorder but is considered a separate disorder.

Specific Phobia

Specific phobia disorder is marked by persistent fear of clearly discernible, circumscribed objects or situations, which often leads to avoidance behaviors. Phobic objects can include animals (e.g., spiders, snakes), natural environment (e.g., heights, storms), blood injection injury (e.g., fear of blood, injections), and situational (e.g., elevators, enclosed spaces). The lifetime prevalence rates range from 7% to 9%, and the disorder generally affects women twice as much as men (APA, 2013). It has a bimodal distribution, peaking in childhood and then again in the 20s. The focus of the fear in specific phobia may result from the anticipation of being harmed by the phobic object. For example, dogs are feared because of the chance of being bitten or automobiles are feared because of the potential of crashing. The focus of fear may likewise be associated with concerns about losing control, panicking, or fainting on exposure to the phobic object.

Anxiety is usually felt immediately on exposure to the phobic object; the level of anxiety is usually related to both the proximity of the object and the degree to which escape is possible. For example, anxiety heightens as a cat approaches a person who fears cats and lessens when the cat moves away. At times, the level of anxiety escalates to a full panic attack, particularly when the person must remain in a situation from which escape is deemed to be impossible. Fear of specific objects is fairly common, and the diagnosis of specific phobia is not made unless the fear significantly interferes with functioning or causes marked distress. Assessment differentiates simple phobia from other diagnoses with overlapping symptoms. Box 27.11 lists a number of specific phobias. Among

---

BOX 27.11
Common Phobias

- Acrophobia: fear of heights
- Agoraphobia: fear of open spaces
- Ailurophobia: fear of cats
- Algophobia: fear of pain
- Arachnophobia: fear of spiders
- Brontophobia: fear of thunder
- Claustrophobia: fear of closed spaces
- Cynophobia: fear of dogs
- Entomophobia: fear of insects
- Hematophobia: fear of blood
- Microphobia: fear of germs
- Nyctophobia: fear of night or dark places
- Ophidiophobia: fear of snakes
- Phonophobia: fear of loud noises
- Photophobia: fear of light
- Pyrophobia: fear of fire
- Topophobia: fear of a place, like a stage
- Xenophobia: fear of strangers
- Zoophobia: fear of animal or animals

---

adult patients who are seen in clinical settings, the most-to-least common phobias are situational phobias, natural environment phobias, blood injection, injury phobia, and animal phobias (APA, 2013).

Blood injection injury phobia merits special consideration because the phobia involves medical treatments. The physiologic processes that are exhibited during phobic exposure include a strong vasovagal response, which significantly increases blood pressure and pulse, followed by deceleration of the pulse and lowering of blood pressure in the patient. Monitor closely when giving required injections or medical treatments.

About 75% of patients with blood injection injury phobia report fainting on exposure. Factors that may predispose individuals to specific phobias may include traumatic events; unexpected panic attacks in the presence of the phobic object or situation; observation of others experiencing a trauma; or repeated exposure to information warning of dangers, such as parents repeatedly warning young children that dogs bite.

Phobic content must be evaluated from an ethnic or cultural background. In many cultures, fears of spirits or magic are common. They should be considered part of a disorder only if the fear is excessive in the context of the culture, causes the individual significant distress, or impairs the ability to function. Psychotropic drugs have not been effective in the treatment of specific phobia. Anxiolytics may give short-term relief of phobic anxiety, but no evidence confirms that they affect the course of the disorder. The treatment of choice for specific phobia is exposure therapy. Patients who are highly motivated can experience success with treatment (Böhnlein et al., 2020).

Social Anxiety Disorder (Social Phobia)

Social anxiety disorder involves a persistent fear of social or performance situations in which embarrassment may occur. Exposure to a feared social or performance situation nearly always provokes immediate anxiety and may trigger panic attacks. People with social anxiety disorder fear that others will scrutinize their behavior and judge them negatively. They often do not speak up in crowds out of fear of embarrassment. They go to great lengths to avoid feared situations. If avoidance is not possible, they suffer through the situation with visible anxiety (APA, 2013).

People with social anxiety disorder appear to be highly sensitive to disapproval or criticism, tend to evaluate themselves negatively, and have poor self-esteem and a distorted view of their personal strengths and weaknesses. They may magnify their personal flaws and underrate any talents. They often believe others would act with more assertiveness in a given social situation. Women are more likely to have social anxiety disorder, but both men and women tend to have difficulties with dating and with sexual relationships (Asher et al., 2017). Children tend to underachieve in school because of test-taking anxiety. This is an important area that should be assessed in all patients. See Box 27.12.

Generalized social anxiety disorder is diagnosed when the individual experiences fears related to most social situations, including public performances and social interactions. These individuals are likely to demonstrate deficiencies in social skills, and their phobias interfere with their ability to function (Asher et al., 2017).

People with social anxiety disorder fear and avoid only one or two social situations. Classic examples of such situations are eating, writing, or speaking in public or using public bathrooms. The most common fears for individuals with social anxiety disorder are public speaking, fear of meeting strangers, eating in public, writing in public, using public restrooms, and being stared at or being the center of attention.

Pharmacotherapy is a relatively new area of research in treating patients with social anxiety disorder. SSRIs are used to treat those with social anxiety disorder because they significantly reduce social anxiety and phobic avoidance. Benzodiazepines are also used to reduce anxiety caused by phobias. Providing referrals for appropriate psychiatric treatment is a critical nursing intervention.

SUMMARY OF KEY POINTS

- Anxiety is an unavoidable human condition. Anxiety becomes an anxiety disorder when anxiety and fear significantly interferes with social and occupational functioning.

- Anxiety-related disorders are the most common of all psychiatric disorders and comprise several disorders, including panic disorder.

- The anxiety disorders share the common symptom of recurring anxiety but differ in symptom profiles. Panic attacks can occur in many different disorders. Physical symptoms can mimic a heart attack.

- Panic disorder can occur throughout the lifespan but is most common in adulthood. Those experiencing anxiety disorders have a high level of physical and emotional illness and often experience dual diagnoses with other anxiety disorders, substance use disorder, or depression. These disorders often render individuals unable to function effectively at home or at a job.

- There appears to be a familial predisposition to panic disorders. Serotonin and norepinephrine are both implicated in panic disorders. The hypothalamic–pituitary–adrenal axis and activation of the stress hormones are also implicated in the expression of this disorder.

- Patients with panic disorder are often seen in various health care settings, frequently in hospital emergency departments or clinics, presenting with a confusing array of physical and emotional symptoms. Skillful assessment is required to eliminate possible life-threatening causes.

- Treatment approaches for all anxiety-related disorders are somewhat similar, including pharmacotherapy, psychological treatments, or often a combination of both.

- Antidepressants are the first-line medication treatment and are often included in psychosocial therapies such as cognitive-behavior therapy, and exposure therapy. Virtual mental health strategies such as telehealth, mobile apps provide most of the same therapies as face-to-face therapies.

- Nursing interventions include helping patients manage a panic attack, promoting healthy diet, exercise and sleep hygiene habits, medication administration and monitoring, psychoeducation, and cognitive interventions.

BOX 27.12
A Mental Health Recovery Journey

Hickmott, J., & Raeburn, T. (2020). Mouse to man, a mental health recovery journey. Journal of Psychiatric and Mental Health Nursing, *27*(6), 844–849. https://doi.org/10.1111/jpm.12621

THE QUESTION: What are the insights that can be gained from narratives written by people with lived experience of mental illness?

METHODS: A lived experience about recovery from a social anxiety disorder that began in childhood is written in first person.

FINDINGS: Recovery is an ongoing process of growth and development. His symptoms began at age 11 years when his parents divorced and he began missing school, not communicating with teachers, and avoiding doctors. The author did not recognize that he needed help until after he attended a clinic at age 16 years. He experienced treatment in a variety of settings for social anxiety. He did not really engage in recovery until he began seeing a nurse who was more like a coach and he was the player. Within this collaborative relationship, he learned a lot about what was going on with him. He gained insight, finished university, and is now a Peer Worker.

IMPLICATIONS FOR NURSING: This narrative supports the need for recovery-oriented mental health nursing and the hypothesis that recovery is possible. Hope was important throughout his journey. Recovery takes time. In this instance, it was 2 years of frequent visits. This narrative emphasizes that individuals with mental health issues are more than symptoms. It is important to see the whole person.

■ Many persons with panic disorders have other health problems that are treated in primary care. Mental and physical health needs should be integrated with both primary and mental health services.

CRITICAL THINKING CHALLENGES

1. A patient is unable to focus on your directions. He does not seem to notice others in the room; instead, he is intent on cutting his food into small pieces. Applying Peplau stages of anxiety, what level of anxiety is he experiencing?

2. Compare and contrast the following treatment modalities for anxiety disorders: systematic desensitization, implosive therapy, exposure therapy, and CBT.

3. Identify the major nursing assessment areas for a person experiencing a panic disorder.

4. A patient asks you how to prevent hyperventilation. How would you answer her question?

5. Delineate the differences in treatment effects of antidepressants versus antianxiety medication in the treatment of panic disorder.

6. Compare the various phobias that people experience. What interventions should a nurse use for a person who has a blood injection injury phobia?

7. How might one differentiate shyness from social anxiety disorder?

A related Psychiatric-Mental Health Nursing video on the topic of Anxiety is available at http://thepoint.lww.com/Boyd7e.

A Practice and Learn Activity related to the video on the topic of Anxiety is available at http://thepoint.lww.com/Boyd7e.

Unfolding Patient Stories: Linda Waterfall • Part 2

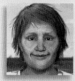

Recall from Unit II Linda Waterfall, a 48-year-old Native American diagnosed with an aggressive form of breast cancer. The recommended treatment is a mastectomy followed by chemotherapy, which she refused. What is the association between her illness and episodes of severe anxiety since diagnosis? How can a secondary mental health disorder contribute to her physical decline from cancer? What psychosocial assessments and interventions should the nurse incorporate into the plan of care to manage her anxiety?

Care for Linda and other patients in a realistic virtual environment: *vSim* for Nursing (thepoint.lww.com/vSimMental Health). Practice documenting these patients' care in DocuCare (thepoint.lww.com/DocuCareEHR).

REFERENCES

Aghayan, S. S., Farajzadeh, A., Bagheri-Hosseinabadi, Z., Fadaei, H., Yarmohammadi, M., & Jafarisani, M. (2020). Elevated homocysteine, as a biomarker of cardiac injury, in panic disorder patients due to oxidative stress. *Brain and Behavior*, e01851. Advance online publication. https://doi.org/10.1002/brb3.1851

American Psychiatric Association. (2013). *Diagnostic and statistical manual of mental disorders DSM-5 (5th ed.)*. Author.

Andreescu, C., & Lee, S. (2020). Anxiety disorders in the elderly. *Advances in Experimental Medicine and Biology*, 1191, 561–576. https://doi.org/10.1007/978-981-32-9705-0_28

Asher, M., Asnaani, A., & Aderka, I. M. (2017). Gender differences in social anxiety disorder: A review. *Clinical Psychology Review*, 56, 1–7. https://doi.org/10/10.1016/f.cpr.05-044

Asok, A., Kandel, E. R., & Rayman, J. B. (2019). The neurobiology of fear generalization. *Frontiers in Behavioral Neuroscience*, 2, 329. https://doi.org/10.3389/fnbeh.2018.00329

Assari, S. (2017). Psychiatric disorders differently correlate with physical self-rated health across ethnic groups. *Journal of Personalized Medicine*, 7(4), e6. https://doi.org/10.3390/jpm7040006

Baker, H. J., & Waite, P. (2020). The identification and psychological treatment of panic disorder in adolescents: A survey of CAMHS clinicians. *Child and Adolescent Mental Health*, 25(3), 135–142. https://doi.org/10.1111/camh.1237210.1097/YIC.0000000000000078

Barkowski, S., Schwartze, D., Strauss, B., Burlingame, G. M., & Rosendahl, J. (2020). Efficacy of group psychotherapy for anxiety disorders: A systematic review and meta-analysis. *Psychotherapy Research*, 30(8), 965–982. https://doi.org/10.1080/10503307.2020.1729440

Barzilay, R., White, L. K., Moore, T. M., Calkins, M. E., Taylor, J. H., Patrick, A., Huque, Z. M., Young, J. F., Ruparel, K., Pine, D. S., Gur, R. C., & Gur, R. E. (2020). Association of anxiety phenotypes with risk of depression and suicidal ideation in community youth. *Depression and Anxiety*, 37(9), 851–861. https://doi.org/10.1002/da.23060

Bilet, T., Olsen, T., Andersen, J. R., & Martinsen, E. W. (2020). Cognitive behavioral group therapy for panic disorder in a general clinical setting: a prospective cohort study with 12 to 31-years follow-up. *BMC psychiatry*, 20(1), 259. https://doi.org/10.1186/s12888-020-02679-w

Böhnlein, J., Altegoer, L., Muck, N. K., Roesmann, K., Redlich, R., Dannlowski, U., & Leehr, E. J. (2020). Factors influencing the success of exposure therapy for specific phobia: A systematic review. *Neuroscience and Biobehavioral Reviews*, 108, 796–820. https://doi.org/10.1016/j.neubiorev.2019.12.009

Bourdon, J. L., Savage, J. E., Verhulst, B., Carney, D. M., Brotman, M. A., Pine, D. S., Leibenluft, E., Roberson-Nay, R., & Hettema, J. M. (2019). The genetic and environmental relationship between childhood behavioral inhibition and preadolescent anxiety. *Twin Research and Human Genetics*. https://doi.org/10.1017/thg.2018.73

Cackovic, C., Nazir, S., & Marwaha, R. Panic disorder. [June 25, 2020]. In: *StatPearls* [Internet]. StatPearls Publishing; January 2020. https://www.ncbi.nlm.nih.gov/books/NBK430973

Carballo, J. J., Llorente, C., Kehrmann, L., Flamarique, I., Zuddas, A., Purper-Ouakil, D., Hoekstra, P. J., Coghill, D., Schulze, U., Dittmann, R. W., Buitelaar, J. K., Castro-Fornieles, J., Lievesley, K., Santosh, P., Arango, C., & STOP Consortium (2020). (2019). Psychosocial risk factors for suicidality in children and adolescents. *European Child & Adolescent Psychiatry*, 1–8. 29(6), 759–776. https://doi.org/10.1007/s00787-018-01270-9

DeMartini, J., Patel, G., & Fancher, T. L. (2019). Generalized anxiety disorder. *Annals of Internal Medicine*, 170(7), ITC49–ITC64. https://doi.org/10.7326/AITC201904020

Forstner, A. J., Awasthi, S., Wolf, C., Maron, E., Erhardt, A., Czamara, D., Eriksson, E., Lavebratt, C., Allgulander, C., Friedrich, N., Becker, J., Hecker, J., Rambau, S., Conrad, R., Geiser, F., McMahon, F. J., Moebus, S., Hess, T., Buerfent, B. C., Hoffmann, P., … Schumacher, J. (2019). Genome-wide association study of panic disorder reveals genetic overlap with neuroticism and depression. *Molecular Psychiatry*, 10.1038/s41380-019-0590-2. Advance online publication. https://doi.org/10.1038/s41380-019-0590-2

Garcia, S. C., Mikhail, M. E., Keel, P. K., Burt, S. A., Neale, M. C., Boker, S., & Klump, K. L. (2020). Increased rates of eating disorders and their symptoms in women with major depressive disorder and anxiety disorders. *The International Journal of Eating Disorders*, 10.1002/eat.23366. Advance online publication. https://doi.org/10.1002/eat.23366

Hamilton, M. (1959). The assessment of anxiety states by rating. *British Journal of Medical Psychology*, 32, 50–55.

Hornboll, B., Macoveanu, J., Nejad, A., Rowe, J., Elliott, R., Knudsen, G. M., Siebner, H. R., & Paulson, O. B. (2018). Neuroticism predicts the impact of serotonin challenges on fear processing in subgenual anterior cingulate cortex. *Scientific Reports*, *8*, 17889. https://doi.org/10.1038/s41598-018-36350-y

Kolek, A., Prasko, J., Ociskova, M., Holubova, M., Vanek, J., Grambal, A., & Slepecky, M. (2019). Severity of panic disorder, adverse events in childhood, dissociation, self-stigma and comorbid personality disorders Part 2: Therapeutic effectiveness of a combined cognitive behavioural therapy and pharmacotherapy in treatment-resistant inpatients. *Neurondocrinology Letters*, *40*(6), 271–283.

Kroenke, K., Krebs, E. E., Turk, D., Von Korff, M., Bair, M. J., Allen, K. D., Sandbrink, F., Cheville, A. L., DeBar, L., Lorenz, K. A., & Kerns, R. D. (2019). Core outcome measures for chronic musculoskeletal pain research: Recommendations from a Veterans Health Administration work group. *Pain Medicine*. https://doi.org/10.1093/pm/pny279

Love, A. S., & Love, R. (2019). Anxiety disorders in primary care settings. *The Nursing Clinics of North America*, *54*(4), 473–493. https://doi.org/10.1016/j.cnur.2019.07.002

Meuret, A. E., Tunnell, N., & Roque, A. (2020). Anxiety disorders and medical comorbidity: Treatment implications. *Advances in Experimental Medicine and Biology*, *1191*, 237–261. https://doi.org/10.1007/978-981-32-9705-0_15

Moitra, E., Duarte-Velez, Y., Lewis-Fernández, R., Weisberg, R. B., & Keller, M. B. (2018). Examination of ataque de nervios and ataque de nervios like events in a diverse sample of adults with anxiety disorders. *Depression and Anxiety*, 1190–1197. https://doi.org/10.1002/da.22853

Olaya, B., Moneta, M. V., Miret, M., Ayuso-Mateos, J. L., & Haro, J. M.. (2018). Epidemiology of panic attacks, panic disorder and the moderating role of age: Results from a population-based study. *Journal of Affective Disorders*, *241*, 627–633. https://doi.org/10.1016/j.jad.2018.08.069

Pace, M., Heckendorn, M., Aouizerate, B., Hanon, C., Seigneurie, A. S., Lavaud, P., Hozer, F., Pascal De Raykeer, R., Guerin-Langlois, C., Cormier, L., Poncelin De Raucourt, H., Limosin, F., & Hoertel, (2020). Management of panic disorder in the elderly. Prise en charge du trouble panique chez le sujet âgé. *Geriatrie et psychologie neuropsychiatrie du vieillissement*, *18*(3), 295–304. https://doi.org/10.1684/pnv.2020.0878

Penninx, B., & Lange, S. (2018). Metabolic syndrome in psychiatric patients: overview, mechanisms, and implications. *Dialogues in Clinical Neuroscience*, *20*(1), 63–73. https://doi.org/10.31887/DCNS.2018.20.1/bpenninx

Peplau, H. (1989). Theoretic constructs: Anxiety, self, and hallucinations. In A. O'Toole & S. Welt (Eds.), *Interpersonal theory in nursing practice: Selected works of Hildegarde E. Peplau*. Springer.

Pera, A. (2020). Cognitive, behavioral, and emotional disorders in populations affected by the COVID-19 outbreak. *Frontiers in Psychology*, *11*, 2263. https://doi.org/10.3389/fpsyg.2020.02263

Quagliato, L. A., Freire, R. C., & Nardi, A. E. (2018). Risks and benefits of medications for panic disorder: A comparison of SSRIs and benzodiazepines. *Expert Opinion on Drug Safety*. *17*(3), 315–324. https://doi.org/10.1080/14740338.2018.1429403

Quagliato, L. A., & Nardi, A. E. (2018). Cytokine alterations in panic disorder: A systematic review. *Journal of Affective Disorders*, *228*, 91–96. https://doi.org/10.1016/j.jad.2017.11.094

Scheer, V., Blanco, C., Olfson, M., Lemogne, C., Airagnes, G., Peyre, H., Limosin, F., & Hoertel, N. (2020). A comprehensive model of predictors of suicide attempt in individuals with panic disorder: Results from a national 3-year prospective study. *General Hospital Psychiatry*, *67*, 127–135. https://doi.org/10.1016/j.genhosppsych.2020.09.006

Stein, L. A., Goldmann, E., Zamzam, A., Luciano, J. M., Messé, S. R., Cucchiara, B. L., Kasner, S. E., & Mullen, M. T. (2018). Association between anxiety, depression, and post-traumatic stress disorder and outcomes after ischemic stroke. *Frontiers in Neurology*, *9*, 890. https://doi.org/10.3389/fneur.2018.00890

Zugliani, M., Cabo, M. C., Nardi, A. E., Perna, G., & Freire, R. C. (2019). Pharmacological and neuromodulatory treatments for panic disorder: Clinical trials from 2010 to 2018. *Psychiatry Investigation*. *16*(1), 50–58. https://doi.org/10.30773/pi.2018.12.21.1

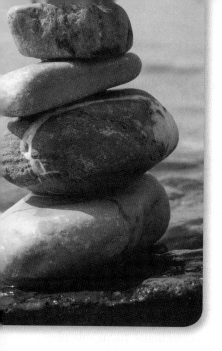

28

Obsessive-Compulsive and Related Disorders

Nursing Care of Persons with Obsessions and Compulsions

Patricia E. Freed

KEYCONCEPTS

- compulsions
- obsessions

LEARNING OBJECTIVES

After studying this chapter, you will be able to:

1. Discuss the role of obsessions and compulsions in mental disorders.

2. Delineate clinical symptoms and course of obsessive-compulsive disorders.

3. Analyze theories of obsessive-compulsive disorders.

4. Develop strategies to establish a patient-centered, recovery-oriented therapeutic relationship with a person with obsessions and compulsions.

5. Apply a person-centered, recovery-oriented nursing process for persons with obsessive-compulsive disorders.

6. Identify medications used to treat people with obsessions and compulsions and evaluate their effectiveness.

7. Develop wellness strategies for persons with obsessions and compulsions.

8. Differentiate the type of mental health care provided in emergency care, inpatient-focused care, community care, and virtual mental health care.

9. Discuss the importance of integrated health care for persons with obsessions and compulsions.

10. Describe other related obsessive-compulsive disorders.

KEY TERMS

- Circumferential speech • Conditioned stimuli • Cyberchondria • Dissociative absorption • Family accommodation
- Isolation • Reaction formation • Rituals • Scrupulosity • Undoing

Case Study: Tim

Tim, a 32-year-old engineer, was diagnosed with OCD as a teenager when his obsession with cleanliness and compulsively washing his hands interfered with his friendships and school work.

INTRODUCTION

Most of us experience times when we are preoccupied with specific thoughts or ideas. Many also find that routines or rituals are important in organizing our work and home life. When these preoccupations and rituals interfere with daily life, they become abnormal and may represent symptoms of a mental disorder. This chapter explains obsessions and compulsions and their role in obsessive-compulsive disorders. Obsessive-compulsive disorder (OCD) is highlighted in this chapter.

OBSESSIONS AND COMPULSIONS

When preoccupied thoughts become excessive, intrusive, or unwanted, such thoughts are considered to be obsessions.

> **KEYCONCEPTS Obsessions** are excessive, unwanted, intrusive, and persistent thoughts, impulses, or images that cause anxiety and distress.
> Obsessions are not under the person's control and are inconsistent with the person's usual thought patterns.

Common obsessions include fears of contamination, pathologic doubt, the need for symmetry and completion, thoughts of hurting someone, and thoughts of sexual images.

Routines are a part of everyday life. Getting up in the morning at the same time and going to work or school structures our lives and helps us be productive. When routines become ritualistic and interfere with normal daily activity, they become compulsions.

> **KEYCONCEPT Compulsions** are repetitive behaviors and mental acts performed in a ritualistic fashion with the goal of preventing or relieving anxiety and distress caused by obsessions.

For example, making sure a stove is turned off before leaving the house can be a safety routine, but being late for work because of making several trips to the stove before leaving the house is a compulsion. Common compulsions include handwashing, excessive cleaning, checking, arranging things, counting, ordering, and hoarding.

OBSESSIVE-COMPULSIVE AND RELATED DISORDERS: OVERVIEW

Obsessions and compulsions are characteristic of obsessive-compulsive and related disorders. These disorders include OCD, body dysmorphic disorder (BDD; perceived flaws or defects in one's physical appearance), hoarding disorder (excessive accumulation and/or difficulty discarding possessions), trichotillomania (i.e., compulsively pulling out one's hair), excoriation disorder (skin picking), and substance/

medication-induced OCD. These disorders are closely related to anxiety disorders (American Psychiatric Association [APA], 2013).

OBSESSIVE-COMPULSIVE DISORDER

In OCD, affected persons may have both obsessions and compulsions and believe that they have no control over them, which results in devastating consequences for affected individuals. Because of the nature of the disorder, nurses who work in settings other than psychiatric settings or in-home health care may be among the first to identify an individual's symptoms as OCD and make the appropriate referrals. Symptoms of OCD can be grouped under four dimensions: contamination and germs, responsibility for unintentional harm, blasphemous or immoral thoughts, and concerns with symmetry, counting, or completion. Many individuals have good or fair insight regarding the accuracy of their beliefs. However, some show an absence of insight, similar to delusional beliefs, which has been linked to worse long-term outcomes (APA, 2013). Though obsessive beliefs may be irrational, they are not as fixed and unyielding as delusions, and insight regarding these beliefs may change over the course of the disorder. Symptoms of OCD are often less severe than those in delusional disorder, and individuals with OCD generally have higher levels of educational attainment and experience higher quality of life (QOL) than those with delusional disorders.

While it may seem that some symptoms of OCD overlap with obsessive-compulsive personality disorder (OCPD), they are separate disorders (OCPD is discussed in Chapter 30). A major difference between these two disorders is that the repeated irrational behaviors of those with OCD are driven by underlying anxiety and have no apparent aim or purpose. OCD symptoms also fluctuate according to the individual's state of anxiety, and the individual is often driven to seek professional help to find relief.

Clinical Course

OCD follows a chronic waxing and waning course. Symptoms of OCD (nonclinical or subclinical) often begin in childhood, but many receive treatment only after the disorder has significantly affected their lives. In preschool-age children, OCD is often misdiagnosed as separation anxiety disorder (Miyawaki et al., 2018). Onset in early or middle childhood is associated with a better outcome than later onset (Sharma & Math, 2019).

Subclinical symptoms can be distressing and cause some impairment. Escalation of subclinical symptoms takes on average 7 years. Predisposition to escalation is associated with being a male, younger age of symptom assessment, being in a new romantic relationship, having more severe sexual/religious symptoms, and having low rates of hoarding (Thompson et al., 2020).

Individuals with OCD may become incapacitated by their symptoms and spend most of their waking hours locked in a cycle of obsessions and compulsions. They may even become unable to complete a task as simple as walking through a door without performing **rituals**. Interpersonal relationships suffer, and the person may actively isolate and withdraw from contact with others. Individuals with OCD often engage in **dissociative absorption**, a tendency to become excessively absorbed in fantasy (movies, online gaming), leading to decreased self-awareness and inattention to their surroundings. Dissociative absorption may predict the onset of obsessive-compulsive symptoms, though this possible link is still being investigated (Soffer-Dudek, 2019).

Remember Tim?

When Tim was in high school, he was unable to eat at the school cafeteria because he was afraid the other students' germs would contaminate his food. He avoided touching doorknobs and would wash his hands for 3 minutes if he inadvertently touched a doorknob.

Diagnostic Criteria

OCD is diagnosed when recurrent obsessions or compulsions (or both) take up more than 1 hour a day or cause considerable stress to the individual. These obsessions or compulsions are not caused by substance or medication use or other disorders. Some individuals recognize that these obsessions or compulsions are excessive and unrealistic; others have limited insight and are unsure whether the obsessive thoughts are true but continue to have the thoughts and feel compelled to perform the actions. Another group of individuals are convinced that their obsessive thoughts are true. These thoughts and compulsive behaviors are stressful and interfere with normal daily routines (APA, 2013).

Obsessions

Obsessions create tremendous anxiety. Some individuals have obsessions surrounding aggressive acts of hurting someone or themselves. After hitting a bump in the road, for example, they may obsess for hours over whether they have hit someone. Parents may have recurrent intrusive thoughts that they may hurt their child. The most common obsession is fear of contamination and results in compulsive handwashing. Fear of contamination usually focuses on dirt or germs, but other materials may be feared as well, such as toxic chemicals, poison, radiation, and heavy metals. Individuals with contamination obsessions report anxiety as their most common effect, but shame and disgust, linked with embarrassment and guilt, also are experienced. Still, others obsess over following the letter of the law, or over the meaning of sin.

Scrupulosity is a specific OCD dimension in which symptoms center on religious or morally intrusive thoughts, followed by repetitive actions, such as going to confession or repeatedly asking for forgiveness. Diagnosis of scrupulosity is not made unless the thoughts or rituals clearly exceed cultural or religious norms, occur at inappropriate times as described by members of the same religion or culture, or interfere with social obligations (APA, 2013). Although it might be difficult to have a conversation centering on religious concerns and family practices, recent findings show that youth with religious obsessions benefit from treatment (Wu et al., 2018b). Somatic obsessions, such as persistent attention to normal bodily processes like breathing, blinking, and swallowing, can also be present and can become intrusive, terrifying thoughts which can interfere with everyday activities.

Compulsions

Compulsions are often performed to relieve the anxiety created by the obsession. Worries about contamination and germs or catching infectious diseases are common. Thoughts about how to protect ourselves should be crossing our minds, especially during the COVID-19 pandemic. For most people, these are fleeting thoughts, and the actions we are taking, via public service announcements, laws, and other friendly reminders, have become part of our expected common-sense approach to public protection. These actions are not pathologic compulsions.

Rituals are common compulsions in which objects must be in a certain order, motor activities are performed in a rigid fashion, or things must be arranged in perfect symmetry. A ritualized behavior may be driven by obsessive thoughts or may be attributed to a distinctive urge that creates tension and pressure throughout the body. A ritual consumes a great deal of time to complete, interfering with even the simplest task. Some individuals experience discontent, rather than anxiety, when things are not symmetrical or perfect. Others think magically and perform compulsive rituals to ward off an imagined disaster, such as repeatedly turning on and off the alarm clock to prevent disaster. Those who hoard are compelled to check their belongings repeatedly to see that all are accounted for and check the garbage to make sure that nothing of value has been discarded.

Cyberchondria, characterized by excessive online searching for health information, is under investigation as another type of compulsive behavior. Excessive searching might provide some temporary reassurance while leading to ever-worsening anxiety and distress (Vismara et al., 2020).

 Concept Mastery Alert

Certain actions, such as making sure that all doors are locked before going to bed, are safety considerations in which the associated anxiety is protective. This is a normal activity and concern, not a pathologic compulsion.

Obsessive-Compulsive Disorder Across the Life Span

Although OCD is relatively common, it is still under-recognized and undertreated. OCD affects people of all ages. Identification, diagnosis, and treatment of OCD are necessary for recovery and optimal functioning.

Disorders Across the Life Span

Children and Adolescents

Because children subscribe to myths, superstition, and magical thinking, obsessive and ritualistic behaviors may go unnoticed. Behaviors such as touching every third tree, avoiding cracks in the sidewalk, or consistently verbalizing fears of losing a parent in an accident may have some underlying pathology but are common behaviors in childhood. Obsessions and compulsions in children are more likely to change/evolve as well as to wax and wane, compared to the course of the disorder in adults. Typically, parents notice that a child's grades begin to fall as a result of decreased concentration and a great amount of time spent performing rituals. Children often have at least one other mental disorder and are less likely than adults to recognize the irrationality of their symptoms. A link between infection with β-hemolytic streptococci and other infections and a subset of acute-onset OCD has been established. The condition is known as pediatric acute-onset neuropsychiatric syndrome. First signs may be the dramatic (2 or 3 days) onset of obsessions and compulsions and overwhelming anxiety (fears). Some children develop sudden eating restrictions and personality changes. Treatments such as antibiotics and immunomodulatory interventions have been suggested, but further study is needed to reach consensus about how best to treat the immunologic response and eliminate (or diminish) the symptoms (Sigra et al., 2018).

Older Adults

Among older adults, OCD most likely began in childhood, but there are some older adults whose onset (beginning of individual distress and interference in work, family, and social activities associated with obsessions and compulsions) began later in life. In the older adult, continuing symptoms are linked to higher rates of depression and poorer mental and social functioning (Dell'Osso et al., 2017). Older adults who engage in checking compulsions and hoarding may have more thought disturbances and communication difficulties than those who engage in other types of compulsive behaviors (Lo Monaco et al., 2020; Box 28.1).

Epidemiology and Risk Factors

The lifetime prevalence of OCD among U.S. adults over 18 was 2.3%, with slightly higher rates in females during adolescence and adulthood (Mathes et al., 2019). Identifying those at risk for more rapid symptom escalation may lessen the heavy public health burden of this chronic disorder for the more than 60 million people in the United States who experience OCD symptoms without meeting the formal criteria for diagnosis (Beyond OCD, 2020). In most people, this chronic condition is associated with moderate to severe disability and carries a heavy health burden for the patient and family. In 2017, the World Health Organization listed this condition among the sixth-largest contributors to nonfatal global health loss (OCD UK, 2020).

Age of Onset

The onset of the illness has a bimodal peak—in early adolescence and early adulthood (Sharma & Math, 2019). Males were thought to have a higher rate of

BOX 28.1 CLINICAL VIGNETTE

Older Adult

Louise, a 76-year-old retired accountant, resides in an assisted living complex with her husband. Always very neat and organized, she recently began cleaning excessively, sometimes in the middle of the night. She developed a routine where she had to have everything cleaned before she could eat. Her husband expressed his concern to their primary care provider, who referred them to a geriatric psychiatrist. A diagnosis of OCD was made. Louise recognizes that her behavior has changed and is interfering with her life but says she gets too nervous if she doesn't carry out her routine.

What Do You Think?

- Are there indications that Louise may have had subclinical OCD symptoms?
- What symptoms of OCD is Louise experiencing?

childhood onset, but it may be that males experience greater symptom severity at a younger age for which they seek treatment (Mathes et al., 2019; Torresan et al., 2013).Occurrence over the age of 35 is rare (APA, 2013). While subclinical symptoms may not lead to a formal diagnosis of OCD, they may still be troubling and contribute to some level of impairment. Obsessional thinking styles might have an effect on cognitive performance, and knowing this could help tailor cognitive-behavior therapy (CBT) for those with subclinical symptoms.

Gender Differences

Gender and age differences in OCD are being clarified and sometimes challenging earlier studies. Female adults are more likely to experience symptoms related to contamination or to have aggressive thoughts toward the child after a birth (Torresan et al., 2013), while males are more likely to report blasphemous obsessions (Mathes et al., 2019). However, these differences may be a product of the way genders report symptoms. Males report a broad range of symptoms, and females tend to report only one or two symptoms (Raines et al., 2015). One study that did consider both age and gender differences found that the risk of OCD in daughters (rather than sons) born to older (rather than younger) parents was higher (Janecka et al., 2019).

A recent literature review found no gender differences in outcomes of behavioral or pharmacologic treatment or in the likelihood of experiencing comorbidities. However, gender may influence the specific type of comorbid condition. Reproductive hormones may play a central role in the differences found between males and females (Karpinski et al., 2017; Mathes et al., 2019).

Family, Ethnicity, and Culture Differences

The core features of OCD are thought to be relatively independent of cultural variation, but there has been little investigation into the impact of culture on symptom expression. An exception is religious affiliation, which appears to influence the content of obsessions and the severity of OCD symptoms. Among individuals who identify as Catholics, there is a higher risk of developing scrupulosity than in persons identifying with other religious affiliations or having no religious affiliation (Buchholz et al., 2019). Other factors related to culture, such as poverty, educational background, and access to health services, have not been investigated (Nicolini et al., 2017).

Culture, ethnic, and family beliefs shape the perception and influence the treatment of OCD. The symptoms are interpreted and manifested within culturally accepted norms. At times, cultural or religious beliefs and practices may be misunderstood and mistaken for obsessions or compulsions. These beliefs and actions must be evaluated in the context of the individual's culture. If these beliefs are consistent with the patient's social, family, or cultural environment; are not harmful to the individual or others; and do not interfere with individual functioning in that environment, they should not be considered symptoms of OCD.

Comorbidity

High rates of comorbid conditions can be found in populations with OCD, most commonly, anxiety disorders, mood disorders, and other related obsessive-compulsive disorders (Brakoulias, 2017). Having any comorbid condition is associated with a longer course of illness, and having two or more contributes to symptom severity and chronicity. Worsening levels of suicidality (thoughts)and suicide attempts are related to the severity of comorbid depression, anxiety and obsessive symptoms, feeling hopeless and to having a history of suicide attempts (Eskander et al., 2020).

OCD and eating disorders (EDs), such as anorexia and bulimia, are highly comorbid and share similarities such as obsessional thinking, ritualized behaviors, and perfectionism (Meier et al., 2020). The presence of an ED complicates the treatment of OCD. In both disorders, individuals have difficulty controlling their thoughts. In OCD, there is difficulty controlling obsessional thoughts and in EDs, there is weight overvaluation, fear of loss of control, and concerns that other see one eats (Meier et al., 2020).

More than half of children with OCD have one or more comorbid conditions and though understudied, Tics/Tourette syndrome, attention deficit hyperactivity disorder (ADHD), and OCD frequently occur together, though symptom severity of each disorder decreases with age (Groth et al., 2017).

Obsessive-compulsive symptoms are common in persons who have migraines and in individuals with schizophrenia, who are experiencing anxiety, mood symptoms, and psychosis. Although treatable, when obsessive-compulsive symptoms appear along with schizophrenia, they often go unrecognized and remain untreated (Bener et al., 2018; Jeyagurunathan et al., 2020).

As a child, Tim frequently went to the school nurse about multiple physical symptoms. Later, he was unable to engage in sexual relations with a long-time girlfriend because the thought of the sex act made him feel nauseous, and twice he experienced severe vomiting. At the time, he sought emergency treatment but ultimately no physical reason was discovered.

Etiology

During the 1990s, research evidence from neuroimaging studies, neurochemical studies, and treatment advances substantiated a predominantly neurobiologic basis for OCD. The following sections provide a brief overview of these findings and evidence pointing to genetic vulnerability. Psychological factors are also discussed because of their contributions to the disorder. Because no single explanation accounts for all aspects of OCD, a combination of factors will probably be found to produce the disorder.

Biologic Theories

Genetic, neuropathologic, and biochemical research, reviewed in this section, suggests that OCD has a biologic basis involving several neuroanatomic structures.

Genetic Factors

Family and twin studies demonstrate that OCD is a multifactorial familial condition that involves multiple genes and environmental risk factors (Pauls et al., 2014; Purty et al., 2019). OCD occurs more often in people who have first-degree relatives with OCD or with Tourette syndrome than it does in the general population. Some studies show an increased prevalence of anxiety and mood disorders in relatives of individuals who have OCD. Twin studies indicate that OCD occurs more frequently in siblings of twins. There appears to be an elevated risk of suicide attempts among the relatives of those with OCD, and the odds increase with closer relationships (Sidorchuk et al., 2021). Some symptom dimensions may have more familiarity than others (hoarding, contamination, symmetry related). These discoveries may lead to breakthroughs in pharmacologic treatments of OCD.

Neuropathologic Theories

Neuroimaging studies of individuals with OCD have shown excessive activity in the frontal cortex and subcortical structures of the brain that correlate with clinical symptoms and cognition and brain function (Nakao et al., 2014). A link between activity in specific brain circuits and reduction of OCD symptoms after successful pharmacologic or psychological treatment has been confirmed via meta-analysis (van der Straten et al., 2017). Because there are broader brain areas involved than originally thought, OCD is assumed to be a heterogenous condition with several abnormal neurobiologic circuits (Nakao et al., 2014).

Currently, OCD has been conceptualized as a dysfunction in stopping the dynamics of normal brain networks, which evolved to handle danger (Woody et al., 2019). Simply put, this means that sufferers may realize there are errors in their behavior but have no inhibitory control (disconnected brakes, metaphorically). Note that these studies don't confirm the neurologic etiology of OCD, but they make it possible to match responders to specific treatments. For instance, in cases of severe, disabling OCD, where neurosurgery is an emerging option, the neurosurgeon will have a better idea of which brain region to target, either by disconnecting an area of the brain with a tiny burst of energy or by inserting a tiny probe to stimulate (activate) a specific area.

Biochemical Theories

Biochemical theories address imbalances of chemicals in the brain, but there is no persuasive evidence that any mental illness is caused by a single biochemical imbalance. Serotonin has been the most extensively studied neurotransmitter in relation to OCD, largely through challenge tests in which serotonin agonists were administered to persons with OCD and with control subjects. The most convincing evidence for serotonin's role is that serotonin-specific antidepressants relieve the symptoms of OCD for about 40% to 60% of those who take them. Conventional and novel antipsychotic medications and mood stabilizers are used in conjunction with serotonin-targeting medications to treat refractory symptoms, indicating that other biochemical processes exist (Del Casale et al., 2019). When chemical balances are identified, it is still difficult to understand how they relate to precise mechanisms of OCD, nor is it possible to know if the chemical changes caused the symptoms or presented because of the symptoms (chicken and egg confound). Prolonged treatment with selective serotonin reuptake inhibitor (SSRI), combined with CBT or with exposure and response prevention (ERP) therapy, is the most effective treatment (Del Casale et al., 2019). New treatments for refractory OCD are needed, and likely candidates will be based on pharmacogenetics (Del Casale et al., 2019).

Psychological and Psychosocial Theories

Although psychological theories of OCD have not been scientifically tested, the rich literature describing clinical examples and case histories helps us understand the symptoms and behaviors related to OCD. In addition, behavioral treatment of individuals with severe compulsions improves symptoms. CBT, which should be considered in every treatment plan, is associated with lower relapse rates (Richter & Ramos, 2018).

Psychosocial Theories

Psychodynamic Factors

The psychodynamic theory hypothesizes that OCD symptoms and character traits arise from three unconscious defense mechanisms: **isolation** (separation of affect from a thought or impulse), **undoing** (an act performed with the goal of preventing consequences of a thought or impulse), and **reaction formation** (behavior and consciously stated attitudes that oppose underlying impulses). Classic psychoanalytic theory describes OCD as regression from the oedipal phase to the anal phase of development, which includes preoccupations with anger and dirt (see Chapter 7). This regression occurs when the patient becomes anxious about retaliation or loss of love.

Behavioral Factors

Behavioral explanations for OCD stem from learning theory. From this viewpoint, obsessions are seen as **conditioned stimuli**. Though being associated with noxious events, stimuli that are usually considered neutral become anxiety provoking. The individual then engages in activities to escape or avoid the anxiety. Compulsions develop as the individual discovers behaviors that successfully reduce the obsessional anxiety. As the principles of operant conditioning indicate, the more the behaviors decrease the anxiety, the more likely the individual is to continue using them. However, the rituals or behaviors preserve the fear response because the person avoids the initial stimuli and thus never extinguishes the compulsion. Interrupting this cycle is the focus of behavioral therapy in treating an individual with OCD. Nurses often use behavioral approaches to reinforce and encourage acceptable behaviors, to set limits, and to impose structure on the environment to make people feel safe, which can reduce anxiety and confusion.

Family Response to Obsessive-Compulsive Disorder

OCD poses a considerable caregiving burden on families, which is heightened by severe symptoms, functional impairment, and comorbid psychopathologies in the child or caregiver (Wu et al., 2018a). Severity of symptoms has been linked to family distress. Families often accommodate a family member's symptoms by taking part in rituals or by modifying their daily routines. Levels of **family accommodation** should be carefully tracked and monitored, because reducing the family's involvement in compulsions may improve treatment outcomes (La Buissonniere-Ariza, et al., 2018).

Family assessment will reveal the amount of education and support needed and will begin the partnership among the individual, family, and treatment team. Evaluate the family's understanding of the disorder and of proposed treatments. Are they able and willing to help the individual practice cognitive and behavioral techniques? Are

they knowledgeable about prescribed medicines? These questions offer a wonderful opportunity for individual and family education.

Family members offer a perspective on the severity of the individual's illness. Family members are experts in the patient's rituals and may observe subtle changes. Evaluate the family's response to changes in the individual's behavior as treatment progresses. You may have to discuss how the family will manage the changes brought about by a decrease in rituals. If obsessions and compulsions make it difficult for the individual to leave home or function at work, financial difficulties may result. These factors should be assessed and appropriate assistance obtained through social services when necessary. Adverse family functioning is strongly associated with pediatric OCD, though its role remains unclear (Murphy & Flessner, 2015).

Tim's Family

Tim's parents recognized their son had unusual behaviors that interfered with his normal growth and development. When he was in high school, his parents took him to a psychiatrist who prescribed medication and offered brief counseling. Tim was able to successfully complete high school with honors and was accepted into a highly respected college. He was able to function when taking medications.

RECOVERY-ORIENTED CARE FOR PERSONS WITH OBSESSIVE-COMPULSIVE DISORDER

Teamwork and Collaboration: Working Toward Recovery

OCD can be difficult to treat because obsessions and compulsions consistently interfere with recovery efforts. OCD is treated with medications, CBT, and supportive therapy. Prolonged treatment with SSRI, combined with CBT or with ERP therapy, is the most effective treatment (Del Casale et al., 2019). The overall goal is for the patient to recover and to decrease the symptoms. Staff may have differing opinions about the amount of control the individual has over the behavior, but these differences of opinion must be resolved. All staff must be consistent in their expectations and acceptance of the patient's behaviors to keep these patients from becoming frustrated or confused regarding expectations during treatment (see Box 28.2).

Electroconvulsive Therapy

The effect of electroconvulsive therapy (ECT) on decreasing obsessions and compulsions cannot be confirmed or refuted. Authors who reviewed the literature concluded that it may have no role in the routine treatment of OCD (Fontenelle et al., 2015). Previous reports of high success may have been compromised by poorly defined treatment resistance, less than optimal treatment, and other specific differences between the population studied (Fontenelle et al., 2015). A recent case report described complete remission after a course of ECT in a patient with anorexia and disabling OCD, which did not recur during the first year of follow-up (Sağlam et al., 2018). Although it is too early to draw a definite conclusion, future research may identify the effectiveness of ECT under certain circumstances or for those with specific comorbid conditions. Nursing's role in caring for the individual undergoing ECT is outlined in Chapter 12.

Transcranial Magnetic Stimulation

Transcranial magnetic stimulation (TMS), a noninvasive procedure that uses magnetic fields to stimulate brain cells, has recently been approved by the U.S. Food and Drug Administration (FDA) for the treatment of OCD. The procedure is contraindicated for patients with implanted metallic objects or implanted stimulator devices in or near the head. Those with a history of seizure disorder may be cautiously considered for treatment.

During treatment, the patient wears earplugs to reduce exposure to the loud noises made by the device. Headache is the most commonly reported side effect of treatment, and other muscle discomforts or pain at the application site resolve shortly after treatment (FDA, 2018). There is emerging evidence that TMS may be effective in treatment-resistant cases of BDD (Hong, 2019).

Psychosurgery

Psychosurgery is sometimes used to treat extremely severe OCD that has not responded to prolonged and intensive drug treatment, behavioral therapy, or a combination of the two. Modern stereotactic surgical techniques that produce lesions of the cingulum bundle (a bundle of connective tissue) or anterior limb of the internal capsule (a region near the thalamus and part of the circuit connecting to the cortex) may bring about substantial clinical benefit in some individuals without causing significant morbidity (Pepper et al., 2019). Other treatment options include radiotherapy and deep brain stimulation, in which electrical current is applied through an electrode inserted into the brain (Szechtman et al., 2020).

Safety Issues

As with any individual with a mental disorder, a suicide assessment must be completed. Although individuals with OCD do not usually become suicidal as a direct result of anxiety, the disorder greatly distresses the person, who realizes the pointlessness and absurdity of the behaviors. Often, the person has tolerated symptoms for quite some time before seeking treatment. The person may feel a sense of hopelessness and helplessness and may contemplate suicide to end the suffering. An additional risk for suicide is created by the high probability of major depression and substance abuse, which often accompanies OCD. Patients may feel a need to punish themselves for their intrusive thoughts (e.g., religious coupled with sexual obsessions). Some persons have aggressive obsessions, so that external limits may have to be imposed for the protection of others.

EVIDENCE-BASED NURSING CARE OF PERSONS WITH OCD

Persons with OCD may be of any age; many have other disorders. Nursing care involves a careful assessment of the impact of the mental health disorder on an individual and a family. Nursing Care Plan 28.1—which sets forth a plan of care for Tim, the case study patient in this chapter—is available at http://thepoint.lww.com/Boyd7e.

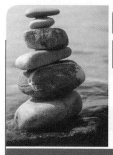

NURSING CARE PLAN 28.1

The Person with Obsessive-Compulsive Disorder (OCD)

Tim, a 32-year-old engineer, is admitted to an inpatient unit for compulsively washing his hands and being unable to go to work. His wife is with him and is quite upset about his behavior. He was being successfully treated for OCD with clomipramine and sertraline but stopped taking his medications 3 months ago, shortly after his marriage. He denies suicidal ideation.

Setting: Acute Mental Health Unit

Baseline Assessment: Tim is a casually dressed, clean-shaven man. Hands are very red with small abrasions. He reports washing his hands several times a day to protect himself from germs. If he does not wash his hands, he gets very anxious. He has a specific routine for washing his hands that has interfered with his job. He stopped taking his medication and does not want to resume taking the same medications. He is concerned that his wife will leave him if he does not get better. He does understand that his behavior is unusual and is symptomatic of his disorder. He denies using alcohol or other substances. He works out regularly at a gym but has been unable to keep up with his routine because of his need to wash his hands. He is 6'2", weighs 190, BMI 24.4; BP 135/70; P70, R 16. His goal is to manage his symptoms and resume his life.

Strengths: Wife wants him to get better and is supportive. He is motivated for change, does not use substances, and wants to return to exercise. Nutrition is excellent.

Associated Psychiatric Diagnosis	Medications
Obsessive-compulsive disorder	None

Priority of Care: Inability to Manage OCD Symptoms

Important Characteristics	Associated Considerations
Acceleration of symptoms of illness Lack of attention to illness Verbalizes desire to manage illness Verbalizes difficulty with prescribed regimen	Discontinuation of medication

Outcomes

Initial	Long term
*Recognize the need to treat symptoms *Identify acceptable strategies for managing symptoms	*Reduce OCD symptoms *Return to work and resume normal lifestyle activities

Interventions

Interventions	Rationale	Ongoing Assessment
*Initiate a nurse–patient relationship by using an accepting, nonjudgmental approach.	A therapeutic relationship will provide an opportunity for Tim to understand the reason for not discontinuing medication.	Determine the extent to which Tim is willing to trust and engage in a therapeutic relationship.
*Encourage Tim to identify OCD symptoms.	By identifying symptoms, Tim will be able to discuss options for treatment.	Assess Tim's recognition of his symptoms and level of understanding of their relationship to his current distress.
*Explore with Tim the reasons he discontinued taking his medications.	There are a variety of reasons individuals stop taking medications. Understanding the reasons will help the nurse explore other alternatives.	Identify the reason(s) Tim discontinued taking his medication.

Continued

Nursing Care Plan 28.1 Continued

* Discuss with Tim the evidence-based options for treating OCD, including other medications, and cognitive-behavior therapy.	Collaboration with patient is important in planning for successful outcomes.	Make sure that Tim takes his medication. Monitor for improvement in OCD symptoms and side effects (e.g., nervousness, nausea).

Priority of Care: Motivated to Learn New Coping Skills

Defining Characteristics	Related Factors
Aware of possible environmental changes Defines stressors as manageable Seeks knowledge of new strategies	Recognition that he needs symptom management

Outcomes

Initial	Long-term
*Commit to strategies to improve symptoms.	*Implement strategies that control symptoms.

Interventions	Rationales	Ongoing Assessment
* Discuss evidence-based strategies for managing OCD, including medications.	Evidence-based strategies include medication and psychotherapy.	*Determine whether Tim discusses all possibilities.
*Based on Tim's medication side effects, discuss other medication options.	Medications have helped Tim in the past and will probably work again.	*Determine whether Tim is open to taking other medications and monitoring side effects.
*Discuss psychotherapy opportunities, including cognitive-behavior therapy (CBT), supportive therapy.	CBT can improve symptoms.	*Determine if Tim has the time and commitment to CBT.

Mental Health Nursing Assessment

The nurse should assess the type and severity of the person's obsessions and compulsions. If the assessment occurs in a hospital, remember that some individuals with OCD experience a transient decrease in symptoms when admitted to a hospital; therefore, sufficient time must be allowed for an accurate assessment. If that time is unavailable, family members or significant others may provide an important source of information, with the individual's permission.

Physical Health and Functioning

Individuals with OCD do not have a higher prevalence of physical disease than others. However, they may report multiple physical symptoms. With late-onset OCD (i.e., after 50 years of age) and with symptoms that occur with a febrile illness, cerebral pathology should be considered. Each person with OCD should be assessed for dermatologic lesions caused by repetitive handwashing, excessive cleaning with caustic agents, or bathing. Osteoarthritic joint damage secondary to cleaning rituals may also be observed. Undetected somatic compulsions, such as persistent nausea and vomiting, can contribute to diminished QOL and pose diagnostic challenges for clinicians.

Nutrition

Unless OCD is accompanied by an ED (which occurs in around 10% to 17%) or another comorbid disorder that interferes with eating or metabolism, nutrition is usually not a recognized problem. Improving eating habits and nutritional status would, however, certainly contribute to overall well-being. Vitamin D and other vitamin deficiencies could be risks for developing OCD (Esnafoğlu & Yaman, 2017) and may play a role in the development of pediatric acute-onset neuropsychiatric syndrome (the pediatric autoimmune disorder), with dramatic onset of obsessive-compulsive symptoms (Çelik et al., 2016).

Medication

A careful assessment of current and past medication helps in understanding and predicting the best medications. Persons with OCD have been prescribed a variety of medications to treat symptoms in addition to over-the-counter vitamins and herbal substances.

Substance Use

Many individuals self-medicate to relieve the anxiety produced by obsessive thoughts. About one-third experience substance abuse or dependence in their lifetime. In addition, some individuals may abuse benzodiazepines and other prescription medications. OCD and substance use disorder are frequently comorbid, but there is a complex relationship between the severity of the illness and the use of substances. Since compulsivity plays a central role in both OCD and addictions, there may be a common brain circuit dysfunction in these two disorders, which can help in identifying appropriate prevention and treatment targets (Figee et al., 2016). Social isolation can also lead to drug use, as sufferers avoid being around others, and avoid social or family events, because they are shamed and embarrassed by behaviors that they realize are irrational.

Psychosocial Assessment

A psychosocial assessment involves gathering by interviewing and talking with the patient, family, and reviewing prior medical records.

Mental Status and Appearance

Most individuals appear neatly dressed and groomed, cooperative, and eager to answer questions. Speech should be at normal rate and volume, but often, individuals with an obsessional, ruminative style of thinking exhibit **circumferential speech**. This speech, loaded with irrelevant details, eventually addresses the question. Listening may be frustrating and require considerable patience, but remember that such speech, which expresses the individual's thinking, is part of the disorder and may be beyond the person's awareness. Continually interrupting and redirecting them can interfere with establishing a therapeutic relationship, especially in the initial assessment. Redirection should be done in a gentle and noncritical manner to allow the patient time to refocus.

Self-Concept

Children and adults with OCD often have low self-concept. Their compulsive behaviors and obsessive thoughts are often internalized as personality quirks instead of understanding them as symptoms. They recognize that others do not have the same types of thoughts and behaviors and want to hide them. Their constant worrying contributes to low self-esteem (Pedley et al., 2019).

Stress and Coping Patterns

An exploration of typical levels of stress and general mood states of the individual is essential. Gather information about the presence of stress in daily life and stress related to OCD symptoms and determine how the individual has coped. Current changes in levels of stress from crisis, life-transitions, or other reasons must also be explored as these can exacerbate symptoms. Be sure to include taking a trauma history, which is often neglected, as a growing body of evidence shows that past traumas can complicate treatment and that some obsessive-compulsive symptoms may have developed as a way of coping with trauma (Tibi et al., 2020).

Social Network/Support Systems

An individual's social networks and support systems should be assessed. While no studies show that lack of social support predicts relapse, empathy and positive interactions are associated with maintenance of gains, while negative family interactions (like anger and criticism) could lead to poorer outcomes. A review of literature found that levels of social support correlated with symptom severity, and in two studies, marital adjustment was correlated with less severe symptoms, though that finding remains inconclusive (Palardy et al., 2018).

Functional Assessment

Identifying the degree to which the OCD symptoms interfere with the patient's daily functioning is important. Several rating scales can be used to identify symptoms and monitor improvement. Some of these scales are to be used by the nurse; others are self-rating scales for the patient, child, or family member. The Maudsley Obsessive-Compulsive Inventory is a 30-item, true–false, self-assessment tool that may help the individual recognize symptoms. See Table 28.1 for more information about psychometrically valid scales, recommended as the cornerstone to evidence-based treatment (Rapp et al., 2016).

It is also important to assess for secondary complications related to compulsive behaviors (like skin chaffing, high use of soap and paper towels, unexplained utility bills, frequent checking on family members) as these factors need to be addressed in planning care. Also, be sure to explore the person's level of insight about the accuracy of their obsessions and feelings about being able to control them as this plays a role in treatment planning and outcomes (see Table 28.1).

Quality of Life

Experiencing comorbid depressive symptoms is a strong predictor of poor QOL in adults with OCD. Children with OCD compared to those without OCD have overall decreased QOL in social and school-related settings (Coluccia et al., 2016). OCD symptoms can impact specific domains of functioning. For example, contamination fears and the need for things to be perfect, exact,

TABLE 28.1	EVIDENCE-BASED ASSESSMENT TOOLS FOR OBSESSIVE-COMPULSIVE DISORDER
Rating Scale	**Description**
Yale-Brown Obsessive Compulsive Scale Y-BOCS/y-BOCS-II/ CY-BOCS	A clinician-rated, 16-item scale with separate subtotals for the severity of obsessions and compulsions. Scoring changes after repeated measurement are used to identify response to treatment.
The Sheehan Disability Scale (SDS)	Brief, self-rated, 3-item, visual analog scale to assess disability. A global measure of functioning can be determined. Recommended for tracking functional changes over time.
Family Accommodation Scale for Obsessive-Compulsive Disorder (FAS-SR)	This self-rated, 19-item rating scale can be used by the parent, child, or others to track and monitor the family's response to symptoms during treatment.
The Brown Assessment of Beliefs Scale (BABS)	A self-rated scale that scores on six dimensions: conviction, perception of other's views, explanation of differing views, idea fixity, attempts to reject beliefs, and insight. Helps rate the degree of conviction and insight patients have concerning their obsessions.

Source: Rapp, et al., 2018.

or symmetrical contribute to lower satisfaction in social relationships. These fears can interfere with leisure activities and sexual functioning which in turn can negatively impact relational intimacy (Schwartzman et al., 2017).

Strengths Assessment

The personal and social strengths of the person should emerge during the assessment interview. Questions to ask could include: Does the child or adult enjoy good physical health? Is the person motivated for treatment? Does the person recognize that obsessions or compulsions are unusual or abnormal? Are there social supports, safe and stable housing? Does the person have unique talents, interests, and character strengths? All this information will be useful in establishing a personalized recovery plan.

CLINICAL JUDGMENT

Patients with OCD may present with various problems, depending on the particular obsession and the compulsions that have evolved to cope with that obsession. As a result, nursing priorities could run the gamut from psychologic issues related to anxiety, poor self-concept,

and loneliness to physical issues such as skin integrity. Outcomes are determined collaboratively after the issues have been identified. Do not forget that a suicide assessment is an essential part of care, and an emergency plan for that contingency as well as for other possible adverse events (medication side effects) should be in place before a client leaves the acute care setting. Recovery plans may take longer to generate, but the acute care nurse can collaborate and begin to develop a recovery plan. The patient should be encouraged to commit to follow-up for long-term treatment and recovery.

THERAPEUTIC RELATIONSHIP

Establishing a therapeutic relationship with a person with OCD requires patience and active listening. The individual may go to great lengths to explain some minute aspect of their life. It is important not to interrupt or rush these explanations. Being unable to finish thoughts increases the patient's anxiety and frustration. See Box 28.3.

MENTAL HEALTH NURSING INTERVENTIONS

Recovery-oriented goals include mental health and wellness components. Goals are collaboratively determined within the context of a therapeutic nurse–client relationship. Ideally the client will want to reduce symptoms, learn about the disorder and treatment, manage health-related issues, and seek a higher level of wellness.

The nurse's interpersonal skills are crucial to successful intervention with the patient who has OCD. Nurses must control their own anxiety. The nurse should interact with the individual in a calm, nonauthoritarian fashion without exhibiting any disapproval of the patient or the patient's behaviors while demonstrating empathy about the distress that the disorder has caused. This approach is one of the most effective means available for communicating appreciation for the individual as separate from the illness.

Establishing Recovery and Wellness Goals

Despite reports of remission rates ranging from 32% to 70%, this disorder is persistent and disabling; but recovery is a realistic goal. Nurses should advocate for policies that facilitate early diagnosis, stepped-care techniques, and a personalized approach that will help in achieving a recovery orientation for persons with OCD L (Burchi et al., 2018).

BOX 28.3 • THERAPEUTIC DIALOGUE: OBSESSIVE-COMPULSIVE DISORDER

Tim is admitted to an inpatient unit; an initial assessment is currently being conducted.

INEFFECTIVE APPROACH

Nurse: Could you tell me what brings you here?

Tim: What? Oh, sorry I get distracted easily. What did you say?

Nurse: I said, why are you here? What do you hope to accomplish while you are here?

Tim: Well, this is how I see it. We need to make sure everyone is healthy, and I want to make sure...

Nurse: (interrupts) No, you don't understand what I am asking. *Why* are you here?

Tim: Forget it. I want to see my wife.

EFFECTIVE APPROACH

Nurse: Tim, how can I help you?

Tim: Well, I am not sure. My wife thinks I am doing strange things. See, I want everyone to be protected, and I think that it is important to stay healthy. There is an outbreak of staph infections, and I want to make sure that my family is safe, and I am just trying to figure things out.

Nurse: OK, it sounds like you are concerned about your family and you are trying to protect them.

Tim: Yes, it is all of the germs. They are everywhere.

Nurse: And you are trying to get rid of them?

Tim: Yes, my wife thinks I am going overboard and wants me to take my medication.

Nurse: Your medication?

Tim: Yes, I used to take medication when I felt like this.

Nurse: You don't take your medication anymore?

Tim: No, I don't need it.

Nurse: I see. But your wife thinks you do?

Tim: Yes, but I don't like the side effects.

Nurse: Such as?

Tim: Well, to tell you the truth, I'd rather not talk about it.

Nurse: OK. While you are here, we can look at different options to help you feel more comfortable.

CRITICAL THINKING CHALLENGE

- How did the first nurse's interaction block communication and increase Tim's frustration?
- What effective communication techniques did the nurse use in the second scenario?

Physical Care

Interventions focus on the physical consequences of the compulsion as well as the psychosocial aspects. The next section provides an overview of biopsychosocial interventions, including medications.

Maintaining Skin Integrity

For the patient with cleaning or handwashing compulsions, attention to skin condition is necessary. Encourage the individual to use tepid water when washing and hand cream after washing. Remove harsh abrasive soaps and replace them with moisturizing soaps. Attempt to decrease the frequency of washing by agreeing on a time schedule and time-limited washing.

Relaxation Techniques

Individuals with OCD experience insomnia because of heightened anxiety levels. Relaxation exercises may be helpful in improving sleep patterns. These exercises do not affect OCD symptoms, but they may be used to decrease anxiety. The nurse may also teach and encourage the person to use other relaxation measures, such as deep breathing, taking warm baths, going for a walk, enjoying music, or engaging in other quiet activities

Wellness Challenges

Healthy living is a challenge for persons who worry excessively, especially about health-related issues or who spend most of their waking hours cleaning. A wellness plan takes into account all of the dimensions of wellness: physical, mental, spiritual, emotional, intellectual, social, occupational, financial, and environmental. Helping the person develop healthy eating habits and exercising regularly should be included in the recovery plan. Obsessional thinking can interfere with sleep and become a major issue for some with OCD. Sleep hygiene habits can help reduce some of the OCD symptoms as well as enhance overall well-being. Some specific challenges people with OCD face and some broad coping directions can be seen in Table 28.2.

Medication Interventions

SSRIs, including fluoxetine, fluvoxamine, paroxetine, sertraline, and clomipramine, a tricyclic antidepressant, are approved by the FDA for treatment of OCD (Del Casale et al., 2019). These drugs are generally recommended along with concurrent CBT consisting of ERP, though if CBT is not accessible, monotherapy with an SSRI is adequate. Clomipramine is approved for children aged 10 years and over, and of the SSRIs, fluoxetine, fluvoxamine, and sertraline are approved for even younger children (Mallinckrodt, 2019). SSRIs or clomipramine lead to improvement in 40% to 60% of people who take them for OCD. SSRIs are recommended over clomipramine because of its unfavorable side effects and over venlafaxine, a serotonin norepinephrine reuptake inhibitor, because there is less support for its effectiveness. Relapse rates vary widely, possibly because of study inconsistencies, but APA practice guidelines recommend that those who respond adequately should continue on the same SSRI for at least 1 to 2 years (see Table 28.3).

Medication Treatment Response

A *successful response* to drug treatment is indicated by a reduction in the baseline score on a standardized instrument like the Yale-Brown Obsessive-Compulsive scale (YBOCS). A 35% or more reduction in YBOC scores indicates a successful response. Switching to another SSRI before an adequate trial can further diminish treatment response (Del Casale et al., 2019).

TABLE 28.3	ADMINISTRATION AND COURSE OF TREATMENT FOR OBSESSIVE-COMPULSIVE DISORDER	
Medications	**Suggested Therapeutic Dose Ranges**
Selective Serotonin Reuptake Inhibitors	
Fluoxetine*	40 to 80 mg/day
Fluvoxamine*	200 to 300 mg/day
Paroxetine*	40 to 60 mg/day
Sertraline*	50 to 200 mg/day
Citalopram**	Up to 40 mg/day; (20 mg in those older than 60)
Escitalopram**	20 to 40 mg/day
Tricyclic Antidepressant	
Clomipramine*	100 to 250 mg/day
Serotonin-Norepinephrine Uptake Inhibitors	
Venlafaxine **	225 to 350 mg/day

SSRI's Administration and Safe Handling

Start at a low dose to enhance tolerability, and the dose can be increased every week or every other week as tolerated. Maintain at therapeutic level for at least 6 weeks before concluding the patient is nonresponsive to the drug.

SSRIs given in higher doses lead to greater response rates and/or greater mean rate of improved compared with lower doses. However, higher doses are associated with higher dropouts due to side effects.

Patients who respond to an adequate trial of a serotonergic antidepressant should stay on that medication for at least 1 to 2 years.

To discontinue, slow taper at 10% to 25% every 1 to 2 months.

Refer to manufacturer's information. In general, tablets are kept dry and stored away from light.

*FDA Approved for OCD; ** Used off-label for OCD.

Source: Forest Laboratories. (2009). Escitalopram Prescribing Information. Retrieved October 10, 2020.

TABLE 28.2	WELLNESS CHALLENGES	
Challenge	**Coping Strategy**
To cope effectively with daily obsessions/compulsions	Practice resisting urges to perform compulsive behaviors such as internet health searching; develop strategies to avoid obsessive thoughts, reframe thoughts
To seek environments that reduce the need for using compulsive behaviors	Seek safe living arrangement; maintain a structured living environment
To find satisfying and enriching work that can accommodate obsessive/compulsive behaviors	Satisfying and enriching work that can accommodate obsessive/compulsive behaviors
To recognize the need for physical activity, healthy foods, and sleep	Balance the need for regular physical activity; discuss healthy diets; encourage establishing healthy sleep hygiene routines
To developing a sense of connection, belonging, and a support system	Explore availability of support groups, family psychoeducation
To expanding a sense of purpose and meaning in life	Focus on goals, values, and beliefs; read inspiring stories or essays

Because patients may become discouraged with a perceived lack of effect, they should be informed that these medications may take 10 to 12 weeks before their effects are realized (Del Casale et al., 2019). All patients should be warned not to stop taking prescribed antidepressant medications abruptly. See Chapter 12 for more information.

Treatment resistance means that there is a minimal or absent response to treatment with an SSRI, and these individuals are given another trial with a different SSRI, clomipramine or venlafaxine, though only about a half respond. A *refractory response* means there has been no response to a trial of two or more SSRIs. For those who are treatment refractory, there are a number of alternatives being trialed. For instance, N-acetyl cysteine along with vitamin D supplementation may be a promising nutraceutical approach that is much more tolerable and is thought to play a protective role against obsessive-compulsive symptoms by modulating inflammatory pathways in the brain (di Michele et al., 2018).

Augmentation with a neuroleptic agent (haloperidol, risperidone, or aripiprazole) can be considered for partial responders (YBOC reductions of 20% to 35%), refractory OCD, and those with psychotic or schizotypal symptoms, rather than switching to a different SSRI (Del Casale et al., 2019), though their use remains off-label. Clozapine, an atypical antipsychotic, and other related drugs are not indicated for OCD, having shown poor efficacy and an association with worsening or new onset of OC symptoms in those with comorbid psychotic disorders (Grover et al., 2015). If neuroleptics are used to augment treatment, they should be prescribed in low doses and administered with careful consideration of the benefits and risks of long-term use (Del Casale et al., 2019; Janardhan Reddy et al., 2017).

Administering and Monitoring Medications

Antidepressants used to treat persons with OCD are often given in higher doses than those normally used to treat depressed patients. The most common route of administration is oral. For refractory OCD, high dose, intravenous treatment with antidepressant drugs may be indicated to bring the symptoms quickly under control. Medication effects must be closely monitored, including being alert to signs of toxicity, to provide safe and adequate care.

Monitoring for Drug Interactions

Because of the extensive list of drug–drug interactions associated with antidepressant medications, a prudent nurse will consult a drug reference or consult with a pharmacist before administering any other medications. As antidepressant treatment occurs over an extended period of time, the probability of a patient experiencing a drug interaction is high. Metabolic drug interactions can result in additive, synergistic, or antagonistic effects. For instance, fluoxetine can cause an increase in plasma concentrations of traditional antipsychotics and may interfere with the elimination of atypical antipsychotics and benzodiazepines. These patients must be monitored for the onset of akathisia or parkinsonian symptoms requiring anticholinergic medication. Quick recognition of signs and symptoms of interactions or toxic reactions is imperative for safe care. Allergic reactions are rare but can occur and can be fatal. Anaphylactic reactions (bronchospasm, angioedema) and/or the presence of urticaria (rash and intense itching) should alert the nurse to hold the next dose of medication and contact the primary care provider.

Management of Complications

Though all antidepressants have a black box warning for suicidality in children, adolescents, and young adults, there is no current evidence to show that adults (over the age of 18) treated with SSRIs are at an increased risk of suicide (Fornaro et al., 2019). Treatment with tricyclic antidepressants and the SSRI, citalopram poses the greatest risk for sudden death related to a specific type of ventricular tachycardia (Rochester et al., 2018). Symptoms include heart palpitations, rapid pulse, dizziness, chest pain, cold sweats, low blood pressure, and shortness of breath. Since other factors may contribute to this life-threatening cardiac condition known as torsade de points, a baseline ECG should be completed prior to initiating any type of antidepressant treatment. Sertraline and paroxetine are usually considered safest for breastfeeding because they have a low level of excretion in breast milk, but any antidepressant taken during pregnancy may endanger the fetus, or cause complications in the newborn, such that the benefits of treatment over the risks should always be carefully weighed. See Chapters 12 and 25 for further discussion. Common side effects of the SSRIs can be seen in Box 28.4.

Psychosocial Nursing Interventions

Psychosocial interventions are crucial to successful treatment of OCD. Nurses engage with patients who are receiving therapy, sit-in on group therapy sessions to provide support and reinforcement, and monitor progress toward outcomes. Nurses can reinforce CBT strategies their patients are learning in therapy and help them practice and use them when anxiety is escalating. Nurses use other complementary strategies to help clients manage anxiety, such as relaxation techniques, mindfulness, cue cards (to help with obsessive thinking), and basic behavioral interventions to reinforce change and avoid adding unnecessary stress to their patient's lives. Nurses are also responsible for providing clients and their families with psychoeducation,

---

BOX 28.4

Common SSRI Side Effects

AUTONOMIC

Dry mouth
Sweating

CENTRAL/PERIPHERAL NERVOUS SYSTEM

Headache
Sedation
Psychiatric
Somnolence
Insomnia
Anorexia
Anxiety
Agitation
Manic Switch
Extrapyramidal symptoms
Nervousness

GASTROINTESTINAL

Nausea/vomiting
Diarrhea

Constipation
Dyspepsia

MUSCULOSKELETAL

Myalgia

UPPER RESPIRATORY

Rhinitis

UROGENITAL/SEXUAL

Ejaculation difficulty
Micturition problems
Impotence
Decreased libido

GENERAL

Drug interactions
Weight gain
Weight loss

Source: Ferguson, J. M. (2001). SSRI antidepressant medications: Adverse effects and tolerability. *Primary Care Companion to the Journal of Clinical Psychiatry, 3*(1), 22–27.

---

which provides information and resource needed to manage the illness in future, establish continuing support, and develop effective coping strategies. Some great sources of self-help for those with OCD are available on the internet. These offer information about treatment, opportunities to be involved in clinical trials, to learn more about the disorders, many self-help strategies, links to support groups, and even events and personal stories about the disorders. See Table 28.4 for some helpful internet resources nurses can share with patients and families.

Therapeutic Interactions

Interactions with persons who are experiencing symptoms of COD require a calm, nonjudgmental approach. It is important to validate the thoughts the person is experiencing and be sensitive to their feelings. If they are experiencing anxiety, they may not be able to concentrate on verbal conversations or able to sit still. The nurse can initiate a discussion about the triggers for the anxiety and the behaviors that the patient is using to control the anxiety. The nurse supports the patient as positive behaviors and thoughts replace the symptomatic obsessions and compulsions.

Enhancing Cognitive Functioning: Cognitive Restructuring

Cognitive restructuring based in CBT is a method of teaching the person to restructure dysfunctional thought processes by defining and testing them. The goal of treatment

TABLE 28.4	INTERNET RESOURCES FOR LIVING WITH OCD
Website	**URL**
The TLC Foundation for Body-focused Repetitive Behaviors	https://bfrb.org
International OCD Foundation	https://iocdf.org/
Body Dysmorphic Disorder Foundation	https://bddfoundation.org/
Peace of Mind Foundation	https://peaceofmind.com/
Psych Central-OCD and Mindfulness	https://psychcentral.com/lib/ocd-and-mindfulness/
Support Groups Online	
Facebook	https://www.facebook.com/Obsessive-compulsive-disorder-OCD-support-site-107975219222496/
TEAM Teens Engaging Anxiety of the Mind) OCD: A Goal Support Group	https://www.facebook.com/Obsessive-compulsive-disorder-OCD-support-site-107975219222496/

is to alter the person's immediate, dysfunctional appraisal of a situation and perception of long-term consequences. The individual is taught to monitor automatic thoughts and then to recognize the connection between thoughts, emotional response, and behaviors. The distorted thoughts are examined and tested by for-or-against evidence presented by the nurse, which helps the individual to realistically assess the likelihood that the feared event will happen if the compulsive behavior is not performed. The person begins to analyze their thoughts as incongruent with reality. For example, even if the alarm clock is not checked 30 times before going to bed, it will still go off in the morning, and the person will not be disciplined for tardiness at work. Maybe it needs to be checked only once or twice.

Personalized Cue Cards/Cognitive Coping Cards

Nurses may introduce clients to the use of cue cards to help restructure thoughts. With the help of the nurse, the client generates cards with a few words on them that pertain specifically to the individual's obsessions and compulsions or other goal statements the patient finds to be inspiring. The cards are ordered to represent least to most anxiety-provoking symptoms, so the patient can use them effectively. The cards can help reinforce positive beliefs or other helpful statements or reminders. Practice is important, and family can help by reminding the person to use them when they are anxious. Some examples of what to write on cue cards can be seen in Box 28.5.

Exposure and Response Prevention

For those who perform ritualized (time-consuming) compulsions, ERP may be a very effective strategy. The person is exposed to situations or objects that are known to trigger (induce) anxiety but is asked to refrain from performing the ritualized behavior. The goal is to help the person understand that resisting the ritual is less anxiety producing and time consuming than performing rituals. Another goal is to confound the expectation of distressing outcomes, which eventually extinguish the compulsive behaviors. About half of those who receive ERP with or without supplemental medication achieve symptom reduction, but because some people do not respond, development of alternative strategies that build

---

BOX 28.5

Examples of Cue Cards/Coping Card Statements

- "It is the OCD, not me:"
- "These are only OC thoughts, OC thoughts don't mean action, I will not act on the thoughts."
- "My anxiety level goes up but will always go down."
- "I never sat with the anxiety long enough to see that it would not harm me."
- "Trust myself."
- "I did it right the first time."
- "Checking the locks again won't keep me safe. I am really safe in the world."

---

on genetic and neurobiologic approaches continues to be needed (Hezel & Simpson, 2019).

Acceptance and Commitment Therapy

Nurses may have clients who are engaged in acceptance and commitment therapy (ACT), which is a form of CBT. ACT is, however, somewhat different than CBT or ERP in that it focuses more on altering obsessional thinking and the way it is experienced. Strategies here help the person accept thoughts and anxiety without allowing them to interfere with life (Roche, 2020). Better functioning can be achieved without changing the frequency or severity of symptoms. ACT was particularly helpful for patients who relapsed after a course of ERP or CBT (Buchholz & Abramowitz, 2019). While reports are positive, this CBT-based therapy is still under investigation.

Behavioral Interventions and Interactions

Although most patients with OCD are treated in outpatient settings, some are hospitalized with comorbidities and are unable to care of themselves or pose a substantial risk of harm to self or others. Some general behavioral-based strategies that can be used in any setting include the following:

- Unit routines must be carefully and clearly explained to decrease fear of the unknown.
- Assess and monitor the level of anxiety and disability.
- Monitor for psychiatric comorbidities and suicide risk.
- At least initially, do not prevent the individual from engaging in rituals because the person's anxiety level will increase.
- Recognize the significance of the rituals to the person and empathize with the person's need to perform them.
- Make reasonable demands and set reasonable limits, avoid situations that provoke or increase frustration.
- Encourage discussions that identify disturbing topics that may relate to underlying anxiety or fear.
- Assist the individual in arranging a schedule of activities that not only incorporates some private time but also integrates the person into normal unit activities.
- Help the person recognize triggers to obsessive thoughts and ritualistic behaviors and the relationship between them.
- Give positive reinforcement for non-ritualistic behavior and to acknowledge the person's progress, strengths, and accomplishments
- Reinforce the use of cognitive strategies, including constructive self-talk and cognitive restructuring.

Mindfulness

Mindfulness means paying attention to the present movement. For persons with OCD, this might be difficult as they struggle with painful, intrusive thoughts and sensations that lend to self-judgment. But nurses can teach patients who are interested in learning as to how to practice mindfulness. In mindfulness, no attempt is made to neutralize internal experiences with compulsions, and the nurse helps the client accept and become aware that these are mental events, capable of being observed (perhaps reframing them as well-intentioned, but "just a thought"). One study found that mindfulness added to traditional CBT produced significantly larger gains in QoL and symptom improvement (at 6 months), compared with a group which received only psychoeducation (Külz et al., 2019). Improvements in this study were self-reported, and clinicians did not rate OC symptoms improvement (Kulz et al., 2019). Perhaps it is more difficult for the therapist to observe improvement when therapy is delivered online. While further study is needed, in general, clients with OCD who learn to use mindfulness find the practice beneficial.

Psychoeducation

Psychoeducation is a crucial nursing intervention for the person with OCD. Knowledge is power; the more the person knows about their disorder, the more control they will have over symptoms. The individual should be instructed not only about the biologic components of OCD but also about its treatments and disease course. Treatment is a shared responsibility between the individual and the health care provider; the individual should be included in the medication and treatment decision-making processes. If local support groups are available, the person should be referred to reduce feelings of uniqueness and embarrassment about the disease. See Box 28.6 for components to include in psychoeducation for those with OCD.

Teaching Strategies

Educating children, youth, and adults who have OCD requires some special consideration. Modifying the environment can help the child manage anxiety, be less distracted, and ultimately prevent disruptions. In a school setting, teachers are encouraged to structure seating arrangements, provide private testing rooms, extend test times, have books on tape, provide access to laptops for writing, and break homework down into small chunks. Teachers should be aware of the child's triggering events, give advance notice of any change whenever possible, and have a plan that the child can use when things become too overwhelming (Child Mind Institute, 2020). These tips translate well to pediatric settings, where nurses

> **BOX 28.6**
>
> **Psychoeducation Checklist: Obsessive-Compulsive Disorder**
>
> When caring for the patient with OCD, be sure to include the family. If appropriate, address the following topic areas in the teaching plan.
> - Explanation of mechanisms underlying OCD and selected therapies including length of treatment and expected outcomes.
> - Psychopharmacologic agents (*SSRIs *MAOIs, lithium, anxiolytics, antipsychotics) as prescribed, including drug actions, dose, frequency, possible side effects, and common interactions with food or other drugs)
> - Skin care measures or problem resolution for other secondary consequences of OCD
> - Alternative to ritualistic behaviors
> - Cognitive restructuring strategies
> - Mindfulness and relaxation techniques
> - Recovery strategies
> - Community resources and supports
>
> *SSRI, selective serotonin reuptake inhibitor; MAOI, monoamine oxidase inhibitor.

frequently work with hospitalized children who have the triad of OCD-ADHD-Tics/Tourette syndrome.

Many of the same strategies can be used for adults. Adults often deal with intrusive thoughts, which makes concentration difficult and frustrating. Avoid overloading them with too much information and keep things short, simple, and well organized.

Another learning consideration involves insight regarding the accuracy of obsessional beliefs. Children's insight into their condition is generally limited, but the same is not usually true of adults. When constructing a teaching plan for adults, be sure to consider their level of insight because it will determine your strategy in discussing and exploring the relationship between obsessions and compulsions. The more insight the person has, the more disclosure and self-analysis can be expected. Adults and children with OCD can learn to re-evaluate their thinking and gain a different perspective on their symptoms.

Wellness Strategies

Wellness strategies for those with OCD are not too different than those for other persons. Stress management, relaxation, and anxiety reduction strategies can best help the person manage day-to-day stress. Structured QOL assessments can give the nurse a more accurate picture of mood states and information about other health domains. Self-help strategies can be introduced to help the person manage symptoms and live with OCD, and these strategies are being identified as helpful in ways not previously known. For instance, running (predetermined bouts of running as exercise) reduced the frequency and intensity of OC symptoms and improved mood (Abrantes et al., 2019).

Providing Family Education

The families of persons with OCD need to be educated about the causes of the disorder and to learn about biologic and psychological treatment approaches. Understanding the biologic basis of the disorder should decrease some of the stigma and embarrassment they may feel about the bizarre nature of the patient's obsessions and compulsions. Families also need to learn how to be supportive and to avoid accommodating to a compulsion to the extent that their good intentions impede the person's recovery. The International OCD Foundation offers families some excellent guidelines on what families can do to help them live with the person who has OCD and to make life better for the whole family as well as how they can contribute to recovery and management of symptoms.

Family assistance in monitoring symptom remission and side effects of the medication is invaluable to mark progress, and family can be enlisted (and taught how) to assist the person with behavioral and cognitive interventions to manage symptoms. Families are likely to be experiencing a heavy stress burden themselves because of the symptoms, and need support and respite to maintain their own mental well-being.

EVALUATION AND TREATMENT OUTCOMES

Several methods can be used to measure the response to treatment, including nursing observations, patient self-reports and changes in YBOC scores or other rating scales, remission of presenting symptoms, and the ability to complete activities of daily living. The individual should be able to participate in social or group activities, with a degree of comfort and without self-harm or aggressive intent. They should also be able to demonstrate common knowledge of OCD by describing its symptoms, biologic basis, and treatments.

Continuum of Care

The symptoms of OCD can become debilitating. The symptoms wax and wane throughout treatment. As the focus of treatment shifts from inpatient to outpatient environments, individuals must be assessed continually to ensure favorable outcomes through early intervention if symptoms resurface.

Emergency Care

Individuals with OCD frequently use medical services long before they seek specialized psychiatric treatment. Therefore, early recognition of symptoms and referral are important concerns for nurses working in primary care and other medical settings. After individuals are referred, most psychiatric treatment of OCD occurs on an outpatient basis. Individuals with severe OCD and/or self-harming thoughts and behaviors are hospitalized for their own safety. In these settings, medications are the primary interventions.

Inpatient-Focused Care

In an inpatient setting, the presence of a person with severe OCD may present a nursing management challenge. These individuals require a significant amount of staff time. They may monopolize bathrooms or showers or have disruptive rituals involving eating. Nurses play an integral role in treating the person with OCD. The nurse should help the individual perform activities of daily living to ensure that they are completed. Monitoring medication effects, teaching psychoeducation groups, ensuring adequate caloric intake, and providing individual patient counseling are additional inpatient interventions.

Community Care

Partial hospitalization programs and day treatment programs help individuals in their quest for recovery. These programs can support independence, while individuals begin medications and behavioral therapies. Some patients require outpatient treatment daily when symptoms increase. Maintenance outpatient therapy may be scheduled weekly or biweekly for several weeks until the symptoms are well controlled. Community agency visits are recommended to monitor medication.

Virtual Mental Health Care

Virtual approaches in the assessment and treatment of OCD and related disorders range from online individual and group psychotherapy (well established) to virtual assessment, online peer-support, and (hypothesized) computerized programs designed to break neurocognitive habits (digital behavior change interventions). As the nation quarantines, virtual mental health care can help individuals cope with mental health issues while staying home. Communication with health professionals via text, audio, or video messaging is available, and there are now easy-to-navigate mental health apps. See Box 28.7 for the expectations of virtual mental health care.

Virtual Assessment and Treatment for Obsessive-Compulsive Disorder (e-OCD)

There are several types of technology-enabled psychotherapy programs available. With increasing demand and an expanding role, evidence about them has been accumulating. Technology programs vary by platform (internet, computerized) type of therapy and the level of clinician involvement (Aboujaoude, 2018.). Computerized

---

BOX 28.7

Expectations for Virtual Service Providers

- Maintain/Update privacy protections for personal health information (PHI).
- Control access without patient's written permission.
- Encrypt patient data in transit and in storage.
- Protect display screens and audio transmissions from 'incidental' viewing or eavesdropping.
- Exchange information with only those who need to access PHI.
- Document rules, policies, and procedures about safeguarding PHI.
- Train all staff and document compliance.
- Negotiate HIPAA compliant business associate agreement (BAA) with cloud hosts.

---

cognitive-behavioral therapy, internet-based CBT are proving to be the most effective (Aboujaoude, 2018 with or without an SSRI (Hirschtritt et al., 2017). Less-studied programs such as virtual reality exposure therapy and mobile therapy are also showing promise (Aboujaoude, 2018). Virtual access to therapy has obvious benefits for consumers and may help reduce stigma as some patients who can't leave their homes can still get treatment. For younger generations who are accustomed to interacting via technology, online models may help normalize mental health care and make the process easier.

Online and Virtual Groups for OCD

Virtual support for OCD has been available for many years. Generally, these are peer support groups that offer advice and support for those living with OCD and related disorders and their families/friends and supporters. CBT or a similarly oriented model ERP are typically the types of therapy offered electronically. Online training for qualified, licensed mental health professionals is available to attain certification and training for the skills they wish to develop in their practices. A caution is called for—training sites found on the internet should be thoroughly investigated and demonstrated as reputable (such as training attained from the National Alliance on Mental Illness) before signing up or paying for the program.

Emerging Technologies

Profound changes are on the horizon for the assessment and management of OCD, which will help tailor treatment, define diagnostic procedures, and improve moment-to-moment condition monitoring for actional outcomes (Ferreri et al., 2019). Some new devices and digital measurement tools are already available, like a smartphone application to log the frequency of compulsive activity, or wearable products like a wrist band that monitors compulsions and minimizes observer influence. More exciting still is the possibility of

programs (digital behavior change interventions) that can modify cognitive behavior. Computerized models of habit alteration (to differentiate habits from goal-directed behavior) with the potential to alter behavior have already been developed (Pinder et al., 2018), and one study using a digital strategy was able to determine that all symptoms dimensions (except hoarding) were associated with bias toward habits at the expense of goal-directed behavior (Snorrason et al., 2016). What this all means and how it impacts the practices of licensed and advance practice psychiatric nurses are yet to be determined, but it may change education, challenge beliefs, and ethics and even alter the professional culture of nursing.

Integration with Primary Care

Effective treatment for those with OCD requires a continuum of preventive and restorative mental health and addiction services, according to changing needs over time and across different levels of the health care system. A team-based approach for individuals and families with OCD and related disorders is best when mental health care and general medical care are offered in the same setting. Currently, there is little articulation between behavioral health and primary care systems. As virtual therapies and treatments become popular, it may be even more difficult to coordinate and integrate care. The goals of primary care in promoting self-care and the recovery and resilient orientation of behavioral health are highly compatible (NCBH, 2020). Policies to promote better integration and collaboration between behavioral health and primary care should be a priority for mental health advocates, like nurses.

OTHER RELATED OBSESSIVE-COMPULSIVE DISORDERS

The other related obsessive-compulsive disorders are grouped together in the *Diagnostic and Statistical Manual (DSM-5)* because evidence has accumulated to show a relationship, such as symptom similarity, presentation, frequent co-occurrence, genetic risks, and other common threads (APA, 2013). Grouping disorders together also allows for more discriminating research, which can improve screening, assessment, and earlier treatment. Trichotillomania, excoriation disorder, BDD, and hoarding disorder are briefly described here.

Trichotillomania and Excoriation Disorder

Trichotillomania is chronic self-destructive hair pulling that results in noticeable hair loss, usually in the crown, occipital, or parietal areas of the head, although sometimes also involves the eyebrows and eyelashes. The individual has an increase in tension immediately before pulling out the hair or while attempting to resist the behavior. After the hair has been pulled, the person feels a sense of relief. Some would classify this disorder as one of self-mutilation. It becomes a problem when accompanied by significant distress or impairment in other areas of function. A hair-pulling session can last several hours, and the individual may either ritualistically eat the hairs or discard them. Hair ingestion may result in the development of a hair ball, which can lead to anorexia, stomach pain, anemia, intestinal obstruction, and peritonitis. Other medical complications include infection at the hair-pulling site. Hair pulling is usually done alone and persons may deny it; for some there is little conscious awareness, and for others active pulling may regulate negative feelings (Lochner et al., 2019).

Clinical Course

The onset of trichotillomania occurs among children before the age of 5 years and in adolescents. For the young child, distraction or redirection may successfully eliminate the behavior. The behavior in adolescents may begin a chronic course that may last well into adulthood.

Diagnostic Criteria

Trichotillomania is diagnosed when recurrent pulling out of hair with hair loss occurs. The individual is unable to reduce or stop such hair pulling, which causes considerable distress (APA, 2013).

Etiology and Treatment

This disorder is poorly understood. An etiologic relationship to OCD has not been established, but support is present for a familial connection (Lochner et al., 2019). The prevalence of trichotillomania is estimated at 1% to 2% of the population (APA, 2013). No particular medication class demonstrates effectiveness in treatment. Studies of individual medications, including olanzapine (antipsychotic) and clomipramine (tricyclic antidepressant), show treatment effectiveness (Baczynski & Sharma, 2020). CBT and habit reversal training, a behavioral intervention, can improve the symptoms.

Evidenced-Based Nursing Care of Persons with Trichotillomania

The assessment includes a review of current problems, developmental history (especially school conflicts and learning difficulties), family and social history, identification of support systems, previous psychiatric treatment, and general health history. The cultural context in which the trichotillomania occurs must be taken into consideration because in some cultures, this behavior may be viewed as socially acceptable. The hair-pulling history and pattern are also used to determine the duration and severity of the disorder. Within the therapeutic relationship, a cognitive-behavioral approach can be used to help the person identify when hair pulling occurs, the precipitating events, and the details of the episode.

Individuals with trichotillomania report that anxiety, loneliness, anger, fatigue, guilt, frustration, and boredom can all trigger the hair-pulling behavior. Persons with chronic hair pulling typically avoid social activities and events. In addition, the economic impact of trichotillomania can be significant in relation to lost work or school days. Teaching about the disorder will help affected individuals understand that they are not alone and that others have also had this problem. The goal of treatment is to help the individual learn to substitute positive behaviors for the hair-pulling behavior through self-monitoring of events that precipitate the episodes.

Excoriation (Skin-Picking) Disorder

Repetitive and compulsive picking of skin causing tissue damage characterizes **excoriation or skin-picking disorder** (APA, 2013). Although face, arms, or hands are the most common sites for picking, it can occur at other body sites. Most affected people pick with their fingers, but tweezers or pins are also sometimes used. Similar to other disorders, skin picking causes significant distress to individuals. Prevalence is estimated at 1.4% to 5%; it occurs more frequently in persons with OCD. Treatment data are limited but include behavioral and pharmacologic interventions. CBT and ACT are highly recommended. SSRIs, topiramate, and N-acetylcysteine are sometimes prescribed for symptom reduction. Antihistamines can be used to reduce pruritus (itch or an unpleasant sensation of the skin that provokes the urge to scratch). It is a characteristic feature of many skin diseases and an unusual sign of some systemic diseases. Nursing care is similar to caring for a person with trichotillomania. Cold compresses or cremes (antibiotics and corticosteroids) can also be applied. These disorders can carry a significant amount of shame and embarrassment, and individuals frequently try to camouflage skin lesions that could be detected. Possible medical sequala, such as infections, lesions, scarring, and even severe physical disfigurement, can result (Torales et al., 2020).

Body Dysmorphic Disorder

Individuals with BDD focus on real (but slight) or imagined defects in appearance, such as a large nose, thinning hair, or small genitals. Preoccupation with the

BOX 28.8 CLINICAL VIGNETTE

Body Dysmorphic Disorder

K, a 16-year-old girl, for about 6 months has believed that her pubic bone is becoming increasingly dislocated and prominent. She believes that everyone stares at it and talks about it. She does not remember a particular event related to the appearance of the symptom but is absolutely convinced that she can be helped only by a surgical correction of her pubic bone.

She was treated recently for anorexia nervosa with marginal success. Although her weight is nearly normal, she continues to be preoccupied with the looks of her body. She spends almost the entire day in her bedroom, wearing excessively large pajamas, and she refuses to leave the house. Once or twice a day, she lowers herself to the ground and measures, with her fingers, the distance between her pelvic girdle and the ground in order to check the position of the pubic bone.

In desperation, her parents called the clinic for help.

The family was referred to a home health agency and a psychiatric home health nurse who arranged for an assessment visit.

What Do You Think?

- How should the nurse approach K? Should an assessment begin immediately?
- From the vignette, identify nursing diagnoses, outcomes, and interventions.

Adapted from Sobanski, E., & Schmidt, M. H. (2000). "Everybody looks at my pubic bone"—a case report of an adolescent patient with body dysmorphic disorder. *Acta Psychiatrica Scandinavica, 101,* 80–82.

perceived defect causes significant distress and interferes with their ability to function socially. They feel so self-conscious that they avoid work or public situations. Some fear that their "ugly" body part will malfunction. Surgical correction of the problem by a plastic surgeon or a dermatologist does not correct their preoccupation and distress. BDD is an extremely debilitating disorder and can significantly impair an individual's QOL. BDD usually begins in adolescence and continues throughout adulthood. These individuals are not usually seen in psychiatric settings unless they have a coexisting psychiatric disorder or a family member insists on psychiatric attention (see Box 28.8).

This disorder occurs in men and women, with a prevalence of 2.4% in the United States (APA, 2013). The risk of depression, suicide ideation, and suicide is high. The suicide risk in BDD is increased by the presence of other disorders such as substance use disorder, major depressive disorder, eating, and personality disorders. People with comorbid OCD-BDD have high morbidity, a decrease in insight, and poor psychosocial functions (Eskander et al., 2020). No single theory explains the cause of BDD. Unrealistic cultural expectations and genetic predisposition most likely underlie this disorder.

Hoarding Disorder

Difficulty parting with or discarding possessions, regardless of actual value, characterize hoarding disorder. Individuals with this disorder have a need to save items

BOX 28.9

The Role of Intrusive Imagery in Hoarding Disorder.

Stewart, N. A. J., Brewin, C.R., & Gregory, J. D. (2020). The role of intrusive imagery in hoarding disorder. Behavior Therapy, 51(1), 42–53.

THE QUESTION: Do people with hoarding disorder (HD) experience intrusive imagery more frequently, and how does it differ from intrusive imagery experienced by individuals without HD (healthy controls)?

METHODS: A semi-structured interview was used in this investigational study. Opportunity sampling was used to identify and screen participants for two groups. Subjects in one group (HD) met the *DSM-5* criteria for HD, and subjects in the second group (CC) had no mental health problems. Semi-structured interview questions explored the presence and characteristics of intrusive images in everyday and in discarding situations, by having the participant identify the intrusive image (frequency) and ranking its valence on six criteria: emotional tone, vividness, realness (happening now), identification (with image), avoidance of the image, and interference of the image with everyday life. Data (mixed) across groups were compared, and narrative descriptions were coded into themes.

FINDINGS: Both groups (96% for the HD group and 86% for the CC) experienced intrusive imagery. Everyday imagery for the HD group was more frequent and more negative; these images were more likely to interfere with their lives, and they tried to avoid them. No differences in vividness or that the images reflected their identity was found. The themes of the HD group (everyday imagery) reflected illness or death to others and negative interpersonal memories, whereas the CC group has themes that were more neutral. During the discarding scenarios, there were significant differences with the HD group reporting more frequent intrusive imagery when discarding low (subjective) value episodes, and (unexpectedly) more positive imagery when discarding (or trying to discard) high-value objects. The authors conclude that mental events have an important role in maintaining HD and that this is the first study of this kind that links imagery to compulsive hoarding.

IMPLICATIONS FOR NURSING: This study highlights the importance of trauma history screening and the unsuspected aftermaths of traumatic events. It also provides nurses with a better understanding of how mental imagery contributes to the inability to discard possessions in HD, which has heretofore remained inexplicable. Better understanding of why discarding objects is so difficult for those with HD may help families address hoarding with more empathy. This study alerts nurses to the need to explore images around discarding possessions and begins to give some direction about how nurses can better help patients with HD rescript the images that keep them living in cluttered, unsafe, and unhealthy environments.

and experience distress if their items are discarded. Most affected individuals with hoarding disorder also exhibit excessive acquisition (excessive purchasing of items or collecting free items).

The prevalence of this disorder is estimated at 2% to 6% (APA, 2013). Hoarding may begin in childhood with an increase in severity throughout a life span. This disorder tends to be familial and present in different generations. Over 50% of the individuals have co-occurring depression or chronic anxiety. See Box 28.9. Treatment includes pharmacologic agents and CBT. There is some evidence that peer-led groups may be effective (Mathews et al., 2018).

Hoarding poses public health and safety risks for individuals, families, and communities. Excessive collection of items not only clutters living areas but can also lead to being trapped in an inaccessible environment and one that is at high risk for fire. Home health nurses are often the first health care providers that recognize the problem and so are a valuable resource in determining the safety hazards and helping the individual become aware of the problem and seek treatment. Currently, treatment includes CBT and medication for co-occurring mental disorders (Mathews et al., 2016).

SUMMARY OF KEY POINTS

- Obsessions are excessive, intrusive, or unwanted thoughts. Compulsions are repetitive behaviors performed in a ritualistic manner.

- The most common obsession is the fear of contamination.

- Compulsions relieve anxiety and should not be interrupted unless the behavior jeopardizes the safety of the person or others. Interrupting compulsive behavior increases the person's anxiety.

- OCD is characterized by obsessions, compulsion, or both. OCD can occur in children and adults.

- Medications and CBT can help affected individuals to get through episodes and reduce the compulsive behavior.

- Nursing care focuses on motivating the person for change, administering and monitoring medication, providing psychoeducation, and supporting positive new behaviors.

- The primary characteristics of trichotillomania and excoriation disorders are compulsive behaviors that damage the hair or skin. Compulsive behaviors of both disorders cause significant distress to the person who cannot stop or decrease the behaviors. Medications and psychotherapy can reduce these behaviors.

- BDD involves excessive focus on slight or imagined defects in appearance. The person with these extreme-

ly distressing defects seeks treatment by plastic surgeons or dermatologists. Correction does not relieve the patient's preoccupation, which continues to interfere with their QOL. These individuals are at high risk for depression and suicide.

- Hoarding disorder can begin in childhood and last a lifetime. Individuals with this disorder need to save things and become very upset if items are removed. When excessive collection leads to extreme clutter, it becomes a safety issue.

CRITICAL THINKING CHALLENGES

1. Differentiate an obsession from a compulsion.

2. List common obsession-compulsion dimensions and their consequences to the individual and family.

3. Jane, a 35-year-old single mother, has been unable to go to work because she fears her apartment will burn down. She is constantly checking the stove and furnace. Her family convinced her to be admitted to a mental health unit. Discuss how you would prioritize her assessment and develop a plan of care.

4. Jon, a 25-year-old man, is admitted to an inpatient unit for depression and extreme anxiety. He was diagnosed with OCD as a child and had been able to function with medication. He recently married and decided to stop taking his medication. When his symptoms recurred, his wife tried to prevent Jon's compulsive behaviors by removing the knobs from the stove. He became more anxious. As Jon's nurse, develop a teaching plan about OCD for his wife.

5. Explain how nurses contribute to treatment using CBT and behavioral strategies.

6. Identify patient teaching strategies for children and adults with OCD, including milieu modifications.

7. Explain the behaviors associated with trichotillomania, excoriation disorder, BDD, and hoarding disorder. What are the similarities and differences?

 Movie Viewing Guides
Aviator: 2004. The movie starring Leonardo DiCaprio depicts the earlier years of film producer, industrialist, and aviator Howard Hughes who suffered from OCD. Hughes' perfectionism in his film making and his need for order related to his food and cleanliness eventually contributed to his functional decline. Several scenes illustrate his obsession and compulsion. Hughes' symptoms eventually take over his life, and he retreats to a self-imposed solitary confinement.

Viewing Points: How does his early life contribute to the development of his OCD symptoms? Identify his obsessions and compulsions. If Howard Hughes were your patient, what nursing diagnoses and interventions would you want to implement? Identify teaching needs related to medication and the obsessions and compulsions.

Related to this chapter are available at http://thepoint. lww.com/Boyd7e.

REFERENCES

Aboujaoude E. (2018). Telemental health: Why the revolution has not arrived. *World Psychiatry, 17*(3), 277–278. https://doi.org/10.1002/wps.20551

Abrantes, A. M., Farris, S. G., Brown, R. A., Greenberg, B. D., Strong, R., McLaughlin, N. C., & Riebe, D. (2019). Acute effects of aerobic exercise on negative affects and obsessions and compulsions in individuals with obsessive-compulsive disorder. *Affective Disorders, 15*(245), 991–997. https://doi.10.1016/j.jad.2018.11.074

American Psychiatric Association. (2013). *Diagnostic and statistical manual of mental disorders (5th ed.)* (DSM-5).Author.

Baczynski, C., & Sharma, V. (2020). Pharmacotherapy for trichotillomania in adults. *Expert Opinion on Pharmacotherapy, 21*(12), 1455–1466. https.//doi.org/10.1080/14656566.2020.1761324

Bener, A., Dafeeah, E. E., Abou-Saleh, M. T., Bhugra, D., & Ventriglio, A. (2018). Schizophrenia and co-morbid obsessive—compulsive disorder: Clinical characteristics. *Asian Journal of Psychiatry, 37*, 80–84. https://doi-org.ezp.slu.edu/10.1016/j.ajp.2018.08.016

Beyond OCD. (2020). *Facts about obsessive compulsive disorder.* https://beyondocd.org/ocd-facts

Brakoulias, V., Starcevic, V., Belloch, A., Brown, C., Ferrao, Y. A., Fontenelle, L. F., Lochner, C., Marazziti, D., Matsunaga, H., Miguel, E. C., Reddy, Y., do Rosario,M. C., Shavitt, R. G., Shyam Sundar, A., Stein, D. J., Torres, A. R., & Viswasam, K. (2017). Comorbidity, age of onset and suicidality in obsessive-compulsive disorder (OCD): An international collaboration. *Comprehensive Psychiatry, 76*, 79–86. https://doi-org.ezp.slu.edu/10.1016/j.comppsych.2017.04.002

Buchholz, J. L., & Abramowitz, J. (2019). Using an Acceptance and Commitment Therapy Approach when exposure and cognitive therapy become rituals in the treatment of obsessive-compulsive disorder. *Journal of Cognitive Psychotherapy, 33*(3), 256–268. https://doi.org/10.1891/0889-8391.33.3.256

Buchholz, J. L., Abramowitz, J. S., Riemann, B. C., Reuman, L., Blakey, S. M., Leonard, R. C., & Thompson, K. A. (2019). Scrupulosity, religious affiliation and symptom presentation in obsessive compulsive disorder. *Behavioural and Cognitive Psychotherapy, 47*(4), 478–492. https://doi-org.ezp.slu.edu/10.1017/S1352465818000711

Burchi, E., Hollander, E., & Pallanti, S. (2018). From treatment response to rRecovery: A realistic goal in OCD. *The International Journal of Neuropsychopharmacology, 21*(11), 1007–1013. https://doi-org.ezp.slu.edu/10.1093/ijnp/pyy079

Çelik, G., Taş, D., Tahiroğlu, A., Avci, A., Yüksel, B., & Çam, P. (2016). Vitamin D deficiency in obsessive-compulsive disorder patients with pediatric autoimmune neuropsychiatric disorders associated with streptococcal infections: A case control study. *Archives of Neuropsychiatry, 53*(1), 33–37. https://do:10.5152/npa.2015.8763

Child Mind Institute. (2020). Teachers guide to OCD in the classroom. https://childmind.org/guide/a-teachers-guide-to-ocd-in-the-classroom

Coluccia, A., Fagiolini, A., Ferretti, F., Pozza, A., Costoloni, G., Bolognesi, S., & Goracci, A. (2016). Adult obsessive-compulsive disorder and quality of life outcomes: A systematic review and meta-analysis. *Asian Journal of Psychiatry, 22*, 41–52. https://doi.org/10.1016/j.ajp.2016.02.001

Del Casale, A., Sorice, S., Padovano, A., Simmaco, M., Ferracuti, S., Lamis,D. A., Rapinesi, C., Sani, G., Girardi, P., Kotzalidis, G. D., & Pompili, M. (2019). Psychopharmacological treatment of obsessive-compulsive disorder (OCD). *Current Neuropharmacology, 17*(8), 710–736. https://doi-org.ezp.slu.edu/10.2174/1570159X16666180813155017

Dell'Osso, B., Benatti, B., Rodriguez,C. I., Arici, C., Palazzo, C., Altamura, A. C., Hollander, E., Fineberg, N., Stein, D. J., Nicolini, H., Lanzagorta, N., Marazziti,D., Pallanti, S., Van Ameringen, M., Lochner, C., Karamustafalioglu, O., Hranov, L., Figee, M., Drummond, L., Grant, J., … Zohar, J. (2017). Obsessive-compulsive disorder in the elderly: A report from the International College of Obsessive-Compulsive Spectrum Disorders (ICOCS). *European*

Psychiatry: The Journal of the Association of European Psychiatrists, 45, 36–40. https://doi-org.ezp.slu.edu/10.1016/j.eurpsy.2017.06.008

di Michele, F., Siracusano, A., Talamo, A., & Niolu, C. (2018). N-Acetyl cysteine and vitamin D supplementation in treatment resistant obsessive-compulsive disorder patients: A general review. *Current Pharmaceutical Design, 24*(17), 1832–1838. https://doi-org.ezp.slu.edu/10.2174/1381612824666180417124919

Eskander, N., Limbana, T., & Khan, F. (2020). Psychiatric comorbidities and the risk of suicide in obsessive-compulsive and body dysmorphic disorder. *Cureus, 12*(8), e9805. https://doi.org/10.7759/cureus.9805

Esnafoğlu, E., & Yaman, E. (2017). Vitamin B12, folic acid, homocysteine and vitamin D levels in children and adolescents with obsessive compulsive disorder. *Psychiatry Research, 254*, 232–237. https://doi-org.ezp.slu.edu/10.1016/j.psychres.2017.04.032

Ferguson, J. M. (2001). SSRI antidepressant medications: Adverse effects and tolerability. *Primary Care Companion to the Journal of Clinical Psychiatry, 3*(1), 22–27. https://doi-org.ezp.slu.edu/10.4088/pcc.v03n0105

Ferreri, F., Bourla, A., Peretti, C. S., Segawa, T., Jaafari, N., & Mouchabac, S. (2019). How new technologies can improve prediction, assessment, and intervention in obsessive-compulsive disorder (e-OCD): Review. *JMIR Mental Health, 6*(12), e11643. https://doi.org/10.2196/11643

Figee, M., Pattij, T., Willuhn, I., Luigjes, J., van den Brink, W., Goudriaan, A., Potenza, M. N., Robbins, T. W., & Denys, D. (2016). Compulsivity in obsessive-compulsive disorder and addictions. *European Neuropsychopharmacology: The Journal of the European College of Neuropsychopharmacology, 26*(5), 856–868. https://doi-org.ezp.slu.edu/10.1016/j.euroneuro.2015.12.003

Fontenclle, L. F., Coutinho, E. S., Lins Martins, N. M., Fitzgerald, P. B., Fujiwara, H., & Yücel, M. (2015). Electroconvulsive therapy for obsessive-compulsive disorder: A systematic review. *The Journal of Clinical Psychiatry, 76*(7), 949–957. https://doi-org.ezp.slu.edu/10.4088/JCP.14r09129

Fornaro, M., Anastasia, A., Valchera, A., Carano, A., Orsolini, L., Vellante, F., Rapini, G., Olivieri, L., Di Natale, S., Perna, G., Martinotti, G., Di Giannantonio, M., & De Berardis, D. (2019). The FDA "Black Box" Warning on antidepressant suicide risk in young adults: More harm than benefits?. *Frontiers in Psychiatry, 10*, 294. https://doi.org/10.3389/fpsyt.2019.00294

Groth, C., Mol Debes, N., Rask, C. U., Lange, T., & Skov, L. (2017). Course of tourettesyndrome and comorbidities in a large prospective clinical study. *Journal of the American Academy of Child and Adolescent Psychiatry, 56*(4), 304–312. https://doi-org.ezp.slu.edu/10.1016/j.jaac.2017.01.010

Grover, S., Hazari, N., Chakrabarti, S., & Avasthi, A. (2015). Relationship of obsessive-compulsive symptoms/disorder with clozapine: A retrospective study from a multispeciality tertiary care centre. *Asian Journal of Psychiatry, 15*, 56–61. https://doi-org.ezp.slu.edu/10.1016/j.ajp.2015.05.002

Hezel, D. M., & Simpson, H. B. (2019). Exposure and response prevention for obsessive-compulsive disorder: A review and new directions. *Indian Journal of Psychiatry, 61*(Suppl 1), S85–S92. https://doi-org.ezp.slu.edu/10.4103/psychiatry.IndianJPsychiatry_516_18

Hirschtritt, M. E., Bloch, M. H., & Mathews, C. A. (2017). Obsessive-compulsive disorder: Advances in diagnosis and treatment. *JAMA, 317*(13), 1358–1367. https://doi-org.ezp.slu.edu/10.1001/jama.2017.2200

Hong, K., Nezgovorova, V., Uzunova, G., Schlussel, D., & Hollander, E. (2019). Pharmacological treatment of body dysmorphic disorder. *Current Neuropharmacology, 17*(8), 697–702. https://doi-org.ezp.slu.edu/10.2174/1570159X16666180426153940

Janardhan Reddy, Y. C., Sundar, A. S., Narayanaswamy, J. C., & Math, S. B. (2017). Clinical practice guidelines for obsessive-compulsive disorder. *Indian Journal of Psychiatry, 59*(Suppl 1), S74–S90. https://doi-org.ezp.slu.edu/10.4103/0019-5545.196976

Janecka, M., Hansen, S. N., Modabbernia, A., Browne, H. A., Buxbaum, J. D., Schendel, D. E., Reichenberg, A., Parner, E. T., & Grice, D. E. (2019). Parental age and differential estimates of risk for neuropsychiatric disorders: Findings from the Danish birth cohort. *Journal of the American Academy of Child and Adolescent Psychiatry, 58*(6), 618–627. https://doi-org.ezp.slu.edu/10.1016/j.jaac.2018.09.447

Jeyagurunathan, A., Abdin, E., Vaingankar, J. A., Chua,B. Y., Shafie, S., Chang, S. H. S., James, L., Tan, K. B., Basu, S., Chong, S. A., & Subramaniam, M. (2020). Prevalence and comorbidity of migraine headache: Results from the Singapore Mental Health Study 2016. *Social Psychiatry and Psychiatric Epidemiology, 55*(1), 33–43. https://doi-org.ezp.slu.edu/10.1007/s00127-019-01755-1

Karpinski, M., Mattina, G. F., & Steiner, M. (2017). Effect of gonadal hormones on neurotransmitters implicated in the pathophysiology of obsessive-compulsive disorder: A critical review. *Neuroendocrinology, 105*(1), 1–16. https://doi-org.ezp.slu.edu/10.1159/000453664

Külz, A. K., Landmann, S., Cludius, B., Rose, N., Heidenreich, T., Jelinek, L., Alsleben, H., Wahl, K., Philipsen, A., Voderholzer, U., Maier, J. G.,

& Moritz, S. (2019). Mindfulness-based cognitive therapy (MBCT) in patients with obsessive-compulsive disorder (OCD) and residual symptoms after cognitive behavioral therapy (CBT): A randomized controlled trial. *European Archives of Psychiatry and Clinical Neuroscience*, *269*(2), 223–233. https://doi-org.ezp.slu.edu/10.1007/s00406-018-0957-4

La Buissonnière-Ariza, V., Schneider, S. C., Højgaard, D., Kay, B. C., Riemann, B. C., Eken, S. C., Lake, P., Nadeau, J. M., & Storch, E. A. (2018). Family accommodation of anxiety symptoms in youth undergoing intensive multimodal treatment for anxiety disorders and obsessive-compulsive disorder: Nature, clinical correlates, and treatment response. *Comprehensive Psychiatry*, *80*, 1–13. https://doi-org.ezp.slu.edu/10.1016/j.comppsych.2017.07.012

Lochner, C., Keuthen, N. J., Curley, E. E., Tung, E. S., Redden, S. A., Ricketts, E. J., Bauer, C. C., Woods, D. W., Grant, J. E., & Stein, D. J. (2019). Comorbidity in trichotillomania (hair-pulling disorder): A cluster analytical approach. *Brain and Behavior*, *9*(12), e01456. https://doi.org/10.1002/brb3.1456

Lo Monaco, Di Stasio, E., Zuccalà, G., Petracca, M., Genovese, D., Fusco, D., Silveri, M. C., Liperoti, R., Ricciardi, D., Cipriani, M. C., Laudisio, A., &Bentivoglio, A. R. (2020). Prevalence of obsessive-compulsive symptoms in elderly parkinson disease patients: A case-control study. *The American Journal of Geriatric Psychiatry: Official Journal of the American Association for Geriatric Psychiatry*, *28*(2), 167–175. https://doi.org/10.1016/j.jagp.2019.08.022

Mathes, B. M., Morabito, D. M., & Schmidt, N. B. (2019). Epidemiological and clinical gender differences in OCD. *Current Psychiatry Report*, *21*(5), 36.https://doi:10.1007/s11920-019-1015-2

Mathews,C. A., Mackin, R. S., Chou, C. Y., Uhm, S. Y., Bain, L. D., Stark, S. J., Gause, M., Vigil, O. R., Franklin, J., Salazar, M., Plumadore, J., Smith, L. C., Komaiko, K., Howell, G., Vega, E., Chan, J., Eckfield, M. B., Tsoh, J. Y., & Delucchi, K. (2018). Randomised clinical trial of community-based peer-led and psychologist-led group treatment for hoarding disorder. *BJPsych Open*, *4*(4), 285–293. https://doi-org.ezp.slu.edu/10.1192/bjo.2018.30

Mathews, C. A., Uhm, S., Chan, J., Gause, M., Franklin, J., Plumadore, J., Stark, S. J., Yu, W., Vigil, O., Salazar, M., Delucchi, K. L., & Vega, E. (2016). Treating Hoarding Disorder in a real-world setting: Results from the Mental Health Association of San Francisco. *Psychiatry Research*, *237*, 331–338. https://doi-org.ezp.slu.edu/10.1016/j.psychres.2016.01.019\

Mallinckrodt. (2019). Anafranil Prescribing Information. https://www.accessdata.fda.gov/drugsatfda_docs/label/2012/019906s037lbl.pdf

Meier, M., Kossakowski, J. J.,Jones, P. J., Kay, B., Riemann, B. C., & McNally, R. J. (2020). Obsessive-compulsive symptoms in eating disorders: A network investigation. *The International Journal of Eating Disorders*, *53*(3), 362–371. https://doi-org.ezp.slu.edu/10.1002/eat.23196

Miyawaki, D., Goto, A., Iwakura, Y., Hirai, K., Miki, Y., Asada, N., Terakawa, H., & Inoue, K. (2018). Preschool-onset obsessive-compulsive disorder with complete remission. *Neuropsychiatric Disease and Treatment*,*14*, 1747–1753. https://doi-org.ezp.slu.edu/10.2147/NDT.S169797

Murphy, Y. E., & Flessner, C. A. (2015). Family functioning in paediatric obsessive compulsive and related disorders. *The British Journal of Clinical Psychology*, *54*(4), 414–434. https://doi-org.ezp.slu.edu/10.1111/bjc.12088

Nakao, T., Okada, K., &Kanba, S. (2014). Neurobiological model of obsessive-compulsive disorder: evidence from recent neuropsychological and neuroimaging findings. *Psychiatry and Clinical Neurosciences*, *68*(8), 587–605. https://doi-org.ezp.slu.edu/10.1111/pcn.12195

National Council of Behavioral Health [NCBH]. (2020). Health Integration and Wellness. NCBH. https://www.thenationalcouncil.org/topics/health-integration-and-wellness/

Nicolini, H., Salin-Pascual, R., Cabrera, B., & Lanzagorta, N. (2017). Influence of culture in obsessive-compulsive disorder and its treatment. *Current Psychiatry Reviews*, *13*(4), 285–292. https://doi-org.ezp.slu.edu/10.2174/2211556007666180115105935

OCD UK. (2020). About OCD https://www.ocduk.org/

Palardy, V., El-Baalbaki, G., Fredette, C., Rizkallah, E., & Guay, S. (2018). Social support and symptom severity among patients with obsessive-compulsive disorder or panic disorder with agoraphobia: A systematic review. *Europe's Journal of Psychology*, *14*(1), 254–286. https://doi-org.ezp.slu.edu/10.5964/ejop.v14i1.1252

Pauls, D. L., Abramovitch, A., Rauch, S. L., & Geller, D. A. (2014). Obsessive-compulsive disorder: An integrative genetic and neurobiological perspective. *Nature Reviews. Neuroscience*, *15*(6), 410–424. https://doi-org.ezp.slu.edu/10.1038/nrn3746

Pedley, R., Bee, P., Wearden, A., & Berry, K. (2019). Illness perceptions in people with obsessive-compulsive disorder: A qualitative study. *PLoSOne*, *14*(3), e0213495. https://doi.org/10.1371/journal.pone.0213495

Pepper, J., Zrinzo, L., & Hariz, M. (2019). Anterior capsulotomy for obsessive-compulsive disorder: A review of old and new literature. *Journal of Neurosurgery*, 1–10. Advance online publication. https://doi.org/10.3171/2019.4.JNS19275

Pinder, C., Vermeulen, J., Cowan, B. R., & Beale, R. (2018) Digital behavior change interventions to break and form habits. *ACM Transactions on Computer-Human Interaction*, *25*(3), 410–424. https://doi.org/10.1145/3196830

Purty, A., Nestadt, G., Samuels, J. F., & Viswanath, B. (2019). Genetics of obsessive-compulsive disorder. *Indian Journal of Psychiatry*,*61*(Suppl 1), S37–S42. https://doi-org.ezp.slu.edu/10.4103/psychiatry.IndianJPsychiatry_518_18

Raines, A. M., Allan, N. P., Oglesby, M. E., Short,N. A., & Schmidt, N. B. (2015). Examination of the relations between obsessive-compulsive symptom dimensions and fear and distress disorder symptoms. *Journal of Affective Disorders*, *183*, 253–257. https://doi-org.ezp.slu.edu/10.1016/j.jad.2015.05.013

Rapp, A. M., Bergman, R. L., Piacentini, J., & McGuire, J. F. (2016). Evidence-based assessment of obsessive-compulsive disorder. *Journal of Central Nervous System Disease*,*8*, 13–29. https://doi-org.ezp.slu.edu/10.4137/JCNSD.S38359

Richter, P., & Ramos, R. T. (2018). Obsessive-compulsive disorder. *Continuum (Minneapolis, Minn.)*, *24*(3, Behavioral Neurology & Psychiatry), 828–844. https://doi-org.ezp.slu.edu/10.1212/CON.0000000000000603

Roche, L. (2020). Using an acceptance and commitment therapy-based intervention for PTSD following traumatic brain injury: A case study. *Brain Injury*, *34*(2), 290–297. https://doi-org.ezp.slu.edu/10.1080/02699052.2019.1683896

Rochester, M. P., Kane, A. M., Linnebur, S. A., & Fixen, D. R. (2018). Evaluating the risk of QTc prolongation associated with antidepressant use in older adults: A review of the evidence. *Therapeutic Advances in Drug Safety*, *9*(6), 297–308. https://doi.org/10.1177/2042098618772979

Sağlam, T., Aksoy Poyraz, C., Poyraz, B. Ç., & Tosun, M. (2018). Successful use of electroconvulsive therapy in a patient with anorexia nervosa and severe acute-onset obsessive-compulsive disorder. *The International Journal of Eating Disorders*, *51*(8), 1026–1028. https://doi-org.ezp.slu.edu/10.1002/eat.22923

Schwartzman,C. M., Boisseau, C. L., Sibrava, N. J., Mancebo, M. C., Eisen, J. L., & Rasmussen, S. A. (2017). Symptom subtype and quality of life in obsessive-compulsive disorder. *Psychiatry Research*, *249*, 307–310. https://doi-org.ezp.slu.edu/10.1016/j.psychres.2017.01.025

Sharma, E., & Math, S. B. (2019). Course and outcome of obsessive-compulsive disorder. *Indian Journal of Psychiatry*, *61*(Suppl 1), S43–S50. https://doi.org/10.4103/psychiatry.IndianJPsychiatry_521_18

Sidorchuk, A., Kuja-Halkola, R., Runeson, B., Lichtenstein, P., Larsson, H., Rück, C., D'Onofrio, B. M., Mataix-Cols, D., & Fernández de la Cruz, L. (2021). Genetic and environmental sources of familial coaggregation of obsessive-compulsive disorder and suicidal behavior: A population-based birth cohort and family study. *Molecular Psychiatry*, *26*(3), 974–985. https://doi.org/10.1038/s41380-019-0417-1

Sigra, S., Hesselmark, E., & Bejerot, S. (2018). Treatment of PANDAS and PANS: A systematic review. *Neuroscience and Biobehavioral Reviews*,*86*, 51–65. https://doi-org.ezp.slu.edu/10.1016/j.neubiorev.2018.01.001

Snorrason, I., Lee, H. J., de Wit, S., & Woods, D. W. (2016). Are nonclinical obsessive-compulsive symptoms associated with bias toward habits? *Psychiatry Research*, *241*, 221–223. https://doi-org.ezp.slu.edu/10.1016/j.psychres.2016.04.067

Soffer-Dudek, N. (2019). Dissociative absorption, mind-wandering, and attention-deficit symptoms: Associations with obsessive-compulsive symptoms. *The British Journal of Clinical Psychology*, *58*(1), 51–69. https://doi-org.ezp.slu.edu/10.1111/bjc.12186

Stewart, N., Brewin, C. R., & Gregory, J. D. (2020). The role of intrusive imagery in hoarding disorder. *Behavior Therapy*, *51*(1), 42–53. https://doi-org.ezp.slu.edu/10.1016/j.beth.2019.04.005

Szechtman, H., Harvey, B. H., Woody, E. Z., & Hoffman, K. L. (2020). The psychopharmacology of obsessive-compulsive disorder: A preclinical roadmap. *Pharmacological Reviews*, *72*(1), 80–151. https://doi.org/10.1124/pr.119.017792

Thompson, E. M.,Torres, A. R., Albertella, L., Ferrão, Y. A., Tiego, J., Shavitt, R. G., Conceição do Rosario, M., Miguel, E. C., & Fontenelle, L. F. (2020). The speed of progression towards obsessive-compulsive disorder. *Journal of Affective Disorders*, *264*, 181–186. https://doi-org.ezp.slu.edu/10.1016/j.jad.2019.12.016

Tibi, L., van Oppen, P., van Balkom, A., Eikelenboom, M., Hendriks, G. J., &Anholt, G. E. (2020). Childhood trauma and attachment style predict the four-year course of obsessive compulsive disorder: Findings from the Netherlands obsessive compulsive disorder study. *Journal of Affective Disorders*, *264*, 206–214. https://doi-org.ezp.slu.edu/10.1016/j.jad.2019.12.028

Torales, J., Díaz, N. R., Barrios, I., Navarro, R., García, O., O'Higgins, M., Castaldelli-Maia, J. M., Ventriglio, A., & Jafferany, M. (2020). Psychodermatology of skin picking (excoriation disorder): A comprehensive review. *Dermatologic Therapy*, *33*(4), e13661. https://doi.org/10.1111/dth.13661

Torresan, R. C., Ramos-Cerqueira, A. T., Shavitt, R. G., do Rosário, M. C., de Mathis, M. A., Miguel, E. C., & Torres, A. R. (2013). Symptom dimensions, clinical course and comorbidity in men and women with obsessive-compulsive disorder. *Psychiatry Research*, *209*(2), 186–195. https://doi-org.ezp.slu.edu/10.1016/j.psychres.2012.12.006

U.S. Food & Drug Administration [FDA], 2018. FDA permits marketing of transcranial magnetic stimulation for treatment of obsessive-compulsive disorder. https://www.fda.gov/newsevents/newsroom/pressannouncements/ucm617244.htm

van der Straten, A. L., Denys, D., & van Wingen, G. A. (2017). Impact of treatment on resting cerebral blood flow and metabolism in obsessive compulsive disorder: a meta-analysis. *Scientific Reports*, *7*(1), 17464. https://doi-org.ezp.slu.edu/10.1038/s41598-017-17593-7

Vismara, M., Caricasole, V., Starcevic, V., Cinosi, E., Dell'Osso, B., Martinotti, G., &Fineberg, N. A. (2020). Is cyberchondria a new transdiagnostic digital compulsive syndrome? A systematic review of the evidence. *Comprehensive Psychiatry*,*99*, 152167. https://doi-org.ezp.slu.edu/10.1016/j.comppsych.2020.152167

Woody, E. Z., Hoffman, K. L., &Szechtman, H. (2019). Obsessive compulsive disorder (OCD): Current treatments and a framework for neurotherapeutic research. *Advances in Pharmacology (San Diego, Calif.)*, *86*, 237–271. https://doi-org.ezp.slu.edu/10.1016/bs.apha.2019.04.003

Wu, M. S., Hamblin, R., Nadeau, J., Simmons, J., Smith, A., Wilson, M., Eken, S., Small, B., Phares, V., & Storch, E. A. (2018a). Quality of life and burden in caregivers of youth with obsessive-compulsive disorder presenting for intensive treatment. *Comprehensive Psychiatry*, *80*, 46–56. https://doi-org.ezp.slu.edu/10.1016/j.comppsych.2017.08.005

Wu, M. S., Rozenman, M., Peris, T. S., O'Neill, J., Bergman, R. L., Chang, S., &Piacentini, J. (2018b). Comparing OCD-affected youth with and without religious symptoms: Clinical profiles and treatment response. *Comprehensive Psychiatry*, *86*, 47–53. https://doi-org.ezp.slu.edu/10.1016/j.comppsych.2018.07.009

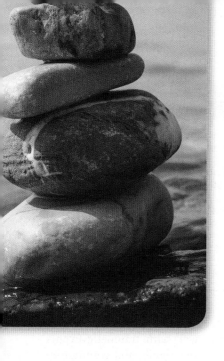

29
Trauma- and Stressor-Related Disorders
Nursing Care of Persons with Posttraumatic Stress and Other Trauma-Related Disorders

Mary Ann Boyd

KEYCONCEPTS

- resilience
- psychological trauma
- traumatic event

LEARNING OBJECTIVES

After studying this chapter, you will be able to:

1. Discuss the role of psychological trauma in mental disorders.

2. Discuss the importance of resilience in prevention of mental disorders.

3. Delineate clinical symptoms and course of posttraumatic stress disorder.

4. Analyze the primary theories related to posttraumatic stress disorder.

5. Develop strategies to establish a patient-centered, recovery-oriented therapeutic relationship with a person with posttraumatic stress disorder.

6. Apply nursing persons-centered, recovery-oriented nursing process for persons with posttraumatic stress disorder.

7. Identify medications used to treat people with posttraumatic stress disorder.

8. Develop wellness strategies for persons with posttraumatic stress disorder.

9. Differentiate the type of mental health care provided in emergency care, inpatient-focused care, community care, and virtual mental health care.

10. Discuss the importance of integrated health care.

11. Describe dissociation and dissociative disorders.

KEY TERMS

- Complex posttraumatic stress disorder (CPTSD) • Depersonalization • Derealization • Dissociation • Emotional reactions • Hyperarousal • Hypervigilance • Intrusion • Numbing • Posttraumatic stress disorder (PTSD) • Trauma-informed care

---

Case Study

Thirty-year-old Susan is admitted to an inpatient mental health unit following a suicide attempt. Her relationship with her husband has deteriorated since she returned from Iraq 6 months ago. She is overwhelmed by her responsibilities as a parent and wife. She has been diagnosed with posttraumatic stress disorder.

INTRODUCTION

All of us experience stress in our daily lives, but our responses vary from person to person. One person may develop a severe **emotional reaction** (strong agitation of feelings), and another resilient individual is hardly aware of a traumatic event. While most stressful events do not lead to mental disorders, sometimes, emotional problems and mental disorders develop as the response to trauma. This chapter explains the role of resilience in buffering the mental health consequences of psychological trauma and the nursing care for those who develop trauma- and stressor-related disorders. **Posttraumatic stress disorder (PTSD)** is highlighted in this chapter.

TRAUMA AND RESILIENCE

Trauma can be viewed from several different perspectives. Physical trauma may result from bodily injury resulting from an accident, self-inflicted damage, or violence perpetrated by others. Falls are a leading cause of accidents in the home. Automobile accidents are a major threat to adolescents. Self-inflicted physical trauma is often associated with mental disorders. Physical abuse of intimate partners and elder abuse are nationwide health problems. Rape and sexual abuse are physically traumatic and produce psychological trauma.

| **KEYCONCEPT Psychological trauma** is an emotional injury caused by an overwhelmingly stressful event that threatens one's survival and sense of security.

Harassment, embarrassment, child abuse, sexual abuse, employment discrimination, police brutality, bullying, and domestic violence are examples of events that can lead to psychological trauma. Family violence, loss of family members, acts of terrorism, and natural disasters are all traumatic events. Exposure to war, natural disasters, and witnessing catastrophic events also may cause psychological trauma.

Not everyone who experiences a traumatic event will be emotionally injured. One explanation for the variability in experiencing psychological trauma is resilience.

Resilience reduces the impact of risk factors and enhances the ability to "bounce back" and recover from stressful experiences. The stronger the resilience, the less likely the individual will experience reactions that lead to maladaptive behaviors and outcomes (Naifeh et al., 2019). An important mental health promotion nursing strategy is enhancing resilience, especially for persons with mental and/or substance abuse problems (see Box 29.1).

Resilience develops in association with a positive self-concept and self-worth, a feeling of being in control one's life, and a feeling of power. Resilience is acquired over time, beginning in early childhood, as positive problem-solving, communication, and coping skills are

---

BOX 29.1

Resilience

Joe, a 22-year-old college student, was a victim of an armed robbery. His companion was shot and killed when Joe refused to give the robbers his money. After the incident, he was preoccupied with thoughts of the murder and felt personally responsible for his friend's death.

Joe sought psychological help from the college counseling center. During weekly counseling sessions, Joe was able to reframe his experience. Although he still has brief periods of sadness, he no longer blames himself for his friend's death. He is now resuming his normal activities and is no longer having intrusive thoughts.

---

learned. Some children seem more resilient to trauma and are able to cope quite well with traumatic events (Mitra & Hodes, 2019). Positive family and community support also play a role in developing resilience.

| **KEYCONCEPT Resilience** is the capacity to withstand stress and catastrophe. It develops over time and is the culmination of multiple internal and external factors.

TRAUMA- AND STRESSOR-RELATED DISORDERS OVERVIEW

Exposure to a traumatic or otherwise stressful event can lead to a trauma- and stressor-related disorder such as reactive attachment disorder, disinhibited social engagement disorder, PTSD, acute stress disorder, and adjustment disorder.

Trauma- and Stressor-Related Disorders Across the Lifespan

Trauma- and stressor-related disorders can develop at any time throughout a lifespan. In children, exposure to trauma can cause enduring emotional problems that lead to any one of these disorders. One of the most traumatic losses for children is an unexpected death of a loved one, which can lead to multiple psychiatric disorders (see Chapter 16) (Atwoli et al., 2017).

Childhood psychological and physical abuse including sexual abuse can lead to a lifelong struggle with a trauma- and stressor-related disorder. Adverse childhood experiences are categorized by the CDC-Kaiser Permanente Adverse Childhood Eperiences (ACE) Study into three groups: abuse (emotional, physical, sexual); household challenges (mother treated violently, household substance abuse, mental illness in household, parental separation or divorce, criminal household member); and neglect (emotional, physical). In this study of 8,667 adult members of a health maintenance organization childhood physical and sexual abuse, as well as witnessing of maternal battering, was common. More than one third of the members experienced more than one type of maltreatment. The more frequent and severe the abuse as a child, the greater the PTSD symptoms as an adult (Chang et al., 2019; Oral et al., 2016).

Military violence is responsible for lifelong effects for deployed service members. There are many reports of older adults who served in World War II developing symptoms of PTSD in later life. There is a growing number of research studies that demonstrate the traumatic impact on children during military deployment and reintegration of their parents (Williamson et al., 2018).

When an older adult experiences trauma, memories of a lifetime of previous traumas and abuse influence the current experience. Loss of partners, friends, and family members through death, marriage, or relocation can add to the trauma. Elder abuse is discussed in Chapter 31.

POSTTRAUMATIC STRESS DISORDER

PTSD occurs following exposure to an actual or threatened traumatic event such as death, serious injury, or sexual violence (American Psychiatric Association [APA], 2013). Traumatic events include those that are directly experienced, witnessed, learned about from others, or repeated exposure to aversive events. Examples of traumatic events are violent personal assault, rape, military combat, natural disasters, terrorist attacks, being taken hostage, incarceration as a prisoner of war, torture, an automobile accident, or being diagnosed with a life-threatening illness.

> **KEYCONCEPT Traumatic events** include those that are directly experienced, witnessed, learned about from others, or repeated exposure to adverse events.

Clinical Course

Most people who experience a traumatic event do not develop PTSD. However, for those who do, the symptoms often develop within several days of the event and must persist for a minimum of 30 days in order for the criteria of the diagnosis to be met. In some cases, the symptoms may initially occur substantially after the event, sometimes up to 6 months later. This is known as delayed-onset PTSD (APA, 2013). About one third of the persons diagnosed with PTSD develop chronic symptoms. For these individuals, symptoms fluctuate in intensity with time and usually are worse during periods of stress. Children with PTSD may react differently than adults (see Box 29.2).

Diagnostic Criteria

PTSD is diagnosed following exposure to a traumatic event when symptoms in four general areas appear:

BOX 29.2

Posttraumatic Stress Disorder Symptoms in Children and Adolescents

PTSD Symptoms in Children
- Bedwetting, after they had learned how to use a toilet
- Forgetting how or being unable to talk
- Acting out the scary event during playtime
  - Being unusually clingy with a parent or other adult

PTSD Symptoms in Adolescents
- May show symptoms similar to adult
- Develop disruptive, disrespectful, or destructive behaviors
  - Feel guilty for not preventing injury or death

Thoughts of revenge. (Source: U.S. Department of Health & Human Services. www.nimh.nih.gov.)

---

(1) intrusive symptoms, avoidance of person(s), places, or objects that are a reminder of the traumatic event; (2) negative mood and cognitions or negative thoughts associated with the event; (3) **hyperarousal** characterized by aggressive, reckless, or self-destructive behavior; and (4) sleep disturbances or **hypervigilance** for at least 1 month (APA, 2013).

Intrusion

In PTSD, **intrusion** is defined as involuntary appearance of thoughts, memories, or dreams of traumatic events that cause psychological and sometimes physiologic distress. Often the intrusive thoughts are associated with cues that symbolize or resemble the original event. Sometimes, the traumatic images, thoughts, or perceptions are reexperienced, known as flashbacks. Nightmares are common. Intrusive symptoms also include dissociative reactions (i.e., feeling or acting as if the event is reoccurring). Sleeping is difficult. Terrifying flashbacks and nightmares often include fragments of traumatic events exactly as they happened. Many stimuli (e.g., loud noises, odors) associated with the trauma cause flashbacks and dreams. Consequently, affected individuals avoid such stimuli (Brooks et al., 2019).

In children, older than 6, repetitive play may occur that expresses the themes or aspects of the traumatic events. They may reenact the specific trauma. Nightmares of these children may not have content (APA, 2013).

Remember Susan?

She suffers from flashbacks of exploding helicopters when she hears loud noises. Her husband tells her she screams while sleeping. She reports frightening nightmares.

Avoidance and Numbing (Dissociative Symptoms)

Individuals with PTSD avoid reminders of the event including people, places, or activities associated with the event (e.g., fireworks may bring back memories of war). Many persons suffering with this disorder escape situations by altering their state of consciousness or **numbing** by dissociating. **Dissociation** is a disruption in the normally occurring linkages among subjective awareness, feelings, thoughts, behavior, and memories (APA, 2013). A person who dissociates is making themselves "disappear." That is, the person has the feeling of leaving their body and observing what happens to them from a distance. During trauma, dissociation enables a person to observe the event while experiencing no pain or only limited pain and to protect themselves from awareness of the full impact of the traumatic event (see Box 29.3). Examples of dissociation include (1) **derealization** (feelings of unreality) and **depersonalization** (the experience of self or the environment as strange or unreal); (2) periods of disengagement from the immediate environment during stress, such as "spacing out"; (3) alterations in bodily perceptions; (4) emotional numbing; (5) out-of-body experiences; and (6) amnesia about abuse-related memories.

Mood and Cognition

After a traumatic event, moods often become more irritable with episodes of explosive anger, fear, guilt, or shame. Individuals with PTSD often have difficulty experiencing positive emotions such as happiness or love. Consequently, they become estranged from loved ones who become frustrated with their family member's unpredictable moods and lack of emotional connection. In PTSD, the thought process becomes distorted with exaggerated negative beliefs or expectations about oneself, others, and the world. They may believe that no one can be trusted or that they are terrible people (APA, 2013).

Hyperarousal and Hypervigilance

After a traumatic experience, the stress system seems to go on permanent alert, as if the danger might return at any time. In this state of physiologic hyperarousal, the traumatized person is hypervigilant for signs of danger, startles easily, reacts irritably to small annoyances, and sleeps poorly. They are looking for physical danger, a repeat of a trauma, or something wrong in a relationship. The state of hyperarousal causes other problems for family members. The affected individual is irritable and overreacts to others, which cause others to avoid the person who in turn maintains a state of continual arousal (Marshall et al., 2019).

Sleep Disturbance

Sleep disturbance is one of the most commonly reported symptoms of PTSD. The disruptions fall into two categories—insomnia (persistent difficulty falling asleep or staying asleep) and nightmares. Many people with PTSD experience both. Sleep disturbances prior to the trauma is believed to be a risk factor for PTSD and insomnia immediately after the trauma is predictive of PTSD developing within 1 year. Improvement in sleep quality is associated with reduction of PTSD symptoms (Maguire et al., 2020).

Susan and Her Family

Susan feels she does not fit into the family and no longer believes she has a role as a wife and mother. She is extremely irritable and argues with her husband constantly. She is suspicious of her neighbors and fearful that her children will be kidnapped.

Complex Posttraumatic Stress Disorder

Complex posttraumatic stress disorder (CPTSD) is a subgroup of PTSD that occurs with severe chronic, repetitive trauma that continues for months or years. While PTSD focuses on the threats and avoidance of harm, CPTSD is understood as a betrayal of trust and occurs in extreme childhood neglect, repeated sexual or physical abuse, domestic abuse, and human trafficking. These traumas result in fundamental damage to one's sense of self, personality changes, and significant impairment in personal, family, social, education, and occupational functioning (Ford, 2019).

This diagnosis is not specified in the *DSM-5* but is accepted by several international organizations. For example, the WHO's *International Classification of Diseases* (ICD-11) differentiates CPTSD from PTSD by symptoms. PTSD core symptoms are intrusion, avoidance, and hyperarousal. CPTSD symptoms include the core

---

BOX 29.3

Dissociation

Carol, a 14-year-old high school student, was brutally raped by an older man. When the accused man was arrested, Carol could not recall any part of the attack. Her last memory was walking home after school and seeing a strange man parked on the street.

PTSD symptoms plus emphasis on symptoms of affective dysregulation, negative self-concept, and interpersonal problems (Böttche et al., 2018; Jowett et al., 2020).

Posttraumatic Stress Disorder Across the Lifespan

Children

In children 6 years and younger, exposure to actual or threatened death, serious injury, or sexual violence may result in PTSD. The symptoms include recurrent, involuntary, and intrusive distressing memories of the evens. These memories may not appear distressing and may be expressed as play. The child may not be able to explain or remember the content of the distressing dreams related to the event. For a child 6 years and under to be diagnosed with PTSD, one of the following symptoms must be present for at least 1 month and not related to physiologic changes caused by medication or illness: avoidance of stimuli or negative cognitions/mood associated with the traumatic event, irritable behavior and angry outbursts after the event with little or no provocation, or clinically significant distress (APA, 2013).

Older Adults

PTSD in older adults can occur following a new trauma or to an event that happened in several years earlier. Since there are multiple possible traumas that can precipitate PTSD, longevity increases the possibility of experiencing a traumatic event. There are many well-published accounts of World War II veterans who first experienced PTSD symptoms when they were in the 1970s. Older adults are also exposed to other traumas associated with physical health issues such as cardiovascular and musculoskeletal conditions, pain, loss of partners, changes in residences, and consequences of the COVID-19 pandemic (González-Sanguino et al., 2020; Pietrzak et al., 2021; Sommer et al., 2021).

Epidemiology and Risk Factors

The lifetime prevalence of PTSD ranges from 6.1% to 9.2% in the United States and Canada. The type of trauma a person experiences is related to the probability of PTSD occurring. For example, in sexual relationship violence, there is a 33% probability that PTSD will occur compared to exposure to organized violence, such as a civilian in a war zone, of 3% (Gradus, 2020).

Risk factors for PTSD include a prior diagnosis of acute stress disorder; the extent, duration, and intensity of trauma involved; and environmental factors. High levels of anxiety, low self-esteem, and existing personality difficulties may increase the likelihood that PTSD

will develop (Sareen et al., 2020). COVID-19 health care workers working in high-risk units are high risk for PTSD related to the perception of risk of infection, job-related stress, direct contact with affected patients, being quarantined, being infected, lack of confidence in equipment and protective measures (Preti et al., 2020).

Gender Differences

PTSD varies among all genders. Women are approximately twice as likely as men to experience PTSD; the median time from onset to remission for women is 4 years compared with 1 year for men. Several factors may contribute to these differences. People experience different types of traumatic events. As reported by Mota, men report exposure to events such as fires or disasters, life-threatening accidents, physical assault, combat, being threatened with a weapon, and being held captive. Women report anxiety and depressive disorders, child abuse, sexual molestation, sexual assault, and traumatic events before the age of 18 years (Mota et al., 2019).

> ### Consider This
>
> Susan was exposed to exploding improvised explosive devices (IEDs) while serving in Iraq. Between the ages of 6 to 9 years old, she was sexually abused by an uncle. She never told anyone.
>
> PTSD symptoms in women who are sexually assaulted may vary based on their age at the time of the first sexual assault. The younger the assault, the more severe the symptoms (Angelone et al., 2018). In a landmark study, childhood cancer survivors have been found to have four times the risk of developing PTSD as their siblings (Oral et al., 2016). Similarly, high rates of PTSD have been reported among patients with alcohol and drug dependence who have experienced childhood abuse (Fitzpatrick et al., 2020).

High rates of PTSD in veterans returning from Iraq and Afghanistan are unprecedented in modern times. PTSD prevalence estimates range from 0% to 48% in males and from 2% to 68% in women (Maguen et al., 2020). PTSD is more prevalent in the Army, among enlisted personnel when compared to officers, and more common among health care occupations, combat specialists, and service and supply personnel. PTSD in veterans is associated with postdeployment violence and alcohol misuse (Kennedy, 2020). Suicide attempts are predicted by pre-deployment history of minor traumatic brain

---

BOX 29.4

PTSD and Risky Sexual Behavior

Weiss, M. H., et al. (2019). A longitudinal examination of posttraumatic stress disorder symptoms and risky sexual behavior: Evaluating emotion dysregulation dimensions as mediators. Archives of Sexual Behavior. https://doi.org/10.1007/s10508-019-1392-y

THE QUESTION: Are PTSD symptoms a predictor of risky sexual behavior among trauma-exposed community women? Is emotional dysregulation a factor in risky sexual behavior?

METHODS: A convenience sample of 491 women 18 to 25 recruited from four sites in the southern and midwestern United States completed 5 assessments every 4 months for a 16-month period. The assessments included (1) traumatic exposure, (2) PTSD symptoms, (3) emotion dysregulation (inability to accept negative emotion ["When upset, I become angry at self for feeling that way"], difficulties engaging in goal-directed behaviors when distressed, difficulties controlling impulsive behaviors, limited strategies to regulate emotion, lack of emotional awareness and clarity), and (4) risky sexual behavior (number of different vaginal sexual partners, number of instances of condomless sex, number of instance of risky/impulsive sexual behavior such as sex in exchange for money, drugs).

FINDINGS: Women who were unable to accept their own negative feelings (i.e., they felt they should not be angry or upset) were more likely to be distressed and engaged in risky sexual behavior to reduce the negative affect of the emotion and PTSD symptoms. Women who experienced difficulties controlling impulsive behavior would be more likely to engage in risky sexual behavior.

IMPLICATIONS FOR NURSING: Early intervention in primary care and school settings for girls and women who are victims of sexual assault may prevent future revictimization and PTSD.

---

injury (TBI), frequent mental health treatment visits, young age, female, and indicators of relationship difficulties (low relationship quality, previously married, not dating) (Zuromski et al., 2019) (see Chapter 40).

Ethnicity and Culture

Discrimination is associated with higher rates of PTSD in minority groups. African American individuals experience higher rates of PTSD than White individuals and are more likely to develop PTSD following trauma exposure. Research shows that discrimination contributes to the disparate rates of PTSD experienced by African Americans (Brooks Holliday et al., 2020). Increasing discrimination since the terrorist attacks (9/11) and the discriminatory climate of the Trump administration are associated with more severed PTSD symptoms experienced by Muslim Americans (Lowe et al., 2019).

Asian Americans experienced increased stress and PTSD during the COVID-19 pandemic because of heightened discrimination related to the initial source of the coronavirus (Liu et al., 2020). Violent victimization of African American and Puerto Rican adolescents contributes to emerging increase in PTSD and comorbid psychiatric disorders (Pahl et al., 2020).

Etiology

A growing body of research postulates that biologic factors, including neurobiology and genetics, interact with environmental factors, such as childhood experiences, and the severity and extent of the traumatic exposure, to affect susceptibility to PTSD. The amygdala and hippocampus appear to be important players in fear conditioning along with the thalamus, locus coeruleus, and sensory cortex. Interaction between the cortex and the amygdala may be necessary for specific stimuli to elicit traumatic memories (Lori et al., 2019).

Several neurochemical systems are involved in regulating fear conditioning, including norepinephrine, dopamine, opiate, and corticotropin-releasing systems. Hyperarousal symptoms are characteristic of increased noradrenergic function, particularly in the locus coeruleus and in the limbic system (hypothalamus, hippocampus, and amygdala), and of increased dopamine activity, particularly in the prefrontal–cortical systems (Malikowsa-Racia & Salat, 2019).

Behavioral sensitization may be one mechanism underlying the hyperarousal seen in PTSD. The sensitized person reacts with a magnified stress response to later, milder stressors. Research shows that traumatic exposure can alter neurotransmitter connectivity in the frontal areas resulting in severe reaction to a minor stressor. This finding would account for the fact that some individuals with PTSD experience intense fear, anxiety, and panic in response to minor stimuli. One example of behavioral sensitization is that PTSD after combat exposure is more likely to develop in veterans who are survivors of childhood abuse than in those who have not experienced prior trauma (Young et al., 2020).

RECOVERY-ORIENTED CARE FOR PERSONS WITH PTSD

Recovery from PTSD takes time and involves support and patience from the family and friends, as well as a team of health care providers. **Trauma-informed care** is important in supporting recovery and includes an understanding of trauma and an awareness of the impact it can have across settings, services, and populations. Early recognition of the symptoms and treatment lead to a more successful outcomes with less likelihood of major complications. It is important to understand that there are several paths to recovery (see Chapter 2).

Teamwork and Collaboration: Working Toward Recovery

Major approaches to the treatment of PTSD include pharmacotherapy and psychotherapy. The selection of treatment is guided by practice guidelines that recommend various interventions based on medical and functional status, preexisting psychiatric and medical conditions, and current mental health assessment. The treatment guidelines, developed by the Department of Veterans Affairs and Department of Defense with the support of the Institute of Medicine, recommend education, brief psychotherapy sessions, and acute symptom management (sleep disturbance, hyperarousal, pain) for an acute reaction. During an acute reaction, psychological debriefing is not recommended. For treatment of more chronic symptoms, trauma-focused therapy and stress management are recommended along with medication (Department of VA & DOD, 2017).

Psychotherapeutic approaches to the treatment of patients with PTSD include psychodynamic psychotherapy; cognitive behavioral therapy (CBT); and eye movement, desensitization, and reprocessing. *Psychodynamic psychotherapy* focuses on different factors that may influence current PTSD symptoms such as early childhood experience and current relationships. There is emphasis on the unconscious mind. *CBTs* focus on the evaluation of situations, thoughts, feelings, and the problematic ways these evaluations cause a person to act (see Box 29.5).

Eye Movement Desensitization and Reprocessing therapy is a process of reviewing and visualizing disturbing memories of traumatic or distressing experiences to reduce the long-term impact of the events. The patient is guided through images of the trauma, allowing for progressive desensitization. Under deep relaxation, the patient maintains an image of the traumatic event while focusing on the lateral movement of the clinician's finger. This recent approach has been successful in minimizing the fear response and avoidance pattern of those with PTSD (Every-Palmer et al., 2019). Virtual Reality Exposure Therapy, the use of a virtual environment to facilitate emotional process of memories related to the trauma, is being used in some treatment settings. It can be used as a part of exposure therapy (Bourassa et al., 2020).

Group therapy and family therapy should also be considered in the treatment of those with PTSD. Sharing the traumatic experiences with family or with others who have experienced trauma can be both supportive and therapeutic. PTSD disrupts both the life of the patient and their

BOX 29.5
Cognitive Behavioral Therapies

Therapy	Purpose
Exposure therapy	Helps people face and control their fear by exposing them to the trauma in a safe way. Strategies are mental imagery, writing, or visits to the place where the event happened.
Cognitive restructuring	Helps people make sense of the bad memories by reframing their experiences in a more realistic way. They may feel guilt or shame about what is not their fault.
Cognitive processing therapy	Helps people understand why recovery from traumatic events has been difficult and how symptoms of PTSD affect daily life. Focus is on identifying how traumatic experiences changed thoughts and beliefs and influenced current feelings and behaviors.
Stress inoculation training	Teaches a person how to reduce anxiety. Like cognitive restructuring, this treatment helps people look at their memories in a healthy way.

significant others. Social support is a protective factor in the development of the disorder, and patients who have PTSD can benefit from tangible social support they receive from spouses, family, and friends (Ahmad et al., 2020).

Safety Issues

PTSD is associated with an increased risk of suicide, suicide attempts, aggression, and substance abuse (Fox et al., 2020; Kehle-Forbes et al., 2019; Miles et al., 2020). The first contact the nurse often has with the patient is after a suicide attempt or an aggressive episode. A careful assessment should include determination of the risk for self-injury or aggression toward others. These individuals are in high risk for substance abuse and suicide, so that a suicide risk assessment should be included in the nursing assessment. Safety measures such as suicide precautions may be needed, particularly if the person is hospitalized.

EVIDENCE-BASED NURSING CARE OF THE PERSON WITH POSTTRAUMATIC STRESS DISORDER

Patients with PTSD receive nursing services in a variety of settings throughout the continuum of care. Many will access care through a primary care setting, and others will seek out services in a mental health or primary health clinic. In many instances, the patient is reluctant to disclose information and has a difficult time trusting others. Distrust is especially common in persons whose trauma is associated with a violation of trust such as a rape. Gaining the patient's trust through a warm, empathic interaction, for example, offering the patient the opportunity to talk about the trauma without pressing them on the details, can lead to a meaningful therapeutic relationship.

Mental Health Nursing Assessment

After the physical health needs are met and suicidal/aggressive safety measures are established, the mental health nursing assessment targets specific areas. These include identification of the original trauma, specific physical symptoms, and the emotional and behavioral consequences of the patient's PTSD. The nursing assessment is best conducted through an interview to identify the impact of the trauma and the individual's physical and psychological strengths. The full assessment may need to take place over the course of one or more meetings, depending on the patient's capacity to discuss the traumatic events and sequelae without emotionally reexperiencing the trauma (retraumatization).

Trauma

Identifying the original trauma establishes the nature of the trauma and the length of time that the patient's PTSD has been present. However, if the person does not want to talk about the details of the trauma, the nurse should not pursue the topic. The meaning of the trauma to the individual is much more important than what happened. The survivor of trauma may be seeking help for the consequences of the trauma and is unable to discuss the original trauma. If the person wants to share information related to the traumatic experience, the following questions can be used in the assessment:

- In what ways has your life been different since the trauma?
- What does the trauma mean to you?
- Do you feel that you are the same person now as you were before the trauma? How are you the same? How are you different?
- Did anyone help you? Who are the supportive people in your life?
- Were you a survivor of trauma or abuse prior to the trauma associated with PTSD?

Physical Health Assessment

The assessment should focus not only on the physical problems but also on healthy aspects. For example,

nutrition, exercise, and self-care, such as hobbies and leisure activities, may be the individual's strengths. The assessment process should be similar to the one described in Chapter 10.

Physical Health

Sleep: In PTSD, sleep is often disrupted or practically nonexistent. Disturbing nightmares are common. The nurse should compare sleep patterns before and after the trauma. Insomnia is typically characterized by difficulty falling asleep, fragmented sleep, or panic like awakenings. The nurse should also assess for nightmares including frequency and intensity. Family members may be able to provide detailed information that is out of the patient's awareness.

Pain: The original trauma may result in chronic pain. For example, physical abuse or wartime injury may result in long-term physical treatment and pain. Prescribed pain medication is often used for reasons other than those for which it was prescribed. For example, a co-occurring traumatic brain injury may be present.

Other Somatic Responses: Patients with PTSD often have multiple unexplained physical problems (e.g., gastrointestinal, cardiovascular, neurologic, and musculoskeletal symptoms). Sometimes, the patient is reluctant to admit a trauma such as a rape or domestic assault and instead seeks out medical care for physical problems. Obtaining a trauma history becomes very important when multiple physical symptoms are present.

Nutrition

The nutritional status of a person with PTSD can be severely compromised by a poor diet following a traumatic event. Over time, a poor diet can increase the risk of other chronic diseases. The unhealthy eating habits usually appear shortly after the trauma. The nurse should assess for changes in diet.

Medication

Taking regularly prescribed medication is often difficult following a trauma. The nurse should determine the medications, vitamins, and herbal supplements the patient was taking prior to the trauma. If the person has been unable to maintain a recommended medication regimen, medication adherence can be addressed when goals are established.

Substance Use

Substance Use: Commonly, individuals with PTSD self-medicate to relieve the discomfort, anxiety, or pain caused by the trauma. The use of alcohol or other drugs is common. Assessment of the use of substances and the frequency will give direction for interventions.

> ## Consider This
> Susan started drinking alcohol regularly in Iraq. After returning home, she continued to drink six to eight cans of beer every day.

Psychosocial Assessment

The focus of the psychosocial assessment is identifying the severity of the PTSD symptoms, the disruptions that these symptoms cause the affected individual and family and current coping approaches. The patient should be asked about intrusive thoughts, irritable moods, negative thoughts, avoidance behaviors, and arousal behaviors, and what impact they have on their daily lives.

Behavioral Responses

Avoidance and isolation are common responses to trauma. The nurse should determine if the person is avoiding others, situations, or environmental reminders of the trauma. Other responses associated with PTSD are agitation and aggression after the event or events. The nurse would want to determine if these behaviors are interfering with functioning and interpersonal relationships.

The nurse should assess for hyperarousal and hypervigilance such as checking surroundings and difficulty focusing on conversations. The person may be easily startled or distracted and overreacts to things happening in the environment.

Self-Concept

In PTSD, guilt, shame, and depression are often present. Guilt may relate to feeling responsible for the events that led up to the trauma. Survivor guilt occurs when one person survives a traumatic event when others do not (see Box 29.6). Assessing self-esteem and self-concept will provide clues to the patient's resilience (see Chapter 10).

Stress and Coping Patterns

The amount of daily stress can impact the ability of the person to manage PTSD symptoms. The individual may notice that the PTSD symptoms are worse on certain days or during certain circumstances. For example, one nurse noticed her hypervigilance was worse after working the night shift for several days. These stresses should be

> ### BOX 29.6
> #### Survivor Guilt
>
> A 92-year-old survivor of World War II concentration camps has suffered from depression most of his adult life. When admitted to a long-term care facility, his daughter told the nurse that her dad often had bouts of depression where he would bemoan the fact that he had lived, and his parents and siblings had not. He often told his daughter that he felt guilty because he had survived the Holocaust.

linked to the person's current coping skills, which may be positive (meditation, relaxation) or negative (use of substances).

As the nurse and patient identify and evaluate to the effectiveness of coping skills, the nurse should determine if the patient is resilient in dealing with stress. Some coping skills may be effective immediately but have negative consequences such as the use of substances. Developing new coping skills may be important in order to enhance resilience and positive consequences.

Functional Status

An important assessment component is determining the impact of the PTSD symptoms on daily functioning. Is the person able to maintain activities of daily living, shopping, and maintaining a household? Are there difficulties in school or work performance? If there are problems in these areas, the nurse will be able to address them during the recovery planning.

Social Network and Systems

A family assessment focusing on any changes in family dynamics that has occurred since the traumatic event should also be included. The availability of a support network should be determined and built into the recovery plan.

Quality of Life

Quality of life is an overall measure of the culmination and impact of these previously discussed changes. The impact of the trauma and PTSD symptoms on overall quality of life should be examined. For example, a rape can leave a person despondent and unable to function. Nightmares and flashbacks impede sleep and physical health.

Strength Assessment

Throughout the assessment, the nurse should be listening for evidence of individual physical and psychosocial strengths. Was the patient physically healthy before the traumatic event occurred? How does the patient cope with the stress of the trauma? Does the patient have family or friends who can support the individual? Is the patient motivated to deal with PTSD symptoms, develop new coping strategies, and engage in a collaborative, therapeutic relationship? Are there financial or social resources available? This information can be used in helping patient develop a safety and recovery plan.

CLINICAL JUDGMENT

The first priority is safety. If there is a risk for suicide, the nurse and patient should first begin to address these ideations and behaviors. For someone who has been traumatized and, as a result, developed PTSD, the nurse

and patient can establish a recovery plan that addresses areas that interfere with coping and functioning such as feelings of anxiety, hopelessness, and powerlessness. For some individuals, a loss of impulse control that results in angry outbursts or aggressive behavior characterizes their difficulty with their quality of life and well-being.

THERAPEUTIC RELATIONSHIP

Establishing a trusting relationship with a person with PTSD is the basis of nurse–patient collaboration. Needs and safety are defined by the survivor who chooses the help that is wanted. Developing a relationship may take time because many survivors have had their trust violated during the traumatic event (see Box 29.7). Trauma can have a lasting effect on the ability to trust others

---

BOX 29.7 • THERAPEUTIC DIALOGUE: APPROACHING SUSAN

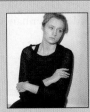

Susan did not want to be admitted to the inpatient unit and reported that she did not want to live. Her husband wants Susan to forget about Iraq and return to her former self. When she arrived on the unit, she was asked several assessment questions. She did not want to tell her story again to the nurse. The nurse needed to complete the admission assessment.

INEFFECTIVE APPROACH

Nurse: Susan, I need to ask you some questions.

Susan: Can't it wait?

Nurse: Oh—unfortunately I have to ask questions.

Susan: I am tired of talking. Everyone is asking the same questions. For the record, I do not have a problem, I do not drink too much, and I wish my husband would go away.

Nurse: Your husband is a nice guy and is only trying to help.

Susan: You do not know what you are talking about. He wants to control me.

Nurse: If you just answer some questions, I can finish my assessment.

Susan: Not now. Go away.

EFFECTIVE APPROACH

Nurse: Hi Susan, my name is Jane, and I am your nurse today.

Susan: What do you want? I don't need a nurse.

Nurse: Well, we can just talk. What brought you here?

Susan: I am tired of talking. Everyone is asking the same questions. For the record, I do not have a problem, I do not drink too much, and I wish my husband would go away.

Nurse: Talking can be tiring. What questions have you been asked?

Susan: My whole life story—where I grew up, when I got married, how do I get along with my husband and children, what happened in Iraq?

Nurse: You have had a lot of questions since you have been here. How were you able to answer all those questions?

Susan: The worst questions were about abuse and Iraq. I don't think I can talk about that yet.

Nurse: Why don't we stick to the easier ones for now?

Susan: OK, I can try.

CRITICAL THINKING CHALLENGE

• What ineffective techniques did the nurse use in the first scenario? Whose needs was the nurse meeting?

• What effective techniques did the nurse use in the second scenario?

and form intimate relationships. Coping behaviors may be misinterpreted as being "noncompliant" and can lead to negative reactions by health care providers.

MENTAL HEALTH NURSING INTERVENTIONS

Trauma is linked to health challenges over the lifespan. Trauma-informed care considers the events and circumstances causing the trauma, the person's experience of these events, and the effects of the trauma (SAMHSA, 2014). Adverse childhood experiences can lead to physiologic changes that lead to long-term health and social problems. When caring for an individual with PTSD, the impact of the trauma should be considered. Survivors of trauma may respond to the present through the lenses of their past.

Establishing Recovery and Wellness Goals

The nurse needs to guide the patient in prioritizing goals. It is unrealistic to expect the patient to work on all goals at a time. Trauma can leave people feeling powerless. For example, one place to start is with reestablishing reasonable eating and sleeping patterns. By introducing small changes, the patient will be able to determine which interventions are likely to be effective.

Physical Care

Many of the same nursing interventions discussed in Chapter 18 are used with the person with PTSD. Proper nutrition and regular exercise can help fortify the resilience.

Sleep Enhancement

Sleep hygiene is also an important strategy because sleep disruption is common in PTSD. Early life adversity and PTSD severity are associated with fewer hours of resting and sleeping when compared to those who had lower early life adversity (see Chapter 28) (Gavrieli et al., 2015). Nurses should collaborate with the patient in finding a strategy that will help the person sleep and manage nightmares. For example, the individual may want to sleep with the lights on because of the nightmares. However, light interferes with nighttime sleep for some people. It may be possible to go to sleep with the lights on but ask a family member to turn off the lights later. Some persons with PTSD find that they cannot sleep in their bed but can sleep in a chair. Some of the following strategies may be helpful:

- Establish and maintain a regular bedtime and rising time.
- Avoid naps.

- Abstain from alcohol. Although alcohol may assist with sleep onset, an alerting effect occurs when it wears off.
- Refrain from caffeine after midafternoon. Avoid nicotine before bedtime and during the night. Caffeine and nicotine are strong stimulants and cause fragmented sleep.
- Avoid exercising 3 hours before bedtime.

Exercise and Yoga

Severe PTSD symptoms are associated with poor physical performance and decreased physical functioning (van den Berk-Clark et al., 2018). Yet, we know that exercise is associated with reduced PTSD symptoms (Hall et al., 2020). Nurses need to encourage patients with PTSD to engage in regular exercise, not only for health promotion but also to reduce symptoms. Practicing yoga may motivate people with PTSD to increase physical activity along with enhancing self-efficacy. Simple stretching and breathing have shown to reduce abnormal cortisol levels and can be taught in many practice settings (Niles et al., 2018).

Nutrition Interventions

PTSD and early life adversity are associated with risk of obesity, diabetes, and cardiovascular disease. The greater the symptoms, the higher the body weight and blood pressure and lower the insulin sensitivity (Kidman et al., 2020). Poor diet quality including the consumption of *trans* fatty acids can be a major health issue with these individuals. Monitoring body weight and blood pressure should be included in the patient's plan of care. If these health issues are present, nurses should encourage patients to make different food choices and to choose healthy foods. Referral to a dietician may be necessary.

Smoking Cessation

Individuals with PTSD have higher smoking rates than others, and fewer have quit than the general population. Smoking serves as a way of coping with the symptoms of PTSD. Smoking often co-occurs with alcohol use disorders and cannabis use. Nurses should discuss the health risks associated with these behaviors and encourage the patient to reduce their use. Smoking cessation programs are readily available in most communities (Homish et al., 2019).

Medication Interventions

The selective serotonin reuptake inhibitors (SSRIs), serotonin-norepinephrine reuptake inhibitors, atypical antipsychotics, and mood stabilizers may be effective in reducing the symptoms of PTSD (see Chapters 12 and 25). Two SSRI antidepressants, sertraline (Zoloft) and paroxetine (Paxil), are approved for PTSD and are used to treat symptoms such as sadness, worry, anger, and feeling numb inside (see Box 29.8). Benzodiazepines are not recommended for persons with PTSD. Recently, off-label use of prazosin, an alpha$_1$ inhibitor, has been shown to be effective in treating nightmares and improving sleep in PTSD (Ehret, 2019). When prescribed in conjunction with psychotherapy, pharmacotherapy can minimize the excessive fear and anxiety of PTSD (Grasser & Javanbakht, 2019).

Because the person with PTSD may take many different types of medication, the nurse needs to monitor for any drug interactions and teach the person about all the medications including expected therapeutic effect(s) and side effects. These individuals often take prescribed or over-the-counter pain medications that may interact with mood stabilizers, antidepressants, antianxiety agents, or antipsychotic agents.

Management of Complications

Substance Abuse Interventions: If the person has been using substances to dull the feelings associated with the trauma, the nurse should educate the individual about the addiction and make a referral to a substance abuse treatment team. It is important for the nurse to use a nonjudgmental approach, recognizing the person is suffering from the trauma and is trying to cope with intrusive thoughts and pain. The nurse should emphasize that there are more effective coping mechanisms and offer hope that the person can find other means of alleviating the PTSD symptoms.

Psychosocial Interventions and Trauma-Informed Care

Many of the same psychosocial interventions discussed in Chapter 27 can be used for persons with PTSD. Relaxation strategies and stress reduction techniques are particularly helpful for these individuals. Encouraging the person to participate in a support group can decrease the isolation that may be present and learn how others deal with their symptoms. Service and companion dogs are also helpful in helping the person address the stress of PTSD.

Therapeutic Interactions

One of the greatest treatment challenges is avoiding secondary trauma. When caring for persons with PTSD, we should assume that they have a history of traumatic stress. Extreme stress occurs when shocking or unexpected events overwhelm a person's ability to cope. The nurse should respect how and when a person chooses to talk about the trauma. Healing from trauma requires finding and maintaining a sense of safety, gaining a sense of control over one's life and environment.

The focus of the interactions should be on understanding "what happened," not on what is wrong with

---

BOX 29.8

Drug Profile: Sertraline (Zoloft)

DRUG CLASS: Antidepressant (SSRI)

RECEPTOR AFFINITY: Blocks the reuptake of serotonin

INDICATIONS: Major depressive disorder, obsessive–compulsive disorder, panic disorder, PTSD, premenstrual dysphoric disorder, social anxiety disorder

ROUTES AND DOSAGES: Available in 25-mg, 50-mg, 100-mg rts, 20 mg/mL

Adults: 50 to 200 mg PO once daily; start 50 mg PO once daily, may increase by 50 mg/day

HALF-LIFE (PEAK EFFECT): 62 to 104 hours

SELECTED ADVERSE REACTIONS: Nausea, headache, insomnia, diarrhea, dry mouth, ejaculatory dysfunction, somnolence, weakness, lack of energy, tremor, dyspepsia, anorexia, constipation, decrease in libido, nervousness, anxiety, rash, visual disturbance

WARNINGS: Increase suicidality risk in children, adolescents, and young adults with major depressive or other psychiatric disorders. Contradicted in persons being treated with monoamine oxidase inhibitors and pimozide, an antipsychotic. Risk for serotonin syndrome.

SPECIFIC PATIENT AND FAMILY EDUCATION
- Take exactly as prescribed.
- Can be taken with or without food.
- If a dose is missed, take missed dose as soon as patient remembers unless time for next dose; then skip missed dose.
- Can cause sleepiness or may affect ability to make decisions, think clearly or react quickly.
- Do not drive, operate heavy machinery until patient knows how medication will affect them.
- Do not drink alcohol while taking medication.
- Report any signs and symptoms of adverse reactions, suicidal thoughts, or actions.
- Notify your health care provider if severe agitation, hallucinations, coordination problems, muscle twitching, racing heartbeat, high or low blood pressure, muscle rigidity, sweating or fever, nausea, vomiting, diarrhea occur.

the person. The nurse seeks to understand the meaning of the experience to the individual. Similar events have different meanings to different people. When patients are describing traumatic events, it is important for the nurse to avoid responding in shock, dismay, or disgust. A welcoming approach creates a safe environment for the person to discuss the trauma. Within a collaborative relationship, coping strategies, not symptoms, are the focus. In a safe environment, the person can develop positive coping skills and make sense of who they are.

Enhancing Cognitive Functioning

There are several approaches to managing the intrusive thoughts, dissociative experiences, and hypervigilance that the person may be experiencing. The intrusive thoughts could be addressed through distraction, thought stopping, meditation, or relaxation. Deep breathing or reframing the situation may reduce the hypervigilance and refocusing may reduce the dissociation. The specific approach will depend on the ability of the person to use the techniques.

Psychoeducation

Teaching About Symptoms

PTSD impacts every aspect of a person's life. Trauma, genetic predisposition, brain changes, risk for multiple health problems, and risk for addiction are a part of PTSD. Education about the disorder, its consequences, health risks, and treatment become key topics for patient and family education. Psychoeducation should be individualized to the person's specific issues. There are general psychoeducation topics that should be considered for patient teaching (see Box 29.9).

BOX 29.9

Posttraumatic Stress Disorder

When caring for a person with a PTSD, be sure to include the following topic areas in the teaching plan:
- Identification of individual triggers and cues that lead to reexperiencing trauma
- Safety plans for stressful periods
- Recovery plans that focus on personal strengths
- Risk factors for reoccurrence of symptoms
- Various treatment options: if one does not help, others exist
- Avoid substances such as alcohol and drugs
- Nutrition
- Exercise
- Sleep hygiene
- Follow-up appointments
- Community services

Wellness Strategies

Many of the wellness strategies are interventions to treatment of the symptoms of PTSD. For example, sleep hygiene is important for those with sleep problems. Managing stress is very important for a person with this disorder. Practicing healthy stress management techniques are critical for handling the events related to hyperarousal. An innocent loud noise may be misinterpreted as a gunshot causing an aggressive response. Exercise helps reduce stress and supports healthy functioning.

Providing Family Education

Families need support as they learn to cope with their family member with PTSD. Family members often feel hopeless in trying to understand the changes that their loved one is undergoing. In many instances, the member with PTSD is unable to share information about the trauma and the symptoms. If alcohol or other drugs are used to self-medicate, the family has additional challenges in dealing with the substance use. Support groups, education about PTSD, and family therapy are helpful.

Promoting Safety

Hospitalization provides a measure of safety for the patient. During hospitalization, the nurse should continue with suicide risk screening as needed and protection from triggering events such as load noises or stimulating activities. A safety plan should be developed if the patient has had thoughts of dying by suicide (see Chapter 22).

Evaluation and Treatment Outcomes

The treatment of PTSD may last several years with changing goals. Early in treatment, the goals may be to reduce the intrusive thoughts and regulate sleep; later goals may include being able to establish a trusting relationship with a partner. The evaluation will be modified as the goals and interventions change.

Continuum of Care

The person with PTSD is primarily treated in the community rather than a medical facility as an inpatient. Short-term hospitalization for safety may be needed if suicidal or homicidal thoughts are strong or for an adjustment of medication.

Emergency Care !

When individuals with PTSD need emergency care, they are usually having suicidal ideation or thoughts to hurt others. Safety interventions should be implemented. It is important for the nurse to know the nature of the trauma to be able to approach the patient. For example, a person previously exposed to combat may be sensitive to loud noises and is more likely to become aggressive when doors slam, whereas a woman who has been raped may not tolerate anyone touching her.

Inpatient-Focused Care

Inpatient settings can provide a safe environment for the person who is tormented with frequent flashbacks, has become depressed and potentially suicidal, or is harboring thoughts about hurting others. Medications may be initiated or adjusted. However, hospitalization and restrictive treatment can also retraumatize the patient. Being locked in a mental health unit or being restrained can be extremely traumatizing to the person who has already been traumatized See the Nursing Care Plan 29.1, which sets forth a plan of care for Susan, the case study patient in this chapter.

Community Care

Treatment mostly occurs in the community with the individual attending group therapy, support groups, individual therapy, and medication management. Most

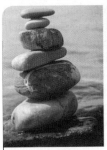

NURSING CARE PLAN 29.1

The Person with Posttraumatic Stress Disorder

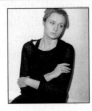

Susan is a 30-year-old woman admitted to an acute mental health unit after a suicide attempt with an overdose of benzodiazepines and alcohol. She was discharged from the Army 6 months ago and returned home to her husband and two children, age 6 and 8. She was sexually assaulted by an uncle when she was 6 years old. While in Iraq, she was exposed to combat and was sexually assaulted by another soldier. She has been drinking alcohol heavily after her return home. She and her husband have been arguing since her return and are now discussing divorce. She decided to end it all.

Setting: Acute Mental Health Unit

Baseline Assessment: Susan is dressed in hospital scrubs following medical treatment of overdose. She is oriented X3. She is gazing downward, with flat affect, shoulders slightly hunched, soft voice. She reports she is no longer having suicidal thoughts but feels very depressed. "I don't know what to do. I don't feel close to my kids and my husband wants a divorce." She reports that she began taking her mother's benzodiazepines to help her sleep. She is having constant thoughts about the killings she saw in Iraq, cannot sleep, often has nightmares when she does sleep, does not want sexual relations with husband, and sleeps on a couch close to the front door. She drinks six to eight beers a day. She has not worked since returning from Iraq. She is 5'5" tall, weighs 140 lbs (BMI 23.3), has BP 120/70; P70, R16. Her goal is to have a normal life.

Strengths: Husband states he does not want a divorce and wants to stay married and is willing to engage in counseling. Mother is very supportive. She has work skills.

Associated Psychiatric Diagnosis	Medications
Posttraumatic Stress Disorder Lorazepam 1 mg every 4 to 6 hours as needed Zolpidem 5 mg PO HS as needed	Sertraline, 25 mg every morning for 1 week, then 50 mg PO every day.

Priority of Nursing Care: Post-Trauma Behaviors

Important Characteristics	Associated Considerations
Depression Flashbacks Intrusive thoughts	Abuse, witnessing violent death Rape Substance abuse

Outcomes

Initial	Long Term
• Motivate patient to reduce use of alcohol and abuse of benzodiazepines for stress reduction. • Discuss original trauma and the more recent trauma in Iraq. • Increase quality of sleep. • Practice stress reduction techniques.	• Engage in psychotherapy to reduce impact of trauma. • Develop positive healthy strategies for managing stress.

Interventions

Interventions	Rationale	Ongoing Assessment
• Initiate a nurse–patient relationship by using an accepting, nonjudgmental approach.	A relationship with a therapist will provide an opportunity for Susan to discuss her trauma and strengths.	Determine the extent to which Susan is willing to trust and engage in a therapeutic relationship.
• Encourage Susan to identify symptoms of PTSD.	By identifying symptoms, Susan will be able to recognize that the intrusive thoughts, insomnia, and other symptoms are related to her traumatic experience.	Assess Susan's recognition of her symptoms and her level of understanding of the symptoms' relationship to her current distress.
• Help Susan develop a plan to address her current marital problems such as counseling or therapy after discharge.	Her marital problems may be related to her sexual assaults and exposure to combat.	Determine Susan's willingness to develop a plan.
• Administer sertraline 50 mg as prescribed. Observe for target effect and side effects. Begin teaching about the medication and the importance of taking the medication as prescribed, avoiding consuming alcohol, and reporting any side effects.	Sertraline is an SSRI that blocks the reuptake of serotonin and is indicated for PTSD.	Make sure that Susan takes her medication. Monitor for improvement in PTSD symptoms and side effects such as nervousness, nausea, and any others.
• Monitor sleep patterns and teach improved sleep hygiene. Administer zolpidem as prescribed.	Disturbed sleep is common in association with PTSD.	If Susan continues to have disturbed sleep or experience side effects from zolpidem therapy, notify the primary care prescriber.
• Support development of resilience by examining Susan's strengths (e.g., social support, nutrition, exercise).	Resilience is important in reducing the impact of previous trauma. Positive social support, nutrition, and exercise help support resilience.	Determine Susan's social support, nutrition, and exercise regimen.

Priority of Nursing Care: Difficulty in Assuming Parenting Responsibilities

Important Characteristics	Associated Considerations
Decreased capacity to parent Inadequate coping to stresses of parenting	Substance use Stress Conflict with husband

Outcomes

Initial	Long Term
• Resume parenting role. • Decrease conflict with husband. • Reduce use of substances.	• Serve as role model to children. • Develop positive relationship with husband. • Eliminate the use of substances as a stress reliever.

Evaluation

Interventions	Rationales	Ongoing Assessment
• Collaborate with Susan in identifying her current role perceptions.	Recovery-oriented nursing care engages the patient in decision-making.	Validate whether her current role perceptions accord with reality.
• Identify the changes that she would like to make in her parenting role. • Discuss her goals for her marriage.	Relationship rebuilding starts with self-awareness of personal goals.	Determine if she needs referral to community resources that can help her with her relationship and role issues.
• Discuss strategies for reducing substance use for stress reduction. • Offer relaxation, meditation, or imagery for stress reduction.	Substance use for stress reduction has negative outcomes with high risk of addiction.	Determine whether strategies are useful to Susan. May need referral to substance abuse counselor if necessary.

appointments will occur after working hours. Nursing care can be delivered in all settings. The community setting is an excellent opportunity for patient and family education.

Virtual Mental Health Care

Virtual strategies are beneficial for the care of individuals with PTSD. Remote access to providers and treatment apps are readily available on cell phones and computers. More sophisticated virtual reality technology is also being used. For example, imagery tasks are used to create safe spaces through the use of Google or Microsoft applications (Frewen et al., 2020).

Integration of Primary Care

The persons with PTSD may first seek help from a primary care provider. For example, sleep problems in adults and behavior problems of children are often treated in a nonmental health environment. Conversely, when mental health clinicians care for persons with PTSD, they must address the physical problems as well as their psychological problems. Because there is no one medication indicated for PTSD, there is a risk of multiple medications being prescribed to treat various physical and mental health problems. Ideally, individuals with PTSD should be treated in an integrated setting where close monitoring of all treatments is possible.

OTHER TRAUMA- AND STRESSOR-RELATED DISORDERS

Acute stress disorder is similar to PTSD except that it is resolved within 1 month of the traumatic event. Acute stress disorder can develop into PTSD if the symptoms last longer than 1 month. Two trauma- and stressor-related disorders typically occurring in childhood are reactive attachment disorder and disinhibited social engagement disorder. *Reactive attachment disorder* is characterized by inhibited, emotionally withdrawn behavior toward an adult caregiver. These children rarely seek or respond to comfort when distressed. This disorder usually occurs when the primary caregiver frequently changes. In *disinhibited social engagement disorder,* the child is overly familiar with others in ways uncharacteristic of cultural norms. For instance, the child does not hesitate to go somewhere with an unfamiliar adult.

One of the most common diagnoses for hospitalized persons is adjustment disorder (APA, 2013). These disorders occur within 3 months of the stressor. Affected individuals experience distress that seems out of proportion to the severity of the stressor and may be unable to function socially. After the situation is resolved, the symptoms subside.

Dissociative Disorders

Dissociative disorders are thought to be responses to extreme external or internal events or stressors where dissociation, or a splitting from the self, occurs as a way of coping with severe anxiety. Prevalence is higher among people who experience childhood physical or sexual abuse than among others. The onset of these disorders may be sudden or may occur gradually; the course of each may be long term or transient. Dissociative disorders include *dissociative amnesia,* the inability to recall important yet stressful information; *depersonalization/derealization disorder,* the feeling of being detached from one's mental processes; and *dissociative identity disorder* (DID) (formerly called multiple personality disorder), presence of at least two distinct personality or identity states.

The essential feature of these disorders involves a failure to integrate identity, memory, and consciousness. That is, unwanted intrusive thoughts disrupt one's contact with the here and now, or memories that are normally accessible are lost. These disorders are closely related to the trauma- and stressor-related disorders but are categorized separately. Persons with dissociative disorders may also have comorbid substance abuse, mood disorders, personality disorders, or PTSD (APA, 2013).

DID has long been a controversial diagnosis, with many skeptics challenging the legitimacy of this disorder. Recent empirical evidence supports DID as a complex, posttraumatic developmental disorder. Once believed to be relatively rare, prevalence rates are reported at approximately 1.1% to 1.5% of community samples. The highest prevalence is found in groups highly exposed to trauma or cultural oppression (Brand et al., 2016). There is also emerging evidence that there are structural brain changes in persons with this disorder (Reinders et al., 2018).

Treatment options include the use of antidepressants to treat the patient's underlying mood and anxiety. Psychotherapy options include CBT and psychodynamic psychotherapy to determine the triggers that lead to heightened anxiety and dissociation.

SUMMARY OF KEY POINTS

- The development of psychological trauma depends on the meaning of the event and the resilience of the individual. The stronger the resilience, the more likely the individual will be able to withstand the negative impact of a potentially traumatic event.

- Resilience develops over time when there are a positive self-concept and measured self-worth, and when problem-solving, communication, and coping skills have been learned.

- PTSD occurs after a traumatic event and is characterized by involuntary intrusive thoughts, avoidance and numbing, negative moods and thoughts, and hyper-arousal. CPTSD develops when there is betrayal of trust and chronic repetitive trauma over months or year.

- Women are twice as likely as men to experience PTSD. Service members returning from Iraq and Afghanistan have high rates of PTSD.

- There are several approaches to the treatment of PTSD including CBT, traditional psychotherapy, and medications.

- Nursing care focuses on assessing symptoms of PTSD, building strengths, enhancing resilience, and collaborating with the patient in counseling interventions, administration of medication, psychoeducation, and family support.

CRITICAL THINKING CHALLENGES

1. What are the various traumatic events that can lead to PTSD? Why do some people develop PTSD and others, who have experienced the same trauma, do not?

2. Identify strategies the nurse can use to support the development of resilience.

3. Differentiate intrusive thoughts from dissociative symptoms.

4. Give examples of derealization and depersonalization.

5. Compare trauma- and stressor-related disorders with dissociative disorders. How are they similar? How are they different?

6. How should a nurse approach a military veteran who is having intrusive thoughts, is having nightmares, and is unable to sleep?

Movie Viewing Guides

The Dry Land: (2010). James (Ryan O'Nan), an Iraq war veteran, returns to his small-town life in Texas. His family quickly realizes that he has changed and has PTSD. He is irritable, anxious, and considers suicide. He keeps a gun at his bedside. He drinks with his friends and is easily provoked into fights. His family cannot truly understand the pain he feels. An award-winning movie, it depicts a veteran's struggle with regaining his life.

VIEWING POINTS: Identify the behaviors that are characteristic of PTSD. Identify the strengths that he demonstrated that represented resilience. Develop a plan of care that includes his family, friends, and community support.

REFERENCES

Ahmad, F., Othman, N., & Lou, W. (2020). Posttraumatic stress disorder, social support and coping among Afghan refugees in Canada. *Community Mental Health Journal*, 56(4), 597–605. https://doi.org/10.1007/s10597-019-00518-1

American Psychiatric Association. (2013). *Diagnostic and statistical manual of mental disorders DSM-5 (5th ed.)*. Author.

Angelone, D. J., Marcantonio, T., & Melillo J. (2018). An evaluation of adolescent and young adult (re)victimization experiences: Problematic substance use and negative consequences. *Violence Against Women, 2018*, 24(5), 586–602. https://doi.org/10.1177/1077801217710001.

Atwoli. L., Stein, D. J., King, A., Petukhova, M., Aguilar-Gaxiola, S., Alonso, J., Bromet, E. J., de Girolamo, G., Demyttenaere, K., Florescu, S., Maria Haro, J., Karam, E. G., Kawakami, N., Lee, S., Lepine, J. P., Navarro-Mateu, F., O'Neill, S., Pennell, B. E., Piazza, M., Posada-Villa, J., ... WHO World Mental Health Survey Collaborators (2017). Posttraumatic stress disorder associated with unexpected death of a loved one: Cross-national findings from the world mental health surveys. *Depression and Anxiety*, 34(4), 315–326. https://doi.org/10.1002/da.22579.

Böttcher, M., Ehring, T., Krüger-Gottschalk, A., Rau, H., Schäfer, I., Schellong, J., Dyer, A., & Knaevelsrud, C. (2018). Testing the ICD-11 proposal for complex PTSD in trauma-exposed adults: Factor structure and symptom profiles. *European Journal of Psychotraumatology*, 9(1), 1512264. https://doi.org/10.1080/20008198.2018.1512264

Bourassa, K. J., Smolenski, D. J., Edwards-Stewart, A., Campbell, S. B., Reger, G. M., & Norr, A. M. (2020). The impact of prolonged exposure therapy on social support and PTSD symptoms. *Journal of Affective Disorders*, 260, 410–417. https://doi.org/10.1016/j.jad.2019.09.036

Brand, B. L., Sar, V., Stavropoulos, P., Krüger, C., Korzekwa, M., Martínez-Taboas, A., & Middleton, W. (2016). Separating fact from fiction: An empirical examination of six myths about dissociative identity disorder. *Harvard Review of Psychiatry*, 24(4), 257–270. https://doi.org/10.1097/HRP.0000000000000100

Brooks Holliday, S., Dubowitz, T., Haas, A., Ghosh-Dastidar, B., DeSantis, A., & Troxel, W. M. (2020). The association between discrimination and PTSD in African Americans: exploring the role of gender. *Ethnicity & Health*, 25(5), 717–731. https://doi.org/10.1080/13557858.2018.1444150

Brooks, M., Graham-Kevan, N., Robinson, S., & Lowe, M. (2019). Trauma characteristics and posttraumatic growth: The mediating role of avoidance coping, intrusive thoughts, and social support. *Psychological Trauma: Theory, Research, Practice, and Policy*, 11(2), 232–238. https://doi.org/10.1037/tra0000372

Chang, X., Jiang, X., Mkandarwire, T., & Shen, M. (2019). Associations between adverse childhood experiences and health outcomes in adults aged 18–59 years. *PLoS One*, 14(2), e0211850. https://doi.org/10.1371/journal.pone.0211850

Department of Veteran Affairs & Department of Defense. (2017). *VA/DoD clinical practice guideline for management of post-traumatic stress*. Version 3.0. Washington, DC: Quality, Safety and Value, VA, & Office of Evidence Based Practice, U.S. Army Medical Command. https://www.healthquality.va.gov/guidelines/MH/ptsd/VADoDPTSDCPGFinal012418.pdf

Ehret, M. (2019). Treatment of posttraumatic stress disorder: Focus on pharmacotherapy. *The Mental Health Clinician*, 9(6), 373–382. https://doi.org/10.9740/mhc.2019.11.373

Every-Palmer, S., Flewett, T., Dean, S., Hansby, O., Colman, A., Weatherall, M., & Bell, E. (2019). Eye movement desensitization and reprocessing (EMDR) therapy for posttraumatic stress disorder in adults with serious mental illness within forensic and rehabilitation services: A study protocol for a randomized controlled trial. *Trials*, 20(1), 642. https://doi.org/10.1186/s13063-019-3760-2

Fitzpatrick, S., Saraiya, T., Lopez-Castro, T., Ruglass, L. M., & Hien, D. (2020). The impact of trauma characteristics on post-traumatic stress disorder and substance use disorder outcomes across integrated and substance use treatments. *Journal of Substance Abuse Treatment*, 113, 107976. https://doi.org/10.1016/j.jsat.2020.01.012

Ford, J. D. (2019). Commentary on the special section on Complex PTSD: Still going strong after all these years. *Journal of Traumatic Stress*, 32(6), 877–880. https://doi.org/10.1002/jts.22474

Fox, V., Dalman, C., Dal, H., Hollander, A. C., Kirkbride, J. B., & Pitman, A. (2020). Suicide risk in people with post-traumatic stress disorder: A cohort study of 3.1 million people in Sweden. *Journal of Affective Disorders*, 279, 609–616. https://doi.org/10.1016/j.jad.2020.10.009

Frewen, P., Mistry, D., Zhu, J., Kielt, T., Wekerle, C., Lanius, R. A., & Jetly, R. (2020). Proof of concept of an eclectic, integrative therapeutic approach to mental health and well-being through virtual reality technology. *Frontiers in Psychology*, 11, 858. https://doi.org/10.3389/fpsyg.2020.00858

Gavrieli, A., Farr, O. M., Davis, C. R., Crowell, J. A., & Mantzoros, C. S. (2015). Early life adversity and/or posttraumatic stress disorder severity are associated with poor diet quality, including consumption of trans fatty acids, and fewer hours of resting or sleeping in a US middle-aged population: A cross-sectional and prospective study. *Metabolism*, 64, 1597–1610.

González-Sanguino, C., Ausín, B., Castellanos, M. Á., Saiz, J., López-Gómez, A., Ugidos, C., & Muñoz, M. (2020). Mental health consequences during the initial stage of the 2020 Coronavirus pandemic (COVID-19) in Spain. *Brain, Behavior, and Immunity, 87,* 172–176. https://doi.org/10.1016/j.bbi.2020.05.040

Gradus, J. L. (2020). Epidemiology of PTSD. PTSD: *National Center for PTSD.* U.S. Department of Veterans Affairs. https://www.ptsd.va.gov/professional/treat/essentials/epidemiology.asp#:~:text=The%20NCS%2DR%20estimated%20the,%25%20among%20women%20(3)

Grasser, L. R., & Javanbakht, A. (2019). Treatments of posttraumatic stress disorder in civilian populations. *Current Psychiatry Reports, 21*(2), 11. https://doi.org/10.1007/s11920-019-0994-3

Hall, K. S., Morey, M. C., Bosworth, H. B., Beckham, J. C., Pebole, M. M., Sloane, R., & Pieper, C. F. (2020). Pilot randomized controlled trial of exercise training for older veterans with PTSD. *Journal of Behavioral Medicine, 43*(4), 648–659. https://doi.org/10.1007/s10865-019-00073-w

Homish, G. G., Hoopsick, R. A., Heavey, S. C., Homish, D. L., & Cornelius, J. R. (2019). Drug use and hazardous drinking are associated with PTSD symptoms and symptom clusters in US Army Reserve/National Guard Soldiers. *The American Journal on Addictions, 28*(1), 22–28. https://doi.org/10.1111/ajad.12829

Jowett, S., Karatzias, T., Shevlin, M., & Albert, I. (2020). Differentiating symptom profiles of ICD-11 PTSD, complex PTSD, and borderline personality disorder: A latent class analysis in a multiply traumatized sample. *Personality Disorders, 11*(1), 36–45. https://doi.org/10.1037/per0000346

Kehle-Forbes, S. M., Chen, S., Polusny, M. A., Lynch, K. G., Koffel, E., Ingram, E., Foa, E. B., Van Horn, D., Drapkin, M. L., Yusko, D. A., & Oslin, D. W. (2019). A randomized controlled trial evaluating integrated versus phased application of evidence-based psychotherapies for military veterans with comorbid PTSD and substance use disorders. *Drug and Alcohol Dependence, 205,* 107647. https://doi.org/10.1016/j.drugalcdep.2019.107647

Kennedy, L. (2020). Postwar interpersonal violence: Reflections and new research directions. *Aggression and Violent Behavior, 53,* https://doi.org/10.1016/j.avb.2020.101429

Kidman, R., Piccolo, L. R., & Kohler, H. P. (2020). Adverse childhood experiences: Prevalence and association with adolescent health in Malawi. *American Journal of Preventive Medicine, 58*(2), 285–293. https://doi.org/10.1016/j.amepre.2019.08.028

Liu, C. H., Zhang, E., Wong, G., Hyun, S., & Hahm, H. C. (2020). Factors associated with depression, anxiety, and PTSD symptomatology during the COVID-19 pandemic: Clinical implications for U.S. young adult mental health. *Psychiatry Research, 290,* 113172. https://doi.org/10.1016/j.psychres.2020.113172

Lori, A., Maddox, S. A., Sharma, S., Andero, R., Ressler, K. J., & Smith, A. K. (2019). Dynamic patterns of threat-associated gene expression in the amygdala and blood. *Frontiers in Psychiatry, 9,* 778. https://doi.org/10.3389/fpsyt.2018.00778

Lowe, S. R., Tineo, P., Bonumwezi, J. L., & Bailey, E. J. (2019). The trauma of discrimination: Posttraumatic stress in Muslim American college students. *Traumatology, 25*(2), 115–123. https://doi-org.libproxy.siue.edu/10.1037/trm0000197

Maguen, S., Holder, N., Li, Y., Madden, E., Neylan, T. C., Seal, K. H., Lujan, C., Patterson, O. V., DuVall, S. L., & Shiner, B. (2020). Factors associated with PTSD symptom improvement among Iraq and Afghanistan veterans receiving evidenced-based psychotherapy. *Journal of Affective Disorders, 273,* 1–7. https://doi.org/10.1016/j.jad.2020.04.039

Maguire, D. G., Ruddock, M. W., Milanak, M. E., Moore, T., Cobice, D., & Armour, C. (2020). Sleep, a Governor of Morbidity in PTSD: A systematic review of biological markers in PTSD-related sleep disturbances. *Nature and Science of Sleep, 12,* 545–562. https://doi.org/10.2147/NSS.S260734

Malikowsa-Racia, N., & Salat, K. (2019). Recent advances in the neurobiology of posttraumatic stress disorder: A review of possible mechanisms underlying an effective pharmacotherapy. *Pharmacological Research,* pii: S1043-6618(18)31172-1. https://doi.org/10.1016/j.phrs.2019.02.001

Marshall, G. N., Jaycox, L. H., Engel, C. C., Richardson, A., Dutra, S. J., Keane, T. M., Rosen, R. C., & Marx, B. P. (2019). PTSD symptoms are differentially associated with general distress and physiological arousal: Implications for the conceptualization and measurement of PTSD. *Journal of Anxiety Disorders, 62,* 26–34. https://doi.org/10.1016/j.janxdis.2018.10.003

Miles, S. R., Dillon, K. H., Jacoby, V. M., Hale, W. J., Dondanville, K. A., Wachen, J. S., Yarvis, J. S., Peterson, A. L., Mintz, J., Litz, B. T., Young-McCaughan, S., Resick, P. A., & STRONG STAR Consortium. (2020). Changes in anger and aggression after treatment for PTSD in active duty military. *Journal of Clinical Psychology, 76*(3), 493–507. https://doi.org/10.1002/jclp.22878

Mitra, R., & Hodes, M. (2019). Prevention of psychological distress and promotion of resilience amongst unaccompanied refugee minors in resettlement countries. *Child: Care Health and Development,* https://doi.org/10.1111/cch.12640

Mota, N. Turner, S., Taillieu, T., Garcés, I., Magid, K., Sethi, J., Struck, S., El-Gabalawy, R., & Afifi, T. O. (2019). Trauma exposure, DSM-5 posttraumatic stress disorder, and sexual risk outcomes. *American Journal of Preventive Medicine, 56*(2), 215–223.

Naifeh, J. A., Mash, H., Stein, M. B., Fullerton, C. S., Kessler, R. C., & Ursano, R. J. (2019). The Army Study to assess risk and resilience in servicemembers (Army STARRS): Progress toward understanding suicide among soldiers. *Molecular Psychiatry, 24*(1), 34–48. https://doi.org/10.1038/s41380-018-0197-z

Niles, B. L., Mori, D. L., Polizzi, C., Pless Kaiser, A., Weinstein, E. S., Gershkovich, M., & Wang, C. (2018). A systematic review of randomized trials of mind-body interventions for PTSD. *Journal of Clinical Psychology, 74*(9), 1485–1508. https://doi.org/10.1002/jclp.22634

Oral, R., Ramirez, M., Coohey, C., Nakada, S., Walz, A., Kuntz, A., Benoit, J., & Peek-Asa, C. (2016). Adverse childhood experiences and trauma informed care: The future of health care. *Pediatric Research, 79*(1), 227–233.

Pahl, K., Williams, S. Z., Lee, J. Y., Joseph, A., & Blau, C. (2020). Trajectories of violent victimization predicting PTSD and comorbidities among urban ethnic/racial minorities. *Journal of Consulting and Clinical Psychology, 88*(1), 39–47. https://doi.org/10.1037/ccp0000449

Pietrzak, R. H., Tsai, J., & Southwick, S. M. (2021). Association of symptoms of posttraumatic stress disorder with posttraumatic psychological growth among US veterans during the COVID-19 pandemic. *JAMA Network Open, 4*(4), e214972. https://doi.org/10.1001/jamanetworkopen.2021.4972

Preti, E., Di Mattei, V., Perego, G., Ferrari, F., Mazzetti, M., Taranto, P., Di Pierro, R., Madeddu, F., & Calati, R. (2020). The psychological impact of epidemic and pandemic outbreaks on healthcare workers: Rapid review of the evidence. *Current Psychiatry Reports, 22*(8), 43. https://doi.org/10.1007/s11920-020-01166-z

Reinders, A. A. T. S., Marquand, A. F., Schlumpf, Y. R., Chalavi, S., Vissia, E. M., Nijenhuis, E., Dazzan, P., Jäncke, L., & Veltman, D. J. (2018). Aiding the diagnosis of dissociative identity disorder: Pattern recognition study of brain biomarkers. *British Journal of Psychiatry, 215*(3), 536–544. https://doi.org/10.1192/bjp.2018.255

Sareen, J., Stein, M. B., & Friedman, M. (2020). Posttraumatic stress disorder in adults: Epidemiology, pathophysiology, clinical manifestations, course, assessment, and diagnosis. *Up to Date.* https://www.uptodate.com/contents/posttraumatic-stress-disorder-in-adults-epidemiology-pathophysiology-clinical-manifestations-course-assessment-and-diagnosis/print

Sommer, J. L., Reynolds, K., El-Gabalawy, R., Pietrzak, R. H., Mackenzie, C. S., Ceccarelli, L., Mota, N., & Sareen, J. (2021). Associations between physical health conditions and posttraumatic stress disorder according to age. *Aging & Mental Health, 25*(2), 234–242. https://doi.org/10.1080/13607863.2019.1693969

Substance Abuse and Mental Health Services Administration. (2014). *SAMHSA's concept of trauma and guidance for a trauma informed approach.* HHS Publication No. (SMA) 14–4884. Rockville, MD. Substance Abuse and Mental Health Services Administration.

van den Berk-Clark, C., Secrest, S., Walls, J., Hallberg, E., Lustman, P. J., Schneider, F. D., & Scherrer, J. F. (2018). Association between posttraumatic stress disorder and lack of exercise, poor diet, obesity, and co-occurring smoking: A systematic review and meta-analysis. *Health Psychology: Official Journal of the Division of Health Psychology, American Psychological Association, 37*(5), 407–416. https://doi.org/10.1037/hea0000593

Weiss, M. H., et al. (2019). A longitudinal examination of posttraumatic stress disorder symptoms and risky sexual behavior: Evaluating emotion dysregulation dimensions as mediators. *Archives of Sexual Behavior.* https://doi.org/10.1007/s10508-019-1392-y

Williamson, V., Stevelink, S., Da Silva, E., & Fear, N. T. (2018). A systematic review of wellbeing in children: A comparison of military and civilian families. *Child & Adolescent Mental Health & Psychiatry, 12,* 46. https://doi.org/10.1186/s13034-018-0252-1

Young, L. B., Timko, C., Pulido, R. D., Tyler, K. A., Beaumont, C., & Grant, K. M. (2020). Traumatic childhood experiences and posttraumatic stress disorder among veterans in substance use disorder treatment. *Journal of Interpersonal Violence,* 886260519900937. Advance online publication. https://doi.org/10.1177/0886260519900937

Zuromski, K. L., Bernecker, S. L., Chu, C., Wilks, C. R., Gutierrez, P. M., Joiner, T. E., Liu, H., Naifeh, J. A., Nock, M. K., Sampson, N. A., Zaslavsky, A. M., Stein, M. B., Ursano, R. J., Kessler, R. C., Site Principal Investigators, Army liaison/consultant, & Other team members. (2020). Pre-deployment predictors of suicide attempt during and after combat deployment: Results from the Army Study to Assess Risk and Resilience in Servicemembers. *Journal of Psychiatric Research, 121,* 214–221. https://doi.org/10.1016/j.jpsychires.2019.12.003

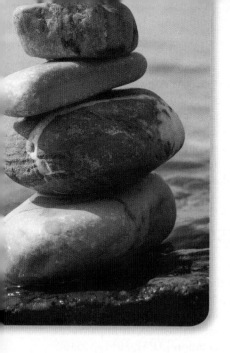

30
Personality and Impulse-Control Disorders
Nursing Care of Persons with Personality and Impulse-Control Disorders

Kimberlee Hansen and Mary Ann Boyd

KEYCONCEPTS

- antisocial personality disorder (ASPD)
- borderline personality disorder (BPD)

- difficult temperament
- emotional dysregulation
- impulse-control disorders
- personality

- personality disorder
- self-harm
- temperament

LEARNING OBJECTIVES

After studying this chapter, you will be able to:

1. Discuss the role of a personality in personality disorders.

2. Delineate the clinical symptoms of borderline personality disorder and antisocial personality disorder, with emphasis on emotional dysregulation, self-harm, temperament, and impulsivity.

3. Analyze the theories explaining personality disorders.

4. Develop strategies to establish a patient-centered, recovery-oriented therapeutic relationship with a person with borderline personality disorder.

5. Apply a person-centered, recovery-oriented nursing process for persons with borderline personality disorder.

6. Identify the role medications play in treating people with borderline and antisocial personality disorders and discuss their effectiveness.

7. Differentiate the type of mental health care provided in emergency care, inpatient-focused care, community care, and virtual mental health care.

8. Develop wellness strategies for persons with borderline personality disorder.

9. Discuss the importance of integrated health care for persons with borderline personality disorder.

10. Describe other personality disorders and relevant nursing care for persons with these disorders.

11. Compare and contrast disruptive impulse-control disorders.

KEY TERMS

- Affective instability • Avoidant personality disorder • Cognitive schemata • Dependent personality disorder
- Dialectical behavior therapy (DBT) • Dichotomous thinking • Dissociation • Histrionic personality disorder
- Identity diffusion • Inhibited grieving • Intermittent explosive disorder • Invalidating environment • Kleptomania
- Mentalization-based therapy (MBT) • Mentalizing • Narcissistic personality • Obsessive-compulsive personality disorder • Paranoid personality disorder • Parasuicidal behavior • Personality traits • Projective identification
- Pyromania • Schizoid personality disorder • Schizotypy • Schizotypal personality disorder
- Separation-individuation • Splitting

Case Study: Rebecca

Rebecca is a 23-year-old single female who lives alone. She has few friends but does attend regular psychotherapy sessions that help her understand her emotions and behaviors. She becomes very upset when her therapist leaves town for a planned vacation. Her family wants to help but is frustrated with Rebecca's inability to deal with everyday stresses.

Case Study: Danny

Danny is a 55-year-old man admitted to the inpatient mental health unit from the county jail after threatening suicide with a plan to hang himself. He was arrested after physically assaulting his girlfriend with whom he lives.

INTRODUCTION

The concept of personality seems deceptively simple but instead is very complex. Historically, the term *personality* was derived from the Greek word *persona*, the theatrical mask used by dramatic players that had the connotation of a projected pretense or allusion. With time, the connotation changed from being an external surface representation to the internal traits of the individual

KEYCONCEPT Personality is a complex pattern of characteristics, largely outside of the person's awareness, which comprise the individual's distinctive pattern of perceiving, feeling, thinking, coping, and behaving.

Personality traits are prominent aspects of personality that are exhibited in a wide range of social and personal contexts. Intrinsic and pervasive, personality traits emerge from a complicated interaction of biologic dispositions, psychological experiences, and environmental situations that ultimately comprise a distinctive personality.

No sharp division exists between normal and abnormal personality functioning. Instead, personalities are viewed on a continuum from normal at one end to abnormal at the other. Many of the same processes involved in the development of a "normal" personality are responsible for the development of a personality disorder.

This chapter provides an overview of personality disorders with borderline personality disorder (BPD) explained in detail and antisocial personality disorder (ASPD) emphasized. Disruptive impulse-control disorders, a closely related group of disorders, are also discussed. Oppositional defiant disorder and conduct disorder, which are childhood diagnoses, are discussed in Chapter 37.

PERSONALITY DISORDERS OVERVIEW

A personality disorder is "an enduring pattern of inner experience and behavior that deviates markedly from the expectations of the individual's culture, is pervasive and inflexible, has an onset in adolescence or early adulthood, is stable over time, and leads to distress or impairment" (American Psychiatric Association [APA], 2013, p. 646).

Historically there has always been the question of the cause of personality disorders. Is it "bad genes" and/or "bad environment"? There appears to be a general agreement that the main etiological factors for personality disorder are heritably heightened affect states (excessive fear, anger, detachment) and adverse environmental factors (substandard parenting, childhood psychological trauma), acting singly or in concert (Svrakic & Divac-Jovanovic, 2019).

KEYCONCEPT A personality disorder diagnosis is based on abnormally inflexible behavior patterns of long duration—traced to adolescence or early adulthood—that deviates from acceptable cultural norms.

Consider Danny
Danny explains that rules are made to be broken.

The prevalence rate of any personality disorder in the adult population is estimated at 12.16% (Volkert et al., 2018). These rates are of public health significance because of the extreme social dysfunction and high health care use of persons with personality disorders. Many others do not seek treatment for the distress or impairment related to their personality disorder because they do not perceive themselves as having a problem. However, they frequently seek help for concurrent medical or mental health disorders.

At present, 10 personality disorders are recognized in the *DSM-5* within three clusters. Cluster A disorders are characterized by odd or eccentric behavior, Cluster B disorders are characterized by dramatic, emotional, or erratic behavior, and in Cluster C disorders, individuals appear anxious or fearful (APA, 2013).

CLUSTER A DISORDERS: PARANOID, SCHIZOID, AND SCHIZOTYPAL PERSONALITY DISORDERS

Paranoid Personality Disorder

Clinical Course and Diagnostic Criteria

Paranoid personality disorder is characterized by a long-standing suspiciousness and mistrust of people in general. Individuals with these traits refuse to assume personal responsibility for their own feelings, assign responsibility to others, and avoid relationships in which they are not in control or power. These individuals are suspicious, guarded, and hostile. They are consistently mistrustful of others' motives, even those of relatives and close friends. Actions of others are often misinterpreted as deception, deprecation, and betrayal, especially regarding loyalty or trustworthiness of friends and associates (APA, 2013).

People with paranoid personality disorder are unforgiving and hold grudges; their typical emotional responses are anger and hostility. They distance themselves from others and are outwardly argumentative and abrasive; internally, they feel powerless, fearful, and vulnerable. Other hallmark features of paranoid personality disorder are persistent ideas of self-importance and the tendency to be rigid and controlling. Blind to their own unattractive behaviors and characteristics, they often attribute these same traits to others. Their outward demeanor often seems cold, sullen, and humorless. They want to appear controlled and objective, yet often they react emotionally, displaying signs of nervousness, anger, envy, and jealousy. Orderly by nature, they are hypervigilant to any environmental changes that may loosen their control of the world. Occupational problems are common. In clinical populations, paranoid personality disorder is one of the strongest predictors of aggressive behavior, often associated with violence and stalking. People with this disorder do not seek mental health care until they have symptoms of comorbid disorders (Lee, 2017).

Epidemiology and Risk Factors

The prevalence estimates for paranoid personality range from 1.2% to 4.4%. Paranoid personality disorder is the second-most prevalent personality disorder after **obsessive-compulsive personality disorder** (OCPD; Lee, 2017).

Etiology

The etiologic factors of paranoid personality remain unclear, but a genetic predisposition for an irregular maturation may be involved. As children, these individuals tend to be active and intrusive, difficult to manage, hyperactive, and irritable and have frequent outbursts of temper.

Evidence-Based Nursing Care of Persons with Paranoid Personality Disorder

Nurses most likely see these patients about other health problems but formulate nursing approaches based on the patient's underlying paranoia. Assessment of these individuals reveals disturbed or illogical thoughts that demonstrate misinterpretation of environmental stimuli. For example, a man was convinced that his wife was having an affair with the neighbor because his wife and the neighbor left their homes for work at the same time each morning. Although the man's beliefs were illogical, he never once considered that he was wrong. He frequently followed them but never caught them together. He continued to believe they were having an affair.

Because of their inability to develop relationships, these patients are often socially isolated and lack social support systems.

Mental health nursing interventions based on the establishment of a therapeutic relationship are difficult to implement because of the patient's mistrust. If a trusting relationship is established, the nurse helps the patient identify problematic areas, such as getting along with others or keeping a job. Through therapeutic techniques such as acceptance, confrontation, and reflection, the nurse and patient examine a problematic area to gain another view of the situation. Changing thought patterns takes time. Patient outcomes are evaluated in terms of small changes in thinking and behavior.

Continuum of Care

Individuals with paranoid personalities are unlikely to participate in treatment or recovery plans. If they have other comorbid disorders and are forced to seek treatment (through loss of their job or being ordered by a court in connection with an offense of a chargeable nature), they may seek help for depression or psychosis.

Schizoid Personality Disorder

Clinical Course and Diagnostic Criteria

People with **schizoid personality disorder** are characterized as being seclusive, isolated, and inept at forming relationships (Fariba & Gupta, 2020). They tend to be unable to experience the joyful and pleasurable aspects of life. They are introverted, reclusive, and clinically seem distant, aloof, apathetic, and emotionally detached. Typically, life-long loners, they have difficulty making friends, seem uninterested in social activities, and appear to gain little satisfaction in personal relationships. In fact, they appear to be incapable of forming social relationships. Their interests are directed at objects, things, and abstractions. They may do well at solitary jobs other people might find difficult to tolerate. Often people with schizoid personality disorders may daydream excessively and become attached to animals, and they frequently do not marry or even form long-lasting romantic relationships. As children, they engage primarily in solitary activities, such as stamp collecting, computer games, electronic equipment, or academic pursuits such as mathematics or engineering. In addition, they seem to have a cognitive deficit characterized by obscure thought processes, particularly about social matters. Communication with others is confused and lacks focus. These individuals reveal minimum introspection and self-awareness, and interpersonal experiences are described in a very mechanical way.

Epidemiology and Risk Factors

Schizoid personality disorder is rarely diagnosed in clinical settings. It is estimated that the prevalence is 3.1% (APA, 2013).

Etiology

The etiologic processes are speculative. There may be neuroanatomical or neurotransmitter changes associated with schizoid disorder (Fariba & Gupta, 2020). The defects of this personality may stem from an adrenergic–cholinergic imbalance in which the parasympathetic division of the autonomic nervous system is functionally dominant. Excesses or deficiencies in acetylcholine and norepinephrine may result in the proliferation and scattering of neural impulses that may be responsible for the cognitive "slippage" or affective deficits.

Evidence-Based Nursing Care of Persons with Schizoid Personality Disorder

Difficulty with social relations and low self-esteem are typical nursing priorities of patients with schizoid personality disorder. Major treatment goals are to enhance the experience of pleasure, prevent social isolation, and increase emotional responsiveness to others. Because these individuals often lack customary social skills, social skills training is useful in enhancing their ability to relate in interpersonal situations. The primary focus is to increase the patient's ability to feel pleasure. The nurse balances interventions between encouraging enough social activity to prevent the individual from retreating into a fantasy world and too much social activity that becomes intolerable to the patient.

The nurse may find working with such individuals unrewarding and as a result, the attending nurses may become

frustrated, feel helpless, or become bored during the interactions. It is difficult to establish a therapeutic relationship with these individuals because they tend to shy away from interactions and are rarely motivated about treatment. Evaluation of outcomes should be in terms of increasing the patient's feelings of satisfaction with solitary activities.

Continuum of Care

People with schizoid personalities are rarely hospitalized unless they have a comorbid disorder. Family members may seek treatment for them in an outpatient setting.

Schizotypal Personality Disorder
Clinical Course and Diagnostic Criteria

Schizotypal personality disorder is characterized by a pattern of social and interpersonal deficits. The term **schizotypy** refers to traits that are similar to the symptoms of schizophrenia but are less severe. Cognitive perceptual symptoms are a primary characteristic and include magical beliefs (similar to delusions) and perceptual aberrations (similar to hallucinations). Other common symptoms include referential thinking (interpreting insignificant events as personally relevant) and paranoia (suspicion of others).

Persons with schizotypal personality disorder are more dramatically eccentric than those with schizoid personality disorder who are characteristically flat, colorless, and dull. These individuals are perceived as strikingly odd or strange in both appearance and behavior, even to laypersons. They may have unusual mannerisms, an unkempt manner of dress that does not quite "fit together," and inattention to usual social conventions (e.g., avoiding eye contact, wearing clothes that are stained or ill fitting, and being unable to join in the give-and-take banter of coworkers). Devoid of any close friends other than first-degree relatives, their mood is constricted or inappropriate, with excessive social anxieties. They usually exhibit an avoidant behavior pattern.

Persons with schizotypal personality disorder may respond to stress with transient psychotic episodes (lasting minutes to hours). Because of their short duration, the symptoms mirror but fall short of features that would justify the diagnosis of schizophrenia. Many individuals (30% to 50%) with schizotypal personality disorder also have a co-occurring major depressive disorder diagnosis when admitted to a hospital (APA, 2013; Racioppi et al., 2018). Schizotypal personality disorders may be slightly more common in males (APA, 2013).

Epidemiology and Risk Factors

The lifetime prevalence of schizotypal personality disorder is 3.9%, with higher rates among men (4.2%) than women. There are cultural variations of traits across countries and cultures. Persons from some cultures express all of the symptoms of schizotypal personality disorder and others only one or two distinct symptoms (Fonseca-Pedrero et al., 2018).

Etiology

Magnetic resonance imaging studies of individuals with schizotypal personality disorder show smaller gray matter volume, which is correlated with negative symptoms. Studies show changes in temporal gyrus volume asymmetry and in the white matter tracts (Chan et al., 2018). There is also evidence that trauma-exposed individuals have a greater risk of developing schizotypal disorder (Quidé et al., 2018).

Evidence-Based Nursing Care of Persons with Schizotypal Personality Disorder

Depending on the amount of decompensation (i.e., deterioration of functioning and exacerbation of symptoms), the assessment of a patient with a schizotypal personality disorder can generate a range of clinical priorities. If a person has severe symptoms, such as delusional thinking or perceptual disturbances, the nursing priorities are similar to those for a person with schizophrenia (see Chapter 24). If symptoms are mild, social isolation, coping with stress and daily living, low self-esteem, and difficult social interactions are the focus of nursing care.

People with schizotypal personality disorder need help in developing recovery-oriented strategies to increase their sense of self-worth and recognize their positive attributes. They can benefit from social skills training and environmental management that increases their psychosocial functioning. Their eccentric thoughts and behaviors alienate them from others. Reinforcing socially appropriate dress and behavior can improve their overall appearance and ability to relate to the environment. Because they have a hard time generalizing from one situation to another, attention to cognitive skills is important.

Continuum of Care

Quality of life for a patient with schizotypal personality disorder can be improved with supportive psychotherapy, but their suspiciousness, lack of trust, or impaired social interactions make it difficult to establish a therapeutic relationship. These individuals do not usually seek treatment unless more serious symptoms appear, such as depression or anxiety. Medications are not generally used unless the individual has coexisting anxiety or depression.

Nursing care is often provided in a home or clinic setting, with the personality disorder being secondary to the purpose of the care. This means that nurses focus on other aspects of patient care and may miss the underlying psychiatric disorder. A psychiatric nursing consult may be needed for these patients to help identify the disorder.

CLUSTER B DISORDERS: BORDERLINE, ANTISOCIAL, HISTRIONIC, AND NARCISSISTIC PERSONALITY DISORDERS

Borderline Personality Disorder

The term *borderline* was first coined by Adolph Stern in 1938 when he identified a "border line group of patients" who "fit frankly neither into the psychotic nor into the psychoneurotic group, and are extremely difficult to handle by any psychotherapeutic method" (Stern, 1938).

People with BPD have problems regulating their moods, developing a self-identity, maintaining interpersonal relationships, maintaining reality-based thinking, and avoiding impulsive or destructive behavior. The severity and difficulty in treating the disorder lead to enormous public health costs from health care utilization and functional disability (Meuldijk et al., 2017).

> **KEYCONCEPT Borderline personality disorder (BPD)** is characterized by a disruptive pattern of instability related to self-identity, interpersonal relationships, and affect, combined with marked impulsivity and destructive behavior. BPD has historically been seen as a lifelong, highly disabling disorder; however, research over the past two decades has challenged that assumption. BPD can be accurately identified in adolescence, and the course of the disorder in adolescence and adulthood is generally similar, with reductions in symptoms over time (Winsper, 2021).

Clinical Course

Individuals with BPD appear more competent than they actually are and often set unrealistically high expectations for themselves. When these expectations are not met, they experience intense shame, self-hate, and self-directed anger. Their lives are like soap operas—one crisis after another. Some of the crises are caused by the individual's dysfunctional lifestyle or inadequate social milieu, but many are caused by fate—the death of a spouse or a diagnosis of an illness. They react emotionally with minimal coping skills. The intensity of their emotions often frightens them and others. Friends, family members, and coworkers limit their contact with the person, which furthers the sense of aloneness, abandonment, and self-hatred. It also diminishes opportunities for learning self-corrective measures.

Remissions from the acute symptoms (e.g., self-injurious behaviors, suicide attempts, or threats about suicide) are fairly common, and the relapse rate is relatively low compared with other disorders. Overall, the prognosis is good for persons with BPD (Chapman et al., 2020). However, psychosocial functioning does not necessarily improve as symptoms decrease (Shah & Zanarini, 2018).

Diagnostic Criteria

BPD is a "pervasive pattern of instability of interpersonal relationships, self-image, and affects, and marked impulsivity beginning by early adulthood and present in a variety of contexts" (APA, 2013, p. 663). See Key Diagnostic Characteristics 30.1. Individuals with BPD also exhibit related cognitive and behavioral dysfunctions.

Unstable Interpersonal Relationships

People with BPD have an extreme fear of abandonment, as well as a history of unstable or insecure attachments (Palihawadana et al., 2019). They suffer from difficulties in emotion regulation, which includes **affective instability**, impulsivity, fear of abandonment, eruptions of rage, feelings of emptiness, unstable interpersonal relationship, chronic dysphoria, or depression, as well as heightened risk-taking behaviors (Grambal et al., 2016). Most have never experienced a consistently secure, nurturing relationship and are constantly seeking reassurance and validation. In an attempt to meet their interpersonal needs, they idealize others and establish intense relationships that violate others' interpersonal boundaries, which leads to rejection. The relationships of individuals with BPD may be chaotic, intense, and marked with difficulties (Grambal et al., 2016).

When these relationships do not live up to their expectations, they devalue the person. Continually disappointed in relationships, these individuals, who are already intensely emotional and have a poor sense of self, feel estranged from others and inadequate in the face of perceived social standards. Intense shame and self-hate follow. These feelings often result in self-injurious behaviors, such as wrist cutting, self-burning, or head banging. BPD is associated with high mortality by suicide. There is also a high risk to die prematurely because of impulsive risk-taking, as well as succumbing to violence from others. Even though the characteristics of BPD are easy to identify, the diagnosis is often overlooked. A key reason for this neglect is the perception that the overemotional, sometimes theatrical, and self-injurious behaviors are signs of willfulness and manipulations rather than signs of an illness (Ekselius, 2018).

> ### Consider Rebecca
> Rebecca hates being alone, but her behaviors drive others away. When she feels rejected, anxious, or angry, she cuts her wrists, which decreases her anxiety.

Unstable Self-Image

These patients appear to have no sense of their own identity and direction; this becomes a source of great distress to them and is often manifested by chronic feelings of emptiness and boredom. It is not unusual for people with BPD to direct their actions in accord with the wishes of other people. For example, one woman with BPD describes herself: "I am a singer because my mother wanted me to be.

KEY DIAGNOSTIC CHARACTERISTICS 30.1 • BORDERLINE PERSONALITY DISORDER 301.83

Diagnostic Criteria

A pervasive pattern of instability of interpersonal relationships, self-image, and diminished affect, and marked impulsivity, beginning by early adulthood and present in a variety of contexts, as indicated by five (or more) of the following:

1. Frantic efforts to avoid real or imagined abandonment. (**Note:** Do not include suicidal or self-mutilating behavior covered in Criterion 5.)
2. A pattern of unstable and intense interpersonal relationships characterized by alternating between extremes of idealization and devaluation.
3. Identity disturbance: markedly and persistently unstable self-image or sense of self.
4. Impulsivity in at least two areas that are potentially self-damaging (e.g., spending, sex, substance use, reckless driving, binge eating). (**Note:** Do not include suicidal or self-mutilating behavior covered in Criterion 5.)
5. Recurrent suicidal behavior, gestures, or threats, or self-mutilating behavior.
6. Affective instability due to a marked reactivity of mood (e.g., intense episodic dysphoria, irritability, or anxiety

usually lasting a few hours and only rarely more than a few days).
7. Chronic feelings of emptiness.
8. Inappropriate intense anger or difficulty controlling anger (e.g., frequent displays of temper, constant anger, recurrent physical fights).
9. Transient stress-related paranoid ideation or severe dissociative symptoms.

Associated Behavioral Findings

- Pattern of undermining self at the moment a goal is to be realized
- Possible psychotic like symptoms during times of stress
- Recurrent job losses, interrupted education, and broken marriages
- History of physical and sexual abuse, neglect, hostile conflict, and early parental loss or separation

I live in the city because my manager thought that I should. I become whatever anyone tells me to be. Whenever someone recommends a song, I wonder why I didn't think of that. My boyfriend tells me what to wear." distress to them and is often manifested by chronic feelings of emptiness and boredom. It is not unusual for people with BPD to direct their actions in accord with the wishes of other people. For example, one woman with BPD describes herself: "I am a singer because my mother wanted me to be. I live in the city because my manager thought that I should. I become whatever anyone tells me to be. Whenever someone recommends a song, I wonder why I didn't think of that. My boyfriend tells me what to wear."

Unstable Affect

Affective instability (i.e., rapid and extreme shift in mood) is a core characteristic of BPD and is evidenced by erratic emotional responses to situations and intense sensitivity to criticism or perceived slights. For example, a person may greet a casual acquaintance with intense affection yet later be aloof with the same acquaintance. Friends describe individuals with BPD as moody, irresponsible, or intense. These individuals often fail to recognize their own emotional responses, thoughts, beliefs, and behaviors and have difficulty interpreting the facial effects of others. In this disorder, recognizing emotions in others is altered (Santangelo et al., 2017).

Cognitive Dysfunctions

People with BPD often have **dichotomous thinking**. That is, they evaluate experiences, people, and objects in terms of mutually exclusive categories (e.g., good or bad, success or failure, trustworthy or deceitful). Their interpretation of normally occurring events is usually extremely positive or extremely negative. Sometimes their thinking becomes disorganized with irrelevant, bizarre notions and vague or scattered thought connections, as well as delusions and hallucinations.

Another cognitive dysfunction common in BPD is **dissociation**, or times when thinking, feeling, or behaviors occur outside a person's awareness. It is a coping strategy for avoiding disturbing events. In dissociating, the person does not have to be aware of or remember traumatic events. There is evidence of functional changes in the fronto-limbic regions (amygdala, anterior cingulate, inferior frontal gyrus, medial, and dorsolateral prefrontal cortices) and temporoparietal areas (Krause-Utz & Elzinga, 2018).

Impaired Problem-Solving

In BPD, affected people often fail to engage in active problem-solving. Instead, problem-solving is attempted by soliciting help from others in a helplessly hopeless manner. Suggestions offered are rarely taken up.

Impulsivity

These individuals often have difficulty delaying gratification or thinking through the consequences before acting on their feelings; their actions are often unpredictable. Essentially, they act in the moment and clean up the mess afterward. Gambling, spending money irresponsibly, binge eating, engaging in unsafe sex, and abusing substances are typical of these individuals. They can also be physically or verbally aggressive. Job losses, interrupted education, and unsuccessful relationships are common.

Self-Harm Behaviors

The turmoil and unsuccessful interpersonal relationships and social experiences associated with BPD may lead the person to undermine him- or herself when a goal is about to be reached. The most serious consequences are suicide attempts or parasuicidal behavior (i.e., deliberate self-injury with intent to harm oneself).

❚ **KEYCONCEPT Self-harm** is deliberate self-injurious behavior.

Self-harm behavior can be compulsive (e.g., hair pulling), episodic, or repetitive (e.g., cutting wrists, arms, other body parts) and is more likely to occur when the individual with BPD is depressed; has highly unstable interpersonal relationships, especially problems with intimacy and sociability; and is paranoid, hypervigilant (i.e., alert, watchful), and resentful. It is not unusual for persons with this disorder to self-harm in unusual ways such as swallowing pens, staples, and even razor blades, or banging one's head against a brick wall. All self-harm behaviors should be considered potentially life threatening and taken seriously.

Borderline Personality Disorder Across the Life Span

Many children and adolescents show symptoms similar to those of BPD, such as moodiness, self-destruction, impulsiveness, lack of temper control, and rejection sensitivity. If a family member has BPD, the adolescent should be carefully assessed for this disorder. Because symptoms of BPD begin in adolescence, it makes sense that some children and adolescents would meet the criteria for BPD even though it is not diagnosed before young adulthood. More likely, some personality traits, such as impulsivity and mood instability, in many adolescents should be recognized and treated whether or not BPD eventually develops.

Epidemiology and Risk Factors

The estimated prevalence of BPD is roughly 1.0% in community settings. In clinical settings, the prevalence of BPD is approximately 12% in outpatient mental health clinics and 22% in inpatient psychiatric settings, with a higher proportion of women. Several studies demonstrated that traumatic life events, such as sexual and physical abuse, parental divorce, or illness or parental psychopathology, are important risk factors for the development of BPD.

Age of Onset and Gender Differences

BPD commonly starts and peaks in early to late adolescence and then largely declines over time (Winsper, 2021). Women are more often diagnosed with BPD, but it is generally believed that it occurs equally in people (Mainali et al., 2020).

One possible explanation for women being diagnosed more often than men is that it is more socially acceptable for women to seek help from the health care system. Another reason is that childhood sexual abuse, which more commonly affects girls, is one of the strongest risk factors for BPD. Still another explanation is that because eating disorders are more common in women with BPD, they have a greater likelihood of also having a mood, anxiety, or posttraumatic stress disorder. Men with BPD are more likely to have a substance use problem and intermittent explosive disorder (IED). Other studies cite parental loss and separation as risk factors. Clearly, more research is needed to identify risk factors for the development of BPD (Ellison et al., 2018).

Ethnicity and Culture

The pattern of behavior seen in BPD has been identified in many settings around the world (Choudhary & Gupta, 2020). Adolescents and young adults with identity problems (especially when accompanied by substance use) may transiently display behaviors that misleadingly give the impression of BPD. Such situations are characterized by emotional instability, "existential" dilemmas, uncertainty, anxiety-provoking choices, conflicts about sexual orientation, and competing social pressures to decide on careers.

Familial Differences

BPD has a clear genetic predisposition, with studies showing over 40% heritability (Amad et al., 2014). BPD has a clear heritability component on self-harm, with estimates ranging from 31% to 41%. There are strong relationships demonstrated in twin studies that demonstrated heritability of impulsive spending, risk of suicide and injury, and other risk-taking behaviors (Schermer et al., 2020).

Comorbidity

Comorbid psychiatric disorders are extremely common in patients with BPD. Mood disorders, particularly MDD and substance use disorder, anxiety disorder, and eating disorder are more frequently seen in patients with BPD, compared with patients with other personality disorders (Chapman et al., 2020). The coexistence of BPD with other disorders presents clinicians with the difficult choice of which disorder receives treatment priority. Symptoms associated with this disorder often provoke negative reactions on the part of clinicians, which interfere with clinicians' ability to provide effective care (Shah & Zanarini, 2018).

Etiology

Evidence supports a biopsychosocial etiology. Studies suggest that BPD traits are heritable, although the specific genetic factors remain unclear. There is clear evidence of differences in brain functioning between those with and without BPD. There is also clear evidence that psychological and social factors contribute to the development of the disorder (Meehan et al., 2018). The following discussion highlights the leading explanations for BPD.

Biologic Theories

Evidence of central nervous system dysfunction in BPD is now clear, including possible structural changes. Biologic abnormalities are associated with three BPD characteristics: affective instability; transient psychotic episodes; and impulsive, aggressive, and suicidal behavior. Associated brain dysfunction occurs in the limbic system and frontal lobe and increases the behaviors of impulsiveness, parasuicide, and mood disturbance (Perez-Rodriguez et al., 2018).

Psychosocial Theories

Psychoanalytic Theories

Using psychoanalytic methodology suggests persons with BPD have not achieved the normal and healthy developmental stage of **separation-individuation**, during which a child develops a sense of self, a permanent sense of significant others (object constancy), and integration of seeing both bad and good components of oneself (Stern et al., 2018). Those with BPD lack the ability to separate from the primary caregiver and develop a separate and distinct personality or self-identity. **Projective identification**, a defense mechanism by which people with BPD protect their fragile self-image, is believed to play an important role in the development of BPD. For example, when overwhelmed by anxiety or anger at being disregarded by another, they defend against the intensity of these feelings by unconsciously blaming others for what happens to them. They project their feelings onto a significant other with the unconscious hope that that person knows how to deal with it. Projective identification becomes a defensive way of interacting with the world, which leads to more rejection.

Maladaptive Cognitive Processes

Cognitive schemata are patterns of thought that determine how a person interprets events. Each person's cognitive schemata screen, code, and evaluate incoming stimuli. In personality disorders, maladaptive cognitive schemata cause misinterpretation of other people's actions or reactions and of events that result in dysfunctional ways of responding. Cognitive schemata are important in understanding BPD (and ASPD as well).

Individuals with BPD develop dysfunctional beliefs and maladaptive schemata early in life, leading them to misinterpret environmental stimuli continuously, which, in turn, leads to rigid and inflexible behavior patterns in response to new situations and people (Esmaeilian et al., 2019). Because those with BPD have been conditioned to anticipate rejection and disappointment in the past, they become entrenched in a pattern of fear and anxiety regarding encountering new people or situations. They have fears that disaster is going to strike at any minute. The work of cognitive therapists is to challenge distortions in thinking patterns and replace them with realistic ones.

Remember Rebecca?

Rebecca does not see herself as contributing to her problem but believes her misfortunes are caused by others. For example, when she encounters new people, she shares too much personal information and is disappointed when they do not respond with the same intensity. She interprets their response as rejection.

Social Theories: Biosocial Theories

The biosocial viewpoint proposed by Marsha Linehan and colleagues sees BPD as a multifaceted problem, a combination of innate emotional vulnerability (sensitivity and reactivity to environmental stress), emotional dysregulation (inability to control emotions in social interactions), and the environment (Linehan, 1993) (Box 30.1).

> **KEYCONCEPT Emotional dysregulation** is the inability to control emotions in social interactions and includes an instability of mood, marked shifts to or from depression, stress-related and transient mood crashes, rejection sensitivity, and inappropriate and intense outbursts of anger.

The emotional dysregulation and aggressive impulsivity entail both social learning and biologic regulation. Much of the neurobiologic research is directed at corticolimbic function and other cerebral functions (Perez-Rodriguez et al., 2018). In fact, restoring balance in these systems permits more consistent neural firing

BOX 30.1

Behavioral Patterns in Borderline Personality Disorder

1. *Emotional vulnerability.* Person experiences a pattern of pervasive difficulties in regulating negative emotions, including high sensitivity to negative emotional stimuli, high emotional intensity, and slow return to emotional baseline.
2. *Self-invalidation.* Person fails to recognize one's own emotional responses, thoughts, beliefs, and behaviors and sets unrealistically high standards and expectations for self. May include intense shame, self-hate, and self-directed anger. Person has no personal awareness and tends to blame social environment for unrealistic expectations and demands.
3. *Unrelenting crises.* Person experiences pattern of frequent, stressful, negative environmental events, disruptions, and roadblocks—some caused by the individual's dysfunctional lifestyle, others by an inadequate social milieu, and many by fate or chance.
4. *Inhibited grieving.* Person tries to inhibit and overcontrol negative emotional responses, especially those associated with grief and loss, including sadness, anger, guilt, shame, anxiety, and panic.
5. *Active passivity.* Person fails to engage actively in solving of own life problems but will actively seek problem-solving from others in the environment, learned helplessness, hopelessness.
6. *Apparent competence.* Tendency for the individual to appear deceptively more competent than they actually are, usually because of failure of competencies to generalize across expected moods, situations, and time. Person fails to display adequate nonverbal cues of emotional distress.

Adapted from Linehan, M. (1993). *Cognitive-behavioral treatment of borderline personality disorder* (p. 10). Guilford Press.

between the limbic system and the frontal and prefrontal cortices. When these circuits are functional, the person has a greater capacity to think about their emotions and modulate behavior more responsibly.

The ability to control emotion is partly learned from private experiences and encounters with the social environment. BPD is believed to develop when emotionally vulnerable individuals interact with an **invalidating environment**, a social situation that negates private emotional responses and communication. When core emotional responses and communications are continuously dismissed, trivialized, devalued, punished, and discredited (invalidated) by respected or valued persons, the vulnerable individual becomes unsure about their feelings. A minor example of an invalidating environment or response follows: The parents of Emily, a 4-year-old girl, tell her that the family is going to grandmother's house for a family meal. The child responds, "I am not going to Gramma's. I hate Stevie (her cousin)." The parents reply, "You don't hate Stevie. He is a wonderful child. He is your cousin, and only a spoiled and selfish little girl would say such a thing." The parents have devalued Emily's feelings and discredited her comments, thereby invalidating her feelings and sense of personal worth.

The most severe form of invalidation occurs in situations of child sexual abuse. Often, the abusing adult has told the child that this is a "special secret" between them. The child experiences feelings of fear, pain, and sadness, yet this trusted adult continuously dismisses the child's true feelings and tells the child what they should feel.

Family Response to Borderline Personality Disorder

Individuals with BPD are typically part of a chaotic family system, but their behavior adds to the chaos. Family members often feel captive to these patients. Family members are afraid to disagree with them or refuse to meet their multiple needs, fearing that self-destructive behavior will follow. During the course of the disorder, family members often get "burned out" and withdraw from the patient, only adding to the patient's fear of abandonment (Kay et al., 2018).

RECOVERY-ORIENTED CARE FOR PERSONS WITH BORDERLINE PERSONALITY DISORDER

Teamwork and Collaboration: Working Toward Recovery

Treatment of BPD requires the collaboration of the entire mental health care team. Because persons with BPD view the world in absolutes, nurses and other treatment team members are alternately categorized as all good or all bad. This defense is called **splitting** and presents clinicians with a challenge to work openly with each other as well as the patient until the issue can be resolved through team meetings and clinical supervision.

People with BPD are inadvertently highly stigmatized by many clinicians. Much of the stigma occurs when clinicians encounter these patients in crisis settings, such as the emergency department, crisis clinics, and general psychiatric inpatient wards. As these are not the settings in which treatment occurs, clinicians develop a biased perspective on these patients. Few clinicians have the opportunity to see these patients improve over time in specialized treatment clinics; nonetheless, these patients improve and are treatable. Staff often accuse these individuals of "manipulation" to get attention and say so in a very derogatory manner. In reality, all of us want attention from significant people in our lives. Most of us have the necessary skills to successfully meet our need for closeness and attention without alienating the very people who are important to us. People with BPD are unsuccessful in developing long-term meaningful relationships or getting

what they want because their approach alienates others. Their need for attention and closeness to others is very normal: It is how they seek attention that is problematic.

Psychotherapy is needed to help the individual with BPD manage the dysfunctional moods, impulsive behaviors, and self-injurious behaviors. Specially trained therapists who are comfortable with the many demands of these patients are needed. These therapists represent a variety of mental health disciplines, including psychology, social work, and advanced practice nursing. This disorder requires ongoing treatment as the individual copes with multiple interpersonal crises. Several types of medications are usually needed, including mood stabilizers, antidepressants, and anxiolytics; careful medication monitoring is necessary.

Dialectical behavior therapy (DBT) combines cognitive and behavior therapy strategies with acceptance-based practice drawn from Zen and humanistic approaches; it was developed for persons with BPD. Core interventions include problem-solving, exposure techniques (i.e., gradual exposure to cues that set off aversive emotions), skills training, contingency management (i.e., reinforcement of positive behavior), and cognitive modification. Skills groups are an integral part of DBT and are taught in group settings in which patients practice emotional regulation, interpersonal effectiveness, distress tolerance, core mindfulness, and self-management skills. Weekly individual therapy sessions focus on enhancing motivation and improving competence (DeCou et al., 2019).

Mentalization-based therapy (MBT) is a psychodynamic psychotherapy that is used in both individual and group formats. In MBT, borderline personality symptoms are viewed as a result of distortion or reduction in **mentalizing**, which is the ability to understand the mental states of oneself and others, including thoughts and feelings, that lead to actions. The goal of MBT is to improve patients' capacity to accurately understand others' actions and develop self-awareness skills through a therapeutic relationship (Levy et al., 2018).

Safety Issues

Persons with BPD can be extremely volatile emotionally. Because they experience emotions so intensely, they are at high risk for self-harm and suicide. Self-harm threats should be taken very seriously.

EVIDENCE-BASED NURSING CARE FOR PERSONS WITH BORDERLINE PERSONALITY DISORDER

Persons with BPD may enter the mental health system early (during young adulthood or even before) because of their chaotic lifestyles. Behavior includes unstable moods, problems with interpersonal relationships, low self-esteem, and self-identity issues. Thinking and behavior are dysregulated (Box 30.2). They have problems in daily living, including maintaining intimate relationships, keeping a job, and living within the law (Box 30.3). Nursing Care Plan 30.1—which sets forth a plan of care for Rebecca, the case study patient in this chapter—is available at http://thepoint.lww.com/Boyd7e.

Mental Health Nursing Assessment

Physical Health

People with BPD are usually able to maintain personal hygiene and physical functioning. Because of the comorbidity of BPD and eating disorders and substance use, however, a nutritional assessment may be needed. The patient should be queried about physiologic responses of emotion. Sleep patterns also should be assessed because sleep alterations may suggest coexisting depression or mania.

Physical Indicators of Self-Injurious Behaviors

Patients with BPD should be assessed for self-injurious behavior or suicide attempts. It is important to ask the patient about specific self-abusive behaviors, such as cutting, scratching, or swallowing foreign objects. The patient may wear long sleeves to hide injury to the arms. Specifically, asking about thoughts of hurting oneself when experiencing a major upset provides an opportunity for prevention and for coaching the patient toward alternative self-soothing measures.

BOX 30.2
Response Patterns of Persons with Borderline Personality Disorder

- Affective (mood) dysregulation
- Mood lability
- Problems with anger
- Interpersonal dysregulation
- Chaotic relationships
- Fears of abandonment
- Self-dysregulation
- Difficulties with sense of self
- Sense of emptiness
- Behavioral dysregulation
- Parasuicidal behavior or threats
- Impulsive behavior
- Cognitive dysregulation
- Dissociative responses
- Paranoid ideation

Courtesy of M. Linehan, Department of Psychology, Box 351525, University of Washington, Seattle, WA 98195-1525, 1993.

BOX 30.3 CLINICAL VIGNETTE
Borderline Personality Disorder

Joanne is a 22-year-old single woman who was recently fired from her job as a data entry clerk. She lives with her mother and stepfather, who brought her to the emergency department after finding her crouched in a fetal position in the bathroom, her wrists bleeding. She seemed to be in a daze. This is her first psychiatric admission although her mother and stepfather have suspected that she has "needed help" for a long time. In high school, she received brief treatment for a potential eating disorder. She remains very thin but is able to eat at least one meal per day. During periods of stress, she will go for days without eating. Joanne is the second of three children. Her parents divorced when she was 3 years old. She has not seen her father since he left. Although she has pleasant memories of her father, her mother has told her that he beat Joanne and her sisters when he was drinking. When Joanne was 6 years old, her older sister died as a result of an automobile accident. Joanne was in the car but was uninjured. As a child, Joanne was seen as a potential singing star. Her natural musical talent attracted her teachers' support, which encouraged her to develop her talent. She took singing lessons and entered statewide competitions in high school. Although she enjoyed the attention, she was never really comfortable in the limelight and felt "guilty" about having a talent that she sometimes resented. She was able to make friends but found that she was unable to keep them. They described her as "too intense" and emotional. She had one boyfriend in high school, but she was very uncomfortable with any physical closeness. After ending the relationship with the boyfriend, she concentrated on dieting to have a "perfect body." When her dieting attracted her parents' attention, she vowed to eat just enough to keep them "off her back about it." She spent much of her leisure time with her grandmother. She attended college briefly but was unable to concentrate. It was during college and after her grandmother's death that Joanne began cutting her wrists during periods of stress. It seemed to calm her.

After leaving college, Joanne returned home. She had several jobs and short-lived friendships. She was usually fired from her job because of "moodiness," and it took her several months before she would again find another. She spent days in her room listening to music. Her recent episode occurred after she was fired from work and spent 3 days in her bedroom.

What Do You Think?
- How would you describe Joanne's mood?
- Are Joanne's losses of her father and sister really severe enough to affect her ability to relate to others now? Do the losses seem to relate to the self-injury?
- What behaviors indicate problems with self-esteem and self-identity are present?

Medication

Patients with BPD may be taking several medications. As mood dysregulation is a primary symptom, treatment with mood stabilizers (e.g., Lithium, Valproate, or Lamotrigene) and/or a low-to-moderate dose of an atypical antipsychotic (e.g., aripiprazole or quetiapine) are common (Svrakic & Divac-Jovanovic, 2019).

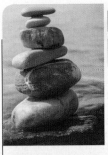

NURSING CARE PLAN 30.1

The Patient with Borderline Personality Disorder

Rebecca is a 23-year-old woman admitted voluntarily to the inpatient mental health unit after cutting her wrists and arriving in the emergency department with blood-soaked towels wrapped around her wrists. She lives alone and has no close friends. Her relationships are intense, which drives people away. She often reveals too much personal information to strangers. Her therapist left town and she believes that she will not return. This admission is one of multiple past admissions.

Setting: Inpatient Psychiatric Unit in a General Hospital

Baseline Assessment: Rebecca's wrists have several fresh lacerations and many older cuts in various stages of healing. She also has several scars from self-harming incidents in the past. Before harming herself, Rebecca reports feeling angry, anxious, numb, empty, or feeling detached from her body. She states that after she cuts herself she feels a sense of relief. She has a poor self-concept and low self-esteem. She says she does not understand why everyone is so mean to her. She has a history of being sexually abused as a child by her uncle following the death of her mother at age 4. BP is 120/70, P72, R 15, Ht. 5'4", Wt. 130, BMI 22.3.

Psychiatric Diagnosis	Medications
Borderline personality disorder	Sertraline (Zoloft) 150 mg daily for anxiety and depression

Priority of Care: Self-Injury

Important Characteristics	Associated Considerations
Cuts and scratches on body	Fears of abandonment secondary to therapist's vacation
Self-inflicted wounds	Inability to handle stress

Outcomes

Initial

Remain safe and not harm herself.

Identify feelings before and after cutting herself.

Agree not to harm herself over the next 24 hours.

Identify ways of dealing with self-harming impulses if they return.

Discharge

Verbalize alternate thinking with more realistic expectations of others.

Identify community resources to provide structure and support while therapist is away.

Interventions

Interventions	Rationale	Ongoing Assessment
Monitor patient for changes in mood or behavior that might lead to self-injurious behavior.	Close observation establishes safety and protection of patient from self-harm and impulsive behaviors.	Document according to facility policy. Continue to observe for mood and behavior changes.
Discuss with patient need for close observation and rationale to keep her safe.	Explanation to patient for purpose of nursing interventions helps her cooperate with the nursing activity.	Assess her response to increasing level of observation.
Administer medication as prescribed and evaluate medication effectiveness in reducing depression, anxiety, and cognitive disorganization.	Allows for adjustment of medication dosage based on target behaviors and outcomes.	Observe for side effects.
After 6 to 8 hours, present written agreement to not harm herself.	Permits patient time to return to more thoughtful ways of responding rather than her previous reactive response. Also permits her to save face and avoid embarrassment of losing a power struggle if presented much earlier.	Observe for her willingness to agree to not harm herself.
Communicate information about patient's risk to other nursing staff.	The close observation should be continued throughout all shifts until patient agrees to resist self-harm urges.	Review documentation of close observation for all shifts.

Continued

Nursing Care Plan 30.1 Continued

Outcomes Evaluation

Outcomes	Revised Outcomes	Interventions
Remained safe without further harming self. Identified fears of abandonment before cutting herself and relief of anxiety afterward.	Use hotlines or call friends if fears to harm self-return.	Give patient hotline number and ask her to record friends' numbers in an accessible place.
She identified friends to call when fears return and hotlines to use if necessary.		
Agreed to not harm herself over the next 3 days.	Does not harm self for 3 days.	Remind her to call someone if urges return.
Enrolled in a day hospital program for 4 weeks.	Attend day hospital program.	Follow-up on enrollment.

Priority of Care: Feeling Abandoned

Important Characteristics	Associated Characteristics
Frequent feelings of abandonment	Therapist's absence

Outcomes

Initial	Discharge
1. Discuss being lonely.	3. Identify strategies to deal with loneliness while therapist is away.
2. Identify previous ways of coping with loneliness.	

Interventions

Interventions	Rationale	Ongoing Assessment
Develop a therapeutic relationship.	People with BPD are able to examine loneliness within the structure of a therapeutic relationship.	Assess her ability to relate and nurse's response to the relationship.
Discuss past experience with therapist being gone with emphasis on how she was able to survive it.	She has survived therapist's absences before. By identifying the strategies she used, she can build on those strengths.	Assess her ability to assume any responsibility for "living through it." This will become a strength.
Acknowledge that it is normal to feel angry when the therapist is gone, but there are other strategies that may help the patient deal with the loneliness besides cutting.	Acknowledging feelings is important. Helping patient focus on the possibility of other strategies for dealing with the anger helps her regain a sense of control over her behavior.	Assess whether she is willing to acknowledge that there are other behavioral strategies to manage her anger.
Begin immediate disposition planning with focus on day hospitalization or day treatment for skills training and management of loneliness.	While patient is in the hospital, she is out of the stressful environment in which she can learn more effective behaviors and use the therapy. Moving out of the hospital and back into outpatient therapy decreases possibility of regression and lost learning (Linehan, 1993).	Assess her willingness to learn new skills within a day treatment setting.
Teach her about stress management techniques. Assign her to anger management group while she is in the hospital.	Learning about ways of dealing with feelings and stressful situations helps the patient with BPD choose positive strategies rather than self-destructive ones.	Monitor whether she actually attends the groups. She should be encouraged to attend.

Continued

Nursing Care Plan 30.1 Continued

Evaluation

Outcomes	Revised Outcomes	Interventions
Rebecca was able to verbalize her anger about her therapist's absence and fears of abandonment. The last two times her therapist went on vacation, the patient became self-injurious and was hospitalized for 2 weeks.	None	
Rebecca was willing to be discharged the next day if she could attend day treatment while her therapist was gone.	Identify other strategies of dealing with her therapist's vacation besides cutting herself.	Attend stress management, communication, and self-comforting classes.

Depressive symptoms are frequently treated with SSRIs, SNRIs, or TCA and may be augmented with atypical antipsychotics and/or lamotrigene. Benzodiazepines should be avoided for anxiety due to habituation and that they are not meant for long-term use. Buspar is considered a safer option for treating anxiety in patients with BPD. Initially, patients may be reluctant to disclose all the medications they are taking because, for many of them, trial and error has led to repeated prescription. They are fearful of having medication taken away from them. Development of rapport with special attention to a nonjudgmental approach is especially important when eliciting current medication practices. The effectiveness of the medication in relieving the target symptom needs to be determined.

Nutrition

A nutritional assessment is important if the person is using food for self-soothing and anxiety control. In some instances, excessive food intake may indicate self-injury or impulse eating may occur. The assessment should also include the use of caffeinated beverages (e.g., coffee, tea, cola, energy drinks). Since there is often a comorbidity with anorexia nervosa and bulimia nervosa, an assessment focusing on eating patterns and food intake is important. In patients who engage in binging or purging, assessment should include examining the teeth for pitting and discoloration, as well as the hands and fingers for redness and calluses caused by inducing vomiting. See Chapter 32.

Substance Use

Since individuals with BPD are at risk for substance use, use of alcohol, OTC medications, and street drugs should be carefully assessed (Rosenström et al., 2020). Use of benzodiazepines (i.e., Xanax, Ativan, or Valium) is contraindicated due to the risk of habituation and abuse. Impulsiveness in patients with BPD must be considered.

Alcohol can lower inhibition and lead to high-risk behaviors (e.g., suicide and parasuicide gestures or accidental overdosing).

Psychosocial Assessment

People with BPD have usually experienced significant losses in their lives that shape their view of the world. They experience **inhibited grieving**, "a pattern of repetitive, significant trauma and loss, together with an inability to fully experience and personally integrate or resolve these events" (Linehan, 1993). They have unresolved grief that can last for years and will avoid situations that evoke those feelings of separation and loss. During the assessment, the nurse can identify the losses (real or perceived) and explore the patient's experience during these losses, paying particular attention to whether the patient has reached resolution. A history of physical or sexual abuse and early separation from significant caregivers may provide important clues to the severity of the disturbances.

Mood fluctuations are common and can be assessed by any number of the depression and anxiety screening scales or by asking the following questions:

- What things or events bother you and make you feel sad or angry?
- Do these things or events trouble you more than they trouble other people?
- Do friends and family tell you that you are moody?
- Do you get angry easily?
- Do you have trouble with your temper?
- Do you think you were born with these feelings or did something happen to make you feel this way?

Mental Status and Appearance

Appearance and activity level generally reflect the person's mood and psychomotor activity. Many of those with BPD have been physically or sexually abused and thus should be assessed for depression. A disheveled appearance can reflect depression or an agitated state. When feeling good, these patients can be very engaging; they tend to be dramatic in their style of dress and attract attention, such as by wearing an unusual hairstyle or heavy makeup. Because physical appearance reflects identity, patients may experiment with their appearance and seek affirmation and acceptance from others. Body piercing, tattoos, and other perceived adornments provide a mechanism to define self.

Rebecca's Assessment

Rebecca loves to project a dramatic appearance when she is feeling good. When she is in a good mood, she projects as an overly confident, engaging person. She has several body piercings. She refuses to discuss any childhood trauma or sexual abuse.

Cognitive Disturbances

The mental status examination of those with BPD usually reveals normal thought processes that are not disorganized or confused except during periods of stress. Those with BPD usually exhibit dichotomous thinking, or a tendency to view things as absolute, either black or white, good or bad, with no perception of compromise. Dichotomous thinking can be assessed by asking patients how they view other people. Evidence of dichotomous thinking is indicated with responses of "good" or "bad," "wonderful" or "terrible."

Self-Concept and Identity Disturbance

Unstable self-image is often manifested as an identity disturbance or **identity diffusion**, a loss of the capacity for self-definition and commitment to values, goals, or relationships. There is not a consistent sense of self, and the process of identity formation is impaired. They have difficulties differentiating themselves from others and defining psychological boundaries. The nurse can recognize identity diffusion if the patient reports an ongoing "emptiness" or contradictory behavior. "I know I should not have gone out with him, but he wanted to see me." The person's thoughts and behavior will seem fragmented and superficial (Bozzatello et al., 2019).

Dissociation and Transient Psychotic Episodes

With BPD, periods of dissociation and transient psychotic episodes may occur. Dissociation can be assessed by asking if there is ever a time when the patient does not remember events or has the feeling of being separate from their body. Some patients refer to this as "spacing out." By asking specific information about how often, how long, and when dissociation first was used, the nurse can get an idea of how important dissociation is as a coping skill. It is important to ask the person what happens in the environment when dissociation occurs. Frequent dissociation indicates a highly habitual coping mechanism that is difficult to change. Because transient psychotic states occur, it is also important to elicit data regarding the presence of hallucinations or delusions and their frequency and circumstances.

Impulsivity

Impulsivity can be identified by asking the patient whether they do things impulsively or at the spur of the moment. For example: "Have there been times when you were hurt by your actions or were sorry later that you acted in the way you did?" Direct questions about gambling, choices in sexual partners, sexual activities, fights, arguments, arrests, and habits related to consumption of alcohol can also help in identifying areas of impulsive behavior.

From a neurophysiologic perspective, impulsively acting before thinking seems to be mediated by rapid nerve firing in the mesolimbic area. This activates psychomotor responses before pathways reach the prefrontal cortex (Perez-Rodriquez et al., 2018). Teaching the patient strategies to slow down automatic responses (e.g., deep breathing, counting to 10) buys time to think before acting.

Interpersonal Skills

Assessment of the person's ability to relate to others is important because interpersonal problems are linked to dissociation and self-injurious behavior. Information about friendships, frequency of contact, and intimate relationships provide data about the person's ability to relate to others. Patients with BPD often are sexually active and may have numerous sexual partners. Their need for closeness clouds their judgment about sexual partners, so it is not unusual to find these patients in abusive, destructive relationships with people with ASPD.

Stress and Coping Skills

Coping with stressful situations is one of the major problems of people with BPD. Assessment of their coping skills and their ability to deal with stressful situations is important. Self-esteem is closely related to identifying with health care workers. Patients with BPD perceive their families and friends as being weary of their numerous crises and their seeming unwillingness to break the vicious self-destructive cycle. Feeling rejected by their natural support system, these individuals create one within the health system. During periods of crisis, especially during the late evening, early morning, or on weekends, they may call or visit various psychiatric units asking to speak to specific personnel who formerly cared for them. They even know different nurses' scheduled days off and make the rounds to several hospitals and clinics. Sometimes they bring gifts to nurses or call them at home. Because their newly created social support system cannot provide the support that is needed, the patient continues to feel rejected. One of the treatment goals is to help the individual establish a more natural support network.

Functional Status

Some individuals with BPD can function very well except during periods when symptoms erupt. They hold jobs, are active in communities, and can perform well. During periods of stress, symptoms often appear. Conversely, some individuals with severe BPD function poorly; they seem to be always in a crisis, which often they have created.

Social Support Systems

Identification of social supports (e.g., family, friends, religious organizations) is the purpose of assessing resources. Knowing how the patient obtains social support is important in understanding the quality of interpersonal relationships. For example, some patients consider as their "best friends" nurses, physicians, and other health care personnel. Because these are false friendships (i.e., not reciprocated), they inevitably lead to frustration and disappointment. However, helping the patient find ways to meet other people and encouraging the patient's efforts are more realistic.

Risk Assessment: Suicide or Self-Injury

It is critical that patients with BPD be assessed for suicidal and self-damaging behavior, including alcohol and drug use (see Chapter 22). The assessment should include direct questions, such as asking whether the patient thinks about or engages in self-injurious behaviors. If so, the nurse should continue to explore the behaviors: what is done, how is it done, how frequently is it done, and what are the circumstances surrounding the self-injurious behavior. It is helpful to explain briefly to the patient that sometimes people cut, scratch, or pick at themselves as a way of bringing some relief and comfort. Although the behavior brings temporary relief, it also places the person at risk for infection. Approaching the assessment in this way conveys a sense of understanding and is more likely to invite the patient to disclose honestly.

Quality of Life

An inferior quality of life is associated with all personality disorders, poor health, and significant suffering (Ekselius, 2018). Persons diagnosed with BPD are predisposed to have a substantial degree of functional impairment through a variety of social and occupational domains, including trouble with finding and maintaining adequate work, housing, or relationships. BPD patients have poor social functioning; they are often socially isolated and unemployed or on long-term sick leave. Many patients with BPD do not finish their education or complete at a minimal level. BPD patients often participate in problematic relationships and practice problematic parenting. Job environment can be one of the areas where patients with BPD struggle for maintaining their identity. Conflicts with boss and colleagues are frequent; individuals with BPD mostly fight against assumed injustice and nepotism and accuse the others of incompetence, lack of diligence, and gaining benefits from their bosses. Occupational patterns are characterized by instability, intense preoccupation, the subsequent loss of interest in the job, lack of job satisfaction, and problems in relationships. Later in life, most of them achieve greater stability in social and work functioning (Grambal et al., 2016).

Strength Assessment

The strength assessment is important because these positive thoughts, skills, and behaviors can be supported as the individuals replace self-defeating behaviors with positive ones. Many of these individuals are extremely resilient despite the trauma that they have often experienced. The person's strength will emerge in the assessment and increase as the nurse gets to know the patient better. Some key questions include the following:

- How do you make yourself feel better?
- How do you resist the urge to hurt yourself?
- How do you make friends?
- What is the most positive thought, skill, or behavior that you have?

CLINICAL JUDGMENT

The first priority in care is safety of the patient. Self-injury and suicide ideation should be considered when establishing recovery goals. If the patient is not experiencing suicidal or self-injury thoughts or behavior, the patient thought processes (dissociation) or ability to cope with everyday stress may emerge as priorities of care, especially if these interfere with daily living. If the individual copes with stressful situations by dissociating or hallucinating, the nurse should begin to help the patient identify other coping strategies. Patients who are very emotional sometimes find that they will be able to cope if they learn emotional regulation strategies. For other patients, identity issues, anxiety, or low self-esteem may become priorities of care.

Identified strengths should be included in the priorities. By including a person's strengths, such as being motivated to manage self-destructive thoughts, the nurse can channel these attributes to deal with specific issues.

THERAPEUTIC RELATIONSHIP

Psychiatric-mental health registered nurses do not function as the patient's primary therapists, but they do need to establish a therapeutic relationship that strengthens the patient's coping skills and self-esteem and also supports individual psychotherapy. The therapeutic relationship helps the patient to experience a model of healthy interaction with consistency, limit setting, caring, and respect (both self-respect and respect for the patient). Patients who have low self-esteem need help in recognizing genuine respect from others and reciprocating with respect for others. In the therapeutic relationship, the nurse models self-respect by observing personal limits, being assertive, and clearly communicating expectations (Box 30.4). The nurse should always avoid using stigmatizing language, such as describing the person's behavior as manipulating instead of reporting or documenting specific behaviors.

Nurses should use their own self-awareness skills to examine their personal response to the patient. How the

---

BOX 30.4 • THERAPEUTIC DIALOGUE: BORDERLINE PERSONALITY DISORDER

INEFFECTIVE APPROACH

Rebecca: Hey, you know what? You are my favorite nurse. That night nurse sure doesn't understand me the way you do.

Nurse: Oh, I'm glad you are comfortable with me. Which night nurse?

Rebecca: You know, Sue.

Nurse: Did you have problems with her?

Rebecca: She is terrible. She sleeps all night or she is on the telephone.

Nurse: Oh, that doesn't sound very professional to me. Anything else?

Rebecca: Yeah, she said that you didn't know what you were doing. She said that you couldn't nurse your way out of a paper bag (smiling).

Nurse: She did, did she? (Getting angry.) She should talk.

Rebecca: Well, I gotta go to group. Where will you be? I feel so much better if I know where you are. I don't know how I can possibly be discharged tomorrow.

EFFECTIVE APPROACH

Rebecca: Hey, you know what? You are my favorite nurse. That night nurse sure doesn't understand me the way you do.

Nurse: I really like you, Rebecca. Tomorrow you will be discharged, and I'm glad that you will be able to return home. (Nurse avoided responding to "favorite nurse" statement. Redirected interaction to impending discharge.)

Rebecca: That night nurse slept all night.

Nurse: What was your night like? (Redirecting the interaction to Sara's experience.)

Rebecca: It was terrible. Couldn't sleep all night. I'm not sure that I'm ready to go home.

Nurse: Oh, so you are not quite sure about discharge? (reflection)

Rebecca: I get so, so lonely. Then, I want to hurt myself.

Nurse: Lonely feelings have started that chain of events that led to cutting, haven't they? (validation)

Rebecca: Yes, I'm very scared. I haven't cut myself for 1 week now.

Nurse: Do you have a plan for dealing with your lonely feelings when they occur?

Rebecca: I'm supposed to start thinking about something that is pleasant—like spring flowers in the meadow.

Nurse: Does that work for you?

Rebecca: Yes, sometimes.

CRITICAL THINKING CHALLENGE

• How did the nurse in the first scenario get sidetracked?

• How was the nurse in the second scenario able to keep the patient focused on herself and her impending discharge?

nurse responds to the patient can often be a clue to how others perceive and respond to the person. For example, if the nurse feels irritated or impatient during the interview that is a sign that others respond to this person in the same way; conversely, if the nurse feels empathy or closeness, chances are this patient can evoke these same feelings in others.

MENTAL HEALTH NURSING INTERVENTIONS

Establishing Recovery and Wellness Goals

Changing or modifying personality traits is difficult. The person has to want to change cognitive, emotional, and behavioral responses that were established in early childhood. The recovery goals should initially focus on the most problematic areas and will shift as outcomes are achieved. The patient and nurse should establish specific wellness goals, such as reducing food intake or increasing exercise. There should be an agreed-upon plan.

Physical Care

Usually, the person can manage hydration and self-care fairly well. This section focuses on those areas that are more likely to be problematic.

Sleep Hygiene

Disturbed sleep patterns are common in BPD. The nurse can intervene by helping the person establish a regular bedtime routine by teaching sleep hygiene strategies such as avoiding foods and drinks that could interfere with sleep. If relaxation exercises are used, they should be adapted to the tolerance of the individual. Special consideration must be made for persons who have been physically and sexually abused and who may be unable to put themselves in a vulnerable position (e.g., lying down in a room with other people or closing their eyes). These patients may need additional safeguards to help them sleep, such as a night light or repositioning the furniture in the room to allow a quick exit.

Teaching Nutritional Balance

The nutritional status of the person with BPD can quickly become a priority, particularly if the patient has coexisting eating disorders, mood disorders, or substance dependence. Eating is often a response to stress, so patients can quickly become overweight. This is especially problematic when the patient has also been taking medications that promote weight gain, such

as antipsychotics, antidepressants, or mood stabilizers. Helping the patient learn the basics of nutrition, make reasonable choices, and develop other coping strategies than eating are important interventions. If patients are engaging in purging or severe dieting practices, teaching the patient about the dangers of both of these practices is important (see Chapter 32). Referral to an eating disorders specialist may be needed.

Medication Interventions

Limiting medication is better for people with BPD. Patients should take medications only for target symptoms for a short time (e.g., an antidepressant for a bout with depression) because they may be taking many medications, particularly if they have a comorbid disorder, such as a mood disorder or substance use. Medications are used to control emotional dysregulation, impulsive aggression, cognitive disturbances, and anxiety as an adjunct to psychotherapy. Recent evidence shows some benefits from atypical antipsychotics, but there is little evidence to support the use of mood stabilizers. There is weak evidence to either support or exclude the SSRIs (Hancock-Johnson et al., 2017).

Administering and Monitoring Medications

In inpatient settings, it is relatively easy to control medications; in other settings, however, patients must be aware that it is their responsibility to take their medication and monitor the number and type of drugs being taken. Patients who rely on medication to help them deal with stress and those who are periodically suicidal are at high risk for abuse of medications. Patients who experience unusual side effects are also at high risk for noncompliance. The nurse must determine whether the patient is actually taking medication, whether the medication is being taken as prescribed, its effect on target symptoms, and the use of any OTC drugs (e.g., antihistamines, sleeping pills, or herbal supplements with similar pharmacologic activity).

Monitoring Side Effects

Patients with BPD appear to be sensitive to many medications, so the dosage may need to be adjusted based on the side effects they experience. Listen carefully to the patient's description of the side effects. Any unusual side effects should be accurately documented and reported to the prescriber.

Teaching Points

Patients should be educated about the prescribed medications and their interactions with other drugs and substances, but they should be encouraged to avoid relying on medication alone. Interventions include teaching patients about the medication and how and where it acts in the brain and body, helping establish a routine for taking prescribed medication, reporting side effects, and facilitating the development of positive coping strategies to deal with daily stresses rather than relying on medications. Eliciting the patient's partnership in care improves adherence and thereby outcomes.

Psychosocial Interventions

Therapeutic Interactions

One key to helping patients with BPD is recognizing their fears of both abandonment and intimacy. Informing the patient of the length of the therapeutic relationship as much as possible allows the patient to engage in and prepare for termination with the least pain of abandonment. If the patient's hospitalization is time limited, it is important to acknowledge the limit overtly and remind the patient with each contact how many sessions remain.

In day treatment and outpatient settings, the duration of treatment may be indeterminate, but the nurse may not be available that entire time. The termination process cannot be casual; this would stimulate abandonment fears. However, some patients end prematurely when the nurse informs them of the impending end as a way to leave before being rejected. The best approach is to explore these anticipated feelings with the patient. After careful planning, the nurse and patient discuss how to cope with anticipated feelings, including the wish to run away, review the progress the patient has made, and summarize what the patient has learned from the relationship that can be generalized to future encounters.

Establishing Personal Boundaries and Limitations

Personal boundaries are highly context specific; for example, stroking the hair of a stranger on the bus would be inappropriate, but stroking the hair and face of one's intimate partner while sitting together would be appropriate. Clarifying limits requires making explicit what is usually implicit. This may mean having a standing time during each shift that the nurse will talk with the patient. The nurse should refrain from offering personal information, which is frequently confusing to the person with BPD. At times, the person may present in a somewhat arrogant and seemingly entitled way. It is important for the nurse to recognize such a presentation as reflective of internal confusion and dissonance. Responding in a very neutral manner avoids confrontation and a power struggle, which might also unwittingly reinforce the patient's internal sense of inferiority.

Some additional strategies for establishing the boundaries of the relationship include the following:

- Documenting in the patient's chart the agreed-on appointment expectations
- Sharing the treatment plan with the patient
- Confronting violations of the agreement in a nonpunitive way
- Discussing the purpose of limits in the therapeutic relationship and applicability to other relationships

When patients violate boundaries, it is important to respond right away but without taking the behavior personally. For example, if a patient is flirtatious, simply say something like, "Mr. J., I feel uncomfortable with your overly friendly behavior. It seems out of place because we have a professional relationship. That would be more fitting for an intimate relationship that we will never have."

Enhancing Cognitive Functioning

The nurse can often challenge the patient's dysfunctional ways of thinking and encourage the person to think about the event in a different way. When a patient engages in catastrophic thinking, the nurse can challenge by asking, "What is the worst that could happen?" and "How likely would that be to occur?" Or in dichotomous thinking, when the patient fixates on one extreme perception or alternates only between the extremes, the nurse should ask the patient to think about any examples of exceptions to the extreme. The point of the challenge is not to debate or argue with the patient but to provide different perspectives to consider. Encouraging patients to keep journals of real interactions to process with the nurse or therapist is another effective way of testing the reality of their thinking and anticipations, affording more choices and flexibility (Box 30.5).

BOX 30.5 **CLINICAL VIGNETTE**

Challenging Dysfunctional Thinking

Ms. S had worked for the same company for 20 years with a good job record. After an accident, she made some minor mistakes in her work that she quickly corrected. She informed her company nurse that her work was "really slipping" and that she was fearful of her coworkers' disapproval and of getting fired from her job. The nurse asked her to keep a journal of coworkers' comments for the next week. At the next visit, the following dialogue occurred:

Nurse: I noticed that you received several compliments on your work. Even a close friend of your boss expressed appreciation for your work.

Ms. S: It was a light week at work. I really don't believe they meant what they said.

Nurse: I can see how you can believe that one or two comments are not genuine, but how do you account for four and five good reports on your work?

Ms. S: Well, I don't know.

Nurse: It looks like your beliefs are not supported by your journal entries. Now, what makes you think that your boss wants to fire you after 20 years of service?

In problem-solving, the nurse might encourage the patient to debate both sides of the problem and then search for common ground. Practicing communication and negotiation skills through role-playing helps the patient make mistakes and correct them without harm to their self-esteem. The nurse also encourages patients to use these skills in their everyday lives and report back on the results, asking patients how they feel applying the skills and how doing so affects their self-perceptions. Success, even partial success, builds a sense of competence and self-esteem (Table 30.1).

Using Behavioral Interventions

The goal of behavioral interventions is to replace dysfunctional behaviors with positive ones. The nurse has an important role in helping patients control emotions and behaviors by acknowledging and validating desired behaviors and ignoring or confronting undesired behaviors. Patients often test the nurse for a response, so nurses must decide how to respond to particular behaviors. This can be tricky because even negative responses can be viewed as positive reinforcement by the patient. In some instances, if the behavior is irritating but not harmful or demeaning, it is best to ignore, rather than focus, on it. However, grossly inappropriate and disrespectful behaviors require confrontation. If a patient throws a glass of water on an assistant because she is angry at the treatment team for refusing to increase her hospital privileges, an appropriate intervention would include confronting the patient with her behavior and issuing the consequences, such as losing her privileges and apologizing to the assistant.

However, such an incident can be used to help the patient understand why such behavior is inappropriate and how it can be changed. The nurse should explore with the patient what happened, what events led up to the behavior, what the consequences were, and what feelings were aroused. Advanced practice nurses or other therapists explore the origins of the patient's behaviors and responses, but the generalist nurse needs to help the patient explore ways to change behaviors involved in the current situation. The laboriousness of this analytic process may be a sufficient incentive for the patient to abandon the dysfunctional behavior.

Psychoeducation

Patient education within the context of a therapeutic relationship is one of the most important, empowering interventions for the generalist psychiatric–mental health nurse to use. Teaching patients skills to resist parasuicidal urges, improve emotional regulation, enhance interpersonal relationships, tolerate stress, and enhance overall quality of life provides the foundation for long-term behavioral changes. These skills can be taught in any treatment setting as a part of the overall facility program (Box 30.6). If nurses are practicing in a facility where DBT is the treatment model, they can be trained in DBT and can serve as group skills leaders.

Teaching Emotional Regulation

A major goal of cognitive therapeutic interventions is emotional regulation—recognizing and controlling

TABLE 30.1	THOUGHT DISTORTIONS AND CORRECTIVE STATEMENTS
Thought Distortion	**Corrective Statement**
Catastrophizing	
"This is the most awful thing that has ever happened to me"	*"This is a sad thing but not the most awful."*
"If I fail this course, my life is over."	*"If you fail the course, you can take the course again. You can change your major."*
Dichotomizing	
"No one ever listens to me."	*"Your husband listened to you last night when you told him ..."*
"I never get what I want."	*"You didn't get the promotion this year, but you did get a merit raise."*
"I can't understand why everyone is so kind at first and then always dumps me when I need them the most."	*"It is hard to remember those kind things and times when your friends have stayed with you when you needed them."*
Self-Attribution Errors	
"If I had just found the right thing to say, she wouldn't have left me."	*"There is not a single right thing to say, and she left you because she chose to."*
"If I had not made him mad, he wouldn't have hit me."	*"He has a lot of choices in how to respond, and he chose hitting. You are responsible for your feelings and actions."*

the expression of feelings. Patients often fail even to recognize their feelings; instead, they respond quickly without thinking about the consequences. Remember, the time needed for taking action is shorter than the time needed for thinking before acting. Pausing makes up for the momentary lag between the limbic and autonomic response and the prefrontal response.

Another element of emotional regulation is learning to delay gratification. When the patient wants something that is not immediately available, the nurse can teach patients to distract themselves, find alternate ways of meeting the need, and think about what would happen if they have to wait to meet the need.

Teaching Effective Ways to Communicate

Patients lack interpersonal skills in relating because they often had inadequate modeling and few opportunities to practice. The goals of relationship skill development are to identify problematic behaviors that interfere with relationships and to use appropriate behaviors in improving relationships. The starting point is with communication. The nurse teaches the patient basic communication approaches, such as making "I" statements, paraphrasing what the other party says before responding, checking the accuracy of perceptions with others, compromising and seeking common ground, listening actively, and offering and accepting reactions. Besides modeling the behaviors, the nurse guides patients in practicing a variety of communication approaches for common situations. When role-playing, the nurse needs to discuss not only what the skills are and how to perform them but also the feelings patients have before, during, and after the role-play.

In day treatment and outpatient settings, the nurse can give the patient homework, such as keeping a journal, applying role-playing skills to actual situations, and observing behaviors in others. In the hospital, the patient can experience the same process, where the nurse is available to offer immediate feedback. Whatever the setting or whatever the specific problems addressed, the nurse must keep in mind and remind the patient that change occurs slowly. Thus, working on the problems occurs gradually, with severity of symptoms as the guide to deciding how fast and how much change to expect.

Wellness Strategies

Whole Health is a cutting-edge approach to care that supports a person's health and well-being. This approach is currently being implemented throughout the U.S. Department of Veterans Affairs. It is a nationally supported, grassroots movement that is bringing about system-wide transformation to health care in VA medical centers across the country. Whole Health centers around **what matters to you**, not what's the matter with you. The health care team gets to know you as a person, and then works with you to develop an individual health plan that is based on your values, needs, and goals. Whole Health is wellness-oriented care. It has been found to be extremely effective for patients with all kinds of health care needs and is a great adjunctive care approach for persons with psychiatric disorders. Whole Health programs like meditation, yoga, acupuncture, Tai Chi, nutrition, and cooking classes serve as nonpharmaceutical approaches to health and wellness. Patients with BPD and depression especially have reported enjoying and benefiting from Whole Health programs.

Although some health care providers have implemented some type of wellness education and training in their practices for many years, the Whole Health approach to care is anticipated to be more formally included in all medical practices in the future.

Building Social Skills and Self-Esteem

In the hospital, the nurse can use group therapy to discuss feelings and ways to cope with them. Women with BPD benefit from assertiveness classes and women's health issues classes. Many of the women are involved in abusive relationships and lack the ability to resolve these relationships because of their extreme anxiety regarding separating from those they love and their extreme need to feel connected. These women verbalize desires to do it, but they do not have the strength and self-confidence needed to leave. Exposing them to a different style of interaction as well as validation from other people increases their self-esteem and ability to get away from negative influences.

Providing Family Education

Caring for or living with a person with BPD is challenging. Families and friends experience high levels of anxiety, depression, and grief. They often feel that they are burdened with the person's problems and crises. These feelings are higher in families with a member with this disorder than families of individuals with other severe mental disorders. Psychoeducation programs are currently being studied to support families and friends in their relationship with the affected person and reduce the feelings of grief, depression, anxiety, and burden (Betts et al., 2018).

The awareness of these caregiver issues affords the nurse the opportunity to provide family educations in several areas:

- Educating the family about the diagnosis of BPD
- Educating the caregiver about mental health and support recourses for the person with BPD
- Educating the caregiver and normalizing their feelings that they too need support and care
- Educating the caregiver on access to mental health care for self-care and access to caregiver support resources (e.g., The National Alliance on Mentally Illness.)

Promoting Safety

Patients with BPD are usually admitted to the inpatient setting because of threats of self-harm. Observing for antecedents of self-injurious behavior and intervening before an episode are important safety interventions. Patients can learn to identify situations leading to self-destructive behavior and develop preventive strategies.

Because patients with BPD are impulsive and may respond to stress by harming themselves, observation of the patient's interactions and assessment of mood, level of distress, and agitation are important indicators of impending self-injury. Remembering that self-harm is an effort to self-soothe by activating endogenous endorphins, the nurse can assist the patient to find more productive and enduring ways to find comfort. Linehan (1993) suggests using the Five Senses Exercise:

- Vision (e.g., go outside and look at the stars or flowers or autumn leaves)
- Hearing (e.g., listen to beautiful or invigorating music or the sounds of nature)
- Smell (e.g., light a scented candle, boil a cinnamon stick in water)
- Taste (e.g., drink a soothing, warm, nonalcoholic beverage)
- Touch (e.g., take a hot bubble bath, pet your dog or cat, get a massage)

Evaluation and Treatment Outcomes

Evaluation and treatment outcomes vary depending on the severity of the disorder, the presence of comorbid disorders, and the availability of resources. For a patient with severe symptoms or continual self-injury, keeping the patient safe and alive may be a realistic outcome. Helping the patient resist parasuicidal urges may take years. In contrast, individuals who rarely need hospitalization and have adequate resources can expect to recover from the self-destructive impulses and learn positive interaction skills that promote a high-quality lifestyle. Most patients fall somewhere in between, with periods of symptom exacerbation and remission. In these patients, increasing the symptom-free time may be the best indicator of outcomes.

Continuum of Care

Treatment and recovery involve long-term therapy. Hospitalization is sometimes necessary during acute episodes involving **parasuicidal behavior**, but after this behavior is controlled, patients are discharged. It is important for these individuals to continue with treatment in the outpatient or day treatment setting. Because these individuals often appear more competent and in control than they are, nurses must not be deceived by these outward appearances. These individuals need continued follow-up and long-term therapy, including individual therapy, psychoeducation, and positive role models (see Box 30.7). There is growing evidence that virtual psychosocial applications for persons with BPD are clinically useful (Frías et al., 2020).

Integration with Primary Care

The mental health team should work closely with the primary care providers and explain the behaviors that interfere with receiving care. People with BPD often have multiple medical problems such as diabetes, obesity, and hyperlipidemia. The person may not show up for appointments yet expect the providers to call and remind them. Their interaction style and need for attention may quickly wear out a busy primary care staff, causing the staff to reject the person. Emotional dysfunction may erupt when the person is confronted with a stressful situation or diagnosis. The mental health team should be available to provide support to the primary care staff and help the patient negotiate the health care system.

ANTISOCIAL PERSONALITY DISORDER

ASPD is defined as "a pervasive pattern of disregard for, and violation of, the rights of others occurring since age 15 years" (APA, 2013, p. 659). This diagnosis is given to individuals 18 years of age or older who fail to follow society's rules—that is, they do not believe that society's rules are made for them and so are

---

BOX 30.7

Research for Best Practice: Brief Admissions During Prolonged Treatment

Helleman, M., Goossens, P. J., Kaasenbrood, A., & van Achterberg, T. (2016). Brief admissions during prolonged treatment in a case involving borderline personality disorder and posttraumatic stress disorder: Use and functions. Journal of the American Psychiatric Nurses Association, 22(3), 215–224.

THE QUESTION: How can brief admissions be used during a long-term treatment process (7 years) for a person suffering from severe symptoms of borderline personality disorder and complex PTSD?

METHODS: A descriptive qualitative case study design explored the usefulness of brief admissions to an acute care setting for a 37-year-old female with borderline personality disorder and PTSD. Multiple sources of data were triangulated to reach convergence on the functions and use of brief admissions across and extended treatment period. Semistructured interviews were conducted with the patient, her husband, psychiatric, community psychiatric nurse, and a clinical nurse involved in her care. Key concepts in the interview transcripts were identified, coded, and analyzed by two researchers.

FINDINGS: Initially, the main goal of the brief admission was to prevent suicide and self-harm. As treatment progressed, the brief admission served other functions such as prevention of long admissions, prevention of dropout from therapy, opportunities to exercise newly acquired skills, opportunities to expand autonomy and self-care, and to establish preconditions needed to maintain social roles.

IMPLICATIONS FOR NURSING: Brief admission can positively influence the treatment course for a patient with diagnoses of borderline personality disorder and PTSD.

---

consistently irresponsible. ASPD has a long history in the psychopathological literature. A condition termed *moral insanity* was first described in the early 19th century. Since then the disorder has also been called psychopathy, and sociopathy (Paris, 1997). The term *psychopath*, or *sociopath*, a person with a tendency toward antisocial and criminal behavior with little regard for others, is often used in describing the behaviors of people with ASPD.

| **KEYCONCEPT Antisocial personality disorder** is characterized by a pervasive pattern of disregard for and violation of the rights of others.

Clinical Course and Diagnostic Criteria

ASPD has a chronic course with antisocial behaviors tending to diminish later in life, particularly after the age of 40 years (APA, 2013). Individuals with ASPD are arrogant and self-centered and feel privileged and entitled. They are self-serving, and they exploit and seek

power over others. They can be interpersonally engaging and charming, which is often mistaken for a genuine sense of concern for other people. In reality, they lack empathy; are unable to express human compassion; and tend to be insensitive, callous, and contemptuous of others. Deceit and manipulation for personal profit or pleasure are central features associated with this disorder. They are behaviorally impulsive and interpersonally irresponsible. Many with this disorder repeatedly perform acts that are grounds for arrest (whether they are arrested or not), such as destroying property, harassing others, stealing, or pursuing other illegal occupations. They act hastily and spontaneously, are temperamentally aggressive and shortsighted, and fail to plan ahead or consider alternatives. They fail to adapt to the ethical and social standards of the community. They lack a sense of personal obligation to fulfill social and financial responsibilities, including those involved with being a spouse, parent, employee, friend, or member of the community. They lack remorse for their transgressions (APA, 2013).

Some of these individuals openly and flagrantly violate laws and end up in jail. But most people with ASPD never come in conflict with the law and instead find a niche in society, such as in business, the military, or politics, which rewards their competitively tough behavior. Although ASPD is characterized by continual antisocial acts, the disorder is not synonymous with criminality. See Key Diagnostic Characteristics 30.2.

Epidemiology and Risk Factors

Twelve-month prevalence rates of ASPD are estimated between 0.2% and 3.3% (APA, 2013). Males with alcohol use disorder and those released from substance abuse clinics, prisons, or other forensic settings have the highest rates. Adverse socioeconomic (i.e., poverty) or sociocultural (i.e., migration) factors also are associated with higher prevalence (APA, 2013). Gender differences also exist in how symptoms are manifest (Key Diagnostic Characteristics 30.2).

Age of Onset

To be diagnosed with ASPD, the individual must be at least 18 years old and must have exhibited one or more childhood behavioral characteristics of conduct disorder before the age of 15 years, such as aggression to people or animals, destruction of property, deceitfulness or theft, or serious violation of rules. The likelihood of developing adult ASPD is increased if onset of conduct disorder is seen before age 10 years as well as an accompanying childhood attention deficit hyperactivity disorder diagnosis (APA, 2013).

Comorbidity

ASPD is associated with several other psychiatric disorders, including mood, anxiety, and other personality disorders. ASPD is strongly associated with alcohol and drug abuse (Tielbeek et al., 2018). However, a diagnosis of ASPD is not warranted if the antisocial behavior occurs only in the context of substance use. For example, some people who misuse substances sometimes engage in criminal behavior, such as stealing or prostitution, only when in pursuit of drugs. Therefore, it is crucial to assess whether the person with possible ASPD has engaged in illegal activities at times other than when pursuing or using substances.

Etiology

Biologic Theories

Perhaps more than any other personality disorder, an extensive number of biologically oriented studies explore the genetic bases, neuropsychological factors, and arousal levels among this group of pathologies. Many of these studies show neurobiological changes associated with personality disorders or characteristics, but the evidence lacks that these changes caused the disorder. These studies often overlap with studies of aggression, temperament, and substance use (Kolla et al., 2018; Tielbeek et al., 2017).

Magnetic resonance imaging studies demonstrate difference in the brain regions that are related to impulsivity and irresponsibility (Deming et al., 2020). These findings support the neural basis of fearlessness in these individuals. Impairment in frontotemporal, cerebellar, limbic, and paralimbic regions are associated with poor moral judgment and introspective abilities (Johanson et al., 2020). In adolescence, antisocial behavior is related to increased amygdala reactivity to interpersonal threats, which may lead to anger-related behavior (Dotterer et al., 2017).

Psychosocial Theories

Temperament

Scientists believe temperament is neurobiologically determined, and many believe that it is central to understanding personality disorders. A temperament, the natural predisposition to express feelings and actions, is evident during the first few months of life and remains stable through development. For example, whereas some infants are more relaxed or calm and sleep a lot, others are extremely alert, startled by the slightest noise, cry more, and are sleepless.

Difficult temperaments are common in ASPD and are often on the basis of their aggression and impulsivity.

> **KEYCONCEPT Temperament** comprises a person's characteristic intensity, rhythmicity, adaptability, energy expenditure, and mood. A **difficult temperament** is characterized by withdrawal from stimuli, low adaptability, and intense emotional reactions. Four key behaviors are present in a difficult temperament: aggression, inattention, hyperactivity, and impulsivity.

Temperaments consist of two behavioral dimensions that interact with each other. The activity spectrum varies from intense to passive. The adaptability spectrum varies from having a positive attitude about new stimuli with high flexibility to withdrawal from new stimuli and minimal flexibility in response to change. A strong relationship is found between difficult temperament and ASPD behaviors (Lennox & Dolan, 2014).

Attachment

One of the leading explanations of ASPD is that unsatisfactory attachments in early relationships lead to antisocial behavior in later life. Attachment, attaining and retaining interpersonal connection to a significant person, begins at birth. In a secure attachment, a child feels safe, loved, and valued and develops the self-confidence to interact with the rest of the world. Experiences within the context of secure relationships enable the child to develop trust in others. Strong attachments between parents and child may lower the risk of delinquency, assault, and other offenses that are characteristic of those who develop antisocial behavior (Christian et al., 2017).

In individuals with ASPD, a failure to make or sustain stable attachments in early childhood can lead to avoidance of future attachments. Risk factors for developing dysfunctional attachments include parental abandonment or neglect, loss of a parent or primary caregiver, and physical or sexual abuse. Parents who lacked secure attachment relationships in their own childhoods may be unable to form secure attachment relationships with their own children.

Family Issues

In many cases, individuals with ASPD come from chaotic families in which alcoholism and violence are the norm. Individuals who have been victims of abuse or neglect, live in a foster home, or had several primary caregivers are more likely to be victimized by antisocial behaviors, especially aggression. Child abuse and growing up in a home with domestic violence increase the risk of antisocial behavior (Green & Browne, 2019). It is difficult to separate the influence of social factors on the development of the disorder because the symptoms of ASPD are expressed as social manifestations, including unemployment, multiple divorces and separations, and violence.

Family Response to Antisocial Personality Disorder

If family members are present in a patient's life, they have probably been abused, mistreated, or intimidated by these patients. For example, one patient sold his mother's possessions while she was at work. Another abused his wife after drinking. However, family members may be fiercely loyal to the patient and blame themselves for their shortcomings.

Men who have ASPD often engage in relationships with women who have BPD. This is known as assortive mating. Assortive mating is a pattern and form of sexual selection in which individual with similar phenotypes or observable physical characteristics, including appearance, development, and behavior, mate with one another more frequently than would be expected under a random matting pattern. Individuals with BPD use coercion and manipulation for emotional closeness, whereas those with ASPD use manipulation in the pursuit of physical sex. Individuals with ASPD often mate with BPD because their cold and manipulative behavior feeds into the fears of abandonment of the BPD, resulting in very dramatic and chaotic relationships for both (Munoz Centifanti et al., 2016).

RECOVERY-ORIENTED CARE FOR PERSONS WITH ANTISOCIAL PERSONALITY DISORDER

Nursing Care Plan 30.2 is available at http://thepoint.lww.com/

Teamwork and Collaboration: Working Toward Recovery

People rarely seek mental health care for ASPD but rather for treatment of depression, substance use, uncontrolled anger, or forensic-related problems. Patients with psychiatric disorders who are admitted through the courts often have a comorbid diagnosis of ASPD. Patients with ASPD usually present for treatment as a result of an ultimatum. Treatment is often a choice between losing a job, being expelled from school, ending a marriage or relationship with children, or giving up on a chance at probation and psychological treatment. Under these circumstances, treatment is usually forced on them. Other times people with ASPD who find themselves in trouble with the law will seek out psychiatric care on their own in an attempt to "prove" to the court they are seeking help for their offenses, when they are actually only manipulating the justice system through deception. Most prisons and other correctional facilities require inmates to attend psychotherapy sessions. In either case, working with people with ASPD is likely to be a frustrating and exasperating experience for the nurse due to the patient's clear lack of insight and/or motivation to change. Treatment is difficult and involves helping the patient alter their cognitive schemata.

Safety Issues

Although they can be interpersonally charming, these patients can become verbally and physically abusive if their expectations are not met. Protection of other patients and staff is a priority.

EVIDENCE-BASED NURSING CARE OF PERSONS WITH ANTISOCIAL PERSONALITY DISORDER

Mental Health Nursing Assessment

Physical Health and Functioning

ASPD does not significantly impair physical functioning except in the presence of coexisting substance use disorder or another psychiatric diagnosis involved. Because substance use is a major problem with this population, the physical effects of chronic use of addictive substances must be considered. If admitted inpatient, the nurse needs to keenly observe for possible withdrawal symptoms from substance use. Conversely, someone who has health problems secondary to chronic substance misuse should also be assessed for concurrent personality disorders. Substance use and ASPD are not mutually exclusive. Some people with substance use disorders are not antisocial but may commit crimes (e.g., selling drugs, robbery, theft) in the context of obtaining drugs for their personal use.

Psychosocial Assessment

Eliciting psychosocial data from persons with ASPD may be difficult because of their basic mistrust of authority figures. Many patients with ASPD are committed to mental health care by the court system. They may not give an accurate history or may embellish aspects to project themselves in a more positive light. They often deny any criminal activity even if they are admitted to police custody.

Behavioral Responses

Key areas of assessment are determining the quality of relationships, impulsivity, and the extent of aggression. These individuals do not assume responsibility for their own actions and often blame others for their misfortune. Their disregard for others is manifested in their interactions. For example, one patient with human immunodeficiency virus was engaging in unprotected sex with several different women because he wanted to "have fun as long as I can." He was completely unconcerned about the possibility of transmitting the virus. These individuals often make good first impressions. Self-awareness is especially important for the nurse because of the initial charming quality of many of these individuals. When these patients realize that the nurse cannot be used or manipulated, they lose interest in the nurse and revert to their normal, egocentric behaviors.

Support Network

Social support for these individuals is often minimal, just as it is for individuals with BPD, but the reasons are different. These individuals have often taken advantage of friends and relatives who, in turn, no longer trust them. Helping the patient build a new support system after new skills are learned is usually the only option. For these individuals to develop friends and re-engage family members, they must learn to interact in new ways, develop empathy, and risk an attachment. For many, this never truly becomes a reality.

Clinical Judgment

People with ASPD are often admitted to psychiatric units following a violent incident, such as a physical confrontation or a suicide attempt. As with any patient, safety is a priority. One of the first priorities is to establish a safe environment for the patient and staff. After safety is established, other mutually agreed-upon priorities can be considered, such as improving interpersonal communication with family members or addressing anger issues.

Outcomes should be short-term and relevant to a specific problem. For example, if a patient has been chronically unemployed, a reasonable short-term outcome is for the patient to set up job interviews rather than obtain a job.

THERAPEUTIC RELATIONSHIP

Therapeutic relationships are difficult to establish because these individuals do not attach themselves to others and are often unable to use a relationship to change behavior. The goal of the therapeutic relationship is to identify dysfunctional thinking patterns and develop new problem-solving behaviors. After the first few meetings with these patients, the nurse may believe that the relationship has a good start, but in reality, a superficial alliance is usually formed. Additional sessions reveal the lack of patient commitment to the relationship. These patients begin to revisit topics discussed in previous sessions or lose interest in trying to work on problems. By using self-awareness skills and accessing supervision regularly, the nurse can identify blocks in the development of a therapeutic relationship (or lack of) and their response to the relationship.

MENTAL HEALTH NURSING INTERVENTIONS

Establishing Recovery and Wellness Goals

Recovery involves changing interpersonal and lifestyle behaviors. The overall treatment goals are to develop a nurturing sense of attachment and empathy for other people and situations and to live within the norms of society. Several current treatment modalities may be helpful in establishing these goals. Harm reduction is a pragmatic approach for managing high-risk behaviors such as substance use or high-risk sexual behaviors that are often characteristic of persons with ASPD. For example, the harm reduction approach recognizes that the reduction of substance use from 7 to 3 days per week is progress. Reducing the harm of substance use is celebrated and built upon for further success. See Chapter 31. Motivational interviewing can help the person explore and resolve ambivalence to change. MBT, discussed earlier in this chapter, can also be for persons with ASPD.

Physical Care

In instances in which there are comorbid disorders, the patient with ASPD may actually interfere with interventions aimed at improving physical functioning. For example, a patient with substance use disorder and ASPD may not develop enough trust within a relationship to examine their delusional thoughts or other aspects of dysfunction, such as alcohol or drug abuse.

In instances in which there are concurrent diagnoses, such as a patient with ASPD with a co-occurring substance use disorder, may actually interfere with interventions aimed at improving his physical functioning. For example, a patient with ASPD who develops a case of pancreatitis may refuse to refrain from abusing alcohol. As a result, he may be hospitalized for multiple episodes of pancreatitis.

Wellness Challenges

Enhancing self-awareness (i.e., exploring and understanding personal thoughts, feelings, motivation, and behaviors) is another nursing intervention that is helpful in developing an understanding about relating peacefully to the rest of the world. Encouraging patients to recognize and discuss their thoughts and feelings helps the nurse understand how the patient views the world. Some evidence indicates that substance misuse can be improved through cognitive-behavioral treatment, but there is little evidence that the core problems of this disorder (aggression, reconviction, global functioning, and social functioning) are improved with psychological interventions (Brazil et al., 2018).

Medication Interventions

There are no medications to treat ASPD, only treatment for symptoms they may experience. For example, impulsive aggression may benefit from the use of lithium,

SSRIs, atypical antipsychotics, gamma-aminobutyric acid enhancers, beta-blockers, MAOIs, or buprenorphine (Svrakic & Dvac-Jovanovic, 2019).

Psychosocial Interventions

Facilitating self-responsibility (i.e., encouraging a patient to assume more responsibility for personal behavior) is an important intervention. The nursing activities that are particularly helpful include holding the patient responsible for the behavior, monitoring the extent that self-responsibility is assumed, and discussing the consequences of not dealing with responsibilities. The nurse needs to refrain from arguing or bargaining about the unit rules, such as time for meals, use of the television room, and smoking. Instead, positive feedback is given to the patient for accepting additional responsibility or changing behavior.

Psychoeducation

Patient education efforts have to be creative and thought provoking. In teaching a person with ASPD, a direct approach is best, but the nurse must avoid "lecturing," which the patient will resent. In teaching the patient about positive health care practices, impulse control, and anger management, the best approach is to engage the patient in a discussion about the issue and then direct the topic to the major teaching points. These patients often take great delight in arguing or showing how the rules of life do not apply to them. A sense of humor is important, as are clear teaching goals and avoiding being sidetracked (see Boxes 30.8, 30.9).

Providing Family Education

Family members of patients with ASPD usually need help in establishing boundaries. Because there is a long-term pattern of interaction in which family members feel responsible for the patient's antisocial behavior, these patterns need to be stopped. Families need help in recognizing the patient's responsibility for their own actions.

Promoting Safety

Aggressive behavior is often a problem for these individuals and their family members. Similar to patients with BPD, people with ASPD tend to be impulsive. Instead of self-injury, these individuals are more likely to strike out at those who are perceived to be interfering with their immediate gratification. Anger control assistance (helping to express anger in an adaptive, nonviolent manner) becomes a priority intervention. Because the expression of anger and aggression develops during a lifetime, these individuals can benefit from anger management techniques.

BOX 30.8 • THERAPEUTIC DIALOGUE: ANTISOCIAL PERSONALITY DISORDER

INEFFECTIVE APPROACH

Danny: Hey, I need a light for my cigarette.

Nurse: Really? You know the rules—no smoking on the unit.

Danny: I'm not going to smoke here. I just need a light so that I can have a cigarette when I leave here.

Nurse: I also need your cigarettes. Cigarettes are contraband.

Danny: You are terrible—just like the bitch who kicked me out. Who do you think you are anyway?

Nurse: You need to quiet down.

Danny: Yeah, says who?

Nurse: I will call security if you don't quiet down.

Danny: Call them, I don't care.

EFFECTIVE APPROACH

Danny: Hey, I need a light for my cigarette.

Nurse: A light? I don't have a light.

Danny: I need a light so that I can smoke later.

Nurse: Oh, I see. Did you have a lighter when you were admitted?

Danny: Yea, they took everything away including my belt and shoelaces.

Nurse: The reason for storing everything is for the safety of everyone. When you are discharged, you can retrieve everything. I also need to store any cigarettes you have.

Danny: What makes you think I have any cigarettes?

Nurse: Well, you asked for a light. Many patients manage to bring cigarettes into the unit. I need to put them with your things. You can retrieve them when you are discharged.

Danny: This place is something.

Nurse: I will put your cigarettes in a bag with your name on them.

Danny: This sucks. But here they are.

CRITICAL THINKING CHALLENGE

• How did the nurse in the first scenario get sidetracked?

• How was the nurse in the second scenario able to convince Danny to give up his cigarettes without escalating his anger?

BOX 30.9

Psychoeducation Checklist: Antisocial Personality Disorder

When caring for the patient with ASPD, be sure to include the following topic areas in the teaching plan:
• Positive health care practices, including substance use control
• Effective communication and interaction skills
• Impulse control
• Anger management
• Group experience to help develop self-awareness and impact of behavior on others
• Analyzing an issue from the other person's viewpoint
• Maintenance of employment
• Interpersonal relationships and social interactions

Group Interventions

Group interventions are more effective than individual modalities because other patients and staff can validate or challenge the patient's view of a situation. Problem-solving groups that focus on identifying a problem and developing a variety of alternative solutions are particularly helpful because patient self-responsibility is reinforced when patients remind each other of better alternatives. Patients are likely to confront each other with dysfunctional schemata or thinking patterns. Teaching patients with ASPD the same communication techniques as those with BPD will also encourage self-responsibility. These patients often attend groups that focus on the development of empathy.

Implementing Milieu Therapy

Milieu interventions, such as providing a structured environment with rules that are consistently applied to patients who are responsible for their own behavior, are important. While living in close proximity to others, the individual with ASPD will demonstrate dysfunctional social patterns that can be identified and targeted for correction. For example, these patients often violate ward rules, such as no smoking or limitations on the number of visitors, and may bring contraband, such as illegal drugs, into the unit.

In an inpatient unit, interventions can be more intense and focus on helping the patient develop positive interaction skills and experience a consistent environment. For example, the focus of nursing interventions may be the patient's continual disregard of the rights of others. On one unit, a patient continually placed orders for pizzas in the name of another patient who had limited intelligence and was genuinely afraid of the person with ASPD. The victimized patient always paid for the pizza. When the nursing staff realized what was happening, they confronted the patient with ASPD about the behavior and revoked his unit privileges.

Evaluation and Treatment Outcomes

The outcomes for patients with ASPD are evaluated in terms of managing specific problems, such as maintaining employment or developing a meaningful interpersonal relationship. The nurse will most likely see these patients for other health care problems, so adherence to treatment recommendations and development of health care practices (e.g., reducing smoking and alcohol consumption) can also be factored into the evaluation of outcomes.

Continuum of Care

People with ASPD rarely seek mental health care unless there is a co-morbid condition, such as depression. Nurses are most likely to see these patients in medical–surgical settings for comorbid conditions. Consistency in interventions is necessary for treating the patient throughout the continuum of care.

OTHER CLUSTER B PERSONALITY DISORDERS

Histrionic Personality Disorder

Clinical Course and Diagnostic Criteria

Attention seeking, *excitable*, and *emotional* are terms used to describe people with **histrionic personality disorder (HPD)**. Histrionic personality disorder is one of the most ambiguous diagnostic categories in psychiatry. HPD made its first official appearance in the *Diagnostic and Statistical Manual of Mental Disorders II (DSM II)* and since its revisions through *DSM-V*. HPD is the only modern category in diagnostic classifications that conserved a derivative of the old concept of Hysteria. Several psychiatric disorders are derived from the original term *hysteria* such as the *conversion disorder*, the *somatization disorder*, *somatoform disorders*, *phobic anxiety*, the term *mass*

hysteria, and finally the *HPD*. The word *hysteria* is derived from the Greek term *hystera*, meaning the womb or uterus. It has been used since ancient times and appears in text of the Egyptians, Greeks, and Romans. In the Old Rome, the word *Histrione* was already used to define the actors that represented coarse farces representing those who are false and theatrical (Novais et al., 2015).

HPD is more likely in women. Affected individuals are lively and dramatic and draw attention to themselves by their enthusiasm, dress, and apparent openness. They are the "life of the party" and, on the surface, seem interested in others. Their insatiable need for attention and approval quickly becomes obvious. Their need to be "center stage" arises in two ways: (1) their interests and topics of conversation focus on their own desires and activities and (2) their behavior, including their speech pattern, continually calls attention to themselves. These needs are inflexible and persistent even after others attempt to meet them. Persons with HPDs are quick to form new friendships and just as quick to become demanding. Because they are trusting and easily influenced by other opinions, their behavior often appears inconsistent. Their strong dependency need makes them overly trusting and gullible. They are moody and often experience a sense of helplessness when others are uninterested in them. They are sexually seductive in their attempts to gain attention and often are uncomfortable within a single relationship. Their appearance is provocative and their speech dramatic. They express strong opinions without supporting facts. Loyalty and fidelity are lacking (Hamlat et al., 2019).

Gender influences the manifestations of this disorder. Women dress seductively, may express dependency on selected men, and may "play" a submissive role. Men may dress in a very masculine manner and seek attention by bragging about athletic skills or successes in their jobs. Individuals with this disorder have difficulty achieving any true intimacy in interpersonal relationships. They seem to possess an innate sensitivity to the moods and thoughts of those they wish to please. This hyperalertness enables them to maneuver quickly to gain their attention. They then attempt to control relationships by their seductiveness at one level but become extremely dependent on their friends at another level. Their demand for constant attention quickly alienates their friends. They become depressed when they are not the center of attention.

Epidemiology and Risk Factors

The prevalence of HPD is estimated at 1.8% of the general population of the United States (Grant et al., 2004). No gender differences arise in the occurrence of this disorder; however, this diagnosis is seen more frequently in women than men clinically. Risk of occurrence of this disorder is greater among African Americans than Whites. Low-income groups and less educated persons are also at higher risk for occurrence of HPD. Widowed, separated, divorced, or people who never married are at greater risk than married ones. This disorder occurs concurrently with other mental disorders; anxiety disorder, obsessive-compulsive syndromes, somatic symptom disorder, substance use disorder, and mood disorders, in which they overplay their feelings of dysthymia by expressing them through dramatic and eye-catching gestures (French & Shrestha, 2020).

Etiology

Research related to this personality disorder is minimal. Some speculate that there is a biologic component and that heredity may play a role but that the biologic influence is less than in some of the previously discussed personality problems. In infancy and early childhood, these individuals are extremely alert and emotionally responsive. The tendencies for sensory alertness may be traced to responses of the limbic and reticular systems. They demonstrate a high degree of dependence on others and a type of dissociation in which they have reduced awareness of their behavior in relation to others (French & Shrestha, 2020).

It is believed that these highly alert and responsive infants seek more gratification from external stimulation during their first few months of life. Depending on the responsiveness of caregivers to them, they develop behavior patterns in response to their caregivers. It is believed that these children experience brief, highly charged, and irregular reinforcement from multiple caregivers (parents, siblings, grandparents, foster parents) who are unable to provide consistent experiences.

Parental behavior and role modeling are also believed to contribute to the development of HPD. Many of the women with this disorder reported that they are just like their mother, who is emotionally labile, bored with the routines of home life, flirtatious with men, and clever in dealing with people. It is believed that through role modeling, these children learn and mimic the behaviors observed in caregivers or adults (French & Shrestha, 2020).

Evidence-Based Nursing Care of Persons with Histrionic Personality Disorder

The ultimate treatment goal for patients with HPD is to correct the tendency to expect others to fulfill all of their needs. When these individuals seek mental health care, they have usually experienced a period of social disapproval or deprivation. Their hope is that the mental health providers will help fulfill their needs. Specific goals are needed to protect the person from becoming dependent on a mental health system. In the nursing assessment, the nurse focuses on the quality of the individual's interpersonal relationships. It is common that the person is dissatisfied with their partner, and sexual relations may be nonexistent.

During the assessment, the patient will make statements that indicate low self-esteem. Because these individuals believe that they are incapable of handling life's demands and have been waiting for a truly competent person to take care of them, they have not developed a positive self-concept or adequate problem-solving abilities.

Priority of care areas for persons with this disorder include focusing on self-esteem and coping patterns. Outcomes focus on helping the patient develop autonomy, a positive self-concept, and mature problem-solving skills.

A variety of interventions support the outcomes. A nurse–patient relationship that allows the patient to explore positive personality characteristics and develop independent decision-making skills forms the basis of the interventions. Reinforcing personal strengths, conveying confidence in the patient's ability to handle situations, and examining the patient's negative perceptions of him- or herself can be done within the therapeutic relationship. Encouraging the patient to act autonomously can also improve the individual's sense of self-worth. Attending assertiveness groups can help increase the individual's self-confidence and improve self-esteem.

Continuum of Care

Patients with HPD do not seek mental health care unless they have a coexisting medical or mental disorder. They are likely to be treated within the community for most of their lives, with the exception of short hospitalizations for nonpsychiatric problems.

Narcissistic Personality Disorder
Clinical Course and Diagnostic Criteria

People with **narcissistic personality disorder** are grandiose, have an inexhaustible need for admiration, and lack empathy. Beginning in childhood, these individuals believe that they are superior, special, or unique and that others should recognize them in this way (Hamlat et al., 2019). They are often preoccupied with fantasies of unlimited success, power, beauty, or ideal love. They overvalue their personal worth, direct their affections toward themselves, and expect others to hold them in high esteem. They define the world through their own self-centered view. Their sense of entitlement is striking. People with narcissistic personality disorder are benignly arrogant and feel themselves above the conventions of their cultural group. They handle criticism poorly and may become enraged if someone dares to criticize them or else they may appear totally indifferent to criticism. They believe they are entitled to be served and that it is their inalienable right to receive special considerations. People with this disorder want to have their own way and are frequently ambitious for fame and fortune. These individuals are often successful in their jobs but may alienate their significant others, who grow tired of their narcissism. They cannot show empathy, and they feign sympathy only for their own benefit to achieve their selfish ends. Clinically, those with narcissistic personality disorder show overlapping characteristics of BPD and ASPD.

Epidemiology and Risk Factors

The prevalence of narcissistic personality disorder is 6.2% of the U.S. general population with rates greater for men (7.7%) than for women (4.8%) according to a recent national epidemiologic survey (Stinson et al., 2008). Narcissistic personality disorder can be found in professionals who are highly respected, such as those in law, medicine, and science and those associated with celebrity status. Persons with this disorder may impart an unrealistic sense of omnipotence, grandiosity, beauty, and talent to their children; therefore, children of parents with a narcissistic personality disorder have a higher than usual risk of developing the disorder themselves. It also commonly occurs in only children and among first-born boys in cultural groups in which males have special privileges (Mitra &Fluyau, 2020).

Etiology

Limited evidence suggests biologic factors contribute to the development of this disorder. One notion about its development is that it is the result of parents' overvaluation and overindulgence of a child. These children are overly pampered and indulged, with every whim catered to. They learn to view themselves as special beings and to expect special treatment and subservience from others. They do not learn how to cooperate, share, or consider others' desires and interests. An alternate explanation is that the child never truly separated emotionally from their primary caregiver and therefore cannot envision functioning independently. According to another set of theories, these individuals try to avoid or reduce intense feelings of shame and engage in diverse strategies to gain attention for themselves (Roepke & Vater, 2014).

Evidence-Based Nursing Care for Persons with Narcissistic Personality Disorder

The nurse usually encounters persons with narcissism in medical settings and in psychiatric settings with a coexisting psychiatric disorder. They are difficult patients who often appear snobbish, condescending, and patronizing in their attitudes. It is unlikely that these individuals are motivated to develop sensitivity to others and socially cooperative attitudes and behaviors. Building a therapeutic relationship is a slow process because these patients avoid self-reflection and often reject the clinician's approaches. It is important not to engage in power struggles with the patient. Nurses need to use their self-awareness skills in interacting with these patients and help the person identify concrete, realistic, and measurable treatment goals that the patient identifies as their own (Weinberg & Ronningstam, 2020).

Continuum of Care

Similar to patients with histrionic disorder, those with narcissistic personality disorder do not seek mental health care unless they have a coexisting medical or mental disorder. They are likely to be treated within the community for most of their lives, with the exception of short hospitalizations for nonpsychiatric problems.

CLUSTER C DISORDERS: AVOIDANT, DEPENDENT, AND OBSESSIVE-COMPULSIVE PERSONALITY DISORDERS

Avoidant Personality Disorder

Clinical Course and Diagnostic Criteria

Avoidant personality disorder (AVPD) is characterized by extensive avoidance of social interaction driven by fears of rejection and feelings of personal inadequacy (Lampe & Malhi, 2018). Individuals with this disorder stay out of social situations in which interpersonal contact with others may be expected. Individuals appear timid, shy, and hesitant; they also fear criticism and feel inadequate. These individuals are extremely sensitive to negative comments and disapproval and appraise situations more negatively than others do. They perceive themselves as unwanted and isolated from others. This behavior becomes problematic when it restricts their social activities and work opportunities because of their extreme fear of rejection. In comparison to other personality disorders, AVPD is associated with the highest level of impairment in daily functioning (Weinbrecht et al., 2016).

Chronic depression is associated with AVPD in persons who have experienced childhood abuse and trauma (Klein et al., 2015). Anxious and avoidant attachments with early caregivers have been shown to contribute to the development of AVPD. Fear, expectations of being shamed, and overuse of cognitive and behavioral avoidance contribute to the vicious cycles of maintenance in AVPD (Lampe & Malhi, 2018).

In childhood, persons with AVPD are shy, but instead of growing out of the shyness, it becomes worse in adulthood. They perceive themselves as socially inept, inadequate, and inferior, which, in turn, justifies their isolation and rejection by others. Vocationally, people with AVPD often take jobs on the sidelines, rarely obtaining personal advancement or exercising much authority, but to employers, they seem shy and eager to please. They are reluctant to enter relationships unless they are given strong assurance of uncritical acceptances, so they consequently often have no close friends or confidants (Fariba & Sapra, 2020).

Epidemiology and Risk Factors

The prevalence of AVPD is 2.4% in the general population (APA, 2013), but it has been reported in 10% of outpatients in mental health clinics (Grant et al., 2004). The problem with examining the epidemiology of AVPD is its potential overlap with social anxiety disorder. Several studies found that a significant portion of the patients with diagnoses of social anxiety disorder also met criteria for AVPD (Carter & Wu, 2010; Cox et al., 2009). More research is needed to clarify the relationship between avoidant personality and anxiety disorders. In light of prevalence rates, societal costs, and the current state of research, it needs to be stated that AVPD qualifies as a neglected disorder. Up to now, the available research has primarily focused on the delineation of social anxiety disorder and AVPD (Weinbrecht et al., 2016).

Etiology

Experts speculate that individuals with AVPD experience aversive stimuli more intensely and more frequently than others do because they may possess an overabundance of neurons in the aversive center of the limbic system (Fariba & Sapra, 2020).

Evidence-Based Nursing Care of Persons with Avoidant Personality Disorder

Assessment of these individuals reveals a lack of social contacts, a fear of being criticized, and evidence of chronic low self-esteem. The focus of nursing care is on increasing self-esteem and decreasing social isolation. The establishment of a therapeutic relationship is necessary to be able to help these individuals meet their treatment outcomes. The development of the nurse–patient relationship is a slow process and requires an extreme amount of patience on the part of the nurse. These

individuals may not have had positive interpersonal relationships and need time to be able to be sure that the nurse will not criticize and demean them. Interventions should focus on refraining from any negative criticism, assisting the patient to identify positive responses from others, exploring previous achievements of success, and exploring reasons for self-criticism. The patient's social dimension should be examined for activities that increase self-esteem and interventions focused on increasing these self-esteem-enhancing activities. Social skills training may help reduce symptoms.

Continuum of Care

Long-term therapy is ideal for patients with AVPD because it takes time to make changes in one's behavior. Mental health nurses may initially see these individuals for other health problems. Encouraging the patient to continue with therapy and contacting the therapist when necessary are important in maintaining continuity of care. These patients are hospitalized only for a coexisting disorder.

Dependent Personality Disorder

Clinical Course and Diagnostic Criteria

People with **dependent personality disorder** cling to others in a desperate attempt to keep them close. Their need to be taken care of is so great that it leads to doing anything to maintain the closeness, including total submission and disregard for themselves.

Decision-making is difficult or nonexistent. They adapt their behavior to please those to whom they are attached. They lean on others to guide their lives. They ingratiate themselves with others and denigrate themselves and their accomplishments. Their self-esteem is determined by others. Behaviorally, they withdraw from adult responsibilities by acting helpless and seeking nurturance from others. In interpersonal relationships, they need excessive advice and reassurance. They are compliant, conciliatory, and placating. They rarely disagree with others and are easily persuaded. Friends describe them as gullible. They are warm, tender, and noncompetitive. They timidly avoid social tension and interpersonal conflicts (Hamlat et al., 2019).

Epidemiology and Risk Factors

A recent study estimates the prevalence at 0.49% (APA, 2013). The diagnosis is made more frequently in women than in men. This gender difference may represent a sex bias by clinicians because when standardized instruments are used, men and women receive diagnoses at equal rates. The risk of dependent personality disorder is greater for the least educated and for widowed, divorced, separated, and never-married women (Disney, 2013).

Etiology

It is likely that a biologic predisposition exists to develop the dependency attachments of this disorder. However, no research studies support a biologic hypothesis. Dependent personality disorder is most often explained as a result of parents' genuine affection, extreme attachment, and overprotection. Children then learn to rely on others to meet their basic needs and do not learn the necessary skills for autonomous behavior. Persons with chronic physical illnesses in childhood may be prone to developing this disorder.

Evidence-Based Nursing Care of Persons with Dependent Personality Disorder

Nurses can determine the extent of dependency by assessment of self-worth, interpersonal relationships, and social behavior. They should determine whether there is currently someone on whom the person relies (parent, spouse) or whether there has been a separation from a significant relationship by death or divorce.

Priorities of care that are usually identified include low self-esteem, difficulties in social situations, and coping with stresses of everyday life. Home management skills may be a priority if the patient does not have these skills and has to make decisions related to finances, shopping, cooking, and cleaning. The challenge of caring for these patients is to help them recognize their dependent patterns; motivate them to want to change; and teach them adult skills that have not been developed, such as balancing a checkbook, planning a weekly menu, and paying bills when they are due. Occasionally, if a patient is extremely fatigued, lethargic, or anxious, the disorder interferes with efforts at developing greater independence; antidepressants or antianxiety agents may be used in therapy.

These patients readily engage in a nurse–patient relationship and initially look to the nurse to make all decisions. The nurse can support patients to make their own decisions by resisting the urge to tell them what to do. Ideally, these patients are in individual psychotherapy and working toward long-term personality changes. The nurse can encourage patients to stay in therapy and to practice the new skills that are being learned. Assertiveness training is helpful.

Continuum of Care

Individuals with dependent personality disorder readily seek out therapy and are likely to spend years seeking

therapy. Hospitalization occurs for comorbid conditions such as depression.

Obsessive-Compulsive Personality Disorder

Clinical Course and Diagnostic Criteria

OCPD stands out because it bears close resemblance to obsessive-compulsive disorder (OCD). Although these disorders have similar names, the clinical manifestations are quite different. A distinguishing difference is that those with OCD tend to use obsessive thoughts and compulsions when anxious but less so when anxiety decreases. Persons with OCPD do not demonstrate obsessions and compulsions but rather a pervasive pattern of preoccupation with orderliness, perfectionism, and control. They also have the capacity to delay rewards, whereas those with OCD do not (Pinto et al., 2013). Individuals with this disorder attempt to maintain control by careful attention to rules, trivial details, procedures, and lists (Thamby & Khanna, 2019). They may be completely devoted to work, which typically has a rigid character, such as maintaining financial records or tracking inventory. They are uncomfortable with unstructured leisure time, especially vacations. Their leisure activities are likely to be formalized (e.g., season tickets to sports, organized tour groups). Hobbies are approached seriously.

Behaviorally, individuals with OCPD are perfectionists, maintaining a regulated, highly structured, strictly organized life. A need to control others and situations is common in their personal and work lives. They are prone to repetition and have difficulty making decisions and completing tasks because they become so involved in the details. They can be overly conscientious about morality and ethics and value polite, formal, and correct interpersonal relationships. They also tend to be rigid, stubborn, and indecisive and are unable to accept new ideas and customs. Their mood is tense and joyless. Warm feelings are restrained, and they tightly control the expression of emotions (APA, 2013).

Epidemiology and Risk Factors

OCPD is one of the most prevalent personality disorders in the general population, with estimated prevalence ranging from 2.1% to 7.9% (APA, 2013). This disorder is associated with higher education, employment, and marriage. Subjects with the disorder had a higher income than did those without the disorder.

Etiology

As with some other personality disorders, evidence for a biologic formulation is scant. The basis of the compulsive patterns that characterize OCPD is parental overcontrol and overprotection that is consistently restrictive and sets distinct limits on the child's behavior. Parents teach these children a deep sense of responsibility to others and to feel guilty when these responsibilities are not met. Play is viewed as shameful, sinful, and irresponsible, leading to dire consequences. They are encouraged to resist the natural inclinations toward play and impulse gratification, and parents try to impose guilt on the child to control behavior.

Nursing Care

These individuals seek mental health care when they have attacks of anxiety, spells of immobilization, sexual impotence, and excessive fatigue. The nursing assessment focuses on the patient's physical symptoms (sleep, eating, sexual), interpersonal relationships, and social problems. There may be multiple nursing care priorities such as anxiety, loneliness, decision-making, sexual problems, insomnia, and interpersonal relationships. People with OCPD realize that they can improve their quality of life, but they find it extremely anxiety provoking to make the necessary changes. To change the compulsive pattern, psychotherapy is needed. There may be short-term pharmacologic intervention with an antidepressant or anxiolytic as an adjunct may take place. A supportive nurse–patient relationship based on acceptance of the patient's need for order and rigidity will help the person have enough confidence to try new behaviors. Examining the patient's belief that underlies the dysfunctional behaviors can set the stage for challenging the childhood thinking. Because the compulsive pattern was established in childhood, it will take a long time to modify the behavior.

Continuum of Care

People with OCPD are treated primarily in the community. If there is a coexisting disorder or the person experiences periods of depression is present, hospitalization may be useful for a short period of time.

DISRUPTIVE, IMPULSE-CONTROL, AND CONDUCT DISORDERS

Disruptive, impulse-control, and conduct disorders are a group of mental conditions that have the essential feature of irresistible impulsivity. Behaviors associated with these disorders violate the rights of others and/or are in conflict with societal norms (APA, 2013). Disorders discussed include IED, kleptomania, and **pyromania**.

> **KEYCONCEPT Impulsivity,** acting without considering consequences or alternative actions, results when neurobiologic overactivity is stimulated by psychological, personality, or social factors related to personal needs of the individual (Tansey, 2010).

> **KEYCONCEPT Impulse-control disorders** often coexist with other disorders and are characterized by an inability to resist an impulse or temptation to complete an activity that is considered harmful to oneself or others.

Tension increases before the individual commits the act and derives excitement or gratification when the act is committed. The release of tension is perceived as pleasurable, but remorse and regret usually follow the act. The disruptive behavior disorders, which include oppositional defiant disorder and conduct disorder, are a group of conditions marked by significant problems of conduct. See Chapter 37.

Intermittent Explosive Disorder

Episodes of aggressiveness that result in assault or destruction of property characterize people with **intermittent explosive disorder**. The severity of aggressiveness is out of proportion to the provocation. The episodes can have serious psychosocial consequences, including job loss, interpersonal relationship problems, school expulsion, divorce, automobile accidents, or jail. This diagnosis is given only after all other disorders with aggressive components (e.g., delirium, dementia, head injury, BPD, ASPD, substance use) have been excluded. Little is known about this disorder, but it is a more common condition than previously thought.

Aggression is a destructive behavior that imposes a considerable burden on individuals and society. In clinical settings, recurrent problematic aggression is identified as IED. Intermittent explosive disorder is associated with significantly more aggression than are BPD or ASPD alone (Fanning et al., 2019).

The prevalence of IED in the United States is about 2.7%. The onset is most common in childhood or adolescence and rarely begins for the first time after the age 40 years. The mean age at onset is 14 years. It is more prevalent in individuals with a high school education or less (APA, 2013). The anger experience and expression of anger contribute to suicidality (McCloskey & Ammerman, 2018).

The treatment of this disorder is multifaceted. Psychopharmacologic agents are sometimes used as an adjunct to psychotherapeutic, behavioral, and social interventions. Serotonergic antidepressants and gamma-aminobutyric acid-ergic mood stabilizers have been used. Anxiolytics are used to treat obsessive patients who experience tension states and explosive outbursts. Medication alone is insufficient, and anger management should be included in the treatment plan.

Kleptomania

In **kleptomania**, individuals cannot resist the urge to steal, so they independently steal items that they could easily afford. These items are not particularly useful or wanted. The underlying issue is the act of stealing. The term *kleptomania* was first used in 1838 to describe the behavior of several kings who stole worthless objects (Aboujaoude & Koran, 2010). These individuals experience an increase in tension and then pleasure and relief at the time of the theft. Kleptomania occurs in about 4% to 22% of individuals arrested for shoplifting. Its prevalence in the general population, however, is very rare, at approximately 0.3% to 0.6%. Kleptomania or compulsive stealing remains poorly understood with limited data regarding its underlying pathophysiology and appropriate treatment choices. Severity of kleptomania behaviors is associated with having more frequent urges to steal, feeling excited by stealing, having a current eating disorder, and having a current diagnosis of OCD. Furthermore, worse symptom severity was associated with a shorter transition time (between first stealing and developing kleptomania), as well as with more chance of stealing from relatives and seeking treatment at some point. The association of worse kleptomania severity with stealing-related reward and disorder of compulsivity (OCD, anorexia nervosa) may provide clues for appropriate targets for cognitive behavioral therapy or pharmacotherapy (Grant & Chamberlin, 2018).

Females outnumber males at a ratio of 3:1 (APA, 2013). Because it is considered a "secret" disorder, little is known about it, but it is believed to last for years despite numerous convictions for shoplifting. It appears that kleptomania often has its onset during adolescence (Grant & Kim, 2005).

Some shoplifting appears to be related to anxiety and stress in that it serves to relieve symptoms. In a few instances, brain damage has been associated with kleptomania (Blum et al., 2018). Depression is the most common symptom identified in a compulsive shoplifter.

Kleptomania is difficult to detect and treat and means of treatment are little known. It appears that behavior therapy is frequently used. Medication that helps relieve the depression has been successful in some cases. Despite being described in the medical literature for nearly two hundred years, kleptomania still remains poorly understood with limited data regarding its underlying pathophysiology, and appropriate treatment choices.

Medications capable of dampening urges (such as naltrexone and others) may be worth exploring in clinical trials. Medication that helps relieve depression has been successful in some cases. Naltrexone is also promising in the treatment of kleptomania. More investigation is needed (Chamberlain & Grant, 2019).

Pyromania

Irresistible impulses to start fires characterize pyromania, repeated fire setting with tension or arousal before setting fires; fascination or attraction to the fires; and gratification when setting, witnessing, or participating in the aftermath of fire. These individuals often are regular "fire watchers" or even firefighters. They are not motivated by aggression, anger, suicidal ideation, or political ideology. Little is known about this disorder because only a small number of deliberate fire starters are apprehended, and of those individuals, only a few undergo a psychiatric evaluation. The prevalence of fire setting in the general population is about 1%, but most fire setting is not done by people with pyromania, which occurs infrequently, mostly in men. However, those with a history of fire setting are most likely male, young, and never married and are more likely to have other psychiatric issues such as ASPD, substance use, and impulsivity (Tanner et al., 2016). Prevalence rates are lower among African Americans and Hispanics (Vaughn et al., 2010).

Early research demonstrated low serotonin and norepinephrine levels associated with arson. Little is known about treatment, and as with the other impulse-control disorders, no approach is uniformly effective. Historically, fire starters generally possess poor interpersonal skills, exhibit low self-esteem, battle depression, and have difficulty managing anger. Education, parenting training, behavior contracting with token reinforcement, problem-solving skills training, and relaxation exercises may all be used in the management of the patient's responses (Tanner et al., 2016).

Continuum of Care for Disruptive, Impulse-Control Disorders

Impulse-control disorders require long-term treatment, usually in an outpatient setting. Group therapy is often a facet of treatment because patients can talk in a community where people share common experiences. Hospitalization is rare except when patients have comorbid psychiatric or medical disorders.

SUMMARY OF KEY POINTS

- A personality is a complex pattern of characteristics, largely outside of the person's awareness, that comprise the individual's distinctive pattern of perceiving, feeling, thinking, coping, and behaving.

- A personality disorder is an enduring pattern of inner experience and behavior that deviates markedly from the expectations of the individual's culture, is pervasive and inflexible, has an onset in adolescence or early adulthood, is stable over time, and leads to distress or impairment.

- For many patients with personality disorders, maintaining a therapeutic nurse–patient relationship can be one of the most helpful interventions. Through this therapeutic relationship, the patient experiences a model of healthy interaction, establishing trust, consistency, caring, boundaries, and limitations that help to build the patient's self-esteem and respect for self and others. In some personality disorders, nurses will find it more difficult to engage the patient in a true therapeutic relationship because of the patient's avoidance of interpersonal and emotional attachment (i.e., ASPD or paranoid personality disorder).

- Patients with personality disorders are rarely treated in an inpatient facility except during periods of destructive behavior or self-injury. Treatment is delivered in the community and over time. Continuity of care is important in helping the individual change lifelong personality patterns.

- People with BPD have difficulties regulating emotion and have extreme fears of abandonment, leading to dysfunctional relationships; they often engage in self-injury.

- Medications, including mood stabilizers, antidepressants, and antipsychotics, are useful in regulating the symptoms. They should, however, only be taken for target symptoms for a short time because patients may already be taking other medications, particularly for a comorbid disorder.

- During hospitalizations, keeping the patients safe by preventing self-harm is priority. Open communication and use of DBT techniques are important interventions.

- Recovery-oriented approaches are grounded in cognitive behavioral therapy. The interdisciplinary treatment or recovery team needs to maintain open communication to work effectively with a person with BPD.

- ASPD, often synonymous with psychopathy, includes people who have no regard for and refuse to conform to social rules.

- The primary characteristic of disruptive, impulse-control disorders is impulsivity, which leads to inappropriate social behaviors that are considered harmful to oneself or others and that give the patient excitement or gratification at the time the act is committed.

CRITICAL THINKING CHALLENGES

1. Define the concepts *personality* and *personality disorder*. When does a normal personality become a personality disorder?

2. Karen, a 36-year-old woman receiving inpatient care, was admitted for depression; she also has a diagnosis of BPD. After a telephone argument with her husband, she approaches the nurse's station with her wrist dripping with blood from cutting. What nursing approach best fits this behavior? What interventions should the nurse use with the patient after the self-injury is treated?

3. A 22-year-old man with BPD is being discharged from the mental health unit after a severe suicide attempt. As his primary psychiatric nurse, you have been able to establish a therapeutic relationship with him but are now terminating the relationship. He asks you to meet with him "for just a few sessions" after his discharge because his therapist will be on vacation. What are the issues underlying this request? What should you do? Explain and justify.

4. Compare the biologic theory with the psychoanalytic and Linehan's biosocial theory. What are the primary differences between these theories?

5. Compare the characteristics, epidemiology, and etiologic theories of antisocial and BPDs.

6. Discuss the differences between histrionic and OCPD.

7. Compare and contrast ASPD with narcissistic personality trait.

8. Define and summarize personality disorders. Compare the following among the Cluster A, B, and C disorders:

   a. Defining characteristics

   b. Epidemiology

   c. Biologic, psychological, and social theories

   d. Key nursing assessment data

   e. Priority of care and outcomes

   f. Specific issues related to a therapeutic relationship

   g. Interventions

9. Define and summarize the impulse-control disorders. Compare the following among kleptomania, pyromania, and conduct disorders:

   a. Defining characteristics

   b. Epidemiology

   c. Biologic, psychological, and social theories

   d. Key nursing assessment data

   e. Nursing priorities and outcomes

   f. Interventions

Movie Viewing Guides

Fatal Attraction: (1987) This award-winning film portrays the relationship between a married attorney, Dan Gallagher (played by Michael Douglas), and Alex Forest, a single woman (played by Glenn Close). Their one-night affair turns into a nightmare for the attorney and his family as Alex becomes increasingly possessive and aggressive, demonstrating behaviors characteristic of borderline personality disorder, including anger, impulsivity, emotional lability, fear of rejection and abandonment, vacillation between adoration and disgust, and self-mutilation.

Viewing Points: Identify the behaviors of Alex that are characteristics of borderline personality disorder. Identify the feelings that are generated by the movie. With which characters do you identify? For which characters do you feel sympathy? If Alex had lived and been admitted to your hospital, what would be your first priority?

Grey Gardens: (1975) This documentary by Albert and David Maysles is the unbelievable true story of Mrs. Edith Bouvier Beale and her daughter Edie, who are the aunt and first cousin of Jacqueline Kennedy Onassis. The film depicts mother and daughter, known as "Big Edie" and "Little Edie," who have descended into a strange life of dependence and eccentricity.

Living in a world of their own in a decaying 28-room East Hampton mansion, their living conditions—infested by fleas, inhabited by numerous cats and raccoons, deprived of running water, and filled with garbage—give viewers a glimpse into schizotypal personality disorder.

Viewing Points: Identify the behaviors of Big Edie and Little Edie that are characteristic of schizotypal personality disorder. Do "Big Edie" and "Little Edie" exhibit a folie à deux (a shared psychotic disorder)? Why or why not?

Related Psychiatric-Mental Health Nursing videos on the topics of Antisocial Personality Disorder and Borderline Personality Disorder are available at http://thepoint.lww.com/Boyd7e.

Related Psychiatric-Mental Health Nursing Practice and Learn Activities related to the videos on the topics of Antisocial Personality Disorder and Borderline Personality Disorder are available at http://thepoint.lww.com/Boyd7e.

REFERENCES

Aboujaoude, E., & Koran, L. M. (2010). *Impulse control disorders*. Cambridge University Press.

Amad, A., Ramoz, N., Thomas, P., Jardri, R., &Gorwood, P. (2014). Genetics of borderline personality disorder: Systematic review and proposal of an integrative model. *Neuroscience and Biobehavioral Reviews,40*, 6–19. https://doi.org/10.1016/j.neubiorev.2014.01.003

American Psychiatric Association. (2013). *Diagnostic and statistical manual of mental disorders* (5th ed.). Author.

Betts, J., Pearce, J., McKechnie, B., McCutcheon, L., Cotton, S. M., Jovey, M., Rayner, V., Seigerman, M., Hulbert, C., McNab, D. & Chanen, A. M. (2018). A psychoeducational group intervention for family and friends of youth with borderline personality disorder features: Protocol for a randomised controlled trial. *Borderline Personality Disorder and Emotion Dysregulation, 5*, 13. https://doi.org/10.1186/s40479-018-0090-z

Blum, A. W., Odlaug, B. L., Redden, S. A., & Grant, J. E. (2018). Stealing behavior and impulsivity in individuals with kleptomania who have been arrested for shoplifting. *Comprehensive Psychiatry,80*, 186–191. https://doi.org/10.1016/j.comppsych.2017.10.002

Bozzatello, P., Morese, R., Valentini, M. C., Rocca, P., Bosco, F., &Bellino, S. (2019). Autobiographical memories, identity disturbance and brain functioning in patients with borderline personality disorder: An fMRI study. *Heliyon, 5*(3), e01323. https://doi.org/10.1016/j.heliyon.2019.e01323

Brazil, I.A., van Dongen, J., Maes, J., Mars, R. B., & Baskin-Sommers, A. R. (2018). Classification and treatment of antisocial individuals: From behavior to biocognition. *Neuroscience & Biobehavioral Reviews, 91*, 259–277. https://doi.org/10.1016/j.neubiorev.2016.10.010

Carter, S. A., & Wu, K. D. (2010). Relations among symptoms of social phobia subtypes, avoidant personality disorder, panic, and depression. *Behavior Therapy, 41*(1), 2–13.

Chamberlain, S. R., & Grant, J. E. (2019). Efficacy of pharmacological interventions in targeting decision-making impairments across substance and behavioral addiction. *Neuropsychology Review*, https://doi-org.libproxy.siue.edu/10.1007/s11065-019-09400-z.

Chan, C. C., Szeszko, P. R., Wong, E., Tang, C. Y., Kelliher, C., Penner, J. D., Perez-Rodriguez, M. M., Rosell, D. R., McClure, M., Roussos, P., New, A. S., Siever, L. J., & Hazlett, E. A. (2018). Frontal and temporal cortical volume, white matter tract integrity, and hemispheric asymmetry in schizotypal personality disorder. *Schizophrenia Research, 197*, 226–232. https://doi.org/10.1016/j.schres.2018.01.025

Chapman, J., Jamil, R. T., & Fleisher, C. Borderline personality disorder. [Updated November 20, 2020]. In: *StatPearls* [Internet]. Treasure Island (FL): StatPearls Publishing; January 2020. Available from: https://www.ncbi.nlm.nih.gov/books/NBK430883/

Choudhary, S., & Gupta, R. (2020). Culture and borderline personality disorder in India. *Frontiers in Psychology, 11*, 714. https://doi.org/10.3389/fpsyg.2020.00714

Christian, E., Sellbom, M., & Wilkinson, R. B. (2017). Clarifying the associations between individual differences in general attachment styles and psychopathy. *Personality Disorders, 8*(4), 329–339. https://doi.org/10.1037/per0000206.

Cox, B. J., Pagura, J., Stein, M. B., & Sareen, J. (2009). The relationship between generalized social phobia and avoidant personality disorder in a national mental health survey. *Depression and Anxiety, 26*(4), 354–362.

De Cou, C. R., Comtois, K. A., & Landes, S. J. (2019). Dialectical behavior therapy is effective for the treatment of suicidal behavior: A meta-analysis. *Behavior Therapy,50*(1), 60–72. https://doi.org/10.1016/j.beth.2018.03.009

Deming, P., Dargis, M., Haas, B. W., Brook, M., Decety, J., Harenski, C., Kiehl, K. A., Koenigs, M., &Kosson, D. S. (2020). Psychopathy is associated with fear-specific reductions in neural activity during affective perspective-taking. *NeuroImage,223*, 117342. https://doi.org/10.1016/j.neuroimage.2020.117342

Disney, K. L. (2013). Dependent personality disorder: A critical review. *Clinical Psychology Review, 33*, 1184–1196.

Dotterer, H. L., Hyde, L. W., Swartz, J. R., Hariri, A. R., & Williamson, D. E. (2017). Amygdala reactivity predicts adolescent antisocial behavior but not callous-unemotional traits. *DevelopmentalCognitive Neuroscience, 24*, 84–92. https://doi.org/10.1016/j.dcn.2017.02.008

Ekselius, L. (2018). Personality disorder: A disease in disguise. *Upsala Journal of Medical Sciences, 123*(4), 194–204.

Ellison, W. D., Rosenstein, L. K., Morgan, T. A., & Zimmerman, M. (2018). Community and clinical epidemiology of borderline personality disorder. *Psychiatric Clinics of North America, 41*, 561–573.

Esmaeilian, N., Dehghani, M., Koster, E. H. W., & Hoorelbeke, K. (2019). Early maladaptive schemas and borderline personality disorder features in a nonclinical sample: A network analysis. *Clinical Psychology Psychotherapy*. https://doi.org/10.1002/cpp.2360

Fanning, J. R., Coleman, M., Lee, R., & Coccaro, E. F. (2019). Subtypes of aggression in intermittent explosive disorder. *Journal of Psychiatric Research*, February; 109, 164–172.

Fariba, K., & Gupta, V. (2020). Schizoid personality disorder. *In StatPearls*. StatPearls Publishing.

Fariba, K., & Sapra, A. (2020). Avoidant personality disorder. *In StatPearls*. StatPearls Publishing.

Fonseca-Pedrero, E., Chan, R., Debbané, M., Cicero, D., Zhang, L. C., Brenner, C., Barkus, E., Linscott, R. J., Kwapil, T., Barrantes-Vidal, N., Cohen, A., Raine, A., Compton, M. T., Tone, E. B., Suhr, J., Muñiz, J., de Albéniz, A. P., Fumero, A., Giakoumaki, S., Tsaousis, I., ... Ortuño-Sierra, J. (2018). Comparisons of schizotypal traits across 12 countries: Results from the International Consortium for Schizotypy Research, Schizophrenia Research, 199, 128–134. https://doi.org/10.1016/j.schres.2018.03.021

French, J. H., & Shrestha, S. (2020). Histrionic personality disorder. *In StatPearls*. StatPearls Publishing.

Frías, Á., Solves, L., Navarro, S., Palma, C., Farriols, N., Aliaga, F., Hernández, M., Antón, M., &Riera, A. (2020). Technology-based psychosocial interventions for people with borderline personality disorder: A scoping review of the literature. *Psychopathology, 53*(5–6), 254–263. https://doi.org/10.1159/000511349

Grambal, A., Prasko, J., Kamaradova, D., Latalova, K., Holubova, M., Sedlackova, Z., & Hruby, R. (2016). Quality of life in borderline patients comorbid with anxiety spectrum disorders - a cross-sectional study. *Patient Preference and Adherence, 10*, 1421–1433. https://doi.org/10.2147/PPA.S108777

Grant, B. F., Hasin, D. S., Stinson, F. D., Dawson, D. A., Chou, S. P., & Ruan, W. J. (2004). Prevalence, correlates, and disability of personality disorders in the United States: Results from the National epidemiologic survey on alcohol and related conditions. *Journal of Clinical Psychiatry, 65*(7), 948–995.

Grant, J. E., & Chamberlain, S. R. (2018). Symptom severity and its clinical correlates in kleptomania. *Annals of Clinical Psychiatry, 30*(2), 97–101.

Grant, J. E., & Kim, S. W. (2005). Quality of life in kleptomania and pathological gambling. *Comprehensive Psychiatry, 46*(1), 34–37.

Green, K., & Browne, K. (2019). Personality disorder traits, trauma, and risk in perpetrators of domestic violence. *International Journal of Offender Therapy & Comparative Criminology, 8*, 306624X19826516. https://doi.org/10.1177/0306624X19826516

Hamlat, E. J., Young, J. F., & Hankin, B. L. (2019). Developmental course of personality disorder traits in childhood and adolescence. *Journal of Personality Disorders, 14*, 1–19. https://doi.org/10.1521/pedi_2019_33_433

Hancock-Johnson, E., Griffiths, C., & Picchioni, M. (2017). A focused systematic review of pharmacological treatment for borderline personality disorder. *CNS Drugs, 31*(5), 345–356. https://doi.org/10.1007/s40263-017-0425-0

Johanson, M., Vaurio, O., Tiihonen, J., & Lähteenvuo, M. (2020). A systematic literature review of neuroimaging of psychopathic traits. *Frontiers in Psychiatry,10*, 1027. https://doi.org/10.3389/fpsyt.2019.01027

Kay, M. L., Poggenpoel, M., Myburgh, C. P., & Downing, C. (2018). Experiences of family members who have a relative diagnosed with borderline personality disorder. *Curationis, 41*(1), e1–e9. https://doi.org/10.4102/curationis.v41i1

Klein, J. P., Roniger, A., Schweiger, U., Spath, C., & Brodbeck, J. (2015). The association of childhood trauma and personality disorder with chronic depression: A cross-sectional study in depressed outpatients. *Journal of Clinical Psychiatry, 76*, e794–e801. https://doi.org/10.4088/JCP.14m09158

Kolla, N. J., Dunlop, K., Meyer, J. H., & Downar, J. (2018). Corticostriatal connectivity in antisocial personality disorder by MAO-A genotype and its relationship to aggressive behavior. *The International Journal of Neuropsychopharmacology*. https://doi.org/10.1093/ijnp/pyy035

Krause-Utz, A., &Elzinga, B. (2018). Current understanding of the neural mechanisms of dissociation in borderline personality disorder. *Current Behavioral Neuroscience Reports, 5*(1), 113–123. https://doi.org/10.1007/s40473-018-0146-9

Lampe, L., & Malhi, G. S. (2018). Avoidant personality disorder:Current insight. *Psychology Research and Behavior Management, 8*, 11, 55–66.10.2147/PRBM.S121073 https://doi.org/10.2147/PRBM.S121073.eCollection 2018.

Lee, R. (2017). Mistrustful and misunderstood: A review of paranoid personality disorder. *Current Behavioral Neuroscience Reports, 4*(2), 151–165.

Lennox, C., & Dolan, M. (2014). Temperament and character and psychopathy in male conduct disordered offenders. *Psychiatry Research, 215*(3), 706–710.

Levy, K. N., McMain, S., Bateman, A., & Clouthier, T. (2018). Treatment of borderline personality disorder. *Psychiatric Clinics of North America, 41*, 711–728.

Linehan, M. (1993). Cognitive-behavioral treatment of borderline personality disorder. Guilford Press.

Mainali, P., Rai, T., &Rutkofsky, I. H. (2020). From child abuse to developing borderline personality disorder into adulthood: Exploring the neuromorphological and epigenetic pathway. *Cureus, 12*(7), e9474. https://doi.org/10.7759/cureus.9474

McCloskey, M. S., & Ammerman, B. A. (2018). Suicidal behavior and aggression-related disorders. *Current Opinion in Psychology, 22*, 54–58. https://doi.org/10.1016/j.copsyc.2017.08.010

Meehan, K. B., Clarkin, J. F., & Lenzenweger, M. F. (2018). Conceptual models of borderline personality disorder, Part 1. *Psychiatric Clinics of North America, 41*, 535–548.

Meuldijk, D., McCarthy, A, Bourke, M. E., & Grenyer, B. F. (2017). The value of psychological treatment for borderline personality disorder: Systematic review and cost offset analysis of economic evaluations. *PLoS One, 12*(3), e0171592. https://doi.org/10.1371/journal.pone.0171592

Mitra, P., &Fluyau, D. (2020). Narcissistic personality disorder. **In StatPearls**. StatPearls Publishing.

Munoz Centifanti, L. C., Thomason, N. D., & Kwok, A. H. (2016). Identifying the manipulative mating methods associated with psychopathic traits and BPD features. *Journal of Personality Disorders, 30*(6), 721–741.

Novais, F., Araujo, A., &Godinho, P. (2015). Historical roots of histrionic personality disorder. *Frontiers in Psychology, 6*, 1463. https://doi.org/10.3389/fpsyg.2015.01463

Palihawadana, V., Broadbear., J. H., & Rao, S. (2019). Reviewing the clinical significance of 'fear of abandonment' in borderline personality disorder. *Australasian Psychiatry, 27*(1), 60–63. https://doi.org/10.1177/1039856218810154

Paris, J. (1997). Antisocial and borderline personality disorder: Two separate diagnoses or two aspects of the same psychopathology? *Comprehensive Psychiatry, 38*(4), 237–242.

Perez-Rodriquez, M. M., Bulbena-Cabré, A., Bassir Nia, A., Zipursky, G., Goodman, M., & New, A. S. (2018). The neurobiology of borderline personality disorder. *Psychiatric Clinics of North America, 41*, 633–650.

Pinto, A., Steinglass, J. E., Greene, A. L., Weber, E. U., & Simpson, H. B. (2013). Capacity to delay reward differentiates obsessive-compulsive disorder and obsessive compulsive personality disorder. *Biological Psychiatry, 75*(8), 653–659.

Quidé, Y., Cohen-Woods, S., O'Reilly, N., Carr, V. J., Elzinga, B. M., & Green, M. J. (2018). Schizotypal personality traits and social cognition are associated with childhood trauma exposure. *The British Journal of Clinical Psychology, 57*(4), 397–419. https://doi.org/10.1111/bjc.12187

Racioppi, A., Sheinbaum, T., Gross, G. M., Ballespí, S., Kwapil, T. R., &Barrantes-Vidal, N.(2018). Prediction of prodromal symptoms and schizophrenia-spectrum personality disorder traits by positive and negative schizotypy: A 3-year prospective study. *PLoS One, 13*(11), e0207150. https://doi.org/10.1371/journal.pone.0207150

Roepke, S., & Vater, A. (2014). Narcissistic personality disorder: An integrative review of recent empirical data and current definitions. *Current Psychiatry Reports, 16*(5), 445–453.

Rosenström, T., Torvik, F. A., Ystrom, E., Aggen, S. H., Gillespie, N. A., Krueger, R. F., Czajkowski, N. O., Kendler, K. S., & Reichborn-Kjennerud, T. (2020). Specific antisocial and borderline personality disorder criteria and general substance use: A twin study. *Personality Disorders, 10.1037/per0000404*. Advance online publication. https://doi.org/10.1037/per0000404

Santangelo, P. S., Reinhard, I., Koudela-Hamila, S., Bohus, M., Holtmann, J., Eid, M., & Ebner-Priemer, U. W. (2017). The temporal interplay of self-esteem instability and affective instability in borderline personality disorder patients' everyday lives. *Journal of Abnormal Psychology, 26*(8), 1057–1065. https://doi.org/10.1037/abn0000288

Schermer, J. A., Colodro-Conde, L., Grasby, K. L., Hickie, I. B., Burns, J., Ligthart, L., Willemsen, G., Trull, T. J., Martin, N. G., &Boomsma, D. I. (2020). Genetic and environmental causes of individual differences in borderline personality disorder features and loneliness are partially shared. *Twin Research and Human Genetics : The Official Journal of the International Society for Twin Studies, 23*(4), 214–220. https://doi.org/10.1017/thg.2020.62

Shah, R., & Zanarini, M. C. (2018). Comorbidity of borderline personality disorder. *Psychiatric Clinics of North America, 41*, 583–593.

Stern, A. (1938). Psychoanalytic investigation of and therapy in the border line group of neuroses. *The Psychoanalytic Quarterly, 7*, 467–489. https://doi.org/0.1080/21674086.1938.11925367

Stern, B. L., Caligor, E., Horz-Sagstetter, S., & Clarkin, J. F. (2018). An object-Relations based model for the assessment of borderline psychopathology, *Psychiatric Clinics of North America, 41*, 595–611.

Stinson, F. S., Dawson, D. A., Goldstein, R. B., Chou, S. P., Huang, B., & Smith, S. M. (2008). Prevalence, correlates, disability, and comorbidity of DSM-IV narcissistic personality disorder: Results from the Wave 2 National Epidemiologic Survey on Alcohol and Related Conditions. *Journal of Clinical Psychiatry, 69*(7), 1033–1045.

Svrakic, D. M., & Divac-Jovanovic, M. (2019). *The fragmented personality: An integrative, dynamic and personalized approach to personality disorder*. Oxford University Press.

Tanner, A., Hasking, P., & Martin, G. (2016). Co-occurring non-suicidal self-injury and firesetting among at-risk adolescents: Experiences of negative life events, mental health problems, substance use, and suicidality. *Archives of Suicide Research, 20*(2), 233–249. https://doi.org/10.1080/1381 1118.2015.1008162

Tansey, T. N. (2010). Impulsivity: An overview of a biopsychosocial model. *Journal of Rehabilitation, 76*(3), 3–9.

Thamby, A., & Khanna, S. (2019). The role of personality disorders in obsessive-compulsive disorder. *Indian Journal of Psychiatry, 61*(Suppl 1), S114–S118. https://doi.org/10.4103/psychiatry.IndianJPsychiatry_526_18

Tielbeek, J. J., Barnes, J. C., Popma, A., Polderman, T., Lee, J. J., Perry, J., Posthuma, D., & Boutwell, B. B. (2018). Exploring the genetic correlations of antisocial behaviour and life history traits, *BJPsych Open, 4*(6), 467–470. https://doi.org/10.1192/bjo.2018.63

Tielbeek, J. J., Tielbeek, J. J., Johansson, A., Polderman, T., Rautiainen, M. R., Jansen, P., Taylor, M., Tong, X., Lu, Q., Burt, A. S., Tiemeier, H., Viding, E., Plomin, R., Martin, N. G., Heath, A. C., Madden, P., Montgomery, G., Beaver, K. M., Waldman, I., Gelernter, J., Kranzler, H. R., … Broad Antisocial Behavior Consortium collaborators. (2017). Genome-Wide Association Studies of a Broad Spectrum of Antisocial

Behavior. *JAMA Psychiatry, 74*(12), 1242–1250. https://doi.org/10.1001/jamapsychiatry.2017

Vaughn, M. G., Fu, Q., Delisi, M., Wright, J. P., Beaver, K. M., & Perron, B. E.(2010). Prevalence and correlates of fire-setting in the United States: Results from the national epidemiological survey on alcohol and related conditions. *Comprehensive Psychiatry, 51*(3), 217–223.

Volkert, J., Gablonski, T. C., & Rabung, S. (2018). Prevalence of personality disorders in the general adult population in Western countries: systematic review and meta-analysis. *The British Journal of Psychiatry, 213*(6), 709–715. https://doi.org/10.1192/bjp.2018.202

Weinberg, I., & Ronningstam, E. (2020). Dos and don'ts in treatments of patients with narcissistic personality disorder. *Journal of Personality Disorders, 34* (Supplement), 122–142. https://doi.org/10.1521/pedi.2020.34.supp.122

Weinbrecht, A., Schulze, L., Boettcher, J., & Renneberg, B. (2016). Avoidant personality disorder: A current review. *Current Psychiatry Reports, 18*, 29. https://doi.org/10.1007/s11920-016-0665-6

Winsper, C. (2021). Borderline personality disorder: Course and outcomes across the lifespan. *Current Opinion in Psychology,37*, 94–97. Advance online publication. https://doi.org/10.1016/j.copsyc.2020.09.010

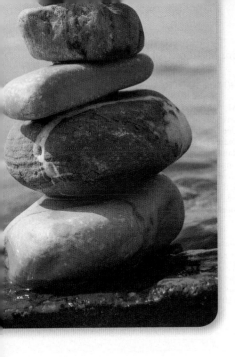

31
Addiction and Substance Use-Related Disorders
Nursing Care of Persons with Alcohol and Drug Use Disorders

Susan Dawson and Patricia E. Freed

KEYCONCEPTS

- addiction
- denial
- motivation

LEARNING OBJECTIVES

After studying this chapter, you will be able to:

1. Discuss the role of addiction in substance-related disorders.

2. Differentiate alcohol effects, overdose and alcohol withdrawal syndrome.

3. Identify prolonged use effects of alcohol, marijuana, stimulants, tobacco, hallucinogens, opioids, and inhalants. Identify medications used to prevent alcohol use relapse.

4. Differentiate the medications used to treat opioid overdose and opioid maintenance treatment.

5. Identify the similarities between a substance-related and non-substance-related disorder.

6. Develop strategies to establish a patient-centered, recovery-oriented therapeutic relationship with a person with a substance-related disorder.

7. Differentiate motivational interviewing, harm reduction, and peer support self-help groups.

8. Apply a person-centered, recovery-oriented nursing process for persons with a substance-related disorder.

KEY TERMS

- Alcohol withdrawal syndrome • Alcoholics Anonymous • Brief interventions • Codependence • Confabulation
- Confrontation • Craving • Delirium tremens • Denial • Detoxification • Gambling disorder • Hallucinogen
- Harm reduction • Inhalants • Intoxication • Korsakoff amnestic syndrome • Methadone maintenance • Motivation
- Motivational interviewing • Opioids • Recovery • Relapse • Substance-induced disorder • Substance use disorder
- Sudden sniffing death • Tolerance • Wernicke–Korsakoff syndrome • Wernicke encephalopathy • Withdrawal

Case Study

Gladys, a 68-year-old widow, lives by herself in a comfortable apartment. She spends her days with friends and visiting her grandchildren. At night, she frequently has an alcoholic drink to relax her and help her sleep. She denies that she has a drinking problem.

INTRODUCTION

The human use and abuse of alcohol and other drugs has been around since the beginning of history; so too have the subsequent social and emotional problems that accompany substance use. This chapter reviews the concept of addiction, types of substance use, biologic and psychological effects, current theories of substance-related disorders, and interventions. Gambling disorder is a non–substance-related disorder that is also discussed in this chapter. Gambling behaviors and their consequences have similar characteristics to the behaviors associated with substance disorders. The nurse's role in helping persons with these disorders recover is discussed. Professional issues related to chemical dependency within the nursing profession are also examined.

SUBSTANCE USE AND ABUSE OVERVIEW

Alcohol, tobacco, marijuana, and illegal prescription drug use has reached epidemic proportions in the United States, with the incidence rising in younger age groups, particularly among adolescents and young adults. One of the goals of *Healthy People 2020* is "to reduce substance abuse to protect the health, safety, and quality of life for all, especially children" (U.S. Department of Health and Human Services, 2020). A major challenge facing our country is the opioid epidemic. The overriding concern about using mind-altering substances is that these substances compromise health, and the continued use will lead to addiction.

> **KEYCONCEPT Addiction** is a condition of continued use of substances (or reward-seeking behaviors) despite adverse consequences.

Many mind-altering substances are physiologically addicting and easily can lead to severe health and legal problems. Use by ingestion, smoking, sniffing, or injection of some mind-altering substances such as alcohol, pain medication, tobacco, or caffeine is legal for adults. State laws on marijuana use are changing rapidly as more states legalize and decriminalize use for medicinal and/or recreational purposes. Other substances such as cocaine and heroin are illegal in the United States. Abuse occurs when a person uses alcohol or drugs for the purpose of intoxication or, in the case of prescription drugs, for purposes other than their intended use. Substance-related disorders involve substances that are commonly abused.

Physiologic dependence can develop with many different types of medications such as beta-blockers, antidepressants, opioids, antianxiety agents, and others. As long as medications are used for their intended purposes and under the supervision of qualified health care providers, physiologic dependence is an expectation of treatment. That is,

dependence can be a normal response to some medications (American Psychiatric Association [APA], 2013).

Diagnostic Criteria

Substance-related disorders are categorized into two categories: substance use disorders and substance-induced disorders. Substance-induced disorders occur when medications used for other health problems or medical/mental health disorders cause intoxication, withdrawal, or other health-related problems. A substance use disorder occurs when an individual continues using substances despite cognitive, behavioral, and physiologic symptoms. The *Diagnostic and Statistical Manual of Mental Disorders (DSM-5)* identifies 10 diagnostic categories of substances including alcohol, caffeine, cannabis (marijuana), hallucinogens, inhalants, opioids, sedative–hypnotics, stimulants, tobacco, and others (APA, 2013). Gambling disorder is included within the substance use disorder category because gambling behaviors can activate the brain's reward system similar to the substance use disorders.

A substance use disorder occurs when there is an underlying change in brain circuitry that may persist after detoxification, the process of safely and effectively withdrawing a person from an addictive substance, usually

---

BOX 31.1

Medical Complications of Alcohol Abuse

- **Cardiovascular system:** Cardiomyopathy, congestive heart failure, hypertension
- **Respiratory system:** Increased rate of pneumonia and other respiratory infections
- **Hematologic system:** Anemias, leukemia, hematomas
- **Nervous system:** Withdrawal symptoms, irritability, depression, anxiety disorders, sleep disorders, phobias, paranoid feelings, diminished brain size and functioning, organic brain disorders, blackouts, cerebellar degeneration, neuropathies, palsies, gait disturbances, visual problems
- **Digestive system and nutritional deficiencies:** Liver diseases (fatty liver, alcoholic hepatitis, cirrhosis), pancreatitis, ulcers, other inflammations of the GI tract, ulcers and GI bleeds, esophageal varices, cancers of the upper GI tract, pellagra, alcohol-amnestic disorder, dermatitis, stomatitis, cheilosis, scurvy
- **Endocrine and metabolic systems:** Increased incidence of diabetes mellitus, hyperlipidemia, hyperuricemia, and gout
- **Immune system:** Impaired immune functioning, higher incidence of infectious diseases, including tuberculosis and other bacterial infections
- **Integumentary system:** Skin lesions, increased incidence of infection, burns, and other traumatic injury
- **Musculoskeletal system:** Increased incidence of traumatic injury, myopathy
- **Genitourinary system:** Hypogonadism, increased secondary female sexual characteristics in men (hypoandrogenization and hyperestrogenization), erectile dysfunction in men, electrolyte imbalances due to excess urinary secretion of potassium and magnesium

under medical supervision. These brain changes lead to pathologic behaviors that occur with repeated relapses and intense drug cravings when exposed to drug-related cues (e.g., a party, emotional experiences) (APA, 2013).

Epidemiology

Age of Onset

In the United States, alcohol is the most abused substance, followed by marijuana. Alcohol use is at historically low levels for adolescents. In 2019, 7.9% of 8th graders, 18.4% of 10th graders, and 29.3% of 12th graders reported getting drunk in the previous month. In 2018, less than 14% of high school seniors reported binge drinking—a drop of a more than one third since the late 1990s—but illicit drug use continues to be a concern. In 2019, 1.3% of 8th graders, 4.8% of 10th graders, and 6.4% of 12th graders used marijuana daily (NIDA, 2019e). Marijuana use reflects a change in attitude and perception that marijuana is a safe drug, especially in light of recent legalization of marijuana in some states (National Institute of Drug Abuse [NIDA], 2019f).

The nonmedical use of prescription and over-the-counter (OTC) medicines continues to represent a significant part of adolescent drug use, but prescription opioids have significantly decreased over the last 5 years. Fewer teens smoke cigarettes daily (1.8% of middle school students and 2.4% high school students). Vaping, on the other hand, has increased, with 35.7% of middle schoolers and 30.95 of high schoolers reporting monthly use (NIDA, 2018f). Thousands of people with serious lung illness and dozens of deaths have been associated with vaping, and a thickening agent, vitamin E acetate, is a prime chemical of concern (NIDA, 2019i).

Diversity and Disparity

Epidemiologic data show that in the United States, sex/race/ethnic groups differ in drug preferences, use, accessibility, and risk (Substance Abuse and Mental Health Services Administration [SAMSHA], 2018a). Such identified differences should be used to direct the service needs for the population. For instance, youth identifying as sexual minorities were found to have higher substance use, experienced more violence victimization, and were at a higher risk for suicide than other teens (Johns et al., 2018). These teens need more access to crisis services, anti-bullying approaches, and more screening for suicide prevention. Furthermore, racial/ethnic minorities are disproportionately incarcerated for drug crimes and placed in facilities that have insufficient substance abuse treatment and follow-up (Sanmartin et al., 2020). Identifying differences and disparities among the diverse US population is essential to the design of programs, services, and policies that can effectively address specific population needs.

Comorbidity

Many people who abuse substances have other mental disorders. Some disorders are in part a byproduct of long-term substance use; others predispose the individual to alcohol or drug abuse. Whatever the reason, nurses should be aware that patients who abuse substances often have psychotic, anxiety, mood, or personality disorders (SAMHSA, 2018). More than 67,300 Americans died from drug-involved overdose in 2018, including illicit drugs and prescription opioids (Fig. 31.1). Individuals who abuse substances are at high risk for death from drug overdoses and are at increased risk for death from other causes, including homicide, suicide,

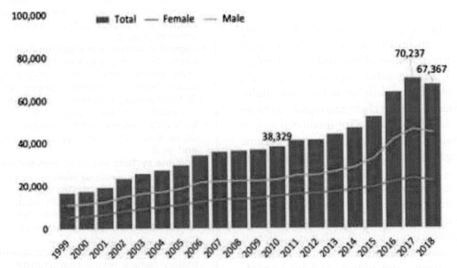

FIGURE 31.1 National drug overdose deaths number among all ages, by gender, 1999–2018. Overdose death rates. National Institute on Drug Abuse. https://www.drugabuse.gov/related-topics/trends-statistics/overdose-death-rates

Consider Gladys

She is also depressed and spends many days in bed. During the last few months, her alcohol consumption has increased significantly.

accidents, and opportunistic infections (such as human immunodeficiency virus [HIV]) secondary to drug injection. Earlier studies have documented the connection between alcohol abuse and increased risk for diabetes mellitus (DM), gastrointestinal (GI) problems, hypertension, liver disease, and stroke (Winhusen et al., 2019).

Etiology

Substance abuse encompasses the body, the mind, and society's influences. Human and animal studies confirm a genetic predisposition for drinking and drug-abusing behaviors and self-administering mind-altering drugs. As yet, no precise genetic marker has been established, though clusters of genes are being identified that may play a role in addictions (NIDA, 2019b). Temperament, stress, self-concept, age, motivation for change, social consequences for problematic behaviors, parental and family relationships, and peer pressure all contribute to expression of substance abuse—a chronic and progressive disorder.

Family Responses to Substance Use and Abuse

Abuse of substances by one or more members has devastating effects on families, their functioning, and the community. Fetal alcohol syndrome (FAS) results from drinking alcohol during pregnancy and is one of the leading causes of irreversible mental retardation. Addictions lead to loss of jobs and family relationships due to behaviors such as lying, stealing, and putting the addiction before the well-being of one's self and family. Use of illegal substances can lead to arrest and prison and heated disputes over child custody.

Many families try to help their family member learn to abstain or reduce the use of substances. Support groups provide education and help in understanding the addiction. Conversely, some persons who recover from substance abuse find that they must distance themselves from families that are actively using and abusing alcohol and drugs. Poor family relationships and dysfunction are important predictors of addictions to all psychoactive substances.

Treatment and Recovery

The goal for persons abusing substances is to recover from the abuse. Recovery involves a partnership between

health care providers and the individual and family. For many individuals, a period of intense treatment is necessary to safely manage the physical and psychological withdrawal symptoms that occur when a substance is no longer used. Specific withdrawal symptoms depend on the addictive substance and are explained in the following sections as the substances are discussed. The withdrawal process usually involves detoxification. After a person has safely withdrawn from the substance of abuse, the real work toward recovery can begin. A primary concern is relapse, the recurrence of alcohol- or drug-dependent behavior in an individual who has previously achieved and maintained abstinence for a significant time beyond the period of detoxification. Relapse is an expected part of the chronic disease of addiction, and the cycle of use-detoxication-sobriety and relapse will likely continue for years.

TYPES OF SUBSTANCES AND RELATED DISORDERS

Alcohol

Alcohol (or ethanol) found in various proportions in liquor, wine, and beer relaxes inhibitions and heightens emotions. Mood swings can range from bouts of gaiety to angry outbursts, aggression, and assaultive behavior. Cognitive impairments can vary from reduced concentration or attention span to impaired judgment and memory. Alcohol ultimately produces a sedative effect by depressing the central nervous system (CNS). Depending on the amount of alcohol ingested, the effects can range from feelings of mild sedation and relaxation to confusion and serious impairment of motor functions and speech to severe intoxication that can result in coma, respiratory failure, and death.

Table 31.1 provides a summary of the effects of abused substances.

All patients should be screened not only for alcohol use disorders but also for drinking patterns or behaviors that may place them at increased risk for experiencing adverse health effects or alcoholism. A frequently used screening tool is the CAGE Questionnaire. This tool consists of four self-report responses to questions about respondents' beliefs of cutting down on their drinking, their experience of others criticizing their drinking, the presence of guilt about drinking, and early morning drinking (Ewing, 1984). People who abuse alcohol exhibit various patterns of use. Some engage in heavy drinking on a regular or daily basis, others may abstain from drinking during the week and engage in heavy drinking on the weekends, and still others experience longer periods of sobriety interspersed with bouts of binge drinking (several days of intoxication). Another early detection

TABLE 31.1		SUMMARY OF EFFECTS OF ABUSED SUBSTANCES, OVERDOSE, WITHDRAWAL SYNDROMES, AND PROLONGED USE		
Substance	**Route**	**Effects (E) and Overdose (O)**	**Withdrawal Syndrome**	**Prolonged Use**
Alcohol	PO	E: Sedation, decreased inhibitions, relaxation, decreased coordination, slurred speech, nausea O: Respiratory depression, cardiac arrest	Tremors; seizures, elevated temperature, pulse, and blood pressure; delirium tremens	Affects all systems of the body. Can lead to other dependencies, and malnutrition
Stimulants (e.g., amphetamines, cocaine)	PO, IV, inhalation, smoking	E: Euphoria, initial CNS stimulation and then depression, wakefulness, decreased appetite, insomnia, paranoia, aggressiveness, dilated pupils, tremors O: Cardiac arrhythmias or arrest, increased or lowered blood pressure, respiratory depression, chest pain, vomiting, seizures, psychosis, confusion, seizures, dyskinesias, dystonias, coma	Depression: psychomotor retardation at first and then agitation; fatigue and then insomnia; severe dysphoria and anxiety; cravings, vivid, unpleasant dreams; increased appetite. Amphetamine withdrawal is not as pronounced as cocaine withdrawal.	Often alternates with use of depressants. Weight loss and resulting malnutrition and increased susceptibility to infectious diseases. May produce schizophrenia-like syndrome with paranoid ideation, thought disturbance, hallucinations, and stereotyped movements Deviated nasal septum, irreversible nasal damage
Cannabis (marijuana, hashish, THC)	Smoking, Ingesting Skin patches	E: Euphoria or dysphoria, relaxation and drowsiness, heightened perception of color and sound, poor physical coordination, spatial perception and time distortion, unusual body sensations (e.g., weightlessness, tingling), dry mouth, dysarthria, and cravings for particular foods O: Increased heart rate, reddened eyes, dysphoria, lability, disorientation		Can decrease motivation and cause cognitive deficits (e.g., inability to concentrate, impaired memory). Lung damage, may precipitate psychosis
Hallucinogens (LSD, MDMA)	PO	E: Euphoria or dysphoria, altered body image, distorted or sharpened visual and auditory perceptions, depersonalization, bizarre behavior, confusion, incoordination, impaired judgment and memory, signs of sympathetic and parasympathetic stimulation, palpitations (blurred vision, dilated pupils, sweating) O: Paranoia, ideas of reference, fear of losing one's mind, depersonalization, derealization, illusions, hallucinations, synesthesia, self-destructive or aggressive behaviors, tremors	"Flashbacks" or Hallucinogenic Persisting perception disorder (HPPD) may occur after termination of use.	
PCP	PO, inhalation, smoking	E: Feeling superhuman, decreased awareness of and detachment from the environment, stimulation of the respiratory and cardiovascular systems, ataxia, dysarthria, decreased pain perception O: Hallucinations, paranoia, psychosis, aggression, adrenergic crisis (cardiac failure, cerebrovascular accident, malignant hyperthermia, status epilepticus, severe muscle contractions)		"Flashbacks," HPPD, organic brain syndromes with recurrent psychotic behavior, which can last up to 6 months after not using the drug, numerous psychiatric hospitalizations and police arrests

Continued

TABLE 31.1	SUMMARY OF EFFECTS OF ABUSED SUBSTANCES, OVERDOSE, WITHDRAWAL SYNDROMES, AND PROLONGED USE (continued)			
Substance	**Route**	**Effects (E) and Overdose (O)**	**Withdrawal Syndrome**	**Prolonged Use**
Opioids (heroin, codeine)	PO, injection, smoking	E: Euphoria, sedation, reduced libido, memory and concentration difficulties, analgesia, constipation, constricted pupils O: Respiratory depression, stupor, coma	Abdominal cramps, rhinorrhea, watery eyes, dilated pupils, yawning, "goose flesh," diaphoresis, nausea, diarrhea, anorexia, insomnia, fever	Can lead to criminal behavior to get money for drugs, risk for infection related to needle use (e.g., HIV, endocarditis, hepatitis, abscesses)
Sedatives, hypnotics, anxiolytics	PO, injection	E: Euphoria, sedation, reduced libido, emotional lability, impaired judgment O: Respiratory depression, cardiac arrest	Anxiety rebound and agitation, hypertension, tachycardia, sweating, hyperpyrexia, sensory excitement, motor excitation, insomnia, possible tonic–clonic convulsions, nightmares, delirium, depersonalization, hallucinations	Often alternated with stimulants, use with alcohol enhances chance of overdose, risk for infection related to needle use
Inhalants (e.g., glue, lighter fluid), gasoline, screen-cleaners, hair spray (other aerosol sprays)	Inhalation	E: Euphoria, giddiness, excitation O: CNS depression: ataxia, nystagmus, dysarthria, coma, and convulsions	Similar to findings with alcohol but milder, with anxiety, tremors, hallucinations, and sleep disturbance as the primary symptoms	Long-term use can lead to hepatic and renal failure, blood dyscrasias, damage to the lungs; CNS damage (e.g., OBS, peripheral neuropathies, cerebral and optic atrophy, parkinsonism)
Nicotine	Smoking	E: Stimulation, enhanced performance and alertness, and appetite suppression O: Anxiety	Mood changes (e.g., craving, anxiety) and physiologic changes (e.g., poor concentration, sleep disturbances, headaches, gastric distress, and increased appetite)	Increased chance for cardiac disease and lung disease (COPD, Cancer)
Caffeine	PO	E: Stimulation, increased mental acuity, inexhaustibility O: Restlessness, nervousness, excitement, insomnia, flushing, diuresis, gastrointestinal distress, muscle twitching, rambling flow of thought and speech, tachycardia or cardiac arrhythmia, agitation	Headache, drowsiness, fatigue, craving, impaired psychomotor performance, difficulty concentrating, yawning, nausea	Physical consequences are under investigation, may have risks and benefits

CNS, central nervous system; CVA, cerebrovascular accident; HIV, human immunodeficiency virus; HPPD, hallucinogen persisting perceptual disorder; LSD, d-lysergic acid diethylamide; MDMA, 3,4-methylenedioxymethamphetamine; OBS, organic brain syndrome; PO, oral; PCP, phencyclidine; THC, D-9-tetrahydrocannabinol.

screening tool commonly used is The Alcohol Use Disorders Identification Test (AUDIT), a 10-item tool developed by the World Health Organization, which has been validated for use across genders and racial groups and is approved for adolescents aged 14 to 18 (Society for Adolescent Health and Medicine [SAHM], 2011).

The level of CNS impairment while under the influence of alcohol depends on how much has been consumed in a given period of time and how rapidly the body metabolizes it. Intoxication is determined by the level of alcohol in the blood, called blood alcohol level (BAL). The body can metabolize 1 oz of liquor, a 5-oz glass of wine, or a 12-oz can of beer per hour without intoxication. Table 31.2 lists behavioral responses at various BALs.

Effects of Long-Term Use

People who use alcohol regularly usually develop alcohol tolerance, the ability to ingest an increasing amount of alcohol before they experience a "high" or a "buzz" and

TABLE 31.2	BLOOD ALCOHOL LEVELS (BAL) AND BEHAVIOR	
Number of Drinks	BAL (mg%)	Behavior
1–2	0.05	Impaired judgment, giddiness, mood changes
5–6	0.10	Difficulty driving and coordinating movements
10–12	0.20	Motor functions severely impaired, resulting in ataxia; emotional lability
15–20	0.30	Stupor, disorientation, and confusion
20–24	0.40	Coma
25	0.50	Respiratory failure, death

Current blood and breath alcohol concentrations (BAC) in all 50 states is .08—Concentrations at or over .08 are considered legally impaired for operating machinery or driving any type of vehicle.
Some states are considering lowering the BAC to .05.

show cognitive and motor effects. The locus coeruleus, which normally inhibits the action of ethanol, is believed to be instrumental in the development of alcohol tolerance. Even though these individuals do not appear intoxicated, their BALs reflect the increased amount of alcohol, which affects their bodies, as described in Table 31.1. Excessive or long-term abuse of alcohol can adversely affect all body systems; the effects can be serious and permanent. Box 31.1 lists the major physical complications of alcohol abuse for the major organ systems.

Alcohol Withdrawal and Detoxification

Withdrawal from alcohol presents many physiologic and psychological challenges. Because of physiologic addiction, abrupt cessation of alcohol ingestion can cause mild-to-severe physical withdrawal symptoms, depending on the length and amount of alcohol use. Alcohol withdrawal syndrome is characterized by an increased heart rate and blood pressure, diaphoresis, mild anxiety, restlessness, and hand tremors. The most severe symptoms are delirium tremens (autonomic hyperarousal, disorientation, hallucinations), grand mal (tonic–clonic) seizures, and even status epilepticus (continuous seizures, lasting more than 30 minutes). These symptoms can be life threatening (Table 31.3). In patients with alcoholism and in chronic drinkers, the alcohol withdrawal syndrome usually begins within 12 hours after abrupt discontinuation or attempt to decrease consumption. If seizures occur, they usually do so within the first 48 hours of withdrawal.

Alcohol withdrawal can be accomplished safely without a person experiencing serious physical consequences. **Detoxification** is period of time where the patient is observed, usually in a hospital setting, and given medications to avoid withdrawal symptoms. Uncomplicated alcohol withdrawal is usually completed within 48 to 96 hours. Assessing for vital sign changes, nausea, vomiting, tremors, perspiration, agitation, headache, and change in mental status are important nursing interventions. The Clinical Institute Withdrawal Assessment for Alcohol Scale (CIWA-Ar) is frequently used for assessment (Box 31.2). Close monitoring continues until there is no indication of withdrawal symptoms.

TABLE 31.3	ALCOHOL WITHDRAWAL SYNDROME		
	Stage I: Mild	Stage II: Moderate	Stage III: Severe
Vital signs	Heart rate elevated, temperature elevated, normal or slightly elevated systolic blood pressure	Heart rate, 100–120 bpm; elevated systolic blood pressure and temperature	Heart rate, 120–140 bpm; elevated systolic and diastolic blood pressures; elevated temperature
Diaphoresis	Slight	Usually obvious	Marked
Central nervous system	Oriented; no confusion; no hallucinations Mild anxiety and restlessness Restless sleep Hand tremors; "shakes"; no convulsions	Intermittent confusion; transient visual and auditory hallucinations and illusions (mostly at night) Painful anxiety and motor restlessness Insomnia and nightmares Visible tremulousness, rare convulsions	Marked disorientation, confusion, disturbing visual and auditory hallucinations, misidentification of objects, delusions related to the hallucinations, delirium tremens, disturbances in consciousness Agitation, extreme restlessness, and panic states Unable to sleep Gross uncontrollable tremors, convulsions common
Gastrointestinal system	Impaired appetite, nausea	Anorexia, nausea and vomiting	Rejecting all fluid and food

BOX 31.2

Clinical Institute Withdrawal Assessment of Alcohol Scale, Revised (CIWA-Ar)

Patient: _____ Date: _____ Time: _____ (24-h clock, midnight = 00:00)

Pulse or heart rate, taken for 1 min: _____ Blood pressure: _____

NAUSEA AND VOMITING – Ask, "Do you feel sick to your stomach? Have you vomited?" Observation.
0 no nausea and no vomiting
1 mild nausea with no vomiting
2
3
4 intermittent nausea with dry heaves
5
6
7 constant nausea, frequent dry heaves and vomiting

TACTILE DISTURBANCES – Ask, "Have you any itching, pins and needles sensations, any burning, any numbness, or do you feel bugs crawling on or under your skin?" Observation.
0 none
1 very mild itching, pins and needles, burning or numbness
2 mild itching, pins and needles, burning or numbness
3 moderate itching, pins and needles, burning or numbness
4 moderately severe hallucinations
5 severe hallucinations
6 extremely severe hallucinations
7 continuous hallucinations

TREMOR – Arms extended and fingers spread apart. Observation.
0 no tremor
1 not visible but can be felt fingertip to fingertip
2
3
4 moderate, with patient's arms extended
5
6
7 severe, even with arms not extended

AUDITORY DISTURBANCES – Ask, "Are you more aware of sounds around you? Are they harsh? Do they frighten you? Are you hearing anything that is disturbing to you? Are you hearing things you know are not there?" Observation.
0 not present
1 very mild harshness or ability to frighten
2 mild harshness or ability to frighten
3 moderate harshness or ability to frighten
4 moderately severe hallucinations
5 severe hallucinations
6 extremely severe hallucinations
7 continuous hallucinations

PAROXYSMAL SWEATS – Observation.
0 no sweat visible
1 barely perceptible sweating, palms moist
2
3
4 beads of sweat obvious on forehead
5
6
7 drenching sweats

VISUAL DISTURBANCES – Ask, "Does the light appear to be too bright? Is its color different? Does it hurt your eyes? Are you seeing anything that is disturbing to you? Are you seeing things you know are not there?" Observation.
0 not present
1 very mild sensitivity
2 mild sensitivity
3 moderate sensitivity
4 moderately severe hallucinations
5 severe hallucinations
6 extremely severe hallucinations
7 continuous hallucinations

ANXIETY – Ask, "Do you feel nervous?" Observation.
0 no anxiety, at ease
1 mild anxious
2
3
4 moderately anxious, or guarded, so anxiety is inferred
5
6
7 equivalent to acute panic states as seen in severe delirium or acute schizophrenic reactions

HEADACHE, FULLNESS IN HEAD – Ask, "Does your head feel different? Does it feel like there is a band around your head?" Do not rate for dizziness or lightheadedness. Otherwise, rate severity.
0 not present
1 very mild
2 mild
3 moderate
4 moderately severe\
5 severe
6 very severe
7 extremely severe

AGITATION – Observation.
0 normal activity
1 somewhat more than normal activity
2
3
4 moderately fidgety and restless
5
6
7 paces back and forth during most of the interview, or constantly thrashes about

ORIENTATION AND CLOUDING OF SENSORIUM – Ask, "What day is this? Where are you? Who am I?"
0 oriented and can do serial additions
1 cannot do serial additions or is uncertain about date
2 disoriented for date by no more than 2 calendar days
3 disoriented for date by more than 2 calendar days
4 disoriented for place/or person

Total **CIWA-Ar** Score _____
Rater's Initials _____
Maximum Possible Score 67

The **CIWA-Ar** is not copyrighted and may be reproduced freely. This assessment for monitoring withdrawal symptoms requires approximately 5 minutes to administer. The maximum score is 67 (see instrument). Patients scoring less than 10 do not usually need additional medication for withdrawal.

Sullivan, J. T., Sykora, K., Schneiderman, J., Naranjo, C. A., & Sellers, E. M. (1989). Assessment of alcohol withdrawal: The revised Clinical Institute Withdrawal Assessment for Alcohol scale (**CIWA-Ar**). *British Journal of Addiction*, *84*, 1353–1357.

Several medications are used to prevent physiologic complications and provide a gradual withdrawal from alcohol. Antianxiety and sedating drugs, such as benzodiazepines, are titrated downwardly over several days as a substitution for alcohol. Chlordiazepoxide (Librium) and diazepam have longer half-lives and smoother tapers. Lorazepam (Ativan) is better for older adults and people with liver impairment. Antidepressants are usually initiated to treat mood states, and sleep medication is used to promote a regular sleep pattern. Anticonvulsive and antipsychotic medications are also used if needed.

Alcohol withdrawal symptoms can occur in any patient who abuses alcohol and is forced to stop drinking because of an admission to a hospital or any alcohol-free environment. Patients who abuse alcohol for long periods of time are at high risk for alcohol withdrawal syndrome. Observing for signs of seizure activity is a priority nursing intervention.

Remember Gladys?

Gladys abruptly stopped her alcohol intake when she was admitted to the hospital for depression and suicidal thoughts. She did not tell her primary care provider that her intake of alcohol was significant. She began to go through withdrawal.

Alcohol-Induced Amnestic Disorders

Although certain alcohol-related cognitive impairments are reversible with abstinence, long-term alcohol abuse can cause specific neurologic complications that lead to organic brain disorders, known as alcohol-induced amnestic disorders. Alcohol is directly toxic to the brain, causing atrophy of the frontal cortex and eventually chronic brain syndrome. Patients with alcohol-induced amnestic disorders usually have a history of many years of heavy alcohol use and are generally older than 40 years. Poor dietary intake leads to deficiencies or insufficiencies in folic acid and thiamine (and other B vitamins), which are particularly important to numerous aspects of brain functioning (Lewis, 2020).

Wernicke encephalopathy, a degenerative brain disorder caused by thiamine deficiency, is characterized by vision impairment, ataxia, hypotension, confusion, and coma. Korsakoff amnestic syndrome, associated with alcoholism, involves the heart and the vascular and nervous systems, but the primary problem is acquiring new information and retrieving memories. Symptoms include amnesia, confabulation (i.e., telling a plausible but imagined scenario to compensate for memory loss), attention deficit, disorientation, and vision impairment. Although Wernicke encephalopathy and Korsakoff amnestic syndrome can appear as two different disorders, they are generally considered to be different stages of the same disorder called Wernicke–Korsakoff syndrome, with Wernicke encephalopathy representing the acute phase and Korsakoff amnestic syndrome the chronic phase. Early symptoms can be reversed, but without long-term treatment, the prognosis is poor (Yoon et al., 2019).

Prevention of Relapse

Relapse prevention is important in the recovery of people with substance-related disorders, and alcohol addiction is no exception. Psychosocial interventions such as self-help groups, psychoeducation, and cognitive behavioral therapy (CBT) are designed specifically for those with alcohol addictions. These interventions are discussed later in this chapter.

Other medications are used for those who are recovering. Disulfiram (Antabuse) is neither a treatment nor a cure for alcoholism, but it can be used to help deter some individuals from drinking while using other treatment modalities to teach new coping skills to alter abuse behaviors. Disulfiram plus even small amounts of alcohol produces episodes of severe nausea and vomiting. These unpleasant reactions are expected to deter drinking. Severe reactions may also occur, and these include respiratory depression, cardiovascular collapse, arrhythmias, myocardial infarction, acute congestive heart failure, unconsciousness, convulsions, and death. Those taking this drug must be informed about consuming unexpected sources of alcohol (wine and malt vinegar, baked goods, nonalcoholic beer, and others) and that alcohol can be absorbed transdermally through the use of aftershaves, or lotions that contain alcohol. Informed consent is required to initiate disulfiram therapy, and there is some conjecture that disulfiram's effectiveness for alcohol aversion is attributable to the patient's awareness of having consumed it (Stokes & Abdijadid, 2020).

Acamprosate calcium is a delayed-release tablet that decreases alcohol intake and reduces the risk of returning to drink alcohol in the person who is alcohol-dependent. It is indicated for the maintenance of abstinence from alcohol in patients who are alcohol-dependent. Acamprosate is effective only if the individual is abstinent from alcohol prior to its initiation 2015). The maintenance dose (333 to 666 mg orally) must be taken with meals three times daily, which can discourage compliance with treatment.

Naltrexone was originally used as a treatment for heroin abuse, but it is now approved for the treatment of alcohol dependence (see Box 31.3). Naltrexone is formulated in a once-daily pill and a monthly injection (Vivitrol). Naltrexone does not treat withdrawal symptoms; its effects are due to blocking the mu receptors (opioid) in the brain. It has no abuse protential and does not result in the development of physical dependence. Reports from successfully treated patients suggest three kinds of effects: (1) it can reduce craving (the urge or desire to drink or use drugs despite negative consequences), (2) it can help maintain abstinence, and (3) it can interfere with the tendency to want to drink more if a recovering patient slips and has a drink. Naltrexone may be particularly useful in patients who continue to drink heavily. Some controversy still remains about the effectiveness of these harm-reduction medications in promoting abstinence or reducing alcohol consumption. Patients have been known to stop using naltrexone if they plan to drink alcohol and restart it later, leaving them open to relapsing. More research considering other harm-reduction outcomes (reduced mortality, reduced incidence of adverse events) and studies that are better controlled to avoid attrition and selection bias are needed (Farhadian et al., 2020).

Naltrexone can also be administered via an intramuscular injection (Vivitrol), which must be given after opioid detoxification and may cause injection site reactions, including intense hip pain, induration, swelling, bruising, and severe reactions such as open wounds or sterile abscesses. Patients must have adequate gluteal muscle mass to support 4cc injection, and nurses must carefully monitor and rotate injection sites. Adverse reactions and pain at the injection site can contribute to nonadherence with therapy.

Promotion of Health: Adequate Nutrition and Supplemental Vitamins

Multivitamins and adequate nutrition are essential for patients who are withdrawing from alcohol. Because malnutrition is common, other vitamin replacement may be necessary for certain individuals. Thiamine (vitamin B_1) is initiated during detoxification, given to decrease ataxia and other symptoms of deficiency. It is usually given orally, 100 mg three to four times daily, but can be given intramuscularly or by intravenous infusion with glucose. Folic acid deficiency is corrected with administration of 1.0 mg orally four times daily. Magnesium deficiency is also found in those with long-term alcohol dependence. Magnesium sulfate, which enhances the body's response to thiamine and reduces seizures, is given prophylactically for patients with histories of withdrawal seizures. The usual dose is 1.0 g intramuscularly, four times daily for 2 days.

Stimulants

Cocaine

Cocaine (also known as coke, snow, nose candy, flake, blow, big c, lady, white, or snowbirds) is made from the leaves of the *Erythroxylon coca* plant, turned into a coca paste that is refined into cocaine hydrochloride, a crystalline form (thus the white powder appearance), which is commonly

---

BOX 31.3

Drug Profile: Naltrexone (Relistor)

DRUG CLASS: Narcotic antagonist

RECEPTOR AFFINITY: Binds to opioid receptors in the CNS and competitively inhibits the action of opioid drugs, including those with mixed narcotic agonist–antagonist properties

INDICATIONS: Adjunctive treatment of alcohol or narcotic dependence as part of a comprehensive treatment program

DOSAGE AND ADMINISTRATION: Available in 50-mg tablets
Adults: For alcoholism: 50 mg/day PO; for narcotic dependence: initial dose of 25 mg PO; if no signs or symptoms seen, complete dose with 25 mg. Usual maintenance dose is 50 mg/day PO.
Injectable intramuscular dose 380 mg/month, rotate and inspect gluteal sites of injection.
Children: Safety has not been established for use in children younger than 18 yrs.

HALF-LIFE (PEAK EFFECT): 3.9–12.9 h (60 min)

SELECTED SIDE EFFECTS: Difficulty sleeping, anxiety, nervousness, headache, low energy, abdominal pain or cramps, nausea, vomiting, delayed ejaculations, decreased potency, rash, chills, increased thirst, joint and muscle pain

WARNINGS: Contraindicated in pregnancy and patients allergic to narcotic antagonists. Use cautiously in narcotic addiction because the drug may produce withdrawal symptoms. Do not administer unless patient has been opioid free for 7–10 days; verify with a negative urine screen. Also, use cautiously in patients with acute hepatitis, liver failure, depression, or suicidal tendencies and in those who are breastfeeding. Must make certain patient is opioid free before administering naltrexone. Always give naloxone challenge test before using, except in patients showing clinical signs of opioid withdrawal.

SPECIFIC PATIENT AND FAMILY EDUCATION

- Understand that this drug will help facilitate abstinence from alcohol and block the effects of narcotics.
- Wear a medical identification tag to alert emergency personnel that you are taking this drug.
- Avoid use of heroin or other opioid drugs; small doses may have no effect, but large doses can cause death, serious injury, or coma.
- Report any signs and symptoms of adverse effects.
- Notify other health care providers that you are taking this drug.
- Keep appointments for follow-up blood tests and treatment program.
- CNS, central nervous system; PO, oral.

inhaled or "snorted" in the nose, injected intravenously (with water), or smoked. The smokable form of cocaine, often called *free-base cocaine*, can be made by mixing crystalline cocaine with ether or sodium hydroxide. Crack cocaine, often simply called "crack," is a form of free-base cocaine produced by mixing the crystal with water and baking soda or sodium bicarbonate and boiling it until a rock precipitant remains. The hardened crystal is then broken into pieces ("cracked") and smoked in cigarettes or water pipes. This extremely potent form produces a rapid high with intense euphoria and a dramatic crash. It is extremely addictive because of the intense and rapid onset of euphoric effects, which leave users craving for more.

After cocaine is inhaled or injected, the user experiences a sudden burst of mental alertness and energy ("cocaine rush") and feelings of self-confidence, being in control, and sociability, which last 10 to 20 minutes. Enhanced sexual experiences and drive can get many started on regular use. This high is followed by an intense let-down effect ("cocaine crash"), in which the person feels irritable, depressed, tired, and craves more of the drug. Users experience a serious psychological addiction and pattern of abuse. Although cocaine users typically report that the drug enhances their feelings of well-being and reduces anxiety, cocaine is also known to bring on panic attacks in some individuals and may also contribute to sexual assault, as the user may not realize how rough they are being. This behavior can also contribute to sexually transmitted infections as condoms break, membranes tear, and blood or body fluids are exchanged. Long-term cocaine use leads to increased anxiety. Increased use of cocaine is associated with stress and drug craving (NIDA, 2018a), and toxic, potentially catastrophic cardiovascular problems, which may become chronic even in those whose exposure to cocaine is limited to occasional, recreational use.

Biologic Responses to Cocaine

Cocaine is absorbed rapidly through the blood–brain barrier and is also readily absorbed through skin and mucous membranes. Rapid intoxication occurs when cocaine is injected intravenously or inhaled. Cocaine increases dopaminergic and serotonergic activity by attaching to transport proteins and, in turn, by blocking neurotransmitter reuptake. Increased dopamine causes euphoria and psychotic symptoms. Cocaine increases norepinephrine levels in the blood, causing tachycardia, hypertension, dilated pupils, and rising body temperatures. Serotonin excess contributes to sleep disturbances and anorexia. With prolonged cocaine use, these neurotransmitters are eventually depleted.

Cocaine Intoxication

Intoxication causes CNS stimulation, the length of which depends on the dosage and route of administration. With steadily increasing doses, restlessness proceeds to

tremors and agitation followed by convulsions and CNS depression. In lethal overdose, death generally results from respiratory failure. Toxic psychosis is also possible; it may be accompanied by physical signs of CNS stimulation (e.g., tachycardia, hypertension, cardiac arrhythmias, sweating, hyperpyrexia, convulsions).

Cocaine and alcohol taken together could cause a potentially dangerous reaction. Taken in combination, the two drugs are converted by the body to cocaethylene, which has a longer duration of action in the brain and is more toxic than either drug individually. Notably, this mixture of cocaine and alcohol is a common two-drug combination that frequently results in drug-related death (Singh, 2019).

Cocaine Withdrawal

Severe anxiety, along with restlessness and agitation, is among the major symptoms of cocaine withdrawal. Users quickly seek more cocaine or other drugs, such as alcohol, marijuana, or sleeping pills, to rid themselves of the terrible effects of crashing. Withdrawal causes intense depression, craving (i.e., a strong desire to use cocaine despite negative consequences), and drug-seeking behavior that may last for weeks. Individuals who discontinue cocaine use often relapse.

Long-term cocaine use depletes norepinephrine, resulting in a "crash" when use of the drug is discontinued that causes the user to sleep 12 to 18 hours. On awakening, withdrawal symptoms may occur, characterized by sleep disturbances with rebound rapid eye movement (REM) sleep, anergia (i.e., lack of energy), decreased libido, depression with possible suicidality, anhedonia, poor concentration, and cocaine craving. Treating individuals with cocaine addiction is complex because it involves assessing the psychobiologic, social, and pharmacologic aspects of abuse.

> **NCLEXNOTE** In cocaine withdrawal, patients are excessively sleepy because of norepinephrine depletion. Recovery is difficult because of the intense cravings. Nursing interventions should focus on helping patients solve problems related to managing these cravings.

Amphetamines

Amphetamines, known on the street as speed, uppers, ups, black beauties, pep pills, or copilots, were first synthesized for medical use in the 1880s. Amphetamines (Biphetamine, Delcobese, dextroamphetamine) and other stimulants, such as phenmetrazine and methylphenidate (Ritalin, Focalin), act on the CNS and peripheral nervous system. They are used to treat ADHD (Attention Deficit Hyperactivity Disorder) in adults and children, narcolepsy, depression, and obesity (on a short-term basis). Some people abuse these drugs to achieve the effects of alertness, increased concentration, a sense of increased energy, euphoria, and appetite suppression. Amphetamines are indirect catecholamine agonists and cause the release of newly synthesized norepinephrine. Similar to cocaine, they block the reuptake of norepinephrine and dopamine, but they do not affect the serotonergic system as strongly. They also affect the peripheral nervous system and are powerful sympathomimetics, stimulating both α- and β-receptors. This stimulation results in tachycardia, arrhythmias, increased systolic and diastolic blood pressures, and peripheral hyperthermia. The effects of amphetamine use, and the clinical course of an overdose, are similar to those of cocaine.

Methamphetamine

Methamphetamine, also known as meth, speed, ice, chalk, crank, fire, glass, and crystal, is an illegal potent CNS stimulant that releases excess dopamine responsible for the drug's toxic effects, including damage to nerve terminals. Highly addictive, it comes in many forms and can be smoked, snorted, orally ingested, or injected. A brief, intense sensation, or rush, is reported by those who smoke or inject methamphetamine. Oral ingestion or snorting produces a long-lasting high instead of a rush, which can continue for as long as half a day. This illegal substance is cheap, easy to make, and has devastating consequences.

High doses can elevate body temperature and stimulate seizures. Methamphetamine has a longer duration of action than cocaine and leads to prolonged stimulant effects. Long-term effects include dependence and addiction psychosis (e.g., paranoia, hallucinations), mood disturbances, violent behavior, repetitive motor activity, stroke, contracting HIV and hepatitis, intense itching leading to skin sores from scratching, weight loss, and extensive tooth decay (Fig. 31.2) (NIDA, 2019g).

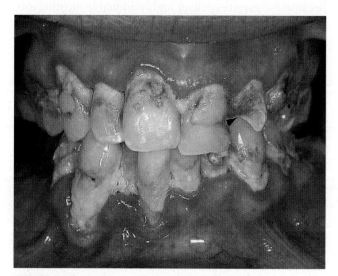

FIGURE 31.2 Severe tooth decay caused by abuse of methamphetamine.

Methamphetamine is often used in a "binge and crash" pattern. Tolerance occurs within minutes, and the pleasurable effect disappears even before the drug concentration in the blood falls significantly. After being assessed, referral of the patient to a drug treatment program is necessary. Long-term meth use can cause cardiac arrhythmias, similar to cocaine use. Babies born to meth-addicted mothers are highly irritable and frequently present with learning or other developmental delays. Parents addicted to methamphetamine often cannot meet parenting responsibilities even after abstaining. They often need continuing support to achieve the parenting role, including interdisciplinary support from child welfare and addiction treatment services (Dyba et al., 2019).

MDMA and Other "Club Drugs"

The drug 3,4-methylenedioxymethamphetamine (MDMA), also known as Ecstasy or Molly, is known as a "club drug" because it is used by teens and young adults as part of the nightclub, bar, and rave scenes. MDMA, chemically similar to both stimulants and hallucinogens, causes activity of dopamine, norepinephrine, and serotonin to increase. It produces feelings of increased energy, pleasure, emotional warmth, and distorted sensory and time perception. MDMA can cause hallucinations, confusion, depression, paranoia, sleep problems, drug craving, severe anxiety, nausea, muscle cramping, involuntary teeth clenching, blurred vision, chills, and sweating. In higher doses, MDMA can sharply increase body temperature (i.e., malignant hyperthermia), leading to muscle breakdown, kidney and cardiovascular failure, and death. MDMA effects last about 3 to 6 hours (NIDA, 2018b).

Other drugs abused, such as Rohypnol gammahydroxybutyrate (GHB) and ketamine, which are predominantly CNS depressants, are also considered to be "club drugs." Often colorless, tasteless, and odorless, the drugs can be ingested unknowingly. Known also as "date rape" drugs when mixed with alcohol, they can be incapacitating, causing a euphoric, sedative like effect and producing an "anterograde amnesia," which means that individuals may not remember events they experience while under the influence of these drugs. Ketamine is associated with an increased heart rate and blood pressure, impaired motor function, memory loss, numbness, and vomiting. At high doses, delirium, depression, respiratory depression, and cardiac arrest can occur (NIDA, 2019a). Ketamine is used as an anesthetic in veterinary practice and is now an accepted treatment for depression related to chronic pain (Humo et al., 2020).

Nicotine

Nicotine, the addictive chemical mainly responsible for the high prevalence of tobacco use, is the primary reason tobacco is named a public health menace. Smoking is more prevalent among people with alcoholism, polysubstance users, and persons with mental disorders than among the general population. Smoking is two to three times more prevalent in persons with mental illnesses than the general population and is two to six times higher among those with schizophrenia, bipolar disorder, post-traumatic stress disorder (PTSD), and alcohol/illicit drug use disorders (Smith et al., 2020).

Biologic Response to Nicotine

Nicotine stimulates the central, peripheral, and autonomic nervous systems, causing increased alertness, concentration, attention, and appetite suppression. Readily absorbed, it is carried in the bloodstream to the liver, where it is partially metabolized. It is also metabolized by the kidneys and excreted in urine (NIDA, 2020a).

Nicotine acts as an agonist of the nicotinic cholinergic receptor sites and stimulates autonomic ganglia in both the parasympathetic and sympathetic nervous systems, resulting in increased release of norepinephrine or acetylcholine. The release of epinephrine by nicotine from the adrenal medulla increases fatty acids, glycerol, and lactate levels in the blood, thereby increasing the risk for atherosclerosis and cardiac muscle pathology.

Other medical complications of nicotine use are numerous. Smoking cigarettes and cigars causes respiratory problems, lung cancer, emphysema, heart problems, and peripheral vascular disease. In fact, smoking is the largest preventable cause of premature death and disability. Cigarette smoking kills at least 480,000 people in the United States each year and makes countless others ill. The use of smokeless tobacco is also associated with serious health problems (NIDA, 2018c).

Repeated use of nicotine produces both tolerance and addiction. Recent research has shown that nicotine addiction is extremely powerful and is at least as strong as addictions to other drugs; most of those who quit relapse within 1 year (NIDA, 2020a).

Nicotine Withdrawal and Smoking Cessation

Nicotine withdrawal is marked by mood changes (e.g., craving, anxiety, irritability, depression) and physiologic changes (difficulty in concentrating, sleep disturbances, headaches, gastric distress, increased appetite). Nicotine replacements, such as nicotine transdermal patches, nicotine gum, nasal spray, and inhalers, have been used successfully to assist in withdrawal by reducing the craving for tobacco. Patches are rotated on skin sites and help maintain a steady blood level of nicotine. They are used daily, with the decrease in strength of nicotine occurring during a period of 6 to 12 weeks.

Successful smoking cessation usually requires more than one type of intervention, including social support and education. However, studies do show that even giving a brief instruction to patients about quitting smoking can be effective. Medications are often used as a smoking cessation strategy. The antidepressant bupropion is marketed as Zyban to help people quit smoking. Another medication, varenicline tartrate (Chantix), reduces the craving and rewarding effects of nicotine by preventing nicotine from accessing one of the acetylcholine receptor sites involved with nicotine dependence, but it can cause depression and related psychiatric symptoms in some people. This side effect may limit its usefulness for some people with psychiatric disorders (Singh & Saadabadi, 2020).

Auricular therapy, or ear acupressure, is being studied as a potential adjunctive treatment for nicotine addiction. Acupressure is based on the principles of an ancient Chinese system of medicine with a goal of returning the body to a harmonic balanced state. Through stimulating acupoints on the ear, endogenous endorphin levels and regulation of the sympathetic nervous system changes the taste for tobacco, suppressing nicotine addiction, decreasing nicotine withdrawal symptoms, reducing the desire to smoke, and promoting cessation for a short period of time. Emerging research into this therapy shows positive effects (Vieira et al., 2018).

Electronic cigarettes (e-cigarettes) were introduced as smoking cessation aids. They are smokeless, battery-operated devices designed to deliver nicotine with flavorings or other chemicals to the lungs without burning tobacco to do so. They resemble regular tobacco cigarettes, cigars, or pipes. More than 250 e-cigarette brands are on the market. E-cigarettes are designed to simulate the act of tobacco smoking without the toxic chemicals produced by burning tobacco leaves. Their safety and effectiveness in smoking cessation are being studied because e-cigarettes deliver highly addictive nicotine into the lungs, and the vapor of some of them contains known carcinogens and toxic chemicals. Additionally, adolescents are increasingly using e-cigarettes believing they are safe, but they may instead serve as a gateway to try other tobacco products. On May 5, 2016, the Food and Drug Administration (FDA) announced that nationwide tobacco regulations now extend to all tobacco products including e-cigarettes and their liquid solutions, cigars, hookah tobacco, and pipe tobacco (NIDA, 2016).

Caffeine

Caffeine is a stimulant found in many drinks (coffee, tea, cocoa, soft drinks), chocolate, and OTC medications, including analgesics, stimulants, appetite suppressants, and cold relief preparations. Metabolism of caffeine is very complicated, involving more than 25 metabolites, and varies among different populations. Recently,

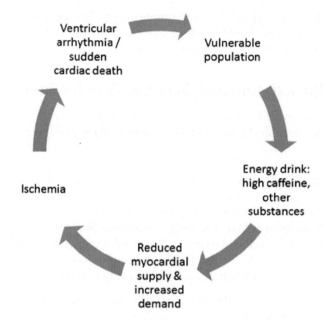

FIGURE 31.3 Possible mechanisms of sudden cardiac death associated with energy drink consumption. https://www.acc.org/latest-in-cardiology/articles/2018/02/28/10/46/stimulant-containing-energy-drinks

high-energy drinks, consisting of alcohol and caffeine, are being marketed to reduce the impairment caused by ingestion of alcohol. The reality is that these energy drinks give a false sense of physical and mental competence and decrease the awareness of impairment. Deaths have been associated with these drinks though causation is difficult to prove (Higgins, 2018)

A suggested relationship between energy drinks and death can be seen in Figure 31.3.

Symptoms of caffeine intoxication can include the following: scattered thoughts, excessive talking, inability to focus on anything, irritability, elevated blood pressure, increased heart rate, nausea, anxiety, heart palpitations (arrhythmias), insomnia, sweating, dizziness, vomiting, cardiac arrest. These may also appear in persons with no tolerance or high caffeine sensitivity (Caffeineinformer, 2020).

Caffeine withdrawal syndrome involves headache, drowsiness, and fatigue, sometimes with impaired psychomotor performance; difficulty concentrating; craving; and psychophysiologic complaints, such as yawning or nausea. Patients with caffeine dependence can be supported in their efforts at withdrawal by learning about the caffeine content of beverages and medication, using decaffeinated beverages, and managing individual withdrawal symptoms.

Cannabis

Marijuana is the common name for the plant *Cannabis sativa*, also known as hemp and many other names. Two main cannabinoids from the marijuana plant are well known: cannabidiol (CBD) and D-9-tetrahydrocannabinol (THC). Hashish, a resin found in flowers of the mature *C. sativa* plant, is its strongest form, containing 10% to 30% THC. Although there are other active ingredients in marijuana, THC gets the most attention because of its psychoactive properties.

Marijuana is fat soluble and is absorbed rapidly after being smoked or taken orally. After ingestion, THC binds with an opioid receptor in the brain—the μ-receptor. This action engages endogenous brain opioid receptors, which are associated with enhanced dopamine activity because THC blocks dopamine reuptake. THC can be stored for weeks in fat tissue and in the brain and is released extremely slowly. Long-term use leads to the accumulation of cannabinoids in the body, primarily the frontal cortex, the limbic areas, and the brain's auditory and visual perception centers. In other areas of the brain, it exerts cardiovascular effects, results in ataxia, and causes increased psychotropic effects. Marijuana use impairs the ability to form memories, recall events, and shift attention from one thing to another. It disrupts coordination of movement, balance, and reaction time. Contrary to popular belief, marijuana is addictive, is an irritant to the lungs, and can produce the same respiratory problems experienced by tobacco users (i.e., daily cough, phlegm). People who smoke marijuana miss work more often than those who do not smoke it, but it is not yet known whether marijuana smoke contributes to the risk of lung cancer (NIDA, 2019g).

Marijuana is usually smoked and causes relaxation, euphoria, at times dyscoria (i.e., abnormal pupillary reaction or shape), spatial misperception, time distortion, and food cravings. It also causes relaxation and drowsiness, unlike other hallucinogens, and is often associated with decreased motivation after long-term use. Effects begin immediately after the drug enters the brain and last from 1 to 3 hours.

The FDA has approved drugs containing marijuana, such as dronabinol (Marinol) and nabilone (Cesamet), which contain THC and are used to treat nausea caused by chemotherapy. The known safety issues related to marijuana include impairment of short-term memory, altered judgment and decision-making, anxiety, and paranoia or psychosis, especially in high doses (NIDA, 2019g). Marijuana is legal as a recreational drug in some states in the United States.

"Spice" and "K2" are terms used for synthetic cannabinoid compounds found in various herbal mixtures that produce an experience similar to that of marijuana. Spice mixtures of this type are illegal to sell in the United States because of their addictive properties. The effects of synthetic cannabinoids can be unpredictable and severe or even life threatening. Some of these compounds bind more strongly to the same receptors as THC and could produce a more powerful and unpredictable effect. Spice products are popular among young people and are second only to marijuana among illegal drugs, used mostly by high school seniors. Emergency departments are seeing an alarming increase in adolescents being treated for severe adverse events related to synthetic cannabinoid use. Fatalities can occur, and there is no antidote available (NIDA, 2018e, 2018i).

Hallucinogens and Dissociative Drugs

The term *hallucinogen* refers to drugs that produce euphoria or dysphoria, altered body image, distorted or sharpened visual and auditory perception, confusion, lack of coordination, and impaired judgment and memory. Hallucinogens cause hallucinations and profound distortions in a person's perceptions of reality. These drugs can be made from plant sources and mushrooms or are man made. They are categorized as hallucinogens and dissociative drugs. When under the influence of either type of drug, people report rapid, intense emotional swings and seeing images, hearing sounds, and feeling sensations that seem real but are not. Severe reactions may cause paranoia, fear of losing one's mind, depersonalization, illusions, delusions, and hallucinations. Hallucinogens typically affect the autonomic and regulatory nervous systems first, increasing heart rate and body temperature, and slightly elevating blood pressure. The individual may experience a dry mouth, dizziness, and subjective feelings of being hot or cold. Gradually, these physiologic changes fade, but then perceptual distortions and hallucinations may become prominent. Intense mood and sexual behavior changes may occur; the user may feel unusually close to others or distant and isolated. Classic hallucinogens include LSD (d-lysergic acid diethylamide), psilocybin (4-phosphoryloxy-*N*, *N*-dimethyltryptamine), Peyote (Mescaline), DMT (dimethyltryptamine), and Ayahuasca (an ethnogenic brew, often used for spiritual ceremonies). Dissociative drugs include PCP (phencyclidine), DXM (dextromethorphan), *Salvia divinorum*, and ketamine (see later). DXM is a cough suppressant and expectorant ingredient in some OTC cold and cough medicines and is commonly abused by adolescents and young adults (NIDA, 2017).

The true content of hallucinogenic drugs purchased on the street is always in doubt; they are often misidentified or adulterated with other drugs. There are more than 100 different hallucinogens with substantially different molecular structures (NIDA, 2019c).

Patients in acute states of intoxication or in dissociated states may become combative. During the acute state, the primary intervention goals are to reduce stimuli, maintain a safe environment for the patient and others, manage behavior, and observe the patient carefully for

medical and psychiatric complications. Instructions to the patient should be clear, short, and simple, and delivered in a firm but nonthreatening tone.

Prescription and Over-the-Counter Drugs

The overall opioid prescribing rate in the United States has been declining since 2012, after peaking and leveling off in 2010–2012, but the amount of opioids prescribed per person is still around three times higher than it was in 1999 (NIDA, 2020b). The United States is still in the midst of an epidemic of prescription opioid overdose deaths. In 2017, an average of 41 persons died each day from an overdose. The highest overdose death rates were in West Virginia, Delaware, Maryland, Pennsylvania, and Ohio (NIDA, 2020). Abuse of prescription and OTC drugs occurs when one of the following criteria is met:

- Taking a medication that has been prescribed for someone else
- Taking a drug in higher quantity or in another manner than prescribed
- Taking a drug for another purpose than prescribed (NIDA, 2018d)

The opioids (e.g., oxycodone, hydrocodone, morphine, fentanyl, codeine) prescribed for pain are some of the more commonly abused prescription medications. The most commonly abused CNS depressants are the benzodiazepines [diazepam, alprazolam, clonazepam, lorazepam]), which are prescribed for anxiety and sleep. The *DSM-5* diagnosis *Sedative, hypnotic, or anxiolytic use disorder* would be given when these drugs are abused. Amphetamines (Adderall, Dexedrine) and methylphenidate (Concerta, Ritalin) are stimulants prescribed for ADHD that are also frequently abused or diverted for illicit purposes. Nurses are well positioned to address the significant public health problem of opioid (and other drug) diversion, through patient education and medication monitoring. Often, patients combine these drugs with alcohol, which is extremely dangerous and can put patients at risk for overdose, causing coma or death.

OTC cough medicine containing DXM can produce the same effects as those of ketamine or PCP, such as impaired motor function, numbness, nausea or vomiting, and increased heart rate and blood pressure. In some cases, severe respiratory depression and hypoxia have occurred (NIDA, 2017).

Opioids and Morphine Derivatives

The term **opioid** refers to any substance that binds to an opioid receptor in the brain to produce an agonist action. Derived from poppies, opioids are powerful drugs that have been used for centuries to relieve pain. They include opium, heroin, fentanyl, morphine, and codeine. Even centuries after their discovery, opioids are still the most effective pain relievers. They also cause CNS depression, sleep, or stupor. Although heroin has no medicinal use, other opioids, such as morphine and codeine, are used to treat pain related to illnesses (e.g., cancer) and during medical and dental procedures. When used as directed by a clinician, opioids are safe and generally do not produce addiction. However, opioids also possess very strong reinforcing properties and can quickly trigger addiction when used improperly.

Two important effects produced by opioids are pleasure (or reward) and pain relief. The brain itself also produces substances known as endorphins that activate the opioid receptors. Opioids cause tolerance and physical dependence that appear to be specific for each receptor subtype. Tolerance develops, particularly to the analgesic, respiratory depression, and sedative actions of opioids. Often, a 100% increase in dose is used to achieve the same physical effects when tolerance exists. Physical dependence can develop rapidly. When the use of the drug is discontinued, after a period of continuous use, a rebound hyperexcitability withdrawal syndrome usually occurs. Table 31.4 describes the onset, duration, and symptoms of mild, moderate, and severe withdrawal symptoms.

Heroin is an illegal, highly addictive drug that is mostly abused and the most rapidly acting of the opioids. Typically sold as a white or brownish powder or as the black sticky substance known as "black tar heroin" on the streets, it is frequently "cut" with other substances, such as sugar, starch, powdered milk, quinine, and strychnine, or other poisons. It can be sniffed, snorted, and smoked but is most frequently injected, which poses risks for transmission of HIV devices and other diseases resulting from the sharing of needles or other injection equipment.

Naturally occurring neurotransmitters normally bind to the μ-opioid receptors, which are involved in pain, hormonal release, and feelings of well-being. When heroin enters the brain, it is converted to morphine and immediately binds to the μ-opioid receptors, stimulating the release of dopamine, which causes an intense pleasurable rush. Usually, the individual also experiences a warm flushing of the skin, dry mouth, and a heavy feeling in the limbs. Side effects include nausea, vomiting, and severe itching. Following these initial side effects, drowsiness, clouded mental function, slowing of the heart rate, and extreme slowing of breathing can occur (NIDA, 2019d).

One of the most detrimental long-term side effects of heroin is addiction itself, which causes neurochemical and molecular changes and profoundly alters brain structure and composition. Enlarged ventricular spaces and loss of frontal volume are reported. Heroin also produces profound degrees of tolerance and physical dependence, which are powerful motivating factors for compulsive use and abuse. After becoming addicted, heroin users gradually spend more and more time and energy obtaining and using the drug until these activities become their primary purpose in life (NIDA, 2019c). Recently, there has been a sharp increase in opioid deaths, attributed to illegally produced fentanyl. While the prescription rates have remained relatively stable, there have been unprecedented increases in the global supply, processing, and distribution of fentanyl by criminal elements beginning in 2013. An urgent, collaborative public health and law enforcement response is recommended by the Centers for Disease Control and Prevention (CDC, 2020). See Figure 31.4.

Opioid Intoxication or Overdose

Emergency treatment of individuals with opioid intoxication is initiated with an assessment of CNS functioning, specifically arousal and respiratory functioning. Naloxone, an opioid antagonist, is given as a rescue drug when extreme drowsiness, slowed breathing, or

TABLE 31.4 SEVERITY OF OPIOID WITHDRAWAL SYNDROME			
Initial Onset and Duration	Mild Withdrawal	Moderate Withdrawal	Severe Withdrawal
Onset: 8–12 h after last use of short-acting opioids. 1–3 days after the last use for longer acting opioids, such as methadone	Physical: yawning, rhinorrhea, perspiration, restlessness, lacrimation, sleep disturbance	Physical: dilated pupils, bone and muscle aches, sensation of "goose flesh," hot and cold flashes	Nausea; vomiting; stomach cramps; diarrhea; weight loss; insomnia; twitching of muscles and kicking movements of legs; increased blood pressure, pulse, and respirations
Duration: Severe symptoms peak between 48 and 72 h. Symptoms abate in 7–10 days for short-acting opioids. Methadone withdrawal symptoms can last several weeks	Emotional: increased craving, anxiety, dysphoria	Emotional: irritability, increased anxiety, and craving	Emotional: depression, increased anxiety, dysphoria, subjective sense of feeling "wretched"

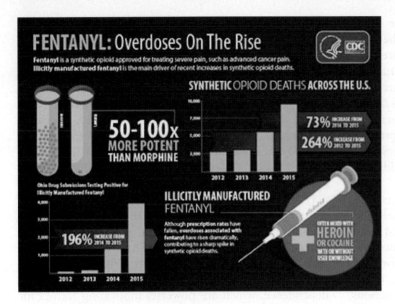

FIGURE 31.4 Fentanyl. https://www.cdc.gov/drugoverdose/data/fentanyl.html

loss of consciousness occurs. It reverses respiratory depression, sedation, and hypotension caused by the opioid agent. Administration of naloxone is life-saving. Naloxone is administered intravenously, intramuscularly, or intranasally. When administered intravenously, the pharmacologic effect is generally apparent within 2 minutes. When administered through other routes, the effect is more prolonged. Naloxone is active for 30 to 81 minutes. Depending upon the strength of the opiate, a second dose is often needed when reversing the overdose.

Initial Opioid Detoxification

Ideally, opioid detoxification is achieved by gradually reducing an opioid dose over several days or weeks. Many treatment programs include administering low doses of a substitute drug, such as buprenorphine, or methadone, which can help satisfy the drug craving without providing the same subjective high. If opioids are abruptly withdrawn ("cold turkey") from someone who is physically dependent on them, severe physical symptoms occur, including body aches, diarrhea, tachycardia, fever, runny nose, sneezing, sweating, yawning, nausea or vomiting, nervousness, restlessness or irritability, shivering or trembling, abdominal cramps, weakness, elevated blood pressure, and severe distress.

Maintenance Treatment

Methadone maintenance is the treatment of people with opioid addiction with a daily stabilized dose of methadone. Methadone is used because of its long half-life of 15 to 30 hours. It is a potent opioid and is physiologically addicting, but it satisfies the opioid craving without producing the subjective high of heroin (Box 31.4).

Detoxification is accomplished by setting the beginning methadone dose and then slowly reducing it during the next 21 days. Treatment programs determine the dose of methadone that will block subjective feelings of craving and will not cause somnolence or intoxication in patients. The initial dose of methadone is determined by the severity of withdrawal symptoms and is usually 20 to 30 mg orally. If symptoms persist after 1 to 2 hours, the dosage can be raised. Dosage should then be re-evaluated daily during the first few days of treatment. Initial doses exceeding 40 mg can cause severe discomfort as the detoxification proceeds.

Patients receive this dose daily in conjunction with regular drug abuse counseling focused on the elimination of illicit drug use; lifestyle changes, such as finding friends who do not use drugs or achieving stability in one's living situation; strengthening social supports; and structuring time into pursuits that do not involve drug use. After illicit drug use ceases for a period of time, major lifestyle changes have been made, and social supports are in place, patients may gradually detoxify from methadone with continuing support through community support groups, such as Narcotics Anonymous.

The length of methadone treatment varies for each patient. The protocol for starting detoxification from methadone varies widely, depending on the patient's commitment to abstinence, lifestyle changes that have occurred, and strong peer group support, all of which are needed to sustain the patient during methadone detoxification when increased cravings often occur. Methadone treatment combined with behavioral therapy and counseling has been used effectively and safely to treat opioid

BOX 31.4

Drug Profile: Methadone (Dolophine)

DRUG CLASS: Narcotic agonist, analgesic

RECEPTOR AFFINITY: Binds to opioid receptors in the CNS to produce analgesia, euphoria, sedation; the receptors mediating the effects of endogenous opioids, which are thought to be enkephalins or endorphins

INDICATIONS: Detoxification and temporary maintenance treatment of narcotic addiction; relief of severe pain

DOSAGE AND ADMINISTRATION: Available in 5-, 10-, and 40-mg tablets; oral concentrate
Adults: Detoxification: Initially 15–30 mg. Increase dosage to suppress withdrawal signs. 40 mg/day in single or divided dose is usually an adequate stabilizing dose; continue stabilizing dose for 2–3 days; then gradually decrease dosage. Usual maintenance dose is 20–120 mg/day in single dosing.

HALF-LIFE (PEAK EFFECT):
PO 90–120 min
IM 1–2 h
SC 1–2 h

SAFE HANDLING: Store in a safe, locked place, use a calibrated measuring device, supervised compliance may continue for at least 6 months or longer. Dispense in a child-resistant container if home consumption is planned.

SELECTED SIDE EFFECTS: Light-headedness, dizziness, sedation, nausea, vomiting, facial flushing, peripheral circulatory collapse, arrhythmia, palpitations, urethral spasm, urinary retention, respiratory depression, circulatory depression, respiratory arrest, shock, cardiac arrest

WARNINGS: Never administer in the presence of hypersensitivity to narcotics, diarrhea caused by poisoning (before toxins are eliminated), bronchial asthma, or chronic obstructive pulmonary disease. Use caution in the presence of acute abdominal conditions and cardiovascular disease. Increased effect and toxicity of methadone are observed if taken concurrently with cimetidine and/or ranitidine. Methadone hydrochloride tablets are for PO administration only and *must not* be used for injection. It is recommended that methadone hydrochloride tablets, if dispensed, be packaged in child-resistant containers and kept out of the reach of children to prevent accidental injection.

SPECIFIC PATIENT AND FAMILY EDUCATION: Avoid use of alcohol in any form.
- Take drug exactly as prescribed.
- Take the drug with food while lying quietly; this should minimize nausea.
- Eat small, frequent meals to treat nausea and loss of appetite.
- If experiencing dizziness and drowsiness, avoid driving a car or performing other tasks that require alertness.
- Administer mild laxative for constipation.
- Report severe nausea, vomiting, constipation, shortness of breath, or difficulty breathing. Methadone products, when used for treatment of narcotic addiction, shall be dispensed only by approved hospital and community pharmacies and maintenance programs approved by the FDA and designated state authority.
- CNS, central nervous system; COPD, chronic obstructive pulmonary disease; IM, intramuscular; FDA, Food and Drug Administration; PO, oral; SC, subcutaneous.

addiction for more than 40 years. Combined with behavioral therapy and counseling, methadone enables patients to stop using heroin.

Naltrexone, similar to naloxone, has been used successfully to treat opioid addiction. It binds to opioid receptors in the CNS and competitively inhibits the action of opioid drugs, including those with mixed narcotic agonist–antagonist properties, thereby blocking the intoxicating effects. It differs from naloxone in that naltrexone is longer acting and is formulated as a 50 mg tablet given once daily. Naltrexone is not used as a rescue drug for respiratory depression associated with an opioid overdose. However, if an opioid-addicted individual takes naltrexone before they are fully detoxified from opioids, withdrawal symptoms may appear (see Table 31.4).

Buprenorphine is a long-acting partial agonist that acts on the same receptors as heroin and morphine, relieving drug cravings without producing the same intense "high" or dangerous side effects. At low doses, buprenorphine produces sufficient agonist effect to enable opioid-addicted individuals to discontinue the misuse of opioids without experiencing withdrawal symptoms. Buprenorphine carries a lower risk of abuse, addiction, and side effects, compared with full opioid agonists. Buprenorphine is highly bound to plasma proteins and metabolized by the liver. The half-life of buprenorphine is 24 to 60 hours. Buprenorphine has poor oral bioavailability and moderate sublingual bioavailability. Formulations for opioid addiction treatment are given as sublingual tablets, skin patches, or buccal films. Patients need careful instructions on handling and applying the films to achieve the correct dosage of medication. Buprenorphine and naloxone are combined into one formulation with a brand name of *Bunavail*, *Suboxone*, or *Zubsolv*, and are indicated for the maintenance treatment of opioid addiction. The medication is administered sublingually as a single dose, which may be repeated up to three times per day. The purpose of adding naloxone to buprenorphine is to protect the patient from an overdose in case the patient has been misusing opiates. Otherwise, naloxone has no beneficial purpose, due to the very low dose within this medication.

Subutex, a buprenorphine-only preparation, is safe in pregnant women and provides consistent support. Fetal exposure to buprenorphine in utero is associated with significantly shorter hospitals stays, shorter length of neonatal abstinence syndrome (NAS), and decreased duration and frequency of pharmacotherapy for NAS (Bivin et al., 2019). There is no need to decrease dosage as delivery nears because there is no evidence of buprenorphine having differential neurodevelopmental outcomes among infants with NAS (Watchman et al., 2018) (see Box 31.5).

Inhalants

Inhalants are organic solvents, also known as *volatile substances* that are CNS depressants. When inhaled, they cause euphoria, sedation, emotional lability, and impaired judgment. Intoxication can result in respiratory depression, stupor, and coma. Inhalants are typically abused by young children, with adolescents using less than younger children. Different inhalants tend to be used by various age groups. New users (ages 12 to 15) are more likely to abuse glue, shoe polish, hair spray, spray paints, gasoline, and lighter fluids. The 16- to 17-year-olds most commonly abuse nitrous oxide or "whippets" and adults a class of nitrites such as amyl nitrites or "poppers." Addiction is rare, but inhalants can be intermediate between legal and illegal drugs, and their use can be fatal (NIDA, 2018g).

Most inhalants are common household or industrial products that give off mind-altering chemical fumes when sniffed. They include the following:

- *Volatile Solvents*: Liquids that vaporize at room temperature, such as paint thinners or removers, degreasers, dry-cleaning fluids, gasoline, and lighter fluid. Office supply solvents include correction fluids, felt-tip marker fluid, electronic contact cleaners, and glue.

- *Aerosols*: Sprays that contain propellant and solvents, such as spray paint, hair spray, fabric protector spray, aerosol computer cleaning products, vegetable oil spray, analgesics, asthma sprays, deodorants, and air fresheners.

- *Gases*: Household or commercial products, such as butane lighters and propane tanks, whipped cream aerosols or dispensers, and refrigerant gases, and medical anesthetics such as ether, chloroform, halothane, and nitrous oxide ("laughing gas").

BOX 31.5

Drug Profile: Buprenorphine (Suboxone, Bunavail, Zubsolv)

DRUG CLASS: Partial opioid agonist/antagonist

RECEPTOR AFFINITY: Partial agonist at the μ-opioid receptor and an antagonist at the kappa receptor. Will displace morphine, methadone, and other opioid full agonists from the receptor

INDICATIONS For pain management and during detoxification and opioid addiction, and long-term maintenance treatment of opioid addiction. May be initiated while the person is actively withdrawing from opioids.

DOSAGE AND ADMINISTRATION: Adults 4 mg to 36 mg/day in divided doses. Dosage level is related to the amount of narcotic and length of time patient has used opioids. The label indicates the dosage of buprenorphine and naloxone (4 mg/1 mg; 8 mg/2 mg, or 12 mg/3 m. Available as a sublingual film or sublingual tablet.

HALF-LIFE (PEAK EFFECT): Buprenorphine can take up to 37 (two days to excrete 50% of the dose) naloxone has a shorter elimination half-life, 2–12 hours,

WARNING: Pregnant women should receive the buprenorphine-only sublingual tablet (Subutex).

SAFE HANDLING: Pill counts may be useful to encourage treatment adherence. Because the injectable is a narcotic, arrangements should be made to have the injection delivered by the pharmacy to the office where it will be administered. Prescribing qualifications are required. Keep out of the reach of children. Store in a closed container at room temperature, away from heat, moisture, and direct light; keep from freezing. Dispose medications in Drug Enforcement Administration (DEA) approved locations.

SELECTED SIDE EFFECTS: Lightheadedness, dizziness or fainting with position changes, cough, feeling of warmth or heat, flushing, headache, painful or difficult urination, slower back or side pain.

DRUG INTERACTIONS:
Multiple drug interactions including antianxiety, antidepressant or antipsychotic medications, and many others. can also cause serious allergic reactions and life-threatening anaphylaxis requiring immediate attention.

SPECIFIC PATIENT AND FAMILY EDUCATION

- Stopping this medication may cause withdrawal symptoms.
- Do not take other medications without first checking with your doctor.
- Tell your provider/dentist that you are using this medicine prior to any procedure
- Notify your physician if you experience darkening or yellowing of the skin, diarrhea, tenderness in the upper stomach, pale stools, loss of appetite, nausea, or vomiting.
- Notify your physician should a rash, hives, hoarseness, trouble breathing or swallowing, swelling of hands, face, or mouth occur while you are using this medication.

- *Nitrites*: Organic nitrites include cyclohexyl, butyl, and amyl nitrites. When marketed for illicit uses, organic nitrates are sold in small brown bottles labeled "video head cleaner," "room odorizer," "leather cleaner," or "room deodorizer" (NIDA, 2012).

Most inhalants other than nitrites depress the CNS in a manner similar to alcohol (e.g., slurred speech, lack of coordination, euphoria, dizziness). They may cause light-headedness, hallucinations, and delusions. The nitrites enhance sexual pleasure by dilating and relaxing blood vessels. They are thought to be antagonistic at the NMDA receptor and may cause neuronal damage in the mesolimbic system (Cruz et al., 2019).

Inhalant Intoxication

Inhalants are easily absorbed through the lungs and are widely distributed in the body, reaching the highest concentrations in fat tissue and the nervous system, where the most profound effects are exhibited. Mild intoxication occurs within minutes and can last as long as 30 minutes. Often, the drugs are inhaled repeatedly to maintain an intoxicated state for hours. Initially, the person experiences a sense of euphoria, but as the dose increases, confusion, perceptual distortions, and severe CNS depression occur. Inhalant users are also at risk for sudden sniffing death, which can occur when the inhaled fumes replace oxygen in the lungs and CNS, causing the user to suffocate. Inhalants can also cause death by disrupting the normal heart rhythm, which can lead to cardiac arrest (NIDA, 2018h).

Long-Term Complications

Chronic neurologic syndromes can result from long-term use, which is linked to widespread brain damage and cognitive abnormalities that can range from mild impairment to severe dementia. In recent studies, considerably more inhalant users than cocaine users had brain abnormalities, and their damage was more extensive. Inhalant users also performed significantly worse on tests of working memory with diminished ability to focus attention, plan, and solve problems. However, inhalants can change brain chemistry and may permanently damage the brain and CNS. Magnetic resonance imaging scans of users demonstrate severe changes in cerebral white matter (NIDA, 2018h).

Steroids

Anabolic steroid is the name for synthetic substances related to the male sex hormones (androgens). Developed in the late 1930s to treat hypogonadism, they are also used to treat delayed puberty, some types of impotence, and wasting of the body caused by HIV infection or other diseases. They promote growth of skeletal muscle and the development of male sexual characteristics. More than 100 different types exist; to be used legally, all require a prescription. Some dietary supplements, such as dehydroepiandrosterone (DHEA) and androstenedione (Andro), can be purchased in commercial health stores. They are often used in the belief that large doses can convert into testosterone or a similar compound in the body that promotes muscle growth. They can be taken orally or intramuscularly. Some are applied to the skin as a cream or gel. When abused, these preparations are taken at 10 to 100 times higher doses than are used for medical disorders. Although use among men is higher than among women, use among women is growing (NIDA, 2018g).

Case reports and small studies indicate that in high doses, anabolic steroids increase irritability and aggression, "roid rage." Some steroid users report that they have committed aggressive acts, such as physical fighting, armed robbery, using force to obtain something, committing property damage, domestic violence, stealing from stores, or breaking into a house or building. Users engage in these behaviors more often when they take steroids than when they are drug free. Other behavioral effects include euphoria, increased energy, sexual arousal, mood swings, distractibility, forgetfulness, and confusion (Ganson & Cadet, 2018.)

Anabolic steroids do not trigger a rapid increase in dopamine or cause the "high" associated with other drugs of abuse. However, long-term use can affect neurotransmitter pathways that regulate mood and behavior. With time, anabolic steroid use is associated with an increased risk for heart attacks and strokes, blood clotting, cholesterol changes, hypertension, depressed mood, fatigue, restlessness, loss of appetite, insomnia, reduced libido, muscle and joint pain, and severe liver problems (including hepatic cancer). Males can have reduced sperm production, shrinking of the testes, and difficulty or pain in urinating. Other undesirable body changes include breast enlargement in men and masculinization of women's bodies. Both sexes may experience hair loss and acne. Intravenous or intramuscular use of the drug and needle sharing put users at risk for HIV, hepatitis B and C, and infective endocarditis, as well as bacterial infections at injection sites (NIDA, 2018g).

EMERGING DRUGS AND TRENDS

New drugs and drug-use trends rapidly enter our communities. The NIDA continuously reports on these drugs. Some of the newer drugs include synthetic cathinones (bath salts, Flakka), Krokodil (toxic homemade opioid), and synthetic hallucinogens (N-bomb).

Bath salts contain cathinone, an amphetamine like stimulant naturally found in the Khat plant (*Catha edulis*). Severe intoxication and dangerous health effects are associated with these drugs. These drugs, which are chemically similar to methamphetamines and MDMA, produce euphoria, increased sociability, and increased sex drive, as well as paranoia, agitation, and hallucinatory delirium. Indication is that they are strongly linked to abuse (NIDA, 2018j).

Synthetic hallucinogens (e.g., the N-bomb) are being sold as substitutes for LSD or mescaline. These chemicals, considered more powerful than LSD, act on serotonin receptors and can cause seizures, heart attack, or respiratory arrest and death (NIDA, 2018j).

NON–SUBSTANCE-RELATED ADDICTIVE DISORDERS

The *DSM-5* reflects developing understandings that certain compulsive behaviors characterized by risky use, urges, cravings, and "highs" make them similar to substance intoxication and dependence. Behavioral addictions may have similar neurocircuitry involved in reward, motivation as substance use disorders. Gambling disorder was included in the *DSM-5* and studies on other addictive behaviors (such as internet addiction, sex addiction, and food addiction) are accumulating (Petry et al., 2018). Gambling addiction is characterized by compulsive and problematic gambling behavior that leads to significant impairments in functioning or distress (APA, 2013). Some evidence shows that changes in the serotonin system are associated with addiction behavior, similar to results reported for nicotine and alcohol dependence (van Timmeren et al., 2018). Individuals with gambling problems are more likely to commit suicide than those who do not have a gambling problem and are less likely to seek mental health treatment (Karlsson & Håkansson, 2018) (Table 31.5).

Compulsive gamblers feel omnipotent in their ability to win back what was lost. This omnipotence serves as self-deception that leads to denial. Care of these patients involves confronting such omnipotent beliefs. These individuals quickly irritate staff with their self-assurance and overbearing attitude. Staff education about the disorder is important. Family involvement is also crucial. Families often have been dealing with the patient in a dysfunctional manner. Relapse prevention involves learning about specific cues that trigger the gambling behavior.

TABLE 31.5	**GAMBLING DISORDER CHARACTERISTICS AND CRITERIA**

The individual with problematic and compulsive gambling leading to significant impairment in functioning or distress exhibits four (4) or more of the following over a 12-month course.

Need to use increasing amounts of money in order to achieve desired level of excitement.

Is restless or excessively irritable when attempting to control or abstain from gambling.

Repeated unsuccessful attempts made to control, reduce, or abstain from gambling.

Regularly preoccupied with gambling.

Seeks out gambling in order to cope with feelings of distress.

Regularly attempts to 'get even' by returning to gamble after losing large quantities of money.

Exhibits erratic behavior, such as lying in order to minimize or conceal gambling involvement.

Impairments noted in terms of interpersonal relationships, functioning at work, or performance in school.

Is reliant on others financially as the result of gambling.

Reprinted with permission from the Diagnostic and Statistical Manual of Mental Disorders, Fifth Edition (Copyright ©2013). American Psychiatric Association. All Rights Reserved.

EVIDENCE-BASED NURSING CARE FOR PERSONS WITH SUBSTANCE-RELATED DISORDERS

The assessment process is, in part, a treatment intervention. Patients are often in denial about the severity of the problem and about its emotional, social, legal, vocational, or other consequences.

Mental Health Nursing Assessment

Assessment is crucial to understanding level of use, abuse, or dependence and to determining the patient's denial or acceptance of treatment. Assessment is often detailed and may involve family members and other loved ones. Along with the psychiatric nursing interview (see Chapter 11), specific areas should be assessed. Box 31.6 gives examples of typical behaviors exhibited by individuals that are associated with each level of use, abuse, and addiction. The nurse can use the Substance Abuse Assessment as a guide in eliciting a substance use history in the assessment process (Box 31.7).

Usually, nurses encounter individuals during crisis when they are seeking professional help. These situations offer an opportunity to explore the denial that keeps their addiction thriving. The nurse's approach should be

BOX 31.6

Behaviors in Substance Use, Abuse, and Addiction

SUBSTANCE USE

- Does not have possible danger or potential legal problems
- Engages in use to enhance social situations and interaction
- Is not intended to result in intoxication
- Has control of the amount and frequency of use
- Exhibits socially acceptable behavior while using

PRESCRIPTION MEDICATION USE

- Use is for the dose, frequency, and indications prescribed.
- Use is for the particular episode of the condition for which it was prescribed.
- Use is coordinated among prescribing physicians.

SUBSTANCE ABUSE

- Use for intoxication or feeling of being "high"
- Use that interferes with normal life functions (e.g., producing sleep when inappropriate, excitability, or irritability interfering with social interaction)
- Potential harm to self or others (e.g., driving while intoxicated, use of injection drug equipment)
- Use that has legal consequences (e.g., all uses of illicit drugs)

- Use resulting in socially unacceptable behavior (e.g., public drunkenness, verbal or physical abuse)
- Use to alter normal feeling states such as sadness or anxiety

PRESCRIPTION MEDICATION ABUSE

- Use is at a higher dose and greater frequency than prescribed
- Use is for indications other than prescribed or for self-diagnosed condition
- Use results in feeling tired, having a clouded mental state, or feeling "hyperactive" or nervous
- Supplementing medication with alcohol or drugs
- Soliciting more than one physician for the same medication
- Inability to control the amount and frequency of use
- Tolerance to larger amounts of the substance
- Withdrawal symptoms when stopping use
- Severe consequences from alcohol or drug use

SUBSTANCE ADDICTION

- Drug craving
- Compulsive use
- Presence of aberrant drug-related behaviors
- Repeated relapse into drug use after withdrawal

BOX 31.7

Substance Abuse Assessment

Drug/Last Use	Pattern of Use (Amount, Route, First Use, Frequency, and Length of Use)
Ask about Alcohol/	
Stimulants/	
Opioids/	
Sedative-hypnotics and anxiolytic agents/	
Hallucinogens/	
Marijuana/	
Inhalants/	
Nicotine/	
Caffeine, other OTC's or herbal products.	

ABUSE INDICATORS

1. Tolerance (increasing use of drug or alcohol with the same level of intoxication): _____
2. Withdrawal symptoms: a. Shakes? _____ b. Tremors? _____ c. Cramps, diarrhea, or rapid pulse? _____ d. Feeling paranoid, fearful? _____ e. Difficulty sleeping? _____
3. Consequences of use (e.g., presenting problems, persistent or recurrent emotional, social, legal, or other problems): _____
4. Loss of control of amount, frequency, or duration of use: _____
5. Desire or efforts to decrease use or control use: _____
6. Preoccupation (increasing focus or time spent on use and obtaining substances): _____
7. Social, vocational, recreational activities affected by use: _____
8. Previous alcohol or drug abuse treatment: _____

caring, matter-of-fact, gentle, and direct. Approaches that are punitive or attempt to elicit feelings of guilt or shame are destructive to the therapeutic relationship. Nursing Care Plan 31.1,which sets forth a plan of care for Gladys.

Denial of a Problem

Denial can be expressed in diverse behaviors and attitudes and may not be expressed as an overt denial of

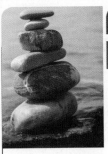

NURSING CARE PLAN 31.1

The Patient with Alcoholism

Gladys is a 68-year-old widow admitted for depression and thoughts of committing suicide by carbon monoxide poisoning. On admission, she denied abuse of alcohol or other substances. She is placed on suicide precautions.

Gladys denies that she currently has suicidal ideation and admits that she was angry with her son, who would not let her see her grandchildren. She reports that she just wanted to go to sleep and not wake up. According to her son, he was concerned about the safety of his children when his mother was intoxicated. He found several wine and liquor bottles in her apartment.

Setting: Inpatient Detoxification Unit, Veterans Administration Medical Center

Baseline Assessment: First admission, last drink 7 PM. Admission vital signs: T 99.2°F, HR 98, R 20, BP 140/88 on admission to the ED. BAL of 0.07 mg%, becoming increasingly anxious and restless. Her CIWA-Ar was 16. She was given chlordiazepoxide 50 mg PO.

Four hours after admission, vital signs were T 99.8°F, HR 110, R 22, BP 152/100. Her CIWA-Ar was 13. She continued to be anxious and was tremulous, diaphoretic, and nauseous. According to CIWA-Ar protocol she was given chlordiazepoxide 25 mg. PO.

Associated Psychiatric Diagnosis	Medications
Alcohol withdrawal	Thiamine
	Folic acid
	Multivitamins
	Chlordiazepoxide according to CIWA-Ar protocol

Priority of Care: Complications of Alcohol Withdrawal

Important Characteristics	Associated Considerations
BAL	Abrupt cessation of alcohol intake
hyperactivity	
History of heavy drinking	

Outcomes

Initial	Discharge
1. Minimize alcohol withdrawal symptoms.	2. Relate an intent to practice selected prevention measures such as maintaining sobriety, removing loose throw rugs, using adequate lighting.

Interventions

Interventions	Rationale	Ongoing Assessment
Implement CIWA-Ar to identify stage of alcohol withdrawal and severity of symptoms. Monitor gait and motor coordination, presence of tremors, mental status, electrolyte balance, and seizure activity.	The more severe the reactions, the more likely that disorientation, confusion, and restlessness increase. As the patient move from stage I to III, he become at higher risk for a fall or injury.	Determine whether Gladys is becoming more disoriented, increasing his risk for injury.
Institute seizure precautions (bed in low position, padded side rails).	Withdrawal seizures usually occur within 48 hours after last drink.	Monitor for seizure activity.

Continued

Nursing Care Plan 31.1 Continued

Interventions	Rationale	Ongoing Assessment
Orient the patient to her surroundings and location of call light; maintain a consistent physical environment.	Disorientation often occurs as BAL drops. These symptoms can last several days.	Determine Gladys's level of orientation to surroundings. Determine whether she can use a call light.
Avoid sudden moves, loud noises, discussion of patient with colleagues at bedside, and lighting that casts shadows downward.	Decreased environmental stimulation helps calm the patient, which, in turn, promotes optimal CNS responses.	Observe reactions to loud noises and monitor room environment.

Evaluation

Outcomes (at 3 Days)	Revised Outcomes	Interventions
Gait steady; patient hydrated. No seizure activity. Gladys is oriented, no increase in CIWA-Ar score.	Maintain current level of orientation.	Continue to monitor for any signs of disorientation.

BAL, blood alcohol level; BP, blood pressure; CNS, central nervous system; GAF, Global Assessment of Functioning; HR, heart rate; IM, intramuscular; PO, oral; PRN, as needed; R, respirations; T, temperature.

the problem. For example, patients may admit to a problem and even thank the nurse for helping them to realize they have a problem but insist they can overcome the problem on their own and do not need outside help.

> **KEYCONCEPT Denial** is the patient's inability to accept their loss of control over substance use or the severity of the consequences associated with the substance abuse or addiction. Remember that denial may appear as confusion, distorted comparisons with other's drinking, difficulty reconciling past positive alcohol experiences with current problems, misunderstanding about the diagnosis of substance use, misguided beliefs that one can overcome an addiction by sheer will power, and refusal to believe that alcohol has had an effect on one's thoughts, feeling, behaviors, or relationships with others.

This quandary about the nature of the problem has often been met with confrontation by nurses and other professionals in the past. But argumentation, presenting evidence of addiction, and lecturing often fail to elicit admission of a problem or induce behavior change.

Gladys and Denial

Gladys continues to deny that she has a drinking problem. She is angry with her son for suggesting that she has a problem and refuses to sign a release of information for him.

Motivation for Change

Motivation is a key predictor of whether individuals will change their substance use behavior, but addiction is a chronic, relapsing biological condition. Motivation alone may be insufficient without additional support and treatment. People can only become addicted to substances that have receptors in the brain, which can be hi-jacked by the substance. This means that in the absence of the substance, the user does not experience pleasure and nothing besides the substance can take its place (not food, sex, or family). Urges to use can be so powerful that they overcome the best of motivations, even the desire to regain custody of one's children or to avoid going to jail. Over time, addiction dominates every aspect of the individual's life. While nurses can capitalize on the individual's motivation to change, they can't really be helpful unless they understand that recovery is a life-long process, requiring dramatic changes at the individual and family level, which must indeed be dealt with, "one day at a time."

> **KEYCONCEPT Motivation** is a goal-oriented attitude that propels action for change and can help sustain the development of new activities and behaviors when additional support and treatment are available

Motivational interviewing is a method of therapeutic intervention that seeks to elicit self-motivational statements from patients, which creates a disconnect between the patient's goals and their continued alcohol and substance use disorder. The acronym FRAMES (which is short form for feedback, responsibility, advice, menu of strategies, empathy, and self-efficacy) summarizes elements of brief interventions with patients using motivational interviewing (Box 31.8).

BOX 31.8

FRAMES—Effective Elements of Brief Intervention

FEEDBACK

Provide patients with personal feedback regarding their individual status, such as personal alcohol and other drug consumption relative to norms, information about elevated liver enzyme values, and other factors.

RESPONSIBILITY

Emphasize the individual's freedom of choice and personal responsibility for change. General themes are as follows:
1. It's up to you; you're free to decide to change or not.
2. No one else can decide for you or force you to change.
3. You're the one who has to do it if it's going to happen.

ADVICE

Include a clear recommendation or advice on the need for change, typically in a supportive and concerned, rather than in a judgmental, manner.

MENU

Provide a menu of treatment options from which patients may pick those that seem more suitable or appealing.

EMPATHIC COUNSELING

Show warmth, support, respect, and understanding in communication with patients.

SELF-EFFICACY

Reinforce self-efficacy or an optimistic feeling that they can change.

NCLEXNOTE Motivational approaches are priority interventions for patients with substance-related disorders. They help patients recognize a problem and begin to develop change strategies for continuing recovery and relapse prevention.

Countertransference

Countertransference is the total emotional reaction of the treatment provider to the patient (see Chapter 10). Patients with substance-related disorders can generate strong feelings and reactions in nurses and other health care providers. These feelings can be generated by overtly unpleasant behaviors of the substance-dependent persons, such as lying, deceit, manipulation, or hostility, or these feelings may be more subconscious and stem from past experiences with people with alcoholism or addicts or even from dealing with situations in the health care provider's own family. To be able to overcome countertransference feelings, nurses must recognize that the patient's behaviors are a part of the disease process involved in addiction. This also requires that nurse reflect on how their own behaviors toward patients with addictions can contribute or detract from the care they wish to provide.

Codependence

The concept of codependence emerged out of studies of women's relationships with husbands who abused alcohol. Today, the scope of codependency includes both men and women who grew up in any type of dysfunctional family system in which substance abuse may or may not have been a problem. Codependence has also been described as "enabling," in which an individual in a relationship with a person who abuses alcohol inadvertently reinforces the drinking behavior of the other person. The codependency label remains controversial and is viewed by some as an oversimplification of complex emotions and behaviors of family members. Mental health professionals should be careful not to use it as a catch-all diagnosis and to take special care to assess and plan interventions that address each person's particular situation, problems, and needs (Mental Health America, 2021).

CLINICAL JUDGMENT

For a hospitalized patient, the first priority is to determine whether the person will be withdrawing. After the person is no longer in danger of withdrawal symptoms, the nurse can discuss the use of substance and encourage the individual to seek help for the addiction. A patient's denial of a problem with substances is common and often a priority.

THERAPEUTIC RELATIONSHIP

It is critical that the nurse establish a therapeutic relationship with patients and families (Box 31.8). Several general guidelines are available for establishing therapeutic interactions with patients in substance abuse treatment programs:

- Encourage honest expression of feelings.
- Listen to what the individual is really saying.
- Express caring for the individual.
- Hold the individual responsible for their behavior.
- Provide fair and consistent consequences for negative behavior.
- Talk about specific objectionable actions.
- Do not compromise your own values or nursing practice.
- Communicate the treatment plan to the patient and to others on the treatment team.
- Monitor your own reactions to the patient.

Confrontation, or pointing out the inconsistencies in thoughts, feelings, and actions, can promote the person's experience of the natural consequences of one's behavior. Learning from previous behavior and its consequences is

BOX 31.9 • THERAPEUTIC DIALOGUE: THE PATIENT WITH ALCOHOLISM

INEFFECTIVE APPROACH

Nurse: I would like to talk with you about your problem with alcoholism.

Gladys: Alcoholism! It's not that bad. Everyone has a few drinks now then!

Nurse: You tell me why you were drinking. Your wife left you. You drink a quart of vodka a day. Your BAL was 0.15% when you were admitted.

Gladys: So, what! I do have some problems, or I wouldn't be here. But, I'm not an alcoholic. (Denial)

Nurse: Do you know what an alcoholic is?

Gladys: Sure, I do. My father was one. He was a useless bum. I'm not anything like him.

Nurse: It sounds like you are a lot like him.

Gladys: I think I need to rest now. My back is killing me (avoidance).

EFFECTIVE APPROACH

Nurse: I would like to talk with you about what happens when you drink.

Gladys: It's not that bad. Everyone has a few drinks now and then!

Nurse: What concerns do you have about your drinking?

Gladys: I'm not really concerned. My son is. He thinks I drink too much.

Nurse: What does he tell you about that?

Gladys: Well, complains about it, but I just have a glass of wine at night.

Nurse: It sounds as if he is concerned about this, but you have your doubts about how serious it is. Your son is invited to our family education group, so he can learn about alcohol abuse.

Gladys: I have a lot of problems besides alcohol. I never use drugs. I only drink because it relaxes me and makes it easier to deal with stress.

Nurse: Many people drink to help them cope with stress. Sometimes the drinking itself can cause stress. While you are here, do you think it would be useful to look at the stress in your life and how it relates to your drinking?

Gladys: Yes. But I only drink when things get too out of hand. My health is pretty good.

Nurse: We can provide information about your health and alcohol use. To evaluate what information may be helpful, I would like to get a little more information about your drinking.

CRITICAL THINKING CHALLENGE

- What effect did the nurse have on the patient in using the word alcoholism in the first interaction?

- Discuss what communication approaches the nurse used in the second scenario to engage the patient in disclosing problems with alcohol and her relationship with her son. How does this nurse's approach vary from the one in the first interaction?

how change occurs. Confrontation can be very threatening to patients and should only occur within the context of a trusting relationship.

MENTAL HEALTH NURSING INTERVENTIONS

Several treatment modalities are used in most addiction treatment (pharmacologic modalities were discussed earlier in this chapter), including 12-step program-focused, cognitive or psychoeducation, behavioral, group psychotherapy, and individual and family therapy. Discharge planning and relapse prevention are also essential components of successful treatment and so are incorporated into most programs. See Table 31.6 for an overview of the different treatment approaches used in drug and alcohol

addiction. Principles of effective treatment for addictions can be seen in Box 31.10.

Because patients with substance-related disorders differ greatly, no single type of treatment program will work for every individual. Often, several approaches can work together, but others may be inappropriate. Treatment programs usually combine many different interventions to provide a comprehensive approach based on the individual's needs. Nursing interventions vary depending on the nature of the current problems and their severity. For a patient who is being detoxified, physical interventions (e.g., monitoring vital signs and neurologic functioning) are necessary. When the substance use disorder is secondary to other physical or psychiatric problems, education of patient and family may be a priority.

Assessment and interventions should include culturally relevant data, such as unique physiologic responses

TABLE 31.6	CHEMICAL DEPENDENCE TREATMENT APPROACHES: PAST AND PRESENT						
Approach	Conception of Etiology	Conception of Patient	Conception of Treatment Outcome	Conception of Treatment Process	Advantages of Approach	Disadvantages of Approach	
Psychiatric	Symptom of underlying emotional problem	Emotionally disturbed	Emotional conflicts are resolved; emotional health improves	Psychotherapy, medication to treat cause of substance abuse	Not punitive, treats comorbidity	Focus is only on treatment of mental disorder	
Social	Society and environment cause dependence	Victim of circumstance	Improved social functioning or improved environment	Removal of environmental influences and increasing coping responses to it	Stresses social supports and coping skills	Blames "ills of society"—the person is not responsible for having an addiction	
Moral	Person is morally weak—can't say "no"	"Hustler," morally deficient Addict	Moral recovery, increased willpower, self-control, and responsible behavior	"Street addict" behavior and manipulation confronted	Holds person responsible for actions and making amends	Punitive, increases low self-esteem and sense of failure. No longer an accepted medical approach.	
Learning	Abuse is a learned, reinforced behavior	Has distorted thinking, poor coping skills	Patient learns new ways of thinking and new coping skills	Cognitive therapy techniques and coping skills taught	Not punitive; teaches new coping skills	Places emphasis on control of use	
Disease	Probably caused by genetic or biologic factors	Has a chronically progressive disease	Abstinence, arresting disease progression, and beginning of recovery process	Is treated as a primary disease, reinforces patient is an addict and is sick	Not punitive, stresses support and education	Minimizes mental health disorders; discounts return to social use	
12-Step	Combination of disease concept and "spiritual bankruptcy"	Has an addiction and is powerless over substances	Abstinence, ongoing spiritual recovery	Use 12 steps, seeking spiritual support, making amends, serving others in need	Widespread success, emphasis is on quality of life and spiritual growth	Self-help group, not a treatment program	
Dual diagnosis	Both a primary substance dependency and a mental health disorder	Has both mental and substance abuse disorder	Improvement in both mental health and substance abuse disorders	Concurrent treatment of both disorders	Treats both mental health disorder and dependency, minimizing relapse potential	Not inclusive enough; does not include social or other issues	
Biopsychosocial	Biologic basis, with social and psychological influences	Has deficiencies in all three interacting areas	Improvement in mental and physical health, utilization of social supports	Concurrent treatment of all issues	Uses different modalities; is more inclusive	Does not match patient and specific interventions	
Multivariant	Many different causes; may be different for each individual	Has multiple issues to be assessed and addressed	Particular issues for individual addressed, so improvement occurs	Treatment strategies are matched with individual patient needs	Treatment matched to individual's needs	Logistical problems can occur during its implementation	
Neurobiological Medication-Assisted Treatment (MAT)	Primarily addiction is a brain-based disorder, involving the neuro-circuitry in the brain associated with memory, reward and motivation and hi-jacking of mu receptors in the brain	Modification of behaviors relat-ed to alcohol or substance use and addictive behaviors	Use of medications to re-es-tablish brain functions and support person through detoxification and recovery to prevent relapse to using	Medication-assisted treatment improves qual-ity of life, allows person to resume functioning and goal-oriented behavior unrelated to drug-seeking.	Controversial Access issues for many; Cost		

BOX 31.10

Principles of Effective Treatment for Addiction

1. Addiction is a complex but treatable disease that affects brain function and behavior.
2. No single treatment is appropriate for everyone.
3. Treatment needs to be readily available.
4. Effective treatment attends to multiple needs of the individual, not just their drug use.
5. Remaining in treatment for an adequate period of time is critical.
6. Behavioral therapies—including individual, family, or group counseling—are the most commonly used forms of drug abuse treatment.
7. Medications are an important element of treatment for many patients, especially when combined with counseling and other behavioral therapies.
8. An individual's treatment and service plan must be assessed continually and modified as necessary to ensure that it meets their changing needs.
9. Many drug-addicted individuals also have concurrent mental disorders.
10. Medically assisted detoxification is only the first stage of addiction treatment and by itself does little to change long-term drug abuse.
11. Treatment does not need to be voluntary to be effective.
12. Drug use during treatment must be monitored continuously because lapses during treatment do occur.
13. Treatment programs should provide assessment for HIV/AIDS, hepatitis B and C, tuberculosis, and other infectious diseases, as well as provide targeted risk-reduction counseling, linking patients to treatment as necessary.

National Institute on Drug Abuse. (2018). Principles of drug addiction treatment: A research-based guide (3rd ed., pp. 3–4). Bethesda, MD. https://www.drugabuse.gov/publications/principles-drug-addiction-treatment-research-based-guide-third-edition/principles-effective-treatment.

---

to substances, behavioral responses to dependence, and social expectations and sanctions. Staff who are knowledgeable about cultural differences and issues are integral to successful treatment.

Brief Intervention

A growing body of evidence indicates that brief interventions are more effective than no treatment, and indications suggest that they are as effective as more intensive interventions. Screening, brief intervention, and referral to treatment (SBIRT) have been shown to be effective in helping individuals with high-risk alcohol use to seek help (Biroscak et al., 2019). Within the alcohol and other drugs field, brief intervention is a highly developed, researched, and widely accepted approach.

Screening and brief intervention are two separate skills that can be used together to reduce risky substance use. Screening involves asking questions about alcohol or drug use. A **brief intervention** is a negotiated conversation between the professional and patient designed to reduce or eliminate alcohol and drug use.

Not everyone who is screened will need a brief intervention, and not everyone who needs a brief intervention will require treatment. In fact, the goals of screening and brief intervention are to reduce risky substance use before people become dependent or addicted.

Brief intervention is effective for several reasons. Research indicates that brief interventions are an appropriate response to patients presenting in a general health or community setting and who are unlikely to need, seek, or attend specialist treatment. Brief intervention—to be given clear concise information by a professional—may be all the patients may want. It is also an important part of the overall approach to harm reduction (discussed later in this chapter).

Brief intervention is most successful when working with people who

- Are experiencing few problems with their drug use
- Have low levels of dependence
- Have a short history of drug use
- Have stable backgrounds
- Are unsure or ambivalent about changing or ending their drug use

It is recommended that brief intervention at a minimum include

- Advising how to reduce patient's drug use
- Providing harm reduction information or self-help manuals relevant to the patient
- Giving the patient relevant information about the following:
  - The consequences of a drug conviction in terms of international travel and employment
  - Consequences of further or heavier drug charges

Discussing harm reduction strategies, especially those relating to the following:

- Overdose
- Violence
- Driving under the influence
- Safe practices (e.g., safe injecting, safe sex)
- Offering and arranging a follow-up visit

Cognitive and Cognitive Behavioral Interventions and Psychoeducation

Cognitive approaches to addiction hypothesize that if a patient can change the way they think about a situation, both the emotional reaction to it and the behavioral response will change. Psychoeducational materials, groups, and one-on-one interactions with nurses also impart information to reduce knowledge deficits related to alcohol and drug dependence (Box 31.11). CBT is a brief structured treatment that focuses on immediate problems. It enables patients to examine the thinking process that leads to decisions to use substances, analyze distortions in thinking, and develop rational responses to these distortions.

Enhancing Coping Skills

Improving coping skills is thought to be one component of preventing relapse into alcohol and drug use. Coping skills include the ability to use thought, emotion, and action effectively to solve interpersonal and intrapersonal problems and to achieve personal goals. Groups in addiction treatment programs that also have a relapse prevention component look at coping. The skills listed in Box 31.12 are often taught as coping strategies for dealing with alcohol and drug cravings. Patients role-play new behaviors and learn from the feedback they receive from other group members. They also increase their sense of competency to use these skills in real-life situations.

Group Interventions and Early Recovery

Isolation and alienation from friends and family are common themes in patients with substance-related disorders. In addition, thinking that has become distorted is left unchallenged without contact with others; thus, change is difficult. When a patient enters a group that is working with the goals of continuing recovery, numerous healing advantages can occur.

Groups in treatment settings focus on immediate goals of maintaining sobriety and not on childhood issues. The emphasis is on using problem solving and other skills to

---

BOX 31.12

Skills Training Group Topics

INTERPERSONAL

Starting conversations
Giving and receiving compliments
Nonverbal communication
Receiving criticism
Receiving criticism about drinking
Drink and drug refusal skills
Refusing requests
Close and intimate relationships
Enhancing social support networks
Recognizing and Expressing Emotions

INTRAPERSONAL

Managing thoughts about alcohol
Problem solving
Increasing pleasant activities
Relaxation training
Awareness and management of anger
Awareness and management of negative thinking
Planning for emergencies
Coping with persistent problems

---

deal with stressful events that threaten abstinence. This type of support group is also extremely effective in outpatient treatment settings. After a period of successful abstinence, group therapy can focus more on traditional psychotherapy work.

Individual Therapy

Often, individual therapy is helpful, particularly in conjunction with group therapy or family therapy. In addiction treatment settings, counselors meet with individuals to maintain focus on the goals and objectives of their treatment, to review the fears and anxieties that often arise in early recovery, and to devise new and healthy responses and solutions to stressful and difficult situations. Therapy shouldn't be considered as one size fits all. For instance, anxiety disorders are common comorbidities in substance abuse, but individuals with social anxiety whose anxiety becomes alarmingly high when they are asked to speak in public shouldn't be expected to participate in groups. Forcing their group participation would be counterproductive not only to the individual but also for others in the group.

Family Interventions

Family therapy, a vital part of addiction treatment, can be used in several beneficial ways to initiate change and help the family when the substance-abusing person is unwilling to seek treatment. Behavioral couples therapy for people with alcoholism can improve family

---

BOX 31.11

Substance Abuse

When caring for the patient and family with substance abuse, be sure to include the following topic areas in the family's teaching plan:

• Psychopharmacologic agents, if used, including drug action, dosage, frequency, and possible side effects
• Manifestations of intoxication, overdose, and withdrawal
• Emergency medical system activation
• Nutrition
• Coping strategies
• Structured planning
• Safety measures
• Available treatment programs
• Family therapy referral
• Self-help groups and other community resources
• Follow-up laboratory testing, if indicated

functioning, reduce stressors, smooth marital adjustment, and lessen domestic violence and verbal conflict. When the substance-abusing person seeks help, family therapy can help stabilize abstinence and relationships. Often, inpatient substance abuse treatment programs have family education and group therapy components that help meet these goals. Family therapy can also help to maintain long-term recovery and prevent relapse. Goals of family therapy should be realistic and obtainable. Action plans must be specific and organized into manageable increments. Target dates should be realistic, so pressure is minimal, yet there is motivation to act in a timely manner. Planning for the future is very difficult as long as alcohol or drug abuse continues.

Harm-Reduction Strategies

Harm reduction, a community health intervention designed to reduce the harm of substance use to the individual, the family, and society, has replaced a moral or criminal approach to drug use and addiction. It recognizes that the ideal is abstinence but works with the individual regardless of their commitment to reduce use. The goal is to reduce the potential harm of the associated behavior. Harm reduction initiatives range from widely accepted designated driver campaigns to controversial initiatives, such as provision of condoms in schools, safe injection rooms, needle exchange programs, and heroin maintenance programs.

Peer Support Self-Help Group

Alcoholics Anonymous (AA) was the first 12-step, self-help program (see Box 31.13 for a list of these steps). AA is a worldwide fellowship of people with alcoholism who provide support, individually and at meetings, to others who seek help. The program steps include spiritual, cognitive, and behavioral components. Many treatment programs discuss concepts from AA, hold meetings at the treatment facilities, and encourage patients to attend community meetings when appropriate. They also encourage continuing use of AA and other self-help groups as part of an ongoing plan for continued abstinence. Twelve-step programs do not solicit members; engage in political or religious activities; make medical or psychiatric diagnoses; engage in education about addiction to the general population; or provide mental health, vocational, or legal counseling (Alcoholics Anonymous, 2020). Using peer support and support groups is an accepted approach with many beneficial outcomes for participants, since nurses are often responsible for the selection and training of individuals who will serve as peer support specialists (PSS). Much can be learned from studies that reveal member's ideas about

---

BOX 31.13

The 12 Steps of Alcoholics Anonymous

1. We admitted we were powerless over alcohol—that our lives had become unmanageable.
2. Came to believe that a Power greater than ourselves could restore us to sanity.
3. Made a decision to turn our will and our lives over to the care of God *as we understood Him.*
4. Made a searching and fearless moral inventory of ourselves.
5. Admitted to God, to ourselves, and to another human being the exact nature of our wrongs.
6. Were entirely ready to have God remove all these defects of character.
7. Humbly asked Him to remove our shortcomings.
8. Made a list of all persons we had harmed, and became willing to make amends to them all.
9. Made direct amends to such people wherever possible, except when to do so would injure them or others.
10. Continued to take personal inventory and, when we were wrong, promptly admitted it.
11. Sought through prayer and meditation to improve our conscious contact with God, as we understood Him, praying only for knowledge of His will for us and the power to carry that out.
12. Having had a spiritual awakening as a result of these steps, we tried to carry this message to alcoholics and to practice these principles in all our affairs.

The Twelve Steps are reprinted with permission of Alcoholics Anonymous World Services, Inc. ("A.A.W.S."). Permission to reprint the Twelve Steps does not mean that A.A.W.S. has reviewed or approved the contents of this publication, or that A.A. necessarily agrees with the views expressed herein. A.A. is a program of recovery from alcoholism only - use of the Twelve Steps in connection with programs and activities which are patterned after A.A., but which address other problems, or in any other non-A.A. context, does not imply otherwise.

---

what works best, and who they can best work with (see Research Update Box 31.14).

Alternative peer support groups differ from these programs in their approach. Four such groups in the United States are Women for Sobriety, Moderation Management, Men for Sobriety, and Self-Management and Recovery Training (SMART) Recovery. These groups are based on harm reduction philosophies and missions. Other harm reduction strategies for prevention of alcohol abuse can be seen in Box 31.15.

Evaluation and Treatment Outcomes

Recovery from alcoholism is a journey, often lasting a lifetime. Recovery involves a change in lifestyle and, often, new relationships. Short-term outcomes can be evaluated within the treatment setting. Long-term outcomes are established and evaluated by the patient who often continues to use professional and nonprofessional support as needed.

BOX 31.14

Research for Best Practices: Peer Support Services for Perinatal Opioid Users

Fallin, Bennett, A., Elswick, A., & Ashfrord, K. (2020). Peer support specialists and perinatal opioid use disorder: Someone that's been there, lived it, seen it. Addictive Behaviors, 102(3), 106–204. doi:10.1016/j.addbeh

QUESTION: How do perinatal women who receive peer support services (PSS) during treatment for their substance use disorders describe the experience, and how can these services be improved?

METHODS: Focus groups were conducted in a clinic that serves postpartum women with perinatal opioid use disorder (OUD) who were parenting a child under the age of 5. From recorded interviews, content themes were analyzed in MAXQDA (software used for analysis of data in qualitative and mixed

FINDINGS: Four themes, 1. Feeling supported by peer support specialists, 2. Qualities of an 'ideal' peer support

specialist, 3. Strategies to improve communication interactions with PSS, and 4. The importance of communication across the perinatal period was identified. Participants reported that PSS had a strong positive influence on their recovery and offered strategies for others to further improve interactions with peer supports.

IMPLICATIONS FOR NURSING: As resources are strained and more women are diagnosed with perinatal opioid use disorder (OUD), nurses must be involved in searching for innovative, cost-effective ways to provide services. Nurses can be involved in selecting and training those who can best offer peer support. This study identified quality improvement ideas directly from service users, highlighting nurse's commitment to patient-centered care, while alerting nurse researchers to design studies that can determine the long-term contributions of peer

BOX 31.15

Harm Reduction Strategies for Alcohol Abuse

Sobriety Homes	Group residence for people who are recovering from addiction; maintain sobriety and live according to residential rules.
Informational Campaigns: SAMSHA's QUICK TIPS	Buy less to use less.
	Set a time limit before your start and then stop drinking at that time.
	Eat a meal before drinking alcohol.
	Choose the least harmful method of use.
	Plan drug/alcohol free-days.
	Use at your own speed.
	Find someone to take with when you are struggling.
	Read self-help books.
	Put condoms in your pocket before you go out!
	www.heretohelp.bc.ca/workbook/you-and-substance-use-harm-reduction-strategies
Expectancy Challenge Interventions	Expectancy challenge interventions do not focus on abstinence or scare tactics but on an individual's perceptions of alcohol's effects and providing accurate information. Negative expectancies are associated with reducing alcohol consumption and other negative consequences of use. This intervention has been delivered in different ways, including experiential learning, informational campaigns, and peer-support sessions.
Resisting Negative Peer Pressure	Strategies to resist peer-pressure for drinking are taught and practices. Strategies include what to say to peers, and what to do under continued pressure. Situations are rehearsed in anticipation of pressure, until the teen feels confident and comfortable using them.

Retrieved March 10, 2020 www.heretohelp.bc.ca/workbook/you-and-substance-use-harm-reduction-strategies

CHEMICAL DEPENDENCY AND PROFESSIONAL NURSES

Although accurate epidemiologic data specific to nursing are scarce, evidence suggests that the prevalence of substance use disorders among nurses is similar to that of the general public (Kunyk, 2015). A nurse is just as susceptible to addiction as any other individual, but additional risk factors exist, such as access and availability of drugs, training in the administration and injection of drugs, and a familiarity with and a frequency of administering drugs. Working conditions may be difficult and involve staffing shortages, acutely ill patients, inadequate patient-to-nurse ratios, shift rotation, shifts lasting longer than 8 hours, and increased overtime all add additional stress to the nurse, which increases the risk of substance abuse. Because of the risk of losing a license to practice, nurses are very reluctant to seek help. To protect patients' safety and maintain the standards of the profession, many states have mandatory reporting laws. According to the nurse practice acts, any nurse who knows of any health care provider's incompetent, unethical, or illegal practice must report that information through proper channels.

In 1982, the American Nurses Association House of Delegates adopted a national resolution to provide assistance to impaired nurses. The peer assistance programs strive to intervene early, reduce hazards to patients, and increase prospects for the nurse's recovery. The program offers consultation, referral, and monitoring for nurses whose practice is impaired, or potentially impaired, because of the use of illicit drugs or alcohol or a psychological or physiologic condition.

A referral can be made confidentially by the employer, Employee Assistance Program, coworker, family member, friend, or the nurse herself or himself. If the nurse is willing to undergo a thorough evaluation to determine the extent of the problem and any treatment needed, all information is kept confidential from the Board of Nursing, so that the nurse does not face disciplinary action against their nursing license.

Some signs of substance abuse in nurses include mood swings, inappropriate behavior at work, frequent days off for implausible reasons, noncompliance with acceptable policies and procedures, deteriorating appearance, deteriorating job performance, sloppy illegible charting, errors in charting, alcohol on the breath, forgetfulness, poor judgment and concentration, lying, and volunteering to act as the medications nurse.

Other characteristics of nurses with substance abuse include high achievement, both as a student and a nurse; volunteering for overtime and extra duties; no drug use unless prescribed after surgery or for a chronic illness; and family history of alcoholism or addiction.

SUMMARY OF KEY POINTS

■ Substance use disorders are categorized according to the following substances: alcohol, caffeine, cannabis (marijuana), hallucinogens, inhalants, opioids, sedative–hypnotics, stimulants, tobacco, and others.

■ Addiction is a condition of continued use of substances despite adverse consequences. Abuse occurs when a person uses alcohol or drugs for the purpose of intoxication or, in the case of prescription drugs, for purposes beyond their use.

■ Accurate and comprehensive assessment is crucial in planning addiction treatment interventions. This assessment should consider all substances for pattern of use, including factors of tolerance; withdrawal symptoms; consequences of use; loss of control over amount, frequency, or duration of use; desire or efforts to cease or control use; and social, vocational, and recreational activities affected by use, history of previous addiction treatment, and family and social support systems.

■ Denial of a substance use disorder is the individual's attempt to avoid accepting the diagnosis; it can be manifest in attempts to rationalize the substance use, minimize the harmful results, deflect attention from one's own problem to society's or someone else's, or blame childhood trauma.

■ Nurses should use a nonconfrontational approach when dealing with patients in denial of their problems. Motivational interviewing approaches are most effective, using empathy and a nonjudgmental approach, to help the patient to realize the discrepancy between life goals and engaging in substance use, thus, motivating patients to change their self-destructive behaviors and make personal choices regarding treatment goals.

■ Several effective modalities are used in addiction treatment, and many programs combine them, which may include 12-step programs, social skills groups, psychoeducational groups, group therapy, and individual and family therapies. No one best treatment method exists for all people.

■ Substance use disorders have many social and political ramifications. No health profession is immune to having members who suffer with substance use disorders.

Unfolding Patient Stories: Andrew Davis

Part 1

Andrew Davis is 56 years old and voluntarily admitted himself to an alcohol rehabilitation facility after his wife asked him to move out of their home. Of his three children, only his son will speak to him. He refuses to attend group therapy and an Alcoholics Anonymous (AA) meeting. How can the nurse establish a therapeutic relationship during the treatment stage of withdrawal and throughout recovery? Why is it important to cultivate trust between the nurse, Andrew, and his family? How can the nurse encourage him to attend group therapy and the AA meeting?

CRITICAL THINKING CHALLENGES

1. Jeff H, a 35-year-old patient who abuses cocaine, has entered a rehabilitation program. What goals do you believe would be realistic to achieve by the end of his projected 30-day inpatient stay?

2. You are working in an orthopedic unit, and Mary L has been admitted for treatment for a fractured femur. She has been drinking recently and has a BAL of 0.08%. What further information in the following areas would you need to plan her care?
   a. Medical
   b. Alcohol and drug use related
   c. Other psychosocial issues

3. Normal adolescent behavior is often similar to that associated with substance abuse. How would you differentiate this normal behavior from possible substance abuse or addiction?

4. John M has sought treatment for depression and job stress. He came to your psychiatric assessment unit smelling of alcohol. He believes that he does not have a drinking problem but a job problem. What interventions would you use for possible alcohol abuse or addiction?

5. Sylvia G has been abusing heroin intravenously heavily for 2 years. She has come into the hospital with an abscess on her leg. What symptoms would you expect to observe as she experiences withdrawal? What medications would likely be used to ease these symptoms?

6. After Sylvia G is free from withdrawal symptoms, she expresses interest in obtaining drug treatment. What are her options? How would you describe them to her?

Raymond L has been treated for hypertension at your clinic. You notice that he complains of peripheral neuropathy and has an unsteady gait. What other medical signs would corroborate alcoholism? What experiences have you had with addictions? What was your response? How do you think those experiences will affect you as your build your practice to help others with addictions and substance misuse?

Movie Viewing Guides
2019: Uncut Gems "Everything I do is not going right," sobs Howard.

This film depicts the experience of a charismatic jeweler named Howard Ratner, who is involved in high-stakes betting scheme that could lead to a lifetime windfall or to the loss of everything he owns, including his family and even his life. The jeweler is entrenched in the fantasy world of gambling addiction, needing high and higher stakes to sustain the pleasure, and ultimately rocketing out of control. Winning or losing doesn't really matter, so long as Howard gets an opportunity to make another bet and get on the roller coaster again. The film unfolds over a couple of days, but tension escalates at a rapid, high-adrenalin pace, that the viewer, for the space of this movie (only 135 minutes), is transported into the world of pathological gambling. When the movie ends, there is an audible sigh of relief on the part of the audience.

VIEWING POINTS: Identify the *DSM-5* criteria associated with behavioral use disorder depicted and alluded to in the film. Notice how the addiction to gambling takes over Howard's life and the costs he is willing to pay in order to experience the high of gaming. Notice his alertness and arousal as he is preoccupied with the bet and notice too, how short the pleasure lasts, before Howard must once again engage in another high-stakes game. Look for Howard's lies, the level of his activity, the extent of measures he takes to hides his addiction. See if you recognize other comorbidities in Howard's behavior. Were you concerned about his safety? What was Howard's level of self-deception and how did he maintain it? Could you identify the phases of gambling addiction:

winning, losing, desperation, and hopelessness? How did you feel as you witness Howard self-destruct? What would it be like to have Howard in treatment?

REFERENCES

Alcoholics Anonymous. (2020). Alcoholics anonymous information on AA [Online]. http://www.aa.org

American Psychiatric Association. (2013). Substance use disorders. In *Diagnostic and statistical manual of mental disorders (5th ed.)*. Arlington, VA: Author.

Biroscak, B. J., Pantalon, M. V., Dziura, J. D., Hersey, D. P., & Vaca, F. E. (2019). Use of non-face-to-face modalities for emergency department screening, brief intervention, and referral to treatment (ED-SBIRT) for high-risk alcohol use: A scoping review. *Substance Abuse*, 40(1), 20–32. https://doi.org/10.1080/08897077.2018.1550465

Bivin, B., Waring, A., & Alves, P. (2019). Buprenorphine compared with methadone in opioid-dependent pregnant women: How does it affect neonatal abstinence syndrome? *Journal of the American Association of Nurse Practitioners*. https://doi.org/10.1097/JXX.0000000000000345

Caffeineinformer. (2020). Top 15 caffeine overdose symptoms. https://www.caffeineinformer.com/caffeine-overdose-facts-and-fiction

Centers for Disease Control and Prevention. (2020). Prescription opioid data. https://www.cdc.gov/drugoverdose/data/prescribing.html.

Cruz, S.L., Torres-Flores, M., & N Galván, E. J. (2019). Repeated toluene exposure alters the synaptic transmission of layer 5 medial prefrontal cortex. *Neurotoxicology and Teratology*, 28(73), 9–14. https://doi.org/10.1016/j.ntt.2019.02.002

Dyba, J., Moesgen, D., Klein, M., & Leyendecker, B. (2019). Mothers and fathers in treatment for methamphetamine addiction Parenting, parental stress, and children at risk. *Child and Family Social Work*, 24, 106–114. https://doi.org/10.1111/cfs12587

Ewing, J. A. (1984). Detecting alcoholism. The CAGE questionnaire. *Journal of the American Medical Association*, 252(14), 1905–1907.

Fallin Bennett, A., Elswick, A., & Ashford, K. (2020). Peer support specialists and perinatal opioid use disorder: Someone that's been there, lived it, seen it. *Addictive Behaviors*, 102(3), 106–204. https://doi.org/10.1016/j.addbeh

Farhadian, N., Moradi, S., Zamanian, M. H., Farnia, V., Rezaeian, S., Farhadian, M., & Shahlaei, M. (2020). Effectiveness of naltrexone treatment for alcohol use disorders in HIV: A systematic review. *Substance Abuse Treatment, Prevention, and Policy*, 15(1), 24. https://doi.org/10.1186/s13011-020-00266-6

Ganson, K. T., & Cadet, T.J. (2018). Exploring anabolic-androgenic steroid use and teen dating violence among adolescent males. *Substance Use & Misuse*, 21, 1–8. https://doi.org/10.1080/10826084.2018.1536723

Higgins, J. P. (2018). Stimulant-containing energy drinks. American College of Cardiology https://www.acc.org/latest-in-cardiology/articles/2018/02/28/10/46/stimulant-containing-energy-drinks

Humo, M., Avazaak, B, Becker, L.J., Waltsiperger, E., Rantamaki, T., & Yalcin, I. (2020). Ketamine induces rapid and sustained antidepressant-like effects in chronic pain induced depression: Role of MPAK signaling pathway. *Progress in Neuropsychopharmacology & Biologic Psychiatry*, 100, 109898. https://doi.org/10.1016/j.pnpbp.2020.109898

Johns, M. M., Lowry, R., Rasbery, C. N., Dunville, R., Robin, L., Pampati S., Stone, D. M., & Mercer Kollar, L. M. (2018). Violence victimization, substance use, and suicide risk among sexual minority high school students- United States, 2015–2017. *MMWR Morbidity and Mortality Weekly Report*, 67(43), 1211–1215. https://doi.org/10.15585/mmwr.mm6743a4

Karlsson, A., & Håkansson, A. (2018). Gambling disorder, increased mortality, suicidality, and associated comorbidity: A longitudinal nationwide register study. *Journal of Behavioral Addictions*, 7(4), 1091–1099. doi: 10.1556/2006.7.2018.112

Kunyk, D. (2015). Substance use disorders among registered nurses: prevalence, risks and perceptions in a disciplinary jurisdiction. *Journal of Nursing Management*, 23(1), 54–64. https://doi.org/10.1111/jonm.12081

Lewis, M. J. (2020). Alcoholism and nutrition: a review of vitamin supplementation and treatment. *Current Opinion in Clinical Nutrition and Metabolic Care*, 23(2), 138–144. https://doi.org/10.1097/MCO.0000000000000622

Mental Health America. (2021). Co-dependency [Online]. Retrieved June 12, 2021 from https://www.mhanational.org/issues/co-dependency

National Institute on Drug Abuse. (2020a). Cigarettes and other tobacco products. National Institutes of Health: U.S. Department of health and Human Services. https://www.drugabuse.gov/publications/drugfacts/cigarettes-other-tobacco-products

National Institute on Drug Abuse. (2020b). Overdose Death Rates. National Institute on Drug Abuse; National Institutes of Health; U.S. Department of Health and Human Services. https://www.drugabuse.gov/related-topics/trends-statistics/overdose-death-rates

National Institute on Drug Abuse. (2019a). Commonly Abused Drug. National Institute on Drug Abuse; National Institutes of Health; U.S. Department of Health and Human Services. https://www.drugabuse.gov/drugs-abuse/commonly-abused-drugs-charts#lsd

National Institute on Drug Abuse. (2019b). Genetics and epigenetics of addiction. https://www.drugabuse.gov/publications/drugfacts/genetics-epigenetics-addiction

National Institute on Drug Abuse. (2019c). Hallucinogens and dissociative drugs. Research Reports. National Institute on Drug Abuse; National Institutes of Health; U.S. Department of Health and Human Services. https://www.drugabuse.gov/publications/research-reports/hallucinogens-dissociative-drugs/what-are-dissociative-drugs

National Institute on Drug Abuse. (2019d). Heroin. Drug Facts. National Institute on Drug Abuse; National Institutes of Health; U.S. Department of Health and Human Services. https://www.drugabuse.gov/publications/drugfacts/heroin

National Institute on Drug Abuse. (2019e). Monitoring Future Study: Trends in Prevalence of Various Drugs (charts) National Institute on Drug Abuse; National Institutes of Health; U.S. Department of Health and Human Services. https://www.drugabuse.gov/trends-statistics/monitoring-future/monitoring-future-study-trends-in-prevalence-various-drugs

National Institute on Drug Abuse. (2019f). What is marijuana? National Institutes of Health: U.S. Department of Health and Human Services. https://www.drugabuse.gov/publications/drugfacts/marijuana

National Institute on Drug Abuse. (2019g). What are marijuana's effects on lung health? National Institutes of Health: U.S. Department of Health and Human Services. https://www.drugabuse.gov/publications/research-reports/marijuana/what-are-marijuanas-effects-lung-health

National Institute on Drug Abuse. (2019h). What is Methamphetamine.? Research Report Series. NIH Publication Number 13-4210. National Institutes of Health. Bethesda, MD:U.S. Department of Health and Human. https://www.drugabuse.gov/publications/drugfacts/methamphetamine

National Institute on Drug Abuse. (2019i). Vaping. Research Report Series. NIH Publication Number 13-4210. National Institutes of Health. Bethesda, MD:U.S. Department of Health and Human. https://www.drugabuse.gov/related-topics/vaping

National Institute on Drug Abuse. (2018a). Cocaine. National Institute on Drug Abuse; National Institutes of Health; U.S. Department of Health and Human Services. https://www.drugabuse.gov/publications/drugfacts/cocaine.

National Institute on Drug Abuse. (2018b). MDMA ("ecstasy" or "Molly"). National Institute on Drug Abuse; National Institutes of Health; U.S. Department of Health and Human Services. https://www.drugabuse.gov/publications/drugfacts/mdma-ecstasymolly

National Institute on Drug Abuse. (2018c). Tobacco, nicotine, and e-cigarettes. *Research Report Series*. National Institute on Drug Abuse; National Institutes of Health; U.S. Department of Health and Human Services. https://www.drugabuse.gov/publications/research-reports/tobacco-nicotine-e-cigarettes/what-scope-tobacco-use-its-cost-to-society

National Institute on Drug Abuse. (2018d). Misuse of prescription drugs. National Institute on Drug Abuse; National Institutes of Health; U.S. Department of Health and Human Services. https://www.drugabuse.gov/publications/misuse-prescription-drugs/overview

National Institute on Drug Abuse. (2018e). Synthetic Cannabinoids (K2/Spice). Drug Facts. National Institute on Drug Abuse; National Institutes of Health; U.S. Department of Health and Human Services. https://www.drugabuse.gov/publications/drugfacts/synthetic-cannabinoids-k2spice

National Institute on Drug Abuse. (2018f). Vaping, Marijuana, and Other Drugs. National Institute on Drug Abuse; National Institutes of Health; U.S. Department of Health and Human Services. https://www.drugabuse.gov/drugs-abuse/vaping-marijuana-other-drugs

National Institute on Drug Abuse. (2018g). What are Anabolic Steroids? National Institute on Drug Abuse; National Institutes of Health; U.S.

Department of Health and Human Services. https://www.drugabuse.gov/publications/drugfacts/anabolic-steroids

National Institute on Drug Abuse. (2018h). What are Inhalants?. Drug Facts. National Institute on Drug Abuse; National Institutes of Health; U.S. Department of Health and Human Services. https://www.drugabuse.gov/publications/drugfacts/inhalants

National Institute on Drug Abuse. (2018i). What are Synthetic Cathinones? (Bath Salts). National Institute on Drug Abuse; National Institutes of Health; U.S. Department of Health and Human Services. https://www.drugabuse.gov/drugs-abuse/synthetic-cathinones-bath-salts

National Institute on Drug Abuse. (2017). What are over-the-counter (OTC) medicines/National Institute on Drug Abuse; National Institutes of Health; U.S. Department of Health and Human Services. https://www.drugabuse.gov/publications/drugfacts/over-counter-medicines

National Institute on Drug Abuse. (2016). New regulations on flavored tobacco products and e-cigarettes will protect public health. National Institute on Drug Abuse; National Institutes of Health; U.S. Department of Health and Human Services. https://www.drugabuse.gov/about-nida/noras-blog/2016/05/new-regulations-flavored-tobacco-products-e-cigarettes-will-protect-public-health

National Institute on Drug Abuse. (2012). Inhalants What are the unique risks associated with nitrite abuse? https://www.drugabuse.gov/publications/research-reports/inhalants/what-are-unique-risks-associated-nitrite-abuse

Petry, N. M., Zajac, K., & Ginley, M. K. (2018). Behavioral addictions as mental disorders: To be or not to be? *Annual Review of Clinical Psychology*, 7(14), 399–423. https://doi.org/10.1146/annurev-clinpsy-032816-045120

Singh, A. K. (2019). Alcohol Interaction with cocaine, methamphetamine, opioids, nicotine, cannabis, and γ-hydroxybutyric acid. *Biomedicines*, 7(10). https://doi.org/10.3390/biomedicines7010016

Singh, D., & Saadabadi, A. (2020). Varenicline. In *StatPearls*. StatPearls Publishing.

Sanmartin, M. X., McKenna, R. M., Ali, M. M., & Krebs, J. D. (2020). Racial disparities in payment source of opioid use disorder treatment among non-incarcerated justice-involved adults in the United States. *The Journal of Mental Health Policy and Economics*,23(1), 19–25.

Smith, P. H., Chhipa, M., Bystrik, J., Roy, J., Goodwin, R. D., & McKee, S. A. (2020). Cigarette smoking among those with mental disorders in the US population: 2012-2013 update. *Tobacco Control*, 29(1), 29–35. https://doi.org/10.1136/tobaccocontrol-2018-054268

Society for Adolescent Health and Medicine [SAHM]. (2011). Screening tools. https://www.adolescenthealth.org/Topics-in-Adolescent-Health/Substance-Use/Clinical-Care-Guidelines/Screening-Tools.aspx

Substance Abuse and Mental Health Services Administration. (2018a). National survey on drug use and health (NSDUH). https://www.samhsa.gov/data/data-we-collect/nsduh-national-survey-drug-use-and-health

Stokes, M., & Abdijadid, S. (2020). Disulfiram. In *StatPearls*. StatPearls Publishing.

U.S. Department of Health and Human Services. (2020). *Healthy People 2020*. Washington, DC: U.S. Government Printing Office. https://www.cdc.gov/nchs/healthy_people/hp2020.htm

van Timmeren, T., Daams, J. G., van Holst, R. J., & Goudriaan, A. E. (2018). Compulsivity-related neurocognitive performance deficits in gambling disorder: A systematic review and meta-analysis. *Neuroscience Biobehavioral Review*, 84, 204–217. https://doi.org/10.1016/j.neubiorev.2017.11.022

Vieira, A., et al. (2018). Does auriculotherapy have therapeutic effectiveness? An overview of systematic reviews. *Complementary Therapies in Clinical Practice*, 33, 61–70. https://doi.org/10.1016/j.ctcp.2018.08.00

Watchman, E. M., Schiff, D. M., & Silverstein, M. (2018). Neonatal abstinence syndrome: Advances in diagnosis and treatment. *Journal of the American Medical Association*, 319(13), 1362–1374. https://doi.org/10.1001/jama.2018.2640

Winhusen, T., Theobald, J., Kaelber, D. C., & Lewis, D. (2019). Medical complications associated with substance use disorders in patients with type 2 diabetes and hypertension: Electronic health record findings. *Addiction*. https://doi.org/10.1111/add.14607

Yoon, C., Gedzior, J., & DePry, D. (2019). Wernicke-Korsakoff syndrome: Focus on low-threshold diagnosis and prompt treatment in the primary care setting. *International Journal of Psychiatry in Medicine*, 1, 91217419832771. https://doi.org/10.1177/0091217419832771

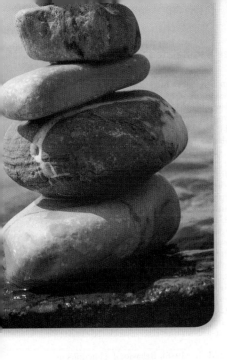

32
Eating Disorders
Nursing Care of Persons with Eating and Weight-Related Disorders

Mary Ann Boyd

KEYCONCEPTS

- body dissatisfaction
- body image distortion
- dietary restraint
- drive for thinness
- emotional dysregulation
- perfectionism

LEARNING OBJECTIVES

After studying this chapter, you will be able to:

1. Discuss the role of body image, body dissatisfaction, and gender identity in eating disorders.

2. Delineate the clinical symptoms of anorexia nervosa (AN) from those of bulimia nervosa (BN).

3. Analyze the primary theories explaining anorexia nervosa and bulimia nervosa.

4. Develop strategies to establish a patient-centered, recovery-oriented therapeutic relationship with a person with anorexia nervosa.

5. Apply a person-centered, recovery-oriented nursing process for persons with anorexia nervosa.

6. Identify medications used to treat people with anorexia nervosa.

7. Develop wellness strategies for persons with anorexia nervosa.

8. Differentiate the type of mental health care provided in emergency care, inpatient-focused care, community care, and virtual mental health care.

9. Discuss the importance of integrated health care for persons with anorexia nervosa.

10. Describe other eating and weight-related disorders.

KEY TERMS

- Anorexia nervosa (AN) • Binge eating • Binge eating disorder (BED) • Bulimia nervosa (BN) • Enmeshment
- Night eating syndrome • Purging disorder • Refeeding • Refeeding syndrome • Self-monitoring

Case Study

Ellen is a 20-year-old college sophomore admitted to an inpatient mental health unit after treatment in a medical unit, where she was admitted for dehydration and electrolyte imbalance. Ellen has been binging and purging while in school to maintain a normal body weight.

INTRODUCTION

Since the 1970s, eating disorders have received national attention, primarily because several high-profile personalities and athletes with these disorders have received front-page news coverage. Since the 1960s, the increased incidence of anorexia nervosa and bulimia nervosa has prompted mental health professionals to address their causes and devise effective treatments.

Wellness depends on good nutritional status and healthy eating. Frequently, nurses will recommend reduction or increase of body to maintain physical health and well-being. In some people, eating and body weight determine their behavior, self-esteem, and self-concept. They strive to reach an unrealistic and unhealthy body weight leading to the development of an eating disorder. Even though eating disorders are defined as mental disorders, the consequences of their disordered eating lead to serious impairment of physical health and sometimes death. All nurses should be able to recognize the symptoms of an eating disorder.

EATING DISORDERS OVERVIEW

Eating disorders are characterized by disturbed eating and eating-related behaviors. The *DSM-5* classification of eating disorders includes pica (eating nonnutritive, nonfood substances), rumination disorder (repeated regurgitation of food), avoidant/restrictive food intake disorder (avoiding food, lack of interest in food), anorexia nervosa, bulimia nervosa, binge eating disorder (BED), and other disorders (APA, 2013). Disordered eating behaviors are often classified as subclinical or subthreshold cases of true eating disorders, such as anorexia nervosa and bulimia nervosa, which are psychiatric diagnoses. These individuals still need treatment despite not meeting the diagnostic criteria.

Even though eating disorders differ in definition, clinical course, etiologies, and interventions, symptoms of these disorders, such as dieting, binge eating, and preoccupation with weight and shape, overlap significantly. Viewing the symptoms along a continuum from less to more severe eating behaviors helps with this conceptualization, as shown in Figure 32.1. There are also common psychological characteristics of people with eating disorders (Box 32.1). This chapter highlights anorexia nervosa (AN), emphasizes bulimia nervosa (BN), and briefly discusses BED.

ANOREXIA NERVOSA

Anorexia Nervosa is a mixture of symptoms that include significantly low body weight, intense fear of gaining weight or becoming fat, and a disturbance in experiencing body weight or shape (undue influence or distorted

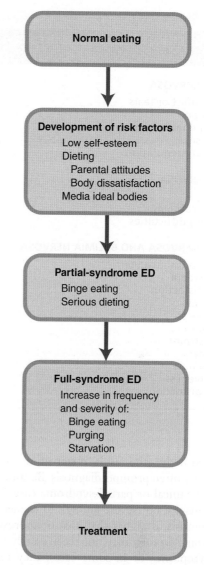

FIGURE 32.1 Progression of symptoms leading to an eating disorder.

self-evaluation of body weight or shape or lack of recognition of the seriousness of low body weight).

Anorexia nervosa is further categorized into two major types: *restricting* (dieting and exercising with no binge eating or misuse of laxatives, diuretics, or enemas) and *binge eating and purging* (binge eating and misuse of laxatives, diuretics, or enemas). Malnutrition and semistarvation result in a preoccupation with food, binge eating, depression, obsession, and apathy, as well as compromising several body systems, leading to medical complications and, in some instances, death (APA, 2013).

Clinical Course

The onset of AN usually occurs in early adolescence. The onset can be slow, with serious dieting occurring before

BOX 32.1

Psychological Characteristics Related to Eating Disorders

ANOREXIA NERVOSA

Sexuality conflict or fears
Maturity fears
Ritualistic behaviors
Perfectionism
Emotional Dysregulation

BULIMIA NERVOSA

Impulsivity
Boundary problems
Limit-setting difficulties

ANOREXIA NERVOSA AND BULIMIA NERVOSA

Difficulty expressing anger
Low self-esteem
Body dissatisfaction
Powerlessness
Ineffectiveness
Perfectionism
Dietary restraint
Obsessiveness
Compulsiveness
Nonassertiveness
Cognitive distortions

an emaciated body—the result of starvation—is noticed. This discovery often prompts diagnosis. Because the incidence of subclinical or partial-syndrome cases, in which the symptoms are not severe enough to use an anorexia nervosa diagnosis, is higher than that of anorexia nervosa, many young women may not receive early treatment for their symptoms, or in some cases, they receive no treatment. The individual's refusal to maintain a normal weight because of a distorted body image and an intense fear of becoming fat make individuals with this disorder difficult to identify and treat.

It can be a chronic condition with relapses characterized by significant weight loss. Reporting conclusive outcomes for anorexia nervosa is difficult because of the variety of definitions used to determine recovery. Although patients considered to have recovered have restored normal weight, menses, and eating behaviors, some continue to have distorted body images and be preoccupied with weight and food; many develop bulimia nervosa, and many continue to have symptoms of other psychiatric illnesses, especially of the anxiety disorders.

Body Distortion

For most individuals, body image (a mental picture of one's own body) is consistent with how others view them.

However, individuals with anorexia nervosa have a body image that is severely distorted from reality. Because of this distortion, they see themselves as obese and undesirable even when they are emaciated. They are unable to accept objective reality and the perceptions of the outside world.

KEYCONCEPT Body image distortion occurs when the individual perceives their body disparately from how the world or society views it.

 Concept Mastery Alert

People with anorexia nervosa have a distorted image of the appearance of their bodies. They can be very thin and still perceive that they are heavy and need to lose weight.

Drive for Thinness

Because of body distortion, individuals with anorexia nervosa have an intense drive for thinness. They see themselves as fat, fear becoming fatter, and are "driven" to work toward "undoing" this fear.

KEYCONCEPT Drive for thinness is an intense physical and emotional process that overrides all physiologic body cues.

The individual with anorexia nervosa ignores body cues, such as hunger and weakness, and concentrates all efforts on controlling food intake. The entire mental focus of the young patient with anorexia nervosa narrows to only one goal: weight loss. Typical thought patterns are as follows: "If I gain a pound, I'll keep gaining." This all-or-nothing thinking keeps these patients on rigid regimens for weight loss.

The behavior of patients with anorexia nervosa becomes organized around food-related activities, such as preparing food, counting calories, and reading cookbooks. Much behavior concerning what, when, and how they eat is ritualistic. Food combinations and the order in which foods may be eaten, and under which circumstances, can seem bizarre. One patient, for example, would eat only cantaloupe, carrying it with her to all meals outside of her home and consuming it only if it were cut in smaller than bite-sized pieces and only if she could use chopsticks, which she also carried with her.

KEYCONCEPT Emotional dysregulation is a difficulty regulating expression of feelings. Emotional dysregulation and increased sensory sensitivity are linked to anorexia nervosa. Emotion dysregulation comprises one's inability to accept one's emotional responses, to accomplish goals in the midst of distress, and to be aware of and acknowledge the significance of developing and implementing coping strategies to influence and manage emotions effectively (Rotella et al., 2018).

NCLEXNOTE The emotional dysregulation model links deficits in emotional regulation with anorexia nervosa, that is, those with anorexia nervosa have deficits in the ability to understand and modulate emotions, which results in experiencing emotions as overwhelming and unmanageable. Consequently, those with anorexia nervosa use disordered eating to regulate their affective state by either reducing negative affect or increasing positive affect, and thus disordered eating, through reinforcement, is maintained (Rotella et al., 2018). Treatment programs that address emotional regulation and focus on teaching skills to regulate emotions may therefore be effective, especially with anorexia nervosa patients.

Guilt and Anger

Patients with anorexia nervosa tend to avoid conflict and have difficulty expressing negative emotions, especially anger (Duarte et al., 2016). They have an overwhelming sense of guilt and anger, which leads to conflict avoidance, which is common in families of those with anorexia nervosa. Because of the ritualistic behaviors, an all-encompassing focus on food and weight, and feelings of inadequacy, social contacts are gradually reduced, and the patient becomes isolated. More severe weight loss is associated with other symptoms, such as apathy, depression, and even mistrust of others.

Perfectionism

Emotional dysregulation is hypothesized to relate to perfectionism. Perfectionistic behavior, such as making sure that everything is symmetrical or that objects are placed at the same distance from each other, or in performance-based tasks, is a typical significant symptom of anorexia nervosa and bulimia nervosa and is hypothesized to develop long before eating symptoms occur. Findings from research demonstrate that perfectionism is a significant personality symptom risk factor in eating disorders (Wagner & Vitousek, 2019).

KEYCONCEPT Perfectionism consists of personal standards (the extent to which the individual sets and tries to achieve high standards for oneself) and concern over mistakes and their consequences for their self-worth and others' opinions.

It is now accepted that perfectionism precedes the development of weight and shape concerns. The more severe the disorder, the more perfectionistic. As symptoms are resolved, perfectionism may decrease (Larsson et al., 2018).

Guilt and Anger

Patients with anorexia nervosa tend to avoid conflict and have difficulty expressing negative emotions, especially anger (Duarte et al., 2016; Monell et al., 2018). They

have an overwhelming sense of guilt and anger, which leads to conflict avoidance, common in these families. Because of the ritualistic behaviors, an all-encompassing focus on food and weight, and feelings of inadequacy, social contacts are gradually reduced, and the patient becomes isolated. More severe weight loss is associated with other symptoms, such as apathy, depression, and even mistrust of others.

Diagnostic Criteria

The diagnosis of anorexia is made when there is a restriction of intake, leading to significantly low body weight. The BMI is used as a measure of severity. Other criteria include an intense fear of gaining weight or becoming fat, and body image issues including an undue influence of body weight on self-concept and lack of recognition of seriousness of low body weight (APA, 2013). See Key Diagnostic Characteristics 32.1 for an overview of diagnostic criteria and associated findings.

Anorexia Nervosa Across the Life Span

Anorexia nervosa is primarily diagnosed in adolescence, with 90% of the cases in women (Andrade et al., 2017). There are reports of AN being diagnosed as young as 8 years old (Kwok et al., 2020). Anorexia nervosa is also the most common eating disorder diagnosed in individuals over 50 years of age. Late-onset AN is mostly diagnosed in women. AN in older adults is associated with significant psychiatric comorbidities and overall morbidity (Zayed & Garry, 2017).

Epidemiology

The 12-month prevalence of anorexia nervosa among young females is approximately 0.4%, but many researchers believe this figure does not reflect the true prevalence of this serious disorder (APA, 2013). Adjusted approximations estimate that eating disorders affect over 13% of adolescents and adult women, and 1% to 2% of men. The age of onset is typically between 14 and 16 years but can occur much earlier. Adolescents are vulnerable because of stressors associated with their development, especially concerns about body image, autonomy, and peer pressure, and their susceptibility to such influences as the media, which extols an ideal body type (Cheng et al., 2019; Mangweth-Matzek & Hoek, 2017).

Gender

Females are 10 times more likely than males to develop anorexia nervosa. This disparity has been attributed to society's influence on females to internalize a thin body

Key Diagnostics Characteristics: Anorexia Nervosa

A. Restriction of energy intake relative to requirements, leading to a significantly low body weight in the context of age, sex, developmental trajectory, and physical health. *Significantly low weight* is defined as a weight that is less than minimally normal or, for children and adolescents, less than that minimally expected.

B. Intense fear of gaining weight or of becoming fat, or persistent behavior that interferes with weight gain, even though at a significantly low weight.

C. Disturbance in the way in which one's body weight or shape is experienced, undue influence of body weight or shape on self-evaluation, or persistent lack of recognition of the seriousness of the current low body weight.

Specify whether:

• **Restricting type:** During the last 3 months, the individual has not engaged in recurrent episodes of binge eating or purging behavior (i.e., self-induced vomiting or the misuse of laxatives, diuretics, or enemas). This subtype describes presentations in which weight loss is accomplished primarily through dieting, fasting, and/or excessive exercise.

• **Binge-eating/purging type:** During the last 3 months, the individual has engaged in recurrent episodes of binge eating or purging behavior (i.e., self-induced vomiting or the misuse of laxatives, diuretics, or enemas).

Specify if:

• **In partial remission:** After full criteria for anorexia nervosa were previously met, Criterion A (low body weight) has not been met for a sustained period, but either Criterion B (intense fear of gaining weight or becoming fat or behavior that interferes with weight gain) or Criterion C (disturbances in self-perception of weight and shape) is still met.

• **In full remission:** After full criteria for anorexia nervosa were previously met, none of the criteria have been met for a sustained period of time.

Specify current severity:

The minimum level of severity is based, for adults, on current body mass index (BMI) (see later) or, for children and adolescents, on BMI percentile. The ranges given next are derived from World Health Organization categories for thinness in adults; for children and adolescents, corresponding BMI percentiles should be used. The level of severity may be increased to reflect clinical symptoms, the degree of functional disability, and the need for supervision.

• **Mild:** BMI ≥17 kg/m^2
• **Moderate:** BMI 16 to 16.99 kg/m^2
• **Severe:** BMI 15 to 15.99 kg/m^2
• **Extreme:** BMI <15 kg/m^2

Reprinted with permission from the Diagnostic and Statistical Manual of Mental Disorders, Fifth Edition (Copyright © 2013). American Psychiatric Association. All Rights Reserved.

BOX 32.2

Adolescent Boys and Young Men with Eating Disorders

Eating disorders in boys and men are becoming more prevalent. Males present with eating disorders between the ages of 16 and 24 with different concerns than females with other specified eating disorders, night eating syndrome, and bulimia nervosa as the most prevalent disorders. Adolescent males are more likely to try to gain weight or bulk up and engage in muscle-enhancing behaviors, such as eating more or differently, using supplements, and taking androgenic-anabolic steroids. Overweight and obesity in males may be associated with disordered eating behaviors, including fasting, skipping meals, vomiting, laxatives, diuretics, or binge-eating. The stigma that eating disorders are a women's disease or the paucity of research related to eating disorders in males may inhibit identification in primary care. Because many of the assessment instruments and treatment protocols are geared toward females, males suffer from a lack of early identification of their disorders and early as well as successful treatment.

Nagata, J. M., Ganson, K. T., & Murray, S. B. (2020). Eating disorders in adolescent boys and young men: an update. *Current Opinion in Pediatrics, 32*(4), 476–481. https://doi.org/10.1097/MOP.0000000000000911

as ideal highlights some of the findings about eating disorders in males. See Box 32.2.

Ethnicity and Culture

In the United States, eating disorders occur in all ethnic and racial groups, and recent studies show there are very few differences in prevalence among European Americans, Latinex Americans, Asian Americans, and African Americans (Cheng et al., 2019). However, research findings demonstrate that Asian Americans have a higher level of belief that the ideal body is thinner than do other groups (Cheng et al., 2019). In Asian countries, eating disorders have risen over the last 10 years, attributed to not only the influence of Western countries' media but also to economic development itself (Pike & Dunne, 2015).

Risk Factors

Research demonstrates that genetic risks play an important role in the development of eating disorders in both men and women. Eating disorders are highly inheritable. Puberty is a risk period for the development of anorexia nervosa. Girls often begin to diet at an early age because of body dissatisfaction, and the need for control of prepubertal weight increases. Restricting food can lead to starvation, binge eating, and purging. Males are more likely to engage in physical activity than dieting. Females demonstrate a drive for thinness; males have increased concern with muscularity and shape (Timko et al., 2019).

Psychiatric disorders increase the risks of eating disorders. Low self-esteem, body dissatisfaction, and feelings of ineffectiveness also put individuals at risk. Bullying and weight teasing are other risk factors for the development of an eating disorder (Lie et al., 2019).

Elite athletes participating in lean sports, such as running and gymnastics, and nonelite athletes taking part in nonlean sports, such as soccer, experience a triad of symptoms (disordered eating, menstrual dysfunction, and osteoporosis). See Box 32.3. Athletes involved in lean sports are at higher risk of developing an eating disorder.

Comorbidity

Depression is common in individuals with anorexia nervosa, and these individuals are at risk for suicide attempts (Sagiv & Gvion, 2020). Anxiety disorders such as obsessive-compulsive disorder (OCD), phobias, and panic disorder are strongly associated with anorexia nervosa. In many individuals with anorexia nervosa, OCD symptoms predate the anorexia nervosa diagnosis by about 5 years, leading many researchers to consider OCD a causative or risk factor for anorexia nervosa (Udo & Gilo, 2019). In fact, perfectionism is an aspect of both OCD and anorexia nervosa and is considered a risk factor for anorexia nervosa (Wagner & Vitousek, 2019). These comorbid conditions may often resolve when anorexia nervosa has been treated successfully. However, in many cases, an anxiety disorder may continue even following successful treatment of anorexia nervosa.

Etiology

The etiology of anorexia nervosa is multidimensional. Some of the risk factors (discussed later) and the etiologic factors overlap. For example, dieting is a risk factor for the development of anorexia nervosa, but it is also an etiologic factor, and in its most serious form—starving—it is also a symptom.

Biologic Theories

There is evidence that the volume of gray and white matter in the brains of persons with anorexia nervosa is reduced but is normalized during weight restoration. These deficits may reflect malnourishment. Other

---

BOX 32.3

Eating Disorders and NCAA Collegiate Athletes

McDonald, A. H., Pritchard, M., & McGuire, M. K. (2020). Self-reported eating disorder risk in lean and non-lean NCAA Collegiate Athletes. Eating and Weight Disorders: EWD, 25(3), 745–750. https://doi.org/10.1007/s40519-019-00681-0

THE QUESTION: Are there gender differences in the overall scores of the Eating Attitudes Test (EAT-26) in National Collegiate Athletic Association (NCAA) college athletes in "lean" sports versus "nonlean" sports.

(Lean sports defined as those for which there is a presumed competitive advantage with a thin shape, lean body, and/or low weight such as aesthetic (i.e., gymnastics, diving, etc.), endurance (i.e., running, cycling, etc.), and weight-class (i.e., wrestling, martial arts, etc.) sports. Nonlean includes all other sports.)

METHODS: Using a self-report survey design, this study examined eating disorder risk in 121 NCAA college athletes, using the EAT-26. A high score (over 20) indicates further investigation is needed.

FINDINGS: Those in lean sport reported higher scores on behavior, whereas those in nonlean sports scored high in attitude. Looking at gender, females scored high on both attitudinal and behavioral sections. Males in lean sports report higher scores than males in nonlean sports.

IMPLICATIONS FOR NURSING: Nurses should be aware that both male and female athletes have higher rates of disordered eating and should be assessed for eating disorders. Nurses can teach parents and adolescents about the value of healthy athletic competition and the need to maintain healthy eating habits. Coaches as well as parents should be involved in educational programs, highlighting the risk factors for eating disorders and symptom identification. An accurate assessment of each young athlete, male or female, is important.

---

studies suggest that there may structural alterations even after long-term recovery (Curzio et al., 2020). Research is ongoing.

Genetic Theories

First-degree relatives of people with anorexia nervosa have higher rates of this disorder. Rates of partial-syndrome or subthreshold cases among female family members of individuals with anorexia nervosa are even higher (Bulik et al., 2019). Female relatives also have high rates of depression, leading researchers to hypothesize that a shared genetic factor may influence development of both disorders.

Genetic research shows that a genetic vulnerability to anorexia nervosa exists, especially in females. Genetic heritability accounts for an estimated 50% to 80% of the risk of developing an eating disorder. Separating genetic influences from environmental influences is difficult when twins share a similar family environment (Bulik et al., 2019).

Neuroendocrine and Neurotransmitter Changes

Several neurobiologic changes occur in an eating disorder. The most common findings are increased activation of the amygdala and changes in the activation of the cingulate cortex. An increase in endogenous opioids (through exercise) contributes to denial of hunger. Malnutrition leads to a decrease in thyroid function. Serotonergic functioning is also blunted in low-weight patients (Foldi et al., 2020; Scharner & Stengel, 2019; Smith et al., 2020).

Psychological Theories

Historically, the most widely accepted explanation of anorexia nervosa was the psychoanalytic paradigm that focused on conflicts of separation–individuation and autonomy. Usually diagnosed between 14 and 18 years of age, anorexia nervosa was thought to occur as a result of a developmental arrest of normal adolescent struggles around identity and role, body image formation, and sexuality (Bruch, 1973). Dieting and weight control were viewed as a means to defend against these feelings of inadequacy and growing into adulthood.

The psychoanalytic paradigm explained the disparity in the prevalence of eating disorders between boys and girls as being related to the development of self-esteem in adolescent girls. It was believed that the normal adolescent increase in self-doubt was linked to naturally occurring pubertal weight gain, which in turn resulted in confusion about one's identity. Unfortunately, this psychoanalytic perspective tended to blame parents, especially mothers, for the development of their child's illness. Today, the psychoanalytic theory is used in some psychotherapies, but it is no longer a competing theory of causation.

Internalization of Peer Pressure

Some adolescents have reported that dieting, binge eating, and purging initially began as a result of peer pressure and a need to conform. Subsequently, many factors then converge that influence the initials behaviors to develop into a full syndrome eating disorder. Peers and friends, as well as peers in the larger school system, influence unhealthy weight-control behaviors among preadolescent and adolescent girls (Smink et al., 2018).

Body Dissatisfaction

Once the body is considered all important, the individual begins to compare their body with others, such as those of celebrities. Images from television and fashion magazines are particularly powerful for young girls and adolescents struggling with the tasks of identity and body image formation. Body dissatisfaction resulting from this comparison, in which one's own body is perceived to fall short of an ideal, may be dissatisfaction about one's weight, shape, size, or even a certain body part. Even in the absence of overweight, most adolescents surveyed in numerous studies were dissatisfied with their bodies (Waszczuk et al., 2019). Because this factor is so prevalent in women and especially adolescents in this country, body dissatisfaction is considered less predictive for a diagnosis of anorexia nervosa (APA, 2013). Yet it remains an important factor that follows the internalizing of an idea body weight.

> **KEYCONCEPT Body dissatisfaction** occurs when the body is viewed negatively and becomes overvalued as a way of determining one's worth.

Many adolescents attempt to overcome this dissatisfaction through dieting and overexercising.

Social Theories

More than with any other psychiatric condition, society plays a significant role in the development of eating disorders with conflicting messages that young women receive from society about their roles in life. Young girls may interpret expectations about how they should look, what roles they should perform, and what they should achieve in society. Exposure to social media sites idealizing excessively thin bodies and glorifying extreme caloric restriction is associated with disordered eating behaviors (Griffiths et al., 2018).

The media, the fashion industry, and peer pressure are significant social influences. Magazines, television, videos, and the Internet depict young girls and adolescents, with thin and often emaciated bodies, as glamorous, successful, popular, and powerful. Girls diet because they want to be similar to these models both in character and appearance.

Preoccupation with body image and weight is also influenced by the obesity epidemic. A study on body dissatisfaction demonstrated that high BMIs and body dissatisfaction were more likely to occur in adolescents who later developed eating disorder symptoms (Goldstein & Gvion, 2019).

Preadolescent children are extremely susceptible to the message to reduce intake and increase exercise as a way to lose weight and maintain health. Coupled with Internet videos that sanction self-starvation, emerging adolescents are already dissatisfied with their bodies and have the tools to lose weight through dieting and exercise.

Feminists have focused on the role of this pressure regarding the female body as one part of an explanation

Since the 1970s, proponents of the feminist cultural model of eating disorders have advanced a position to explain the higher prevalence of these disorders in women. Feminists believe there is a struggle women have today similar to ones they believe women have had in history. They believe that during the Victorian era, "hysteria," a well-known emotional illness, developed as a result of oppression when women were not allowed to express their feelings and opinions and were "silenced" by a male-dominated society. Feminist scholars today have advanced the feminist relational model to understand the development of eating disorders. They view a major issue in development that causes conflict for young girls as the need to be connected versus society's view of the importance of separation. This confusion can be a stress that may be converted into disordered eating. Often at the base of symptoms such as severe food restriction is the gaining of power, lost possibly because of this confusion in one's development (Holmes, Drake, Odgers, Wilson, 2017).

for the significant increase in eating disorders and for the greater prevalence in females. Box 32.4 outlines some feminist assumptions regarding role, feminism, and the development of eating disorders.

Family Response to Disorder

Historically, the family of the patient with anorexia was labeled as overprotective, enmeshed, being unable to resolve conflicts, and being rigid regarding boundaries. Although an uninformed family can delay and complicate treatment, there is no evidence that family interactions are the cause of eating disorders but can contribute to its development (Kluck et al., 2017). Some family interactions can be problematic for the adolescent with an eating disorder. For example, when conflict erupts between two family members and direct communication is blocked, interaction patterns are changed that may result in a dysfunction relay of messages through other family members.

Enmeshment refers to an extreme form of intensity in family interactions and represents low individual autonomy in a family. In an enmeshed family, the individual gets lost in the family system. The boundaries that define individual autonomy are weak. This excessive togetherness intrudes on privacy (Minuchin et al., 1978).

Overprotectiveness is defined as a high degree of concern for one another and can be detrimental to children at high risk for anorexia nervosa. The parents' overprotectiveness retards the child's development of autonomy and competence (Minuchin et al., 1978). *Rigidity* refers to families that are heavily committed to maintaining the status quo and find change difficult. Conflict is avoided, and a strong ethical code or religious orientation is usually the rationale.

The family, often unwittingly, can transmit unrealistic attitudes about weight, shape, and size. Adolescents are particularly sensitive to comments about their bodies because this is the stage for body image formation. Parental attitudes about weight have been found to influence body dissatisfaction and dieting; parental comments about weight or shape or even parents' worrying about their own weight can influence adolescents in much the same way as the media does. See Box 32.5.

Hurtful weight-related comments by family members and significant others have been associated with disordered eating in both females and males. Adolescents' perceived family functioning and the quality of their relationship with each parent have been shown to positively influence body image dissatisfaction and disordered eating. Therefore, healthy family relationships are believed to be a protective factor for developing an eating disorder and support research findings linking parental-focused treatment programs to positive outcomes for those with eating disorders (Wallis et al., 2018).

Handford, C. M., Rapee, R. M., Fardouly, J. (2018). The influence of maternal modeling on body image concerns and eating disturbances in preadolescent girls. Behaviour Research and Therapy, 00:17-23. doi: 10.1016/j.brat.2017.11.001.

THE QUESTION: Do maternal attitudes and behavior about their daughter's weight and eating habits influence body esteem, body satisfaction, eating attitudes, and eating behaviors of young girls?

METHODS: Fifty mother-daughter pairs were recruited from the community and allocated to one of two conditions: maternal modeling (self-critical remarks about their own weight, shape, and diet) or no modeling. Daughters were then asked to complete body esteem, body satisfaction, and eating attitudes questionnaires (pre- and post-maternal modeling).

FINDINGS: Girls whose mothers made self-critical comments about their own appearance and diet reported lower body esteem, lower body satisfaction, more problematic eating attitudes, and ate significantly fewer sweets than girls whose mothers had not made self-critical comments.

IMPLICATIONS FOR NURSING: Families should be cautioned that self-critical statements can lead to daughters' lower esteem, body dissatisfaction, and more problematic eating attitudes.

RECOVERY-ORIENTED CARE FOR PERSONS WITH ANOREXIA NERVOSA

Teamwork and Collaboration: Working Toward Recovery

Treatment for the patient with anorexia nervosa focuses on initiating nutritional rehabilitation to restore the individual to a healthy weight, resolving psychological conflicts around body image disturbance, increasing effective coping, addressing the underlying conflicts related to maturity fears and role conflict, and assisting the family with healthy functioning and communication. Several methods are used to accomplish these goals during the stages of illness and recovery.

The medical complications presented in Table 32.1 influence the decision to hospitalize an individual with an eating disorder. Suicidality is another reason for hospitalization. The criteria for hospital admission vary, and there is a lack of evidence-based studies determining when adolescents with anorexia nervosa should be hospitalized. The APA criteria are outlined in Box 32.6.

After an acceptable weight (at least 85% of ideal) is established, the patient is discharged to a partial hospitalization program or an intensive outpatient program. The intensive therapies needed to help patients with their underlying issues (e.g., body distortion and maturity fears) and to help families with communication and enmeshment usually begin after refeeding because concentration is usually impaired in severely undernourished patients with anorexia.

Family therapy typically begins while the patient is still hospitalized. Recently family-based therapies and caregiver-based approaches have shown promise in the treatment of eating disorders. These assist in improving overall communication within the family and helps members understand the disorder (Wong et al., 2019).

Interpersonal therapy (IPT) is a type of treatment that focuses on uncovering and resolving the developmental and psychological issues underlying the disorder. Role transitions and negative social evaluations typically are the focus (Miniati et al., 2018). IPT and family-based therapies are sometimes combined.

TABLE 32.1	COMPLICATIONS OF EATING DISORDERS
Body System	**Symptoms**
From Starvation to Weight Loss	
Musculoskeletal	Loss of muscle mass, loss of fat (emaciation), osteoporosis
Metabolic	Hypothyroidism (symptoms include lack of energy, weakness, intolerance to cold, and bradycardia), hypoglycemia, decreased insulin sensitivity
Cardiac	Bradycardia; hypotension; loss of cardiac muscle; small heart; cardiac arrhythmias, including atrial and ventricular premature contractions, prolonged QT interval, ventricular tachycardia, sudden death
Gastrointestinal	Delayed gastric emptying, bloating, constipation, abdominal pain, gas, diarrhea
Reproductive	Amenorrhea, low levels of luteinizing hormone and follicle-stimulating hormone, irregular periods
Dermatologic	Dry, cracking skin and brittle nails caused by dehydration, lanugo (fine, baby like hair over the body), edema, acrocyanosis (bluish hands and feet), thinning hair
Hematologic	Leukopenia, anemia, thrombocytopenia, hypercholesterolemia, hypercarotenemia
Neuropsychiatric	Abnormal taste sensation (possible zinc deficiency) Apathetic depression, mild organic mental symptoms, sleep disturbances, fatigue
Related to Purging (Vomiting and Laxative Abuse)	
Metabolic	Electrolyte abnormalities, particularly hypokalemia, hypochloremic alkalosis; hypomagnesemia; increased blood urea nitrogen
Gastrointestinal	Salivary gland and pancreatic inflammation and enlargement with increase in serum amylase, esophageal and gastric erosion (esophagitis) rupture, dysfunctional bowel with dilation, superior mesenteric artery syndrome
Dental	Erosion of dental enamel (perimylolysis), particularly of the frontal teeth, with decreased decay
Neuropsychiatric	Seizures (related to large fluid shifts and electrolyte disturbances), mild neuropathies, fatigue, weakness, mild organic mental symptoms
Cardiac	Ipecac cardiomyopathy arrhythmias

BOX 32.6

Criteria for Hospitalization of Patients with Eating Disorders

MEDICAL

- Acute weight loss, <85% below ideal
- Heart rate near 40 beats/min
- Temperature, <36.1°C
- Blood pressure, <80/50 mm Hg
- Hypokalemia
- Hypophosphatemia
- Hypomagnesemia
- Poor motivation to recover

PSYCHIATRIC

- Risk for suicide
- Severe depression
- Failure to comply with treatment
- Inadequate response to treatment at another level of care (outpatient)

Adapted from American Psychiatric Association (2006). Treatment of patients with eating disorders, third edition. *American Journal of Psychiatry, 163*(7 suppl), 4–54.

Dialectic behavioral therapy specifically designed for patients with anorexia nervosa has shown positive results. This skills training type of intervention focuses on emotional dysregulation, viewed as a key symptom in anorexia nervosa (Accurso et al., 2018).

Safety Issues

Mortality is high among patients with anorexia nervosa, especially when compared with other mental illnesses, and is reported to be 3% to 7% with a longer duration of the disorder predicting the higher range of the mortality rate (Chidiac, 2019). Suicide and cardiopulmonary arrest are the leading cause of death for individuals with anorexia nervosa (Goldstein & Gvion, 2019). These individuals tend to die by suicide with highly lethal means in which rescue is unlikely. Nurses need to pay special attention to the risk of suicide with these individuals (see Chapter 21). A significant number of individuals with eating disorders also self-injure without suicide attempts (Sagiv & Gvion, 2020).

EVIDENCE-BASED NURSING CARE FOR PERSONS WITH ANOREXIA NERVOSA DISORDER

Mental Health Nursing Assessment

Physical Health Assessment

A thorough evaluation of body systems is important because many systems are compromised by starvation. A careful history from both the patient with anorexia

nervosa and the family, including the length and duration of symptoms, such as fasting, avoiding meals, and over-exercising, is necessary to assess altered nutrition. Nursing management involves various biopsychosocial assessments and interventions.

Patients with longer durations of these maladaptive behaviors typically have more difficult and prolonged recovery periods.

NCLEXNOTE Eating disorders are serious psychiatric disorders that threaten life. Careful assessment and referral for treatment are important nursing interventions.

The patient's weight is determined using the BMI and a scale. Currently, criteria for discharge require patients to be at least 85% of ideal weight according to height and weight tables. BMI, thought to reflect weight most accurately because exact height is used, is calculated by dividing weight in kilograms by height in meters squared. An acceptable BMI is between about 19 and 25.

Menses history also must be explored in that it provides information about possible estrogen depletion. However, it is often difficult to conclude that amenorrhea is present due to starvation because females in this age group often have irregular periods, and some are on oral contraceptives. However, if menses was regular prior to anorexia nervosa, a return to regular menses after treatment can signify substantial body fat restoration. Fat and weight restoration have been hypothesized to aid in the loss of bone mineral density (Karageorgiou et al., 2020).

Psychosocial Assessment

Mental Status and Appearance

Behavioral Responses

The psychological symptoms that patients with anorexia experience are listed in Box 32.1. The classic symptoms of body distortion—fear of weight gain, unrealistic expectations and thinking, and ritualistic behaviors—are easily noted during a clinical interview. Often, people with anorexia nervosa avoid conflict and have difficulty expressing negative emotions, such as anger. Other conflicts, such as sexuality fears and feelings of ineffectiveness, may underlie this disorder. These symptoms may not be apparent during a clinical interview; however, a variety of instruments is available to clinicians and researchers for determining their presence and severity. There is a high rate of nonsuicidal self-injury in patients with eating disorders, and the type and frequency of these behaviors should be assessed (Sagiv & Gvion, 2020).

The Eating Attitudes Test is frequently used in community samples (Garner et al., 1982). There is also a child version of this test, the CHEAT. The results of these paper-and-pencil tests can help identify the most significant symptoms for an individual patient and indicate a focus for interventions, especially therapy. In clinical settings, the Eating Disorder Examination Questionnaire (EDEQ) is most often used (Hilbert et al., 2012).

Self-Concept

Individuals with eating disorders are usually struggling with their self-concept. It is important to determine their self-concept and self-esteem. In many instances, these individuals appear to be very competent, but when queried about their views, they often feel that they are not good enough and will describe their perceived faults in great detail.

Stress and Coping Patterns

Individuals with an eating disorder are often coping with stress and anxiety through controlling eating. In times of perceived stressful events, the dysfunctional eating pattern often becomes worse. An assessment of the stress the person is experiencing and coping patterns is important because a part of successful treatment is developing healthy coping skills.

Social Assessment

The assessment should also focus on family interaction, influence, and peer relationships. The role of the patient in the family and community should be considered, as well as the person's ability to cope in social situations. For adolescents who are attending school, a conference with the teacher or counselor provides information regarding the amount and frequency of social contacts.

Quality of Life

Persons with anorexia nervosa have a lowered quality of life than others with psychiatric disorders or those without psychiatric disorders. Behaviors associated with AN such as low body mass index, depression, anxiety, and purging are associated with lower quality of life. Individuals with AN often recall selective events and focus on negative aspect of the event, which, in turn, contributes to a low quality of life (Hamatani et al., 2017).

Strengths Assessment

Strengths such as motivation to eat differently and have a more normal life may emerge during the interview. The following questions could be asked to elicit personal strengths:

- Do you remember a time when you did not have to worry about what you ate? If so, how old were you and what did you like to do?

- Have you found any strategy that prevented you from worrying about what you hate?
- Are you ready to change your eating patterns? What do you think will help you change your eating patterns?
- When you are successful in other areas (school, athletics), how do you reward yourself?

CLINICAL JUDGMENT

Medical complications and suicide ideation are the two top priorities. Bradycardia and hypotension are well-established responses to starvation. Cardiac issues should be treated before the psychological issues can be meaningfully addressed. Normal electrolyte balance should be restored. Suicidality is also a high priority of nursing care and should be carefully assessed.

THERAPEUTIC RELATIONSHIP

Establishing a therapeutic relationship with individuals with anorexia nervosa may be difficult initially because they tend to be suspicious and mistrustful, especially of authority figures and health personnel, who they believe will intervene to disrupt their restricting and starvation behaviors, placing them in a position of extreme fear of becoming fat. At the time they are hospitalized, mistrust can almost reach a state of paranoia. Because of their low body weight and starvation, they are often impatient and irritable. A firm, accepting, and patient approach is important in working with these individuals. Providing a rationale for all interventions helps build trust, as does a consistent, nonreactive approach. Power struggles over eating are common, and remaining nonreactive is a challenge. During such power struggles, the nurse should always think about their own feelings of frustration and need for control.

MENTAL HEALTH NURSING INTERVENTIONS

Establishing Mental Health and Wellness Goals

The mental health and wellness goals are very closely aligned for people with eating disorders. Successful recovery from an eating disorder involves establishing positive wellness habits of nutrition, physical activity, sleep, coping with stress, and developing a support system. The nurse and patient should prioritize long- and short-term goals. For example, a long-term goal is to maintain a normal weight through healthy eating and exercise. A short-term goal is to increase food intake by 300 calories per day.

NCLEXNOTE Setting realistic eating goals is one of the most helpful interventions for patients with eating disorders. Because individuals with anorexia nervosa are often perfectionistic, they often set unrealistic goals.

One of the most helpful skills the nurse can teach is to set realistic goals around food and around other activities or tasks. Because of perfectionism, patients with anorexia often set unrealistic goals and end up frustrated. The nurse can help them establish smaller, more realistic, and attainable goals.

Physical Care

The person with anorexia can usually perform self-care activities. They may actually be overly perfectionistic regarding daily self-care activities. If symptoms become severe, hospitalization may be necessary to re-establish a healthy body weight.

Nutritional Rehabilitation

Refeeding, the most important intervention during the hospital or initial stage of treatment, is also the most challenging. In anorexia nervosa, there is a shift from carbohydrate to fat and protein utilization, placing the body in a catabolic state. In this state, there is an altered insulin response and increased glucagon secretion. As nutritional balance is re-established, anabolic metabolism is restored and the body switches back to carbohydrate metabolism leading to lower levels of phosphate.

The refeeding protocol typically starts with 1,500 calories a day and is increased slowly until the patient is consuming at least 3,500 calories a day in several meals. The higher the initial number of calories prescribed has been demonstrated to influence a shorter length of hospital stay and recovery (Garber et al., 2016). The usual plan for patients with very low weights is a weight gain of between 1 and 2 lb. a week. In severe malnourished adolescents, and especially those resisting refeeding, nasogastric tube feeding of supplements alone, or combined with meals, may be instituted (Garber et al., 2016).

There is controversy regarding aggressive refeeding. To prevent further weight loss, rapid increase of calories provides the best result. However, food anxiety is commonly experienced by people with AN, especially if there is a co-morbid disorder such as depression, obsessive-compulsive disorder, or PTSD. Increased anxiety can exacerbate the symptoms, making recovery more difficult. It is important that benefits of refeeding be weighed against the risk of increasing anxiety (Levinson et al., 2019).

The person will be fearful of weight gain and may refuse to eat. The nurse must monitor and record all intake carefully as part of the weight gain protocol. Weight-increasing protocols usually include behavioral plans using positive reinforcements (i.e., excursion passes) and negative reinforcements (i.e., returning to bed rest) to encourage weight gain. The nurse should help patients to understand that these actions are not punitive. When all staff members agree on a clear protocol for behaviors related to eating and weight gain, reactivity of the staff to the patient is greatly reduced. These protocols provide ready-made, consistent responses to food-refusal behaviors and should be carried out in a caring and supportive context. On rare occasions when the patient is unable to recognize or accept their illness (denial) and their malnutrition is life-threatening, nasogastric tube feedings may be necessary.

Electrolytes may be completely depleted in anorexia nervosa, so nursing care involves stabilizing electrolyte balance. Potassium depletion usually results from use of diuretics, diarrhea, and vomiting. Calcium depletion is related to large intake of dietary fiber, which decreases calcium absorption. Many individuals also need phosphorus replacement (Peebles et al., 2017). During hospitalization, these electrolytes, if warranted, are replaced through oral or intravenous therapy.

A complication of refeeding is the development of **refeeding syndrome** (severe electrolyte disturbances). This condition can develop during the refeeding process and include circulatory fluid overload, respiratory failure, and cardiac failure. Hypophosphatemia is a precursor to refeeding syndrome, which can result in sudden death (Parker et al., 2020).

Promotion of Sleep

Sleep disturbance is also common, and these individuals are viewed as hyperkinetic. They sleep little, but they usually awaken in an energized state. A structured, healthy sleep routine must be established immediately to conserve energy and calorie expenditure because of low weight. To further conserve energy, patients are often relegated to bed rest until a certain amount of weight is regained. Exercise is generally not permitted during refeeding and only with caution after this phase. Inpatients must be closely supervised because they are often found exercising in their rooms, running in place, and doing calisthenics.

Medication Interventions

Selective serotonin reuptake inhibitors (SSRIs) are useful in the treatment of AN, especially regarding comorbid influences and symptoms such as OCD. The SSRI fluoxetine (Prozac) is approved by the Food and Drug Administration for the treatment of anorexia nervosa. Of course, comorbid conditions such as depression or OCD should be treated with appropriate medication. The nurse may be responsible for administering medications or providing patient and family teaching. See Box 32.7.

BOX 32.7

Fluoxetine Hydrochloride (Prozac)

DRUG CLASS: Selective serotonin reuptake inhibitor

RECEPTOR AFFINITY: Inhibits central nervous system neuronal uptake of serotonin with little effect on norepinephrine; thought to antagonize muscarinic, histaminergic, and α-adrenergic receptors

INDICATIONS: Treatment of depressive disorders, obsessive-compulsive disorder, bulimia nervosa, and panic disorder

ROUTES AND DOSAGE: Available in 10- and 20-mg capsules and 20-mg/5-mL oral solution

ADULTS: 20 mg/d in the morning, not to exceed 80 mg/d. Full antidepressant effect may not be seen for up to 4 weeks. If no improvement, dosage is increased after several weeks. Dosages greater than 20 mg/d are administered twice daily. For eating disorders: typically, 60 mg/d is recommended.

GERIATRIC: Administer at lower or less frequent doses; monitor responses to guide dosage.

CHILDREN: Safety and efficacy have not been established.

HALF-LIFE (PEAK EFFECT): 2 to 3 days (6 to 8 hours)

SELECTED ADVERSE REACTIONS: Headache, nervousness, insomnia, drowsiness, anxiety, tremors, dizziness, lightheadedness, nausea, vomiting, diarrhea, dry mouth, anorexia, dyspepsia, constipation, taste changes, upper respiratory infections, pharyngitis, painful menstruation, sexual dysfunction, urinary frequency, sweating, rash, pruritus, weight loss, asthenia, and fever

BOXED WARNING: Increased risk of suicidal thoughts and behaviors in children, adolescents, and young adults.

WARNINGS: Avoid use in pregnancy and while breastfeeding. Use with caution in patients with impaired hepatic or renal function and diabetes mellitus. Possible risk for toxicity if taken with tricyclic antidepressants.

SPECIAL PATIENT AND FAMILY EDUCATION
- Be aware that the drug may take up to 4 weeks to get a full antidepressant effect.
- Take the drug in the morning or in divided doses, if necessary.
- Families and caregivers of pediatric patients being treated with antidepressants should monitor patients for agitation, irritation, and unusual changes in behavior.
- Report any adverse reactions.
- Avoid driving a car or performing hazardous activities because the drug may cause drowsiness or dizziness.
- Eat small, frequent meals to help with complaints of nausea and vomiting.

Management of Complications

Anorexia nervosa has the highest mortality rate of any mental illness. Every organ system can be adversely affected by AN—metabolic, cardiopulmonary, endocrine, gastrointestinal, and hematological. Laboratory tests that are typically ordered include CBC, calcium, magnesium, and phosphorus, liver function and albumin, vitamin D, serum BUN, creatinine, blood glucose, and TSH. Other tests usually included are stool examination for occult blood, ECG, bone densitometry, and abdominal x-ray. Results of all tests should be monitored frequently.

Some patients may have dysphagia as a result of malnutrition and will need to modify diet texture. Low fiber diets that are soft and easy to digest are recommended to reduce the feeding volume and the symptoms of early satiety. The patient may need tube feedings.

SMA (superior mesenteric artery) syndrome is a rare disorder in which acute angulation of the SMA causes compression of the third part of the duodenum between the SMA and the aorta. SMA syndrome can lead to obstruction of the duodenum and can occur in AN, causing patients to have epigastric abdominal pain and a need for a liquid diet or tube feeding.

Multiple musculoskeletal complications are associated with AN, including sarcopenia, which can result in functional weakness and balance impairments that increase fall risks. Physical therapy evaluation and treatment are important when bone mineral density is decreased. Even though falls are not usually associated with a young age group, fall risk evaluation should be conducted for a person with AN.

Psychosocial Interventions

Therapeutic Interactions

Identifying feelings, such as anxiety and fear, and especially negative emotions, such as anger, is the first step in helping patients to decrease conflict avoidance and develop effective strategies for coping with these feelings.

Do not attempt to change distorted body image by merely pointing out that the patient is actually too thin. This symptom is often the last to resolve itself, and some individuals may take years to see their bodies realistically. However, although this symptom is difficult to abate, patients can continue to fear becoming fat but not be driven to act on the distortion by starving. The fear of becoming fat eventually lessens with time.

Enhancing Cognitive Functioning

The nurse can help individuals with cognitive distortions and unrealistic assumptions to restructure the way they view the world, especially relative to food, eating, weight, and shape. Faulty ways of viewing these situations result in ineffective coping. Table 32.2 lists some distortions commonly experienced by individuals with eating disorders and some typical restructuring responses or statements that challenge the distortion, which the nurse can present as more realistic ways of perceiving situations. Imagery and relaxation are often used to overcome distortions and to decrease anxiety stemming from a distorted body image.

Using Behavioral Intervention

Many of the same behavioral interventions used in the care of persons who are depressed or anxious are also implemented in the care of persons with AN. See Chapter 7. Reinforcing and rewarding positive eating behaviors and avoiding reinforcement of perfectionistic and ritualistic behaviors can help the patient re-focus on meaningful, healthy behaviors.

Psychoeducation

When weight is restored and concentration is improved, patients with anorexia nervosa can benefit from psychoeducation. Although these individuals have a wealth of knowledge about food and calories, they also have misinformation that needs clarifying. For example, they are often unclear about the role of "fats" in a healthy diet and try to be as "fat free" as possible. A thorough assessment of their knowledge is important because they seem to be "walking calorie books" with little information on the role of all of the nutrients and the importance of including them in a healthy diet. There are several topic areas that should be included in a teaching plan. See Box 32.8.

Teaching Strategies

Several factors influence the outcome of treatment for individuals with anorexia nervosa. Particularly long duration of symptoms and low weight when treatment begins predict poor outcomes, but family support and involvement generally improve outcomes. Comorbid conditions and their severity also influence recovery, especially anxiety disorders. Although patients are discharged from the hospital when their weight has reached 85% of what is considered ideal, restoration of healthy eating and changes in maladaptive thinking may not have yet occurred. Individuals often continue to restrict foods. Therefore, without intensive outpatient treatment, including nutritional counseling and support, they are unlikely to recover fully. Distorted thinking and eating patterns can set the stage for a relapse and later for the possible development of bulimia nervosa.

TABLE 32.2	COGNITIVE DISTORTIONS TYPICAL OF PATIENTS WITH EATING DISORDERS, WITH RESTRUCTURING STATEMENTS
Distortion	**Clarification or Restructuring**
Dichotomous or All-or-Nothing Thinking	
"I've gained 2 lb., so I'll be up to 100 lb. soon."	"You have never gained 100 lb., but I understand that gaining 2 lb. is scary."
Magnification	
"I binged last night, so I can't go out with anyone."	"Feeling bad and guilty about a binge are difficult feelings, but you are in treatment, and you have been monitoring and changing your eating."
Selective Abstraction	
"I can only be happy 10 lb. lighter."	"When you were 10 lb. lighter, you were hospitalized. You can choose to be happy about many things in your life."
Overgeneralization	
"I didn't eat anything yesterday and did okay, so I don't think not eating for a week or two will harm me."	"Any starvation harms the body, whether or not outward signs were apparent to you. The more you starve, the more problems your body will encounter."
Catastrophizing	
"I purged last night for the first time in 4 months—I'll never recover."	"Recovery includes up and downs, and it is expected you will still have some mild but infrequent symptoms."

BOX 32.8

Anorexia Nervosa

When caring for a patient with anorexia nervosa, be sure to include the following topic areas in the teaching plan:

- Psychopharmacologic agents, if used, including drug, action, dosage, frequency, and possible adverse effects
- Nutrition and eating patterns
- Effect of restrictive eating or dieting
- Weight monitoring
- Safety and comfort measures
- Avoidance of triggers
- Self-monitoring techniques
- Trust
- Realistic goal setting
- Resources

Wellness Challenges and Strategies

Individuals with AN are very aware of wellness recommendations related to nutrition and exercise. Since they focus on nutrition, exercise, and weight control, their real challenge is to focus less on nutrition and exercise and more on developing positive self-concept and emotional wellness. They often ignore the other wellness dimensions, such as developing positive coping skills for stress management, developing a sense of connection with others, and searching for meaning or a purpose in life. See Box 32.9.

Providing Family Education

Denial, guilt, and subsequent greater overprotectiveness are common reactions of the family, especially when hospitalization has been necessary. In addition to family therapy with a skilled therapist, the nurse can help family members express their feelings, increase effective communication, decrease protectiveness, and resolve guilt. Often, siblings become resentful of the patient with an eating disorder because of the significant amount of attention they get from their parents. Having siblings discuss these feelings and the effect the illness has had on them is helpful. Families and friends are eager to help the patient with anorexia but often need direction. Box 32.10 provides a list of strategies that may assist them.

BOX 32.9

Wellness Challenges and Strategies

- Recognizing the need for moderate physical activity, healthy foods, and sleep
- Strategies: Limit physical activity to a reasonable schedule
- Practice increasing amounts of healthy food
- Track sleep and increase amount of sleep (if needed) and engage sleep hygiene techniques
- Coping effectively with drive for thinness.
- Strategies: Identify times when the need to restrict diet occurs; Examine other strategies in dealing with the situation
- Stress management
- Strategies: Practice meditation, use cognitive strategies to examine beliefs and thoughts
- Increase self-concept
- Strategies: Keep a list of accomplishments, help others; keep busy; counseling or therapy
- Developing a sense of connection, belong, and a support system
- Strategies: Develop a plan to increase social contact
- Expanding a sense of purpose and meaning in life
- Strategies: Pray, meditate, help others, volunteer

BOX 32.10

What Family and Friends Can Do to Help Those with Eating Disorders

- Tell the person you are concerned, you care, and you would like to help. Suggest that the person seek professional help from a physician or therapist.
- If the person refuses to seek professional help, encourage reaching out to an adult, such as a teacher, school nurse, or counselor.
- Do not discuss weight, the number of calories being consumed, or particular eating habits.
- Do try to talk about things other than food, weight, counting calories, and exercise.
- Avoid making comments about a person's appearance. Concern about weight loss may be interpreted as a compliment; comments regarding weight gain may be felt as criticism.
- It will not help to become involved in a power struggle. You cannot force the person to eat.
- You can offer support. Ultimately, however, the responsibility and the decision to accept help and to change rest with the person.
- Read and educate yourself regarding these disorders.

Promoting Safety

If hospitalized, the patient's systems are monitored closely because at the time of admission, most patients are severely malnourished (see Table 32.1). Patients usually are placed on a privilege-earning program in which privileges, such as having visitors and receiving passes to go outside the hospital, are earned based on weight gain. See Chapter 10.

Developing Recovery-Oriented Rehabilitation Strategies

Recovery of persons with anorexia nervosa focuses on physical, psychological, and social aspects. Maintaining a normal weight and nutrition will require resisting urges to diet and overexercise. Motivation to continue to work toward recovery should be supported throughout recovery. Development of cognitive strategies to address these issues will need to be reinforced through attending support groups and maintaining a treatment alliance with a provider.

Relapse prevention plays a major role in recovery. The patient and family should work closely with a clinician to understand the patient's individual relapse process. Together, they identify the triggers and early warning signs of relapse and agree upon a relapse prevention plan that responds to the triggers (Berends et al., 2018).

Evaluation and Treatment Outcomes

Short-term outcomes for individuals with anorexia nervosa after hospitalization are generally poor. Poor outcomes are related to lower body mass indices (BMI) at the beginning of treatment, the level of impulsivity, self-induced vomiting, and higher trait anxiety purging (vomiting and laxative use). Long-term outcomes are more positive than short-term outcomes, but remission rates vary from 20% to 70%, depending on the criteria used in the studies. Many individuals do recover, but recovery often takes years and can be characterized by residual symptoms (Fichter et al., 2017).

Continuum of Care

Emergency Care

Emergency care is not usually needed for individuals with anorexia nervosa. Family members and peers usually notice the weight loss and emaciation before patients' systems are compromised to the degree that they require emergency treatment. If systems are compromised enough to warrant emergency treatment, patients usually are admitted immediately for medical-surgical inpatient care.

Inpatient

Hospitalization is required based on criteria noted in Box 32.6. Because of its life-threatening nature, anorexia nervosa in its very acute stage is unlikely to be manageable in outpatient settings.

Community Care

After refeeding, treatment of anorexia nervosa takes place on an outpatient basis and involves individual and family therapy, nutrition counseling to reinforce healthy eating patterns and attitudes, and physician visits to monitor weight and evaluate somatic recovery. Support groups, which are often suggested, should not be substituted for therapy. Following an inpatient treatment program, many anorexia nervosa patients are referred for intensive outpatient therapy or day treatment programs prior to the usual outpatient therapy of 1 or 2 hourly sessions a week. In intensive outpatient therapy, patients may return to school but participate four to five evenings a week in a 4- to 5-hour structured program that includes group therapy, meeting with a dietician, and individual therapy. After full recovery, support groups are useful in maintaining recovery.

School Interventions

Younger patients with anorexia nervosa may have lost some school time because of hospitalization. Integrating back into a school and classroom setting is difficult for most. Shame and guilt about having an eating disorder and being hospitalized must be addressed. Because these patients typically have isolated themselves before hospitalization and treatment, renewing friendships and relationships with peers may provoke anxiety. Involving school nurses and teachers in the reentry process may help.

Prevention and early detection strategies for parents and schoolteachers are often the focus of school nurses and mental health nurses who work in the community. Some of these strategies appear in Box 32.11 and are based on the research on risk factors and protective factors.

National eating disorder awareness and advocacy groups work toward educating the general public, those at risk, and those who work with groups at risk, such as teachers and coaches. They also monitor the media and work to remove unhealthy advertisements and articles that appear in magazines appealing to young girls. Policies, both health and social, can decrease the prevalence of eating disorders. Strategies include improving school-based curriculum to include content on prevention of Eds, implementing school-based anti-bullying policies that protect students from being bullied about their weight, and training educators including coaches and health providers on prevention and early identification.

BOX 32.11

Eating Disorder Prevention Strategies for Parents and Children

EDUCATION FOR PARENTS
- Real versus ideal weight
- Influence of attitudes, behaviors, teasing
- Ways to increase self-esteem
- Role of media: TV, magazines
- Signs and symptoms
- Interventions for obesity
- Boys at risk also
- Observe for rituals
- Supervision of eating and exercise

STRATEGIES FOR CHILDREN
Education
- Peer pressure regarding eating, weight
- Menses, puberty, normal weight gain
- Strategies for obesity
- Ways to develop or improve self-esteem
- Body image traps: media, retail clothing
- Adapting and coping with problems
- Reporting friends with signs of eating disorders
  Screening: Screen for risk factors
  Assessment: Assess for treatment
  Follow-up: Monitor for relapse

Virtual Mental Health Care

Virtual mental health care is available through electronic applications available for downloading on a cell phone from national helplines such as the National Eating Disorders Association and the National Association of Anorexia and Associated Disorders. Virtual applications are also being used in treatment of distorted body image to help the person receive realistic representation of body size (Irvine et al, 2020).

Integration With Primary Care

Persons with eating disorders are frequently treated in primary care for medical issues related to their eating disorder. Care in the mental health and primary care services should be coordinated with the mental health service providing care focusing on mental health issues and primary care treating the medical issues. When there are few psychiatric services available, eating disorders are treated and monitored by the primary care provider. The patient should have access to a therapist and dietitian in any treatment setting. Due to the fast-paced nature of primary care, eating disorders are not as easily recognized in a general health care setting and are often missed.

BULIMIA NERVOSA

Bulimia nervosa was once thought to be a type of anorexia nervosa. However, findings from extensive investigations have identified its characteristics as a separate entity. It is more prevalent than anorexia nervosa. Individuals with bulimia nervosa are usually older at onset than are those with anorexia nervosa. The disorder generally is not as life threatening as anorexia nervosa. The usual treatment is outpatient therapy. Outcomes are better for bulimia nervosa than for anorexia nervosa, and mortality rates are lower.

Clinical Course

Few outward signs are associated with bulimia nervosa. Individuals binge (eating an excessive amount, usually at one sitting) and purge (purposeful initiation of stomach or bowel evacuation through artificial means such as vomiting or laxatives) in secret and are typically of normal weight; therefore, it does not come to the attention of parents and peers as readily as does anorexia nervosa. Treatment consequently can be delayed for years as individuals attempt on their own to get their eating under control. Patients usually initiate their own treatment when control of their eating becomes impossible. When treatment is undertaken and completed, patients

typically recover completely, except in cases in which personality disorders and comorbid serious depression are also present.

Patients with bulimia nervosa present as overwhelmed and overly committed individuals, "social butterflies" who have difficulty with setting limits and establishing appropriate boundaries. They have an enormous number of rules regarding food and food restriction, and they feel shame, guilt, and disgust about their binge eating and purging. They may also be impulsive in other areas of their lives, such as spending.

Diagnostic Criteria

Bulimia nervosa involves eating a large amount of food within a discrete period of time (e.g., 2 hours) and engaging in recurrent episodes of binge eating and compensatory purging in various forms such as vomiting or using laxatives, diuretics, or emetics or in nonpurging compensatory behaviors, such as fasting or over-exercising in order to avoid weight gain. These episodes must occur at least once a week for a period of at least 3 months to meet the *DSM-5* criteria. Self-evaluation is excessively and inappropriately influenced by body weight and shape. Unlike anorexia nervosa, there is little or no weight loss. See Box 32.1 for characteristics related to bulimia nervosa.

Remember Ellen?

She is of normal weight but has been vomiting one to two times a week for several months after binging. She has callouses on her hands from her teeth when she gagged herself. She sees herself as very overweight.

Does Ellen have characteristics of bulimia nervosa? If she did not know that these behaviors were symptoms of bulimia, how would you explain to her what her symptoms might mean?

Binge eating is defined as rapid, episodic, impulsive, and uncontrollable ingestion of a large amount of food during a short period of time, usually 1 to 2 hours. Eating is followed by feelings of guilt, remorse, and often self-contempt, leading to purging. To assuage the out-of-control feeling, severe dieting is instituted, and these restrictions, referred to as *dietary restraint*, precipitate the next binge. The restrictions are viewed as "rules," such as no sweets, no fats, and so forth. The rules may be about what one can and cannot eat. Each binge sets up an out-of-control feeling, and thus the individual then sees the need for even stricter rules about what can and cannot be consumed, leading to more frequent binge eating. This cycle has prompted clinicians to focus treatment primarily on interventions related to dietary restraint. When dietary restraint is resolved, binge eating is decreased, and generally the purging that follows binge eating also is decreased. Feeling out of control with food is often the major complaint when individuals seek treatment for bulimia nervosa.

> **KEYCONCEPT Dietary restraint** has been described by researchers in the field of eating disorders as a way to explain the relationship between dieting and binge eating.

Dieters' deprivation, or restraint, whether real or imagined, contributes to overeating and binging. Genetic predisposition for binge eating and deprivation may make dieters more prone to feel distressed over their dietary "failures," especially if dieting has become a way to overcome body dissatisfaction and to compensate for distress through dietary restraint that leads to overeating (Castillo & Weiselberg, 2017). Whether the eating is influenced by the attraction of forbidden foods or by internal needs to assuage failure, there is significant evidence that restraining one's intake is a precondition for bouts of overeating.

Bulimia Nervosa Across the Lifespan

Bulimia nervosa occurs in all age groups. It is not as common in children as in adolescents and adults; children appear more likely to have BED, discussed later. This finding has only recently been reported, and more data are needed to substantiate this finding.

Epidemiology and Risk Factors

Recent epidemiologic data report the lifetime prevalence of bulimia nervosa to be as high as 2.3% depending on whether clinical or community populations are sampled, but it is estimated that less than one third of the cases have been detected. Strict criteria are used when clinical groups are studied as opposed to self-reported symptoms in community surveys, making the community sample prevalence rates higher (Wade, 2019).

Age of Onset

Typically, the age of onset is between 15 and 24 years, which is later than the typical onset of anorexia nervosa. Some women older than the typical age of onset have developed bulimia nervosa and symptom cases have been identified as subsequent to life stressors such as a loss (Silén et al., 2020).

Gender Differences

As with anorexia nervosa, females are 10 times more likely than males to experience bulimia nervosa. Box 32.2 highlights boys and men with eating disorders.

Ethnicity and Culture

Bulimia nervosa is related to culture in the same way as anorexia nervosa. In western cultures and those becoming westernized in their norms, the focus on achieving a thin body ideal underlies the dieting and dietary restraint that set up the trajectory toward a diagnosable eating disorder. Any ethnic differences have to do with the degree to which individuals from specific cultural backgrounds internalize the thin ideal.

Comorbidity

The most common comorbid conditions are anxiety disorders, mood disorders, self-harm, and substance use. If a comorbid condition occurs before the eating disorder develops, it may actually have a role in precipitating the disorder (Wade, 2019). The suicide rate for bulimia is around 7.5%, with suicide attempts and ideation ranging from 15% to 40%.

There are several medical complications affecting those with bulimia. Electrolyte imbalance can lead to cardiac arrhythmia, seizure, and death. Self-induced vomiting with loss of stomach acid can result in hyperchloremic alkalosis and hypokalemia. Chronic vomiting can result in subconjunctival hemorrhages, esophageal damage, acid reflux, and dental lesions (Castillo & Weiselberg, 2017).

Risk Factors

There are numerous risk factors associated with bulimia nervosa, including genetic risk, female gender, obstetric complication and perinatal factors, higher body mass index, frequent dieting, over-exercising, and concern about body weight. Childhood sexual abuse and/or neglect has often been suggested as a risk factor for eating disorders. The beginning of puberty and the start of early adulthood are high-risk periods when adverse life events or peer teasing about appearance may trigger bulimic behavior, particularly if there is genetic susceptibility (Wade, 2019).

Etiology

As with anorexia nervosa, theories do not individually explain the development of bulimia nervosa. Rather, the convergence of many of these factors at a vulnerable stage of individual development best explains causality.

Some of the predisposing or risk factors for anorexia nervosa and bulimia nervosa overlap with theories of causality. For example, dieting puts an individual at risk for the development of bulimia nervosa. The dieting can turn into dietary restraint, a symptom that leads to binge eating and purging. However, not all individuals who diet experience bulimia nervosa. The interplay of other risk factors (e.g., body dissatisfaction and separation–individuation issues) most likely explains the development of this disorder.

Biologic Theories

Some progress has been made in understanding the biologic changes in bulimia nervosa. Dieting and binging can affect brain function. Dieting is believed to affect serotonergic regulation, and binging affects the dopamine (DA), acetylcholine (ACh), and opioid reward-related systems. The changes are the result of eating dysregulation rather than the cause. As with anorexia nervosa, these changes often disappear when symptoms such as dietary restraint, binge eating, and purging remit (Wade, 2019).

Genetic and Familial Predispositions

Bulimia nervosa runs in families, with an increased risk for individuals if family members are diagnosed with this disorder. Although anorexia and bulimia are both strongly related to genetics, it is believed that only bulimia has genetic specificity—that is, if one twin has bulimia nervosa, the other twin is at higher risk for developing that disorder (Bulik et al., 2019).

Psychosocial Theories

Symptoms of bulimia nervosa develop when psychological, sociocultural, or environmental events occur. Because the age of onset for bulimia nervosa is late adolescence—going away to college, for example—may represent the first physical separation for some adolescents, who are unprepared for the emotional separation. In addition, an inability to set limits and develop healthy boundaries leads to a sense of being overwhelmed and "drained." Overwhelming feelings often lead to binge eating, either to avoid or to distract oneself from feelings such as resentment, or binge eating can serve to assuage emptiness or to fill up a "drained" self with food.

Cognitive Theory

Many experts view bulimia nervosa as a disorder of thinking in that distortions are the basis for behaviors such as binge eating and purging. Psychological triggering mechanism models explain that cues such as stress, negative emotions, and even environmental cues (e.g., the presence of attractive food) play a role in etiology. However, today these cognitive and triggering theories are viewed as an explanation for maintaining the binge eating after it has been established rather than an explanation of causality.

The same sociocultural factors that underlie anorexia nervosa play a significant role in the development of bulimia nervosa.

Ellen's Triggers

Some of Ellen's triggers are anxiety, boredom, alcohol use, exhaustion, anger, and social situations where food is readily available.

What are the theoretical explanations that relate her triggers to bulimia behavior? What interventions would you suggest for these triggers?

Family Factors

Dysfunctional family relationships of persons with eating disorders have been implicated for years. Current research indicates that perceived lack of cohesion in a family relates to depressive and bulimic behaviors. That is, if a person is depressed and views family members as less cohesive, close, or supportive, the individual would be more likely to have depression and/or bulimia (Kluck et al., 2017).

RECOVERY-ORIENTED CARE FOR PERSONS WITH BULIMIA NERVOSA

Teamwork and Collaboration: Working Toward Recovery

Individuals with bulimia nervosa benefit from a comprehensive multimodal treatment approach. The goals for treatment for individuals with bulimia nervosa focus on stabilizing and then normalizing eating, which means stopping the binge–purge cycles; restructuring dysfunctional thought patterns and attitudes, especially about eating, weight, and shape; teaching healthy boundary setting; and resolving conflicts about separation–individuation. Treatment usually takes place in an outpatient setting except when the patient is suicidal or when past outpatient treatment has failed (see Box 32.6).

Pharmacologic interventions paired with cognitive behavioral therapy (CBT) or interpersonal psychotherapy are also effective. Antidepressants demonstrate effectiveness in treating binge eating and purging even without comorbid depression. Nutrition counseling is an important part of outpatient treatment to stabilize and normalize eating. Some mental health professionals, psychologists, advanced practice psychiatric nurses, and social workers specialize in treating eating disorders, often working with nutritionists who also have expertise with this population. Group psychotherapy and support groups are also used. Family therapy is not usually a part of the treatment because many people with bulimia nervosa live on college campuses away from home or are older and live on their own. Usually, treatment becomes less intensive as symptoms remit. Therapy focuses on psychological issues, such as boundary setting and separation–individuation conflicts and on changing problematic behaviors and dysfunctional thinking using CBT.

Safety Issues

Bulimia nervosa is associated with a high risk of suicide, independent of other comorbid disorders. Individuals with bulimia nervosa are also often at risk for self-harm. Because they display high levels of impulsivity, shoplifting, and overspending, financial and legal difficulties have been associated with this disorder (Wade, 2019).

EVIDENCE-BASED NURSING CARE FOR PERSONS WITH BULIMIA NERVOSA DISORDER

Mental Health Nursing Assessment

Physical Health and Functioning

Even though most individuals with bulimia nervosa maintain normal weights, the physical ramifications of this disorder may be similar to those of anorexia nervosa. Hypokalemia can contribute to muscle weakness and fatigability, as well as to the development of cardiac arrhythmias, palpitations, and cardiac conduction defects. Patients who purge as well as abuse laxatives risk fluid and electrolyte abnormalities that can further compromise cardiac status. Tooth enamel erosion because of frequent purging is also a consequence of bulimia nervosa. Neuropsychiatric disturbances, such as poor concentration and attention, and sleep disturbances, are common.

The nurse should assess current eating patterns, determine the number of times a day the individual binges and purges, and note dietary restraint practices. Sleep patterns and exercise habits are also important.

Psychosocial Assessment

For the individual with bulimia nervosa, psychological assessment focuses on cognitive distortions—cues or stimuli that lead to dysfunctional behavior affecting symptom development—and knowledge deficits. The psychological characteristics typical of patients with bulimia nervosa are presented in Box 32.1.

Individuals with bulimia nervosa display a significant number of cognitive distortions, examples of which are found in Table 32.2. These thought patterns form the basis for "rules" and lead the way to destructive eating patterns. During routine history taking, patients relate many of these erroneous assumptions. Situations that produce feelings of being overwhelmed and powerless need to be explored, as does the patient's ability to set boundaries, control impulsivity, and maintain quality relationships. These underlying issues precipitate binge eating. Body dissatisfaction should be openly explored. Mood is an important area for evaluation because many people with bulimia nervosa also have depression. Symptoms of depression should be thoroughly explored (see Chapter 23). See Nursing Care Plan 32.1—which sets forth a plan of care for Ellen, the case study patient in this chapter.

Quality of Life

Quality of life is negatively impacted by bulimia nervosa as well as AN. In bulimia nervosa, binging and purging are related to poor quality of life and are associated with alcohol binging (Escrivá-Martínez et al., 2020; van Hoeken & Hoek, 2020).

Strengths Assessment

Persons with bulimia can usually identify periods of time when they were able to resist binging and purging. They are usually motivated to reduce or eliminate the binging and purging. The following questions can be used if the strengths do not emerge during the assessment interview.

- How have you curtailed the binging and purging behavior in the past?
- What do you do to reduce your anxiety (instead of binging)?
- Is there anyone in your life that you feel understands your situation?
- How motivated are you to change your eating behaviors and work on body image issues?

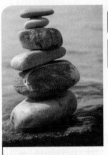

NURSING CARE PLAN 32.1

The Patient With Bulimia Nervosa

Ellen is a 20-year-old female admitted to the inpatient eating disorders unit for treatment of bulimia nervosa. She was discharged from a medical unit where she was treated for electrolyte imbalance and dehydration. She started binging and purging when she left home for college. She was introduced to Ipecac but found that she could force herself to vomit through sticking her hand in her throat. She has agreed to admission in order to learn how to change her behavior.

Setting: Inpatient Psychiatric Unit

Baseline Assessment: Ellen wants to maintain a normal weight but believes that she is overweight. She has been binging and purging for 2 years. When she is dieting, she becomes very hungry and binges on as many as 10,000 calories at once. She then becomes angry with herself and purges through vomiting. She feels better temporarily, but soon feels out of control, guilty, and remorseful. She does not use laxatives or diuretics to lose weight. She has dental problem, bilateral parotid enlargement, and tenderness. Her menstrual periods are irregular; cardiac arrhythmias related to electrolyte imbalance noted in chart. BP 110/60; P 70, R 16, Ht. 5 ft 3 in, Wt. 125, BMI 22.9.

Associated Psychiatric Diagnosis	Medications
Bulimia Nervosa	None

Priority of Nursing Care: Body Image Disturbance

Important Characteristics	Associated Considerations
Considers herself too fat and unattractive despite contrary evidence	Inaccurate perceptions of body size
	Believes that she is too fat despite evidence that she is normal weight.

Outcomes

Initial	Long Term
Verbalizes feelings related to changing body shape and weight.	Identifies positive aspects of her body and its ability to function.
Identifies beliefs about controlling body size.	

Interventions

Interventions	Rationale	Ongoing Assessment
Explore Ellen's beliefs and feelings about body. Maintain a nonjudgmental approach.	To help patient gain a more positive body image, an understanding of her own views is important.	Monitor for statements that identify perceptions of her body. Is her view *distorted* or *dissatisfied*?
Assist patient in identifying positive physical characteristics.	In anorexia, the body is viewed negatively. By focusing on parts of the body that are positive, such as eyes or hands, the patient can begin to experience a positive image of her body.	Observe for patient's reaction to her body. Which areas are viewed positively? Observe for negative statements related to body size and self-esteem.
Clarify patient's views about an ideal body.	Many societal cues idealize an unrealistically thin female body.	Monitor for statements indicating external pressures to lose weight, experiences of teasing about body changes, or evidence of sexual abuse from others.
Provide education related to normal growth of women's bodies, role of fat in protection of body.	Providing education will help in reinforcing a broader view of the importance of a healthy body.	Assess patient's willingness to learn information.

Continued

Nursing Care Plan 32.1 Continued

Evaluation

Outcomes	Revised Outcomes	Interventions
Ellen revealed that she believes that she is too fat but does have positive physical traits—eyes. She believes that those who are overweight have lost control of their lives. She knows some models who are 6 ft and weigh barely 100 lb. Willing to read information about normal body functioning.	Accept alternative beliefs related to her own body. Accept a new view of body functioning as a complex phenomenon.	Gradually, focus on other positive physical aspects of Ellen's body. Discuss grooming that encourages a more attractive look. Challenge her beliefs about body weights of models. Discuss the biologic aspect of the development of body weight. Emphasize multiple factors determine body weight.

Priority of Care: Motivated for change

Important Characteristics	Associated Considerations
Expresses willingness to change binging and purging behavior	History of dieting and purging.
Choices of daily living are appropriate for meeting treatment goals.	Wanting to resume normal eating patterns without purging.

Outcomes

Initial	Long Term
Desires to move to a higher level of wellness. Identify two new strategies to enhance management of bulimia nervosa.	Develop positive eating patterns.

Interventions

Interventions	Rationale	Ongoing Assessment
Encourage Ellen to discuss her strategies to meet higher wellness goals.	Patient needs to identify specific goals to meet wellness goals.	Determine if she is able to articulate realistic goals.
Help Ellen identify two new strategies to avoid dieting and purging.	Identification of specific, realistic plans to meet needs increases possibility of carrying out strategies.	Determine if goals are doable.

Evaluation

Evaluation	Revised Outcomes	Interventions
Met new wellness goals.	Completed	
Able to use new strategies to resist dieting and purging.	Completed	

CLINICAL JUDGMENT

The first priority is to address emerging medical problems such as electrolyte imbalances. Suicide or self-harm behaviors should also be addressed.

THERAPEUTIC RELATIONSHIP

Individuals with bulimia nervosa experience a great deal of shame and guilt. They also often have an intense need to please and be liked and may approach the nurse–patient relationship in a superficial manner. They are too ashamed to discuss their symptoms but do not want to disappoint others, so they may discuss more social or unrelated issues in an attempt to engage the nurse (Box 32.12). A nonjudgmental, accepting approach, stressing the importance of the relationship and outlining its purpose, is important at the outset. Explaining the nature of the relationship and the goals of therapy will help clarify the boundaries.

BOX 32.12 • THERAPEUTIC DIALOGUE: THE PATIENT WITH AN EATING DISORDER

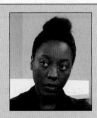

INEFFECTIVE APPROACH

Nurse: Ellen, I am glad to see that you ate your lunch.

Ellen: Thanks, I feel so fat after I eat.

Nurse: I will lock the bathroom so you are not tempted to purge.

Ellen: What, don't you trust me?

Nurse: It is not about trust, but I don't feel comfortable leaving you alone with bathroom access.

Ellen: Really? You have your nerve.

Nurse: We are just trying to help.

Ellen: Some help you are. I know you don't trust me.

Nurse: Now, Ellen that is not what I said.

Ellen: No, but that is what you meant.

EFFECTIVE APPROACH

Nurse: Ellen, how was your lunch.

Ellen: I was ok. I always feel so fat after I eat.

Nurse: That is understandable. How long does that feeling last.

Ellen: Well, it depends on how much I have eaten. Since I didn't eat much, it will last for about an hour?

Nurse: Oh, I see. For many people with bulimia, the urges to purge are strongest after a meal? Is this a hard time for you?

Ellen: Sometimes it is.

Nurse: How can I help you resist the urges? Would you like me to stay with you until group time?

Ellen: That would be great.

CRITICAL THINKING CHALLENGE

- What effect did the first interaction have on Ellen's behavior? Why?
- In the second interaction, what theories and interventions regarding eating disorders did the nurse use in her approach to Ellen?

Consider This

Ellen feels shame and guilt over her binging and purging. She does not like to talk about it and is very reluctant to talk to the nurse about the behavior.

Which interventions would be helpful to help Ellen deal with her guilt? Would she be a candidate for a support group?

MENTAL HEALTH NURSING INTERVENTIONS

Establishing Recovery and Wellness Goals

Important goals for a person with bulimia are to establish a normal eating/elimination pattern and to develop positive self-esteem and positive body image. Since these individuals are not likely to be over-exercising, helping them normalize physical activities and develop healthy sleep patterns are two possible wellness goals.

Physical Care

If the patient is admitted to the hospital, meals and all food intake are strictly monitored to normalize eating. Bathroom visits may also be supervised to prevent purging. Outpatients are asked to record their intake, binges, and purges. Because individuals with bulimia nervosa have chaotic lifestyles and are often overcommitted, sleep may be a low priority. Sleep-deprived individuals may assume that food would be helpful, and they begin to eat, triggering a binge. To encourage regular sleep patterns, sleep hygiene strategies are implemented.

Medication Interventions

Fluoxetine is approved by the FDA for treating bulimia nervosa. This SSRI has been shown to reduce vomiting and binging episodes (Bello & Yeomans, 2018).

Using Cognitive and Behavioral Interventions

The behavioral techniques, such as cue elimination and response prevention, require self-monitoring to individualize the therapy. Self-monitoring is accomplished using a diary in which the patient records binges and purges and precipitating emotions and environmental cues. Emotional and environmental cues are identified, and alternative responses are suggested, tried, and reinforced. When a cue or stimulus leads to a dysfunctional or unhealthy response, the response can be eliminated or an alternate, healthier response to the cue can be substituted, tried, and then reinforced. Figure 32.2 gives two examples of behavioral interventions. In Example 1, for the patient with anorexia nervosa, the response is modified or altered to a healthier one; in Example 2, for the patient with bulimia nervosa, the cue is changed to produce a different, healthier response. Other techniques, such as postponing binges and purges through distraction, a technique to interrupt the cycle, are also effective.

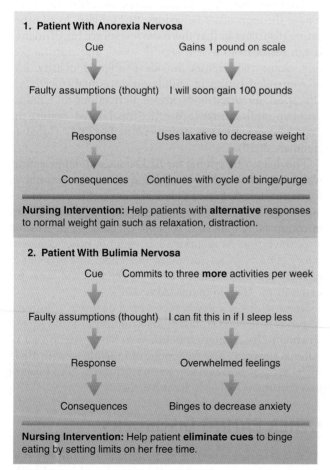

1. Patient With Anorexia Nervosa

Cue	Gains 1 pound on scale
↓	↓
Faulty assumptions (thought)	I will soon gain 100 pounds
↓	↓
Response	Uses laxative to decrease weight
↓	↓
Consequences	Continues with cycle of binge/purge

Nursing Intervention: Help patients with **alternative** responses to normal weight gain such as relaxation, distraction.

2. Patient With Bulimia Nervosa

Cue	Commits to three **more** activities per week
↓	↓
Faulty assumptions (thought)	I can fit this in if I sleep less
↓	↓
Response	Overwhelmed feelings
↓	↓
Consequences	Binges to decrease anxiety

Nursing Intervention: Help patient **eliminate cues** to binge eating by setting limits on her free time.

FIGURE 32.2 Examples of the relationship of cues, thoughts, responses, and behavioral interventions.

NCLEXNOTE Cognitive nterventions within the context of a therapeutic relationship are a priority in the nursing care of patients with eating disorders.

Psychoeducation

Teaching Strategies

In addition to cognitive and behavioral techniques, educational strategies are also incorporated into treatment. For individuals with bulimia nervosa, psychoeducation focuses on setting boundaries and healthy limits, developing assertiveness, learning nutritional concepts related to healthy eating, and clarifying the many misconceptions they have about food and its influence on weight. Rules that result from dichotomous thinking mustalso be addressed because of their role in dietary restraint and resulting binge eating.

Teaching About Symptoms

The nurse can assist patients in understanding the binge–purge cycle and the role of rigid rules in contributing to this cycle. The value of eating meals regularly to ward off hunger and reduce the possibility of a binge is also important. Patients who abuse laxatives must be taught that although these drugs produce water-weight loss, they are ineffective for true, lasting weight loss because they work on the colon and not the small intestine or stomach where food is absorbed. Patients also need information about potassium depletion, electrolyte imbalances, dehydration, and the medical consequences of binge eating and purging. Other topics for psychoeducation are included in Box 32.13.

BOX 32.13

Bulimia Nervosa

When caring for the patient with bulimia nervosa, be sure to include the following topic areas in the teaching plan:

- Psychopharmacologic agents, if used, including drug, action, dosage, frequency, and possible adverse effects
- Binge–purge cycle and effects on the body
- Nutrition and eating patterns
- Hydration
- Avoidance of cues
- Cognitive distortions
- Limit setting
- Appropriate boundary setting
- Assertiveness
- Resources
- Self-monitoring and behavioral interventions
- Realistic goal setting

Convening Support Groups

Group interventions are cost effective and increase learning more effectively than does individual treatment because patients learn from each other as well as from the nurse, therapist, or leader. Some experts have recommended 12-step programs for treating bulimia nervosa. However, many clinicians who work in this specialty have noted that these programs, with their strict rules, can be counterproductive for patients with bulimia nervosa, who already have rigid rules and are "abstinent" in many ways that lead to binge eating. Broad parameters regarding food choices (e.g., all foods allowed in moderation), in combination with knowledge about healthy eating, should be encouraged instead.

After symptoms subside, patients can concentrate on interpersonal issues in therapy, such as a fused relationship with their mothers or feelings of inadequacy and low self-esteem, which often underlie their lack of assertiveness.

Developing Recovery-Oriented Rehabilitation Strategies

Strategies used for AN can also be applied to BN. There is emerging research that shows that physical exercise and dietary therapy may be a realistic approach that supports recovery (Mathisen et al., 2020).

Evaluation and Treatment Outcomes

Most people recover from bulimia nervosa over time. Rates of recovery from bulimia peak within the first 10 years. Patients with bulimia nervosa have better and quicker recovery than do those with anorexia nervosa (Eddy et al., 2017).

Continuum of Care

Emergency and Inpatient-Focused Care

Although patients with bulimia nervosa are less likely than those with anorexia nervosa to require hospitalization, those with extreme dehydration and electrolyte imbalance, depression and suicidality, or symptoms that have not remitted with outpatient treatment need hospitalization.

However, most treatment takes place in outpatient settings. After treatment, referrals to recovery groups and support groups are important to prevent relapse. Rarely do patients with bulimia nervosa require emergency care.

Community Care

As with anorexia nervosa, preventing bulimia nervosa requires effort on the part of teachers, school nurses, parents, and society as a whole. Because many of the risk factors are seen early in children attending elementary school, educating school nurses and teachers is an important focus for psychiatric–mental health nurses working in the community. Protective factors that mediate between risk factors and the development of an eating disorder must be emphasized and developed. Box 32.11 covers important prevention strategies for parents and their children or adolescents.

Society has begun to engage in an effort to help young girls. The federal government has developed a website called *girlshealth* that is devoted to areas such as body changes, body image, relationships, and self-confidence.

BINGE EATING DISORDER

BED is characterized by episodes of consuming large amounts of foods in a short period of time. These individuals binge in the same way as those with bulimia nervosa do, but they do not purge or compensate for binges through other behaviors. BED differs from other eating disorders in that there are few severe impairments. It can result from psychological, social, and cultural factors. Some risk factors include childhood obesity, loss of controlled eating in childhood, intestinal microbiota alteration, distorted body image, perfectionism, conduct problem, and substance use. In the United States, the prevalence of BED is estimated to be 2.6% (Iqbal & Rehman, 2020).

The diagnostic criteria for BED consist of binge eating, which includes both the ingestion of a large amount of food in a short period of time and a sense of loss of control during the binge, distress regarding the binge; eating until uncomfortably full, and feelings of guilt or depression after the binge. As mentioned, purging or other compensatory behavior does not follow the binge. The prevalence of BED is estimated to be 1.6% for females and 0.8% for males in the United States (APA, 2013).

Because this is a newly recognized disorder, additional research is needed to clarify its symptoms, etiology, and treatment. Its etiology is believed to be similar to that of bulimia nervosa. The treatment of individuals with BED includes psychotherapy, pharmacotherapy, and weight loss treatment (Iqbal & Rehman, 2020).

OTHER EATING DISORDERS

A complete discussion of all the eating disorders is outside the scope of this text. Purging disorder and night eating are briefly described here.

Purging Disorder

In purging disorder, there is frequent purging, but not binging. Individuals with this disorder purge at least once a week and have an intense fear of gaining weight or becoming fat (APA, 2013). They restrict their dietary intake and purge after eating normal amounts of food due to the fear of eating, gaining weight, and/or appearing "fat." These individuals have increased levels of body image disturbance, higher levels of general psychopathology, distress, eating pathology, and personality disorders when compared to a comparable group of persons without purging disorder. While individuals with this disorder do not overeat as those with bulimia nervosa, they do report more dietary restraint, greater fear of losing control, and greater guilt over eating than control groups. On a continuum of bulimic symptomatology, purging disorder may be the midpoint with bulimia nervosa the more severe (Forney et al., 2020).

Night Eating Syndrome

In night eating syndrome, the individual eats after awakening from sleep or consumes an excessive amount of food after the evening meal (APA, 2013). The person is aware of overeating, which causes significant distress or impairment to the individual. There is a feeling of loss of control over consumption, sleep fragmentation, and morning anorexia. Night eating syndrome is conceptualized as a disorder of circadian modulation of food intake and sleep. It is mainly attributed to an endocrine metabolic or psychological trigger factor. These individuals typically experience insomnia and nighttime awakenings (Haraguchi et al., 2019).

SUMMARY OF KEY POINTS

* Anorexia nervosa and bulimia nervosa have some common symptoms but are classified as discrete disorders.
* Eating disorders are best viewed along a continuum that includes subclinical or partial-syndrome disorders; because these disorders occur more frequently than full syndromes, they are often overlooked but, after they are identified, they can be prevented from worsening.
* Similar factors predispose individuals to the development of anorexia nervosa and bulimia nervosa, and these factors represent a biopsychosocial model of risk. These disorders are preventable, and identifying risk factors assists with prevention strategies.
* Etiologic factors contribute in combination to the development of eating disorders; no one factor provides an explanation.

* Treatment of anorexia nervosa frequently includes hospitalization for refeeding; bulimia nervosa is treated primarily on an outpatient basis.
* Cognitive-behavioral therapy and medications improve the symptoms. Individual and group interpersonal psychotherapy are also effective in self-evaluation and communication.
* The outcomes for bulimia nervosa are better than those for anorexia nervosa. The type and severity of comorbid conditions and the length of the illness influence outcomes.
* BED is characterized by periods of binge eating not followed by purging or any other compensating behaviors.

CRITICAL THINKING CHALLENGES

1. Discuss the potential difficulties and risks in attempting to treat a patient with anorexia nervosa in an outpatient setting.
2. Parents are often in need of support and suggestions for how to help prevent eating disorders. Develop a teaching program and include the topics and rationale for suggestions chosen.
3. Identify the important nursing management components of a refeeding program for a hospitalized patient with anorexia nervosa.
4. Bulimia nervosa is often described as a closet disorder with secretive binge eating and purging. Identify the signs and symptoms of each system involved for someone with this disorder.
5. Positive outcomes for the recovery of bulimia nervosa and anorexia nervosa depend on many factors. Identify the factors that promote positive outcomes and those related to poorer outcomes and prognosis.

A related Psychiatric–Mental Health Nursing video on the topic of Eating Disorder is also available at http://thePoint.lww.com/Boyd7e.

A Psychiatric–Mental Health Nursing Practice and Learn Activity related to the video on the topic of Eating Disorder is also available at http://thePoint.lww.com/Boyd7e.

REFERENCES

Accurso, E. C., Astrachan-Fletcher, E., O'Brien, S., McClanahan, S. F., & Le Grange, D. (2018). Adaptation and implementation of family-based treatment enhanced with dialectical behavior therapy skills for anorexia nervosa in community-based specialist clinics. *Eating Disorders*, 26(2), 149–163. https://doi.org/10.1080/10640266.2017.1330319
American Psychiatric Association. (2013). *Diagnostic and statistical manual of mental disorders* (5th ed.). American Psychiatric Association.
Andrade, R., Gonçalves-Pinho, M., Roma-Torres, A., & Brandão, I. (2017). Treatment of anorexia nervosa: The importance of disease progression

in the prognosis. *Acta Medica Portuguesa, 30*(7-8), 517–523. https://doi.org/10.20344/amp.8963

Berends, T., van de Lagemaat, M., van Meijel, B., Coenen, J., Hoek, H. W., & van Elburg, A. A. (2018). Relapse prevention in anorexia nervosa: Experiences of patients and parents. *International Journal of Mental Health Nursing, 27*(5), 1546–1555. https://doi.org/10.1111/inm.12456.

Bulik, M., Bade, L., & Austin, J. (2019). Genetics of eating disorders, *Psychiatric Clinics of North America, 42,* 50–73.

Bruch, H. (1973). *Eating disorders: Obesity, anorexia nervosa and the person within.* Basic Books.

Castillo, M., & Weiselberg, E. (2017). Bulimia nervosa/purging disorder. *Current Problems in Pediatric & Adolescent Health Care, 47*(4), 85–94. https://doi.org/10.1016/j.cppeds.2017.02.004

Cheng, Z. H., Perko, V. L., Fuller-Marashi, L., Gau, J. M., & Stice, E. (2019). Ethnic differences in eating disorder prevalence, risk factors, and predictive effects of risk factors among young women. *Eating Behaviors, 32,* 23–30. https://doi.org/10.1016/j.eatbeh.2018.11.004

Chidiac, C. W. (2019). An update on the medical consequences of anorexia nervosa. *Current Opinion in Pediatrics.* https://doi.org/10.1097/MOP.0000000000000755

Curzio, O., Calderoni, S., Maestro, S., Rossi, G., De Pasquale, C. F., Belmonti, V., Apicella, F., Muratori, F., & Retico, A. (2020). Lower gray matter volumes of frontal lobes and insula in adolescents with anorexia nervosa restricting type: Findings from a Brain Morphometry Study. *European Psychiatry: The Journal of the Association of European Psychiatrists, 63*(1), e27. https://doi.org/10.1192/j.eurpsy.2020.19

Duarte, C., Ferreira, C., & Pinto-Gouveia J. (2016). At the core of eating disorders: Overvaluation, social rank, self-criticism and shame in anorexia, bulimia and binge eating disorder. *Comprehensive Psychiatry, 66,* 123–131.

Eddy, K. T., Tabri, N., Thomas, J. J., Murray, H. B., Keshaviah, A., Hastings, E., Edkins, K., Krishna, M., Herzog, D. B., Keel, P. K., & Franko, D. L. (2017). Recovery from anorexia nervosa and bulimia nervosa at 22-year follow-up. *The Journal of Clinical Psychiatry, 28*(2), 184-189.

Escrivá-Martínez, T., Herrero, R., Molinari, G., Rodríguez-Arias, M., Verdejo-García, A., & Baños, R. M. (2020). Binge eating and binge drinking: A two-way road? An integrative review. *Current Pharmaceutical Design, 26*(20), 2402–2415. https://doi.org/10.2174/1381612826666200316153317

Fichter, M. M., Quadflieg, N., Crosby, R.D., & Koch, S. (2017). Long-term outcome of anorexia nervosa: Results from a large clinical longitudinal study. *International Journal of Eating Disorders, 50*(9), 1018–1030. https://doi.org/10.1002/eat.22736

Foldi, C. J., Liknaitzky, P., Williams, M., & Oldfield, B. J. (2020). Rethinking therapeutic strategies for anorexia nervosa: Insights from psychedelic medicine and animal models. *Frontiers in neuroscience, 14,* 43. https://doi.org/10.3389/fnins.2020.00043

Forney, K. J., Crosby, R. D., Brown, T. A., Klein, K. M., & Keel, P. K. (2020). A naturalistic, long-term follow-up of purging disorder. *Psychological Medicine,* 1–8. Advance online publication. https://doi.org/10.1017/S0033291719003982

Garber, A. K., Sawyer, S. M., Golden, N. H., Guarda, A. S., Katzman, D. K., & Kohn, M. R. (2016). A systematic review of approaches to refeeding in patients with anorexia nervosa. *International Journal of Eating Disorders, 49*(3), 293–310.

Garner, D. M., Olmsted, M. P., Bohr, Y., & Garfinkel, P. E. (1982). The eating attitudes test: Psychometric features and clinical correlates. *Psychological Medicine, 12*(4), 871–878. https://doi.org/10.1017/S0033291700049163

Goldstein, A., & Gvion, Y. (2019). Socio-demographic and psychological risk factors for suicidal behavior among individuals with anorexia and bulimia nervosa: A systematic review. *Journal of Affective Disorders, 15,* 245, 1149–1167. https://doi.org/10.1016/j.jad.2018.12.01

Griffiths, S., Castle, D., Cunningham, M., Murray, S. B., Bastian, B., & Barlow, F. K. (2018). How does exposure to thinspiration and fitspiration relate to symptom severity among individuals with eating disorders? Evaluation of a proposed model. *Body Image, 27,* 187–195. https://doi.org/10.1016/j.bodyim.2018.10.002

Hamatani, S., Tomotake, M., Takeda, T., Kameoka, N., Kawabata, M., Kubo, H., Tada, Y., Tomioka, Y., Watanabe, S., Inoshita, M., Kinoshita, M., Ohta, M., & Ohmori, T. (2017). Influence of cognitive function on quality of life in anorexia nervosa patients. *Psychiatry and Clinical Neurosciences, 71*(5), 328–335.https://doi.org/10.1111/pcn.12491

Haraguchi, A., Komada, Y., Inoue, Y., & Shibata, S. (2019). Correlation among clock gene expression rhythms, sleep quality, and meal conditions in delayed sleep-wake phase disorder and night eating syndrome. *Chronobiology International, 28,* 1–14. https://doi.org/10.1080/07420528.2019.1585366

Hilbert, A., de Zwaan, M., & Braehler, E. (2012). How frequent are eating disorders in the population? Norms of the eating disorder examination questionnaire. *PLoS One, 7*(1), e29125.

Holmes, S., Drake, S., Odgers, K., & Wilson, J. (2017). Feminist approaches to Anorexia Nervosa: A qualitative study of a treatment group. *Journal of Eating Disorders, 13,* 5, 36. https://doi.org/10.1186/s40337-017-0166-y

Irvine, K. R., Irvine, A. R., Maalin, N., McCarty, K., Cornelissen, K. K., Tovée, M. J., & Cornelissen, P. L. (2020). Using immersive virtual reality to modify body image. *Body Image, 33,* 232–243. https://doi.org/10.1016/j.bodyim.2020.03.007

Iqbal, A., & Rehman, A. (2020). Binge eating disorder. In *StatPearls.* StatPearls Publishing.

Joy, E., Kussman, A., & Nattiv, A. (2019). 2016 update on eating disorders in athletes: A comprehensive narrative review with a focus on clinical assessment and management. *British Journal of Sports Medicine, 50*(3), 154–162. https://doi.org/10.1136/bjsports-2015-095735

Karageorgiou, V., Furukawa, T. A., Tsigkaropoulou, E., Karavia, A., Gournellis, R., Soureti, A., Bellos, I., Douzenis, A., & Michopoulos, I. (2020). Adipokines in anorexia nervosa: A systematic review and meta-analysis. *Psychoneuroendocrinology, 112,* 104485. https://doi.org/10.1016/j.psyneuen.2019.104485

Kwok, C., Kwok, V., Lee, H. Y., & Tan, S. M. (2020). Clinical and socio-demographic features in childhood vs adolescent-onset anorexia nervosa in an Asian population. *Eating and Weight Disorders: EWD, 25*(3), 821–826. https://doi.org/10.1007/s40519-019-00694-9

Larsson, E., Lloyd, S., Westwood, H., & Tchanturia K. (2018). Patients' perspective of a group intervention for perfectionism in anorexia nervosa: A qualitative study. *Journal of Health Psychology, 23*(12), 1521–1532. https://doi.org/10.1177/1359105316660183

Levinson, C. A., Sala, M., Murray, S., Ma, J., Rodebaugh, T. L., & Lenze, E. J. (2019). Diagnostic, clinical, and personality correlates of food anxiety during a food exposure in patients diagnosed with an eating disorder. *Eating and Weight Disorders: EWD, 24*(6), 1079–1088. https://doi.org/10.1007/s40519-019-00669-w

Lie, S.Ø., Rø, Ø., & Bang, L. (2019). Is bullying and teasing associated with eating disorders? A systematic review and meta-analysis. *International Journal of Eating Disorders.* https://doi.org/10.1002/eat.23035

Mangweth-Matzek, B., & Hoek, H.W. (2017). Epidemiology and treatment of eating disorders in men and women of middle and older age. *Current Opinion in Psychiatry, 30*(6), 446–451. https://doi.org/10.1097/YCO.0000000000000356

Mathisen, T. F., Rosenvinge, J. H., Friborg, O., Vrabel, K., Bratland-Sanda, S., Pettersen, G., & Sundgot-Borgen, J. (2020). Is physical exercise and dietary therapy a feasible alternative to cognitive behavior therapy in treatment of eating disorders? A randomized controlled trial of two group therapies. *The International Journal of Eating Disorders, 53*(4), 574–585. https://doi.org/10.1002/eat.23228

Miniati, M., Callari, A., Maglio, A., & Calugi, S. (2018). Interpersonal psychotherapy for eating disorders: Current perspectives. *Psychology Research & Behavior Management, 11,* 353–369. https://doi.org/10.2147/PRBM.S120584

Minuchin, S., Rosman, B., & Baker, L. (1978). *Psychosomatic families.* Harvard University Press.

Monell, E., Clinton, D., & Birgegård, A. (2018). Emotion dysregulation and eating disorders-Associations with diagnostic presentation and key symptoms. *International Journal of Eating Disorders, 51*(8), 921–930. https://doi.org/10.1002/eat.22925

Parker, E., Flood, V., Halaki, M., Wearne, C., Anderson, G., Gomes, L., Clarke, S., Wilson, F., Russell, J., Frig, E., & Kohn, M. (2020). Study protocol for a randomised controlled trial investigating two different refeeding formulations to improve safety and efficacy of hospital management of adolescent and young adults admitted with anorexia nervosa. *BMJ open, 10*(10), e038242. https://doi.org/10.1136/bmjopen-2020-038242

Peebles, R., Lesser, A., Park, C. C., Heckert, K., Timko, C. A., Lantzouni, E., Liebman, R., & Weaver, L. (2017). Outcomes of an inpatient medical nutritional rehabilitation protocol in children and adolescents with eating disorders. *Journal of Eating Disorders, 5,* 7. https://doi.org/10.1186/s40337-017-0134-6

Pike, K., & Dunne, P. E. (2015). The rise of eating disorders in Asia: A review. *Journal of Eating Disorders, 3,* 33.

Plana, M. T., Torres, T., Rodríguez, N., Boloc, D., Gassó, P., Moreno, E., Lafuente, A., Castro-Fornieles, J., Mas, S., & Lazaro, L (2019). Genetic variability in the serotoninergic system and age of onset in anorexia nervosa and obsessive-compulsive disorder. *Psychiatry Research, 271,* 554–558. https://doi.org/10.1016/j.psychres.2018.12.019

Rotella, F., Mannucci, E., Gemignani, S., Lazzeretti, L., Fioravanti, G., & Ricca, V. (2018). Emotional eating and temperamental traits in Eating Disorders: A dimensional approach. *Psychiatry Research, 264,* 1–8. https://doi.org10.1016/j.psychres.2018.03.066

Sagiv, E., & Gvion, Y. (2020). A multi factorial model of self-harm behaviors in Anorexia-nervosa and Bulimia-nervosa. *Comprehensive Psychiatry*, *96*, 152142. https://doi.org/10.1016/j.comppsych.2019.152142

Scharner, S., & Stengel, A. (2019). Alterations of brain structure and functions in anorexia nervosa. *Clinical Nutrition Experimental*. https://doi.org.libproxy.siue.edu/10.1016/j.yclnex.2019.02.001

Shu, C. Y., Limburg, K., Harris, C., McCormack, J., Hoiles, K. J., & Hamilton, M. J. (2015). Clinical presentation of eating disorders in young males in a tertiary setting. *Journal of Eating Disorders*, *3*, 39. https://doi.org/10.1186/s40337-015-0075-x

Silén, Y., Sipilä, P. N., Raevuori, A., Mustelin, L., Marttunen, M., Kaprio, J., & Keski-Rahkonen, A. (2020). DSM-5 eating disorders among adolescents and young adults in Finland: A public health concern. *The International Journal of Eating Disorders*, *53*(5), 520–531. https://doi.org/10.1002/eat.23236

Smink, F., van Hoeken, D., Dijkstra, J. K., Deen, M., Oldehinkel, A. J., & Hoek, H. W. (2018). Self-esteem and peer-perceived social status in early adolescence and prediction of eating pathology in young adulthood. *The International Journal of Eating Disorders*, *51*(8), 852–862. https://doi.org/10.1002/eat.22875

Smith, K. E., Martínez-Zalacaín, I., Mestre-Bach, G., Sánchez, I., Riesco, N., Jiménez-Murcia, S., Fernández-Formoso, J. A., Veciana de Las Heras, M., Custal, N., Menchón, J. M., Soriano-Mas, C., & Fernandez-Aranda, F. (2020). Dorsolateral prefrontal cortex and amygdala function during cognitive reappraisal predicts weight restoration and emotion regulation impairment in anorexia nervosa. *Psychological Medicine*, 1–9. Advance online publication. https://doi.org/10.1017/S0033291720002457nalysis. *Journal of Abnormal Psychology*, *126*(5), 565–592.

Timko, C., DeFilipp, L. & Dakanalis, A. (2019). Sex differences in adolescent anorexia and bulimia nervosa: beyond the signs and symptoms. *Current Psychiatry Reports*, *21*(1). https://doi-org.libproxy.siue.edu/10.1007/s11920-019-0988-1

Udo, T., & Grilo, C. M. (2019). Psychiatric and medical correlates of DSM-5 eating disorders in a nationally representative sample of adults in the United States. *International Journal of Eating Disorders*, *52*(1), 42–50. https://doi.org/10.1002/eat.23004

van Hoeken, D., & Hoek, H. W. (2020). Review of the burden of eating disorders: Mortality, disability, costs, quality of life, and family burden. *Current Opinion in Psychiatry*, *33*(6), 521–527. https://doi.org/10.1097/YCO.0000000000000641

Wade, T. D. (2019). Recent research on bulimia nervosa. *Psychiatric Clinics of North America*, *42*, 21–32.

Wagner, A. F., & Vitousek, K. M. (2019). Personality variables and eating pathology. *Psychiatric Clinics of North America*, *42*(1), 105–119. https://doi.org10.1016/j.psc.2018.10.012

Wallis, A., Miskovic-Wheatley, J., Madden, S., Rhodes, P., Crosby, R. D., Cao, L., & Touyz, S. (2018). Family functioning and relationship quality for adolescents in family-based treatment with severe anorexia nervosa compared with non-clinical adolescents. *European Eating Disorders Review*, *6*(1), 29–37. https://doi.org10.1002/erv.2562

Waszczuk, M. A., Waaktaar, T., Eley, T. C., & Torgersen, S. (2019). Etiological influences on continuity and co-occurrence of eating disorders symptoms across adolescence and emerging adulthood. *International Journal of Eating Disorders*, https://doi.org/10.1002/eat.23040

Wong, L., Goh, L. G., & Ramachandran, R. (2019). Family-based therapy for anorexia nervosa: Results from a 7-year longitudinal Singapore study. *Eating & Weight Disorders*, *16*, https://doi.org/10.1007/s40519-019-00654-3

Zayed, M., & Garry, J. P. (2017). Geriatric anorexia nervosa. *Journal of the American Board of Family Medicine: JABFM*, *30*(5), 666–669. https://doi.org/10.3122/jabfm.2017.05.170182

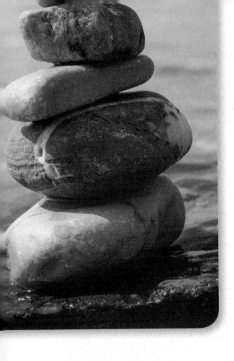

33
Somatic Symptom and Dissociative Disorders
Nursing Care of Persons with Somatization

Mary Ann Boyd and Victoria Soltis-Jarrett

KEYCONCEPT

- somatization

LEARNING OBJECTIVES

After studying this chapter, you will be able to:

1. Discuss the role of somatization in somatic symptom and related disorders in people with mental health problems.

2. Delineate the clinical symptoms and course of somatic symptom disorder (SSD).

3. Analyze the prevailing theories related to somatic symptoms and related disorders.

4. Develop strategies to establish a patient-centered, recovery-oriented therapeutic relationship with a person with somatization and cognitive distortions.

5. Apply a person-centered, recovery-oriented nursing process for persons with somatic symptoms and related disorders.

6. Identify the role of medications for people with SSD.

7. Develop wellness strategies for persons with SSD.

8. Differentiate the type of mental health care provided in emergency care, inpatient-focused care, community care, and virtual mental health care.

9. Discuss the importance of integrated health care for persons with SSD.

10. Describe other disorders related to somatic symptom and dissociative disorders.

KEY TERMS

- Alexithymia • Conversion disorder • Factitious disorder • Factitious disorder imposed on another • Illness anxiety disorder • Pseudologia fantastica • Psychosomatic • Somatic symptom disorder (SSD)

Case Study

Carol is a 48-year-old woman with obesity who is very angry at being forced to see a mental health care provider. She has had multiple surgeries, including hysterectomy, gastric bypass, and carpal tunnel release. She suffers from shoulder and neck pain and from vertigo. She takes multiple medications.

INTRODUCTION

The connection between the "mind" and "body" has been hypothesized and described for centuries. The term **psychosomatic** has been traditionally used to describe, explain, and predict the psychological origins of illness and disease. Unfortunately, this notion perpetuates the stigma that certain disorders are purely "psychological" in nature and thus are not real or valid. For example, it was formerly believed that people with asthma were behaviorally "acting out" their anger, fear, or emotional pain and were seeking attention rather than experiencing an alteration in their respiratory status.

In contrast, the concept of *somatization* acknowledges and respects that bodily sensations and functional changes are expressions of health and illness, and, even though they may be unexplained, they are not imaginary or "all in the head" (Marek et al., 2020).

> **KEYCONCEPT Somatization** (from *soma*, meaning body) is the manifestation of psychological distress as physical symptoms that may result in functional changes, somatic descriptions, or both.

Whereas some evidence suggests that somatization is a result of abnormally high levels of physiologic response (Guo et al., 2019), other evidence supports the idea that somatization is the physical expression of personal problems or the internalization and expression of stress through physical symptoms (Astill Wright et al., 2020). For example, a woman quits her job because of chronic fatigue syndrome rather than recognizing that she is emotionally stressed from the constant harassment of a coworker.

Historically, the concept of somatization was linked to women and was related to a woman's body, mind, or even her soul. For example, the term *hysteria*, frequently associated with somatization, actually comes from ancient times when it was believed that a woman's unfounded physical symptoms were related to her "wandering or discontented uterus." Because *hystera* is the Greek word for "uterus," the terms *hysteria* and *hysterical* were used to describe a woman whose physical or emotional symptoms could not be substantiated by physicians at that time.

We now understand that somatization is not linked to the uterus, nor is it just a problem for women. Men also are affected by somatization. Much research is still needed in this area to be able to make any valid and reliable conclusions about gender and somatization (Shangguan et al., 2020). Somatization also crosses all cultures and is recognized in almost every society (de la Torre-Luque et al., 2020). In many cultures, the expression of physical discomfort is more acceptable than acknowledging psychological distress. The disruption of routine body cycles, such as digestion, menstruation, or sleep, is more socially acceptable than having emotional responses related to

interpersonal relationships, economic crises, adjustment to marriage, infertility, or the death of a spouse.

SOMATIC SYMPTOM AND RELATED DISORDERS OVERVIEW

This chapter explores the holistic evidence-based nursing care for people experiencing the *DSM-5* group of disorders with the prominent symptom of somatization (American Psychiatric Association [APA], 2013). SSD is highlighted and **illness anxiety disorder**, conversion disorder, and factitious disorders are discussed.

SOMATIC SYMPTOM DISORDER

Nurses in primary care and medical–surgical settings are more likely than mental health nurses to encounter persons with these problems. It must be noted that the term *somatoform* is no longer used in the *DSM-5* to describe these disorders (APA, 2013).

Clinical Course

Somatic symptom disorder (SSD) is one of the most difficult disorders to manage because its symptoms tend to change, are diffuse and complex, and vary and move from one body system to another. For example, initially gastrointestinal (e.g., nausea, vomiting, diarrhea) and neurologic (e.g., headache, backache) symptoms may be present that change to musculoskeletal (e.g., aching legs) and sexual issues (e.g., pain in the abdomen, pain during intercourse). Physical symptoms may last for more than 5 years (D'Souza & Hooten, 2020).

Individuals with SSD perceive themselves as being "sicker than the sick" and report all aspects of their health as poor. Many eventually become disabled and unable to work. They typically visit health care providers many times each month and quickly become frustrated because their primary health care providers do not understand their level of suffering and are unable to validate that a particular problem accounts for their extreme discomfort. Consequently, individuals with SSD tend to "provider shop," moving from one to another until they find one who will give them new medication, hospitalize them, or perform surgery. Because the source of worrisome physical symptoms cannot be determined through medical or laboratory tests, medical or psychiatric interviews, or medical imaging, they repeatedly seek a medical reason for their discomfort and ask for relief from suffering. Depending on the severity, these individuals undergo multiple surgeries and even develop iatrogenic illnesses. People with SSD often evoke negative subjective responses in health care providers, who usually wish that the patient would go to someone else.

The following are the most common characteristics:

- Reporting the same symptoms repeatedly
- Receiving support from the environment that otherwise might not be forthcoming (e.g., gaining a spouse's attention because of severe back pain)
- Expressing concern about the physical problems inconsistent with the severity of the illness (being "sicker than the sick")

NCLEXNOTE Patients with SSD seek health care from multiple providers but often avoid mental health specialists.

Diagnostic Criteria

The diagnostic criteria of SSD include one or more symptoms that cause persistent distress or significant disruption in daily lives for at least 6 months and excessive thoughts about the seriousness of the symptoms, feelings (such as anxiety about the symptoms or overall health), or behaviors related to the symptoms or health concerns (e.g., spending excessive time and energy focusing on these symptoms or health) (APA, 2013). These symptoms may or may not be explained by medical evidence. The expression of the symptoms varies from population to population.

SSD Across the Life Span

SSD is found in most populations and cultures even though its expression may vary from population to population. In cultures that highly stigmatize mental illness, somatic symptoms are more likely to appear (Horsfield et al., 2020).

Children and Adolescents

Although many children have somatic symptoms, SSD is not usually diagnosed until adolescence. However, when children have medical symptoms, further evaluation is needed so they are often referred to specialists to rule out physical, sexual, or emotional abuse or a comorbid psychiatric illness, such as depression or anxiety. In children, the most common symptoms are frequent abdominal pain, headache, fatigue, and nausea. Expression of somatic symptoms in children tend to be overlooked or minimized when it needs to be identified as a risk factor for follow-up (Boerner et al., 2020). In adolescents, initial symptoms are typically menstrual difficulties, and pelvic or abdominal pain. Risk factors for both children and adolescents need to be taken seriously. Research has shown a link between childhood sexual abuse and somatization, substance use, and depression in adults (Ibeziako et al., 2020).

Older Adults

SSD can involve a lifelong pattern of symptoms that persists into old age. The symptoms of SSD, however, are often unrecognized by health care providers who tend to accept and minimize them as a part of the natural aging process after no medical cause is found.

Epidemiology and Risk Factors

The estimated prevalence of SSD ranges from 5% to 7% (APA, 2013). Millions of dollars of lost revenue and the increased use of short- and long-term disability have prompted employers to study this unique population of employees. This disorder is believed to be higher than reported. In persons with fibromyalgia syndrome, nearly 35% meet the criteria for SSD (Axelsson et al., 2020).

Age of Onset

SSD usually begins before the age of 30 years, with the first symptom often appearing during adolescence. Rarely diagnosed until several years later, seeking help can last for many years, with the individual frequently going from one health care provider to another to no avail. The use of specific assessment instruments is increasing the likelihood of earlier diagnosis and treatment (Toussaint et al., 2019).

Gender, Ethnic, and Cultural Differences

Epidemiologic studies have reported that SSD occurs primarily in non-White, less educated women, particularly those with a lower socioeconomic status and high emotional distress (Granot et al., 2018). Men are less likely to be diagnosed with SSD, partly because of stereotypic male traits, such as a disinclination to admit discomfort or seek help for their symptoms (APA, 2013).

Familial Differences

SSD tends to run in families, and children of parents with multiple unexplained somatic complaints are more likely to have somatic problems. Individuals with a tendency toward heightened physiologic arousal and a tendency to amplify somatosensory information have a greater risk of developing this disorder. Data have also confirmed a strong association between sexual trauma exposure and somatic symptoms, illness attitudes, and health care utilization in women (Granot et al., 2018).

Comorbidity

SSD frequently coexists with other psychiatric disorders, most commonly depression and anxiety. Others include post-traumatic stress disorder, panic disorder, social phobia, obsessive-compulsive disorder (OCD), psychotic disorders, and personality disorders (Newby et al., 2017). Older adults are at particularly high risk for comorbid depression (Johnson et al., 2017).

Ultimately, numerous unexplained medical problems also coexist with this disorder because many patients have received medical and surgical treatments, often unnecessarily, and are plagued with side effects. A disproportionately high number of women who eventually receive diagnoses of SSD have been treated for irritable bowel syndrome (IBS), polycystic ovary disease, and chronic pain.

Etiology

Biologic Theories

The cause of SSD is unknown. General agreement exists that somatization has a biopsychosocial basis, with the possibility of biologic dysfunction common in depression and chronic fatigue syndrome. There are data to support the presence of anatomical and functional deficits in the cortico-limbic-cerebellar circuit (Li et al., 2018).

Although SSD has been shown to run in families, the exact transmission mechanism is unclear. Strong evidence suggests an increased risk for SSD in first-degree relatives, indicating a familial or genetic effect. Because many individuals with SSD live in chaotic families, the high prevalence in first-degree relatives could be explained by environmental influence.

Psychological Theories

Somatization has been explained as a form of social or emotional communication, meaning that the bodily symptoms express an emotion that cannot be verbalized by the individual. An adolescent who experiences severe abdominal pain after her parents argue or a wife who receives nurturing from her husband only when she has back pain are two examples. From this perspective, somatization may be a way of communicating and maintaining relationships. Following this line of reasoning, an individual's physical problems may also become a way of controlling relationships, so somatization becomes a learned behavior pattern. With time, physical symptoms develop automatically in response to perceived threats. Finally, SSD develops when somatizing becomes a way of life (Davoodi et al., 2018).

Consistent with a communication explanation, cognitive behaviorists explain somatization symptoms as an interaction of negative views of the world with physical factors (e.g., pain, discomfort). In this model, individuals have a heightened response based on their experiences with a stressor, especially if the stressor is uncontrollable and unpredictable. Over time, their exaggerated responses become an automatic pattern, resulting in "sick role" behavior, which in turn provokes either a negative or positive response in others (Bilsky et al., 2018; Mik-Meyer & Obling, 2012).

Another theoretical explanation for somatization is the personality trait **alexithymia**, which is associated with SSD. Individuals with alexithymia have difficulty identifying and expressing their emotions. They have a preoccupation with external events and are described as concrete externally oriented thinkers (de Vroege et al., 2018). Credible evidence suggests a link between a history of childhood sexual abuse, rape, and domestic violence, and subsequent lifetime sequelae of somatic symptoms and somatic disorders (Granot et al., 2018).

Social Theories

SSD has been reported globally even though its conceptualization is primarily Western. The symptoms may vary from culture to culture. For example, studies in China have identified and discussed the notion of somatization as a moral issue rather than a medical problem. Somatization is a more socially acceptable way to express behavior in lieu of being diagnosed as depressed because in China, where mental illness is perceived as a character flaw. In many non-Western societies, where the mind–body distinction is not made and symptoms have different meanings and explanations, these physical manifestations are not labeled as a psychiatric disorder (Zhou et al., 2016) (Box 33.1). In Latin American countries, depression is more likely described in somatic symptoms,

---

BOX 33.1

Somatization in Chinese Culture

In Chinese tradition, the health of the individual reflects a balance between positive and negative forces within the body. Five elements at work in nature and in the body control health conditions (e.g., fire, water, wood, earth, metal), five viscera (e.g., liver, heart, spleen, kidneys, lungs), five emotions (anger, joy, worry, sorrow, fear), and five climatic conditions (e.g., wind, heat, humidity, dryness, cold). All illness is explained by imbalances among these elements. Because emotion is related to the circulation of vital air within the body, anger is believed to result from an adverse current of vital air to the liver. Emotional outbursts are seen as results of imbalances among the natural elements rather than the results of behavior of the person.

The stigma of mental illness in the Chinese culture is so great that it can have an adverse effect on a family for many generations. If problems can be attributed to natural causes, the individual and family are less responsible, so that stigma is minimized. The Chinese have a culturally acceptable term for symptoms of mental distress—the closest translation of which would be *neurasthenia*—which comprises somatic complaints of headaches, insomnia, dizziness, aches and pains, poor memory, anxiety, weakness, and loss of energy (Bhola & Chaturvedi, 2020).

such as headaches, gastrointestinal disturbances, or complaints of "nerves," rather than sadness or guilt (Schantz et al., 2017).

Family Response to Disorder

Family dynamics are shaped by all members, including the person with SSD. When one member has several ongoing chronic health issues, family members' activities and interactions are affected. The physical symptoms of the individual become the focus of family life, so activities are planned around that person. Because so much time and so many resources are used trying to discover an underlying illness, resources to other family members are reduced. Because the person is always sick, expressing anger about the situation is difficult. The family members need support as they learn to understand the seriousness and difficulty of experiencing an SSD.

RECOVERY-ORIENTED CARE OF PERSONS WITH SSD

Teamwork and Collaboration: Working Toward Recovery

The care of patients with SSD involves three approaches:

- Providing long-term supportive general management of the chronic condition
- Treating symptoms of comorbid psychiatric and physical problems
- Providing care in special settings, including individual and group treatment and the use of complementary and alternative medicine.

The cornerstones of management are trust and believing. Ideally, the patient should see only one health care provider at regularly scheduled visits. During each primary care visit, the provider should conduct a holistic assessment, including a partial physical examination of the organ system, focusing on the areas where the patient has complaints. Physical symptoms are treated conservatively using the least intrusive approach. The provider should also assess for any stressors, life changes, and/or a history of trauma that has been linked to the excessive expression of somatic symptoms. In the mental health setting, the use of cognitive-behavioral therapy (CBT) can be effective (Liu et al., 2019).

Safety Issues

SSD and related disorders are associated with a risk of suicide. If depression and anxiety are present, the risk is greater. Safety becomes even more of a concern because these individuals are not usually treated in a mental health setting where suicide assessments are routine (Torres et al., 2021).

EVIDENCE-BASED MENTAL HEALTH NURSING CARE OF THE PERSON WITH SSD

Mental Health Nursing Assessment

During the assessment interview, the nurse should allow enough time for the patient to explain all medical problems; a hurried assessment interview blocks communication. Nursing Care Plan 33.1—which sets forth a plan of care for Carol, the case study patient in this chapter.

> **NCLEXNOTE** Encourage and allow patients with SSD to discuss their physical problems before focusing on psychosocial issues.

Physical Health Assessment

Psychiatric–mental health nurses typically see these patients for problems related to coexisting psychiatric disorders, such as depression, not SSD. While taking the patient's history, the nurse may discover that the individual has had multiple surgeries or medical problems, making SSD a strong possibility. If the patient has not already received a diagnosis of SSD, the nurse should screen for it by determining the presence of the most commonly reported problems associated with this disorder, which include dysmenorrhea, a lump in the throat, vomiting, shortness of breath, burning sensation in the sex organs, painful limbs, and amnesia. If the patient has these symptoms, they should be seen by a mental health provider qualified to make the diagnosis. Box 33.2 presents the Health Attitude Survey, which can be used as a screening test for somatization.

Review of Systems

Although these patients' symptoms have usually received considerable attention from the medical community, a careful review of systems is important because the appearance of physical problems is usually related to psychosocial problems. Even as the patient continues to be seen for mental health problems, an ongoing awareness of biologic symptoms is important, particularly because these symptoms are de-emphasized in the overall case management.

Pain is the most common finding in people with this disorder. Because the pain is usually related to symptoms of all the major body systems, it is unlikely that a somatic intervention such as an analgesic will be effective on a

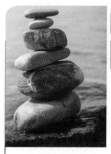

NURSING CARE PLAN 33.1

The Patient with Somatic Symptom Disorder

Carol is a 48-year-old woman who is making her weekly visit to her primary care physician for unexplained multiple somatic problems. This week, her concern is reoccurring abdominal pain that fits no symptom pattern. Upon physical examination, a cause for her abdominal pain could not be found. She is requesting a refill of alprazolam (Xanax), which is the only medication that relieves her pain. She is in the process of applying for disability income because of being completely disabled by neck and shoulder pain. The physician and office staff avoid her whenever possible. The physician will not refill the prescription until Carol is evaluated by the consulting mental health team that provides weekly evaluations and services.

Setting: Primary Care Office

Baseline Assessment: Forty-eight-year-old White woman with obesity who appears very angry. She resents being forced to see a mental health provider for the only medication that works. She denies any psychiatric problems or emotional distress. Carol is wearing a short black top and slacks. Her hair is in curlers, and she says that it is too much trouble to comb her hair. Her mental status is normal, but she admits to being slightly depressed and takes alprazolam for her nerves. She says that sometimes she feels like going to sleep and not waking up, but denies any thoughts of killing herself. She depends on her children for everything and feels very guilty about doing so. She spends most of her waking hours going to various doctors and taking combinations of medications to relieve her pains. She has no friends or nonfamily social contacts because they would not be able to stand her. BP 144/80, P 80, R 18, Ht. 5'2"; Wt. 190; BMI 34.7.

Associated Psychiatric Diagnosis	Medications
R/O depression; SSD	Premarin, 0.625 mg every day
S/P hysterectomy	Alprazolam (Xanax), 25 mg tid
S/P gastric bypass	Ranitidine HCL (Zantac), 150 mg with meals
S/P carpel tunnel release	Simethicone, 125 mg four times daily with meals
Chronic shoulder, neck pain, vertigo	Calcium carbonate, 1,200 mg every day
	Multiple vitamin, every day
	Zolpidem tartrate (Ambien), 10 mg at bedtime PRN
	Ibuprofen, 600 mg q 4 h PRN pain
	Simethicone 125 mg, PRN for indigestion
	phenylephrine topical suppositories PRN for hemorrhoid pain

Priority of Care: Negative Self-Esteem

Important Characteristics	Associated Considerations
Slight depressions	Feels she is a burden to family
Dependency on others	Thinks about going to sleep and not waking up
Expresses guilt	Constant physical problems that interfere with normal social activities
Expresses feelings of helplessness	

Outcomes

Initial	Long-term
Identify need to increase self-esteem	Participate in individual or group therapy for esteem building

Interventions

Interventions	Rationale	Ongoing Assessment
Establish rapport with patient.	Individuals with low self-esteem are reluctant to discuss true feelings.	Examine feelings provoked by patient (discuss with supervisor if interfering with care). Determine whether patient is beginning to engage in a relationship.

Continued

Nursing Care Plan 33.1 Continued

Encourage patient to spend time dressing and grooming appropriately.	Confidence and self-esteem improve when a person looks well-groomed.	Monitor response to suggestions.
Encourage patient to discuss various somatic problems but allow some time to discuss psychological and interpersonal issues.	Patients with SSD need time to express their physical problems. It helps them feel valued. The best way to build a relationship is to acknowledge physical symptoms.	Monitor time that patient spends explaining physical symptoms.
Explore opportunities for Carol will meet other people with similar, nonmedical interests.	Focusing Carol on meeting others will improve the possibilities of increasing contacts.	Observe willingness to identify other interests besides physical problems.

Evaluation

Outcomes	**Revised Outcomes**	**Interventions**
Carol admitted to having low self-esteem but was very reluctant to consider meeting new people.	Focus on building self-esteem.	Identify activities that will enhance personal self-esteem.

Priority of Care: Using Medication Inappropriately

Important Characteristics	**Associated Considerations**
Lack of medication effectiveness. Verbalizes difficulty with prescribed regimens.	Uses medication for other conditions than prescribed.

Outcomes

Initial	**Long-term**
Discuss the use of medications honestly.	Use nonpharmacologic means for stress reduction, especially avoiding continued use of antianxiety medications.

Interventions

Interventions	**Rationale**	**Ongoing Assessment**
Clarify the frequency and purpose of taking alprazolam.	Unsupervised polypharmacy is very common with these patients. Further clarification is usually needed.	Carefully track self-report of medication use; determine if patient is disclosing the use of all medications.
Educate patient about the effects of combining medications, emphasizing side effects.	Education about combining medication is the beginning of helping patient become effective in medication regimen.	Observe patient's ability and willingness to consider negative effects.
Recommend that patient gradually reduce number of medications and problem-solve other means of managing physical symptoms.	Giving patients clear directions about managing health care regimens needs to be followed up with specific strategies to change behavior.	Evaluate patient's ability to solve problems.

Evaluation

Outcomes	**Revised Outcomes**	**Interventions**
Carol disclosed use of medications but was unwilling to consider changing ineffective use of medication.	Identify next step if primary care physician does not refill prescription.	Discuss the possibility of not being able to obtain alprazolam. Refer patient to mental health clinic for further evaluation.

BOX 33.2
Health Attitude Survey

On a scale of 1 to 5, please indicate the extent to which you agree (5) or disagree (1).

DISSATISFACTION WITH CARE

1. I have been satisfied with the medical care I have received. (R)
2. Doctors have done the best they could to diagnose and treat my health problems. (R)
3. Doctors have taken my health problems seriously.
4. My health problems have been thoroughly evaluated. (R)
5. Doctors do not seem to know much about the health problems I have had.
6. My health problems have been completely explained. (R)
7. Doctors seem to think I am exaggerating my health problems.
8. My response to treatment has not been satisfactory.
9. My response to treatment is usually excellent. (R)

FRUSTRATION WITH ILL HEALTH

10. I am tired of feeling sick and would like to get to the bottom of my health problems.
11. I have felt ill for quite a while now.
12. I am going to keep searching for an answer to my health problems.
13. I do not think there is anything seriously wrong with my body. (R)

HIGH UTILIZATION OF CARE

14. I have seen many different doctors over the years.
15. I have taken a lot of medicine recently.
16. I do not go to the doctor often. (R)
17. I have had relatively good health over the years.

EXCESSIVE HEALTH WORRY

18. I sometimes worry too much about my health.
19. I often fear the worst when I develop symptoms.
20. I have trouble getting my mind off my health.

PSYCHOLOGICAL DISTRESS

21. Sometimes, I feel depressed and cannot seem to shake it off.
22. I have sought help for emotional or stress-related problems.
23. It is easy to relax and stay calm. (R)
24. I believe the stress I am under may be affecting my health.

DISCORDANT COMMUNICATION OF DISTRESS

25. Some people think that I am capable of more work than I feel able to do.
26. Some people think that I have been sick just to gain attention.
27. It is difficult for me to find the right words for my feelings.

(R) indicates items reversed for scoring purposes. Scoring—The higher the score, the more likely somatization is a problem.

Reprinted from Noyes, R., Jr, Langbehn, D. R., Happel, R. L., Sieren, L. R., & Muller, B. A. (1999). Health Attitude Survey: A scale for assessing somatizing patients. *Psychosomatics, 40*(6), 470–478. Copyright © 2011 The Academy of Psychosomatic Medicine. With permission.

long-term basis. Remember that although no medical explanation exists for the pain, the patient's pain is real and has serious psychosocial implications. A careful assessment should include the following questions:

- What is the pain like?
- What is the extent of the pain?
- What helps the pain get better?
- When is the pain at its worst?
- What has worked in the past to relieve the pain?

Physical Functioning

The actual physical functioning of these individuals is often marginal. They usually have problems with sleep, fatigue, activity, and sexual functioning. Assessment of these areas generates data to be used in planning interventions. The amount and quality of sleep are important, as are the hours when the individual sleeps. For example, an individual may sleep a total of 6 hours each diurnal cycle but only from 2:00 to 6:00 AM plus an afternoon nap.

Fatigue is a constant problem for many people with SSD, and because various physical problems interfere with normal activity. These patients report an overwhelming lack of energy, which makes maintaining usual routines or accomplishing daily tasks impossible. Fatigue is accompanied by the inability to concentrate on simple functions, leading to decreased performance and disinterest in surroundings. Patients tend to be lethargic and listless and often have little energy (Box 33.3).

Female patients with this disorder usually have had multiple gynecologic problems, so that the physical manifestations of SSD often lead to altered sexual behavior. Symptoms of dysmenorrhea and painful intercourse may indicate a history of sexual abuse and sexual trauma. Physiologic indicators, such as those produced by laboratory tests, are not available. However, a careful assessment of the patient's menstrual history, gynecologic problems, and sexual functioning is important. It is also important to assess whether abuse or trauma has occurred in the past or continues in the present, and whether such abuse is sexual, physical, or emotional.

Nutrition

Nutrition assessment is important because gastrointestinal disorders are highly comorbid with psychiatric disorders, especially SSD. Psychological distress and poorer psychosocial functioning associated with SSD contribute to the severity of IBS (Porcelli et al., 2020). In IBS, there is a disordered communication between the gut and brain that results in motility disturbances, visceral hypersensitivity, and altered CNS processing. The primary treatment of IBS includes dietary changes, soluble fiber, and antispasmodic drugs (Ford et al., 2020).

Somatic Symptom Disorder and Stress

Ms. J, age 42 years, has been coming to the mental health clinic for 2 years for her nerves. She has seen only the physician for medication but now has been referred to the nurse's new stress management group because she is experiencing side effects to all the medications that have been tried. The psychiatrist has diagnosed SSD and wants her to learn to manage her "nerves" without medication.

At the first meeting with the nurse, Ms. J was preoccupied with chest pain and bloating that had lasted for the past 6 months. Her chest pain is constant and sharp at times. The pain does not prevent her from going to her job as a waitress but does interfere with meal preparation at night for her family and her ability to have sexual intercourse. She has numerous other physical problems, including allergies to certain perfumes, dysmenorrhea, ovarian polycystic disease (ovarian cysts), chronic urinary tract infections, and rashes. She is constantly fatigued and has frequent leg cramps. She states that she is too tired to fix dinner for her family. On days off from work, she takes a nap in the afternoon, sleeping until evening. She is unable to fall asleep at night.

She believes that she will soon have to have her gallbladder removed because of occasional referred pain to her back and nausea that occurs a couple hours after eating. She is not enthusiastic about a stress management group and does not believe it will help her problems. However, she has agreed to consider it for as long as the psychiatrist will continue prescribing diazepam (Valium).

What Do You Think?
• How would you prioritize Ms. J's physical symptoms?
• What are some possible explanations for Ms. J's fatigue?

Furthermore, the quality of the diet is associated with medically unexplained gastrointestinal symptoms. Diet patterns loaded with fruits, vegetables, low-fat diary, dried fruits, and whole grains have fewer reported gastrointestinal disturbances than diets loaded with vegetable oil, meat, salt, french fries, hydrogenated oils, onions, egg, poultry, fish, and refined grains or diets loaded with processed meats, sweet deserts, high-fat dairy (Haghighatdoost et al., 2020).

Medication

A medication assessment of these patients can be challenging. Patients with SSD frequently seek help from numerous providers because they do not feel that they are believed, or they think that providers don't care about their suffering. Because they often receive medications from each provider, they usually take a large number of drugs. A medication assessment is needed not only because of the number of medications but also because these individuals frequently experience unusual side effects, or they report that they are "sensitive" to medications. Because of their somatic sensitivity, they often overreact to medication. Developing a therapeutic

relationship promotes trust and can minimize these patients' search for a health care professional who believes their symptoms and suffering.

Substance Use

These patients spend much of their lives trying to find out what is wrong with them. When one health care provider after another can find little if any explanation for their symptoms, many patients become anxious and/or depressed. To alleviate their symptoms of anxiety, they sometimes self-medicate with over-the-counter (OTC) medications and/or substances of abuse (e.g., alcohol, marijuana), or they seek a health care provider who prescribes a benzodiazepine such as alprazolam. Because symptoms associated with their disorder cannot be treated within a few weeks with a benzodiazepine, they can become dependent on medication that should not have been prescribed in the first place.

Although benzodiazepines have a place in therapeutics, they are not recommended for long-term use and only complicate the treatment of individuals with SSD. These medications should also be avoided because of their addictive qualities, which place patients at risk of addiction. Unfortunately, by the time patients with SSD see a mental health provider, they often have already begun taking the medications for anxiety. Many times, they only agree to see a mental health provider because the last provider would no longer prescribe an anxiolytic without a psychiatric evaluation.

Remember Carol?

Carol has been taking alprazolam for stress for years. Her primary health care provider is refusing to prescribe it again until she has a complete mental health examination. No other health care providers will prescribe alprazolam for her.

Psychosocial Assessment

The mental status of individuals with SSD can be within normal limits, although most patients report frustration, depression, and hopelessness about their situation. What is most noticeable is their intense focus on their bodies and the physical symptoms that are causing them distress and disability.

Cognitive and Behavioral Responses

Generally, cognition is not impaired in people with SSD, but it may be distorted, such as believing the pain means a life-threatening condition. These individuals seem preoccupied with the signs and symptoms of their illnesses and may even keep a record of their experiences. Living with illness, diseases, and suffering truly becomes a way of life.

Self-Concept

People with SSD usually have a negative self-concept of physical weakness and illness-related symptom evaluation. The self-concept can be determined by physical appearance, affect, and explanation of the current situation. Negative self-concept usually begins in childhood or adolescence when the child begins to see themselves as ill and cannot participate in normal school or recreational activities. Parents who focus on protecting children from illness can inadvertently reinforce the self-concept of being ill.

Stress and Coping Patterns

Some individuals with SSD have intense emotional reactions to life stressors and have led or are leading traumatic or chaotic lives. These patients usually have had a series of personal crises beginning at an early age. Examples include severe sexual and physical abuse and psychological trauma. Typically, a new symptom or medical problem develops during times of emotional stress, as well as during anniversaries of losses or traumas that have occurred in the patient's lifetime. It is critical that the link between the physical assessment data and the patient's psychological and social history are considered. A thorough history of major psychological events should be compared with the chronology of physical problems. Special attention should be paid to any history of sexual abuse or trauma in the patient's younger years. Early sexual abuse may also prevent the individual from being able to perform sexually or to endure chronic abdominal pain or discomfort during sexual relations.

The individual's mood is usually labile, often shifting from extremely excited or anxious to being depressed and hopeless. Response to physical symptoms is usually magnified, such as interpreting a simple cold as pneumonia or a brief chest pain as a heart attack. Family members may not believe the physical symptoms are real and may view them as attention-getting behavior because symptoms often improve when the patient receives attention. For example, a woman who has been in bed for 3 weeks with severe back pain may suddenly feel much better when her children visit her.

Social Network

People with this disorder spend excessive time seeking medical care and treating their multiple illnesses. Because they believe themselves to be very sick, they also believe that they are disabled and cannot work. Many are unemployed, so frequently these individuals have changed jobs, had multiple positions over their lifetimes or careers, or have had absences or gaps in employment (Sharma & Manjula, 2013).

Because their symptoms are often inconsistent with any identifiable medical diagnosis, these individuals are rarely satisfied with their health care providers, who can find nothing wrong. However, their social network often consists of a series of health care providers, rather than peers or family members, who can also become weary of the individual's constant complaints of physical problems. Identifying a support network requires sorting out the health care providers from family and friends.

Consider Carol's Limited Social Network
Carol has no friends and spends her time going from provider to provider. Her anxiety about her symptoms has impacted her ability to maintain friendships and other close relationships.

Family Issues

Individuals with SSD sometimes live in chaotic families with multiple problems. In assessing the family structure, other members with psychiatric disorders must be identified. Women may be married to abusive men who have antisocial personality disorders; substance use disorders are common. Identifying the positive and negative relationships within the family is important.

SSD is particularly problematic because it disrupts the family's social life. Changes in routine or major life events often precipitate the appearance of a symptom. For example, a person may be planning a vacation with the family but at the last minute decides they cannot go because the back pain has returned, and they will be unable to sit in the car. These family disruptions are common. In addition, as already noted, employment history for the person with SSD may be erratic.

Quality of Life

SSD has a negative impact on the quality of life. Since many of the physical symptoms (25% to 50%) are unexplained, the person is continually told that there are no medical explanations, which leads to frustration and seeking out additional medical opinions. The pain or discomfort interferes with daily activities and prevents the person from participating fully with family and friends (van Westrienen et al., 2020).

Strengths Assessment

A person with SSD may have difficulty identifying *any* personal strengths. The nurse should help the person focus on daily activities and suggest strengths that emerge. For example, some strengths might be that the person has a place to live, has a caring family, or some educational attainment. The nurse also elicits motivation to feel better.

CLINICAL JUDGMENT

The physical issues dominate the individual's concern and should not be dismissed. They may have a variety of health issues to discuss, including fatigue, pain, and insomnia. Psychologically, depression and suicidal behavior should always be considered. Social isolation may be an outward expression of depression.

THERAPEUTIC RELATIONSHIP

The most difficult aspect of nursing care is developing a sound, positive, nonjudgmental nurse–patient relationship, yet this relationship is crucial. Without it, the nurse is just one more provider who fails to meet the patient's expectations. Developing this relationship requires time and patience. Therapeutic communication techniques should be used to refocus the patient on psychosocial problems related to the physical manifestations (Box 33.4).

During periods when symptoms of other psychiatric disorders surface, additional interventions are needed. For example, if depression occurs, additional supportive or cognitive approaches may be needed.

Carol's Behavior on the Mental Health Unit
Carol felt she was tricked into agreeing to be admitted to a mental health unit for medication evaluation. She believes she should be on a medical unit for her constant pain.

MENTAL HEALTH NURSING INTERVENTIONS

Establishing Recovery and Wellness Goals

Establishing recovery and wellness goals may seem to be out of the question with individuals who defines themselves as "ill," "sick," and/or in "chronic pain." However, helping such individuals define their symptoms and validate them is a start to recovery. Nurses are poised to educate individuals with multiple somatic problems to better understand their symptoms (e.g., what triggers them) and to define short-term goals for recovery. The notion of recovery itself is patient centered and focused on what the patient believes is realistic and possible. For example, some patients with this disorder may choose to learn to live with their symptoms (e.g., pain) and find alternative ways of coping. Nursing interventions can focus on individuals learning the triggers in their lives that worsen their symptoms as well as those activities that lessen them. Even though a patient may suffer from multiple somatic symptoms and/or this chronic illness, together the nurse and the patient can work toward setting short- and long-term goals that promote health and wellness.

Physical Health Interventions

Nursing interventions that focus on physical health become especially important because medical treatment must be conservative; aggressive pharmacologic treatment must be avoided. Each time a nurse sees the patient, some of that time should be spent respectfully discussing physical complaints and validating the patient's distress. During the discussion, it is important that the nurse project the belief that the patient is truly experiencing the symptoms. Several physically focused interventions, including pain management, activity enhancement, nutrition regulation, relaxation, and pharmacologic interventions, may be useful in caring for patients with SSD.

Pain Management

In pain management, a single approach rarely works. Pain is a primary issue and was previously considered a separate disorder. Nursing care focuses on helping patients identify strategies to relieve pain and to examine stressors in their lives. After a careful assessment of the pain, nonpharmacologic strategies should be developed to reduce it. If gastrointestinal pain is frequent, eating and bowel habits should be explored and modified as needed. For back pain, exercises and consultation from a physical therapist may be useful. Headaches are a challenge. Self-monitoring and tracking them engages the patient in the therapeutic process and helps to identify psychosocial triggers. In addition, suggesting or referring the individual for complementary and alternative treatments may be useful. Relaxation techniques, identifying thoughts and feelings about pain or discomfort, and including family members in the intervention have also been shown to be useful.

Activity Enhancement

Helping the patient establish a daily routine may alleviate some of the difficulty with sleep but doing so may be difficult because most of these patients are not employed.

BOX 33.4 • THERAPEUTIC DIALOGUE: ESTABLISHING A RELATIONSHIP

INEFFECTIVE APPROACH

Nurse: Good morning, Carol.

Carol: I'm in so much pain. Take that breakfast away.

Nurse: You don't want your breakfast?

Carol: Can't you see? I hurt! When I hurt, I can't eat!

Nurse: If you don't eat now, you probably won't be able to have anything until lunch.

Carol: Who cares? I have no intention of being here at lunchtime. I don't belong here.

Nurse: Carol, I don't think that your doctor would have admitted you unless there were a problem. I would like to talk to you about why you are here.

Carol: Nurse, I'm just here. It's none of your business.

Nurse: Oh.

Carol: Please leave me alone.

Nurse: Sure, I will see you later.

EFFECTIVE APPROACH

Nurse: Good morning, Carol.

Carol: I'm in so much pain. Take that breakfast away.

Nurse: (Silently removes tray. Pulls up chair and sits down.)

Carol: My back hurts.

Nurse: Oh, when did the back pain start?

Carol: Last night. It's this bed. I couldn't get comfortable.

Nurse: These beds can be pretty uncomfortable.

Carol: My back pain is shooting down my leg.

Nurse: Does anything help it?

Carol: Sometimes, if I straighten out my leg it helps.

Nurse: Can I help you straighten out your leg?

Carol: Oh, it's OK. The pain is going away. What did you say your name is?

Nurse: I'm Susan Miller, your nurse while you are here.

Carol: I won't be here long. I don't belong in a psychiatric unit.

Nurse: While you are here, I would like to spend time with you.

Carol: OK, but you understand, I do not have any psychiatric problems.

Nurse: We can talk about whatever you want. But because you want to get out of here, we might want to focus on what it will take to get you ready for discharge.

CRITICAL THINKING CHALLENGE

- What communication mistakes did the nurse in the first scenario make?
- What communication strategies helped the patient feel comfortable with the nurse in the second scenario?
- How is the first scenario different from the second?

Encouraging the patient to get up in the morning and go to bed at night at specific times can help the patient to establish a routine. These patients should engage in regular exercise to improve their overall physical state, although they often have numerous reasons why they cannot. This is where the nurse's patience is tested; the nurse ultimately needs to remember that the patient's symptoms are an expression of suffering. Agreeing that daily exercise is difficult but continuing to emphasize the importance of exercise can counter some of the reluctance to exercise.

Nutrition Regulation

Patients with SSD often have gastrointestinal problems and may have special nutritional needs. The nurse should discuss the nutritional value of foods with the patient. Discussing the use of whole healthy food sources rather than processed or "junk" food is a strategy nurses can use to assist the patient with gastrointestinal distress to consider dietary changes. The act of talking with patients about ways that they can exert some control of their bodies can have a positive effect and assist them with managing some of their symptoms. If patients are being prescribed medications that promote weight gain, weight control strategies may be discussed, including exercise or increasing movement with physical therapy.

Relaxation

Patients taking anxiety-relieving medication can be taught relaxation techniques to alleviate stress. It is a challenge to help these patients really use these strategies. The nurse should consider various techniques, including simple relaxation techniques, distraction, and guided imagery (see Chapter 11).

Wellness Challenges

Individuals with SSD focus on signs of illness, not behaviors supporting wellness. Because these individuals have intense bodily sensations that are associated with illness, it is difficult to help them re-focus on wellness.

Medications Interventions

No medication is specifically recommended for patients with SSD; however, psychiatric symptoms of comorbid disorders, such as depression and anxiety, should be treated pharmacologically as appropriate. Usually, patients who are depressed or anxious take an antidepressant to treat their symptoms (see Chapter 25).

Multiple antidepressants have been shown to be effective for treating pain and the symptoms of depression. Duloxetine—a serotonin and norepinephrine (NE) reuptake inhibitor that is indicated for neuropathy, depression, and anxiety—is also used to manage pain (Brammer, 2018). See Box 33.5.

Patients who report symptoms of anxiety are treated pharmacologically, similar to those with depression. The first line of treatment for all anxiety disorders is with an SSRI. Doses for SSD are usually higher than those prescribed for depression to relieve and manage the symptoms of the anxiety disorders, including panic, social

---

BOX 33.5

Drug Profile: Duloxetine

DRUG CLASS: Serotonin and norepinephrine reuptake inhibitor (SNRI)

RECEPTOR AFFINITY: Binds selectively and has a high affinity to both NE and serotonin (5-HT) transporters yet lacks affinity for monoamine receptors within the central nervous system.

INDICATIONS: Treatment of depression, generalized anxiety disorder, chronic musculoskeletal pain, diabetic peripheral neuropathic pain, fibromyalgia

ROUTE AND DOSAGE: Available as capsules: 30 mg, 60 mg

Adults: Initially, 60 mg daily and increasing to 90 mg/d consistent with patient tolerance. Therapy at 120 mg/d may be necessary before response occurs. Can be given in divided doses for individuals who are used to taking pain medication twice a day.

Geriatric: Adjust dosage as needed because older patients—particularly those on other medications—are more prone to develop side effects. May initiate dose of 30 mg daily for 2 weeks.

Pediatric: Not recommended for children younger than 18 years of age

HALF-LIFE (PEAK EFEECTS): Duloxetine has an elimination half-life of about 12 hours (the range is 8 to 17 hours). Steady state is usually achieved after 3 days.

SELECTED SIDE EFFECTS: Nausea, dry mouth, constipation, diarrhea, fatigue, difficulty sleeping, and dizziness. Increased blood pressure can occur and should be monitored. Seizures have been reported. Sexual dysfunction (decreased sex drive and delayed orgasm and ejaculation) has been associated with duloxetine.

BOXED WARNING: Suicidal thoughts and behaviors

WARNINGS: Screen for bipolar disorder, monitor for serotonin syndrome; monitor blood pressure before and after dosage is initiated (e.g., weekly for one month), screen for medication-to-medication interactions.

SPECIFIC PATIENT/FAMILY EDUCATION

- Take drug exactly as prescribed; do not stop taking it abruptly or without consulting your health care provider.
- If patients wish to stop the medication, they need to consult with their provider about tapering the dose due to discontinuation syndrome, a cluster of physical and emotional symptoms that are associated with decreasing SNRIs and SSRIs too quickly. Symptoms of abrupt discontinuation can include the following: Symptoms of withdrawal include dizziness, anxiety, nausea, vomiting, nervousness, and diarrhea.
- Families and caregivers of patients should be advised to observe for the emergence of anxiety, agitation, panic attacks, insomnia, irritability, hostility, aggressiveness, impulsivity, hypomania, mania, other unusual changes in behavior, worsening of depression, and suicidal ideation. Such symptoms should be reported to the patient's prescriber or health professional, especially if side effects are severe, abrupt in onset, or were not part of the patient's presenting symptoms.
- Report any signs and symptoms of side effects.
- Combining duloxetine with aspirin, nonsteroidal anti-inflammatory drugs (NSAIDs), warfarin (Coumadin), or other drugs that are associated with bleeding may increase the risk of bleeding.

phobia, generalized anxiety, OCD, and post-traumatic stress disorder.

Nonpharmacologic approaches, such as biofeedback and relaxation, are also quite useful in conjunction with pharmacologic treatment. Benzodiazepines may be used initially in the treatment of those with anxiety but should be slowly decreased and discontinued because of the psychological and physiologic dependence associated with these medications. Buspirone (BuSpar), a nonbenzodiazepine, does not lead to tolerance or withdrawal and may be useful for relief of acute anxiety. BuSpar should be used cautiously with other serotonin-related medications (such as SSRIs) because of its high affinity for serotonin receptors. If panic disorder is present, it should be treated aggressively with SSRIs and frequently at higher doses.

Pain medication should be prescribed conservatively. If mood disorders are also present, some mood stabilizers not only treat the depression but also may treat the pain. An example is gabapentin, another frequently prescribed medication for neuropathic pain experienced during and after herpes zoster (also commonly known as shingles).

Administering and Monitoring Medications

In SSD, patients are usually treated in the community, where they commonly self-medicate. Carefully question patients about self-administered medicine and determine which medicines or substances they are currently using to relieve their pain and/or discomfort (including OTC, herbal supplements, and/or illicit substances). Also listen carefully to determine any side effects the patient attributes to the medication. This information should be documented and reported to the rest of the team. The patient should be encouraged to continue taking only prescribed medication and to seek approval before taking any additional OTC or other prescribed medications. SSD patients are at high risk for prescription drug misuse and abuse, as well as for purchasing substances illicitly. The recent trends of prescription drug misuse have been linked to opioid use disorder and overdose.

Managing Side Effects

These individuals often have atypical reactions to their medications. Side effects should be assessed, but the patient should be encouraged to compare the benefits of the medication with any problems related to side effects. Patients should also be encouraged to give the medications enough time to be effective because many medications require up to 6 weeks before the patient has a response or experiences a relief of symptoms. This is especially true for patients who are prescribed some of the antidepressants that have been in use the longest, such as fluoxetine.

Management of Complications

In working with patients with SSD, always be on the lookout for drug–drug interactions. Medications these patients take for physical problems could interact with psychiatric medications. Patients may be taking alternative medicines, such as herbal supplements, but they usually willingly disclose doing so. The patient should be encouraged to use the same pharmacy for filling all prescriptions so possible interactions can be checked and monitored.

Psychosocial Interventions

The choice of psychosocial intervention depends on the specific problem the patient is experiencing. The most important and ongoing intervention is the maintenance of a therapeutic relationship.

Therapeutic Interactions

Nursing care should include listening to the patient's report of symptoms and fears, validating it by acknowledging that the fears may be real, asking the patient to monitor symptoms in a journal, and encouraging the patient to bring the journal to the next visit. By reviewing the symptom pattern, it is possible to continue to educate the patient and assess for significant symptoms. The outcome of this approach should be a decrease in fears and better control of the symptoms.

Using Cognitive Behavioral Interventions

Several interventions are effective in reducing patients' fears of experiencing serious illnesses. Cognitive-behavioral therapy (CBT), stress management, and group interventions can decrease the intensity and increase the control of symptoms (Wortman et al., 2018). Whether the positive outcomes result from the intervention itself or from the symptom validation and increased attention given to the patient remains unknown.

Counseling

Counseling with a focus on problem-solving is needed from time to time. These patients often have chaotic lives and need support through the multitude of crises. Although they may appear fascinating and at times self-assured, they can easily irritate others because of their constant complaints. The consequences of their impaired social interaction with others must be examined within a counseling framework. It will become evident that the patient's problem-solving and decision-making skills could be improved. Identifying stresses and strengthening positive coping responses helps the patient deal with a chaotic lifestyle.

Psychoeducation

Teaching About Symptoms

Health teaching is useful throughout the nurse–patient relationship. These patients have many questions about illnesses, symptoms, and treatments. Emphasize positive health care practices and minimize the effects of serious illness. Because of problems in managing medications and treatment, the therapeutic regimen needs constant monitoring, resulting in ample opportunities for teaching. (Box 33.6).

Wellness Strategies

Wellness strategies should be included in the discussion of the interventions. The same interventions that were discussed in reducing the symptoms of SSD are also used as wellness strategies. Patients with SSD should focus on "staying healthy" instead of focusing on their illnesses. For these individuals, approaching the topic of health promotion usually has to be within the context of preventing further problems. Setting aside time for themselves and identifying activities that meet their psychological and spiritual needs, such as going to church or synagogue, are important in maintaining a healthy balance.

Social Relationships

Patients with SSD are usually isolated from their families and communities. Strengthening social relationships and activities often becomes the focus of nursing care. The nurse should help the patient identify individuals with whom contact is desired, ask for a commitment to contact them, and encourage them to reinitiate the

relationship. The nurse should counsel patients about talking too much about their symptoms with these individuals and emphasize that medical information should be shared with the nurse instead. The nurse must also ensure that patients know when their next appointments are scheduled.

Providing Family Education

The results of a family assessment often reveal that families of these individuals need education about the disorder, helpful strategies for dealing with the multiple complaints of the patient, and usually help in developing more effective communication patterns. Because of the chaotic nature of some of the families and the lack of healthy problem solving, physical, sexual, and psychological abuse may be evident. It is important to be particularly sensitive to any evidence of current physical or sexual abuse because this may lead to a need for additional interventions.

Promoting Safety

Individuals with SSD can benefit from a crisis safety plan that could be used during times of stress or depression. The safety plan would list triggers for anxiety, suicidal ideation, and mood changes with specific behavioral strategies for each trigger. See Chapters 11 and 22.

Group Interventions

Although these patients may not be candidates for insight group psychotherapy, they do benefit from cognitive-behavioral groups that focus on developing coping skills for everyday life (Liu et al., 2019). Because most are women, participation in groups that address feminist issues should be encouraged to strengthen their assertiveness skills and improve their generally low self-esteem.

When leading a group that has members with this disorder, redirection can keep the group from giving too much attention to a person's illness. However, these individuals need reassurance and support while in a group. They may say that they do not fit in or belong in the group. In reality, they are feeling insecure and threatened by the situation. The group leader needs to show patience and understanding to engage the individual effectively in meaningful group interaction.

Evaluation and Treatment Outcomes

Recovery outcomes for patients with SSD should be realistic. Because this is a lifelong disorder, small successes should be expected. Specific outcomes should be identified, such as gradually increasing social contact.

BOX 33.6

Somatic Symptom Disorder

When caring for a patient with SSD, be sure to include the following topic areas in the teaching plan:

- Psychopharmacologic agents (anxiolytics) if ordered, including drug, action, dosage, frequency, and possible side effects
- Nonpharmacologic pain relief measures
- Exercise
- Nutrition
- Social interaction
- Appropriate health care practices
- Problem-solving
- Relaxation and anxiety-reduction techniques
- Sexual functioning

Over time, a gradual reduction in the number of health care providers the individual contacts should occur and a slight improvement in the ability to cope with stresses should follow.

Continuum of Care

Emergency Care

The emergencies these individuals experience may be physical (e.g., chest pain, back pain, gastrointestinal symptoms) or stress responses related to a psychosocial crisis. Occasionally, these individuals become suicidal and require an intensive level of care. Generally speaking, nonpharmacologic interventions should be tried first, with very conservative use of antianxiety medications. All attempts should be made to retrieve records from other facilities.

Inpatient Care

Ideally, individuals with SSD spend minimal time in the hospital for treatment of their medical or comorbid mental disorders. While an inpatient, the patient should have consistency in providers who care or oversee all nursing care. Therapeutic interactions and relationships are very important and can help move the individual toward recovery.

Community Care

Patients with SSD can spend a lifetime in the health care system and still have little continuity of care. Switching from one health care provider to others is detrimental to their long-term care. Most are outpatients. When they are hospitalized, it is usually for evaluation of medical problems or to receive care for comorbid disorders.

Virtual Mental Health Care

Digital applications provide immediate access to self-health programs such as relaxation, stress reduction, sleep, and imagery. Using these tools can reduce the intensity of the distress and discomfort. Virtual primary care visits and health education sessions provide opportunities for patient–clinician interactions within a safe environment.

Integration with Primary Care

Primary care is the main treatment setting for persons with SSD. With the exception of a severe depression or comorbid mental health disorder, mental health specialists serve primarily as supportive consultants to primary care clinicians. The role of the mental health clinician is

---

BOX 33.7

Psychoeducational Intervention in Primary Care

Johnson, K. K., Bennett, C., & Rochani, H. (2020). Significant improvement of somatic symptom disorder with brief psychoeducational intervention by PMHNP in primary care. Journal of the American Psychiatric Nurses Association, 1078390320960524. Advance online publication. https://doi.org/10.1177/1078390320960524

THE QUESTION: Does a psychoeducation intervention by a psychiatric mental health nurse practitioner that explains the HPA axis response to acute and chronic stress reduce anxiety and stress in persons diagnosed with SSD?

METHOD: Thirty-four primary care patients (24 females, 9 males) participated in a 30-minute psychoeducational intervention following their medical visit. A visual analog scale consisting of SSD symptoms and the Patient Health Questionnaire (PHQ-15) were use pre- and post-intervention. The intervention included open-ended questions about their visit to establish rapport, education on the release of the cortisol hormone by the HPA axis, stress responses, symptom pathways, benefits of wellness strategies, problem-solving strategies, and information about other psychotherapeutic interventions.

FINDINGS: Following the brief intervention, the participants rated the overall health significantly better than prior to the intervention. Anxiety, fearfulness, and worry about their health, loneliness, and pain were significantly less at the completion of the intervention. At 3-week follow-up, the participates continued to experience less distress about their health.

IMPLICATIONS FOR NURSING: Persons with SSD can benefit from early intervention in a primary care setting. A psychoeducational intervention can significantly reduce the anxiety and distress associated with health concerns.

---

to validate the diagnosis in order to avoid unnecessary treatments. SSD will most likely be diagnosed if the primary care provider is aware of the patient medical and social history, recognizes a discrepancy between the symptoms presented by the patient and objective findings, and identifies the lack of clarity about the nature of the patient symptoms (Patel et al., 2020).

Health education in a familiar environment can help protect the patient from unnecessary procedures and use of resources. Education can improve perceptions of pain, views of health, and decrease feelings of loneliness (Johnson et al., 2020). See Box 33.7.

OTHER DISORDERS

Illness Anxiety Disorder

Illness anxiety disorder is a new classification in the *DSM-5*. Previously, the term *hypochondriasis* (or hypochondria) was used to designate this disorder. Most of the persons with hypochondriasis were also diagnosed with SSD. However, there are some individuals who either do not have somatic symptoms or have only very mild symptoms, but who remain preoccupied with having or developing a medical illness (APA, 2013). These individuals would receive the diagnosis of illness anxiety disorder and would be encouraged to seek mental health treatment for their anxiety and preoccupation.

Individuals with illness anxiety disorder are fearful about developing a serious illness based on their misinterpretation of body sensations. The fear of having an illness continues despite medical reassurance and interferes with psychosocial functioning. They spend time and money on repeated examinations looking for feared illnesses. For example, an occasional cough or the appearance of a small sore results in the person making an appointment with an oncologist. An illness anxiety disorder sometimes appears if the person had had a serious childhood illness or if a family member has a serious illness.

It is important to understand that the lack of physical sensation and movement is real for the patient. In approaching this patient, the nurse treats conversion symptoms as real symptoms that may have distressing psychological aspects. Acknowledging the symptoms helps the patient deal with them. As trust develops within the nurse–patient relationship, the nurse can help the patient develop problem-solving approaches to everyday problems.

Conversion Disorder (Functional Neurologic Symptom Disorder)

Conversion disorder is a psychiatric condition in which severe emotional distress or unconscious conflict is expressed through physical symptoms (APA, 2013). Patients with conversion disorder have neurologic symptoms that include impaired coordination or balance, paralysis, aphonia (i.e., inability to produce sound), difficulty swallowing or a sensation of a lump in the throat, and urinary retention. They may also have loss of touch, vision problems, blindness, deafness, and hallucinations. In some instances, they may have seizures (Peeling & Muzio, 2020). However, laboratory, electroencephalographic, and neurologic test results are typically negative. The symptoms, different from those with an organic basis, do not follow a neurologic course but rather follow the person's own perceived conceptualization of the problem. For example, if the arm is paralyzed and will not move, reflexes and muscle tone may still be present.

Some evidence suggests that there are neurobiologic changes in the brains of people with this disorder that may be responsible for the loss of sensation or control of movement. Stress may also be a contributing factor. Published reports state that childhood trauma (e.g., sexual abuse) is associated with the later development of conversion disorder (Hailes et al., 2019).

It is important to understand that the lack of physical sensation and movement is real for the patient. In approaching the patient, the nurse treats conversion symptoms as real symptoms that may have distressing psychological aspects. Acknowledging the symptoms helps the patient deal with them. As trust develops within the nurse–patient relationship, the nurse can help the patient develop problem-solving approaches to everyday problems.

Factitious Disorders

Factitious disorders are very different from SSDs. Persons with factitious disorders intentionally cause an illness or injury to receive the attention of health care workers. These individuals are motivated solely by the desire to become a patient and develop a dependent relationship with a health care provider. There are two types of factitious disorders: factitious disorder and factitious disorder imposed on another.

Factitious Disorder

Although feigned illnesses have been described for centuries, it was not until 1951 that the term *Münchausen's* [sic] *syndrome* was used to describe the most severe form of this disorder, which was characterized by fabricating a physical illness, having recurrent hospitalizations, and going from one health care provider to another (Asher, 1951). This disorder is now called *factitious disorder* and is differentiated from malingering, in which the individual who intentionally produces symptoms of illness and is motivated by another specific self-serving goal, such as being classified as disabled or avoiding work.

Clinical Course and Diagnostic Criteria

Unlike people with borderline personality disorder, who typically injure themselves overtly and readily admit to self-harm, patients with factitious disorder injure themselves covertly. The illnesses are produced in such a manner that the health care provider is tricked into believing that a true physical or psychiatric disorder is present (Carnahan & Jha, 2020).

The self-produced physical symptoms appear as medical illnesses and involve all body systems. They include seizure disorders, wound-healing disorders, the abscess processes (i.e., introduction of infectious material below the skin surface), and feigned fever (rubbing the thermometer). These patients are extremely creative in simulating illnesses. They tell fascinating but false stories of personal triumph. These tales are referred to as pseudologia fantastica and are a core symptom of the disorder. **Pseudologia fantastica** are stories that are not entirely improbable and often contain a mixture of truth and falsehood. These patients falsify blood, urine, and other samples by contaminating them with protein or fecal matter. They self-inject anticoagulants to receive diagnoses of "bleeding of undetermined origin" or ingest thyroid hormones to produce thyrotoxicosis. They also inflict injury on themselves by inserting objects or feces into body orifices, such as the urinary tract, open wounds, or even intravenous tubing. They produce their own surgical scars, especially abdominal, and when treated surgically, they delay wound healing through scratching, rubbing, or manipulating the wound and introducing bacteria into the wound. These patients put themselves in life-threatening situations through actions such as ingesting allergens known to produce an anaphylactic reaction.

Patients who manifest primarily psychological symptoms produce psychotic symptoms such as hallucinations and delusions, cognitive deficits such as memory loss, dissociative symptoms such as amnesia, and conversion symptoms such as pseudoblindness or pseudoparalysis. These individuals often become psychotic, depressed, or suicidal after an unconfirmed tragedy. When questioned about details, they become defensive and uncooperative. Sometimes these individuals have a combination of both physical and psychiatric symptoms.

Epidemiology and Risk Factors

The prevalence of factitious disorder is unknown because diagnosing it and obtaining reliable data are difficult. The prevalence was reported to be high when researchers were actually looking for the disorder in specific populations. Within large general hospitals, factitious disorders are diagnosed in about 1% of patients with whom mental health professionals consult. The age range of patients with the disorder is between 19 and 64 years. The median age of onset is the early 20s. Formerly thought to occur predominantly in men, this disorder is now reported predominantly in women. No genetic pattern has been identified, but it does seem to run in families. The presence of comorbid psychiatric disorders, such as mood disorders, personality disorders, and substance-related disorders, is common. Health care professionals, nurses, pharmacists, and physicians are over-represented in the occurrence of this disorder (Jimenez et al., 2019).

Etiology

Many people with factitious disorder have experienced severe sexual abuse, trauma, and/or distress before the development of the disorder. The psychodynamic explanation is that these individuals, who were often abused as children, received nurturance only during times of illness; thus, they try to recreate illness or injury in a desperate attempt to receive love and attention. During the actual self-injury, the individual is reported to be in a trancelike, dissociative state. Many patients report having an intimate relationship with a health care provider, either as a child or as an adult, and then experiencing rejection when the relationship ended. The self-injury and subsequent attention is an attempt by the individual to re-enact those experiences and gain control over the situation and the other person (Jimenez et al., 2019).

These patients are usually discovered in medical–surgical settings. They are hostile and distance themselves from others. Their network is void of friends and family and usually consists only of health care providers, who change at regular intervals. In factitious disorder, the patient fabricates a detailed and exaggerated medical history. When the interventions do not work and the fabrication is discovered, the health care team feels manipulated and angry. When the patient is confronted with the evidence, they become enraged and often leave that health care system, only to enter another. Eventually, the person is referred for mental health treatment. The course of the disorder usually consists of intermittent episodes.

Evidence-Based Nursing Care for Persons with Factitious Disorder

The overall goal of treatment for a patient with factitious disorder is to replace the dysfunctional attention-seeking behaviors with positive behaviors. To begin treatment, the patient must acknowledge the deception. Because the pattern of self-injury is well established and meets overwhelming psychological needs, giving up the behaviors is difficult. The treatment is long-term psychotherapy. The psychiatric–mental health nurse will most likely care for the patient during or after periods of feigned illnesses.

Mental Health Nursing Assessment

A nursing assessment should focus on obtaining a history of medical and psychological illnesses. Physical disabilities should be identified. Early childhood experiences, particularly instances of abuse, neglect, or abandonment, should be identified to understand the underlying psychological dynamics of the individual and the role of self-injury. Family assessment is important because family relationships become strained as the members become aware of the self-inflicted nature of this disorder.

Clinical Judgment

The consequences of self-injury are the first priority. Medical treatment may be needed. The patient is at high risk for self-abuse as discovery unfolds. Any nursing intervention must be implemented within the context of a strong nurse–patient relationship. A nonjudgmental attitude is imperative. Desired outcomes include decreased self-injurious behavior and increased positive coping behaviors.

Mental Health Nursing Interventions

The fabrications and deceits of patients with factitious disorder provoke anger and a sense of betrayal in many nurses. To be effective with these patients, it is important to be aware of these feelings and resolve them by developing a better understanding of the underlying psychodynamic issues. Confronting the patient has been reported to be effective only if the patient feels supported and accepted and if there is clear communication among the patient, the mental health care team, and family members. All care should be centralized within one facility. The patient should see health care providers regularly even when not in active crisis. Offering the patient a tactful way of giving up the behaviors is often crucial. Behavioral techniques that shape new behaviors help the patient move forward toward a new life.

The health care team that knows the patient, agrees on a treatment approach, and follow-up is crucial to the patient's eventual recovery. For this to happen, the medical, psychiatric, inpatient, and outpatient teams need to communicate with each other on a regular basis. Family members must also be aware of the need for consistent treatment.

Factitious Disorder Imposed on Another

A rare but dramatic disorder, **factitious disorder imposed on another** (previously *factitious disorder by proxy* or *Münchausen's* [sic] *by proxy*), involves a person who inflicts injury on another person. It is commonly a mother, who inflicts injuries on her child to gain the attention of the health care provider through her child's injuries. These actions include inducing seizures, poisoning, or smothering. This most severe form of child abuse is usually identified in the emergency department. The mother rarely admits injuring the child and thus is not amenable to treatment; the child is frequently removed from the mother's care. This form of child abuse is distinguished from other forms by the routine unwitting involvement of health care workers, who subject the child to physical harm and emotional distress through tests, procedures, and medication trials. Some researchers suspect that children who are abused in this way may later experience factitious disorder themselves (Abeln & Love, 2018).

SUMMARY OF KEY POINTS

- Somatization is affected by sociocultural and gender factors. It occurs more frequently in women than men

and in those who are less educated. It also has been strongly associated with individuals who have been sexually abused as children.

- SSD is a chronic relapsing condition characterized by multiple physical symptoms of unknown origin that develop during times of emotional distress.

- Conversion disorder is a condition of neurologic symptoms (e.g., impaired voluntary muscles or sensory stimulation) that is associated with severe emotional distress.

- Factitious disorders include two types, factitious disorder and factitious disorder imposed on another. In factitious disorder, physical or psychological symptoms (or both) are fabricated to assume the sick role. In factitious disorder imposed on another, the intentional production of symptoms is in others, usually children.

- Identifying SSDs is very complex because patients with these disorders refuse to accept any psychiatric basis to their health problems and often go for years moving from one health care provider to another to receive medical attention and avoid psychiatric assessment.

- These patients are often seen on the medical–surgical units of hospitals and go years without receiving a correct diagnosis. In most cases, they finally receive mental health treatment for comorbid conditions, such as depression, anxiety, and panic disorder.

- The development of the nurse–patient relationship is crucial to assessing these patients and identifying appropriate interventions. Because these patients deny any psychiatric basis to their problem and continue to focus on their symptoms as being medically based, the nurse must take a flexible, relaxed, and nonjudgmental approach that acknowledges the symptoms but focuses on new ways of coping with stress and avoiding recurrence of symptoms.

- Health teaching is important to help the individual develop positive lifestyle changes in place of somatization responses. Identifying personal strengths and supporting the development of positive skills improve self-esteem and personal confidence. Teaching the use of stress management provides the patient with positive coping skills.

CRITICAL THINKING CHALLENGES

1. A depressed young woman is admitted to a psychiatric unit in a state of agitation. She reports extreme abdominal pain. Her admitting provider tells you that she has a classic case of somatization disorder and to de-emphasize her physical symptoms. Under no circumstances can she have any more pain medication. Conceptualize the assessment process and how you would approach this patient.

2. Develop a continuum of "self-injury" for patients with borderline personality disorder, SSD, factitious disorder, and factitious disorder imposed on another.

3. Develop a teaching plan for an individual who has a long history of somatization but who recently received a diagnosis of breast cancer. How will the patient be able to differentiate the physical symptoms of somatization from those associated with the treatment of her breast cancer?

4. A Chinese American patient was admitted for panic attacks and numerous somatic problems, ranging from dysmenorrhea to painful joints. The results of all medical examinations have been negative. She truly believes that her panic attacks are caused by a weak heart. What approaches should the nurse use in providing culturally sensitive nursing care?

5. A person with depression is started on a regimen of phenelzine, 15 mg three times a day. She believes that she is allergic to most foods but insists on having wine in the evenings because it helps digest her food. Develop a teaching plan that provides the knowledge that she needs to prevent a hypertensive crisis caused by excessive tyramine but that is sensitive to the patient's food preferences.

Movie Viewing Guidelines

Safe: 1995. This is a story of Carol White (Julianne Moore), a married stay-at-home mother who appears to have everything. She begins having headaches that lead to a grand mal seizure. As the movie unfolds, she becomes sicker and sicker as she reports she is allergic to environmental toxins. She seeks help from an allergist and psychiatrists. She eventually leaves her husband for a retreat that is actually a scam.

SIGNIFICANCE: The film depicts the pain and suffering that is characteristic of somatization and its impact on the family. It also shows how desperate a person can be to seek out relief of symptoms.

VIEWING POINTS: Identify the mistakes in recognizing and treating the somatic disorder.

REFERENCES

Abeln, B., & Love, R. (2018). An overview of Munchausen syndrome and Munchausen syndrome by proxy. *Nursing Clinics of North America, 53*(3), 375–384. https://doi.org/10.1016/j.cnur.2018.04.005

American Psychiatric Association (APA). (2013). *Diagnostic and statistical manual of mental disorders* (5th ed.). American Psychiatric Association.

Astill Wright, L., Roberts, N. P., Barawi, K., Simon, N., Zammit, S., McElroy, E., & Bisson, J. I. (2020). Disturbed sleep connects symptoms of posttraumatic stress disorder and somatization: A network analysis approach. *Journal of Traumatic Stress.* https://doi.org/10.1002/jts.22619

Asher, R. (1951). Münchausen's syndrome. *Lancet, 1,* 339–341.

Axelsson, E., Hedman-Lagerlöf, M., Hedman-Lagerlöf, E., Ljótsson, B., & Andersson, E. (2020). Symptom preoccupation in fibromyalgia: Prevalence and correlates of somatic symptom disorder in a self-recruited sample. *Psychosomatics, 61*(3), 268–276. https://doi.org/10.1016/j.psym.2020.01.012

Bhola, P., & Chaturvedi, S. K. (2020). Neurasthenia: Tracing the journey of a protean malady. *International Review of Psychiatry (Abingdon, England), 32*(5-6), 491–499. https://doi.org/10.1080/09540261.2020.1758638

Bilsky, S. A., Cloutier, R. M., Bynion, T.-M., Feldner, M. T., & Leen-Feldner, E. W. (2018). An experimental test of the impact of adolescent anxiety on parental sick role reinforcement behavior. *Behaviour Research and Therapy, 109,* 37–48. https://doi-org.libproxy.siue.edu/10.1016/j.brat.2018.07.009

Boerner, K. E., Green, K., Chapman, A., Stanford, E., Newlove, T., Edwards, K., & Dhariwal, A. (2020). Making sense of "somatization": A systematic review of its relationship to pediatric pain. *Journal of Pediatric Psychology, 45*(2), 156–169. https://doi.org/10.1093/jpepsy/jsz102

Brammer, S. V. (2018). What interventions improve outcomes for the patient who is depressed and in pain. *Pain Management Nursing, 19*(6), 580–584. https://doi.org/10.1016/j.pmn.2018.06.006

Carnahan, K. T., & Jha, A. (2020). Factitious disorder. In *StatPearls.* StatPearls Publishing.

Davoodi, E., Wen, A., Dobson, K. S., Noorbala, A. A., Mohammadi, A., & Farahmand, Z. (2018). Early maladaptive schemas in depression and somatization disorder. *Journal of Affective Disorders, 35,* 82–89. https://doi.org/10.1016/j.jad.2018.04.017

de la Torre-Luque, A., Ojagbemi, A., Caballero, F. F., Lara, E., Moreno-Agostino, D., Bello, T., Olaya, B., Haro, J. M., Gureje, O., & Ayuso-Mateos, J. L. (2020). Cross-cultural comparison of symptom networks in late-life major depressive disorder: Yoruba Africans and the Spanish Population. *International Journal of Geriatric Psychiatry, 35*(9), 1060–1068. https://doi.org/10.1002/gps.5329

de Vroege, L., Emons, W. H. M., Sijtsma, K., & van der Feltz-Cornelis, C. M. (2018). Alexithymia has no clinically relevant association with outcome of multimodal treatment tailored to needs of patients suffering from somatic symptom and related disorders A clinical prospective study. *Frontiers in Psychiatry, 9.* https://doi-org.libproxy.siue.edu/10.3389/fpsyt.2018.00292

D'Souza, R. S., & Hooten, W. M. (2020). Somatic syndrome disorders. In *StatPearls.* StatPearls Publishing.

Ford, A. C., Sperber, A. D., Corsetti, M., & Camilleri, M. (2020). Irritable bowel syndrome. *Lancet (London, England), 396*(10263), 1675–1688. https://doi.org/10.1016/S0140-6736(20)31548-8

Granot, M., Yovell, Y., Somer, E., Beny, A., Sadger, R., Uliel-Mirkin, R., & Zisman-Ilani, Y. (2018). Trauma, attachment style, and somatization: A study of women with dyspareunia and women survivors of sexual abuse. *BMC Women's Health, 18*(1), 29. https://doi.org/10.1186/s12905-018-0523-2

Guo, D., Kleinstäuber, M., Johnson, M. H., & Sundram, F. (2019). Evaluating commonalities across medically unexplained symptoms. *International Journal of Environmental Research and Public Health, 16*(5), pii: E818. https://doi.org/10.3390/ijerph16050818

Haghighatdoost, F., Feizi, A., Esmaillzadeh, A., Hassanzadeh Keshteli, A., Roohafza, H., Afshar, H., & Adibi, P. (2020). Dietary patterns in relation with psychosomatic complaints profile: Results from SEPAHAN study among a large sample of general adults. *Nutritional neuroscience, 23*(3), 190–200. https://doi.org/10.1080/1028415X.2018.1485611

Hailes, H. P., Yu, R., Danese, A., & Fazel, S. (2019). Long-term outcomes of childhood sexual abuse: An umbrella review. *The Lancet Psychiatry, 6*(10), 830–839. https://doi.org/10.1016/S2215-0366(19)30286-X

Horsfield, P., Stolzenburg, S., Hahm, S., Tomczyk, S., Muehlan, H., Schmidt, S., & Schomerus, G. (2020). Self-labeling as having a mental or physical illness: The effects of stigma and implications for help-seeking. *Social Psychiatry and Psychiatric Epidemiology, 55*(7), 907–916. https://doi.org/10.1007/s00127-019-01787-7

Ibeziako, P., Randall, E., Vassilopoulos, A., Choi, C., Thomson, K., Ribeiro, M., Fernandes, S., Thom, R., & Bujoreanu, S. (2020). Prevalence, patterns, and correlates of pain in medically hospitalized pediatric patients with somatic symptom and related disorders. *Psychosomatics, S0033-3182*(20), 30146–3048. https://doi.org/10.1016/j.psym.2020.05.008

Jimenez, X. F., Nkanginieme, N., Dhand, N., Karafa, M., & Salerno, K. (2019). Clinical, demographic, psychological, and behavioral features of factitious disorder: A retrospective analysis. *General Hospital Psychiatry, 31.* pii: S0163-8343(19)30005-2. https://doi.org/10.1016/j.genhosppsych.2019.01.009

Johnson, K., Nkanginieme, N., Dhand, N., Karafa, M., & Salerno, K. (2017). It is a painful somatic symptom, not the history of cancer/

malignancy that is associated with depression: Findings from multiple national surveys. *Pain*, *158*(4), 740–746. https://doi.org/10.1097/j.pain.0000000000000826

Johnson, K. K., Bennett, C., & Rochani, H. (2020). Significant improvement of somatic symptom disorder with brief psychoeducational intervention by PMHNP in primary care. *Journal of the American Psychiatric Nurses Association*, 1078390320960524. https://doi.org/10.1177/1078390320960524

Li, R,. Liu, F., Su, Q., Zhang, Z., Zhao, J., Wang, Y., Wu, R., Zhao, J., & Guo, W. (2018). Bidirectional causal connectivity in the cortico-limbic-cerebellar circuit related to structural alterations in first-episode, drug-naive somatization disorder. *Frontiers in Psychiatry*, *26*(9), 162. https://doi.org/10.3389/fpsyt.2018.00162

Liu, J., Gill, N. S., Teodorczuk, A., Li, Z. J., & Sun, J. (2019). The efficacy of cognitive behavioural therapy in somatoform disorders and medically unexplained physical symptoms: A meta-analysis of randomized controlled trials. *Journal of Affective Disorders*, *5*(245), 98–112. https://doi.org/10.1016/j.jad.2018.10.114

Marek, R. J., Anderson, J. L., Tarescavage, A. M., Martin-Fernandez, K., Haugh, S., Block, A. R., Heinberg, L. J., Jimenez, X. F., & Ben-Porath, Y. S. (2020). Elucidating somatization in a dimensional model of psychopathology across medical settings. *Journal of Abnormal Psychology*, *129*(2), 162–176. https://doi.org/10.1037/abn0000475

Mik-Meyer, N., & Obling, A. R. (2012). The negotiation of the sick role: General practitioners; classification of patients with medically unexplained symptoms. *Sociology of Health & Illness*, *34*(7), 1025–1038.

Newby, J. M., Hobbs, M. J., Mahoney, A., Wong, S. K., & Andrews, G. (2017). DSM-5 illness anxiety disorder and somatic symptom disorder: Comorbidity, correlates, and overlap with DSM-IV hypochondriasis. *Journal of Psychosomatic Research*, *101*, 31–37. https://doi.org/10.1016/j.jpsychores.2017.07.010

Noyes, R. Jr., Langbehn, D., Happel, R., Sieren, L., & Muller, B. (1999). Health attitude survey: A scale for assessing somatizing patients. Psychosomatics, 40(6), 470–478.

Schantz, K., Reighard, C., Aikens, J. E., Aruquipa, A., Pinto, B., Valverde, H., & Piette, J. D. (2017). Screening for depression in Andean Latin America: Factor structure and reliability of the CES-D short form and the PHQ-8 among Bolivian public hospital patients. *International Journal of Psychiatry in Medicine*, *52*(4-6), 315–327. https://doi.org/10.1177/0091217417738934 Survey: A scale for assessing somatizing patients. *Psychosomatics*, *40*(6), 470–478.

Patel, M., James, K., Moss-Morris, R., Ashworth, M., Husain, M., Hotopf, M., David, A. S., McCrone, P., Landau, S., Chalder, T., & PRINCE Primary trial team (2020). BMC family practice integrated GP care for patients with persistent physical symptoms: Feasibility cluster randomised trial. *BMC Family Practice*, *21*(1), 207. https://doi.org/10.1186/s12875-020-01269-9

Peeling, J. L., & Muzio, M. R. (2020). Conversion disorder. In *StatPearls*. StatPearls Publishing.

Porcelli, P., De Carne, M., & Leandro, G. (2020). Distinct associations of DSM-5 somatic symptom disorder, the diagnostic criteria for psychosomatic research-revised (DCPR-R) and symptom severity in patients with irritable bowel syndrome. *General Hospital Psychiatry*, *64*, 56–62. https://doi.org/10.1016/j.genhosppsych.2020.03.004

Shangguan, F., Quan, X., Qian, W., Zhou, C., Zhang, C., Zhang, X. Y., & Liu, Z. (2020). Prevalence and correlates of somatization in anxious individuals in a Chinese online crisis intervention during COVID-19 epidemic. *Journal of Affective Disorders*, *277*, 436–442. https://doi.org/10.1016/j.jad.2020.08.035

Sharma, M. P., & Manjula, M. (2013). Behavioural and psychological management of somatic symptom disorders: An overview. *International Review of Psychiatry*, *25*(1), 116–124.

Torres, M. E., Löwe, B., Schmitz, S., Pienta, J. N., Van Der Feltz-Cornelis, C., & Fiedorowicz, J. G. (2021). Suicide and suicidality in somatic symptom and related disorders: A systematic review. *Journal of Psychosomatic Research*, *140*, 110290. https://doi.org/10.1016/j.jpsychores.2020.110290

Toussaint, A., Hüsing P., Kohlmann, S., & Löwe, B. (2019). Detecting DSM-5 somatic symptom disorder: Criterion validity of the Patient Health Questionnaire-15 (PHQ-15) and the Somatic Symptom Scale-8 (SSS-8) in combination with the Somatic Symptom Disorder—B Criteria Scale (SSD-12). *Psychological Medicine*, 7, 1–10. https://doi.org/10.1017/S003329171900014X

van Westrienen, P. E., Pisters, M. F., Toonders, S., Gerrits, M., de Wit, N. J., & Veenhof, C. (2020). Quality of life in primary care patients with moderate medically unexplained physical symptoms. *Quality of Life Research: An International Journal of Quality of Life Aspects of Treatment, Care and Rehabilitation*, *29*(3), 693–703. https://doi.org/10.1007/s11136-019-02358-8

Wortman, M. S. H., Lokkerbol, J., van der Wouden, J. C., Visser, B., van der Horst, H. E., & Hartman, T. C. O. (2018). Cost-effectiveness of interventions for medically unexplained symptoms: A systematic review. *PLoS One*, *13*(10), e0205278. https://doi.org/10.1371/journal.pone.0205278

Zhou, X., Zhou, X., Peng, Y., Zhu, X., Yao, S., Dere, J., Chentsova-Dutton, Y. E., & Ryder, A. G. (2016). From culture to symptom: Testing a structural model of "Chinese somatization". *Transcultural psychiatry*, *53*(1), 3–23. https://doi.org/10.1177/13634615155897008(2016). From culture to symptom: Testing a structural model of "Chinese somatization". *Transcultural psychiatry*, 53(1), 3–23. https://doi.org/10.1177/1363461515589708

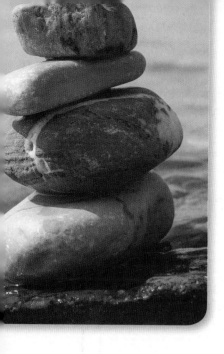

34
Sleep–Wake Disorders
Nursing Care of Persons with Insomnia and Sleep Problems

Sheri Compton-McBride

KEYCONCEPTS

- sleep
- sleep–wake cycle
- insomnia
- rhythm

LEARNING OBJECTIVES

After studying this chapter, you will be able to:

1. Describe the role of the sleep–wake cycle in mental disorders.

2. Delineate the clinical symptoms and course of insomnia disorder.

3. Analyze the primary theories of insomnia disorder.

4. Develop strategies to establish a patient-centered, recovery-oriented therapeutic relationship with a person with insomnia disorder.

5. Apply a person-centered, recovery-oriented nursing process for persons with insomnia disorder.

6. Identify medications used to treat people with insomnia disorder and evaluate their effectiveness.

7. Develop wellness strategies for persons with insomnia disorder.

8. Discuss the treatment setting for insomnia disorder.

9. Discuss the importance of integrated health care for persons with insomnia disorder.

10. Describe other sleep–wake disorders.

KEY TERMS

• Chronotherapy • Circadian rhythm • Insomnia disorder • Non–rapid eye movement (NREM) • Rapid eye movement (REM) sleep • Sleep architecture • Sleep debt • Sleep diary • Sleep efficiency • Sleep homeostasis • Sleep–wake disorders • Sleep latency • Slow-wave sleep • Somnambulism

Case Study

Michael is a 20-year-old student who is majoring in nursing. He presents himself at Student Health Services with a complaint of insomnia. In assessing his problem, the nurse ascertains that he falls asleep 2 to 3 hours after turning lights out.

INTRODUCTION

Sleep is a recurrent, altered state of consciousness that occupies nearly one third of our lives and occurs for sustained periods. Unlike a coma, sleep can be disrupted and reversed quite easily. Sleep is usually preceded by a period of sleepiness or the urge to fall asleep.

> **KEYCONCEPT Sleep,** which is necessary for human survival, is a state of decreased awareness of environmental stimuli and a relative state of unconsciousness with no memory of the state.

Sleep is important to our development, functioning, and health. Sleep has identifiable cycles and a variety of cognitive experiences, ranging from memory recall to feeling energetic. The consequences of disturbed sleep include impaired alertness and performance.

This chapter presents a discussion of normal sleep rhythms and patterns, sleep–wake disorders, and nursing care for persons with sleep problems. Insomnia disorder is highlighted.

SLEEP AND WELLNESS

Adequate sleep is a critical aspect of wellness. Sleeping less than the recommended 7 hours per night is associated with obesity, diabetes, high blood pressure, coronary heart disease, stroke, and mental distress (Centers for Disease Control and Prevention [CDC], 2017). More than one third of Americans report sleeping less than 7 hours per night (CDC, 2017), with the average sleep duration of U.S. adults being between 6 and 6.5 hours from a high of 8.5 hours in 1960. Sleepiness has been linked to catastrophic disasters, such as the Exxon Valdez oil spill, the nuclear meltdown at Chernobyl in Ukraine, the space shuttle *Challenger* accident, and the Three Mile Island disaster in the United States (Mitler et al., 1988; Rajaratnam & Arendt, 2001).

Biologic Theories

The biology of sleep appears to involve dopamine, gamma-aminobutyric acid (GABA), adenosine, histamine, hypocretin, melatonin, and cortisol, which play roles in changing sleep states (Herrera-Solis et al., 2019). Wakefulness is maintained by the reticular activating system in the brain. As the cycle of the reticular activating system dwindles, neurotransmitters that promote sleep take over (see Chapter 8).

Psychosocial Theories

Sleep is also related to psychosocial factors, such as lifestyle, stress, and work- and school-related factors. Underrepresented groups have short sleep duration (Johnson et al., 2019). Short sleep duration is associated with lower socioeconomic groups and the unemployed (Guglielmis et al., 2019).

Pattern of Sleep

Sleep is a patterned activity and is one component of the biphasic 24-hour sleep–wake cycle.

> **KEYCONCEPT** The **sleep–wake cycle** is an endogenously generated rhythm close to 24 to 25 hours synchronized with the day–night cycle. The sleep–wake cycle is regulated by circadian rhythms and sleep homeostasis (Zisapel, 2018).

Sleep latency, the amount of time it takes to fall asleep, is measured from "lights out," or bedtime, to initiation of sleep. Sleep architecture is the pattern of non–rapid eye movement (NREM) and rapid eye movement (REM) that are in about a 90- to 110-minute cycle. Sleep occurs in stages, and the timing of sleep is regulated by circadian rhythms. Sleep efficiency is the ratio of total sleep time to time in bed.

Circadian Rhythms

> **KEYCONCEPT Rhythm** is movement with a cadence, a measured flow that occurs at regular intervals, with a cycle of coming and going, ebbing and rising, to return at the start point and begin again.

Nearly all physiologic and psychological functions fluctuate in a pattern that repeats itself in a 24-hour cycle, called circadian rhythms (Fig. 34.1). The biologic clock that regulates our circadian rhythms is located in the *suprachiasmatic nucleus,* an area of the hypothalamus that lies on top of the optic chiasm. However, it is now recognized that almost all cells and tissues in the body are circadian clocks (Reinke & Asher, 2019). When two or more rhythms reach their peak at the same time, they are

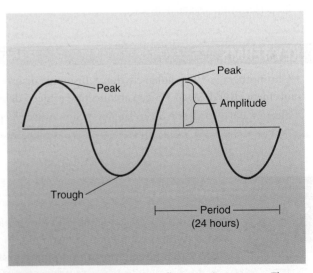

FIGURE 34.1 Circadian rhythms fluctuate in patterns. The peak is the point at which the rhythm reaches its maximum, and the trough is the point at which the rhythm reaches its minimum. The period is the time it takes to complete a cycle. The amplitude is the extent of the peak and is half the distance from peak to trough.

synchronized; if they reach their peak at different times, they are desynchronized.

Most physiologic functions reach their lowest levels during the middle of the sleep period. For example, body temperature follows a predictable pattern from lowest, in the early morning, to highest, in the mid-evening. Manual dexterity, reaction time, and simple recognition appear to coincide with the circadian rhythm of body temperature. Most circadian rhythms continue even when humans are unaware of the time of day. Natural age-related changes in circadian sleep rhythms generally regulate people as they get older, toward morning alertness and productivity and sleepiness at night (Hood & Amir, 2017).

Sleep Homeostasis

The circadian rhythms are not the only processes that regulate sleep. Sleep homeostasis is an internal biochemical system that operates as a timer or counter that generates pressure to sleep and regulates sleep intensity. This process reminds the body to sleep after a certain time. The longer we have been awake, the stronger the desire and need for sleep becomes and the likelihood of falling asleep increases. The longer we sleep, the pressure to sleep decreases and we are more likely to wake (Frank & Heller, 2019).

Stages of Sleep

Sleep is biphasic, cycling between NREM and REM (Fig. 34.2). During an 8-hour sleep period, the cycle of NREM and REM repeats itself. This duration of the cycles may change as the night progresses. In the first cycle, the amount of REM sleep is brief. With each succeeding cycle, the amount of time spent in REM

lengthens. Conversely, NREM is most prominent during the initial cycle but declines as total sleep time progresses (Fig. 34.3).

Non–Rapid Eye Movement Sleep

NREM sleep occurs about 90 minutes after falling asleep and consists of four substages. Light sleep is characteristic of stages 1 and 2, in which the person is easily aroused. A person aroused from stage 1 sleep may even deny having been asleep, such as dozing while watching television and awakening minutes later during a loud commercial. Stage 1 accounts for only 2% to 5% of a night's sleep and is a transition between relaxed wakefulness and sleep. Stage 2 comprises about 45% to 55% of sleep. During phases 1 and 2, an electroencephalogram (EEG) shows an alpha rhythm gradually being replaced by a theta rhythm. Sleep spindles or "k complexes" occur in stage 2 (see Fig. 34.3).

Slow-wave sleep, or the deepest state of sleep, characterizes stages 3 and 4. Slow-wave sleep is believed to have a restorative function, although the exact mechanism for this is unclear. It may serve to conserve energy because metabolism and body temperature decrease during this part of sleep. These stages make up 10% to 23% of sleep. EEG findings show high-amplitude waves, slow waves, or delta waves. The difference between stages 3 and 4 is the amount of delta waves seen, with stage 3 demonstrating 20% to 50% of delta waves and stage 4 showing more than 50% of delta waves.

Rapid Eye Movement Sleep

Rapid eye movement (REM) sleep is a state characterized by bursts of rapid eye movements. REM sleep occurs in four to six separate episodes and makes up about 20% to 25% of a night's sleep. Although REM sleep is a deep sleep and muscles seem to be at rest, EEG findings

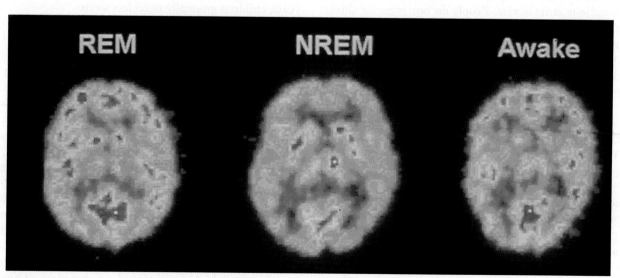

FIGURE 34.2 Brain activity during the sleep–wake cycle. The brain is as active in rapid eye movement (REM) or dreaming sleep as when awake but is metabolically less active in slow-wave or non–rapid eye movement (NREM) sleep. (Courtesy of Monte S. Buchsbaum, MD, the Mount Sinai Medical Center and School of Medicine, New York.)

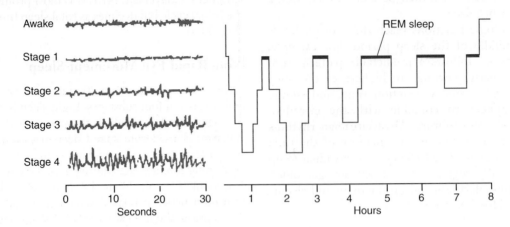

FIGURE 34.3 Brain waves during wakefulness and stages. Brain waves during wakefulness and stages 1, 2, 3, and 4 sleep on the *left* and duration of wakefulness, rapid eye movement (REM), and non–rapid eye movement (NREM) sleep on the *right*. In typical sleep architecture in normal young adults, NREM and REM sleep stages cycle every 90 to 110 minutes through the night. Wakefulness accounts for less than 5% of the night's sleep pattern. Slow-wave sleep dominates the first third of the night during NREM stages 3 and 4. REM sleep occurs in four to six separate episodes throughout the night (20% to 25% of sleep) and dominates the last third of the night's sleep. Reprinted with permission from Norris, T. L.. (2019). *Porth's Pathophysiology: Concepts of altered health states* (10th ed.). Philadelphia, PA: Wolters Kluwer.)

demonstrate an active brain. Brain waves resemble a mixture of wakeful and drowsy patterns. Although vivid dreaming is the outstanding feature reported by adults when awakened out of REM sleep, people also report dreams when they awaken from NREM sleep.

During REM sleep, nerve impulses are blocked within the spinal cord. Muscle tone diminishes to the point of paralysis. Only stronger impulses are relayed, producing muscular twitches, eye movements, and impulses controlling heart rate and respiration. Breathing and heart rate may become irregular.

This type of sleep has a circadian rhythm that closely coincides with the body temperature rhythm. The greatest amount of REM sleep is seen when the body temperature cycle is at its lowest. People do not sweat or shiver during REM sleep because temperature regulation is impaired. Patterns of hormone release, kidney function, and reflexes change. Women have clitoral engorgement and an increase in blood flow to the vagina. Men have penile erections.

Factors Affecting Sleep Pattern and Quality

Gender

Sleep problems and poorer quality sleep are reported more often by women than men. Disturbed sleep and daytime sleepiness have a cumulative effect on mental health (Thomas et al., 2017). Women are at greater risk for insomnia and other sleep problems. Sleep in women is influenced by the sex hormones, which vary throughout the life cycle (Perger et al., 2019). Socioeconomic factors

contribute to poor sleep quality and daytime sleepiness in American women (Xiao & Hale, 2018). Sleep deprivation and sleep quality in transgender and gender nonconforming adults (TGNC) have been reported and are compounded when TGNC individuals experience sexual victimization (Kolp et al, 2020).

Age

Sleep patterns change dramatically over the course of the life span. Newborns need 17 to 18 hours of sleep each day, which occurs in 3- to 4-hour episodes throughout the day. By age 6 months, 12 hours of sleep at night and two 1- to 2-hour naps each day are needed. After age 5 years, children gradually need less sleep.

Preadolescents need about 10 hours of sleep each night, and napping is rare. A teenager's sleep need is only slightly less, at about 9 hours. During young adulthood, about 8 hours of sleep is needed. The amount of sleep required and sleep architecture typically remain unchanged during the middle-aged years. Poor sleep in women is associated with hormonal changes, such as during the menstrual cycle, pregnancy, and menopause.

For older adults, the need for sleep does not decrease, but the ability to sustain sleep changes. Older people spend more time in bed, sleep less, wake more often during the night, and take longer to fall asleep than younger adults. For some, sleep requirements are met by daytime napping. Furthermore, temperature rhythm in older people peaks earlier; early morning arousals may reflect early rise of body temperature. Older people are at higher risk for sleep disorders (Thomas et al., 2017).

Environment

Sleep-related problems have multiple factors that make up the clinical picture. Whereas some are external, such as the noise and temperature, others are internal (e.g., stress and pain). A person can be sleepy but may stay awake if in a stimulating environment with bright lights or a lot of activity. In contrast, a sleepy person in a quiet place or engaged in sedentary activity cannot resist the urge to fall asleep. Sleepiness is a physiologic state, and although a stimulating environment can temporarily forestall it, when these stimuli are removed, the urge to sleep will persist. Even when someone who is chronically sleep deprived does not feel sleepy, the tendency to fall asleep is much greater and may manifest by causing the person to doze off while sitting in lectures or during the monotonous operation of machinery or driving.

Lifestyles

Many factors can cause disrupted sleep patterns, such as travel across time zones, stress or anxiety, and changes in the sleep–wake pattern because of shift work. When traveling across time zones or working night shifts (and sleeping during the day), one's regular sleepiness–alertness rhythm may persist for several days. Even when daytime sleep is improved with a pharmacologic agent, sleepiness in the early morning hours usually continues for the first 2 to 3 nights. This extreme sleepiness often decreases after a 4- to 6-day reversal of the sleep–wake cycle (see Box 34.1).

BOX 34.1

Nurses' Sleep, Fatigue, and Sleepiness Impact on Cognitive Performance

Wolf, L. A., & Perhats, C. (2017). The effect of reported sleep, perceived fatigue, and sleepiness on cognitive performance in a sample of emergency nurses. The Journal of Nursing Administration, 47(1), 44–49.

THE QUESTION: Is there a relationship between the emergency nurses reported sleep, perceived fatigue and sleepiness, and cognitive performance?

METHODS: A quantitative correlational design was used in the study. In each of seven different statistical models, zero-order relationships between predictors and the dependent variable were examined with appropriate inferential tests.

FINDINGS: Participants reported high levels of sleepiness and chronic fatigue that impeded full functioning both at work and at home. Although high level of self-reported fatigue did not show any effects on cognitive function, others factors in the environment may contribute to delayed, missed, or inappropriate care.

IMPLICATIONS FOR NURSING: Nurses are at high risk for sleep deprivation and fatigue. Self-care and patient can be negatively impacted by fatigue associated with variable shifts, long work hours, and chaotic environments.

Changes in Normal Sleep

Normal sleep is sensitive to changes, and the body responds when deprived of certain phases of sleep, particularly REM sleep and slow-wave sleep. Certain activities, such as early rising, alcohol intake before bedtime, or consumption of certain medications, can suppress REM sleep. One example is the use of central nervous system (CNS)–acting medications. Fragmented sleep interrupts the restorative function of a good night's sleep. Not only does insufficient sleep cause daytime sleepiness, but disturbed sleep also affects daytime alertness and performance. A sleep debt occurs when there is recurrent long-term sleep deprivation.

When individuals are deprived of REM sleep, there is a subsequent "rebound effect," wherein the lost REM sleep is made up during the next sleep period. The body makes up for this lost REM sleep by earlier occurrence of REM sleep during the next night. The presence of REM at sleep onset implies REM deprivation.

Slow-wave sleep does not appear to have a circadian determinant, but it is more sensitive to the amount of previous sleep obtained. When one is deprived of both REM and slow-wave sleep, the body prefers to make up the slow-wave before the REM sleep.

SLEEP–WAKE DISORDERS OVERVIEW

Sleep–wake disorders are diagnosed when an individual is dissatisfied about the quality, timing, and amount of their sleep, which is causing daytime distress and impairment. Sleep problems are more common in women, and prevalence increases with age in both genders. Sleep–wake disorders occur independently of the diagnosis of other mental disorders, but they are also seen in people with mental disorders. For example, a core feature of posttraumatic stress disorder (PTSD) is sleep disturbance.

An occasional change in sleep pattern becomes a sleep disorder when mental and physical health is compromised as a result of problems in the sleep–wake cycle. Sleep–wake disorders include insomnia, hypersomnolence, and narcolepsy. Other disorders include breathing-related sleep disorders (such as obstructive sleep apnea [OSA] and circadian rhythm disorders) and parasomnias.

INSOMNIA DISORDER

KEYCONCEPT Insomnia, which is Latin for "no sleep," refers to difficulty falling asleep or maintaining sleep when opportunity and circumstances are adequate for sleep. Dissatisfaction with sleep quantity or quality may also be present (Khoury & Doghramji, 2015).

Clinical Course

Few studies describe the course of insomnia disorder, which can last for short periods in some patients and for decades in others. Since ancient times, physicians noted individuals having difficulty falling asleep, staying asleep, and early morning awakenings (Riemann et al., 2020). Acute insomnia is described as 3 or more nights per week with symptoms occurring in a 2- to 12-week timeframe, whereas chronic insomnia has a longer duration (Perlis et al., 2020).

Diagnostic Criteria

Insomnia disorder is characterized by dissatisfaction with sleep quantity or quality and difficulty initiating or maintaining sleep, or in waking early in the morning, and being unable to return to sleep (APA, 2013).

Children and Adolescents

Sleep issues in children can occur in the presence of attention deficit hyperactivity disorder (ADHD), epilepsy, and autism spectrum disorder or independently of a neurologic or psychiatric diagnosis (Maski & Owens, 2016). Up to 66% of children are experiencing anxiety disorders, such as separation anxiety disorder or specific phobias, including social anxiety disorder, and experience insomnia (Khurshid, 2018). Not unlike adults, cognition and emotional regulation are impacted when sleep quality and/or sleep quantity are impacted.

Older Adults

Cognitive impairment, depression, anxiety, and increased risk of falls are linked to insomnia in those 65 years and older. Increased rates of insomnia are seen in those residing in institutions versus those in a community setting. Older adults should be educated about the impact of poor quality sleep on daily functioning as well as vital organs, including cardiovascular, neurologic, and mental health implications (Berkley et al., 2020).

Epidemiology and Risk Factors

Age of Onset

Age of onset for insomnia varies and may be impacted by physical health issues and psychological and environmental experiences that impact sleep. Older adults and those with health problems are reportedly more likely to experience insomnia (Grewal & Doghramji, 2017).

Gender Differences

Women report a higher prevalence of insomnia as compared to men within the United States and across countries in Europe and Asia (Grewal & Doghramji, 2017).

Ethnicity and Culture

There is not an equal distribution of sleep disorders among race and ethnicity. Underrepresented groups experience less optimal sleep compared to those populations less impacted by health disparities. In addition to poor sleep quality and quantity, underrepresented groups are at increased risk for adverse mental and physical health outcomes, such as diabetes, hypertension, cardiovascular disease, mood disorders, and occupational accidents (Johnson et al., 2019).

Familial Differences

Fatal familial insomnia is characterized by not only insomnia but also dysautonomia, changes to motor function, neuropsychiatric disorders, and myoclonic limb activity. Rarely does clinical onset occur before the age 32, with the average at 51 years of age, with the majority of cases reported from Italy, Spain, and Germany. Genetically, the disorder is of autosomal dominant pattern (Llorens et al., 2017).

The most widely regarded predictor of a familial risk for insomnia is a maternal history. It is challenging to distinguish differences among families and support systems due to the web of intricacies that can impact sleep, specifically insomnia. Known medical disorders and treatment regimens can impact sleep architecture whereby making it challenging to determine if insomnia is idiopathic or a consequence of another component of overall health wellness management or treatment.

Of all sleep-related problems, insomnia is the most prevalent. Thirty percent to 50% of the population experiences short-term, occasional insomnia (Sateia et al, 2017). The prevalence of chronic or severe insomnia (occurring for at least 3 months and a minimum of three times per week) is estimated to range from 10% to 15% (Chen et al., 2017). Insomnia is one of the most prevalent complaints in primary health care.

Insomnia has a greater prevalence among older people and among divorced, separated, and widowed adults. Increasing age, female sex, and comorbid disorders (e.g., medical, mental disorders, and substance use) are all risks for developing insomnia disorder.

Comorbidity

Sleep–wake disorders occur independently of the diagnosis of other mental disorders, but they are also seen in people with mental disorders, such as PTSD and depression. Insomnia often increases the risk for relapse of the mental disorder. Documented comorbid conditions include cardiovascular disorders, diabetes, musculoskeletal disorders (e.g., arthritis, chronic back/neck pain), respiratory disorders (e.g., chronic obstructive pulmonary disease [COPD], seasonal allergies, chronic bronchitis, emphysema), digestive disorders (e.g., gastroesophageal reflux disease, irritable bowel syndrome), pain conditions, and mental disorders including depression, PTSD, and other sleep disorders such as sleep apnea, and restless legs syndrome (RLS) (Kessler et al., 2012).

Etiology

Many factors affect sleep, but one of the major reasons for insomnia is depression, which accounts for most cases. However, most people with insomnia do not have a psychiatric diagnosis (Riemann et al., 2020).

Family Response to Disorder

Living with a family member with insomnia disorder is challenging. Irritability, complaints of sleeplessness, and chronic fatigue interfere with quality of interpersonal relationships. Family members become "exhausted" by living with someone who never sleeps.

RECOVERY-ORIENTED CARE FOR PERSONS WITH INSOMNIA

Teamwork and Collaboration: Working Toward Recovery

Sleep disorders are best treated by clinicians specializing in this area, but primary and mental health care professionals should be able to identify sleep disturbances and provide education and interventions for normalizing sleep. However, because sleep disorders are common in individuals with mental health problems, psychiatric–mental health nurses should be prepared to provide care for those with sleep disorders. Optimal management and treatment of insomnia have been linked to improved outcomes in those with coexisting psychiatric disorders (Khurshid, 2018).

Safety Issues

Safety is a priority for people with insomnia disorder. Sleep deprivation can lead to accidents, falls, and injuries, especially in older patients. Sedating medication could potentially increase falls (Kessler et al., 2012).

EVIDENCE-BASED NURSING CARE FOR PERSONS WITH INSOMNIA

Nursing assessment for the patient with insomnia focuses on difficulty falling asleep, staying asleep, and/or early morning awakenings. The following are examples of assessment questions.

* What time do you go to bed? In your estimation, how long does it take you to fall asleep?
* When did your symptoms begin? Did anything unusual or stressful precipitate the sleep disturbance pattern?

   Does anyone in your family experience the same symptoms?

   Do you find yourself awakening feeling sluggish or refreshed?
* Does your reported sleep issue impact your daily activities or ability to function?
* Do you nap? If so, what time and for how long?

Interventions stress the importance of sleep hygiene and helping the patient establish normal sleep patterns. If medications are given, the commonly prescribed over-the-counter (OTC) medications and supplements include diphenhydramine and melatonin. Prescription medications used for insomnia include Benzodiazepine Receptor Agonists (BzRAs), Melatonin Receptor Agonist, and Orexin Receptor Antagonist.

Mental Health Nursing Assessment

Assessment of a patient's sleep pattern is a part of every psychiatric nursing assessment (see Chapter 11). If a patient has a sleep disorder, a detailed sleep history should be included in the assessment process. See Nursing Care Plan 34.1.

Physical Health and Functioning

During the patient interview, the description, duration (when problem began), stability (every night?), and intensity (how bad is it?) should be determined (Box 34.2). A sleep history includes current sleeping patterns, medical problems, current medications (including OTC and dietary supplements), current life events, use of alcohol and caffeine, and emotional and mental status that might be affecting sleep (see Boxes 34.3 and 34.4). A sleep diary is a person's subjective written account of their sleep experience (Short et al., 2017). The diary may cover a few days to several weeks. A simple diary is a record of the patient's daily, estimated bedtime, rise time, total sleep time, estimated time to fall asleep, number and length of awakenings, and naps. More complicated sleep diaries involve recording the amount and time of alcohol and caffeine ingestion, activity level, ratings of fatigue, medication, and stressful events.

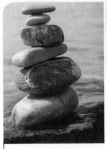

NURSING CARE PLAN 34.1

Insomnia

Michael is a 20-year-old student who is majoring in nursing. He presents himself at Student Health Services with a complaint of insomnia. In assessing his problem, the nurse ascertains that Michael takes 2 to 3 hours to fall asleep. During this interim of wakefulness, he lies in bed, calm but somewhat restless. He has had no prior difficulty with insomnia. His problem falling asleep occurs 3 nights a week—Monday, Wednesday, and Friday. He exercises vigorously during his physical education class (7–9 PM) on these three evenings. He denies any sleep problems during spring break, when he took a trip. The patient drinks 1 cup of coffee in the morning and denies the use of other stimulants. He reports that as a consequence he has had some irritability and difficulty concentrating on the days following a "bad night." He has tried an OTC sleep medication, but does not remember the name of it. When he took these sleeping pills, he was able to fall asleep better, but found them to be costly. He would like a prescription for sleeping medication that would be covered by student health insurance.

Setting: Outpatient Student Health Service

Baseline Assessment: A 20-year-old man who presents with difficulty initiating sleep. After vigorous evening exercise, he takes 2–3 hours to fall asleep. Strengths: intelligence, motivated for treatment, adequate insurance coverage, good physical health.

Associated Psychiatric Diagnoses	Medications
Primary insomnia	None

Priority of Care: Insomnia

Important Characteristics	Associated Considerations
Difficulty falling asleep, estimated sleep latency of 2–3 hours, three nights a week Changes in usual sleep environment Poor sleep hygiene	Mood alterations Poor concentration

Outcomes

Initial	Discharge
1. Describe factors that prevent or inhibit sleep. 2. Identify strategies to improve sleep hygiene.	3. Report an optimal balance of rest and activity.

Interventions

Interventions	Rationale	Ongoing Assessment
Teach patient good sleep hygiene habits.	Discussion of good sleep hygiene is the first treatment strategy.	Monitor Michael's reports of estimated sleep latency.
Instruct patient to keep a sleep diary for 1 week—including bedtime, sleep latency, rising time, naps, caffeine intake, time of exercise.	Keeping a sleep diary can give insight into insomnia problems by identifying alerting influences in relation to disturbed sleep. Exercise before sleep appears to be the primary factor that could be causing insomnia on Monday, Wednesday, and Friday.	Monitor other sleep hygiene issues.
Reassure patient that short-term insomnia will resolve when the factors that caused the problem are eliminated.	Anxiety about insomnia is a predisposing factor to the development of primary insomnia.	Determine Michael's level of anxiety about insomnia.
Determine whether it is possible to adjust schedule so that vigorous exercise occurs several hours before sleep.	Physical exercise raises basal metabolism, which may interfere with sleep.	Determine whether it is possible to adjust course schedule.
Problem solve with Michael how to adjust sleep schedule to avoid insomnia.	Problem-solving allows the patient to learn how to consider alternative strategies.	Evaluate whether strategies are reasonable.

Evaluation

Outcomes	Revised Outcomes	Interventions
After readjustment of exercise schedule, Matthew was able to resume normal sleep.	None	None

BOX 34.2 • SLEEP ASSESSMENT

INEFFECTIVE APPROACH

Nurse: What time do you go to bed at night?

Michael: Oh, my bedtime varies between 10 PM and 2 AM.

Nurse: What time do you get up?

Michael: I get up anywhere between 6 AM and noon.

Nurse: How do you sleep during the night?

Michael: OK.

Nurse: OK?

Michael: Yeah, no problems sleeping.

EFFECTIVE APPROACH

Nurse: What time do you go to bed at night and what time do you get up?

Michael: Oh, my bedtime varies between 10 PM and 2 AM. I get up anywhere between 6 AM and noon.

Nurse: Let's be more specific. During a week's time, what time do you go to bed each night?

Michael: Well, this semester I have a morning clinical rotation Monday through Thursday. I'm usually up till 11 or midnight preparing for the next day. On Friday and Saturday nights, I typically go out with my friends and get to bed around 2 AM. On Sunday night, I get on to bed around 10 PM.

Nurse: What time do you get up each day of the week?

Michael: On the mornings that I have clinicals, I have to get up around 6 AM to be at the hospital by 6:45 AM. On Friday, I get up at 8 AM for a 9 o'clock class. Saturday morning, I get up around 8 AM so I can go to my part-time job. On Sunday, I get up by noon.

Nurse: How long do you take to fall asleep?

Michael: That's gotten much better. I fall asleep in 15 minutes or so.

Nurse: Do you take any naps?

Michael: Outside of class, I don't have time to nap. I'm just too busy with my classes, clinical, homework, job, and social life.

Nurse: Before this semester, how much sleep did you get?

Michael: That was last summer; I had a job that started at 1:30 PM, so I could sleep as late as I wanted. I bet I got 8 or even 9 hours of sleep every night. I don't remember being sleepy then.

CRITICAL THINKING CHALLENGE

- Compare the quality and quantity of elicited data in the two scenarios.
- What conclusions could be drawn from the first scenario?
- Are the conclusions different for the second scenario? Explain.

BOX 34.3

Sleep History

- Perception of sleep problem
- Sleep schedule (bedtime and rise time)
- Difficulty falling asleep or maintaining sleep
- Quality of sleep
- Daytime sleepiness and impact of the sleep disorder on daytime functioning
- General emotional and physical problems (e.g., stress)
- Sleep hygiene (e.g., consuming caffeine immediately before bed)
- Sleep environment (e.g., room temperature, noise, light)

Adapted from Kessler, T. A., & Kurtz, C. P. (2019). Sleep and sleep-wake disorders. In Norris, T.L (Ed.). *Porth's Pathophysiology: Concepts of altered health states*, 10th ed. (pp. 505–523). Philadelphia, PA: Wolters Kluwer.

Consider Michael

His problem falling asleep occurs three nights a week—on Mondays, Wednesdays, and Fridays. He exercises vigorously during his physical education class (7 to 9 PM) on these 3 evenings. He denies any sleep problems during a spring break trip.

Should Michael keep a sleep diary? How would exercise impact his sleep? What does it mean that he has no problem sleeping during spring break?

Substance Use and Medication

The bidirectionality of insomnia and substances must be acknowledged as substances impact the receptors and neurotransmitters directly involved with sleep–wake regulation. The development of sleep-related issues can be associated with the use of OTC products, such as nicotine and caffeine. Those who use products that are stimulating need to be informed about not only the effects on overall health but also the timing of consumption as it relates to initiating sleep and maintaining sleep and the impact on sleep quality. OTC and prescription medications that have a stimulating effect need to be avoided within 4 hours of sleep initiation. Though alcohol consumption may initially assist in helping individuals fall asleep, ultimately alcohol use impacts sleep architecture and leads to disrupted, poor sleep quality; increases the likelihood of snoring or sleep apnea; and due to the diuretic effects increases restroom visits (Krystal et al., 2019).

Psychosocial Assessment

The assessment also includes evaluating the behavioral and social factors related to sleep problems. Though we each respond differently, stressful life events impact the quality and quantity of our sleep. Factors to consider include gender, coping skills, timing and perception of the stressor, and substance use or misuse. Recent changes in relationships, particularly a divorce or death of a loved one, can interfere with sleep significantly. A recent move, travel, and addition of a new family member can impact sleep.

Fatigue and stress increase when individuals assume the role of a caregiver in their personal lives and in those with occupations as professional health care providers. A rotating or variable work schedule compromises the circadian rhythm and contributes to insomnia (Kalmbach et al., 2018).

Quality of Life

Health-related quality of life is decreased in adults who experience insomnia. There are numerous studies showing the quality of life is negatively impacted in people with insomnia. While insomnia has a negative effect on quality of life in both genders, women report a lower quality of life than men (Lucena et al., 2020).

BOX 34.4

Medications and Other Substances and Their Effects on Sleep

ALCOHOL
- Increases TST (total sleep time) during the first half of the night
- Decreases TST during the second half
- Decreases REM sleep during the first half of the night
- Withdrawal from long-term use of alcohol decreases TST, increased wakefulness after sleep onset, and REM rebound

AMPHETAMINES
- Disrupt sleep–wake cycle during acute use
- Decrease TST
- Decrease REM sleep
- Withdrawal may cause REM rebound

ANTIDEPRESSANTS (TRICYCLICS AND MAOIS)
- Sleep effects vary with sedative potential
- Increase slow-wave sleep (i.e., a recurrent period of very deep sleep, typically totaling 5 or 6 hours a night)
- Decrease REM sleep

BARBITURATES
- Increase TST
- Decrease WASO
- Decrease REM sleep
- Withdrawal may cause a decrease in TST and REM rebound

BENZODIAZEPINES
- Drugs vary in onset and duration of action
- Decrease SL
- Increase TST
- Decrease WASO
- Decrease REM sleep
- Daytime sedation may occur with long-acting drugs

BETA-ADRENERGIC BLOCKERS
- Decrease REM sleep
- Increase WASO, nightmares
- Daytime sedation may occur

CAFFEINE
- Increases SL
- Decreases TST
- Decreases REM sleep

L-DOPA
- Vivid dreams and nightmares

LITHIUM
- Increases slow-wave sleep
- Decreases REM sleep

OPIOIDS
- Effects vary with specific agents
- Increase WASO
- Decrease REM sleep
- Decrease slow-wave sleep

PHENOTHIAZINES
- Increase TST
- Increase slow-wave sleep

STEROIDS
- Increase WASO
- MAOI, monoamine oxidase inhibitor; REM, rapid eye movement; SL, sleep latency; TST, total sleep time; WASO, wake after sleep onset.

CLINICAL JUDGMENT

The primary concern is sleep deprivation or insomnia, which can result in depression, cognitive dysfunction, and suicide ideation. It is important to help the patient learn about sleep hygiene and the role that sleeps plays in maintaining health and well-being.

MENTAL HEALTH NURSING INTERVENTIONS

Establishing Recovery and Wellness Goals

Sleep problems impact all aspects of health and wellness. Helping a person examine current sleep patterns and their impact on any mental health issues is a beginning step in establishing wellness goals. Depending on the sleep problem, the nurse and patient should collaborate on establishing realistic goals. For example, going to bed at a regular hour each night or omitting caffeine after a set time of day could be a realistic goal.

Wellness Challenges

Wellness activities are especially challenging because of the negative impact lack of sleep has on daily life. Wellness can be severely compromised because the person is tired and irritable from lack of sleep. The lack of energy can lead to poor nutrition and inadequate performance at work or school. Coping with everyday stress can be difficult (see Box 34.5).

The nurse can help the patient develop bedtime rituals and good sleep hygiene. Bedtime should be at a regular hour, and the bedroom environment should be conducive to sleep. Preferably, the bedroom should not be where the individual watches television or does work-related activities. The bedroom should be viewed as a room for either resting or sleep (see Box 34.6).

Nonpharmacologic health-promoting interventions are the first choice before administering pharmacologic agents (Khoury & Doghramji, 2015). Sleep hygiene strategies can be effective and should be encouraged (Box 34.6). The goal is to normalize sleep patterns to improve well-being.

Activity, Exercise, Nutrition, and Thermoregulation Interventions

With the emergence of smartphones and other portable devices, limiting screen time to within 1 hour of bedtime has been found to improve sleep quality and positively impact daytime vigilance (Perrault et al., 2019). Exercise promotes sleep, but regular exercise should be planned to end 3 hours before bedtime. Routines are important, especially when preparing your body to sleep. Engaging in a quiet relaxing activity, such as listening to soft music or reading nonstimulating material, is often suggested. Additional interventions include avoiding eating a heavy

---

BOX 34.5

Wellness Challenges and Strategies

- Coping effectively with daily stresses when not getting adequate sleep.
  - Strategies: Reduce number of activities that require intense concentration
- Seeking pleasant environments that support well-being
  - Strategies: Arrange for short periods of "quiet time" throughout the day.
- Recognizing the need for physical activity, healthy foods, and sleep
  - Strategies: Encourage regular physical activity, discuss healthy diets, encourage establishing healthy sleep hygiene routines
- Developing a sense of connection, belong, and a support system
  - Strategies: Seek positive relationships and reduce number of unpleasant interactions.

BOX 34.6

Sleep Hygiene Tips

Nurses are often involved in helping patients develop and maintain good sleep habits. Teaching tips include the following:
1. The most important healthy sleep habit is to *establish and maintain a regular bedtime and rising time.* Even if you awaken feeling unrefreshed, get up and out of bed at a regular, consistent time. "Sleeping in" can disturb sleep on the subsequent night. For most, time in bed should be limited to 8 hours.
2. Avoid naps.
3. Abstain from alcohol. Although alcohol may assist with sleep onset, there is an alerting effect when it wears off.
4. Refrain from caffeine after midafternoon. Avoid nicotine before bedtime and during the night. Caffeine and nicotine are strong stimulants and fragment sleep.
5. Exercise regularly, avoiding the 3 hours before bedtime. Exercising 6 hours before bedtime tends to strengthen the circadian rhythms of body temperature and sleepiness.
6. Use the bedroom only for sleep and sex. Promote the bedroom as a stimulus for sleep, not for studying, watching television, or socializing on the telephone.
7. Set a relaxing routine to prepare for sleep. Avoid frustrating or provoking activities before bedtime.
8. Provide for a comfortable environment. A cool room temperature, minimal light, and limiting noise are suggested.

meal, and avoiding drinking alcohol or caffeinated beverages. Patients should be encouraged to evaluate the temperature of the room. Generally, a cooler environment enhances sleep.

Medication Interventions

Types of drugs used to treat symptoms of insomnia include benzodiazepine receptor agonists, melatonin receptor agonists, sedating antidepressants, and OTC medications and dietary supplements.

Remember Michael?

Michael has tried OTC sleep medication but does not remember the name of it. When he took these pills, he was able to fall asleep better but found the pills to be costly. He wants a medication that will be covered by his student health insurance.

What nonpharmacologic interventions would you suggest before exploring less costly medications? Which sleeping medications requiring a prescription have the least side effects?

Benzodiazepine Receptor Agonists

The BzRA hypnotics have U.S. Food and Drug Administration (FDA) approval for insomnia. They include the benzodiazepines (e.g., triazolam, temazepam, estazolam, quazepam, and flurazepam) and the nonbenzodiazepines (e.g., zolpidem, zolpidem extended release, zaleplon, and eszopiclone) (Table 34.1). All these medications bind to benzodiazepine receptors and exert their effects by facilitating GABA effects. GABA, the most common inhibitory neurotransmitter, must be present at the benzodiazepine receptor for the BzRA to exert its effect. These medications are all absorbed rapidly and reduce sleep latency (the amount of time it takes to fall asleep after the lights have been turned off) with medication at recommended doses (Pillai et al., 2017). Nonbenzodiazepine hypnotics, which provide immediate relief, are often used for short-term treatment of insomnia. The most common side effects are headache, dizziness, and residual sleepiness (Box 34.7).

The BzRAs are Schedule IV–controlled substances by federal regulation, have abuse and dependence potential, and produce withdrawal signs and symptoms after abrupt discontinuation. The risk for residual sedation on the day after using hypnotic medication is determined

TABLE 34.1   HYPNOTICS: BENZODIAZEPINE RECEPTOR AGONISTS

	Dosage (mg)	Half-life (h)
Estazolam	1–2	10–24
Flurazepam	15–30	48–120
Temazepam (Restoril)	15–30	8–20
Triazolam (Halcion)	0.125–0.25	2.4
Quazepam (Doral)	7.5–15	48–120
Zolpidem (Ambien)	5–10	1.4–3.8
Zolpidem ER (Ambien)	6.25–12.5	2.8
Zaleplon (Sonata)	5–20	1
Eszopiclone (Lunesta)	1–3	6

by the dose and rate of elimination (Pillai et al., 2017). The recommended therapeutic dose for using zolpidem (immediate release) is 5 mg and zolpidem CR is 6.25 mg.

Melatonin Receptor Agonist

Melatonin is a hormone, released from the pineal gland that aids in the regulation of the sleep–wake cycle through activation of MT_1 and MT_2 receptors.

BOX 34.7

Zaleplon (Sonata)

DRUG CLASS: Sedative–hypnotic (pyrazolopyrimidine nonbenzodiazepine hypnotic). It is readily absorbed and metabolized with only about 1% of zaleplon eliminated in urine.

RECEPTOR AFFINITY: Zaleplon acts at the GABA–benzodiazepine receptor complex.

INDICATION: Treatment of onset or maintenance insomnia

ROUTES AND DOSING: Zaleplon is available in 5- and 10-mg capsules. It should be taken at bedtime or after a nocturnal awakening with difficulty falling back to sleep (but at least 4 hours before the desired rise time).

Adults: The recommended starting dose is 10 mg with a maximum of 20 mg. An initial dose of 5 mg should be considered in adults with low body weight. Doses of over 20 mg have not been sufficiently studied.

Geriatric: Initially, 5 mg is recommended as a starting dose. Older adults should not exceed a 10-mg dose.

HALF-LIFE (PEAK PLASMA CONCENTRATION): 1 hour

SELECTED SIDE EFFECTS: Abdominal pain, headache, dizziness, depression, nervousness, difficulty concentrating, back pain, chest pain, migraine, conjunctivitis, bronchitis, pruritus, rash, arthritis, constipation, and dry mouth

WARNINGS: Zaleplon should not be administered to patients with severe hepatic impairment. Zaleplon potentiates the psychomotor impairments of ethanol consumption.

BOX 34.8

Ramelteon (Rozerem)

DRUG CLASS: Sedative–hypnotic. It is readily absorbed and metabolized with median peak concentrations occurring 0.5–1.5 hours after fasted oral administration.

RECEPTOR AFFINITY: Ramelteon is a melatonin receptor agonist with high affinity for MT_1 and MT_2. No appreciable affinity for the GABA receptor complex.

INDICATION: Treatment of insomnia characterized by difficulty with sleep onset.

ROUTES AND DOSING: The recommended dose is 8 mg. It should be taken 30 minutes before bedtime.

It should not be taken with or immediately after a high fat meal. Patients should be advised to use caution if they consume alcohol in combination with ramelteon.

Adolescents and Children: Ramelteon has been associated with an effect on reproductive hormones in adults, for example, decreased testosterone levels and increased prolactin levels.

Geriatric: No overall differences in safety or efficacy were observed between older and younger adult subjects.

HALF-LIFE (PEAK PLASMA CONCENTRATION): 1–2.6 hours

SELECTED ADVERSE REACTIONS: Somnolence, dizziness, nausea, fatigue, headache, and insomnia

WARNINGS: Ramelteon should not be used by patients with severe hepatic impairment. It should not be used in combination with fluvoxamine.

Melatonin has been shown to shift circadian rhythm, decrease body temperature, alter reproductive rhythm, enhance immune function, and decrease alertness. Normally, levels of melatonin increase with decreasing exposure to light. Ramelteon (Rozerem), indicated for insomnia, is a melatonin receptor agonist with high affinity for melatonin receptors MT_1 and MT_2. This pharmacologic activity is believed to be related to its sleep-promoting properties (Box 34.8). Ramelteon has a low abuse potential and is not a controlled substance (Neubauer et al., 2018).

Orexin Receptor Antagonist

Orexins (also known as hypocretins) are neurotransmitters produced in the hypothalamus that trigger wakefulness, while low levels result in sleep. A deficiency is associated with narcolepsy. Suvorexant (Belsomra) is an orexin receptor antagonist approved for the treatment of insomnia. Blocking the binding of orexins to receptors is thought to suppress the wake drive. This antagonism may also trigger signs of narcolepsy/cataplexy. There is emerging evidence that this group of medications is effective for other psychiatric disorders (Han et al., 2020).

Over-the-Counter Medications and Dietary Supplements

OTC sleeping pills are usually antihistamines. The most common agents are doxylamine and diphenhydramine. These histamine-1 antagonists have a CNS effect that includes sedation, diminished alertness, and slowing of reaction time. These drugs also produce anticholinergic side effects, such as dry mouth, accelerated heart rate, urinary retention, and dilated pupils. Drowsiness lasts from 3 to 6 hours after a single dose. Next-morning hangover can be a problem. Diphenhydramine decreases sleep latency and improves quality of sleep for those with occasional sleep problems but is not as effective as benzodiazepines for chronic sleep disturbances (Neubauer et al., 2018).

Melatonin has long been an available OTC and has been shown to have mild sleep-promoting properties when given outside the period of usual secretion. That is, melatonin can advance the sleep–wake cycle by making it easier to fall asleep earlier than usual. Some evidence suggests that in young and older individuals with insomnia, melatonin can be beneficial in ameliorating the symptoms (Neubauer et al., 2018).

Valerian, a dietary supplement, is used as a medicinal herb in many cultures. The mechanism of action is not fully understood and is believed to inhibit GABA reuptake. Valerian may be useful for sleeplessness, but not enough evidence from double-blind studies exists to confirm this. The American Academy of Sleep Medicine recommended against using valerian for chronic insomnia in adults. Mild side effects include headaches, dizziness, upset stomach, and tiredness the morning after its use (National Center for Complementary and Alternative Medicine, 2020b).

Administering and Monitoring Medication

Sleeping medications are commonly used in all settings. They are usually given nightly for a short period of time to establish a wake–sleep pattern. Rebound insomnia can occur if a drug is abruptly discontinued. This side effect can be minimized or prevented by giving the lowest effective dose and tapering before discontinuing. Nurses should assess for confusion, memory problems, excessive sedation, and risk of falls.

Monitoring for Drug-to-Drug Interactions

Sleep medications generally have increased depressive effects when given with other CNS depressants. Sleep medications can interact with oral contraceptives, isoniazid (an antibiotic), fluvoxamine (a serotonin reuptake inhibitor [SSRI]), and verapamil (a calcium channel blocker) (see Chapter 12). Grapefruit juice should be avoided when taking these drugs. Ramelteon should not be given with fluvoxamine.

Teaching Points

Pharmacologic agents should complement sleep hygiene practices. These medications can be useful on a short-term basis. Alcohol use should be avoided when taking sleeping medications. Patients should use these medications when time for sleeping is adequate (at least 8 hours). Most sleep-related medications should be taken at bedtime. Patients should be instructed about the safe use of these medications and possible side effects.

Psychosocial Interventions

Enhancing Cognitive Functioning

Cognitive-behavioral therapy (CBT) is useful in changing negative learned responses that perpetuate insomnia. This approach is especially helpful for those who also have comorbid depression or anxiety. The objective of CBT is to change the belief system that results in improvement of the self-efficacy of the individual (Khoury & Doghramji, 2015) (see Chapter 13).

Using Behavioral Interventions

Stimulus control is a technique used when the bedroom environment no longer provides cues for sleep but has become the cue for wakefulness. Patients are instructed to avoid behaviors in the bedroom incompatible with sleep, including watching television, doing homework, and eating. This allows the bedroom to be reestablished as a stimulus for sleep.

Another behavioral intervention is sleep *restriction*. Patients often increase their time in bed to provide more opportunity for sleep, resulting in fragmented sleep and irregular sleep schedules. Patients are instructed to spend less time in bed and avoid napping.

Relaxation training is used when patients complain of difficulty relaxing, especially if these patients are physically tense or emotionally distressed. Various procedures to reduce somatic arousal can be used, including progressive muscle relaxation, autogenic training, and biofeedback. Imagery training, meditation, and thought stopping are attention-focusing techniques that center on cognitive arousal (see Chapter 13).

Psychoeducation

Teaching Strategies

Education regarding interventions is crucial for patients with sleep disorders. An explanation of the sleep cycle and the factors that influence sleep are important for

---

BOX 34.9

Sleep Disorders

When teaching patients with sleep disorders, be sure to include the following topics:

- Maintenance of a sleep log
- Foods to avoid before going to bed
- Importance of developing a bedtime ritual and good sleep habits
- Use of sleep medications as prescribed
- Avoidance of caffeine and rigorous exercise within the 6 hours before bedtime
- Avoidance of cigarette smoking 1 hour before bedtime and during nighttime awakenings
- Allowing for 8 hours of sleep per night
- Maintenance of a regular sleep schedule, specifically a routine rise time
- An occasional "bad night" happens to nearly everyone
- Avoidance of alcohol because it disrupts sleep and is a poor hypnotic
- Daytime sleepiness as a symptom of sleep disorders
- How to do relaxation exercises
- Bedroom rituals
- Appropriate family support

---

these patients. For those with insomnia, teaching about avoiding foods and beverages that might interfere with sleep should be highlighted (Box 34.9).

Wellness Strategies

There are sleep hygiene strategies that specifically promote sleep (Box 34.6), but there are many other activities associated with physical and psychological well-being that should also be considered. Eating a healthy diet, avoiding excessive weight gain, and identifying and managing psychological and physical stressors are examples of wellness strategies that promote sleep. Yoga is associated with improvement in sleep quality (Wang et al., 2020). Other strategies include relaxation, massage therapy, and meditation (National Center for Complementary and Integrative Health, 2020a).

Providing Family Education

Family and friends should be encouraged to support the new habits the patient is trying to establish. Patients, spouses, and friends must understand that activities engaged in just before sleep can greatly affect sleep patterns and sleep difficulties, such as socializing, alcohol consumption, use of caffeine, and engaging in stimulating activities. Relaxing activities before bedtime are vital contributors to establishing a routine conducive to sleep. Family and friends can help create a positive environment with an emphasis on sleep as a priority.

Evaluation and Treatment Outcomes

The primary treatment outcome is establishing a normal sleep cycle. Changes in diet and behavior (e.g., initiation of an exercise program) should be evaluated for their impact on the individual's sleep. Environmental modifications, such as a change in the level of lighting in the bedroom, decreased stimulation (e.g., turning off cell phone or moving the television out of the bedroom), or modification in room temperature, can be monitored for any changes affecting the sleep cycle.

Integration with Primary Care

Sleep problems are usually treated in the primary care setting. Cardiovascular and metabolic disorders are associated with sleep disturbances. Sleep deprivation is associated with obesity and hypertension (Matenchuk et al., 2020; Thomas & Calhoun, 2016). If a sleep disorder is being treated by a mental health specialist, it is important that the mental health specialists communicate with the primary care provider.

OTHER DISORDERS

Hypersomnolence Disorder

The essential characteristic of hypersomnolence disorder is excessive sleepiness at least three times a week for at least 3 months. Sleepiness occurs on an almost daily basis and causes significant impairment in social and occupational functioning. They have an excessive quantity of sleep, deteriorated quality of wakefulness, and sleep inertia (a period of impaired performance occurring during the sleep–wake transition characterized by confusion, ataxia, or combativeness) (Cook et al., 2019). This diagnosis is reserved for individuals who have no other causes of daytime sleepiness (e.g., narcolepsy, OSA syndrome).

Clinical Course

People with hypersomnolence typically sleep 8 to 12 hours per night. They fall asleep easily and sleep through the night, often having difficulty awakening in the morning. They often have difficulty meeting morning obligations. They exhibit poor concentration and memory. Excessive sleepiness may not be impacted by napping because they may awaken from a nap feeling unrefreshed. They may even describe dangerous situations, such as being sleepy while driving or operating heavy machinery.

Diagnosis

On the day after overnight polysomnography, a multiple sleep latency test (MSLT) may be used. The MSLT is a standardized procedure that measures sleep variables during a 20-minute period. The process is repeated every 2 hours, occurring approximately five times during the day (Arand & Bonnet, 2019). The faster a person falls asleep during testing, the greater the physiologic sleep tendency. The presence of sleep-onset REM (SOREM) during the MSLT and a report of cataplexy assist providers in determining a sleep diagnosis. Polysomnography shows short sleep latency, a normal-to-long sleep duration, and normal sleep architecture. Subjective symptoms of sleepiness are recognized as heavy eyelids, loss of initiative, reluctance to move, and yawning or slowed speech. Sleepiness is unique to the person and situation, varying from mild to severe.

Evidence-Based Nursing Care of Persons with Hypersomnolence Disorder

Nursing assessment for the patient with hypersomnolence focuses on excessive sleepiness. The following are examples of assessment questions.

* Have you ever nodded off unintentionally?
* When did your sleepiness begin?
* Does anyone in your family experience the same sleepiness symptoms?
* Do you suddenly find yourself awakening feeling refreshed?

Interventions stress the importance of sleep hygiene and helping the patient establish normal sleep patterns. If medications are given, the most commonly prescribed stimulants for treating excessive daytime sleepiness are dextroamphetamine and amphetamine mixtures (Adderall), modafinil (Provigil), methylphenidate (Ritalin, Concerta), and pemoline (Cylert). These agents increase the patient's ability to stay awake and perform. Abuse of these medications should be assessed. In some cases, serotonin antagonists are used off-label.

Sleepy people often self-medicate with caffeine. A cup of brewed coffee contains about 100 to 150 mg of caffeine. A 12-oz can of Mountain Dew contains 54 mg of caffeine. Caffeine contents of popular "energy" drinks range from 80 to 300 mg. Peak plasma concentration is reached 30 to 60 minutes after consumption, and the duration of effect is 3 to 5 hours in adults. Caffeine improves psychomotor performance, particularly tasks involving endurance, vigilance, and attention. High doses, especially in people who are not habitual users, may exhibit side effects such as irritability and anxiety.

Narcolepsy

The overwhelming urge to sleep is the primary symptom of narcolepsy. This irresistible urge to sleep occurs at any time of the day, regardless of the amount of sleep. Falling asleep often occurs in inappropriate situations, such as while driving a car or reading a newspaper. These sleep episodes are usually short, lasting 5 to 20 minutes, but may last up to an hour if sleep is not interrupted. Individuals with narcolepsy may experience sleep attacks and report frequent dreaming. They usually feel alert after a sleep attack, only to fall asleep unintentionally again several hours later.

Clinical Course

Narcolepsy is a chronic disorder that usually begins in young adulthood between the ages of 15 and 35 years. Excessive sleepiness is the first symptom to appear. The severity of sleepiness may remain stable over the lifetime. Narcolepsy has no cure. Treatment is designed to control symptoms based on clinical presentation and severity. A secondary sleep disorder should be considered if the level of sleepiness changes.

Narcolepsy is distinguished by a group of symptoms, including daytime sleepiness, cataplexy, hypnagogic hallucinations, and sleep paralysis. The symptom of daytime sleepiness is found in all individuals with narcolepsy, but existence of the other three symptoms varies.

- Cataplexy is the bilateral loss of muscle tone, triggered by a strong emotion, such as anger or laughter. This muscle atonia can range from subtle (drooping eyelids) to dramatic (buckling knees). Respiratory muscles are not affected. Cataplexy usually lasts for seconds. Individuals are fully conscious, oriented, and alert during the episode. Prolonged episodes of cataplexy may lead to unintentional sleep episodes. The frequency and severity of events generally increase when the individual is sleep deprived.

- Hypnagogic hallucinations are intense dreamlike images that occur at sleep onset and usually involve the current environment. Hallucinations can be visual or auditory, such as hearing one's name called or a door slammed.

- Sleep paralysis, the inability to move or speak when falling asleep or waking up, is often described as terrifying and is accompanied by a sensation of struggling to move or speak. Although the diaphragm is not involved, patients may also complain of not being able to breathe or feeling suffocated. These episodes are typically brief in duration and usually terminate spontaneously or when the individual is touched.

Diagnosis

Excessive daytime sleepiness and the presence of cataplexy are diagnostic of narcolepsy. It is possible to have narcolepsy without cataplexy. The diagnosis should be confirmed by an in-lab polysomnogram demonstrating at least 6 hours of sleep, followed by the MSLT showing a sleep latency of less than or equal to 8 minutes and two or more SOREM periods. The diagnosis can also be confirmed by a cerebrospinal fluid hypocretin-1 level less than or equal to 110 mg/mL (Rosenberg et al., 2019).

Epidemiology and Etiology

The prevalence of narcolepsy is between 20 and 50 per 100,000 people in the United States (Dye et al., 2018). The etiology of most cases of narcolepsy is unknown, but it is thought that there are many triggers such as head trauma, viral illness, exposure to toxins, and development factors. In some patients, there is a deficiency of hypocretin, a hypothalamic peptide that may be linked to chromosome 6 in class II human leukocyte antigen. Hypocretin neurons are part of the neurologic system that wakes and maintains wakefulness (Rosenberg et al., 2019).

Evidence-based Nursing Care of Persons with Narcolepsy

Nursing assessment is similar to that for insomnia. In general, sleepiness is treated with CNS stimulants. Methylphenidate, dextroamphetamine, modafinil, and pemoline are the most frequently prescribed stimulants. Cataplexy may be treated with tricyclic antidepressants because these drugs suppress REM. Sodium oxybate (Xyrem), classified as a Schedule II drug, is indicated for excessive sleepiness and cataplexy. Because of its high abuse potential, patients who are prescribed this medication are closely monitored.

Patient education focuses on factors that can make symptoms worse, such as sleep deprivation. Patients need to develop strategies to manage symptoms. Naps can be integrated into their daily routines such as during work breaks or before engaging in activities that require sustaining alertness.

Breathing-Related Disorders

The *DSM-5* identifies three breathing disorders, including OSA–hypopnea, central sleep apnea, and sleep-related hypoventilation. This section will discuss OSA–hypopnea disorder (OSA syndrome) (APA, 2013). The term *obstructive sleep apnea syndrome* is more commonly used in nonpsychiatric areas and will be used in this section instead of the term *obstructive apnea–hypopnea disorder*. Central sleep apnea and sleep-related hypoventilation will not be discussed.

Obstructive Sleep Apnea Syndrome

OSA syndrome, the most commonly diagnosed breathing-related sleep disorder, OSA is characterized by snoring during sleep and episodes of sleep apnea (cessation of breathing) that fragments sleep and contribute to daytime sleepiness. The hallmark symptoms are snoring and daytime sleepiness. Often, snoring is so loud and disturbing that partners choose separate bedrooms for sleeping. On physical examination, an enlarged, elongated uvula is associated with increased severity of snoring and apneic events (Chang et al., 2018). Snoring affects 57% of men, 40% of women, and 27% of children (National Sleep Foundation, 2020).

Clinical Course

Apneic episodes, which last from 10 seconds up to several minutes, cause disrupted sleep and abrupt awakenings with feelings of choking or falling out of bed; some people even leap out of bed to restore breathing. The person may not later recall the awakening. These brief awakenings deprive essential sleep, resulting in excessive daytime sleepiness that may reach the same degree of pathologic sleepiness found in narcolepsy. Unlike narcolepsy, naps tend to be unrefreshing.

Esophageal reflux, or heartburn, is a common complaint. Genitourinary symptoms include nocturia (three to seven trips to the bathroom), nocturnal enuresis, and erectile dysfunction. Bradycardia, in association with tachycardia, is often seen with apneic events. Other cardiac arrhythmias are also seen, including sinus arrest. The onset of symptoms and sleepiness may coincide with weight gain. Obesity is a major risk factor for apnea and predictor across populations (Sutherland et al., 2019).

Diagnosis

Polysomnography, usually performed at night during sleep, monitors many body functions, including brain wave activity, eye movements, muscle activity, heart rhythm, breathing function, and respiratory effort. Polysomnography may show poor sleep continuity, increased stage 1 and decreased slow-wave and REM sleep, and an increased amount of EEG alpha wave activity while the individual is asleep. Clinical evaluation includes oral and nasal airflow, respiratory effort, oxyhemoglobin saturation, and electromyogram of limb muscle activity. Typically, patients with OSA demonstrate numerous respiratory events per night,

resulting in intermittent hypoxemia and changes in intrathoracic pressure during polysomnographic measurement (Sutherland et al., 2019).

Epidemiology and Risk Factors

The prevalence of OSA is worldwide and is said to impact up to one billion adults globally, between the ages of 30 and 69 years (Benjafield et al., 2018), affecting both men and women. OSA is most common in men aged 45 to 65 who are overweight. The female-to-male ratio is estimated to be 1:8, with women becoming more likely to develop this syndrome after menopause. Men are twice as likely to snore as women (APA, 2013).

Research supports ethnic and racial differences in sleep disturbances. African American individuals and Hispanic individuals have an increased frequency of snoring as compared with White individuals, but the increase may be related to poorer physical health (Petrov & Lichstein, 2016). Lost workplace productivity, motor vehicle accidents, workplace injuries, and increased use of health care services account for some of the societal consequences of untreated OSA (Wickwire et al., 2019). OSA is a risk factor for cardiac events and is commonly associated with metabolic syndrome disorders (Li et al., 2020). OSA is more prevalent in people with mental health disorders than in the general population. Depression, anxiety, PTSD, and bipolar disorder are associated with OSA. The symptoms of depression, such as fatigue, irritability, depressed mood, and poor concentration, are similar to the symptoms of OSA. Evidence suggests that the successfully treated OSA may improve depressive symptoms (Edwards et al., 2020).

Etiology

An obstruction or collapse of the airway causes apnea, or cessation of breathing. In most cases, the site of obstruction is in the pharyngeal area. Vibrations of the soft, pliable tissues found in the pharyngeal airway cause the snoring sounds that occur during breathing.

Teamwork and Collaboration: Working Toward Recovery

There are nonsurgical and surgical options for the treatment of patients with OSA. Nonsurgical options vary based on the severity of the obstructive breathing. For obese patients with less severe OSA, weight loss may help. For others, whose apnea is mild, changing sleeping position from supine to lateral can help control the severity of OSA. There has also been some effort in devising an oral appliance to reduce snoring and the occurrence of apnea. Currently, the most effective nonsurgical treatment is continuous positive airway pressure. This treatment takes place during sleep and involves wearing a nose mask that is connected by a long tube to an air compressor. Airway patency is maintained with air pressure. Although this method of treatment is highly effective, compliance can be a problem. Individuals who have severe OSA symptoms and daytime sleepiness are more compliant with CPAP (continuous positive airway pressure) treatment and report an improved quality of life (Bue et al., 2019).

The most commonly performed surgical procedure to treat patients with OSA is uvulopalatopharyngoplasty. This procedure involves the removal of redundant soft palate tissue, uvula, and tonsillar pillars. The surgery usually eliminates snoring and is judged to be about 50% effective in reducing the amount of sleep apnea. Severity of OSA, body mass index, and pharyngeal anatomic features are factors that impact surgical outcomes (He et al., 2019).

Circadian Rhythm Sleep Disorder

The chief feature of a circadian rhythm sleep disorder is the mismatch between the individual's internal sleep–wake circadian rhythm and the timing and duration of sleep (Burgess & Emens, 2018). People with these disorders complain of insomnia at particular times during the day and excessive sleepiness at others. This diagnosis is reserved for those individuals who present with marked sleep disturbance or significant social or occupational impairment.

Diagnosis and Clinical Course

- *Delayed sleep phase type:* Individuals with delayed sleep phase type, or "night owls," tend to be unable to fall asleep before 2 AM to 6 AM; hence, their whole sleep patterns shift, and they have difficulty rising in the morning.
- *Advanced sleep phase type:* Opposite of the night owls, these individuals are "larks" or earlier risers. They are unable to stay awake in the evening and consistently wake up early.
- *Irregular sleep–wake type:* People with this type have a temporarily disorganized sleep pattern that varies in a 24-hour period.
- *Non–24-hour sleep–wake type:* Individuals with this type have an abnormal synchronization between the 24-hour light–dark cycle and their endogenous circadian rhythm, which leads to periods of insomnia, excessive sleepiness, or both. This type is most common among blind or visually impaired individuals.
- *Shift work type:* The endogenous sleep–wake cycle is normal but is mismatched to the imposed hours of

shift work. Rotating shift schedules are disruptive because any consistent adjustment is prevented. Compared with day and evening shift workers, night and rotating shift workers have a shorter sleep duration and poorer quality of sleep. They may also be sleepier while performing their jobs. This disorder is further exacerbated by insufficient daytime sleep resulting from social and family demands and environmental disturbances (i.e., traffic noise, telephone). Because of the job requirements of the profession, nurses often experience this disorder. Furthermore, 20% of the U.S. workforce is engaged in shift work and thereby at risk for circadian rhythm disorders.

- *Jet lag type:* This type of sleep disturbance occurs after travel across time zones, particularly in coast-to-coast and international travel. The normal endogenous circadian sleep–wake cycle does not match the desired hours of sleep and wakefulness in a new time zone. Individuals traveling eastward are more prone to jet lag because it involves resetting one's circadian clock to an earlier time—it is easier to delay the endogenous clock to a later time period than adjust it to an earlier one.

Epidemiology and Etiology

There are no data regarding the prevalence of circadian rhythm disorders in the general population. The prevalence of circadian rhythm disorders among patients diagnosed at sleep disorder centers accounts for 2% or less of the total patients diagnosed. However, this is a gross underestimate, given that jet lag, a circadian rhythm disorder, affects nearly everyone traveling over three time zones.

Circadian rhythm disorders are caused by the dissociation of the internal circadian pacemaker and conventional time. The cause might be intrinsic, such as genetic factors called "clock genes" or extrinsic, as in jet lag and shift work. Each result is overwhelming daytime sleepiness and overflowing wakefulness at night.

Teamwork and Collaboration: Working Toward Recovery

The goals of treatment of circadian rhythm disorder are to strengthen timed clues (when to go to sleep), timed bright or blue light (stay awake during the day), and timed exogenous melatonin (initiate melatonin secretion at bedtime). Melatonin is often helpful in initiating sleep (Pavlova & Latreille, 2019).

Chronotherapy, timed interventions, manipulates the sleep schedule by progressively delaying bedtime until an acceptable bedtime is attained. Chronopharmacotherapy resets the biologic clock by using medications to induce sleep. Tasimelteon (Hetlioz) is a melatonin receptor agonist that is approved for the treatment of this disorder. Small amounts of hypnotics can also produce high-quality sleep in people who wish to reset their circadian schedules after long transmeridian flights. Conversely, for night shift workers, caffeine taken while working at night improves alertness and performance. However, caffeine should be used judiciously by night shift workers because they become quickly tolerant to the effects after a few nights (Burgess & Emens, 2018).

Luminotherapy (light therapy) is used to manipulate the circadian system. Timing, wavelength intensity and prior light exposure are key factors when considering light therapy (Pavlova & Latreille, 2019). Commercially prepared light boxes produce therapeutic light at 2500 to 10,000 lux. In contrast, indoor light is about 150 lux (Burgess & Emens, 2018).

Parasomnias

Parasomnias are sleep–wake disorders that occur in association with sleep, specific sleep stages, or sleep–wake transitions. The person experiences abnormal behavioral, experiential, or physiologic events. Parasomnias are divided into two primary categories: NREM-related and rapid eye movement (REM)-related NREM sleep arousal disorders, including sleepwalking and sleep terror types, which usually occur during the first third of the major sleep episode. Nightmare disorder is a REM disorder that generally occurs during the second half of the major sleep episode. RLS is considered a sleep disorder and is classified as a sleep-related movement disorder (Carter & Wrede, 2017).

Sleep Terrors and Sleepwalking

In sleep terrors (also called night terrors or pavor nocturnes), there are episodes of screaming, fear, and panic, causing clinical distress or impairing social, occupational, or other areas of functioning. Sleep terrors usually last 1 to 10 minutes, are frightening to the person and to anyone witnessing them. Often, individuals abruptly sit up in bed screaming; others have been known to jump out of bed and run across the room. Other symptoms include a rapid heart rate and breathing, dilated pupils, and flushed skin. Usually, the person having a sleep terror is inconsolable and difficult to awaken completely. Efforts to awaken the individual may prolong the episode. Once awake, most are unable to recall the dream or event that precipitated such a response. A few report a fragmentary image. Often, the individual does not fully awaken and cannot recall the episode the next morning (Ellington, 2018).

In sleepwalking or somnambulism, there are repeated episodes of complex motor behavior during sleep that may involve getting out of bed and walking around. While sleepwalking, people typically have a blank stare and are difficult to awaken. Often, they awaken to find themselves in a different place from where they went to sleep. If awakened during the episode, there is a brief period of confusion.

Clinical Course

Polysomnography shows that these disorders usually begin when slow-wave NREM sleep predominates during the first third of the night. They rarely occur during daytime naps.

Epidemiology and Etiology

The prevalence of sleep terrors is estimated at 6.5% in children and 2.2% in adults. Males and females are affected equally. The prevalence of sleepwalking is 30% in children and 4% in adults. Sleepwalking peaks between 8 and 12 years of age and is more common in males (Ellington, 2018). Fever, stress, and sleep deprivation can increase the frequency of episodes. There appears to be some genetic predisposition for disorders of arousal, and they tend to run in families.

Teamwork and Collaboration: Working Toward Recovery

Learning about parasomnias and the need for safety precautions for patient and family should be the focus of patient education. Hypnosis supplemented by psychotherapy may be considered. Treatment might also include medications, such as benzodiazepines. These disorders usually resolve by adolescence.

Evidence-Based Nursing Practice for the Persons with Parasomnias

Although polysomnography may be used to diagnose or confirm a sleep disorder, the evaluation of a response to an NREM disorder involves a careful sleep history. Episodes of sleep terrors or sleepwalking are often unrealized by the patient but can be described in detail by the parent or partner. Support persons should be advised to avoid attempting to wake the person/child and ensure a safe environment surrounds the individual. Safety features may include a sleep space absent of stairs, as well as securing windows and doors with locks. Sleep diaries should focus on the person's bedtime activities, time of sleep onset and wake up, time to prepare for bed and fall asleep, use of medications, number of awakenings, subjective assessment of quality of sleep, and daytime naps. Sleep hygiene and a routine, to avoid insufficient sleep, should be promoted (Manni et al., 2018).

Nursing interventions range from referring to sleep specialists to patient education about the disorder and strategies in dealing with the disorder. In some instances, nurses care for patients in the inpatient setting who have arousal disorders. In these instances, nurses should develop care plans that address the individual patient's needs. In instances of sleepwalking, staff should be alert to the safety issues and protect the patient from injury (see Box 34.10).

Nightmare Disorder

The repeated occurrence of frightening dreams that occur during REM sleep and often awaken an individual is the essential characteristic of nightmare disorder. Typically, the individual can recall detailed dream content that involves physical danger (e.g., attack or pursuit) or perceived danger (e.g., embarrassment or failure). On awakening, the individual is fully alert and experiences a persisting sense of anxiety or fear. Many people have difficulty returning to sleep. Multiple same-night nightmares may be reported. Some people avoid sleep because of their fear of nightmares. Consequently, people may report that excessive sleepiness, poor concentration, and irritability disrupt their daytime activities. The occurrence of nightmares may be more serious than previously suspected. Nightmares are commonly experienced by military combat personnel who have PTSD (see Chapter 29).

Diagnosis and Clinical Course

Nightmares occur in REM sleep almost exclusively. They most often occur during the second half of the night when REM sleep dominates. Polysomnography demonstrates abrupt awakenings from REM sleep. In most cases, the REM sleep episode lasts for at least 10 minutes. Tachycardia and tachypnea may be evident.

Etiology and Epidemiology

The cause and prevalence of nightmares are unknown. Intriguing evidence provokes a debate as to whether nightmares are a symptom or an adaptive reaction to pathophysiologic factors. Negative emotions, primarily fear, are the most common dream emotions. Brain imaging demonstrates increased metabolic activity during REM sleep in the most primitive regions of the brain, the paralimbic and limbic regions. Many classes of drugs trigger nightmares, including catecholaminergic agents, beta-blockers, some antidepressants, barbiturates, and alcohol. Additionally, withdrawal from barbiturates and alcohol causes REM rebound and more vivid dreaming.

Nightmares often begin in children between the ages of 3 and 6 years, and most children outgrow them. In adults, at least 50% of the population reports occasional nightmares. Women are more likely to report nightmares than men.

Teamwork and Collaboration: Working Toward Recovery

If the nightmares cause significant distress, a person will be treated by multiple providers. Traditionally, psychotherapy aimed at conflict resolution has been the treatment of choice. Today, CBT is recommended, specifically imagery rehearsal therapy, a technique in which patients change the endings of the nightmares while they are awake. After rehearsing new, nonthreatening images and changing the content of the nightmare while awake, a reduction in the frequency of nightmares and associated distress has been shown (Levrier et al., 2016). Pharmacologically, the best studied and most effective medication to treat nightmares with PTSD is prazosin (Minipress), a centrally active alpha-1 adrenergic antagonist indicated for hypertension (El-Solh, 2018). It does not have FDA approval for use with nightmares, but prazosin is recommended by the Standards of Practice Committee of the American Academy of Sleep Medicine for PTSD-associated nightmares (Morgenthaler et al., 2018).

Evidenced-Based Nursing Care

While caring for patients with other disorders, the nurse often is the first health professional to identify nightmares as a problem in a patient. Sleep assessment is vital in every nursing assessment. If nightmares are causing distress, a referral for a sleep evaluation should be made. Sleep hygiene techniques and education about the

---

BOX 34.10

General Safety Precautions for Sleepwalkers and Their Families

- Ensure adequate sleep. The occurrence of sleepwalking dramatically increases after sleep loss.
- Anticipate sleepwalking. Family members should be aware of the likelihood of sleepwalking for the first 2–3 hours after the sleepwalker goes to bed.
- Keep a sleep log to assist in identifying how much sleep is needed to prevent a sleepwalking event.
- Consider use of a noise device on the door of the sleepwalker's room to alert others that the sleepwalker is up.
- Deadbolt locks should be installed on doors leading outside. Windows should be secured to limit their opening.
- When the sleepwalker is spending the night away from home, alert appropriate individuals to the possibility that sleepwalking may occur. Ensure adequate sleep on the preceding nights.

treatment of nightmares should be included in patient teaching. During hospitalization, the nurse should document that the patient has nightmares, and the nurses on the night shift should monitor for them.

Restless Legs Syndrome

RLS is a sleep–wake disorder characterized by an urge to move the legs, which begins or worsens at rest or periods of inactivity, typically in the evening or at night. The urge to move legs is reduced or relieved by movement.

Diagnostic Criteria and Clinical Course

RLS is a sensorimotor, neurologic disorder described as the intense desire to move legs accompanied by uncomfortable sensations such as creeping, crawling, tingling, burning, or itching. The diagnosis is made on the basis of self-report. These symptoms can interfere with sleep and cause considerable clinical distress or functional impairment. RLS is usually diagnosed in the second and third decade of life and can get progressively worse later in life.

Epidemiology and Etiology

RLS affects approximately 2.5% of adults in the United States. The prevalence is about twice higher in women than in men and increases with age in North America and Europe, but not observed in Asian countries. Comorbid conditions of insomnia, excessive sleepiness, and depressive and/or anxiety symptoms are consistently associated with RLS. RLS is the most common movement disorder occurring during pregnancy, usually developing in the third trimester and impacting 1 in 5 women (Esposito et al., 2019; Steinweg et al., 2020).

The etiology of RLS remains unclear, but genetic predisposition, dopaminergic dysfunction, and deficiencies in iron metabolism partially explain the underlying causes. RLS is linked to cardiovascular disease and metabolic syndrome (diabetes, obesity, hypertension, and dyslipidemia) (Yatsu et al., 2019). There is emerging evidence that suggests inflammation and/or immunologic disorders have a role in RLS. Recent studies show an increased prevalence of small intestinal bacterial overgrowth, HIV infection, systemic lupus erythematosus, and cases of hepatitis C (Trenkwalder et al., 2017).

Teamwork and Collaboration: Working Toward Recovery

The treatment of RLS involves a biopsychosocial approach using pharmacologic and nonpharmacologic treatment options. In cases of mild and intermittent RLS, behavioral therapy, sleep hygiene, and lifestyle interventions (avoiding caffeine, alcohol, and heavy meals) help reduce the likelihood of having an episode. If serum ferritin is <50 mcg/L, supplementation with ferrous sulfate is initiated (Khoury & Doghramji, 2015). For moderate-to-severe RLS, there is strong evidence to support the use of pramipexole, rotigotine, cabergoline, and gabapentin enacarbil. There is moderate evidence to support the use of ropinirole, pregabalin, and IV FCM. Augmentation, also diagnosed as refectory RLS, with use of dopaminergic drugs occurs in approximately 7% of clients and can occur after multiple years of use. Assessment for augmentation, sleepiness, and compulsive behaviors are factors of focus for the health care team. The evidence to support the use of levodopa is weak (Winkelman et al., 2016).

Evidence-based Nursing Practice for Persons with Restless Legs Syndrome

A thorough nursing assessment will provide direction for the nursing interventions for a person with RLS. In many instances, there are underlying medical conditions such as diabetes or peripheral neuropathy, which contribute to the severity of RLS, particularly for the older adult. If the underlying medical condition is being treated adequately, the patient can be encouraged to engage in moderate regular physical activity 3 days a week or taking a hot bath before going to sleep. If medication is prescribed, the patient and family will benefit from medication education. If iron supplement is given, follow-up testing should be monitored to prevent overload. Sleep hygiene and encouragement to avoid exacerbating factors should be recommended (Steinweg et al., 2020).

SUMMARY OF KEY POINTS

- The normal sleep–wake cycle runs in a pattern called circadian rhythm. Most body systems follow a circadian rhythm and are often associated with the sleep–wake cycle. Hormones, such as melatonin and cortisol, help promote wakefulness during the day and sleepiness at night.

- Assessment is key. Information should focus on a comprehensive sleep history, including specific details of the sleep complaint, current sleep patterns, and sleep patterns before sleep difficulties, medical problems, current medications, current life events, and emotional and mental status.

- Nursing interventions for sleep disorders focus on nonpharmacologic approaches (e.g., exercise, nutrition, activity, thermoregulation) and pharmacologic interventions.

- Psychosocial nursing interventions for sleep disorders include educating patients about good sleep habits, instructing patients in relaxation exercises and sleep-promoting activities, providing patients with nutritional suggestions regarding foods and substances to avoid, and educating family members and friends regarding the importance of supporting the need for making high-quality sleep a priority.

- Insomnia disorder is characterized by difficulty falling asleep or difficulty maintaining sleep. Insomnia is often precipitated by feelings of stress or tension, with associations and behaviors persisting after the crisis or stressful situation has passed.

- OSA syndrome is a diagnosed breathing-related sleep disorder characterized by excessive snoring and episodes of apnea (i.e., cessation of breathing). These episodes disrupt sleep and may cause daytime sleepiness.

- In circadian rhythm sleep–wake disorders, a mismatch takes place between the individual's internal sleep–wake circadian rhythm and the timing and duration of sleep.

- Parasomnias occur in association with sleep, specific sleep stages, or sleep–wake transitions and include sleepwalking, sleep terrors, nightmare disorders, and RLS. They are characterized by abnormal behavioral, experiential, or physiologic events. The etiology is unknown but appears to be of genetic predisposition. Unrestorative sleep, excessive sleepiness, poor concentration, and irritability are often the result.

CRITICAL THINKING CHALLENGES

1. Describe the sleep hygiene interventions that would be useful for the person with insomnia disorder.

2. Identify the primary problems related to the sleep–wake disorders.

3. A 25-year-old woman reports that she has not slept for 3 days. What are the primary assessment questions for her?

4. A 55-year-old truck driver presents reporting excessive daytime sleepiness. Develop a list of assessment questions that could be used to investigate his chief complaint.

5. Outline nursing interventions and educational highlights for the parents of a 12-year-old child diagnosed with sleepwalking disorder.

Movie View Guides
Insomnia: (1997). This movie is a compelling thriller that occurs in a state of perpetual light.

The setting is north of the Arctic Circle in the middle of summer, where it is daylight 24 hours a day. Jonas Engström (Stellan Skarsgård) and Erik Vik (Sverre Anker Ousdal) are cops from Oslo brought into a small town to help with a murder investigation. Things go wrong, and Engström finds himself trapped in a web of deceit. His guilty conscience and the never-ending light keep him awake at night, and the lack of sleep makes him increasingly desperate and error prone.

VIEWING POINTS: How did the lack of sleep have an impact on Engström's ability to make sound decisions? If the setting of this movie were in an area that had normal nighttime darkness, would the outcome have been different? If you were conducting a sleep assessment, what priorities of care would be generated from the data?

REFERENCES

American Psychiatric Association [APA]. (2013). *Diagnostic and Statistical Manual of Mental Disorders (5th ed.)* Arlington, VA: Author.

Arand, D. L., & Bonnet, M. H. (2019). The multiple sleep latency test. In *Handbook of clinical neurology* (Vol. 160, pp. 393–403). Elsevier.

Benjafield, A., Valentine, K., Ayas, N., Eastwood, P. R., Heinzer, R. C., Ip, M. S., ... & Nunez, C. (2018). Global prevalence of obstructive sleep apnea in adults: estimation using currently available data. In *B67. Risk and prevalence of sleep disordered breathing* (pp. A3962–A3962). American Thoracic Society.

Berkley, A. S., Carter, P. A., Yoder, L. H., Acton, G., & Holahan, C. K. (2020). The effects of insomnia on older adults' quality of life and daily functioning: A mixed-methods study. *Geriatric Nursing*, 1–7.

Bue, A. L., Salvaggio, A., Isidoro, S. I., Romano, S., & Insalaco, G. (2019). OSA and CPAP therapy: Effect of gender, somnolence, and treatment adherence on health-related quality of life. *Sleep and Breathing*, 1–8.

Burgess, H. J., & Emens, J. S. (2018). Drugs used in circadian sleep-wake rhythm disturbances. *Sleep Medicine Clinics*, 13(2), 231–241.

Carter, J. C., & Wrede, J. E. (2017). Overview of sleep and sleep disorders in infancy and childhood. *Pediatric Annals*, 46(4), e133–e138.

Centers for Disease Control and Prevention. (2017). Short sleep duration among US adults. Sleep and Sleep Disorders, https://www.cdc.gov/sleep/data_statistics.html#:~:text=Short%20Sleep%20Duration%20Among%20US,sleep%20per%2024%2Dhour%20period

Chang, E. T., Baik, G., Torre, C., Brietzke, S. E., & Camacho, M. (2018). The relationship of the uvula with snoring and obstructive sleep apnea: A systematic review. *Sleep and Breathing*, 22(4), 955–961.

Chen, T. Y., Lee, S., & Buxton, O.M. (2017). A Greater extent of insomnia symptoms and physician-recommended sleep medication use predict fall risk in community-dwelling older adults. *Sleep*, 40(11). https://doi.org/10.1093/sleep/zsx142

Cook, J. D., Rumble, M. E., & Plante, D. T. (2019). Identifying subtypes of hypersomnolence disorder: A clustering analysis. *Sleep Medicine*, 64, 71–76.

Dye, T. J., Gurbani, N., & Simakajornboon, N. (2018). Epidemiology and pathophysiology of childhood narcolepsy. *Paediatric Respiratory Reviews*, 25, 14–18. https://doi.org/10.1016/j.prrv.2016.12.005

Edwards, C., Almeida, O. P., & Ford, A. H. (2020). Obstructive sleep apnea and depression: A systematic review and meta-analysis. *Maturitas*, 142, 45–54. https://doi.org/10.1016/j.maturitas.2020.06.002

Ellington, E. (2018). It's not a nightmare: Understanding sleep terrors. *Journal of Psychosocial Nursing & Mental Health Services*, 56(8), 11–14. https://doi.org/10.3928/02793695-20180723-03

El-Solh, A. A. (2018). Management of nightmares in patients with posttraumatic stress disorder: Current perspectives. *Nature and Science of Sleep*, 10, 409–420. https://doi.org/10.2147/NSS.S166089

Esposito, G., et al. (2019). Prevalence and risk factors for restless legs syndrome during pregnancy in a Northern Italian population. *Journal of Obstetrics & Gynaecology*, 39(4), 480–484. https://doi.org/10.1080/014436 15.2018.1525341

Frank, M. G., & Heller, H. C. (2019). The function(s) of sleep. *Handbook of Experimental Pharmacology*. https://doi.org/10.1007/164_2018_140

Grewal, R. G., & Doghramji, K. (2017). Epidemiology of insomnia. In *Clinical handbook of insomnia* (pp. 13–25). Springer.

Guglielmis, O., Lanteri, P., & Garbarino, S. (2019). Association between socioeconomic status, belonging to an ethnic minority and obstructive sleep apnea: A systematic review of the literature. *Sleep Medicine*, 57,100106. https://doi.org/10.1016/j.sleep.2019.01.042

Han, Y., Yuan, K., Zheng, Y., & Lu, L. (2020). Orexin receptor antagonists as emerging treatments for psychiatric disorders. *Neuroscience Bulletin*, 36(4), 432–448. https://doi.org/10.1007/s12264-019-00447-9

He, M., Yin, G., Zhan, S., Xu, J., Cao, X., Li, J., & Ye, J. (2019). Long-term efficacy of uvulopalatopharyngoplasty among adult patients with obstructive sleep apnea: A systematic review and meta-analysis. *Otolaryngology–Head and Neck Surgery*, 161(3), 401–411.

Herrera-Solis, A., Herrera-Morales, W., Nunez-Jaramillo, L., & Arias-Carrion, O. (2019). Dopaminergic modulation of sleep-wake states. *CNS & Neurological Disorders Drug Targets*, 16(4), 380–386. https://doi.org/10.2174/1871527316666170320145429

Hood, S., & Amir, S. (2017). The aging clock: Circadian rhythms and later life. *Journal of Clinical Investigation*, 127(2), 437–446. https://doi.org/10.1172/JCI90328

Johnson, D. A., Jackson, C. L., Williams, N. J., & Alcántara, C. (2019). Are sleep patterns influenced by race/ethnicity–a marker of relative advantage or disadvantage? Evidence to date. *Nature and Science of Sleep*, 11, 79.

Kalmbach, D. A., Anderson, J. R., & Drake, C. L. (2018). The impact of stress on sleep: Pathogenic sleep reactivity as a vulnerability to insomnia and circadian disorders. *Journal of Sleep Research*, 27(6), e12710.

Kessler, R., Berglund, P. A., Coulouvrat, C., Fitzgerald, T., Hajak, G., Roth, T., et al. (2012). Insomnia, comorbidity and risk of injury among insured Americans: Results from the America Insomnia survey. *Sleep*, 35(6), 825–834.

Khoury, J., & Doghramji, K. (2015). Primary sleep disorders. *Psychiatric Clinics of North America*, 38, 638–704.

Khurshid, K. A. (2018). Comorbid insomnia and psychiatric disorders: an update. *Innovations in Clinical Neuroscience*, 15(3–4), 28.

Kolp, H., Wilder, S., Andersen, C., Johnson, E., Horvath, S., Gidycz, C. A., & Shorey, R. (2020). Gender minority stress, sleep disturbance, and sexual victimization in transgender and gender nonconforming adults. *Journal of Clinical Psychology*, 76(4), 688–698. https://doi.org/10.1002/jclp.22880

Krystal, A. D., Prather, A. A., & Ashbrook, L. H. (2019). The assessment and management of insomnia: an update. *World Psychiatry*, 18(3), 337–352.

Levrier, K., Marchand, A., Belleville, G., Dominic, B. P., & Guay, S. (2016). Nightmare frequency, nightmare distress and the efficiency of trauma-focused cognitive behavioral therapy for post-traumatic stress disorder. *Archives of Trauma Research*, 5(3), e33051.

Li, X., Wang, F., Xu, H., Qian, Y., Zou, J., Yang, M., ... & Yin, S. (2020). Interrelationships among common predictors of cardiovascular diseases in patients of OSA: A large-scale observational study. *Nutrition, Metabolism and Cardiovascular Diseases*, 30(1), 23–32.

Llorens, F., Zarranz, J. J., Fischer, A., Zerr, I., & Ferrer, I. (2017). Fatal familial insomnia: Clinical aspects and molecular alterations. *Current Neurology and Neuroscience Reports*, 17(4), 30.

Lucena, L., Polesel, D. N., Poyares, D., Bittencourt, L., Andersen, M. L., Tufik, S., & Hachul, H. (2020). The association of insomnia and quality of life: Sao Paulo epidemiologic sleep study (EPISONO). *Sleep Health*, 6(5), 629–635. https://doi.org/10.1016/j.sleh.2020.03.002

Manni, R., Toscano, G., & Terzaghi, M. (2018). Therapeutic symptomatic strategies in the parasomnias. *Current Treatment Options in Neurology*, 20(7), 26.

Maski, K., & Owens, J. A. (2016). Insomnia, parasomnias, and narcolepsy in children: Clinical features, diagnosis, and management. *The Lancet Neurology*, 15(11), 1170–1181.

Matenchuk, B. A., Mandhane, P. J., & Kozyrskyj, A. L. (2020). Sleep, circadian rhythm, and gut microbiota. *Sleep Medicine Reviews*, 53, 101340. https://doi.org/10.1016/j.smrv.2020.101340

Mitler, M. M., Carskadon, M. A., Czeisier, C. A., Dement, W. C., Dinges, D. F., & Graeber, R. C. (1988). Catastrophes, sleep, and public policy: Consensus report. *Sleep*, 11(1), 100–109.

Morgenthaler, T. I., et al. (2018). Position paper for the treatment of nightmare disorder in adults: an American Academy of Sleep Medicine position paper. *Journal of Clinical Sleep Medicine*, 14(6), 1041–1055.

National Center for Complementary and Integrative Health. (2020a). Sleep disorders: In depth. Washington, DC: National Institutes of Health, U.S. Department of Health and Human Services. https://www.nccih.nih.gov/health/sleep-disorders-in-depth

National Center for Complementary and Integrative Health. (2020b). Valerian. Washington, DC: National Institutes of Health, U.S. Department of Health and Human Services. https://www.nccih.nih.gov/health/valerian

National Sleep Foundation. (2020). "Snoring and Sleep. Snoring solutions, aids & remedies" [Online]. https://sleepfoundation.org/sleep-disorders-problems/other-sleep-disorders/snoring

Neubauer, D. N., Pandi-Perumal, S. R., Spence, D. W., Buttoo, K., & Monti, J. M. (2018). Pharmacotherapy of insomnia. *Journal of Central Nervous System Disease*, 10, 1179573518770672.

Perrault, A. A., Bayer, L., Peuvrier, M., Afyouni, A., Ghisletta, P., Brockmann, C., Spiridon, M., Hulo Vesely, S., Haller, D. M., Pichon, S., Perrig, S., Schwartz, S., & Sterpenich, V. (2019). Reducing the use of screen electronic devices in the evening is associated with improved sleep and daytime vigilance in adolescents. *Sleep*, 42(9), zsz125.

Pavlova, M. K., & Latreille, V. (2019). Sleep disorders. *The American Journal of Medicine*, 132(3), 292–299.

Perger, E., Mattaliano, P., & Lombardi, C. (2019). Menopause and sleep apnea. *Maturitas*, 124, 35–38. https://doi.org/10.1016/j.maturitas.2019.02.011

Perlis, M. L., Vargas, I., Ellis, J. G., Grandner, M. A., Morales, K. H., Gencarelli, A., Khader, W., Kloss, J., Goonerantne, N., & Thase, M. E. (2020). The Natural History of Insomnia: The incidence of acute insomnia and subsequent progression to chronic insomnia or recovery in good sleeper subjects. *Sleep*, 43(6), zsz299.

Petrov, M. E., & Lichstein, K. L. (2016). Differences in sleep between black and white adults: An update and future directions. *Sleep Medicine*, 18, 74–81.

Pillai, V., Roth, T., Roehrs, T., Moss, K., Peterson, E. L., & Drake, C. L. (2017). Effectiveness of benzodiazepine receptor agonists in the treatment of insomnia: an examination of response and remission rates. *Sleep*, 40(2), zsw044.

Riemann, D., Krone, L. B., Wulff, K., & Nissen, C. (2020). Sleep, insomnia, and depression. *Neuropsychopharmacology*, 45(1), 74–89. https://doi.org/10.1038/s41386-019-0411-y

Rajaratnam, S. M., & Arendt, J. (2001). Health in a 24-h society. *Lancet (London, England)*, 358(9286), 999–1005. https://doi.org/10.1016/S0140-6736(01)06108-6

Reinke, H., & Asher, G. (2019). Crosstalk between metabolism and circadian clocks. *Nature Reviews: Molecular Cell Biology*, 20(4), 227–241. https://doi.org/10.1038/s41580-018-0096-9

Rosenberg, R., Hirshkowitz, M., Rapoport, D. M., & Kryger, M. (2019). The role of home sleep testing for evaluation of patients with excessive daytime sleepiness: Focus on obstructive sleep apnea and narcolepsy. *Sleep Medicine*, 56, 80–89. https://doi.org/10.1016/j.sleep.2019.01.014

Sateia, M. J., Buysse, D. J., Krystal, A. D., Neubauer, D. N., & Heald, J. L. (2017). Clinical practice guideline for the pharmacologic treatment of chronic insomnia in adults: An American Academy of Sleep Medicine clinical practice guideline. *Journal of Clinical Sleep Medicine*, 13(2), 307–349.

Short, M. A., Arora, T., Gradisar, M., Taheri, S., & Carskadon, M. A. (2017). How many sleep diary entries are needed to reliably estimate adolescent sleep? *Sleep*, 40(3), zsx006.

Steinweg, K., Nippita, T., Cistulli, P. A., & Bin, Y. S. (2020). Maternal and neonatal outcomes associated with restless legs syndrome in pregnancy: A systematic review. *Sleep Medicine Reviews*, 101359.

Sutherland, K., Keenan, B. T., Bittencourt, L., Chen, N. H., Gislason, T., Leinwand, S., ... & Mindel, J. (2019). A global comparison of anatomic risk factors and their relationship to obstructive sleep apnea severity in clinical samples. *Journal of Clinical Sleep Medicine*, 15(4), 629–639.

Thomas, K. M., Redd, L. A., Wright, J. D., & Hartos, J. L. (2017). Sleep and mental health in the general population of elderly women. *Journal of Primary Prevention*, 38(5), 495503. https://doi.org/10.1007/s10935-017-0484-5

Thomas, S. J., & Calhoun, D. (2016). Sleep, insomnia, and hypertension: Current findings and future directions. *Journal of American Society of Hypertension*. https://doi.org/10.1016/j.jash.2016.11.008

Trenkwalder, C., et al. (2018). Comorbidities, treatment, and pathophysiology in restless legs syndrome. *The Lancet Neurology*, 17(11), 994–1005. https://doi.org/10.1016/S1474-4422(18)30311-9

Wang, W. L., Chen, K. H., Pan, Y. C., Yang, S. N., & Chan, Y. Y. (2020). The effect of yoga on sleep quality and insomnia in women with sleep problems: A systematic review and meta-analysis. *BMC Psychiatry*, 20(1), 195. https://doi.org/10.1186/s12888-020-02566-4

Winkelman, J. W., Armstrong, M. J., Allen, R. P., Chaudhuri, K. R., Ondo, W., Trenkwalder, C., et al. (2016). Practice guideline summary: Treatment of restless legs syndrome in adults: Report of the Guideline Development, Dissemination, and Implementation Subcommittee of the American Academy of Neurology. *Neurology, 87*, 2585–2593.

Wickwire, E. M., Albrecht, J. S., Towe, M. M., Abariga, S. A., Diaz-Abad, M., Shipper, A. G., ... & Scharf, S. M. (2019). The impact of treatments for OSA on monetized health economic outcomes: A systematic review. *Chest, 155*(5), 947–961.

Xiao, Q., & Hale, L. (2018). Neighborhood socioeconomic status, sleep duration, and napping in middle-to-old aged US men and women. *Sleep, 41*(7). https://doi.org/10.1093/sleep/zsy076

Yatsu, S., et al. (2019). Prevalence and significance of restless legs syndrome in patients with coronary artery disease. *American Journal of Cardiology, 123*(10), 1580–1586. https://doi.org/10.1016/j.amjcard.2019.02.017

Zisapel, N. (2018). New perspectives on the role of melatonin in human sleep, circadian rhythms and their regulation. *British Journal of Pharmacology, 175*(16), 3190–3199. https://doi.org/10.1111/bph.14116

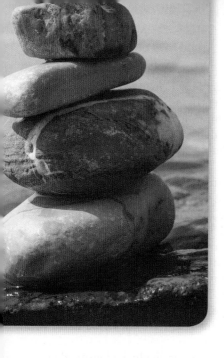

35
Sexual Disorders
Nursing Care of Persons with Sexual Dysfunctions and Paraphilias

Mary Ann Boyd

KEYCONCEPTS

- sexual arousal
- sexual disorders

- sexuality

- sexual health

LEARNING OBJECTIVES

After studying this chapter, you will be able to:

1. Discuss the role of sexuality in mental disorders.

2. Analyze sexual response and theoretical models.

3. Analyze primary theories of female orgasmic and erectile disorders and their relationships to comorbidities.

4. Apply a person-centered, recovery-oriented nursing process for persons with sexual disorders.

5. Identify medications used to treat people with sexual disorders.

6. Discuss the importance of integration of primary care for persons with sexual disorders.

7. Describe other sexually related situations that impact mental health.

KEY TERMS

- Anorgasmia • Biosexual identity • Cisgender • Dyspareunia • Erectile dysfunction (ED) • Excitement phase • Gender identity • Gender dysphoria • Genderqueer identity • Human sexual response cycle • LGBTQ • Non-binary identity • Orgasmic disorder • Orgasmic phase • Paraphilias • Plateau phase • Premature ejaculation • Resolution • Sensate focus • Sex role identity • Sex therapist • Sexual desire • Sexual maturation • Sexual orientation • Vaginismus

Case Study

Alice is a 35-year-old woman diagnosed with multiple sclerosis 3 years ago. She experiences transitory visual blurring, weakness of the lower limbs, and mood swings. She also has problems with urinary leakage and occasional bowel incontinence.

INTRODUCTION

Sexuality is associated with sensuality, pleasure and pleasuring, intimacy, trust, communication, love and affection, attractiveness, affirmation of one's masculinity and femininity, and reverence for life. Sexuality influences how we view ourselves (self-concept) and consequently how we relate to others.

Sexuality is influenced by a person's emotional and physiologic status, beliefs and values, and morals and laws of society. Barriers to sexual fulfillment can arise from medical problems (e.g., neurologic, musculoskeletal, cardiovascular, respiratory, renal, hepatic, and cognitive impairments); from pain, weakness, and fatigue; and from sequelae of surgical procedures and drugs. More often, sexual problems are a result of the interplay of multiple causes that can include intrapsychic, interpersonal, and sociocultural factors. This chapter focuses on sexuality and sexual functioning and discusses nursing care for persons experiencing sexual dysfunction.

> **KEYCONCEPT Sexuality** is a life force that encompasses all that is male or female and how these characteristics relate to all that is human.

SEXUAL DEVELOPMENT

All of us are sexual beings, whether we are or are not sexually active. Sex is what we are, not what we do—the sum total of all of our biologic and experiential influences. **Sexual maturation** encompasses four areas: **biosexual identity**, **gender identity**, **sex role identity**, and **sexual orientation**. Although bisexual identity refers to the anatomic and physiologic states of being male or female, gender identity refers to an individual's identification with maleness/masculinity, femaleness/femininity, neither or both, and it does not always correspond with sex or biology. The innermost concept of self as male or female, neither nor both can be different than physical state.

Sex role identity (or gender role) is the outward expression of gender, including behaviors, feelings, and attitudes. Gender identity is a component of gender that describes a person's psychological sense of their gender. Gender is a set of social, cultural, psychological, and/or emotional traits or norms, often influenced by societal expectations, that classify an individual along a spectrum of man, woman, neither nor both. **Cisgender** is a term used to describe a gender identity that aligns with the same sex that was assigned at birth. **Non-binary** gender (e.g., **genderqueer**, gender-nonconforming, gender neutral, agender, gender-fluid) may or may not correspond to a person's sex assigned at birth, presumed gender based on sex assignments, or primary or secondary sex characteristics (Amherst College Resource Center, 2020). Individuals may identify as lesbian, gay, bisexual, transgender, and questioning or queer (LGBTQ) or as having two or more genders and move between genders, or having no gender (Amherst College Resource Center, 2020).

Other gender identities are also recognized. Intersexual is a term used in which a person's sexual or reproductive anatomy does not fit the definition of male or female. Asexual is an identity term used for a person with little or no sexual attraction. Pansexual or pan refers to a person who is sexually attracted to people of all and/or many gender identities (Amherst College Resource Center, 2020). An in-depth discussion of gender identity is beyond the scope of this chapter. LGBTQ will be used in this chapter to describe multiple gender identities.

Sexual orientation is part of individual identity that refers to the physical and emotional attraction to another person. Sexual orientation is determined early in development because of the influence of genetic factors and the interactions between sex hormones and the developing brain. There is no evidence that interventions can change sexual orientation (Grabowska, 2017; Roselli, 2018; SAMHSA, 2015).

Genes and Determination of Sex

As a result of the sex-determining genes on the Y chromosome, testosterone is present in male fetuses and, by weeks 6 to 12, is responsible for the formation of the penis, prostate, and scrotum. The formation of ovaries in female fetuses depends on the absence of this male hormone. After the male sex organs are formed, testosterone levels temporarily rise, causing a permanent sexual organization of the brain that is different than that of females. Testosterone is also elevated during the first 3 months after birth, causing the brain's structures and circuits to be fixed for the rest of a male's life.

These structural differences are thought to be the basis of sex differences that are reflected in behavior from birth. For example, female newborns are more likely to watch human faces; male infants look more at mobiles. During puberty, rising hormones stimulate these structures and circuits that were set up many years earlier to further respond in feminine or masculine directions. Since the sexual differentiation of the genitals takes place earlier (during the first 2 months of pregnancy) than the sexual differentiation of the brain (second half of pregnancy), these two processes may be influenced differently. In such cases, individuals with male sexual organs may experience their identity as female (Eid & Biason-Lauber, 2016; Ristori, et al., 2020).

Sexual Behaviors in Children and Adolescents

In infants, sexual behaviors are rare with the exception of hand-to-genital contact. As children become more aware of their body parts and the physical sensations deriving from their genitals, they become more interested in gender differences. For 2- to 5-year-old children, sexual behaviors are varied and more common than in older children, who are more aware of the social norms of concealing sexual behaviors. For example, young children observe and comment on body differences, demonstrate interest in bathroom habits and urination, and handle their genitals for pleasure and comfort. Their curiosity leads them to want to look at and touch adult bodies and breasts. Mutual genital exploration or urination among children may be seen at this time along with questions about where babies come from.

Age-appropriate solitary sexual behaviors (i.e., touching one's own genitals) are also common. At this early age, these behaviors do not have the sexualized meaning they do in adults. However, if young children are exposed to sexually explicit material (internet, movies, observation of parental sexual activities) or if their parents overreact to age-appropriate behaviors, these activities can take on additional, more adult like, meanings. If preoccupation with the sexual behaviors interferes with the child's ability to grow and function, then the behaviors are problematic. For example, an 8-year-old boy sneaking to the bathroom several times a day to touch his genitals needs help in addressing this behavior.

Sexual behaviors are common and occur in 42% to 73% of children by the time they reach 13 years of age. Generally, the frequency of overt sexual behaviors decrease with age. These behaviors may not be as obvious because as children mature, they become increasingly more covert in their sexual behavior. For example, whereas 6- to 9-year-old boys and girls often touch their genitals at home, stand too close to others, and try to look at persons when they are nude, 10- to 12-year-old children, who are actually more interested in and know more about sex, limit their behavior to looking at nudity in magazines, television, and the internet (Lussier et al., 2018; Miragoli et al., 2017).

Sexual contact with others occurs at a relatively early age in the United States. In 2015 to 2017, 42% of never-married female teenagers aged 15 to 19 and 38% of never-married male teenagers had had sexual intercourse (Martinez & Abma, 2020). A variety of circumstances lead to this sexual activity. Sex may be engaged in because of peer pressure or because friends or social groups condone sex. The need to be convinced of being in love, wanting to feel loved, and fear of rejection all precipitate risk-taking behavior. Depending on the family environment, stresses, and observation of adult sexual activities, children may exhibit more adult sexual behaviors, which may be considered normal for the environment in which they live. For children and adolescents, sexual behavior (usually involving other people) is considered abnormal when it occurs at a greater frequency or at a much earlier age than would be developmentally or culturally expected.

Sexual Behaviors in Adulthood

Sexual activities occur throughout young adulthood and continue through middle and late adulthood. Although the frequency and types of sexual encounters may change, the quality need not change. During the fourth to fifth decades of life, physical changes become more obvious, and so various chronic illnesses, such as hypertension or arthritis, may also develop. As a result of decreased endocrine production, gradual changes to body tissues occur over a 15- to 20-year span. Most physical symptoms arise from vasomotor instability, which can include morning fatigue, vague pains, hot flashes, dizziness, chills, sweating, nervousness, crying spells, decreased sexual potency, and palpitations.

In women, estrogen deficiency during menopause affects the sexual system by causing a gradual thinning of the vaginal mucosa, decreasing the elasticity of muscles and orgasmic force, and increasing breast involution (sagging of breast tissue). Vaginal lubrication decreases, which may cause dyspareunia (i.e., pain during intercourse), often requiring the use of a water-soluble lubricant or saliva. Although many women experience little or no change in sexual function, both decreased and increased sexual activity and interest are possible. In some women, more time is required to lubricate the vulvovaginal areas and to strengthen clitoral response. Orgasmic capacity and breast response remain fairly constant in appropriately stimulated women.

In men, decreasing testosterone production is responsible for sexual changes. The amount and viability of sperm decrease, erections become less firm, and more direct sexual stimulation is needed. The testicles begin to decrease in elasticity and size, ejaculation time increases, and the force of ejaculation decreases. Spermatogenesis decreases, although viable sperm, capable of impregnation, continue to be produced. Seminal fluid is less voluminous and viscous, and ejaculatory force is decreased. Older men, however, are capable of sustaining erection much longer with decreased ejaculatory demand, potentially benefiting older partners, who may require increased time to reach orgasm. Sexual activity is often perceived as more satisfactory than previously experienced.

Sexual continuity depends to a great extent on good physical health, activity, and regular opportunities for sexual expression and sexual activity in all forms, including masturbation and same-gender behavior. An important influence on sexuality is the attitudes of others, especially attitudes that define specific behaviors as acceptable or unacceptable. This is especially true in later life (Miragoli, et al., 2017; Syme & Cohn, 2016). In healthy adults, sexual function, although modified by the aging process, should remain satisfying despite a differently timed sequence. Frequent sexual activity, whether by coitus, masturbation, or other practices, usually preserves sexual potency.

SEXUAL RESPONSES

Understanding normal sexual responses helps when discussing this very personal, but important, aspect of being human with patients. The following section provides an overview of major concepts and theories related to sexual responses.

Sexual Desire and Arousal

Sexual desire is the ability, interest, or willingness to receive or a motivational state to seek sexual stimulation. In healthy adults, the sex drive is integrated through the central nervous system (CNS) with the autonomic nervous system governing extragenital changes (increased respiration and heart rate). The parasympathetic nervous system largely controls arousal; the sympathetic nervous system largely controls orgasmic discharge. Sexual stimulation brings about a total-body response with dramatic changes seen in the genitals and breasts. Sex hormones, particularly androgen, influence desire in individuals, but less is known about hormonal influence in women. That the higher centers of the brain apparently mediate the lower reflex response centers supports the relationship between cognitive and affective states and sexual function.

During sexual arousal, individuals experience an increased heart rate, blood pressure, respiration, and myotonia.

> **KEYCONCEPT Sexual arousal** is state of mounting sexual tension characterized by vasoconstriction and myotonia.

In men, visual stimulation (i.e., seeing a naked person), fantasies, memories, or physical stimulation of the genitals or other regions (e.g., nipples) causes the parasympathetic system to involuntarily release chemicals that dilate penile arteries. A rapid inflow of arterial blood to the cavernous spaces of corpora cavernosa, facilitated by high levels of intrapenile nitric oxide, causes stiffening and elongation of the penis. With continued stimulation, an emission of semen and an ejaculation occurs. Subcortical structures (hypothalamus, brainstem, spinal cord) and cortical area regulate sexual response. Dopaminergic and serotonergic systems play an important role along with other neurotransmitter systems such as the adrenergic and cholinergic systems (Calabrò, et al., 2019). Testosterone is involved throughout the male sexual response (Rastrelli et al., 2018).

Fantasies, visual stimuli, and physical stimulation are also important for sexual arousal in women, but physical stimulation seems more important for women and visual stimuli for men. The parasympathetic nervous system increases blood flow to the female genitalia, lubricating the vagina and enlarging the breast and clitoris. Estrogens and progestins are involved in female sexual functioning, but androgens are needed by people to maintain arousal.

Theoretical Models of Sexual Response

In 1966, Masters and Johnson described the classic **human sexual response cycle** as consisting of four phases: excitement, plateau, orgasm, and **resolution**. In the **excitement phase**, erotic feelings lead to a penile erection in men and vaginal lubrication in women. Heart rate and respirations also increase. The **plateau phase** is represented by sexual pleasure and increased muscle tension, heart rate, and blood flow to the genitals. For men, the **orgasmic phase** is ejaculation of semen, and for women, it consists of rhythmic contractions of the vaginal muscles. For most men, immediately after orgasm and before resolution, a refractory period occurs when no response is possible. Resolution is the gradual return of the organs and body systems to the nonaroused state. Muscle tension and vasocongestion subside. Breathing and heart rate gradually return to normal rates. Usually, the person feels a sense of relaxation, relief of tension, and satisfaction (Masters & Johnson, 1966, 1970).

After publication of Masters and Johnson's works, Kaplan (1979) proposed a three-phase model of sexual response—desire, excitement, and orgasm—and identified low-desire states as a frequent cause of sexual dysfunction.

This linear approach is criticized as being primarily a biologic model and does not account for nonbiologic experiences such as pleasure, satisfaction, and the context of the relationship. To account for emotional and psychological aspects of sexual response, a circular model focusing on women's sexual responses was developed by Basson (2001). This model proposes that nonsexual interpersonal factors, such as a desire for physical connection and intimacy needs, also motivate women to engage in sexual relations, not only sexual release. Arousal and desire appear to be interchangeable and inseparable from one another, with one reinforcing the other. Subjective feelings of interest may follow the sensation of arousal, and sexual satisfaction may be experienced without orgasm.

These two models—linear and circular—have been debated for years. Both models are supported empirically as being relevant to sexual responses in women. Women report that sexual experiences are at times consistent with the linear and circular models at other times (Ferenidou, et al., 2016; Meston, & Stanton, 2019). There is emerging evidence that the circular model is a better fit for men than the linear model (Connaughton et al., 2016).

Dual-Control Model

Another conceptualization, the dual-control model, focuses on individual variability and proposes that sexual responses involve an interaction between sexual excitement and sexual inhibition (Bancroft et al., 2009). This model assumes that (1) neurobiologic inhibition of sexual response is adaptive and occurs in situations when sexual activity would be a disadvantage, dangerous, or distracting; (2) individuals vary in their propensity for sexual excitation and inhibition; and (3) the context and cultural meaning attributed to the interaction of the individuals are important stimuli for both excitatory and inhibitory processes. Emerging research is showing that the dual-control model is an important framework in understanding how mood influences both subjective and genital sexual in individuals (Hodgson et al., 2016; Turner et al., 2019; Velten et al., 2019).

SEXUAL HEALTH AND WELLNESS

Sexual health is an important aspect of wellness. Sexual health is viewed holistically and positively and is relevant throughout the individual's lifespan. Influenced by gender norms, expectations, and power dynamics, sexual health is understood within specific social, economic, and political contexts (WHO, 2017). Major health threats related to sexuality are human immunodeficiency virus (HIV)/acquired immunodeficiency syndrome (AIDS), hepatitis, and sexually transmitted diseases.

KEYCONCEPT According to the working definition of the World Health Organization (WHO), **sexual health** is "a state of physical, emotional, mental and social well-being in relation to sexuality; it is not merely the absence of disease, dysfunction or infirmity. Sexual health requires a positive and respectful approach to sexuality and sexual relationships, as well as the possibility of having pleasurable and safe sexual experiences, free of coercion, discrimination and violence. For sexual health to be attained and maintained, the sexual rights of all persons must be respected, protected and fulfilled" (WHO, 2021).

The mental health of the **LGBTQ** community is at risk due to discrimination in environments where they live, learn, and work (Vargas et al., 2020). Sexual orientation discrimination is most prevalent in early young adulthood, but it occurs in all ages. Higher risks for alcohol, tobacco, and drug use disorders are associated with discrimination at the older ages (Evans-Polce, et al., 2019). One of the goals of *Healthy People 2030* is to improve the health, safety, and well-being of LGBTQ individuals (Healthy People 2030, 2021). Nurses are in a unique position to provide gender-affirming care in order to improve the safety and well-being of the LGBTQ communities.

SEXUAL DYSFUNCTIONS AND PROBLEMATIC BEHAVIORS OVERVIEW

Sexual dysfunctions are a group of disorders that are characterized by clinically significant disturbances in the person's ability to respond sexually or to experience sexual pleasure (American Psychiatric Association [APA],

2013). Unhealthy lifestyle and obesity contribute to the development of sexual dysfunctions, due to their negative impact on cardiovascular and metabolic functions. Tobacco smoking, alcohol-use and substance-use disorders, and chronic stress lead to the development of sexual dysfunction (Mollaioli et al., 2020).

The *DSM-5* identifies the following as sexual disorders: delayed ejaculation (DE), erectile disorder, female **orgasmic disorder**, female sexual interest/arousal disorder, genito-pelvic pain/penetration disorder, male hypoactive sexual desire disorder, and **premature ejaculation (PE)**. These dysfunctions can be lifelong or acquired and are categorized as mild, moderate, or severe. An occasional episode is not considered dysfunctional (APA, 2013). In this chapter, female orgasmic disorder is highlighted because it is among the most commonly occurring sexual disorders in women, and **anorgasmia** (the inability to achieve an orgasm) is a frequent medication side effect. Male PE and erectile disorder are emphasized. **Paraphilias** and gender dysphoria are included in the discussion.

KEYCONCEPT Sexual disorders are clinical disturbances caused by the inability to respond sexually or to experience sexual pleasure.

FEMALE ORGASMIC DISORDER

A female orgasm is the least understood of all sexual responses; no universal definition exists (Bancroft & Graham, 2011). Women's descriptions of the orgasmic experience vary from altered consciousness to focused sensation. Many women require clitoral stimulation to reach orgasm and only a small group of women report that they always experience orgasm during intercourse. According to the *DSM-5*, an orgasmic disorder is the inability to reach orgasm by any means, either alone or with a partner and/or markedly reduced intensity of orgasmic sensations for at least 6 months. The inability to experience an orgasm must cause clinically significant distress to be considered a disorder (Wheeler & Guntupalli, 2020).

Diagnostic Criteria

Female orgasmic disorder is characterized by the inability of a woman to experience orgasm or the intensity of the orgasm is markedly reduced at least 75% of the time. If other explanations for the anorgasmia exist, such as substance use, medications, or interpersonal issues, the diagnosis is not used.

Epidemiology and Risk Factors

Debate about the issue of female orgasms is considerable. Estimated prevalence of women's inability to reach orgasm ranges from 9% (in the United States) to 41.2% in Southeast Asia (Bancroft & Graham, 2011).

Poor physical health, mental health, and relationship issues, especially partner difficulties, are the primary risk factors. Age, arousal difficulty, and lubrication difficulty are related to difficulty reaching orgasm (Rowland et al., 2018).

Etiology

In general, any local genital or pelvic pathology, trauma, or surgery that causes pain on intercourse can produce impaired response to sexual stimulation. Spinal cord damage, endocrine disorders, systemic diseases, chronic pain, and general debility can interfere with sexual responses. CNS depressants (e.g., alcohol, barbiturates, narcotics), psychiatric disorders, infections, inflammatory disorders, and pregnancy have all been associated with female orgasmic disorder. Additionally, many medications such as antidepressants, antihypertensives, and substances (e.g., alcohol) can also affect the sexual response (Thomas et al., 2018).

Consider Alice.

Alice admits that her sexual activity is far less frequent than before her illness. She feels she is no longer attractive or able to fulfill her functions as a wife.

How would you discuss her feelings? What information would you give her to help her look at her situation realistically?

Sexual responses can be inhibited by many different emotional and cognitions, including sexual anxiety and guilt, anger or hostility toward one's partner, indifference toward one's partner, depression, or excessive and intrusive thoughts. Misinformation or lack of information contributes to the inhibition. Cultural expectations also play an important role in the sexual experience. Religious prohibitions and cultural taboos often contribute to a woman's view of her sexuality. If a woman believes that sexual relationships are sinful or "a woman's duty," she is not as likely to explore her own sexual potential.

RECOVERY-ORIENTED CARE FOR PERSONS WITH FEMALE ORGASMIC DISORDER

Teamwork and Collaboration: Working Toward Recovery

The treatment of the person with an orgasmic disorder is best left to clinicians who specialize in this area, but other health care providers can first treat underlying health,

mental health, and relationship issues. If the orgasmic problem is not related to any of these areas, she should be referred to a qualified **sex therapist**, who blends education and counseling with psychotherapy and specific sexual exercises. For example, **sensate focus** is a method for partners to learn what each finds arousing and to learn to communicate those preferences. It begins with nongenital contact and gradually includes genital touch and sexual intercourse.

Safety Issues

Low sexual functioning is linked to suicide ideation in female service members and veterans. The low sexual functioning is associated with probable depression and posttraumatic stress disorder. It is important to include a suicide screening when caring for persons with sexual dysfunction (Blais et al., 2018).

EVIDENCE-BASED NURSING CARE FOR A PERSON WITH FEMALE ORGASMIC DISORDER

The psychiatric–mental health nurse has a responsibility to conduct an assessment to determine the presence of any sexual issues or problems. The scope of practice dictates the level of assessment and interventions. The nurse will most likely be seeing the patient for a different problem (e.g., psychiatric problem, acute or chronic physical health problem) and will discover a sexual problem during a health assessment. Patients are sometimes reluctant to discuss sexual problems, especially those who are socially stigmatized (same-sex couples, developmentally disabled people, and old people).

Attention should be paid to special populations' high risk for sexual problems, such as those with mental illnesses or chronic health problems. For older adults, poor

---

Remember Alice?

Alice believed that she could not have sexual relations with her husband because of her physical problems. Her nurse practitioner provided education and hope.

What information would you reinforce through discussion? What would you say to reinforce her self-esteem and hope for sexual relations?

If sexual dysfunction exists, one of the most important questions is does the individual want to change sexual functioning? Many women may not see a need to pursue therapy even if a sexual problem exits. See Box 35.1.

BOX 35.1 • THERAPEUTIC DIALOGUE: ASSESSING INTEREST IN SEXUAL ACTIVITY

INEFFECTIVE APPROACH

Nurse: Alice, are you currently sexually active?

Alice: Once in a while.

Nurse: How would you describe your sexual activity?

Alice: How would you feel if you were in my condition?

Nurse: Well, you could still have sexual relations.

Alice: Sure thing. (Getting irritated)

Nurse: Is there a problem?

Alice: Look, I just don't want to talk about it.

EFFECTIVE APPROACH

Nurse: Alice are you currently sexually active?

Alice: Once in a while.

Nurse: Once in a while?

Alice: Yeah, I really don't feel like it anymore.

Nurse: Oh (Silence)

Alice: My illness is messing up things in the bedroom.

Nurse: How so?

Alice: Well, I just feel so ugly—I have to urinate, my legs are weak.

Nurse: Are you feeling that you want to have sex?

Alice: Sometimes I think about it, but then I remember my illness. My poor husband. He should find someone else.

Nurse: Have you talked with him about your feelings?

Alice: Well, no. He is so patient.

Nurse: There are many women who have similar feelings but are able to begin to enjoy sex again. Is that something that you would like to consider?

Alice: Well, maybe.

Nurse: We can talk more about this. There are resources that can help you and your husband.

Alice: OK, sounds good.

CRITICAL THINKING CHALLENGE

• Compare the course of the first dialogue with the second one. What did the second nurse do differently to elicit information about Alice's feelings and concerns?

• What is problematic about the first dialogue?

physical health and lack of a partner are common barriers to sexual continuity. Other barriers include a lack of privacy or institutionalization. Lack of knowledge about the impacts of aging or health conditions on sexuality, the normality of continued sexual desire and interest, and the alternatives for sexual gratification may also inhibit sexual activity.

Mental Health Nursing Assessment

Current sexual functioning, age, physical health, and the presence of any medical or psychiatric and substance use problems as well as factors that contribute to sexual functioning (e.g., rest, nutrition, personal hygiene) are considered in the sexual assessment (Box 35.2). A careful medication history is important because so many medications have a negative effect on sexual performance (see Chapter 12).

Physical Health

Adults with chronic medical illnesses and disabilities who have problems with sensation, movement, body structure, fertility, or energy should be asked about the impact of the medical problems on their sexual function. Diabetes mellitus, heart disease, hormonal imbalances, menopause, and chronic illness such as kidney disease or liver failure are associated with sexual dysfunction in women (Scavello et al., 2019). Sexual activity often changes after a cardiac event because of fear about causing another attack (Mornar et al., 2018). Obesity and pregnancy can both compromise sexual responses (Sarwer et al., 2018).

The woman's sexual knowledge should also be determined. Does she understand the sexual responses, effects of medications, hormonal changes that occur during the woman's life cycle (e.g., adolescence, menstruation, pregnancy, menopause, aging), and the importance of adequate rest and nutrition?

BOX 35.2

Medical Conditions and Substances Affecting Sexual Function

- Cardiovascular conditions and vascular conditions
- Endocrine conditions, particularly diabetes mellitus, which cause gradual impotence in half of men and orgasmic dysfunction in one third of women
- Cancer or cancer treatments, such as radiation
- Surgery, particularly hysterectomy, mastectomy, prostatectomy, and bowel surgery
- Arthritis and neuromuscular disorders
- Spinal cord injury
- Head injury
- Cerebrovascular accident (stroke)
- Organic brain syndrome (senile dementia, Alzheimer disease)
- Cerebral palsy
- Asthma, emphysema, and chronic obstructive pulmonary disease
- Chronic renal failure
- Obesity
- Localized genital conditions, such as Sjögren syndrome, balanitis, vulvar ulcers, and psoriasis
- Prescription medications (e.g., antihypertensive drugs, anticholinergic drugs, some antidepressants)
- Chronic use of most recreational drugs
- Chronic alcohol abuse

Self-Concept

The assessment also includes the woman's self-concept and body image and her relationship with her partner. A poor self-concept can prevent a woman from engaging in sexual relationships. Mood states, such as chronic depression and grief, also seriously affect the woman's ability to have an orgasm.

Stress and Coping

The amount of stress and the ability to relax and focus on her sexuality are important assessment data. An unsatisfactory partner relationship may be at the core of the sexual problem.

Social Network and Support Systems

Cultural and family values play an important role in understanding a patient's response to orgasmic dysfunction and should be considered. Lifestyle disruptions, a birth of a child, a move to another city, or a change in financial or social status may coincide with sexual dysfunction. See Nursing Care Plan 35.1.

NURSING CARE PLAN 35.1

The Person with Multiple Sclerosis and Sexual Dysfunction

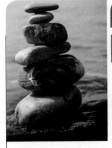

Alice, a 35-year-old woman, happily married for 11 years and the mother of two children, was diagnosed with multiple sclerosis 3 years ago. She is being seen for a periodic checkup by the nurse practitioner. Some of Alice's present symptoms include transitory visual blurring, weakness of the lower extremities, and mood swings. She also has had problems with urinary leakage and occasional bowel incontinence. She admits, with some obvious discomfort, that she is experiencing sexual difficulty and that her sexual activity is far less frequent than before her illness. Although Alice claims her husband has remained attentive and affectionate, she feels she is no longer attractive or able to fulfill her functions as a wife. She says she wouldn't blame her husband if he found someone else.

Setting: Outpatient Clinic

Baseline Assessment: The physical examination has demonstrated decreased sensation and reflexes in the lower extremities, decreased hand grasp, slight delayed blink response and nystagmus, clear speech pattern, nondistended bladder, normal bowel sounds, BP 124/76, P 76, and R 24. The patient wears an absorbent pad for urinary incontinence with a slight odor of urine. She is weepy and wrings her hands, and her eyes are downcast when discussing marital relationship. Alice's husband accompanied her to the appointment, holding her hand in the waiting room. He offered to be present during the examination or answer questions if desired. Alice has had difficulty experiencing orgasm for 2 years. She has difficulty communicating her needs.

Associated Diagnosis	Medications
Rule out: female orgasmic disorder Multiple sclerosis	Interferon-β (Betaseron) 22 mcg three times per week Oxybutynin (Ditropan) 5 mg three times a day

Continued

Nursing Care Plan 35.1 Continued

Priority of Nursing Care; Low Self-esteem and Poor Body Image

Important Characteristics	Associated Considerations
Feels unattractive, can't fulfill matrimonial roles, would understand husband finding another woman. "How would you feel if you had an 'accident' right before you were supposed to make love?" States husband has remained attentive and considerate but believes it's because he feels pity. States she has moods, "… really feeling sorry for myself. I suppose … I'm depressed … frustrated … MS affects you that way."	States she often feels tired and weak. Has some difficulty with mobility, requires assistance with bathing in tub and fastening back buttons and hooks. Frequently has urinary incontinence and occasional loss of bowel control. States she is usually unable to hold urine and sometimes bowels. Satisfactory sexual relationship before onset of illness, although had difficulty verbalizing sexual needs. Altered self-esteem Chronic illness

Outcomes

Initial	Discharge
Alice and her husband will identify three barriers and three enhancers to effective communication regarding their sexual needs and problems.	Alice will adapt to limitations and regain a positive body image. Alice and her husband will experience comfortable and satisfactory sexual expression.

Interventions

Interventions	Rationale	Ongoing Assessment
Lack of Knowledge		
Educate Alice and family; provide written materials; encourage questions.	Patients and families need factual information on the trajectory, treatment, and impact of multiple sclerosis.	Alice and her husband correctly explain the emotional aspects and pathophysiology of multiple sclerosis.
Communication		
Demonstrate empathy for Alice's difficulty in communicating sexual needs.	Talking about sex makes some people embarrassed.	Alice and her husband correctly identify factors that promote or impede their communication.
Explain common reasons for experiencing difficulty when discussing sexual issues.	Individuals may not know how to phrase what they mean. They may be afraid of insulting their partner or have a religious or cultural taboo.	The couple increases comfort in discussing sexual needs.
Emphasize the importance of being able to tell each other what is personally satisfying.	Clear communication is more successful than "telepathy."	Alice is able to identify her need for more time and foreplay.
Help Alice establish effective communication patterns by using role play or teaching assertive communication skills (e.g., beginning statements with "I really like it when you …").	Becoming assertive often requires changing male/aggressive and female/passive learned behavior patterns. Use of a fictional situation that can be role-played and analyzed is an instructive nonthreatening model for learning new behaviors.	Alice and her husband report more open communication, which allows more sharing of true feelings and fears.
Encourage the establishment of a consistent, mutually agreeable, relaxed time to talk.	Communication is easier when it is planned and viewed as a value.	Alice and her husband report that communication is improved by allotting a half hour for "together time" each evening.
Encourage the use of support or self-help groups.	Communication can be enhanced through sharing thoughts, feelings, and experiences with others.	Has contacted Multiple Sclerosis Society.
Describe sexual concerns commonly identified by partners.	Partner may feel guilty about sexual desire when mate is ill; fear of harming, increasing discomfort, or overburdening mate; difficulty when mate assumes caretaking and lover role, often helped by use of a home health aide.	The couple is beginning to address their issues; express difficulty in adapting to the current and inevitable changes of the disease; express fear of complete loss of function in all aspects of function, not just sexuality.

Continued

Nursing Care Plan 35.1 Continued

Interventions	Rationale	Ongoing Assessment
Body Image Disturbance		
Related to illness and change in function	Common sequela of chronic illness.	Alice is able to express her thoughts and feelings about the effects of the disease.
Help Alice confront reality but identify positive aspects of her personality.	Allows Alice to focus on health function and inner being.	Sees herself as a good mother and wife.
Encourage Alice to maintain good hygiene, dress attractively, use grooming aids such as perfume, and treat herself to manicures.	Optimizing appearance is a mood enhancer.	Alice states she is having a friend take her to hairdresser every other week; bought a new outfit through a catalogue.
Fatigue and Weakness		
Identify optimal time for sexual interaction.	Decreases stress; increases relaxation.	Reports using time when children are with grandparents for intimacy.
Do not eat or drink before activity.	Decreases expenditure of energy and potential for incontinence.	Able to cite correct rationale for food and fluid limitations.
Teach use of side lying or rear entry position during intercourse.	Decreases energy expenditure of Alice.	Reports ability to use these positions.
Use pillows to support weakened limbs.	Assists positioning when there is muscle weakness.	Reports increased satisfaction in sexual activity when pillows are used for positioning.
Inform Alice of side effects of medications being taken.	Some drugs cause impaired sexual response and fatigue.	Not applicable at this time.
Impaired Mobility		
Teach active or passive range-of-motion exercises.	Helps to prevent contractures.	Has been evaluated by physical therapist; reports range of motion exercises done twice daily.
Consider use of a waterbed.	Assists with movement.	
Teach possibility and treatment of contractures or adductor spasms.	Antispasmodics may be needed and are effective when taken 10 to 15 min before sexual activity.	Not applicable at this time.
Bladder Incontinence		
For urinary leakage, teach Alice to empty her bladder in accordance with prescribed bladder training program.	To maximize urinary function, bladder training should be initiated as early as possible.	Reports following bladder training program.
Discuss decreasing fluids a few hours before sexual activity and having padding or towels on hand.	These techniques decrease urinary leakage or incontinence; protect bed linens if an accident occurs.	Alice empties her bladder and decreases fluid before attempting sexual intercourse; pads on bed. If using an indwelling catheter, tapes the catheter over her abdomen.
Before sexual activity, void on cue or via intermittent catheterization. If using an indwelling catheter, may advise temporary removal or moving the clamp and taping the catheter to one side.	Permits Alice to have coitus despite urinary retention or indwelling catheter.	
Bowel Incontinence		
Establish a regular bowel program.	Helps decrease the occurrence of accidental bowel elimination; may require preparatory use of a suppository or enema.	Reports following a regulated bowel training program.
Cover bed linens with towels.	Helps prepare for accidents.	

CLINICAL JUDGMENT

Low self-esteem and depression are nursing care priorities for a woman with a sexual disorder. The nurse should determine the significance of this disorder to the person. For some women, this problem may not be a major concern; for others, it may represent loss of femininity.

MENTAL HEALTH NURSING INTERVENTIONS

Establishing Mental Health and Wellness Goals

Sexual problems impact all aspects of health and wellness. The nurse should help a person examine current sexual needs. The nurse can help the person identify ways to enhance sexual health. If there is a sexual problem, the nurse and patient can collaborate on establishing realistic goals. For example, encouraging patient to discuss sexual needs with partner is a beginning step.

Physical Care and Wellness Challenges

Wellness activities are especially challenging because of the importance of sexual health to a person's well-being. Co-occurring illnesses may interfere with sexual functioning. Feeling unattractive or stigmatized can compromise the willingness to discuss sexual needs. Wellness strategies can support sexual health (see Box 35.3).

Psychosocial Interventions

Nursing interventions include providing counseling, sex education, problem-solving opportunities, or referrals.

BOX 35.3

Wellness Challenges

- Feeling positive about sexuality and sexual health
  - Strategies: Discuss the importance of sexual health to wellness
- Seeking pleasant environments that support sexual activities
  - Strategies: Discuss realistic environmental changes that are conducive to sexual activity.
- Recognizing the need for physical activity, healthy foods, and sleep
  - Strategies: Encourage regular physical activity, discuss healthy diets, encourage establishing healthy sleep hygiene routines
- Developing a sense of connection, belong, and a support system
  - Strategies: Seek positive relationships and reduce number of unpleasant interactions.

Several health care practices are also known to promote sexual health such as getting adequate rest, maintaining optimal nutrition, and exercising regularly. Explaining the dynamics of sexual responses is another important nursing action. Individuals who report difficulties with sexual response often benefit from factual information and helpful suggestions and do not need sex therapy. However, when long-standing or highly complex problems emerge in the assessment, it is better to refer the individual or couple to a formally trained, certified, sex therapist. Nurses should be aware that certain processes, techniques, and adaptive devices can improve sexual functioning.

Psychoeducation

Unless the nurse has had additional preparation in sexual counseling, simply providing factual information and helping patients identify issues related to sexual problems and develop problem-solving skills are the primary psychosocial interventions. Patients often benefit from learning how to communicate their sexual needs better in such areas as type of stimulation desired, positioning, and the amount of time required for maximum sexual pleasure. Resource materials and referral sources can be recommended. Box 35.4 outlines topics for patient education.

Support groups

Women with orgasmic dysfunction can also benefit from a support group that includes women with similar problems. Group modalities are useful in helping patients decrease their embarrassment and uneasiness about sexual topics and increase their knowledge. Partner support is critical and should be encouraged throughout treatment.

Evaluation and Treatment Outcomes

Outcomes related to improved sexual functioning are developed with the patient and may vary from acquiring knowledge to increasing communication with her partner and to deciding about a referral for specialized treatment.

BOX 35.4

Female Orgasmic Disorder

When caring for the patient with female orgasmic disorder, be sure to include the following topics in your teaching plan for the patient and partner:

- Possible etiologic factors
- Anxiety reduction techniques
- Communication skills
- Impact of medication on orgasm

Integration with Primary Care

Sexual disorders are treated by specialists, but often the patient's initial concern is shared with a nurse. It is important that mental and health problems are treated from a holistic perspective. Mental health and primary health clinicians should be monitoring the sexual health of the patient and provide appropriate, evidence-based interventions.

EJACULATORY DYSFUNCTIONS

Ejaculatory dysfunction is one of the most common male sexual disorders and ranges from PE, inability to control ejaculation before or shortly after penetration to DE, delay or absence of ejaculation. These dysfunctions cause negative personal consequences, clinical distress, frustration, and the avoidance of sexual intimacy (Stephenson et al., 2018). The dysfunction needs to be present for 6 months to be diagnosed as a sexual dysfunction and is not diagnosed in a man whose difficulty is caused by drug or alcohol abuse. In those cases, a substance abuse diagnosis is made, with the sexual disorder generally resolving when the substance abuse is treated (APA, 2013).

Epidemiology

Based on patient self-report, PE is viewed as the most common male sexual dysfunction, with prevalence rates of up to 30% of men with an ED. It is estimated that about 27% of men seeking treatment report PE as a problem. Most men with PE, however, do not seek treatment (Rastrelli, et al., 2019).

Etiology

The etiology of PE is unknown with few data to support suggested biologic or psychological theories such as anxiety, penile hypersensitivity, and serotonin receptor dysfunction. Age does not seem to an etiologic factor or a risk (El-Hamd et al., 2019).

RECOVERY-ORIENTED CARE FOR PERSONS WITH EJACULATORY DYSFUNCTIONS

Teamwork and Collaboration: Working toward Recovery

The treatment of PE involves medication and behavioral strategies. Men with PE are usually treated by specialists. Nurses are instrumental in teaching patients about the disorder and potential treatments and facilitating decision-making about seeking treatment.

BOX 35.5

Premature Ejaculation

When caring for the patient with PE, be sure to include the following topics in your teaching plan for the patient and partner:

- Possible etiologic factors
- Pharmacologic agents, if indicated, including drug, dosage, action, frequency, and possible side effects
- Measures to decrease anxiety performance
- Communication skills
- Sexual counseling
- Sensate focus
- Sex therapy

EVIDENCE-BASED NURSING CARE FOR PERSONS WITH EJACULATORY DYSFUNCTIONS

The problem of PE may become apparent during a health history that includes specific sexual data. Patients need assurance that many men have similar problems and that treatment is possible (Box 35.5). Patients can be referred to specialists for behavioral strategies. Younger men may find that masturbation before anticipation of sexual intercourse may help.

Integration with Primary Care

Treatment of PE should be coordinated within the context of primary care. Since medications and medical illness can impact sexual functioning, it is important that one provider coordinates care. There is emerging evidence that alternative treatments, such as acupuncture, may be helpful (Dai et al., 2019).

ERECTILE DYSFUNCTION

Erectile dysfunction (ED) refers to the inability of a man to achieve or maintain an erection sufficient for satisfactory completion of the sexual activity.

Diagnostic Criteria

Although most men experience an occasional lack of erection, intervention is required when there is consistent (more than 6 months) erectile inefficiency during masturbation, intercourse, or on awakening (APA, 2013).

Epidemiology

Estimates of ED vary 5% to 20% of men. ED may occur at any age, although incidence increases with aging. Men with diabetes mellitus, cardiovascular disease, or chronic renal failure also have a higher incidence of ED. For those undergoing treatment for prostate cancer, there is a high probability of ED (Vernooij, et al, 2020). ED increases with age with and comorbidities such as diabetes, cardiovascular disease, depression, anxiety, obesity, metabolic syndrome, smoking, and substance use. Single men are more likely to experience ED than those with stable partners (Colson, et al., 2018). Although less common in younger men, ED still affects 5% to 10% of men below the age of 40. Findings from these studies show that ED impacts significantly on mood state, interpersonal functioning, and overall quality of life (Nguyen et al., 2017).

Etiology
Biologic Theories

Common biologic causes of ED include genital trauma, vascular insufficiency, renal disease, hormonal deficiencies, Parkinson disease, diabetes mellitus, multiple sclerosis, surgical procedures, use of antihypertensive and antidepressant drugs, and heavy cigarette smoking. Long-term alcohol or cocaine consumption can affect the erectile response. It is also more common with the aging process (Mollaioli, et al., 2020).

Many men with mental disorders attribute their ED to their psychiatric medication. Consequently, these individuals stop taking their medications. Within a few weeks to months, they have a psychiatric relapse.

Psychological Theories

ED may also have a psychogenic basis. Numerous psychosocial etiologies have been identified. Fear of failure, relationship stress, poor body image, fear of rejection, partner hostility, guilt, cultural taboos, religious proscriptions, lack of knowledge, and negative attitudes are some of the identified related factors (Balon, 2017; Chen, et al., 2018).

RECOVERY-ORIENTED CARE FOR PERSONS WITH ERECTILE DYSFUNCTION

Teamwork and Collaboration: Working toward Recovery

The treatment of men with ED is usually managed in primary care setting except for those with mental disorders, who may seek treatment within the mental health system. Since the introduction of the phosphodiesterase 5 (PDE5) inhibitors, pharmacologic agents such as sildenafil citrate, tadalafil, and vardenafil, many men choose the convenience of medication. For persons with psychiatric disorders, monitoring medications and their potential interaction is important. However, behavioral interventions have also been shown to be useful.

EVIDENCE-BASED NURSING CARE FOR THE PERSON WITH ERECTILE DYSFUNCTION

Mental Health Nursing Assessment

Some men are not comfortable discussing sexuality and sexual problems. The assessment should be conducted in an atmosphere of trust and understanding. In many cultures, male self-esteem is related to the ability to perform sexually. When a man has problems maintaining an erection, it is embarrassing and demeaning to him. Sensitivity to the patient's feelings should be reflected throughout the assessment.

Many medical problems are reported that compromise male sexual activity and responses. Obesity, smoking, diabetes mellitus, hypertension, hyperlipidemia, cardiovascular disease, and obstructive sleep disorder are a few (Akdemir, et al., 2019). In addition, low testosterone, chronic kidney disease, and some neurologic disorders also associated with male sexual dysfunction (Costa, et al., 2018; Huang, et al., 2019; Zamorano-Leon, et al., 2018.).

Assessment should include a discussion about the impact of sexual dysfunction on the quality of the relationship with the partner. If a mental disorder, such as depression or posttraumatic stress disorder, is present, comparing the timing of the dysfunction with the onset of symptoms and prescribed medication can determine whether the ED is related to the disorder and medication.

CLINICAL JUDGMENT

ED affects men differently, and the priorities of care will depend on its meaning to the patient. Low self-esteem and self-identity are two priorities that should be considered. ED may indicate an undiagnosed medical disorder such as diabetes or a medication side effect. There may be wellness priorities such as diet and exercise modifications that emerge.

MENTAL HEALTH NURSING INTERVENTIONS

Wellness Strategies

Promotion of positive health practices that focus on adequate nutrition, rest, and exercise is important in promoting erectile functioning. Weight loss may improve overall health and enhance the strength of the erection. Regular exercise is also related to sexual health. Helping the patient develop a better lifestyle is important in promoting sexual functioning. Reducing alcohol consumption can also improve sexual performance.

Medication Interventions

PDE5 inhibitors are the treatment of choice. With sexual stimulation, nitric oxide is released into the nerve terminations and endothelial cell, stimulating the production of cyclic guanosine monophosphate (cGMP), a substance that enables the smooth muscle cells of the corpora cavernosa to relax. The PDE enzymes are involved in the breakdown of cGMP. The PDE inhibitors inactivate PDE5, thereby enabling the buildup of cGMP, sustaining relaxation of the corpora cavernosa.

Approved PDE5 inhibitors include sildenafil citrate (Viagra), vardenafil HCl (Levitra), tadalafil (Cialis), and avanafil (Stendra). These medications enhance the effect of nitric oxide, which is released in the corpora cavernosa during sexual stimulation. These medications are rapidly absorbed, with maximum observed plasma concentrations reached within 30 to 120 minutes of oral dosing in the fasted state. Cialis acts for up to 36 hours. Although these medications are approved for the treatment of ED in men, they have not been shown to be efficacious in sexual arousal disorders in women.

Before the introduction of PDE5 inhibitors, intracavernosal pharmacotherapy was the treatment of choice for ED. A vascular smooth muscle relaxant such as papaverine hydrochloride, phentolamine mesylate, or prostaglandin is directly injected into the corpora cavernosa by the patient or partner. This increases arterial flow of blood into the corpora cavernosa and decreases venous outflow. Neurogenic, rather than vascular, ED appears to respond better. Complications can include excessive bleeding, scarring and priapism, and potential hepatic involvement. Counseling, strict monitoring, and specific teaching are required (Balon, 2019a).

Another treatment is the use of alprostadil (prostaglandin) in microsuppository form inserted into the urethra using a special applicator. The system called MUSE (Medicated Urethral System for Erections) causes a rapid absorption of the medication through the urethral mucosa into the corpus spongiosum. It is particularly useful for men who are unable to inject themselves (Balon, 2019a).

Other Interventions

When erection is determined to be permanently impaired, several options may be considered to facilitate intercourse. An external penile prosthesis can be placed over the flaccid penis, although some find this esthetically displeasing. A pumping device that creates a vacuum can be used for blood entrapment followed by placement of a rubber band at the base of the penis. Surgical techniques for improving vascular sufficiency are also showing promising results.

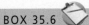

BOX 35.6

Male ED

When caring for the patient with male erectile disorder, be sure to include the following topics in your teaching plan for the patient and partner:

- Possible etiologic factors
- Psychopharmacologic agents (e.g., intracavernosal therapy, yohimbine), including drug, action, frequency, administration technique, and possible side effects
- Alternative methods of sexual expression
- Prosthesis use
- Sexual education and counseling
- Communication skills
- Sex therapy

Psychoeducation

Education is important for the patient with ED. Teaching the patient about positive health practices and treatment options (i.e., mechanical devices, medications, surgical procedures) is usually needed (Box 35.6). The patient's concern about his partner's satisfaction needs to be explored. Many times, men believe that partner satisfaction is related only to penile penetration and their ability to sustain an erection. Encouraging the patient to talk with his partner about her (or his) sexual needs and other aspects of their sexual experience (physical closeness, kissing, hugging, mutual exploration of their bodies) helps him broaden his understanding of the sexual experience.

Evaluation and Treatment Outcomes

The primary outcome for ED is improved sexual functioning. Acceptance of change of physical status is an outcome that is difficult to obtain. Improvement in sexual satisfaction may include increasing the ability for erectile functioning. If ED is permanent, exploration of other avenues of sexual expression may indicate a successful outcome. In this disorder, partner satisfaction is usually of prime concern. Improved communication with the man's partner may also be a positive outcome.

FEMALE SEXUAL INTEREST/AROUSAL DISORDER

A female sexual interest/arousal disorder may occur at any age and may cause relationship difficulties and personal stress along with avoidance of sexual activity and impaired communication. Other etiologic factors, such as anxiety, guilt, and history of sexual abuse, and changes in androgen levels during the menstrual cycle, have been shown to affect arousal. Aging also affects sexual arousal because vasocongestion develops more slowly in older women, so vaginal lubrication decreases after menopause; lower estrogen levels at this life stage may affect sexual arousal.

Intervention focuses on treating factors that contribute to the lack of arousal. Flibanserin, a medication designed and studied for premenopausal women with sexual desire disorder, is approved by the US Food and Drug Administration (FDA) generalized hypoactive sexual desire disorder. The primary side effects of the daily pill are dizziness, sleepiness, and fatigue (Sprout Pharmaceuticals, 2021). Cognitive behavioral therapy is recommended for psychosocial issues. For hormonal changes, a referral to a women's health provider is useful (Balon, 2019a).

MALE HYPOACTIVE SEXUAL DESIRE DISORDER

Male hypoactive sexual desire disorder is a recurrent deficiency or absence of sexual fantasies and desire for sexual activity. Individuals with this disorder are not interested in sex, do not or cannot get "turned on," and require no sexual gratification. Active avoidance of potential sexual relationships may exist. The prevalence is unknown, but it is believed to affect only a small proportion of men. Often, the disorder develops in adulthood after a period of adequate sexual interest and is associated with psychological distress, stressful life events (e.g., childbirth), or relationship difficulties (Balon, 2019a; Parish & Hahn, 2016).

Therapy for psychological issues related to hypoactive sexual desire aims at helping the patient understand the problem and develop strategies to enhance sexual arousal. Treatment approaches may include individual and couples therapy, sex-therapy techniques, clinical hypnosis, cognitive behavioral therapy, guided fantasy exercises, and sexual assertiveness training. If the problem is related to medication, changing to another classification of medication, giving drug holidays, or lowering the dose may help.

GENITO-PELVIC PAIN/PENETRATION DISORDER

Genito-pelvic pain/penetration disorder is characterized by persistent or recurrent difficulties with vaginal penetration during intercourse, marked vulvovaginal or pelvic pain during vaginal intercourse or penetration attempts, or significant fear or anxiety about the vulvovaginal or pelvic pain in anticipation of, during, or as a result of vaginal penetration (APA, 2013).

Dyspareunia is a term used to describe the genital pain associated with sexual intercourse that may be caused by **vaginismus**, which is spastic involuntary constriction of the perineal and outer vaginal muscles fostered by imagined, anticipated, or real attempts at vaginal penetration. This disorder may be related to interpersonal or emotional factors such as sexual dissatisfaction or poor technique leading to inadequate relaxation and lubrication. Biologic etiologies include intact or biperforate hymen, postmenopausal atrophic changes, trauma, malignancy, intestinal disease, or other pelvic disorders (Balon, 2019a).

PARAPHILIAS

Paraphilias are described as "intense and persistent sexual interest other than sexual interest in genital stimulation or preparatory fondling with phenotypically normal, physically mature, consenting human partners characterized by recurrent, intense sexual urges, fantasies, or behaviors involving unusual objects, activities, or situations" (APA, 2013, p. 685). These interests cause significant distress to the individual or impair social or occupational functioning. The paraphilias include voyeurism, exhibitionism, frotteurism, sexual masochism, sexual sadism, pedophilia, and fetishism, disorders (APA, 2013).

Paraphilias are rarely diagnosed; the situation is complicated across cultures because acceptability of sexual practices varies across cultures. Although very few studies exist, some assert that comorbid mood disorders are often associated with paraphilia disorders (Balon, 2019b). These disorders often come to the attention of mental health professionals within the context of illegal sexual activity or sexually violent predators. Treatment of paraphilias is rarely sought by the individual; rather, it is a result of the psychosocial or criminal ramifications.

Certain behaviors and fantasies associated with paraphilias are said to begin in childhood and become more elaborate and better defined during adolescence and early adulthood. The disorders are often found to be chronic and lifelong, with the fantasies and behavior finally diminishing with aging. Table 35.1 includes the different categories of paraphilias along with their descriptions.

GENDER DYSPHORIA

Gender dysphoria is not classified as a sexual dysfunction. *Gender dysphoria* is the term used to describe a person's discomfort or distress regarding the gender that is assigned by society. These symptoms occur because of the way society labels and responds to gender-diverse people. If society were more open to a spectrum of gender expression, these symptoms might not be present (Yarbrough, 2019).

TABLE 35.1	PARAPHILIAS
Paraphilia	Description
Exhibitionism	The behavior involves exposing one's genitals to strangers, with occasional masturbation. There may be an awareness of the desire to shock the individual or the fantasy that the individual will become sexually aroused on observation of the exposure.
Fetishism	An object such as women's undergarments or foot apparel is used for sexual arousal. The individual usually masturbates while holding, rubbing, or smelling the item, or it is worn by a partner during sexual activity. Fetishism usually begins in adolescence and continues throughout life.
Frotteurism	Sexually arousing urges, fantasies, and behaviors occur when touching or rubbing one's genitals against the breasts, genitals, or thighs of a nonconsenting person. This paraphilia usually begins in early adolescence or young adulthood and diminishes with age.
Pedophilia	Sexual activity occurs with a child usually 13 yrs of age or younger by an individual at least 16 yrs of age or 5 yrs older than the child. Pedophilic acts include fondling, oral sex, and anal or vaginal intercourse with the penis, fingers, or objects, with varying amounts of force.
Sexual masochism	This behavior involves the act of being humiliated, beaten, bound, or made to suffer. Self-induced masochistic acts include use of electric shock, pin sticking, restraints, and mutilation; partner-induced acts may include bondage, whipping, being urinated or defecated on; and being forced to crawl, bark, or wear diapers. One dangerous form of sexual masochism that may be practiced alone or with a partner is "hypoxyphilia." Oxygen deprivation by means of a noose, plastic bag, chest compression, or drug effect is used during sexual activity to heighten orgasmic sensation. Deaths have occurred as a result of these techniques.
Sexual sadism	Sexual excitement occurs when causing physical or psychological suffering to another individual. Commonly, the individual with sadistic behavior interacts with a masochistic partner. Sadistic behavior includes various forms of physical punishment, use of restraints, rape, burning, stabbing, strangulation, torture, and murder. This is usually a chronic paraphilia that begins as early sexual fantasies and increases in severity over time.
Voyeurism	This behavior involves "peeping," for the purpose of sexual excitement, at unsuspecting people who are nude, undressing, or engaged in sexual activity.
Other paraphilias	Sexual fantasies, urges, and activities involving animals (zoophilia), corpses (necrophilia), feces (coprophilia), urine (urophilia), body parts (partialism), and obscene telephone calls (telephone scatalogia).

Wellness Challenges

One of the biggest issues facing the gender-diverse community is lack of access to competent gender-affirming care. Gender-diverse individuals face discrimination and health care disparities within the context of a western history of pathologizing a whole group of people.

RECOVERY-ORIENTED CARE FOR PERSONS WITH GENDER DYSPHORIA

Teamwork and Collaboration: Working toward Recovery

For non-binary individuals with gender dysphoria, moving toward gender affirmation requires support and care from gender-affirming clinicians. Some individuals may decide to align their physical state to their true gender identity. Hormones may be used to feminize (estrogen) or masculinize (testosterone) the body. For those that want to feminize their bodies, a testosterone blocker is usually given along with estrogen. The changes that occur takes months to years. Others may decide on

surgical procedures that are increasing in possibility as third-party payers are starting to cover the cost. There is much to learn about gender and its expression (Yarbrough, 2019).

SUMMARY OF KEY POINTS

- Female orgasmic disorder is a common disorder affecting women; ED and PE are the most common disorders affecting men.

- Nursing interventions for people experiencing sexual dysfunction include (but are not limited to) counseling, education, and referral to sex therapists.

- Various medical conditions, psychological states, and medications negatively affect the sexual response cycle. Education about medication side effects and sexual experiences is important in maintaining health.

- Paraphilias are rarely diagnosed, but the prevalence may be higher than usually presented.

- Gender dysphoria occurs when the individual is distressed with assigned sex or gender role.

CRITICAL THINKING CHALLENGES

1. A 36-year-old woman was recently diagnosed with depression and treated with a selective serotonin reuptake inhibitor (an antidepressant). Her depression is improving, but she has not been interested in sexual relations with her husband. Her lack of sexual interest is beginning to cause problems in her marriage. What could account for the changes in sexual interest?

2. A 52-year-old married man who is being successfully treated with lithium carbonate for his bipolar disorder was recently diagnosed with diabetes mellitus. He was told that his diabetes mellitus could be controlled by weight loss and diet. His major worry is that the disease and lithium are causing his impotence. He casually mentions that he is considering stopping the lithium. What issues should the nurse explore with the patient? What actions could the patient begin that would improve his sexual health?

3. During a nursing assessment, a young woman reveals that she identifies as a lesbian and that she is currently living with her partner. She has not yet told her parents about her sexual identification and is experiencing some anxiety about sharing this part of her life with her family. Her partner is supportive and encourages the young woman to take her time in telling her family members. Is this patient experiencing symptoms of a gender dysphoria? Explain.

Movie Viewing Guides

Kinsey: (2004). This critically acclaimed, American biographical drama describes the life of Alfred Charles Kinsey, a pioneer in the area of sexology. Professor Kinsey is being interviewed about his sexual history. During the interview, he has flashbacks to his childhood and young adulthood. His father, a minister, denounces modern inventions as leading to sexual sin and is shown as humiliating his young son. Kinsey, a biologist at Indiana University, marries a student in his class. He comes to terms with his own sexual needs and realizes that sexuality is more varied than originally thought. He publishes books on sexual habits and debunks many 1950s-era myths.

VIEWING POINTS: How did Dr. Kinsey's work contribute to normalizing same-sex relationships and premarital sex? Identify the sexual myths that Dr. Kinsey was able to challenge.

movie: Moonlight (2016) This movie depicts three periods—young adolescence, mid-teen, and young adult—in the life of Chiron, a child who was born to a single mother, Paula, who was addicted to crack. Chiron is a shy withdrawn child with a small for his age. He is bullied and experiences discrimination because of his race, poverty, and identity. Chiron has a sexual encounter with a classmate Kevin, who is a part of Chiron's story throughout the three time periods.

VIEWING POINTS: How did the discrimination that Chiron experience during his childhood impact his development? Speculate on the role of Chiron's sexual encounters in his gender identify.

REFERENCES

Akdemir, A. O., Karabakan, M., Aktas, B. K., Bozkurt, A., Ozgur, E. G., Akdogan, N., & Yarıs, M. (2019). Visceral adiposity index is useful for evaluating obesity effect on erectile dysfunction. *Andrologia, 2*, e13282. https://doi.org/10.1111/and.13282.

American Psychiatric Association (APA). (2013). *Diagnostic and statistical manual of mental disorders* (5th ed.). Author.

Amherst College Resource Center. (2020). *Terms, definition, & labels.* Queer Resource Center. https://www.amherst.edu/campuslife/our-community/queer-resource-center/terms-definitions.

Balon, R. (2017). Burden of sexual dysfunction. *Journal of Sex and Marital Therapy, 43*(1), 49–55. https://doi.org/10.1080/0092623X.2015.1113597.

Balon, R. (2019a). Sexual dysfunctions. In L. W. Roberts, (Ed.), *The American psychiatric publishing textbook of psychiatry* (7th ed.). American Psychiatric Association.

Balon, R. (2019b). Paraphilic disorders. In L.W. Roberts (Eds.), *The American psychiatric publishing textbook of psychiatry* (7th ed.). American Psychiatric Association.

Bancroft, J., & Graham, C. A. (2011). The varied nature of women's sexuality: Unresolved issues and a theoretical approach. *Hormones and Behavior, 59*(5), 717–729.

Bancroft, J., Graham, C. A., Janssen, E., & Sanders, S. A. (2009). The dual control model: Current status and future directions. *Journal of Sex Research, 46*(2–3), 121–142.

Basson, R. (2001). Female sexual response: The role of drugs in the management of sexual dysfunction. *Obstetrics & Gynecology, 98*(2), 350–353.

Blais, R. K., Monteith, L. L., & Kugler, J. (2018). Sexual dysfunction is associated with suicidal ideation in female service members and veterans. *Journal of Affective Disorders, 226*, 52–57. https://doi.org/10.1016/j.jad.2017.08.079.

Calabrò, R. S., Cacciola, A., Bruschetta, D., Milardi, D., Quattrini, F., Sciarrone, F., la Rosa, G., Bramanti, P., & Anastasi, G. (2019). Neuroanatomy and function of human sexual behavior: A neglected or unknown issue? *Brain and Behavior, 9*(12), e01389. https://doi.org/10.1002/brb3.1389.

Chen, J., Chen, Y., Gao, Q., Chen, G., Dai, Y., Yao, Z., & Lu, Q. (2018). Impaired prefrontal-amygdala pathway, self-reported emotion, and erection in psychogenic erectile dysfunction patients with normal nocturnal erection. *Frontiers in Human Neuroscience, 12*, 157. https://doi.org/10.3389/fnhum.2018.00157

Colson, M. H., Cuzin, B., Faix, A., Grellet, L., & Huyghes, E. (2018). Current epidemiology of erectile dysfunction, an update. *Sexologies, 37*(1), e7–e13.

Connaughton, C., McCabe, M., & Karantzas, G. (2016). Conceptualization of the sexual response models in men: Are there differences between sexually functional and dysfunctional men? *The Journal of Sexual Medicine, 13* (3), 453–463.

Costa, M. R., Ponciano, V. C., Costa, T. R., Gomes, C. P., & de Oliveira, E. C. (2018). Stage effect of chronic kidney disease in erectile function. *International Brazilian Journal of Urology, 44*(1), 132–140. https://doi.org/10.1590/S1677-5538.IBJU.2017.0228.

Dai, H., Li, H., Wang, J., Bao, B., Yan, Y., Wang, B., & Sun, S. (2019). Effectiveness comparisons of acupuncture for premature ejaculation: Protocol for a network meta-analysis. *Medicine, 98*(5), e14147. https://doi.org/10.1097/MD.0000000000014147.

Eid, W., & Biason-Lauber, A. (2016). Why boys will be boys and girls will be girls: Human sex development and its defects. *Birth Defects Research (Part C), 108*, 365–379.

El-Hamd, M. A., Saleh, R., & Majzoub, A. (2019). Premature ejaculation: an update on definition and pathophysiology. *Asian Journal of Andrology*, https://doi.org/10.4103/aja.aja_122_18.

Evans-Polce, R. J., Veliz, P. T., Boyd, C. J., Hughes, T. L., & McCabe, S. E. (2019). Associations between sexual orientation discrimination and substance use disorders: differences by age in US adults. *Social Psychiatry and Psychiatric Epidemiology*, *55*(1), 101–110.

Ferenidou, F., Kirana, P. S., Fokas, K., Hatzichristou, D., & Athanasiadis, L. (2016). Sexual response models: Toward a more flexible patter of women's sexuality. *The Journal of Sexual Medicine*, *13*(9), 1569–1576.

Grabowska, A. (2017). Sex on the brain: Are gender-dependent structural and functional differences associated with behavior? *Journal of Neuroscience Research*, *95*, 200–212.

Healthy People 2030. (2021). *Lesbian, gay, bisexual, and transgender health*. U.S. Department of Health and Human Services, Office of Disease Prevention and Health Promotion. https://health.gov/healthypeople/objectives-and-data/browse-objectives/lgbt.

Huang, Y. P., Liu, W., Chen, S. F., Liu, Y. D., Chen, B., Deng, C. H., & Lu, M. J. (2019). Free testosterone correlated with erectile dysfunction severity among young men with normal total testosterone. *International Journal of Impotence Research*, *31*(2), 132–138. https://doi.org/10.1038/s41443-018-0090-y.

Hodgson, B., Kukkonen, T. M., Binik, Y. M., & Carrier, S. (2016). Using the dual control model to investigate the relationship between mood, genital, and self-reported sexual arousal in men and women. *The Journal of Sexual Research*, *4*(8), 1–15.

Lussier, P., McCuish, E., Mathesius, J., Corrado, R., & Nadeau, D. (2018). Developmental trajectories of child sexual behaviors on the path of sexual behavioral problems: Evidence from a prospective longitudinal study. *Sexual Abuse*, *30*(6), 622–658. https://doi.org/10.1177/1079063217691963.

Kaplan, H. S. (1979). *Disorders of sexual desire and other concepts and techniques in sex therapy*. Simon & Schuster.

Martinez, G. M., & Abma, J.C. (2020). Sexual activity and contraceptive use among teenagers aged 15–19 in the United States, 2015–2017. *NCHS Data Brief*, no 366. National Center for Health Statistics.

Masters, W. H., & Johnson, V. E. (1966). *Human sexual response*. Little, Brown.

Masters, W. H. & Johnson, V. E. (1970). *Human sexual inadequacy*. Little, Brown.

Meston, C. M., & Stanton, A. M. (2019). Understanding sexual arousal and subjective-genital arousal desynchrony in women. *Nature Reviews. Urology*, *16*(2), 107–120. https://doi.org/10.1038/s41585-018-0142-6.

Miragoli, S., Camisasca, E., & Di Blasio, P. (2017). Child sexual behaviors in school context: Age and gender differences. *Journal of Child Sexual Abuse*, *26*(2), 213–231. https://doi.org/10.1080/10538712.2017.1280866.

Mollaioli, D., Ciocca, G., Limoncin, E., Di Sante, S., Gravina, G. L., Carosa, E., Lenzi, A., & Jannini, E. (2020). Lifestyles and sexuality in men and women: the gender perspective in sexual medicine. *Reproductive Biology and Endocrinology: RB&E*, *18*(1), 10. https://doi.org/10.1186/s12958-019-0557-9.

Mornar, J. M., Krstačić, G., Perenčević, A., & Pintarić, H. (2018). Sexual activity in patients with cardiac diseases. *Acta Clinica Croatica*, *57*(1), 141–148. https://doi.org/10.20471/acc.2018.57.01.18.

Nguyen, H. M. T., Gabrielson, A. T., & Hellstrom, W. J. G. (2017). Erectile dysfunction in young men-A review of the prevalence and risk factors. *Sexual Medicine Review*, *5*(4):508–520. doi: 10.1016/j.sxmr.2017.05.004.

Parish, S. J., & Hahn, S. R. (2016). Hypoactive sexual desire disorder: A review of epidemiology, biopyschology, diagnosis, and treatment. *Sexual Medicine Reviews*, *4*(2), 103–120.

Rastrelli, G, Cipriani, S., Corona, G., Vignozzi, L., & Maggi, M. (2019). Clinical characteristics of men complaining of premature ejaculation together with erectile dysfunction: A cross-sectional study. *Andrology*, *7*(2), 163–171. https://doi.org/10.1111/andr.12579.

Rastrelli, G., Corona, G., & Maggi, M. (2018). Testosterone and sexual function in men. *Maturitas*, *112*, 46–52. https://doi.org/10.1016/j.maturitas.2018.04.004.

Ristori, J., Cocchetti, C., Romani, A., Mazzoli, F., Vignozzi, L., Maggi, M., & Fisher, A. D. (2020). Brain sex differences related to gender identity development: Genes or hormones? *International Journal of Molecular Sciences*, *21*(6), 2123. https://doi.org/10.3390/ijms21062123.

Roselli, C. E. (2018). Neurobiology of gender identity and sexual orientation. *Journal of Neuroendocrinology*, *30*(7), e12562. https://doi.org/10.1111/jne.12562.

Rowland, D. L., Cempel, L. M., & Tempel, A. R. (2018). Women's attributions regarding why they have difficulty reaching orgasm. *Journal of Sex & Marital Therapy*, *44*(5), 475–484. https://doi.org/10.1080/0092623X.2017.1408046.

Sarwer, D. B., Hanson, A. J., Voeller, J., & Steffen, K. (2018). Obesity and sexual functioning. *Current Obesity Reports*, *7*(4), 301–307. https://doi.org/10.1007/s13679-018-0319-6.

Scavello, I., Maseroli, E., Di Stasi, V., & Vignozzi, L. (2019). Sexual health in menopause. *Medicina (Kaunas, Lithuania)*, *55*(9), 559. https://doi.org/10.3390/medicina55090559.

Sprout Pharmaceuticals. (2021). *FDA Advisory Committee recommends approval for sprout Pharmaceuticals' ADDYI*^{TM} *(flibanserin) to treat hypoactive sexual desire disorder in premenopausal women*. https://www.sproutpharma.com.

Stephenson, K. R., Truong, L., & Shimazu, L. (2018). Why is impaired sexual function distressing to men? Consequences of impaired male sexual function and their associations with sexual well-being. *Journal of Sexual Medicine*, *15*(9), 1336–1349. https://doi.org/10.1016/j.jsxm.2018.07.014.

Substance Abuse and Mental Health Services Administration (SAMHSA). (2015). *Ending conversion therapy: Supporting and affirming LGBTQ youth* (HHS Publication No. (SMA) 15–4928). Substance Abuse and Mental Health Services Administration.

Syme, M. L., & Cohn, T. J. (2016). Examining aging sexual stigma attitudes among adults by gender, age, and generational status. *Aging & Mental Health*, *20*(1), 36–45.

Thomas, H.N., Neal-Perry, G.S., Hess. (2018). Female sexual function at midlife and beyond. *Obstetrics & Gynecology Clinics of North America*, *45*(4), 709–722. https://doi.org/10.1016/j.ogc.2018.07.013.

Turner, D. Wittekind, C. E., Briken, P., Fromberger, P., Moritz, S., & Rettenberger, M. (2019). Approach and avoidance biases toward sexual stimuli and their association with the Dual Control Model of Sexual Response in heterosexual men. *Archives Sexual Behavior*, *48*(3), 867–880. https://doi.org/10.1007/s10508-018-1289-1.

Vargas, S. M., Huey, S. J., & Miranda, J. (2020). A critical review of current evidence on multiple types of discrimination and mental health. *The American Journal of Orthopsychiatry*, *90*(3), 374–390. https://doi.org/10.1037/ort0000441.

Velten, J., Zahler, L., Scholten, S., & Margraf, J. (2019). Temporal stability of sexual excitation and sexual inhibition in women. *Archives of Sexual Behavior*, *48*(3), 881–889. https://doi.org/10.1007/s10508-018-1323-3.

Vernooij, R. W., Lancee, M., Cleves, A., Dahm, P., Bangma, C. H., & Aben, K. K. (2020). Radical prostatectomy versus deferred treatment for localised prostate cancer. *The Cochrane Database of Systematic Reviews*, *6*(6), CD006590. https://doi.org/10.1002/14651858.CD006590.pub3.

Wheeler, L. J., & Guntupalli, S. R. (2020). Female sexual dysfunction: pharmacologic and therapeutic interventions. *Obstetrics and Gynecology*, *136*(1), 174–186. https://doi.org/10.1097/AOG.0000000000003941.

World Health Organization (WHO). (2021). Sexual and reproductive health. *The World Health Organization's department of reproductive health and research*, Geneva. http://www.who.int/reproductivehealth/topics/sexual_health/sh_definitions/en/.

World Health Organization (WHO). (2017). Sexual health and its linkages to reproductive health: an operational approach. Department of Reproductive Health and Research, World Health Organization, Geneva, Switzerland. Retrieved June 22, 2021 from https://www.who.int/health-topics/sexual-health#tab=tab_1

Yarbrough, E. (2019). Gender dysphoria. In L.W. Roberts (Eds.), *The American psychiatric publishing textbook of psychiatry* (7th ed.). American Psychiatric Association.

Zamorano-Leon, J.J., Segura, A., Lahera, V., Rodriguez-Pardo, J. M., Prieto, R., Puigvert, A., & Lopez-Farre, A. J. (2018). Relationship between erectile dysfunction, diabetes and dyslipidemia in hypertensive-treated Men. *Urology Journal*, *15*(6), 370–375. https://doi.org/10.22037/uj.v0i0.4068.

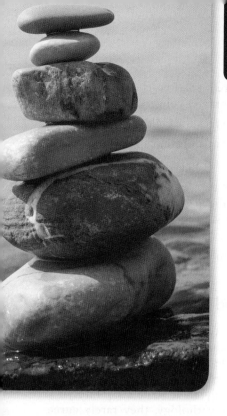

Care of Children and Adolescents

36
Mental Health Assessment of Children and Adolescents

Rebecca Luebbert

KEYCONCEPTS

- assortative mating
- comprehensive assessment

LEARNING OBJECTIVES

After studying this chapter, you will be able to:

1. Define the assessment process for children and adolescents.

2. Discuss techniques of data collection used with children and adolescents.

3. Delineate important areas of assessment for children and adolescents.

KEY TERMS

- Attachment • Attachment disorganization • Developmental delays • Egocentrism • Maturation • Temperament

INTRODUCTION

The mental health assessment of children and adolescents is a specialized process that considers their unique problems and responses within the context of their development. Any nurse who cares for a child should be comfortable with conducting a mental health nursing assessment because the emotional and psychological aspects are central to understanding health needs and behaviors.

The assessment of children and adolescents generally follows the same format as for adults (see Chapter 11), but there are significant differences. Children think in more concrete terms; thus, the nurse needs to ask more specific and fewer open-ended questions than would typically be asked of adults. The nurse should use simple phrasing because children have a narrower vocabulary than do adults. Examples include saying "sad" instead of "depressed" or "nervous" instead of "anxious." The nurse needs to corroborate information that children offer with more sources (e.g., parents, teachers) than they would for adults. The nurse may want to use artistic and play media (e.g., puppets, family drawings) to engage children and evaluate their perceptions, inner worlds, fine motor skills, and intellectual functions. Children have a less specific sense of time and a less developed memory than do adults. When children are asked about a sequence of events or specific times when events occurred, they may not be able to provide accurate information.

A comprehensive evaluation includes a history, mental status examination, additional testing (e.g., cognitive or neuropsychological), if necessary, records of the child's school performance and medical–physical history, and information from other agencies that may be providing services (e.g., Department of Child and Family services [DCF], juvenile court). The nurse may use various assessment tools, including the Child Attention Profile (CAP) and the Devereux Childhood Assessment (DECA), the Behavior Assessment System for Children (BASC), the Child Behavior Checklist (CBCL), or the Children's Depression Inventory (CDI).

NCLEXNOTE Whenever assessing children or adolescents, developmental level will frame the assessment and implementation of the management plan.

TECHNIQUES FOR DATA COLLECTION: THE CLINICAL INTERVIEW

The clinical interview is the primary assessment tool used in child and adolescent psychiatry. A unique set of skills is necessary for interviewing children and adolescents. How the nurse obtains mental health information depends on the developmental level of each child, specifically considering the child's language, cognitive, social, and emotional skills. For example, the nurse should simplify questions for young children or children with developmental delays so they can understand and respond appropriately.

The assessment interview may be the initial contact between the child and parent or guardian and the nurse. The first step is to establish a therapeutic alliance with both the child and parent, and the second is to assess the interactions between the child and parent.

Establishment of a Therapeutic Alliance

The nurse can establish rapport by greeting the child or adolescent in a friendly, polite, open manner and putting them at ease. Speaking clearly and at a normal volume and using friendly, reassuring tones are essential measures. The nurse can establish a treatment alliance by recognizing the child's individuality and showing respect and concern for them. The nurse should demonstrate sensitivity, objectivity, and confidentiality. The child will be more forthcoming if they feel that the nurse is listening carefully and is interested in what they have to say.

Child and Parent Observation

Because the child's primary environment is with the parent or guardian, child–parent interactions provide important data about the child–parent attachment and parenting practices. The nurse's observations focus on both the child alone and the child within the family. The nurse can actually make some of these observations while the family is in the waiting area, including:

- How the child and parent talk to each other, including how frequently each initiates conversation
- How the parent disciplines the child
- How attached the parent and child appear
- How the child and parent separate
- If the parent and child play together
- How the child gets the parent's attention and how responsive the parent is to the child's attention-seeking initiatives
- How the parent and child show affection to each other

Separate Child and Parent Interviews

To get an accurate picture of the child, the nurse should interview the child and parent individually because each can provide unique meaningful information. Research has shown that when parent and child are interviewed separately in a structured interview about the child's psychopathology, they rarely agree on the presence of diagnostic criteria, particularly regarding depression and anxiety (Baumgartner et al., 2020; Orchard et al., 2019; Popp et al., 2017). Generally, there is greater child–parent agreement on external symptoms and behaviors than on non-observable symptoms, such as mood, feelings, and emotions (Hemmingsson et al., 2017).

Discussion with the Child

After talking with the parent and child together, the nurse should ask to speak with the child alone for a while. Young children may fear separating from their parents. The nurse can reassure children by showing them where the waiting area is and telling them that if they get scared, the nurse will accompany them to check on their parents. Introducing a toy or game or allowing the child to hold a transitional object may help. Remember that observing how the child separates from the parent is part of the data needed to complete the assessment.

Adolescents may act indifferent or even hostile when the nurse asks to speak with them alone. Teens tend to be skeptical that adults can really understand their experience, suspicious that they will be blamed for their problems, and fearful that their thoughts and feelings are abnormal. The nurse should convey their genuine interest in wanting to hear the adolescent's perspective. The nurse should be patient with adolescents and say something like, "I can see you're pretty angry about being here. What are you particularly angry about? Perhaps there is some way I can help you." Another useful and reassuring question is, "During the last few minutes, you've been quiet. I'm wondering what you are feeling." Or the nurse may ask, "It can be uncomfortable to tell personal information to someone you don't know. Do you feel this way?" (Frick, Barry, & Kamphaus, 2020).

To begin the initial assessment of a child, the nurse introduces themself and explains briefly what they will be doing. For children younger than 11 years of age, the nurse should explain that they help worried or upset children by talking, playing, and giving advice to them and their parents. The nurse should then ask about the child's understanding of why they are there. This question often helps to identify children's misperceptions (e.g., believing the nurse is going to give them an injection, thinking they have done something bad) that could create barriers to working with them. When conducting the child interview, the nurse needs to get several releases of information from the child's guardian to obtain the corroborating reports, such as the child's physical assessment from the pediatrician or pediatric nurse practitioner; the school's report about the child's academic and behavioral performance, including the child's report card, behavior at school, peer interactions, and adult interactions; and records of diagnosis and treatment from any previous psychiatric provider.

The nurse must adapt communication to the child's age level (Box 36.1). The challenge is to avoid using overly complex vocabulary or talking down to children. Young children often express themselves more easily in the context of play than through adult like conversation. For example, a child may reenact a conversation that he had with a sibling or parent using puppets. Children

---

BOX 36.1

Strategies for Interviewing Children

- Use a simple vocabulary and short sentences tailored to the child's developmental and cognitive levels.
- Be sure that the child understands the questions and that you do not lead the child to give a particular response. Phrase your questions so the child does not receive any hint that one response is more acceptable than another.
- Select the questions for your interview on an individual basis using judgment and discretion and considering the child's age and developmental level.
- Be sure that the manner and tone of your voice do not reveal any personal biases.
- Speak slowly and quietly and try to allow the interview to unfold, using the child's verbalizations and behavior as guides.
- Use simple terms (e.g., "sad" for "depressed") in exploring affective reactions and ask the child to give examples of how they behave or how other people behave when emotionally aroused.
- Assume an accepting and neutral attitude toward the child's communications.
- Learn about children's current interests by looking at Saturday morning television programs, talking with parents, visiting toy stores, looking at children's books, and visiting day care centers and schools to observe children in their natural habitats.

---

respond well to third-person conversation prompts, such as "Some kids don't like being compared with their brothers and sisters," or "I know a kid who was so sad when he lost his dog that he thought he would never be happy again."

Early in the interview, the goal is to explain the nurse's purpose, elicit any concerns the child may have about what is happening, and establish rapport with the child by engaging in unthreatening discussion. Many adults rarely ask children about things that truly interest them but expect children to respond readily to adult conversation. The nurse can establish a high degree of credibility simply by taking note of and asking about things that are obviously important to children (e.g., a sport the child participates in, a rock group displayed on a shirt, a toy a child has brought with her). However, children have an uncanny natural "radar" for phony adult behavior. Attempts to establish rapport work only when the nurse is genuinely interested in the child's life.

Discussion with the Parents

After meeting alone with the child, the nurse should spend some time alone with the parents and ask for a detailed description of their view of the problem. When alone, parents may feel comfortable discussing their children in depth and sharing frustrations with their behavior. Parents need this opportunity to speak freely without being constrained by concern for the child's feelings. In some cases, it would be detrimental for the child to hear the full force of the parents' complaints and feelings, such as helplessness, anger, or disappointment. Parents need the nurse to allow them to express their feelings without passing judgment. This is the nurse's opportunity to enlist the help of parents as partners in the child's evaluation and treatment. This time is also good for filling in any gaps in the history and clarifying the data obtained from the interview with the child.

Parents need the chance to describe the presenting problem in their own words. The nurse can encourage them by asking general questions, such as, "What brings you here today?" or "How have things been in your family?" The nurse should then reflect their understanding of the problem, showing empathy and respect for both the parent and child. Asking any other family members about their view of the problem is always a good idea to clarify discrepant points of view, obtain additional data, and communicate awareness that different family members experience the same problem in different ways.

Development of Rapport

To reduce anxiety about the evaluation, the nurse must develop rapport with the family members. Establishing rapport can be facilitated by maintaining appropriate eye contact; speaking slowly, clearly, and calmly with friendliness and acceptance; using a warm and expressive tone; reacting to communications from interviewees objectively; showing interest in what the interviewees are saying; and making the interview a joint undertaking (see Chapter 10). Suggestions for building rapport with children and adolescents are also addressed in each of the developmental sections that follow. The information in Box 36.2 can serve as a guide to asking specific questions during a comprehensive assessment.

BOX 36.2

Semi-structured Interview with School-Aged Children

Precede the following questions with a preliminary greeting, such as the following: "Hi, I am (your name and title). You must be (child's name). Come in."

FOR ALL SCHOOL-AGED CHILDREN

1. Has anyone told you about why you are here today?
2. (If yes) Who?
3. (If yes) What did they tell you?
4. Tell me why *you* think you are here. (If child mentions a problem, explore it in detail.)
5. How old are you?
6. When is your birthday?
7. Your address is …?
8. And your telephone number is …?

School

9. Let's talk about school. What grade are you in?
10. What is your teacher's name?
11. What grades are you getting?
12. What subjects do you like the best?
13. And what subjects do you like least?
14. What subjects give you the most trouble?
15. And what subjects give you the least trouble?
16. What activities are you in at school?
17. How do you get along with your classmates?
18. How do you get along with your teachers?
19. Tell me how you spend a usual day at school.

Home

20. Now let's talk about your home. Who lives with you at home?
21. Tell me a little about each of them.
22. What does your father do for work?
23. What does your mother do for work?
24. Tell me what your home is like.
25. Tell me about your room at home.
26. What chores do you do at home?
27. How do you get along with your father?
28. What does he do that you like?
29. What does he do that you don't like?
30. How do you get along with your mother?
31. What does she do that you like?
32. What does she do that you don't like?
33. (When relevant) How do you get along with your brothers and sisters?
34. What do they do that you like?
35. What do they do that you don't like?
36. Who handles the discipline at home?
37. Tell me about how they handle it.

Interests

38. Now let's talk about you. What hobbies and interests do you have?
39. What do you do in the afternoons after school?
40. Tell me what you usually do on Saturdays and Sundays.

Friends

41. Tell me about your friends.
42. What do you like to do with your friends?

Moods and Feelings

43. Everybody feels happy at times. What things make you feel happiest?
44. What are you most likely to get sad about?
45. What do you do when you are sad?
46. Everybody gets angry at times. What things make you angriest?
47. What do you do when you are angry?

Fears and Worries

48. All children get scared sometimes about some things. What things make you feel scared?
49. What do you do when you are scared?
50. Tell me what you worry about.
51. Any other things?

Self-Concerns

52. What do you like best about yourself?
53. Anything else?
54. What do you like least about yourself?
55. Anything else?
56. Tell me about the best thing that ever happened to you.
57. Tell me about the worst thing that ever happened to you.

Somatic Concerns

58. Do you ever get headaches?
59. (If yes) Tell me about them. (How often? What do you usually do?)
60. Do you get stomach aches?
61. (If yes) Tell me about them. (How often? What do you usually do?)
62. Do you get any other kinds of body pains?
63. (If yes) Tell me about them.

Thought Disorder

64. Do you ever hear things that seem funny or usual?
65. (If yes) Tell me about them. (How often? How do you feel about them? What do you usually do?)
66. Do you ever see things that seem funny or unreal?
67. (If yes) Tell me about them. (How often? How do you feel about them? What do you usually do?)

Memories and Fantasy

68. What is the first thing you can remember from the time you were a very little baby?
69. Tell me about your dreams.
70. Which dreams come back again?
71. Who are your favorite television characters?

BOX 36.2

Semi-structured Interview with School-Aged Children *(Continued)*

72. Tell me about them.
73. What animals do you like best?
74. Tell me about these animals.
75. What animals do you like least?
76. Tell me about these animals.
77. What is your happiest memory?
78. What is your saddest memory?
79. If you could change places with anyone in the whole world, who would it be?
80. Tell me about that.
81. If you could go anywhere you wanted to right now, where would you go?
82. Tell me about that.
83. If you could have three wishes, what would they be?
84. What things do you think you might need to take with you if you were to go to the moon and stay there for 6 months?

Aspirations

85. What do you plan on doing when you become an adult?
86. Do you think you will have any problem doing that?
87. If you could do anything you wanted when you become an adult, what would it be?

Concluding Questions

88. Do you have anything else that you would like to tell me about yourself?

89. Do you have any questions that you would like to ask me?

FOR ADOLESCENTS

These questions can be inserted after number 67.

Sexual Relations

1. Do you have any special girlfriend (boyfriend)?
2. (If yes) Tell me about her (him).
3. What kind of sexual concerns do you have?
4. (If present) Tell me about them.

Drug and Alcohol Use

5. Do your parents drink alcohol?
6. (If yes) Tell me about their drinking. (How much, how frequently, and where?)
7. Do your friends drink alcohol?
8. (If yes) Tell me about their drinking.
9. Do you drink alcohol?
10. (If yes) Tell me about your drinking.
11. Do your parents use drugs?
12. (If yes) Tell me about the drugs they use. (How much, how frequently, and for what reasons?)
13. Do your friends use drugs?
14. (If yes) Tell me about the drugs they use.
15. Do you use drugs?
16. (If yes) Tell me about the drugs you use.

KEYCONCEPT A **comprehensive assessment** includes a very detailed, focused interview that elicits all aspects of the responses and health promotion information that provides direction for care.

Preschool-Aged Children

When interviewing preschool-aged children, the nurse should understand that they may have difficulty putting their feelings into words and that their thinking is very concrete. For example, a preschool-aged child might assume that a tall container holds more water than a wide container even if both containers hold the same amount of fluid.

The nurse can achieve rapport with preschool-aged children by joining their world of play. Play is an activity by which children transform an experience from real life into a symbolic, nonliteral representation (Sezici, Ocakci, & Kadioglu, 2017). As a natural form of expression, play encourages verbalizations, promotes manual strength, teaches rules and problem solving, and helps children master control over their environment (Al-Yateem & Rossiter, 2016; Boyle-Toledo, 2019). With children younger than 5 years of age, the nurse may conduct the assessment in a playroom. Useful materials are

paper, pencils, crayons, paints, paint brushes, easels, clay, blocks, balls, dolls, doll houses, puppets, animals, dress-up clothes, and a water supply. The nurse must inform preschool-aged children about any rules for the play. For example, the nurse must tell the child that the nurse must ensure safety, so there will be no hitting in the playroom.

When observing the child in a free play setting, the nurse should pay attention to initiation of play, energy level, manipulative actions, tempo, body movements, tone, integration, creativity, products, age appropriateness, and attitudes toward adults. In addition, themes of play, expression of emotions, and temperament are important to observe. The nurse must allow children to direct and initiate these themes. When evaluating a young child's peer relationships through play therapy in a playgroup or school setting, observe play settings and themes, initiation of play, response to peer initiations of play, integration of affect and action during play, resolution of conflicts, responses to suggestions of others during play, and the ability to engage in role taking and role reversals.

The nurse's roles are to be a good listener; use appropriate vocabulary; tolerate a child's anxious, angry, or sad behavior; and use reflective comments about the child's play. Through play, the nurse can assess the

BOX 36.3

LIDZ Assessment Tool

Child's Name: _____ Birth Date: _____ Age: _____

Assessor: _____ Date of Assessment: _____

Describe typical play style/sequence.

Describe range of levels of play from lowest to highest level with age estimates and within contexts of independent/facilitated, familiar/unfamiliar, single/multiple toys.

Describe language and evidence of self-talk and internalized speech.

Describe interpersonal interactions with assessor and facilitator (if not assessor).

Describe content of any play themes.

What held the child's attention the longest? (For how long?) And what were the child's toy/play preferences?

Describe the child's affective state during play.

Implications of aforementioned for intervention.

Republished with permission of John Wiley & Sons from Lidz, C. S. (2003). Early childhood assessment (p. 92). Hoboken, NJ: John Wiley & Sons, Inc.; permission conveyed through Copyright Clearance Center, In

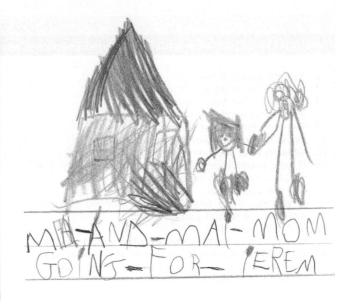

FIGURE 36.1   Me and my mom going for ice cream. Drawing and writing by a 5-year-old girl.

child's sensorimotor skills, cognitive style, adaptability, language functioning, emotional and behavioral responsiveness, social level, moral development, coping styles, problem-solving techniques, and approaches to perceiving and interpreting the surrounding world. Lidz (2003) developed a tool that clinicians can use to assess preschoolers' play (Box 36.3). Analyzing children's perceptions of fairy tales can provide clinicians with clues to culture, problems, solutions, and elements of mental functioning (Raufman & Weinberg, 2016).

Drawings may be used in conjunction with other assessment strategies, and are especially useful when assessing children who are less able to articulate their thoughts and emotions verbally. Through drawings, children can depict basic emotions such as happiness, sadness, fear, and anger. Social emotions, such as pride, shame, and jealousy, can also be conveyed through drawings (Fig. 36.1). Clinicians including child drawings in their assessments should note verbal, paraverbal, and nonverbal observations during the drawing activity. Assessment of human figure drawings generally include facial expressions, posture, and context included in the drawing (Kotroni, Bonoti, & Mavropoulou, 2019; Stauffer, 2019).

School-Aged Children

Unlike preschool-aged children, school-aged (5–11 years) children can use more constructs, provide longer descriptions and make better inferences of others, and acquire more complete conceptions of various social roles. Children in middle school are more capable of verbal exchange and can tolerate limited periods of direct questioning (Box 36.4). The nurse can establish rapport with school-aged children by using competitive board games, such as checkers and playing cards. A therapeutic

game helpful in assessing the child's perceptions, cognition, and emotions and in establishing rapport between a clinician and child is the thinking–feeling–doing game. In this game, the clinician and child take turns drawing cards that pose hypothetical situations and ask what a person might think, feel, or do in such scenarios. For example, one card might say, "A boy has something on his mind that he is afraid to tell his father. What is he scared to talk about?" Another might read, "A girl heard her parents fighting. What were they fighting about? What was the girl thinking while she listened to her parents?"

Adolescents

Adolescents have an increased command of language concepts and have developed the capacity for abstract and formal operations thinking. Their social world is also more complex. Some early adolescents tend to assume that their subjective experiences are real and congruent with objective reality, which can lead to egocentrism. Egocentrism includes the concepts of the imaginary audience (others are watching them) and the personal fable (they are special and unique and omnipotent) (Rycek et al., 1999). Egocentrism is a preoccupation with one's own appearance, behavior, thoughts, and feelings. For example, a preteen may think that he caused his parents to divorce because he fought with his father the day before the parents announced their decision to separate. Egocentrism is increased when emotions associated with uncertainty increase (Todd et al., 2016). Because teenagers have a heightened sense of self-consciousness, they may be preoccupied during the interview with applying makeup or other self-grooming tasks.

BOX 36.4

Psychiatric-Mental Health Nursing Assessment of Children and Adolescents

1. **Identifying information**
   Name
   Sex
   Date of birth
   Age
   Birth order
   Grade
   Ethnic background
   Religious preference
   List of others living in household
2. **Major reason for seeking help**
   Description of presenting problems or symptoms
   When did the problems (symptoms) start?
   Describe both the child's and the parent's perspective.
3. **Psychiatric history**
   Previous mental health contacts (inpatient and outpatient)
   Other mental health problems or psychiatric diagnosis (besides those described currently)
   Previous medications and compliance
   Family history of depression, substance abuse, psychosis, etc., and treatment
4. **Current and past health status**
   Medical problems
   Current medications
   Surgery and hospitalizations
   Allergies
   Diet and eating habits
   Sleeping habits
   Height and weight
   Hearing and vision
   Menstrual history
   Immunizations
   If sexually active, birth control method used
   Date of last physical examination
   Pediatrician or nurse practitioner's name and telephone number
5. **Medications**
   Prescription (dosage, side effects)
   Over-the-counter drugs
6. **Neurologic history**
   Right handed, left handed, or ambidextrous
   Headaches, dizziness, fainting
   Seizures
   Unusual movement (tics, tremors)
   Hyperactivity
   Episodes of weakness or paralysis
   Slurred speech, pronunciation problems
   Fine motor skills (eating with utensils, using crayon or pencil, fastening buttons and zippers, tying shoes)
   Gross motor skills and coordination (walking, running, hopping)
7. **Responses to mental health problems**
   What makes problems (symptoms) worse or better?
   Feelings about those experiences (what helped and did not help)
   What interventions have been tried so far?
   Major loss or changes in past year
   Fears, including punishment
8. **Mental status examination**
   See Box 36.5.
9. **Developmental assessment**
   Mother's pregnancy, delivery
   Child's Apgar score
   Physical maturation
   Psychosocial
   Language
   Developmental milestones: walking, talking, toileting
10. **Attachment, temperament or significant behavior patterns**
    Attachment
    Concentration, distractibility
    Eating and sleeping patterns
    Ability to adjust to new situations and changes in routine
    Usual mood and fluctuations
    Excitability
    Ability to wait, tendency to interrupt
    Responses to discipline
    Lying, stealing, fighting, cruelty to animals, fire setting
11. **Self-concept**
    Beliefs about self
    Body image
    Self-esteem
    Personal identity
12. **Risk assessment**
    History of suicidal thoughts, previous attempts
    Suicide ideation, plan, lethality of plan, accessibility of plan
    History of violent, aggressive behavior
    Homicidal ideation
13. **Family relationships**
    Relationship with parents
    Deaths or losses
    Family conflicts (nature and content)
    Disciplinary methods
    Quality of sibling relationship
    Sleeping arrangements
    Who does the child relate to or trust in the family?
    Relationships with extended family
14. **School and peer adjustment**
    Learning difficulties
    Behavior problems at school
    School attendance
    Relationship with teachers
    Special classes
    Best friend
    Relationships with peers
    Dating Drug and alcohol use
    Participation in sports, clubs, other activities
    After-school routine
15. **Community resources**
    Professionals or agencies working with child or family
    Day care resources
16. **Functional status**
    Global Assessment of Functioning Scale (GAF)
17. **Stresses and coping behaviors**
    Psychosocial stresses
    Coping behaviors (strengths)
18. **Summary of significant data**

During early adolescence, cognitive changes include increased self-consciousness, fear of being shamed, and demands for privacy and secrecy. An adolescent's willingness to talk to a nurse will depend partly on their perception of the degree of rapport between them. The nurse's ability to communicate, respect, cooperation, honesty, and genuineness is important. Rejection by the adolescent, even outright hostility, during the first few interactions is common, especially if the teen is having behavior problems at home, at school, or in the community. The nurse should be patient and avoid jumping to conclusions. Hostility or defiance may be a test of how much the teen can trust the nurse, a defense against anxiety, or a transference phenomenon (see Chapter 7).

Adolescents are likely to be defensive in front of their parents and concerned with confidentiality. At the start of the interview, the nurse should clearly convey to the adolescent what information will and will not be shared with parents. Adolescents generally prefer a straightforward, candid approach to the interview because they often distrust those in authority. Mentioning to adolescents that they do not have to discuss anything that they are not ready to reveal is also a good idea, so they will feel in control while they gradually build trust.

Mental Health Nursing Assessment of Children and Adolescents

As discussed, the comprehensive assessment of the child or adolescent includes interviews with the child and parents, child alone, and parents alone. After completing these components, the nurse should bring the child and parents back together to summarize their view of their concerns and to ask for feedback regarding whether these perceptions agree with theirs. The nurse must give the family a chance to share additional information and ask questions. Then the nurse should thank them for their willingness to talk and give them some idea of the next steps. Use of an assessment tool is helpful in organizing data for mental health planning and intervention.

When interviewing both a child and parents, directly asking the child as many questions as possible is generally the best way to get accurate, firsthand information and to reinforce interest in the child's viewpoint. Asking the child questions about the history of the current problem, previous psychiatric experiences (both good and bad), family psychiatric history, medical problems, developmental history (to get an idea of what the child has been told), school adjustment, peer relationships, and family functioning is particularly important. If necessary, the nurse can ask some or all of these same questions of the parents to verify the accuracy of the data, attain supplemental information, or both. Keep in mind that developmental research shows moderate to low correlation between parent and child reports of family behavior.

Children's Rating Scales for Psychiatric Disorders

A number of children's rating scales can assist in the assessment of various psychiatric disorders. The BASC, developed by Reynolds and Kamphouse (1998), is a tool used to measure behaviors and emotions in children aged 2 to 18 years. The scales include a teacher rating scale, a parent rating scale, and a 180-item self-report of personality. The scale evaluates several dimensions, including attitude to school, attitude toward teachers, sensation seeking, atypicality, locus of control, somatization, social stress, anxiety, depression, sense of inadequacy, relations with parents, interpersonal relations, self-esteem, and self-reliance. The CBCL, developed by Achenbach and Edelbrock (1983), is a 113-item self-report tool used to identify forms of psychopathology and competencies that occur in children aged 4 to 16 years. This instrument provides scores on internalizing and externalizing behaviors.

Several scales are useful for diagnosing specific problems in children and adolescents. The CDI, developed by John March (1997), is a 27-item self-rated symptom orientation scale for children aged 7 to 17 years that is useful for diagnosing physical symptoms, harm avoidance, social anxiety, and separation and panic disorder. The pediatric anxiety rating scale (PARS) developed by the Rupp Anxiety Study Group, is a clinician-administered, 50-item semi-structured interview used to assess severity of anxiety in children aged 6 to 17 years (Riddle et al., 2001). The Swanson, Nolan, and Pelham Scale, fourth revision (SNAP_IV), is a 90-item teacher and parent rating scale containing items from the Conners questionnaire for measuring inattention and overactivity (Swanson, 1983); it is useful for diagnosing ADHD (inattentive and impulsive types) and oppositional defiant disorder. The Children's Yale-Brown Obsessive Compulsive Scale, developed by Goodman et al. (1989), is a 19-item scale that can help diagnose childhood obsessive–compulsive disorder in children 6 to 17 years of age.

Safety Issues

The nurse must ask the child about any suicidal or violent thoughts. The best way to assess these areas is to ask straightforward questions, such as, "Have you ever thought about hurting yourself? Have you ever thought about hurting someone else? Have you ever acted on these thoughts? Have you thought about how you would do it? What did you think would happen if you hurt yourself? Have you ever done anything to hurt yourself before?" Contrary to popular belief, even young children attempt suicide, and they are capable of violent acts toward other children, adults, and animals. When a child shares the intent to commit a suicidal or violent act, the nurse must remind them that they will have to discuss this concern with the parent to keep the child and others safe.

Physical Health and Functioning

Nurses should include a thorough history of psychiatric and medical problems in any comprehensive assessment. A physical assessment is necessary to rule out any medical problems that could be mistaken for psychiatric symptoms (e.g., weight loss resulting from diabetes, not depression; substance-induced psychosis).

Genetic Vulnerability

The line between nature and nurture is not always clear. Characteristics that appear to be inborn may influence parents and teachers to respond differently toward different children, thus creating problems in the family environment. A phenomenon called **assortative mating** may contribute to the genetic transmission of psychiatric disorders.

Research increasingly shows that major psychiatric disorders (e.g., depression, anxiety disorder, schizophrenia, bipolar disorder, substance abuse) run in families. Thus, having a parent or sibling with a psychiatric disorder usually indicates an increased risk for the same or another closely related disorder in a child or adolescent. In addition, many childhood psychiatric disorders, such as autism, intellectual disability, developmental learning disorders, some language disorders (e.g., dyslexia), attention-deficit hyperactivity disorder (ADHD), and Tourette syndrome, appear to be genetically transmitted (Polimanti & Gelernter, 2017; Tsetsos et al., 2016).

> **KEYCONCEPT Assortative mating** is the tendency of individuals to select mates who are similar in genetically linked traits such as intelligence and personality style.

Neurologic Examination

A full neurologic evaluation is beyond the scope of practice for a baccalaureate-level or master's-level nurse without specific neuropsychiatric training. However, a screening of neurologic soft signs can help establish a database that will clarify the need for further neurologic consultation. The nurse should ask the brief neurologic screening questions suggested in Box 36.4 directly of the child and should also note any soft signs of neurologic dysfunction, such as slurred speech, unusual movements (e.g., tics, tremors), hyperactivity, and coordination problems. The nurse can ask young children to hop on one foot, skip, or walk from toe to heel to assess their gross motor coordination and to draw with a crayon or pencil or play pickup sticks or jacks to assess their fine motor coordination.

Medication

Pharmacologic assessment should include prescription and over-the-counter medications. Nurses should ask about any allergies to food, medications, or environmental triggers. Compliance with the prescribed regimen should be assessed. Specifically, the nurse should assess whether the medication is producing the desired effect, the presence of adverse effects, and logistical barriers associated with obtaining or administering the medication (Brinkman, Simon, & Epstein, 2017). Individuals taking medications requiring dosing during school hours may find administration to be disruptive to their day, thus individualized treatment options should be considered (Aston, Wilson, & Terry, 2019).

Substance Use

Substance abuse disorders across the life span account for more deaths, illness, and disabilities than any other preventable health condition. Screening for potential use and abuse of substances is becoming a priority in mental health assessment of adolescents. House (2002) developed an interview protocol that can be useful in identifying substance abuse problems in youth (Box 36.6). It is important to determine the use of substances, including prescription drugs and polysubstance use. The child and family should be referred to community resources. The *Adolescent Screening, Brief Intervention and Referral for Treatment for Alcohol and other Drug Use (SBIRT) Toolkit for Providers* is a useful resource (Levy & Shrier, 2015).

Psychological Assessment

Children can usually identify and discuss what improves or worsens their problems. The assessment may be the first time that someone has asked the child to explain their view of the problem. It is also a perfect opportunity to discuss any life changes or losses (e.g., death of grandparents or pets, parental divorce) and fears, especially of punishment.

Mental Status Examination

As discussed in Chapter 11, the mental status examination is an organized systematic approach to assessment of an individual's current psychiatric condition. It is essential in formulating a diagnosis. It can provide initial data that alert the clinician to obtain further cognitive, neurologic, or psychological testing. The mental status examination of children combines observation and direct questioning (Box 36.5). The nurse should note any areas where the child or adolescent is symptomatic or has difficulty with the task. A mental status examination should be obtained

BOX 36.5

Mental Status Examination

APPEARANCE

Provide a head-to-toe assessment: Describe head shape and size (Down syndrome, fragile X syndrome, Turner syndrome, fetal alcohol syndrome), eyes (clarity, gaze, glasses, eye contact), height, weight, cleanliness, facial expressions, mannerisms, ears, hearing, skin (bruising could indicate physical abuse), gait, posture, nutritional status (possible eating disorder).

Evaluate dress: Is it appropriate for the weather? Does the child wear shirts with logos or groups? Does the child appear older or younger looking? Inquire about symptoms of physical illness.

MOTOR ACTIVITY

Use the following descriptors to assess motor activity: calm, psychomotor retardation, akathisia, agitated, hyper-alertness, tics, muscle spasms, nail biting, hyperactivity, anxiety, restlessness, or compulsions.

SELF-CONCEPT

Ask about play, favorite stories, and three wishes. Ask the child to draw a self-portrait, describe best-liked and least-liked qualities. Ask what they imagine doing for an occupation when grown up. Also evaluate planning ability and sense of a future.

BEHAVIOR

Observe for temper tantrums, attention span, separation from family member, self-care activities, dressing, toileting, feeding, oppositionality, compliance, and so on.

SOCIAL INTERACTION

How does the child relate to the examiner? Is the child wary, submissive, attentive, friendly, manipulative, approval seeking, conforming, hostile, or guarded? Assess the child's relationships with the child's parent or guardian, siblings, and friends.

GENERAL INTELLIGENCE

Assess the child's general vocabulary, fund of knowledge, alertness, orientation, concentration, memory, calculations, organization, abstract reasoning creativity, spontaneity, and frustration tolerance. Ask about school, including regular or special education, grades, and grade retention.

FUND OF KNOWLEDGE

Ask child the following: How many legs does a dog have? How many pennies in a nickel? Have child identify body parts, draw a person, name colors, count as high as possible, and inquire about letter identification (younger children).

Inquire about the time. How many states are in the United States? Who was George Washington? How many days are in a week? What are the seasons of the year? (middle schoolers) What does the stomach do? Who is Charles Darwin? (teenagers)

ORIENTATION

Ask questions such as the following: How old are you? Who is the current president of the United States? Do you know who was the president before our current president?

What are two major news events in the past month? (older children)
What are the year, seasons, date, day, and month?
Where are we? (country, state, city, clinic)

RECENT MEMORY

Ask the child to repeat a memory phrase; remember three to five objects that you say or show and then recall them in a few minutes. Ask the following: What school do you currently attend? What did you have for breakfast or lunch today?

REMOTE MEMORY

Ask questions such as the following: What did you do last weekend? What was your last birthday like? What is your address and telephone number? Who is your first best friend? How old were you when you learned to ride a bike? What was the name of your kindergarten teacher?

ABSTRACT REASONING AND ANALOGIES

Ask what is meant by a stitch in time saves nine; a rolling stone gathers no moss; a bird in the hand is worth two birds in a tree; too many cooks spoil the broth.

Which object does not belong in this group: fish, tree, rock? Why?

Assess the similarity about objects such as peaches and lemons, oceans and lakes, a pencil and typewriter, a bicycle and a bus.

To evaluate comparative ability complete this sentence: An engine is to an airplane as an oar is to a _____.

ARITHMETIC CALCULATIONS

Provide simple addition and subtraction questions based on the child's age. Ask older children multiplication and division problems. Count backward 20 to 1 for younger children. Ask how many quarters are in $3.50 or if you buy something that cost $2.50 and you have $5, how much change you will receive.

WRITING AND SPELLING ABILITY

Ask a first or second grader to spell *cat*, *hat*, *bad*, *old*, *dog*. Ask a third or fourth grader to spell words such as *clock*, *face*, *house*, or *flower*. Ask older children to write a sentence such as: "The grass is greener on the mountains."

READING

Have the child read a paragraph from an age-appropriate book? Reading begins in first grade. Children should demonstrate basic reading skills by the end of second grade.

GROSS MOTOR SKILLS

Assess level of activity, type of activity, and any unusual gestures or mannerisms and compulsions.

Have the patient walk, jump, hop on one foot, and walk heel to toe, throw a ball, balance and climb stairs.

By age 3 years, a child should walk up stairs with alternating feet, pedal a tricycle, jump in one place, and broad jump.

By age 4 years, a child can balance on one foot for 5 seconds, and catch a bounced ball two of three times.

By age 5 years, a child can do heel-to-toe walking.

(Continued)

BOX 36.5

Mental Status Examination *(Continued)*

By age 6 years, a child should jump, tumble, skip, hop, walk a straight line, skip rope with practice, and ride a bicycle.

By age 7 years, a child should skip and play hopscotch, and run and climb with coordination.

By age 9 years, a child should have highly developed eye–hand coordination.

FINE MOTOR SKILLS

Have the child draw a picture or self-portrait as well as pickup sticks.

Have the child copy a design that you have drawn. Ask the child to draw a circle (age 3 years), an X (age 3 to 4 years), a square (age 5 years), a triangle (age 6 years), a diamond (age 7 years), and connecting diamonds (age 8 years).

At age 3 years, a child should unbutton front buttons, copy a vertical line, copy a circle, and build an eight-block tower.

By age 4 years, a child should copy a cross and button large buttons.

By age 5 years, a child should dress themselves with minimal assistance, color within lines, and draw a three-part human.

By age 6 years, a child should be able to draw a six-part human.

By age 7 years, a child should print well and begin to write script.

By age 8 years, a child should demonstrate mature handwriting skills.

ATTENTION SPAN

Ask the patient to follow a series of short commands. Observe motor activity, attention, concentration, impulsivity, hyperactivity, outbursts, and organization.

Observe the child's ability to stay on task and focus during the course of the interview. Tasks include counting backward by seven, spelling the word "world" backward, and saying the letters of the alphabet backward.

INSIGHT AND JUDGMENT

Ask the child to provide a solution to a hypothetical situation such as what would you do if you found a stamped envelope lying on the ground? What would you do if a policeman stopped you for driving your bike through a red light? What would you do if you saw two children fighting on the school ground? Assess the child's ideas about the current problem and the solutions tried so far. Assess if child can make use of assistance. Evaluate how impaired child is in activities of daily living, including attending school, attending recreational activities, making friends, self-care activities, and so on.

COMPREHENSION

Read a few pages or paragraphs from a short book or newspaper article and ask the child to relate what happened in the story.

MOOD AND FEELINGS

Affect is the child's emotional tone. Evaluate the child's range of emotions, intensity, and appropriateness.

Assess for any mood swings, crying, anxiety, depression, anger, hostility, hyperalertness, lability, or pressured speech. Assess mood by asking how many times a week do you feel sad and how often do you cry? What makes you sad, angry, anxious, and so on? Risk assessment questions include the following: Have you ever felt like hurting yourself or someone else? Do you have a plan to hurt yourself? Have you ever done anything to hurt yourself in the past?

THOUGHT PROCESS AND CONTENT

Were there any recurrent themes?

Observe the child's patterns of thinking for appropriateness of sequence, logic, coherence, and relevance to the topics discussed. Does the child talk about age-appropriate topics; is there any thought blocking, or disturbance in the stream of thinking, repetition of words, circumstantial or tangential thinking, perseverations, preoccupations, obsessive thoughts, actions, or compulsive behaviors, any grandiose reasoning, ideas of reference, or paranoia (feelings of being watched or followed, controlled, manipulated, and ritual or checking routines)?

Evaluate the child's perceptions for hallucinations (false perceptions or false impressions or experiences) and delusions (false beliefs that contradict social reality, such as hears voices, sees images or shadowy figures, smells offensive odors, tastes offensive flavors, feels worms crawling on skin). Assess hallucinations in all five senses: auditory, visual, tactile, gustatory, and olfactory. Assess for command hallucinations, which tell the patient to do something.

SPEECH AND LANGUAGE

Note any speech impediments and incongruence between verbal and nonverbal communication. Show a pencil and a watch and ask the patient to name them. Have the patient repeat "no ifs, ands, or buts."

Assess communication skills, including expressive language, vocabulary, and the ability to understand what you are saying (receptive language). Check voice quality, articulation, pronunciation, fluency, rhythm, rate, and ease of expression and volume.

Assess comprehension by giving the child a task. Assess coherence for flight of ideas, loose associations, word salad (meaningless, disconnected word choices), neologisms, clang associations (words that rhyme in a nonsensical way), echolalia (repetition of another person's words), thought blocking, perseveration, irrelevance, and vagueness. Check for aphasia by listening for an omission or addition of letters, syllables, and made-up words or misuse or transposition of words.

BOX 36.6

Practice Note: An Interview Protocol for Reviewing Chemical Use in Youths

As with other topics, questions about substance use are interactive—the answers given determine to some extent the subsequent questions. However, certain topics and areas should be addressed irrespective of the previous responses. In the following sample questions, those marked with an asterisk should always be asked.

- Now I'd like to ask you about your experience with cigarettes, alcohol, and other drugs.
- When was the last time you smoked tobacco?
- Have you ever smoked? Tell me about that.
- How old were you when you first smoked a cigarette?
- How many cigarettes do you smoke a day now?
- How long have you smoked this much?
- Where do you usually do your smoking?
- Where do you usually get your cigarettes from?
- What kind of problems has smoking caused for you?
- How do your parents feel about your smoking?
- Have you gotten into trouble at school for smoking?
- Have you lost any friends or had problems with friends over smoking?
- What other tobacco products have you used?
- When was the last time you drank any alcohol?
- How much alcohol did you drink? What kinds of alcohol were you drinking? What happened afterward?
- Who was with you the last time you were drinking? What happened?
- How about the time before that? Tell me about that.
- What is the most alcohol you have ever drunk? What happened?
- How do you get alcohol?
- What kinds of problems have drinking caused for you?
- How do your parents feel about your drinking?
- Have you ever gotten into problems at school because of drinking?
- Have you ever gotten into legal problems because of drinking?
- Have you had problems with your friends because of drinking?

- What is the worst thing that has happened while you were drinking?
- How old were you the first time you drank alcohol? When did most of your friends start drinking? How does your drinking compare with other kids in your classes at school or other kids your age?
- How has your drinking changed over the past year?
- When was the last time you used any marijuana?
- How old were you when you first tried marijuana?
- How often have you used marijuana in the past month?
- What's usually going on when you use marijuana?
- What other drugs have you used?
- When was the first time you used _____?
- When was the last time you used _____?
- How many times have you used _____?
- Where did you get the _____? How did you know that's what it was?
- How did _____ affect you?
- What has been the biggest effect you have gotten using _____?
- What has been the worst thing about using _____?
- Have you ever 'huffed' or inhaled something to get high? Tell me about that.
- Have you ever used another person's prescription medications? Tell me about that.
- How many people do you regularly do things with—hang out, party with, talk to?
- How many of your friends smoke tobacco occasionally?
- How many of your friends smoke tobacco regularly?
- How many of your friends drink alcohol occasionally?
- How many of your friends drink alcohol regularly?
- How many of your friends smoke marijuana occasionally?
- How many of your friends smoke marijuana regularly?
- What other drugs do your friends use?
- How has drug use affected your friends?

The first session with children and adolescents: conducting a comprehensive mental health evaluation by House, Alvin E. Reproduced with permission of Guilford via Copyright Clearance Center.

---

on subsequent visits so improvements or changes in the patient's functioning can be noted.

The nurse should note the child's general appearance, including the level of attractiveness. Although it perhaps should not be so, social–psychological research shows that the appearance and attractiveness of both children and adults strongly influence their social relationships (Jacobson, Trivers, & Palestis, 2020). The nurse also should note the following:

- Do they seem to have difficulty focusing on the interview, sitting still, refraining from impulsive behavior, and listening without interrupting? (possible signs of ADHD)
- Does the child seem underactive, lethargic, distant, or hopeless? (possible signs of depression)

- Are there problems with speech patterns, such as rate (overly fast or slow), clarity, and volume, or any speech dysfluencies (e.g., stuttering, halting)?
- Are there possible mood disorders (e.g., depression, mania), language disorders, or psychotic processes?

When assessing thought processes, keep in mind that whereas young children are in the concrete operations stage, middle schoolers can begin to use logic and understand conversations. Adolescents should be able to demonstrate abstract thinking and think hypothetically, although they may appear to be self-conscious and introspective. Assessment of preteens and adolescents should address substance use and sexual activity because responses may provide useful information about high-risk behavior or substance abuse. In addition, the nurse should inquire about any obsessions or compulsions (e.g., worries about germs, severe handwashing).

Temperament and Behavior

Temperament is a person's characteristic intensity, activity level, threshold of responsiveness, rhythmicity, adaptability, energy expenditure, and mood. According to research findings, temperamental differences can be observed early in life, suggesting that they are at least partly biologically determined, and patterns of temperament can be correlated with emotional and behavioral problems (Van Heel et al., 2020). When looking at the cerebral activity in 9-month-old infants, consistent with early development of externalizing behaviors, electro-encephalographic activity increased in response to fear rather than love and comfort (Santesso, Schmidt, & Trainor, 2007).

The classic *New York Longitudinal Study* (Thomas, Chess, & Birch, 1968) identified three main patterns of temperament seen in infancy that often extend into childhood and later life:

- *Easy temperament* characterized by a positive mood, regular patterns of eating and sleeping, positive approach to new situations, and low emotional intensity
- *Difficult temperament* characterized by irregular sleep and eating patterns, negative response to new stimuli, slow adaptation, negative mood, and high emotional intensity
- *Slow-to-warm-up temperament* characterized by a negative, mildly emotional response to new situations that is expressed with intensity and initially slow adaptation but evolves into a positive response

On the positive side, an easy temperament can serve as a protective factor against the development of psychopathology. Children with easy temperaments can adapt to change without intense emotional reactions. Difficult temperament places children at high risk for adjustment problems, such as with adjustment to school or bonding with parents.

Temperament has a major influence on the chances that a child may experience psychological problems; however, temperament is not unchangeable, and environmental influences can change or modify a child's emotional style (Miller et al., 2020). Children who respond positively to the environment continue in this pattern. Children who have other temperaments may develop positive temperaments at a later time.

The concept of temperament provides an excellent example of the interaction between biologic–genetic and environmental factors in producing child psychopathology. Although a child may be born with a particular temperament, longitudinal studies show that the temperament can be influenced by other factors such as parental

control (Elizur, Somech, & Vinokur, 2017). However, difficult children, in particular, may evoke negative reactions in parents and teachers, thereby creating environments that exacerbate their biologically based behavior problems, initiating a vicious cycle. Difficult temperament that persists beyond 3 years of age is correlated with the development of child psychopathology (Kushner, 2015). The nurse can help parents accept biologically based differences in their children and learn to adapt their behavior to each child's needs.

Developmental Assessment

Children respond to life's stresses in different ways and in accord with their developmental level. Knowing the difference between normal child development and psychopathology is crucial in helping parents view their children's behavior realistically and respond appropriately. The key areas for assessment include maturation, psychosocial development, and language.

Maturation

Healthy development of the brain and nervous system during childhood and adolescence provides the foundation for successful functioning throughout life. Such development, called maturation, unfolds through sequential and orderly growth processes. These processes are biologically and genetically based but depend on constant interactions with a stimulating and nurturing environment. If trauma or neglect impairs the process of normal biologic maturation, developmental delays and disorders that may not be fully reversible can result. For example, babies born with fetal alcohol syndrome experience permanent brain damage, often resulting in intellectual disability, learning disabilities, behavior disorders, and delays in language (Patel et al., 2020). A pregnant woman's use of crack cocaine deprives the fetus of nutrients and oxygen, leading to developmental delays, speech and language problems, deformities, and behavior disorders (e.g., impulsivity, withdrawal, hyperactivity). The nurse can assess for developmental delays by asking questions from specific sections of the mental status examination:

- *Intellectual functioning:* Evaluate the child's creativity, spontaneity, ability to count money and tell time, academic performance, memory, attention, frustration tolerance, and organization.
- *Gross motor functioning:* Ask the child to hop on one foot, throw a ball, walk up and down the hall, and run.
- *Fine motor functioning:* Ask the child to draw a picture or pick up sticks.
- *Cognition:* The nurse can evaluate the child's general level of cognition by assessing the child's vocabulary, level of comprehension, drawing ability,

and responsiveness to questions. Testing, such as the Wechsler Intelligence Scale for Children (WISC-III), provides measures of intelligence quotient (IQ). A psychologist usually performs such tests. The nurse can request cognitive testing if they have concerns about a child's developmental delays or learning disabilities.

- *Thinking and perception:* Evaluate level of consciousness; orientation to date, time, and person; thought content; thought process; and judgment.
- *Social interactions and play:* Assess the child's organization, creativity, drawing capacity, and ability to follow rules. Children experiencing developmental delays may remain engaged solely in parallel play instead of moving to reciprocal play. They may consistently play with toys designed for younger children, draw crude body pictures, or display receptive or expressive language problems.

Psychosocial Development

Assessment of psychosocial development is very important for children with mental health problems. Various theoretical models are available from which to choose; the most commonly used model is Erikson stages of development. When considering this model, the nurse should examine the child's gender and cultural background for appropriateness. The nurse also may use the Gilligan model (see Chapter 7).

Language

At birth, infants can emit sounds of all languages. Maturation of language skills begins with babbling, or the utterance of simple, spontaneous sounds. By the end of the first year, children can make one-word statements, usually naming objects or people in the environment. By age 2 years, they should speak in short, telegraphic sentences consisting of a verb and noun (e.g., "want cookie"). Between ages 2 and 4 years, vocabulary and sentence structure develop rapidly. In fact, a preschooler's ability to produce language often surpasses motor development, sometimes causing temporary stuttering when the child's mind literally works faster than their mouth.

Language development depends on the complex interaction of physical maturation of the nerves, development of head and neck musculature, hearing abilities, cognitive abilities, exposure to language, educational stimulation, and emotional well-being. Social needs create a natural inclination toward communication, but children need reinforcement to develop correct pronunciation, vocabulary, and grammar.

Before a diagnosis of a communication disorder (i.e., impairment in language expression, comprehension, or both) can be made, the child must be tested to rule out hearing, visual, or other neurologic problems. Brain damage, especially to the left hemisphere (dominant for language in most individuals), can seriously impair the development of communication abilities in children. Any child who has experienced brain damage from anoxia at birth, congenital trauma, head injury, infection, tumor, or drug exposure should be closely monitored for signs of a communication disorder. Before the age of 5 years, the brain has amazing plasticity, and sometimes other intact areas of the brain can take over functions of damaged areas, especially with immediate speech therapy. Genetically based disorders such as autism cause language delays that are sometimes permanent and severe.

The nurse must recognize normal variations in child development and assess lags in the development of vocabulary and sentence structure during the critical preschool years. Delays in this area can seriously affect other areas, such as cognitive, educational, and social development. Many children who receive psychiatric treatment have speech and language disorders that are sometimes undetected, either leading to or compounding their emotional problems (Koomar & Michaelson, 2020).

Self-Concept

For young children, eliciting their view of themselves and the world is helpful. One technique is asking them what they would wish for if they had three wishes. Answers can be revealing. Whereas an inability to wish for anything beyond a nice meal or place to live may reflect hopelessness, wishes to conquer the world or put one's teacher in jail may indicate feelings of grandiosity. Another technique is to tell a story and ask the child to make up an ending for it. For example, a baby bird fell out of a nest—what happened to it? The nurse may design stories to elicit particular fears or concerns that may be relevant for the individual child.

Drawings also provide an excellent window into the child's internal world (Fig. 36.2). Asking the child to draw a picture of a person can provide data about the child's self-concept, sexual identity, body image, and developmental level. By age 3 years, children should be able to draw some facial features and limbs, but their drawings may have an "X-ray" quality, in which clothing is transparent and the body can be seen underneath. Older children should produce more sophisticated drawings unless they are resistant to the task. After the child has finished the drawing, the nurse can ask what the person in the drawing is thinking and feeling, using this device to assess the child's mental processes. For example, one adolescent with school phobia drew a person fully dressed, in great detail, but with no feet. When asked about the drawing, he said that the boy could not go anywhere because his mother was afraid to let him leave home.

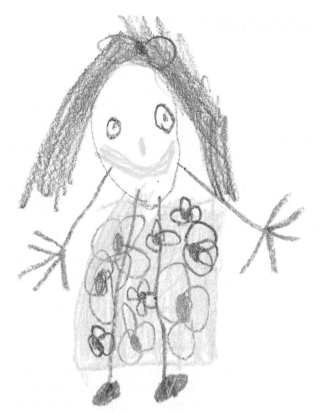

FIGURE 36.2   Self portrait of a girl, age 5 years.

Other ways to assess children's self-concepts include asking them what they want to do when they grow up, what their best subjects are in school, what things they are really good at, and how well-liked they are at school. Before concluding the individual interview with a child, the nurse should always ask if the child has any other information to share and whether they have any questions.

Stress and Coping Behaviors

Physical, behavioral, and personality predispositions; family; and community environment may affect a child's ability to cope with stressful life events. Stressful experiences for children include the death of a loved person or pet, parental divorce, violence, physical illness (especially chronic illness), mental illness, social isolation, racial discrimination, neglect, and physical and sexual abuse.

The number of stressful events that a child experiences (including trauma), the supports that the child has in place, and the child's developmental stage may also influence their ability to cope with stressors. Children who appear to have experienced early life stress may manifest posttraumatic stress symptoms (Lee & Oswald, 2018). It is important to consider a stressful situation within the context of each child's support system and developmental stage.

Attachment

Attachment is the emotional bond between an infant and their parental figure. Studies of attachment show that the quality of the emotional bond between the infant and parental figures provides the groundwork for future relationships. The need to touch and be close to a parental figure appears biologically driven and has been demonstrated in classic studies of monkeys who bonded with a terry-cloth surrogate mother (Harlow, Harlow, & Suomi, 1971). A secure attachment is based on the caretaker's consistent, appropriate response to the infant's attachment behaviors (e.g., crying, clinging, calling, following, protesting). Children who have developed a secure attachment protest when their parents leave them (beginning at about age 6 to 8 months), seek comfort from their parents in unfamiliar situations, and playfully explore the environment in the parent's presence. Mother–child separation for 1 week or longer within the first 2 years of life has been shown to be related to higher levels of child negativity (at age 3 years) and aggression (at ages 3 to 5 years) (Martin et al., 2011).

Secure attachments in early childhood produce cooperative, harmonious parent–child relationships in which the child is responsive to the parents' socialization efforts and likely to adopt the parents' viewpoints, values, and goals. Securely attached young children also socialize competently, are popular with well-acquainted peers during the preschool years, and have warm relationships with important adults in their lives. Securely attached children see themselves and others constructively and have relatively sophisticated emotional and moral understanding (Behrendt et al., 2019).

Although the importance of the parent's responsiveness is unquestionable in determining the development of a secure attachment, the process works both ways. Some babies seem to encourage attachment naturally with their parents by responding positively to holding, cuddling, and comforting behaviors. Others, such as those with developmental delays or autistic disorders, may respond less readily and even reject parental attempts at bonding.

Attachment Theories

Bowlby's early studies (1969) of maternal deprivation formed the initial framework for attachment theory based on the notion that the infant tends to bond to one primary parental figure, usually the mother. Although this pattern is common, recent studies show that children make multiple attachments to parents and other caregivers, but high-quality, intense bonds remain essential for healthy development. Contemporary nursing theories, such as Barnard parent–child interaction model, have stressed the importance of the interaction between the child's spontaneous behavior and biologic rhythms and the mother's ability to respond to cues that signal distress (Barnard & Brazelton, 1990). Whereas a positive attachment is likely to result in a happy child with a sense of self-worth, insecure attachment is associated with depressive symptoms (Spruit et al., 2020). Although most attachment research has been done with mothers, the father's role in child development has become better understood through research done during the past two decades. Fathers' emotional support tends to enhance the quality of mother–child relationships and facilitates positive adjustment by children. When fathers are unsupportive and marital conflict is high, children suffer (Silva & Calheiros, 2018).

Fathers play an important role in children's play, which affects the quality of the child's attachment. Playful interactions involving emotional arousal provide an especially good opportunity to learn how to get along with peers by reinforcing turn taking, affect regulation, and acceptable ways of competing. Fathers are important as role models who assist in their sons' identity formation and serve as models of gender-appropriate behavior, particularly around aggressive behavior. Evidence supports the importance of including the father in the mental health assessment of his child (Verschueren, 2020).

Disrupted Attachments

Disrupted attachments may result from deficits in infant attachment behaviors, lack of responsiveness by caregivers to the child's cues, or both and may lead to reactive attachment disorder, feeding disorder, failure to thrive, or anxiety disorder. A reactive attachment disorder is a state in which a child younger than 5 years of age fails to initiate or respond appropriately to social interaction and the caregiver subsequently disregards the child's physical and emotional needs. Attachment disorder behaviors are related to attention and behavior problems (Bizzi & Pace, 2020).

Attachment disorganization is a consequence of extreme insecurity that results from feared or actual separation from the attached figure. Disorganized infants appear to be unable to maintain the strategic adjustments in attachment behavior represented by organized avoidant or ambivalent attachment strategies, with the result that both behavioral and physiologic dysregulation occurs. Preschoolers with disorganized attachment manifest behaviors of fear, contradictory behavior, or disorientation or disassociation in the caregivers' presence. Attachment disorganization appears moderately stable over time and has been associated with distinct, apparently genetically based, physiologic profiles (Golds, de Kruiff, & MacBeth, 2020).

Social Network

Family Relationship

Children depend on adults to create a safe, nurturing, and appropriate environment to support their development. The nurse should assess the quality of the home, including living space, sleeping arrangements, safety, cleanliness, and child care arrangements, either through a home visit or by discussing these issues with the family. When gathering a family history, a genogram and timeline are useful tools to map family members' birth order and medical and psychiatric histories; family roles, norms, boundaries, strengths, and family subgroups; birth dates, deaths, and relationships; stage in the family cycle; and critical events. To understand fully the family's values, goals, and beliefs, the nurse must consider the family's ethnic, cultural, and economic background throughout the assessment. A comprehensive family assessment should be considered (see Chapter 15).

School and Peer Adjustment

The child's adjustment to school is also significant. Often, children are referred for a mental health assessment as a result of changes in behavior at school. Falling grades, loss of interest in normal activities, decreased concentration, or withdrawal from or aggression toward peers may indicate that the child is experiencing emotional problems. It is very important that the nurse obtain signed permission from the parents to talk to the child's teacher for their observations of the child. The nurse may want to observe the child in school, if feasible, to see how the child functions there. The parent can request a treatment planning conference in which the teacher, parent, and nurse discuss the child's school performance and plan ways to promote the child's emotional, cognitive, and social functioning in school. Suggestions may range from having the child tested for learning disabilities to designing behavior plans that include rewards for improved functioning, such as computer time at the end of the day.

Peers are an important aspect of child and adolescent social development. Assessment of peer relationships and activities with friends provides a rich source of information about the adolescent. Assessment of victimization by peers in the form of bullying is important because it can have a negative impact on social development and self-esteem.

Children and Adolescents Who Identify as LGBTQ

Children and adolescents who identify as Lesbian, gay, bisexual, transgender, questioning/queer (LGBTQ) are highly stigmatized and often face discrimination and victimization because they do not adhere to conventional gender expectations. Transgender children and youth are especially affected by lack of understanding and social support. The health and mental health care needs of these children and adolescents are unique, and they often have difficulty accessing health care services (Romanelli & Lindsey, 2020).

Mental health problems are the leading causes of morbidity and mortality in this population. LGBTQ youth have a higher risk for depression, suicide, and substance use than other adolescents. They are also at increased risk for violence, including being targeted with bullying, teasing, harassment, and physical assault (Centers for Disease Control and Prevention [CDC], 2021). Social prejudice, family rejection, and self-nonacceptance are major risk factors. Protective factors include self-esteem, social support at home, positive relationships with peers, and positive school climates. It is important that the nurse inquire about anti-LGBTQ experiences that could lead to increased mental health problems. For children and adolescents to thrive, it is essential that they feel socially, emotionally, and physically safe and supported. Nurses can contribute to creating safe spaces by helping to create policies that support LGBTQ youth, participating in LGBTQ-related trainings, incorporating inclusive language in their communication, normalizing the use of pronouns, and providing an environment (physical or digital) where the individual can freely seek care without stigma (Advocates for Youth, 2021).

Functional Status

Functional status is evaluated in children and adolescents using the Global Assessment of Functioning (GAF) scale, which tallies behaviors related to school, peers, activity level, mood, speech, family relationships, behavioral problems, self-care skills, and self-concept. The GAF scale ranges from 0 to 100; the lower the score, the higher the level of impairment, indicated by psychiatric symptoms and level of general functioning. For example, a score of 30 may indicate that the child is severely homicidal or suicidal and has made previous attempts, that hallucinations or delusions influence the child's behavior, or that the child has serious impairment in communication or judgment. Moderate impairment scores usually fall in the range of 51 to 69. Indications of moderate impairment include difficulty in one area, such as school phobia, that hinders school attendance or performance, while the child is functioning well within other areas, such as with family and peers. Children in this category are not homicidal or suicidal and usually respond well to outpatient interventions. A score of 70 to 100 usually indicates that the child is functioning well in relation to school, peers, family, and community. The GAF is always measured at the initial assessment so treatment can be evaluated for symptom improvement.

Social Systems

Youth in healthy communities have been shown to be more likely to attend religious services, to believe their schools were places of caring and encouragement, to be involved in structured activities, and to remain committed to their own learning. Assessing the child's economic status, access to medical care, adequate home environment, exposure to environmental toxins (e.g., lead), neighborhood safety, and exposure to violence is important because these community factors place the child at risk (Pearce et al., 2019).

Children and adolescents function better if they are linked to community supports, such as churches, recreational programs, park district programming, and after-school programming. The Big Brother/Big Sister program fosters mentoring relationships for children. A parent or child may call the local Big Brother/Big Sister organization to request a mentor for the child. The mentor may perform a wide range of services, from taking a child to community events, helping with homework, or talking about how the child can achieve their dreams and goals. Some towns offer community-based juvenile justice programs to rehabilitate children who have had altercations with the legal system. Juvenile justice programs provide support, such as individual and family counseling and prosocial recreational activities; teach children how to make positive choices about spending free time; and closely monitor their behaviors.

Religious and Spiritual Assessment

Spiritual assessment is an integral part of a mental health assessment. There is a growing body of research suggesting that religious and spiritual practices may promote both physical and mental health (Gwin et al., 2020). The Joint Commission requires that each psychiatric evaluation include spiritual assessment questions.

Questioning about a patient's spiritual life should include interviewing strategies that are unbiased and facilitate understanding of the client's spiritual values. Questions can include but are not limited to the child's and family's specific faith background, level of activity with that group, support received from spiritual practices, religious rituals of importance, and religious influences on lifestyle and health choices. During a child interview, appropriate questions include, "Where is God?" or asking if the child could talk to God.

Childhood Sexual Abuse

There are several special considerations in interviewing an abused child. First, the nurse must establish a safe and supportive environment in which to conduct the evaluation. Second, the nurse needs to understand the forensic implications of assessment so that the interview format will be acceptable for disclosure in a court hearing. The American Academy of Pediatrics offers practice guidelines for evaluating children who may have been abused (Adams et al., 2016). If the child reports abuse, the nurse has a legal responsibility to report the abuse to child protection agencies. The nurse must use the same language and vocabulary that the child uses to describe the abuse or anatomical terms and ask nonleading questions. Nursing professionals who regularly interview children who have been abused may have special training in the use of anatomically correct dolls to obtain information about the abuse.

SUMMARY OF KEY POINTS

- Mental health assessment of children and adolescents includes evaluating the child's biologic, psychological, and social factors, primarily through interviewing and observation.

- Assessment of children and adolescents differs from assessment of adults in that the nurse must consider the child's developmental level, specifically addressing the child's language, cognitive, social, and emotional skills. Establishing a treatment alliance and building rapport are essential to obtaining a good mental health history.

- The mental status examination includes observations and questions about the child's appearance, motor activity, self-concept, behavior, social interaction, general intelligence, fund of knowledge, attention span, insight and judgment, comprehension, mood and feelings, thought process and content, speech and language, orientation, memory, reasoning, writing and spelling, reading, and motor skills. Assessment of the child and caregiver together provides important information regarding child–parent attachment and parenting practices.

- The three main types of temperament include the easy temperament, difficult temperament, and slow-to-warm-up temperament. Temperament can be evaluated by assessing the child's sleep and eating habits, mood, emotional intensity, and responses to new stimuli.

- A child's self-concept can be evaluated using tools such as play, stories, asking three wishes, and asking the child to draw a picture of themselves.

- If a child reveals suicidal ideation in the interview, the nurse must determine whether the child has a plan; let the parent know the child is suicidal; and make a plan to keep the child safe, such as inpatient hospitalization.

- If a child reports to the nurse neglect or physical or sexual abuse, the nurse must by law report the child's disclosure to the state's DCF.

CRITICAL THINKING CHALLENGES

1. An adolescent is hostile and refuses to talk in an interview. How would you respond?

2. What are some strategies for building rapport with children?

3. A child reports that he is suicidal. What would be your next question? What measures would you take next?

4. What are some techniques and media for obtaining information about a child's inner world, such as self-concept, sexual identity, body image, and developmental level?

5. Explain why it may be detrimental to interview a child in front of their parent. Why may it be detrimental to interview a parent in front of their child?

6. Why is obtaining the mental health histories of parents relevant to the child's mental health assessment?

7. What assessment questions would be important for a transgender child?

8. What are useful tools in obtaining a family history from the child and parent?

9. What types of questions would you ask to inquire about a child's spiritual life?

REFERENCES

Achenbach, T. M., & Edelbrock, C. (1983). *The child behavior checklist: Manual for the child behavior checklist and revised child behavior profile*. Burlington, VT: Queen City Printers.

Adams, J. A., Kellogg, N. D., Farst, K. J., Harper, N. S., Palusci, V. J., Frasier, L. D., et al. (2016). Updated guidelines for the medical assessment and care of children who may have been sexually abused. *North American Society for Pediatric and Adolescent Gynecology, 29*(2), 81–87.

Advocates for Youth (2021). Creating safer spaces for LGBTQ youth: A toolkit for education, healthcare, and community-based organizations. https://advocatesforyouth.org/wp-content/uploads/2020/11/Creating-Safer-Spaces-Toolkit-Nov-13.pdf#:~:text=To%20ensure%20a%20safer%20environment%20for%20LGBTQ%20youth,,progress%20toward%20inclusion%20of%20LGBTQ%20youth%20in%20programs.

Al-Yateem, N., & Rossiter, R. C. (2016). Unstructured play for anxiety in pediatric inpatient care. Journal of Specialists in Pediatric Nursing, 22(1). https://doi.org/10.1111/jspn.1216

Aston, J., Wilson, K. A., & Terry, D. R. P. (2019). The treatment-related experiences of parents, children and young people with regular prescribed medication. *International Journal of Clinical Pharmacy, 41*, 113–121.

Barnard, K. E., & Brazelton, T. B. (1990). *Touch: The foundation of experience*. Madison, CT: International Universities Press.

Baumgartner, N., Haberling, N., Emery, S., Strumberger, M., Nalani, K., Erb, S... Gerger, G. (2020). When parents and children disagree: Informant discrepancies in reports of depressive symptoms in clinical interviews. *Journal of Affective Disorders, 1*(272), 223–230.

Behrendt, H. F., Scharke, W., Herpertz-Dahlmann, B., Konrad, K., & Firk, C. (2019). Like mother, like child? Maternal determinants of children's early social-emotional development. *Infant Mental Health Journal, 40*(2), 234–247.

Bizzi, F., & Pace, C. S. (2020). Attachment representations in children with disruptive behavior disorders: A special focus on insecurity in middle childhood. *Clinical Child Psychology & Psychiatry*, 25(4), 833–846.

Bowlby, J. (1969). *Attachment (Vol. 1 of Attachment and loss)*. New York: Basic Books.

Boyle-Toledo, K. (2019). Why play? Thoughts on evidence-based treatments and why play therapy is still relevant. *The Brown University Child and Adolescent Behavior Letter*, 35(2), 1058–1073.

Brinkman, W. B., Simon, J. O., Epstein, J. N. (2017). Reasons why children and adolescents with Attention-Deficit/ Hyperactivity Disorder stop and restart taking medication. *Academic Pediatrics*, 18, 273–280.

Centers for Disease Control and Prevention (2021). Lesbian, Gay, Bisexual, and Transgender Health. https://www.cdc.gov/lgbthealth/youth.htm

Elizur, Y., Somech, L. Y., & Vinokur, A. D. (2017). Effects of Parent Training on Callous-Unemotional Traits, Effortful Control, and Conduct Problems: Mediation by Parenting. Journal of Abnormal Child Psychology, 45(1), 15–26.

Frick, P. J., Barry, C. T., & Kamphaus, R. W. (2020). *Clinical assessment of child and adolescent personality and behavior (4th ed.)*. New York: Springer.

Golds, L., deKruiff, K., & MacBeth, A. (2020). Disentangling genes, attachment, and environment: A systematic review of the developmental psychopathology literature on gene-environment interactions and attachment. *Development and Psychopathology*, 32(1), 357–381.

Goodman, W. K., Price, L. H., Rasmussen, S. A., Mazure, C., Fleischmann, R. L., Hill, C. L., et al. (1989). The Children's Yale-Brown Obsessive Compulsive Scale (CYBOCS) I. Development, use, and reliability. *Archives of General Psychiatry*, 46(11), 1006–1011.

Gwin, S., Branscum, P., Taylor, L., Cheney, M., Maness, S. B., Frey, M., & Zhang, Y. (2020). Associations between depressive symptoms and religiosity in young adults. *Journal of Religion and Health*, 59(6), 3193–3210.

Harlow, H. F., Harlow, M. K., & Suomi, S. J. (1971). From thought to therapy: Lessons from a private laboratory. *American Scientist*, 59(5), 538–549.

Hemmingsson, H., Olafsdottir, L. B., & Egilson, S. T. (2017). Agreements and disagreements between children and their parents in health-related assessments. *Disability & Rehabilitation*, 39(11), 1059–1072.

House, A. (2002). *The first session with children and adolescents: Conducting a comprehensive mental health evaluation*. New York: Guilford Press.

Jacobson, A. S., Trivers, R., & Palestis, B. G. (2020). Number of friends and self-perception among Jamaican children: The role of attractiveness and fluctuating asymmetry. *Journal of Biosocial Science*, 52(2), 184–197.

Koomar, T., & Michaelson, J. J. (2020). Genetic intersections of language and neuropsychiatric conditions. *Current Psychiatric Reports*, 22(1), 4.

Kotroni, P., Bonoti, F., & Mavropoulou, S. (2019). Children with autism can express social emotions in their drawings. *International Journal of Developmental Disabilities*, 65(4), 248–256.

Kushner, S. C. (2015). A review of the direct and interactive effects of life stressors and dispositional traits on youth psychopathology. *Child Psychiatry & Human Development*, 46(5), 810–819.

Lee, R. S., & Oswald, L. M. (2018). Early life stress as a predictor of co-occurring alcohol use disorder and post-traumatic stress disorder. *Alcohol Research: Current Reviews*, 39(2), e1–e13.

Levy, S., & Shrier, L. (2015). Adolescent SBIRT Toolkit for Providers. Massachusetts Department of Mental Health, Boston Children's Hospital, Massachusetts Department of Public Health, Massachusetts Child Psychiatry Access Project, SA3541, https://massclearinghouse.ehs.state.ma.us/PROG-BSAS-SBIRT/SA1099.html

Lidz, C. S. (2003). *Early childhood assessment*. Hoboken, NJ: John Wiley & Sons, Ltd.

March, J. (1997). *Multidimensional anxiety scale for children*. North Tonawanda, NY: Multi-Health Systems, Inc.

Martin, H. K., Martin, A., Berlin, L. J., & Brooks-Gunn, J. (2011). Early mother-child separation, parenting, and child well-being in early head start families. *Attachment & Human Development*, 13(1), 5–26.

Miller, J. R., Cheung, A., Novilla, L. K., & Crandall, A. (2020). Childhood experiences and adult health: The moderating effects of temperament. *Heliyon*, 6(5), e03927.

Orchard, F., Pass, L., Cocks, L., Chessell, C., & Reynolds, S. (2019). Examining parent and child agreement in the diagnosis of adolescent depression. *Child and Adolescent Mental Health*, 24(4), 338–344.

Patel, M., Agnihotri, S., Hawkins, C., Levin, L., Goodman, D., & Simpson, A. (2020). Identifying fetal alcohol spectrum disorder and psychiatric comorbidity for children and youth in care: A community approach to diagnosis and treatment. *Children and Youth Services Review*, 108, ISSN: 0190-7409.

Pearce, A., Dundas, R., Whitehead, M., & Taylor-Robinson, D. (2019). Pathways to inequalities in child health. *Archives of Disease in Childhood*, 104(10), 998–1003.

Polimanti, R., & Gelernter, J. (2017). Widespread signatures of positive selection in common risk alleles associated to autism spectrum disorder. *PLoS Genetics*, 13(2), e1006618.

Popp, L., Neuschwander, M., Mannstadt, S., In-Albon, T., & Schneider, S. (2017). Parent-child diagnostic agreement on anxiety symptoms with a structured diagnostic interview for mental disorders in children. *Frontiers in Psychology*, 8, 404.

Raufman, R., & Weinberg, H. (2016). Early mother–son relationships, primary levels of mental organization and the foundation matrix as expressed in fairy tales: The case of the 'Jewish mother'. *Group Analysis*, 49(2), 149–163.

Reynolds, C. R., & Kamphouse, R. W. (1998). *Behavior assessment system for children (BASC)*. Circle Pines, MN: American Guidance Service.

Riddle, M. A., Reeve, E. A., Yaryura-Tobias, J. A., Yang, H. M., Claghorn, J. L., Gaffney, G., et al. (2001). Fluvoxamine for children and adolescents with obsessive-compulsive disorder: A randomized, controlled, multicenter trial. *Journal of the American Academy of Child and Adolescent Psychiatry*, 40(2), 222–229.

Romanelli, M., & Lindsey, M. A. (2020). Patterns of healthcare discrimination among transgender help-seekers. *American Journal of Preventative Medicine*, 58(4), e123–131.

Rycek, R., Stuhr, S. L., McDermott, J., Benker, J., & Swartz, M. D. (1998). Adolescent egocentrism and cognitive functioning during late adolescence. *Adolescence*, 33(132), 745–749.

Santesso, D. L., Schmidt, L. A., & Trainor, L. J. (2007). Frontal brain electrical activity (EEG) and heart rate in response to affective infant-directed (ID) speech in 9-month-old infants. *Brain & Cognition*, 65(1), 14–21.

Sezici, E., Ocakci, A. F., & Kadioglu, H. (2017). Use of play therapy in nursing process: A prospective randomized controlled study. *Journal of Nursing Scholarship*, 49(2), 162–169.

Silva, C. S., & Calheiros, M. M. (2018). Stop yelling: Interparental conflict and adolescents' self-representations as mediated by their perceived relationships with parents. *Journal of Family Issues*, 39(7), 2174–2204.

Spruit, A., Goos, L., Weenink, N., Rodenburg, R., Niemeyer, H., Stams, G. J., & Colonnes, C. (2020). A relation between attachment and depression in children and adolescents: A multilevel meta-analysis. *Clinical Child and Family Psychology Review*, 23(1), 54–69.

Stauffer, S. (2019). Ethical use of drawings in play therapy: Considerations for assessment, practice, and supervision. *International Journal of Play Therapy*, 28(4), 183–194.

Swanson, J. M. (1983). *The SNAP-IV*. Irvine, CA: University of California.

Thomas, A., Chess, S., & Birch, H. G. (1968). *Temperament and behavior disorders in childhood*. New York: University Press.

Todd, A. R., Forstmann, M., Burgmer, P., Brooks, A. W., & Galinsky, A. D. (2015). Anxious and egocentric: How specific emotions influence perspective taking. *Journal of Experimental Psychology: General*, 144(2), 374–391.

Tsetsos, F., Padmanabhuni, S. S., Alexander, J., Karagiannidis, I., Tsifintaris, M., Topaloudi, A., et al. (2016). Meta-analysis of Tourette syndrome and attention deficit hyperactivity disorder provides support for a shared genetic basis. *Frontiers in Neuroscience*, 10, 340.

Van Heel, M., Bijttebier, P., Claes, S., Colpin, H., Goossens, L., Hankin, B... Van Leeuwen, K. (2020). Parenting, effortful control, and adolescents' externalizing problem behavior: Moderation by dopaminergic genes. *Journal of Youth and Adolescence*, 49, 252–266.

Verschueren, K. (2020). Attachment, self-esteem, and socio-emotional adjustment: There is more than just the mother. *Attachment and Human Development*, 22(1), 105–109.

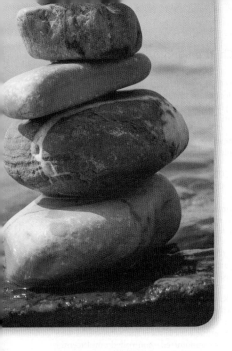

37
Mental Health Disorders of Childhood and Adolescence

Rebecca Luebbert

KEYCONCEPTS

- Attention
- Neurodevelopmental delay
- Hyperactivity
- Impulsiveness
- Tics

LEARNING OBJECTIVES

After studying this chapter, you will be able to:

1. Describe mental disorders usually diagnosed in childhood or adolescence.

2. Discuss prevailing theories relevant to the mental health disorders in childhood and adolescence.

3. Discuss the nursing care of children with neurodevelopmental disorders.

4. Analyze the nursing assessment, diagnosis, intervention, and evaluation processes in caring for a child or adolescent with attention-deficit hyperactivity disorder.

5. Describe the nursing care of children and adolescents with disruptive behavior disorders.

6. Discuss the epidemiology, etiology, medications, and nursing care of children with tic disorders.

7. Discuss the nursing care of children and adolescents with separation anxiety and obsessive–compulsive disorders (OCDs).

8. Compare the nursing care of children and adolescents with mood disorders and schizophrenia with that for adults with similar disorders.

9. Discuss the significance of behavioral intervention strategies for children who have elimination disorders.

KEY TERMS

- Adaptive behavior • Attention-deficit hyperactivity disorder (ADHD) • Autism spectrum disorder (ASD)
- Communication disorders • Conduct disorder • Disruptive behavior disorders • Dyslexia • Encopresis • Enuresis
- Intellectual disability • Learning disorder • Motor tics • Oppositional defiant disorder • Phonic tics • Phonologic processing • Separation anxiety disorder • Tourette Syndrome

INTRODUCTION

Psychiatric problems are less easily recognized in children than in adults. Normal growth and development behaviors of one age group may be a symptom of a disorder in another age group. For example, an imaginary friend is age appropriate for a 4-year-old child but not for an adolescent. Despite the difficulty in diagnosis, an estimated one in six youth in the United States experiences a mental disorder in a given year (National Alliance on Mental Illness [NAMI], 2021). Among the most commonly diagnosed disorders in children and adolescents are

attention-deficit hyperactivity disorder (ADHD) (in 9.4%, approximately 6.1 million), behavior problems (in 7.4%, approximately 4.5 million), anxiety (7.1%, approximately 4.4 million), and depression (3.2%, approximately 1.9 million) (CDC, 2020b). Unfortunately, despite this prevalence, significant gaps in treatment exist, particularly for children in low-income families (Ghandour et al., 2019).

This chapter presents an overview of selected childhood disorders and discusses nursing care for children and their families with these problems. Because it is beyond the scope of this text to present all child psychiatric disorders, this chapter discusses selected ones, including neurodevelopmental disorders (**intellectual disability, autism spectrum disorder (ASD)**, ADHD, and tic disorders), **separation anxiety disorder**, obsessive–compulsive disorder (OCD), mood disorders, childhood schizophrenia, and elimination disorders (**enuresis** and **encopresis**). Oppositional defiant and conduct disorders are discussed in Chapter 30.

> **NCLEXNOTE** All psychiatric disorders of childhood and adolescence should be viewed within the context of growth and development models. Safety and self-esteem are priority considerations.

The **neurodevelopmental disorders** occur early in a child's development, often before grade school. These disorders include developmental deficits that range from very specific limitations of learning to global impairments of social skills. They impact personal, social, academic, or occupational functioning. Under the primary influences of genes and environment, neurodevelopment of attention, cognition, language, affect, and social and moral behavior proceeds along several pathways. Developmental pathways and developmental delays are closely interwoven. For example, a language delay can interfere with a child's social development and contribute to behavior problems (Matte-Landry et al., 2020). This section discusses neurodevelopmental disorders of childhood that include several conditions that are etiologically unrelated; however, their common feature is a significant delay in one or more lines of development.

> **KEYCONCEPT Neurodevelopmental delay** means that the child's development in attention, cognition, language, affect, and social or moral behavior is outside the norm and is manifested by delayed socialization, communication, peculiar mannerisms, and idiosyncratic interests.

INTELLECTUAL DISABILITY

Intellectual disability is defined as a disability characterized by significant limitations in both intellectual function and in **adaptive behavior** that covers many everyday social and practical skills (American Association on Intellectual and Developmental Disabilities [AAIDD], 2021). The disability begins before the age of 18 years.

Diagnostic Criteria and Clinical Course

The diagnosis of intellectual disability involves an assessment of intellectual function such as reasoning, problem-solving, and adaptive function in personal independence and social responsibility (American Psychiatric Association [APA], 2013). A diagnosis is made through clinical assessment of behavioral features; historical accounts from parents and teachers; and performance on standardized tests such as the Stanford–Binet or the Wechsler Intelligence Scales for Children. The usual threshold for intellectual disability is an intelligence quotient (IQ) of 70 or less (i.e., two standard deviations below the population mean).

Adaptive behavior is composed of three skill types: *conceptual skills* (e.g., language and literacy, money, time, number concepts, and self-direction); *social skills* (e.g., interpersonal skills, social responsibility, self-esteem, gullibility, social problem-solving, and the ability to follow rules and obey laws and to avoid being victimized); and *practical skills* (e.g., activities of daily living [ADLs], occupational skills, health care, travel and transportation, schedules and routines, safety, use of money, use of telephone) (AAIDD, 2021). Impaired adaptive functioning is primarily a clinical judgment based on the child's capacity to manage age-appropriate ADLs. However, standardized assessment instruments are available to assist with determination of the child's capabilities (Shields et al., 2020; Verdugo et al., 2020).

An intellectual disability is not necessarily lifelong. Some children may be diagnosed at school age as having an intellectual disability, but with guidance and education, they may no longer meet the criteria as adults.

Epidemiology and Etiology

Data from the 2017 Global Burden of Disease Study estimated the prevalence of intellectual disabilities to be about 3% in the United States and worldwide. A considerable variability worldwide exists, with low- and middle-income countries reporting significantly higher rates of disability than high-income countries (Olusanya et al., 2020). Children and adolescents with intellectual disabilities are at higher risk for other mental disorders than in those without an intellectual disability (Buckley et al., 2020; Mazza et al., 2020). The rate of co-occurring psychiatric disorders is estimated between 38% and 49%, with the most commonly reported disorders including ADHD (39%), anxiety disorders (7% to 34%), conduct disorders (3% to 21%), and depressive disorder (3% to 5%) (Buckley et al., 2020).

Intellectual disabilities result from a variety of causes with the most common etiology related to genetic syndromes. Chromosomal changes or defects (e.g., Down syndrome) and exposure to toxins during prenatal development (e.g., fetal alcohol syndrome), heredity, pregnancy and perinatal complications, medication conditions, and environmental influences are all associated with intellectual disabilities. The cause is unknown in many of the cases (Walkley et al., 2019).

Nursing Care of Children with Intellectual Disability

Assessment of a child with an intellectual disability focuses on current adaptive skills, intellectual status, and social functioning. A developmental history is a useful way to gather information about past and current capacities (Box 37.1). The nurse compares these data with normal growth and development. Developmentally delayed children who have not had a psychological evaluation should be considered for referral. These children also require evaluation for other comorbid psychiatric disorders, which may be a challenge because of the child's cognitive limitations. Discussions about feelings and behavior may be too complex for these children. If children or adolescents with intellectual disabilities have a comorbid mental disorder or serious behavioral problems, a carefully constructed interdisciplinary behavioral plan will guide care and treatment.

The nurse also assesses the child's support systems (family, school, rehabilitative, and psychiatric) to ensure that the child's special needs have been identified and are being addressed. For example, occupational therapy may be recommended to improve motor coordination, but

the family may not have transportation to these services available, so availability to alternative services should be explored.

The child and family's response to intellectual disability and other comorbid conditions will determine the nursing interventions. Interventions most often include promoting coping skills (i.e., interventions directed at building strengths, adapting to change, and maintaining or achieving a higher level of functioning), patient education, and parent education.

The overall goals of treatment and nursing care are an optimal level of functioning for the family and eventual independent functioning within a normal social environment for the child. For many children with intellectual disability, achieving independence in adulthood will be delayed but not impossible.

Continuum of Care

Children and families may require varying levels of interventions at different times throughout the life cycle. When a child is young, the family requires special educational support and, for some, residential services. The need for psychiatric intervention varies according to the severity of disability, family functioning, and the coexistence of other disorders. Feelings of grief and loss in family members (especially parents) related to having a child with a disability may be relieved through family therapy. More specific parent training may be needed to deal with emerging maladaptive behaviors. See Nursing Care Plan 37.1.

AUTISM SPECTRUM DISORDER

ASD is characterized by persistent impairment in social communication and social interaction with others (APA, 2013). Children with ASD may or may not have an intellectual disability, but they commonly show an uneven pattern of intellectual strengths and weaknesses. This condition may be a lifelong pattern of being rigid in manner, intolerant of change, and prone to behavioral outbursts in response to environmental demands or changes in routine. Two conditions, autism disorder and Asperger syndrome, were previously diagnosed as separate disorders. However, because they have many overlapping symptoms and are difficult to differentiate from each other, the *DSM-5* no longer considers autism and Asperger syndrome as separate disorders, but considers both as an ASD differentiated by language or intellectual impairment (APA, 2013).

ASD with restricted repetitive patterns of behavior such as stereotypic or repetitive motor movement, use of objects, inflexible adherence to routine or ritualized patterns, and fascination with lights or movement has

---

BOX 37.1

History and Hallmarks of Childhood and Adolescent Disorders

- Maternal age and health status during pregnancy
- Exposure to medication, alcohol, or other substances during pregnancy
- Course of pregnancy, labor, and delivery
- Infant's health at birth
- Eating, sleeping, and growth in first year
- Health status in first year
- Interest in others in first 2 years
- Motor development
- Mastery of bowel and bladder control
- Speech and language development
- Activity level
- Response to separation (e.g., school entry)
- Regulation of mood and anxiety
- Medical history in early childhood
- Social development
- Interests

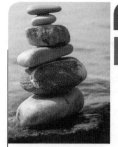

NURSING CARE PLAN 37.1

The Patient with Attention-Deficit Hyperactivity Disorder

Jamie, age 6 years, comes to the primary health care clinic with his mother Lillian because of motor restlessness, distractibility, and disruptive behavior in the classroom. According to Lillian, Jamie had a reasonably good year in kindergarten, but early in the first grade, the teacher began to report disruptive behavior. On reflection, Lillian recalls that kindergarten was a half-day program with more activity. By contrast, Jamie is expected to sit in his seat and pay attention for longer periods in first grade.

Jamie's medical history is unremarkable. Lillian's pregnancy with Jamie was her first and was unplanned. Although there were no complications during the pregnancy, the period was marked by significant marital discord, culminating in divorce before Jamie's first birthday. Jamie was born by cesarean section after a long, unproductive labor. He was healthy at birth and grew normally, with no developmental delays. Despite genuine interest in other children, his intrusive style and inability to wait his turn resulted in frequent conflicts with them. The family history is positive for substance abuse in his father. In addition, Lillian reports that her ex-husband was disruptive in school, had trouble concentrating, and was highly impulsive. These problems have continued into adulthood.

During the two evaluation sessions, Jamie is active but cooperative. His speech is fluent and normal in tone and tempo but somewhat loud. His discourse is coherent, but at times, he makes rather abrupt changes in conversation without warning his listeners. Psychological testing done at the school revealed average to above-average intelligence. Parent and teacher questionnaires concurred that Jamie was overactive, impulsive, inattentive, and quarrelsome but not defiant.

Setting: Psychiatric Home Care Agency

Baseline Assessment: Jamie is a 6-year-old boy with prominent hyperactivity and disruptive behavior. He lives with Lillian, his single mother. These problems interfere with his interpersonal relationships and academic progress. Lillian is discouraged and feels unable to manage Jamie's behavior.

Associated Psychiatric Diagnosis	Medications
Attention-deficit hyperactivity disorder (ADHD)	Methylphenidate 7.5 mg at breakfast and lunch (i.e., at 8 AM and 12 noon) and then adding 5 mg at 7 PM.

Priority of Care: Difficulty in Social Relationships

Important Characteristics	Associated Considerations
Cannot establish and maintain developmentally appropriate social relationships Has interpersonal difficulties at school Is not well accepted by peers Is easily distracted Interrupts others Cannot wait his turn in games Speaks out of turn in the classroom	Impulsive behavior Overactive Inattentive Risk-taking behavior (tried to climb out the window to get away from his mother) Failure to recognize effects of his behavior on others

Outcomes

Initial	Discharge
Decrease hyperactivity and disruptive behavior. Improve attention and decrease distractibility. Decrease frequency of acting without forethought.	Improve capacity to identify alternative responses in conflicts with peers. Improve capacity to interpret behavior of age mates.

Interventions

Intervention	Rationale	Ongoing Assessment
Educate mother and teach about ADHD and use of stimulant medication.	Better understanding helps to ensure adherence; also parents and teachers often miscast children with ADHD as "troublemakers."	Determine the extent to which parent or teacher "blames" Jamie for his problems.

Continued

Nursing Care Plan 37.1 Continued

Intervention	Rationale	Ongoing Assessment
Monitor adherence to medication schedule.	Uneven compliance may contribute to failed trial of medication.	Administer parent and teacher questionnaires; inquire about behavior across entire day.
Ensure that medication is both effective and well tolerated.	Stimulants can affect appetite and sleep.	Administer parent and teacher questionnaires; check height and weight; ask about sleep and appetite.

Evaluation

Outcomes	Revised Outcomes	Interventions
Jamie shows decreased hyperactivity and less disruption in the classroom.	Improve ability to identify disruptive classroom behavior.	Initiate point system to reward appropriate behavior.
Jamie shows improved attention and decreased distractibility.	Improve school performance.	Move to front of classroom as an aid to attention.
Mother and teacher attest to Jamie's decreased impulsive behavior.	Increase Jamie's capacity to recognize the effects of his behavior on others.	Encourage participation in structured activities.
Jamie identifies alternative responses such as walking away until it is his turn.	Increase frequency of acting on these alternative approaches.	Inquire about social skills group at school, if available.
Jamie improves interpretation of motives and behaviors of others.	Improve acceptance by peers.	Encourage participation in community activities.

Priority of Care: Difficulty Parenting

Important Characteristics	Associated Considerations
Verbalizes discouragement and inability to handle situation with Jamie	Chronicity of ADHD More than average childrearing problems

Outcomes

Initial	Discharge
Verbalize frustration at trying to raise a child with ADHD alone. Identify positive methods of interacting and disciplining Jamie that will support the parent–child relationship as well as meet Jamie's development needs.	Identify coping patterns that decrease the sense of frustration and increase parental competence. Initiate a collaborative relationship with the school teacher. Identify sources of support in the community and begin to access these resources.

Interventions

Intervention	Rationale	Ongoing Assessment
Assess mother's discouragement and feelings about parenting, identifying specific problem areas.	Helping the mother verbalize her feelings and identifying problem areas help in formulating problem-solving strategies.	Assess the severity of the problems with which she is living.
Refer mother to Community Mental Health Center for free parenting class.	Parent training based on clear directives and rewards can be effective for decreasing impulsive and disruptive behavior.	Monitor mother's level of confidence and perceived change in Jamie's behavior.

Continued

Nursing Care Plan 37.1 Continued

Intervention	Rationale	Ongoing Assessment
Refer mother to self-help organization.	Parent groups such as Children and Adults with Attention-deficit Disorder (CHAAD) can be sources of support and information.	Determine whether contact was made and whether it was helpful.
Make contact with school to enhance collaboration with mother.	Assess effectiveness of medication and other interventions; need feedback from teachers.	Determine whether mother has been able to contact teacher.

Evaluation

Outcomes	Revised Outcomes	Interventions
After four sessions, Lillian expresses her frustrations, but she has begun to identify different ways of relating to Jamie and his developmental needs.	None	None
Through attending the parenting class and joining a support group, Lillian begins to change her coping patterns, decrease her frustrations, and increase her parental competence.	Complete parenting class; attend at least two support group meetings each month.	If necessary, refer for additional parent counseling.
Lillian initiates a collaborative relationship with Jamie's teacher.	Lillian and teacher mutually develop and implement behavior plans for home and school.	Have mother observe in the classroom; have mother visit highly structured classroom.

been a subject of considerable interest and research effort since its original description more than 70 years ago. Leo Kanner (1943) described the profound isolation of these children and their extreme desire for sameness. These children appear aloof and indifferent to others and often seem to prefer inanimate objects.

Impairment in communication is severe and affects both verbal and nonverbal communication. Children with ASD may manifest delayed and deviant language development, as evidenced by echolalia (repetition of words or phrases spoken by others) and a tendency to be extremely literal in interpretation of language. Pronoun reversals and abnormal intonation are also common. Other common features of ASD are stereotypic behavior, self-stimulating, nonfunctional repetitive behaviors, such as repetitive rocking, hand flapping, and an extraordinary insistence on sameness. These children may also engage in self-injurious behavior, such as hitting, head banging, or biting. In some children, their unusual interests may evolve into fascination with specific objects, such as fans or air conditioners, or a particular topic, such as U.S. Civil War generals.

A child with ASD may have age-appropriate language and intelligence but also have severe and sustained impairment in social interaction and restricted, repetitive patterns of behavior, interests, and activities. This type of ASD was previously known as Asperger syndrome and appears to be a milder form of ASD. These children have social deficits marked by inappropriate initiation of social interactions, an inability to respond to normal social cues, and a tendency to be literal in their interpretation of language (APA, 2013). They may also display stereotypic behaviors, such as rocking and hand flapping, and have highly restricted areas of interest, such as train schedules, fans, air conditioners, or dogs. Signs of developmental delay may not be apparent until preschool or school age, when social deficits become evident (Box 37.2).

Epidemiology and Etiology

Recent studies by the CDC find that approximately 1 in 54 children has been identified with ASD. It is 4.3 times as prevalent among boys as among girls, and is found in all racial, ethnic, and socioeconomic groups (Maenner et al., 2020). Intellectual disability and seizures often occur in ASD (Strasser et al., 2018). Published claims that the prevalence of autism is increasing are confounded by improved methods of diagnosis (Myers et al., 2019).

While research has not identified an exclusive cause for ASD, evidence has identified many likely contributing factors, including environmental, biologic, and genetic factors. There is strong evidence supporting the majority of risk for ASD is from genetic factors. In a multinational cohort study of over 2 million individuals, of whom 22,000 were diagnosed with ASD, the heritability rate

BOX 37.2 CLINICAL VIGNETTE

Frank (Autism Spectrum Disorder Asperger Syndrome)

A pediatrician refers Frank, age 5 years, 6 months, for an evaluation because of Frank's unusual preoccupation with ceiling fans and lawn sprinklers. According to his mother, Frank became interested in ceiling fans at age 3 years when he began drawing them, tearing pictures of them out of magazines, and engaging others in discussions about them. In the months before the evaluation, Frank also became fascinated by lawn sprinklers. These preoccupations so dominated Frank's interactions with others that he was practically incapable of discussing any other topics. He remained on the periphery of his kindergarten class and had few friends. Although he tried to make friends, his approaches were inept and he had trouble reading others.

Frank was the product of a full-term uncomplicated pregnancy, labor, and delivery to his then 25-year-old mother. It was her first pregnancy, and both parents eagerly anticipated Frank's birth. As an infant, Frank was healthy but seemed to cry a lot and was difficult to comfort, causing his mother to feel inadequate and depleted. His motor development was also delayed, and at age 3 years, nonfamily members had difficulty understanding his speech. His articulation, however, was within normal limits at the time of consultation. Frank received regular pediatric care and had no history of serious illness or injury. There was no family history of intellectual disability or psychiatric illness; results of genetic testing for chromosomal abnormality were negative.

In addition to his unusual preoccupations and social deficits, Frank resisted any change in his routine, was easily frustrated, and was prone to temper tantrums. His parents sharply disagreed about the nature of and appropriate response to his problems.

What Do You Think?

- What effect do you think Frank's preoccupation may have on his family and their relationships?
- What kind of teaching program would you develop if you were the nurse assigned to this family?

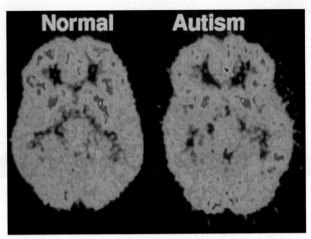

FIGURE 37.1 Patients with autism (*right*) may have decreased metabolic rates in the cingulate gyrus and other associated areas; however, wide heterogeneity in brain metabolic patterns is seen in patients with autism. (Courtesy of Monte S. Buchsbaum, MD, The Mount Sinai Medical Center and School of Medicine, New York.)

was estimated to be approximately 80% (Bai et al., 2020). Other risk factors identified by the CDC as possible contributors to ASD include having a sibling with ASD, children born to older parents, individuals with certain genetic or chromosomal conditions, such as fragile X syndrome or tuberous sclerosis, and the use of prescription drugs valproic acid and thalidomide taken during pregnancy. Studies have shown that there is no link between receiving vaccines and developing ASD (CDC, 2020d) (Figure 37.1).

Teamwork and Collaboration: Working toward Recovery

ASDs require long-term care at various levels of intensity. The total costs per year for children living with ASD in the United States is estimated to be between $11 billion and $61 billion due to a culmination of direct and indirect costs. Youth with ASD have an average of $4,000 to $6,000 additional medical expenditures as compared to youth without ASD, and children needing intensive behavioral interventions incur an additional $40,000 to $60,000 cost per year (CDC, 2020d). Treatment consists of designing academic, interpersonal, and social experiences that support the child's development. Children with autism, even those who are severely affected, may be able to live at home and attend special schools that use behavioral techniques. Other outpatient services may include family counseling, home care, and medication. As the child moves toward adulthood, living at home may become more difficult given the appropriate need for greater independence. The level of structure required depends primarily on IQ and adaptive functioning.

Planning interventions for children with an ASD consider the child, family, and community supports, such as schools, rehabilitation centers, or group homes. First and foremost, the clinicians involved in the child's treatment should collaborate with the family toward the same general goals. As the number of clinicians and educators involved increases, the chance of fragmentation in treatment planning also increases. The nurse can serve as a case coordinator.

Residential care may be necessary in some cases. After making the decision to place a child into a residential facility, family members may experience guilt, loss, and a sense of failure concerning their inability to care for the child at home.

Evidence-Based Nursing Care for Children with ASD

Mental Health Nursing Assessment

Physical Health Assessment

Physical health assessment should include a review of physical health and neurologic status, giving particular attention to coordination, childhood illnesses, injuries, and hospitalizations. The nurse should assess sleep, appetite, and activity patterns because they may be disturbed in affected children. Lack of adequate sleep can increase irritability. Comorbid seizure disorders are common in those with autism; depression is often seen concurrently even when no intellectual or language impairment is evident. Thus, the nurse should consider these conditions in the assessment.

Children with additional psychiatric disorders or seizures may be receiving multiple medications and require the care of several clinicians. Therefore, assessment should include a careful review of current medications and treating clinicians.

Psychosocial Assessment

Communication, behaviors, and flexibility are critical assessment areas. Direct behavioral observation is important to evaluate the child's ability to relate to others, to verify the selection of age-appropriate activities, and to watch for stereotypic behaviors. Assessment of the child with ASD can be based on the following categories:

- Communication
  - Verbal and nonverbal
  - Use of picture cards, writing, or drawing
  - Comfortable with eye contact
  - Understand emotional cues
  - Presence of pain
  - Preoccupation with restricted interests
- Behaviors
  - Items of fixation (how does family manage?)
  - Triggers for agitation
  - Early signs that indicate beginning of agitation
  - Interventions that work when child is overstimulated or agitated
  - Repetitive behaviors
- Flexibility or adherence to routine
  - Home schedule
  - What aggravates or irritates the person
  - Early warning signs of agitation

- When overagitated, what interventions work best The child's behavior, need for structure, and communication style can affect family functioning. Having a child with ASD is bound to influence family interaction; responding to the child's needs may adversely affect family functioning. For example, sleep disruption in family members who care for these children may increase family stress.

Clinical Judgment

Treatment outcomes need to be individualized to the child, family, and social environment and may change with time. Ensuring physical safety is a priority for the nurse. The nurse will need to develop a plan of care that takes into consideration the child's ability to communicate effectively with others. The child may also have difficulty completing ADLs and may demonstrate poor coping and impaired skills. Determining the need for predictability and stability in routine for the child is also important.

Mental Health Nursing Interventions

Physical Health Interventions

In teaching self-care skills, the nurse needs to consider the child's current adaptive skills and language limitations. Developing a list of activities for the child to post in their bedroom may be effective for some children. Drawings or symbols may be useful for nonverbal children. Physical safety is an important concern for children who are cognitively delayed and may have impaired judgment.

No medication has proved effective at changing the core social and language deficits of autism. However, some atypical antipsychotics (i.e., risperidone, aripiprazole) are approved for the treatment of irritability associated with autism. Weight gain and metabolic syndrome are concerns with these agents. Evidence is minimal that anticonvulsants and traditional mood stabilizers are useful in managing mood lability and aggression (Davico et al., 2018).

Psychosocial Interventions

When working with children with neurodevelopmental disorders, building on their strengths and using positive reinforcement are very important. If these children feel that they are constantly criticized or need "fixing," their self-esteem will be eroded and they will be unlikely to cooperate and learn.

Promoting Interaction

Structuring interventions for social isolation should fit the child's cognitive, linguistic, and developmental levels. Interventions fostering nonverbal social interactions may be more useful than those based on speech. For higher-functioning children, activities such as getting the mail, passing out snacks, or taking turns in the context of simple games can engage them in social activities without requiring the use of their limited language skills. Structuring social interactions so that the child shares a task with another, such as carrying a load of books, may help boost confidence in relating to others.

ASDs call for extraordinary patience and determination. With help, these children can learn social and communication skills, such as taking turns in conversation and warning the listener before changing the subject in the context of milieu.

Ensuring Predictability and Safety

When children with ASDs are hospitalized, milieu management—a consistent, structured environment with predictable routines for activities, mealtimes, and bedtimes—is necessary for successful treatment. Changes in routine may provoke disorganization in the child, leading to emotional disequilibrium and explosive behavior. The safety of the inpatient unit offers an opportunity to try behavioral strategies, such as rewards for managing transitions. Health care professionals can pass on successful strategies to parents or primary caretakers (Quiban, 2020).

A structured physical environment will most likely be important to a child with a development disorder. Keeping furniture, dishes, and toys in the same place helps ease anxiety and fosters secure feelings. The nurse should identify the child's individually specific needs for structure.

Behavioral Interventions

Children with ASDs often need specific behavioral interventions to reduce the frequency of inappropriate or aggressive behavior (Kodak & Bergmann, 2020). For example, a child may have angry outbursts in response to routine transitions. If the tantrum is dramatic, the consequence may be that the transition does not take place. By structuring the environment and using visual cues to signal the end of one activity and the start of another, it may be possible to reduce the number and intensity of responses to transitions. Safety is always a concern. Self-injury and aggression are sometimes present, so children may need to be protected from hurting themselves and others. If aggressive or assaultive behavior is a problem, a brief "time out" followed by prompt reentry into activities is usually effective.

Managing the repetitive behaviors of these children depends on the specific behavior and its effects on others or the environment. If the behavior, such as rocking, has no negative effects, ignoring it may be the best approach.

If the behavior, such as head banging, however, is unacceptable, redirecting the child and using positive reinforcement are recommended. In some cases, especially in severely delayed children, these strategies may not work, and environmental alterations and perhaps protective headgear will be needed.

Supporting Family

Unfortunately, lack of integration of medical, psychiatric, social, and educational services can add to the family's burden. Parents may manifest denial, grief, guilt, and anger at various points as they adjust to their child's disability. The nurse can offer parents the opportunity to express their frustrations and disappointments and can be alert for indications that parents are in need of additional assistance, such as parent support groups or respite care.

Family interventions include support, education, counseling, and referral to self-help groups. Whenever possible, the nurse provides education to help parents determine appropriate expectations for their child and to meet the child's special needs. The following are examples of potentially useful nursing interventions focusing on the family:

- Interpreting the treatment plan for parents and child
- Modeling appropriate behavior modification techniques
- Including the parents as co-therapists for the implementation of the care plan
- Assisting the family in identifying and resolving their sense of loss related to the diagnosis
- Coordinating support systems for parents, siblings, and family members
- Maintaining interdisciplinary collaboration

Evaluation and Treatment Outcomes

Evaluation of patient and family outcomes is an ongoing process. Short-term outcomes might consist of discrete behavioral improvements, such as reducing self-injurious behavior by 50%. The long-term goal is for the patient to achieve the highest level of functioning.

ATTENTION-DEFICIT HYPERACTIVITY DISORDER

ADHD is one of the most commonly diagnosed disorders in school-aged children (CDC, 2020c). It is almost certainly a heterogeneous disorder with multiple etiologies. The relatively high frequency of ADHD and associated behavior problems virtually guarantees that nurses will meet affected children in all pediatric treatment settings. ADHD is also diagnosed in adults, but it is less common than in children (Weibel et al., 2020).

Diagnostic Criteria and Clinical Course

A persistent pattern of inattention, hyperactivity, and impulsiveness that interferes with functioning characterizes ADHD (APA, 2013). A diagnosis is made based on school behavior, parents' reports, and direct observation of inattention and hyperactivity–impulsivity that are inconsistent with developmental level. Parents and teachers describe children with ADHD as restless, always on the go, highly distractible, unable to wait their turn, heedless, and frequently disruptive. Indeed, it is often disruptive behavior that brings these children into treatment.

> **KEYCONCEPT Attention** involves concentrating on one activity to the exclusion of others, as well as the ability to sustain focus.

In ADHD, the person finds it difficult to attend to one task at a time and is easily distracted. For some, the lack of attention is related to being unable to filter incoming information, which leads to being unable to screen and select the important information. That is, all incoming stimuli are treated the same (e.g., directions from a teacher elicit the same importance as noise in the hallway). For others, the distractibility may be related to stimuli-seeking behavior. Given the heterogeneity of ADHD, either of these models may explain problems of attention for subgroups of affected children.

Children with ADHD are prone to impulsive, risk-taking behavior and often fail to consider the consequences of their actions (CDC, 2020c). They tend to exercise poor judgment and seem to have more than the usual lumps, bumps, and bruises because of their risk-taking behavior. They often require a high degree of structure and supervision (Daley et al., 2018).

> **KEYCONCEPT Impulsiveness** is the tendency to act on urges, notions, or desires without adequately considering the consequences.

Although hyperactivity is a characteristic often associated with ADHD, controversy is long standing about whether attention-deficit disorder can occur without overactivity. In many cases, the hyperactivity prompts the search for treatment. Parents typically report that a child's hyperactivity was manifested early in life and is evident in most situations (APA, 2013). Hyperactivity and impulsivity in childhood are associated with conduct disorder (Chapter 30) and intimate partner violence perpetration in adults (Buitelaar et al, 2020).

> **KEYCONCEPT Hyperactivity** is excessive motor activity, as evidenced by restlessness, an inability to remain seated, and high levels of physical motion and verbal output.

ADHD across the Lifespan

ADHD is usually diagnosed in childhood and was traditionally viewed as a problem of children. We now understand that ADHD persists into adulthood and it is sometimes first diagnosed later than in childhood. In adults, symptoms of hyperactivity and impulsivity tend to decline with age and deficit of attention persist and become more varied (Torgersen et al., 2016). However, the majority of the adults with ADHD are undiagnosed and untreated (Ginsberg et al., 2014). Many of the adults with ADHD become the parents of children with the same disorder (Uchida et al., 2020).

Epidemiology and Risk Factors

Although prevalence estimates vary depending on the diagnostic criteria used, the sources of data, and the sampling procedure, ADHD has been diagnosed in as many as 9.4% of children aged 2 to 17 (Danielson et al., 2018). Boys are more likely to be diagnosed than girls (12.9% compared to 5.6%) (CDC, 2020c). Researchers believe that several risk factors may contribute to the development of ADHD, including a family history of ADHD, substance use during pregnancy, exposures to environmental toxins (such as lead) during pregnancy and/or at a young age, low birth weight, and brain injuries (Donzelli et al., 2019; Kim et al., 2020; National Institute of Mental Health [NIMH], 2019a).

Etiology

No single explanation for the occurrence of ADHD exists; instead, this disorder is viewed as having multiple causes. Genetic factors are implicated in the etiology of ADHD. They clearly play a fundamental role in the manifestation of the ADHD behavior (Sciberras et al., 2017). In some children, diet during childhood has been investigated as a potential contributing factor to the development of ADHD, specifically a dietary pattern characterized by high consumption of refined sugars and saturated fat (Del-Ponte et al., 2019).

Biologic Theories

Although the etiology of ADHD is uncertain, evidence about neurobiologic dysfunction is pervasive. Several lines of research have shown that the frontal lobe and functional connections impacted with specific subcortical structures also are dysregulated. One clearly dysfunctional area is the dorsolateral prefrontal cortex, the center of directed attention and the ability to manage emotions or delay emotional reactions. Several neurotransmitters (e.g., dopamine, serotonin) are dysregulated (Hou et al., 2018; Klein et al., 2019; Nilsen & Tulve, 2020). Clinically, the hyperactive-impulsive behavior characteristic of ADHD has been shown to be predominantly related to biologic factors, not psychosocial factors (Nilsen & Tulve, 2020).

Psychosocial Theories

Although genetic endowment is clearly a fundamental element in the etiology of ADHD, psychosocial factors are also important risk factors. Family stress, marital discord, and parental substance use are also associated with exacerbation of ADHD behaviors (Sigfusdottir et al., 2017). Other implicated psychosocial factors are poverty, overcrowded living conditions, and family dysfunction.

Family Response to ADHD

Living with a child who has ADHD is a challenge for all family members, particularly those members who also have issues similar to those of the affected child. The family will not only be raising a child who needs a structured environment that helps support focus and attention, but the parents have to partner with their children's school system. For some families, the relationship with the school is positive and supportive. For others, the relationship with the school can be strained and lead to additional stress. It is important that the teachers and parents work together and provide consistent directions to the child.

If parents also have problems related to attention, impulse, and hyperactivity, home chaos and ineffective parenting practices can occur (Deater-Deckard, 2017). If the parents also have ADHD, they might not be able to provide a calm structured environment for the child. Effective parenting requires the ability to resist overreacting emotionally, to focus on the child, to keep track of activities, and to provide consistency in discipline (Bowling et al., 2019).

Teamwork and Collaboration: Working toward Recovery

Children with ADHD and their families benefit from symptom management, education, and support from various disciplines to have a high-quality life. Successful recovery efforts involve early recognition and treatment. By recognizing the problem early, family members and teachers can structure the child's interactions, develop meaningful discipline strategies, and modify the physical environment so the child can learn coping skills to

deal with impulsivity, distractibility, and hyperactivity. Evidence has accumulated over the years that medication is helpful, especially in the early years, but for long-term effects, a combination of medication management and behavioral approaches results in the best outcomes for the children and their families (Feldman et al., 2018).

ADHD is not an easy disorder to treat or manage. Comorbidity complicates successful recovery. Children with ADHD have more behavior or conduct problems (e.g., run-ins with police), **learning disorders**, anxiety, and depression (CDC, 2020c). Many other problems interfere with recovery efforts, such as family disruptions and economic problems, as well as naturally occurring changes such as maturational issues during their adolescent years. Additionally, children from disadvantaged backgrounds fare worse than those children who have socioeconomic and educational support (Huang et al., 2018).

Safety Issues

Due to increased impulsivity and inattention, children and adolescents with ADHD are at greater risk for injury than those without ADHD. Research finds that children with ADHD are significantly more likely to experience injury when riding a bike, have more head injuries and injuries to multiple body parts, and are more likely to be hospitalized for unintentional poisoning. Teenagers with ADHD are more likely to break traffic rules and are more likely to be involved in a car accident than those without ADHD (CDC, 2020c).

Individuals of all ages with ADHD are at high risk for mood changes that could lead to risk-taking behavior and suicidal ideation or attempts. Mood lability, the presence of depression, and potential for self-harm should be carefully assessed in these individuals (Claudius & Axeen, 2020; Giupponi et al., 2020; Levy et al., 2020). The risk of suicide attempts in children and adolescents with ADHD may be increased due to possible exposure to certain environmental risk factors, such as poor performance in school, impaired interpersonal relationships, socioeconomic hardship, depression, and substance use (Liu et al., 2020). In a study comparing youth presenting to an emergency department (ED) with suicide attempts versus suicidal ideation, youth with ADHD were more likely to have made an attempt as compared to youth without ADHD (Claudius & Axeen, 2020).

Evidence-Based Nursing Care for Children with Attention-Deficit Hyperactivity Disorder

The planning of nursing interventions must be done within the context of the family, treatment setting, and school environment. With the parents, clinical team members, and school personnel, the nurse participates in designing a plan of care that fits the child's and family's needs. Persons with ADHD and their families will benefit from nursing care at many different times in the course of the disorder. Unless hospitalized for a comorbid mental health problem, most treatment will occur outside the mental health system. School nurses often provide most of the nursing care and family education.

Mental Health Nursing Assessment

In the school setting, the primary focus of the assessment is the impact of ADHD on classroom behavior and school performance. In the hospital, the nurse tries to determine the contribution of ADHD to the acute psychiatric problem. In both cases, the nurse collects assessment data through direct interview, observation of the child and parent, and teacher ratings. Because children with ADHD may have difficulty sitting through long sessions, interviews are typically brief. Parents and teachers are extremely important sources for assessment data. To this end, the nurse can make use of several standardized instruments (Box 37.3).

BOX 37.3

Standardized Tools for Attention-Deficit Hyperactivity Disorder Diagnosis[1]

CONNERS QUESTIONNAIRES

The Conners Parent Questionnaire is a 48-item scale that a parent completes about their child. Each item is a statement that the parent rates on a 4-point scale from 0 (not at all) to 3 (very much). The Conners Teacher Questionnaire is a 28-item questionnaire that the child's teacher completes according to the same 4-point scale as the Parent Questionnaire. Both questionnaires have been standardized by age and gender for a mean of 50 and a standard deviation of 10 (Conners, 1989; Goyette et al., 1978).

CHILD BEHAVIOR CHECKLIST

The Child Behavior Checklist (CBCL) is a 118-item questionnaire that a parent completes. In addition to the 118 questions about specific behaviors and psychiatric symptoms, the CBCL also includes questions concerning the child's competence in social and academic spheres as well as age-appropriate activities. Normative data are available, allowing the conversion of raw scores to standard scores for age and gender. A teacher version of this scale is also available.

[1]Note that the diagnosis of ADHD is not made on the basis of questionnaires alone. Data from these rating scales augment the information gathered through interview and observation. These questionnaires can be especially useful before and after initiating a treatment plan to measure change.

Physical Health Assessment

As with other psychiatric disorders with onset in childhood, the nursing assessment of children with ADHD begins with identification and exploration of the presenting problems, usually hyperactivity, impulsivity, and inattention. This typically entails a review of the child's developmental course, the onset and pattern of the current symptoms, factors that have worsened or improved the child's problems, and prior treatment or self-initiated efforts to remedy the situation. Medical history is also essential, consisting of perinatal course, childhood illnesses, hospital admissions, injuries, seizures, tics, physical growth, general health status, and date of the child's last physical examination.

The behavior of these children is characteristically very active and can often be observed in the office. They cannot sit still. They fidget. Even in sleep, they may be more active than normal children. Thus, a careful assessment of eating, sleeping, and activity patterns is essential. Assessing daily food intake, typical diet, and frequency of eating will help identify any nutritional problems. Caffeinated products can contribute to hyperactivity in some children. Sleep is often disturbed for children with ADHD and consequently also the family. A detailed sleep assessment can provide points for interventions and help the interpretation of drug effects.

Psychosocial Assessment

Data regarding school performance, behavior at home, and comorbid psychiatric disorders are essential for developing school interventions and behavior plans and establishing the baseline severity for medication. Children with ADHD are more likely to have problems with their cognitive process during changing demands of teachers and parents (cognitive processing, attention, language, and memory) (Korrel et al., 2017; Tamm et al., 2020; Yang et al., 2017). Consequently, they may have more difficulty in school with decision-making. These children are often behind in their work at school because of poor organization, off-task behavior, and impulsive responses.

Dysfunctional interactions can develop within the family. Discipline is frequently an issue because parents may have difficulty controlling their child's behavior, which is disruptive and occasionally destructive. They can exhaust their parents, aggravate teachers, and annoy siblings with their intrusive and disruptive actions. Reviewing the problem behaviors and the situations in which they occur is a way to identify negative interaction patterns.

Because ADHD often occurs in the context of psychosocial adversity, it is important to review the family situation, including parenting style, stability of household membership, consistency of rules and routines, and life events (e.g., divorce, moves, deaths, job loss). Identification of these factors can be useful in shaping a care plan that builds on potential strengths and mitigates the effects of environmental factors that may perpetuate the child's disruptive behavior.

Clinical Judgment

Priorities of nursing care will depend on the severity of the responses, family situation, and school environment. Increased impulsivity and intention puts the child or adolescent at greater risk for injury. Comorbid disorders, such as mood or conduct disorders, may also be present. Sleep deprivation, inadequate nutrition, and the inability to carry out daily routines may require intervention. The child may demonstrate poor coping skills and may not function well in social settings or in structured activities (such as in the school environment). Outcomes should be individualized to the child. Short-term outcomes, such as decreasing the number of classroom ejections within a 2-week period, may be useful for one child, but reducing the frequency and amplitude of angry outbursts at home may be relevant to another child.

Mental Health Nursing Interventions

Physical Health Interventions

Modifying Nutrition

A link between adverse reaction to food (e.g., dietary salicylates and artificially added food colors, flavors, preservatives) and ADHD was suggested many years ago when the Feingold diet was introduced (Feingold, 1975). Over the years, interest in the link between food and behavior continues to spark interest in ADHD as a problem related to food. Agreement exists that in some children the behaviors associated with ADHD can be decreased with diet changes (Uldall & Thomsen, 2020). Study outcomes are mixed. A review of the artificial food color elimination diet (restricted elimination diet), few foods diet, and polyunsaturated fatty acid supplementation diet indicates that the free foods diet provides a contribution to ADHD treatment. The others did not have the research to support their efficacy.

The *few foods diet* includes basic foods that are not likely to produce adverse effects such as lamb, chicken, potatoes, bananas, and apples. Grains, dairy products, and processed foods are avoided in the few foods diet. The *restricted elimination diet* includes all-natural, chemical-free foods. Fruits, vegetables, nuts, nut butters, beans, seeds, gluten-free grains such as rice and quinoa, fish, lamb, wild game meats, organic turkey, and large amounts of water are consumed. This diet is very restricted and consequently difficult to follow all of the time. The *polyunsaturated diet* suggests that children with

ADHD have low levels of omega-3 polyunsaturated fatty acids. Supplements are encouraged for these individuals (Pelsser et al., 2017).

Supplementation with free fatty acids has been shown to be helpful for children who have deficiencies in free fatty acid such as omega-3 free fatty acid, omega-6 free fatty acid, and linolenic acid. This supplementation is usually achieved with capsule-containing oils or diets rich in fish products.

If patients adhere to any of these diets, the nurse should support the patient and family in providing the nutritional information needed for the diet. Additionally, the patient and family will need education regarding those foods that are chemical free. A referral to a dietitian will benefit both patient and family.

Children with ADHD seem to be more susceptible to being overweight and developing obesity (Fuemmeler et al., 2020). An estimated 35% of individuals with ADHD are either obese or overweight (Li et al., 2020). Because of the impulsivity and inattention characteristic of ADHD, these children may be unable to self-regulate and engage in healthy eating behaviors. The nurse can help the family and patient structure the external environment so the child has healthy choices available.

Promoting Sleep

Sleep can be a problem for children with ADHD for many reasons. The overactivity of the disorder itself and the side effects of the psychostimulants contribute to sleep problems. A sleep history should be taken before medications are prescribed. If problems exist, atomoxetine (Strattera) should be considered before the psychostimulants (see next section). If sleep problems arise while taking medications, sleep diaries should be kept. Sleep hygiene and behavior therapy techniques should be implemented (Um et al., 2017). See Chapter 34.

Using Pharmacologic Interventions

Approved medications for ADHD in children as young as 6 years of age include stimulants and nonstimulants. Psychostimulants, including methylphenidate (Ritalin), dextroamphetamine, and mixed amphetamine salts (see Chapter 12), are by far the most commonly used medications for the treatment of ADHD and are found to effective in reducing ADHD symptoms in 70% to 80% of children. These medications enhance dopamine and norepinephrine activity which and thereby improve attention and focus, decrease hyperactivity and impulsivity, and decrease disruptive behaviors (CDC, 2020c; Chang et al., 2020; Feldman et al., 2018; NIMH, 2019a).

Methylphenidate has a total duration of action of about 4 hours (Box 37.4). Thus, parents or teachers often describe a return of overactivity and distractibility as the

---

BOX 37.4

Methylphenidate (Ritalin)

DRUG CLASS: Central nervous system stimulant

RECEPTOR AFFINITY: The mechanisms of pharmacologic effect are not completely clear. At low doses, it provides mild cortical stimulation similar to that of amphetamines. This stimulation results from methylphenidate's ability to promote release and interfere with the reuptake of dopamine in the synaptic cleft. Main sites appear to be the brain stem arousal system and cortex to produce its stimulant effect.

INDICATIONS: Treatment of narcolepsy, attention-deficit disorders, and hyperkinetic syndrome.

ROUTES AND DOSAGE: Available in 5- to 10-mg immediate-release tablets and 20-mg sustained-release tablets (Ritalin-SR). Newer long-acting preparations such as Concerta and Metadate, in various dose strengths, are also available.

Adult Dosage: Must be individualized; range from 10 to 60 mg/day orally in divided doses bid (twice a day) to tid (three times a day), preferably 15 to 30 minutes before meals. If insomnia is a problem, drug should be administered before 6 PM.

Child Dosage: The immediate-release formulation can be started at 5 mg twice or three times daily on a 4-hour schedule with weekly increases depending on response. Starting doses of the long-acting preparations are equivalent to the total tid dose (e.g., 5 TID of short acting would translate into 18 mg of Concerta). Usually given on a tid schedule, with the last dose being roughly half that of the first and second dose. Daily dosage of more than 60 mg is not recommended. Discontinue after 1 month if no improvement is seen.

PEAK EFFECT: 1 hour; half-life: 3 to 4 hours for the immediate-release preparations

SELECT SIDE EFFECTS: Nervousness, insomnia, dizziness, headache, dyskinesias (including tics), toxic psychosis, anorexia, nausea, abdominal pain, increased pulse and blood pressure, palpitations, tolerance, psychological dependence.

WARNING: The drug is discontinued periodically to assess the patient's condition. Contraindications include marked anxiety, tension and agitation, glaucoma, severe depression, and obsessive–compulsive symptoms. Use cautiously in patients with a personal or family history of tic disorders, seizure disorders, hypertension, drug dependence, alcoholism, or emotional instability.

SPECIFIC PATIENT AND FAMILY EDUCATION

- Do not chew or crush sustained-release tablets; they must be swallowed whole.
- Take the drug exactly as prescribed; if insomnia is a problem, the time and dose may need adjustment. The drug is rarely taken after 5 PM.
- Avoid alcohol and over-the-counter products, including decongestants, cold remedies, and cough syrups; these could accentuate side effects of the stimulant.
- Keep appointments for follow-up, including evaluations for monitoring the child's growth and use of parent and teacher ratings to monitor benefit.
- Note that the prescriber may discontinue the drug periodically to confirm effectiveness of therapy.

---

first dose of medication wears off. This "rebound effect" can often be managed by moving the second dose of the day slightly closer to the first dose. Longer-acting preparations of methylphenidate, such as Concerta, Ritalin LA, and Metadate ER or amphetamine–dextroamphetamine (Adderall XR), do not require such frequent dosing and may be a better fit with a school day schedule. The most common side effects associated with stimulants for ADHD include appetite suppression, insomnia, dry mouth, and nausea (Posner et al., 2020). Drug holidays are sometimes implemented to determine the need for continued medication and to manage side effects (Chang et al., 2020).

One major concern with the psychostimulants is the potential for abuse. With the increase in recognition of ADHD, psychostimulant prescriptions have increased, as well as an increase in diversion for cognitive enhancement or appetite suppression. These abused prescription medications are most often acquired from peers who share, sell, or trade their medication. Nurses should caution parents about the potential for abuse and prevent their child's medication from being a source of recreational use (Chaplin, 2018; Molina et al., 2019).

Nonstimulant medications do not work as quickly as stimulants, though they are an alternative for those who

do not tolerate stimulants well, when a stimulant is ineffective, or in combination with a stimulant to increase effectiveness. The three Food and Drug Administration (FDA)-approved non-stimulants for ADHD are a norepinephrine update inhibitor (atomoxetine [Strattera]), and alpha-2 receptor agonists (guanfacine [Intuniv] and clonidine [Kapvay] (CDC, 2020c; NIMH, 2019a; Posner et al., 2020). Nonstimulants are less likely to be abused or misused than stimulant medications due to a lack of immediacy of effect (a lower speed of action and feeling stimulated) and therefore are often used for those who are more likely to be substance dependent (Feldman et al., 2018). These medications are generally well tolerated in children and adults. Common side effects associated with atomoxetine include gastrointestinal (GI) symptoms, somnolence, headaches, moodiness, and irritability. The more commonly reported adverse effects by individuals taking the alpha-2 receptor agonists include fatigue, sedation, and somnolence (Chang et al., 2020; Feldman et al., 2018).

Teaching Points

Medication can help the child's hyperactivity, impulsiveness, and inattention; therefore, teaching the parent, child, and school personnel about the importance of the medication in ADHD and the potential side effects is a place to begin. Explaining to the child that the medication improves concentration and the ability to sit still can help strengthen patient motivation.

Many times parents are reluctant to initiate treatment with psychostimulants because of the fear that their use in childhood will increase the risk of using substances in adulthood. Studies show that children and adolescents who have taken simulants medications for ADHD are no more likely to develop later substance use than those who did not take stimulant medications (National Institute on Drug Abuse [NIDA], 2018). Teaching patients and families about the biologic basis of ADHD helps parents understand that these children are not "bad" kids but that they have problems with impulse control and attention. It may be helpful to review the purposes of the medications and assure parents that evidence shows medications help most affected children.

Psychosocial Interventions

Behavioral programs based on rewards for positive behavior, such as waiting turns and following directions, can foster new social skills. Behavioral parent training, behavioral classroom management, and behavioral peer interventions are well-established treatments. Specific cognitive behavioral techniques are helpful in which the child learns to "stop, look, and listen" before doing. These approaches have been refined and several useful recommendations are available (Chang et al., 2020; Feldman et al., 2018; Posner et al., 2020). In general, interactions with children can be guided by the following:

- Set clear limits with clear consequences. Use few words and simplify instructions.

- Establish and maintain a predictable environment with clear rules and regular routines for eating, sleeping, and playing.

- Promote attention by maintaining a calm environment with few stimuli. These children cannot filter out extraneous stimuli and react to all stimuli equally.

- Establish eye contact before giving directions; ask the child to repeat what was heard.

- Encourage the child to do homework in a quiet place.

- Help the child work on one assignment at a time (reward with a break after each completion).

Family treatment is nearly always a component of cognitive behavioral treatment approaches with the child. This may involve parent training that focuses on principles of behavior management, such as appropriate limit setting and use of reward systems, as well as revising expectations about the child's behavior. School programming often involves increasing structure in the child's school day to offset the child's tendency to act without

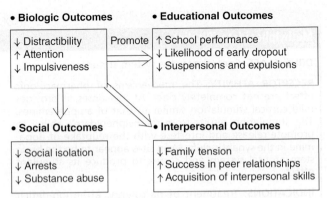

FIGURE 37.2 Long-term outcomes of optimal treatment for patients with attention-deficit hyperactivity disorder.

forethought and to be easily distracted by extraneous stimuli. Specific remediation is required for the child with comorbid deficits in learning or language. Some children may require small self-contained classrooms.

Evaluation and Treatment Outcomes

Children may not notice any effects after taking medication, but people in their environment do. Often, within 1 to 2 weeks of initiating therapy, children with ADHD become more attentive, less impulsive, and less active. Parents and teachers are often the first to notice improvement. With time, academic achievement also may improve (Figure 37.2).

Continuum of Care

Treatment of ADHD typically is conducted in outpatient settings. Optimal treatment is multimodal (i.e., includes several types of interventions), encompassing four main areas: individual treatment for the child, family treatment, school accommodations, and medication. Parent training and social skills training also help diminish disruptive and defiant behavior.

DISRUPTIVE BEHAVIOR DISORDERS

The **disruptive behavior disorders**, which include oppositional defiant disorder and conduct disorder, are a group of conditions marked by significant problems of conduct. Behaviors associated with these disorders violate the rights of others and/or are in conflict with societal norms (APA, 2013).

Oppositional defiant disorder is characterized by a persistent pattern of disobedience, argumentativeness, angry outbursts, low tolerance for frustration, and tendency to blame others for misfortunes, large and small. Children with oppositional defiant disorder have trouble making friends and often find themselves in conflict with adults. See Box 37.5.

BOX 37.5 CLINICAL VIGNETTE

Leon (Conduct Disorder)

- Leon, a 14-year-old Puerto Rican boy, was admitted to the child psychiatric inpatient service from the emergency department (ED) after a fight with his mother. His mother reported that she and Leon had argued earlier in the evening and that he stormed out of the house screaming and vowing he would never return. Several hours later, Leon came back, yelling and demanding entry into the apartment. Leon's father was working. While his mother was getting up to open the door, Leon continued to yell and scream, waking the neighbors. This led to further arguing between Leon and his mother. Before long, the police were called, and Leon was taken to the ED.

- The admission interview revealed that Leon had run away on several occasions and had even stayed away overnight. Although he strongly denied drug use, he had gotten drunk on several occasions. He had also been in several fights, the latest of which resulted in an expulsion from school. Three months before admission, he was caught trying to steal a CD from a music store. More recently, he boasted that he and his friends had snatched a purse at an outdoor concert and had broken into a car to steal its contents. Leon's school performance has been declining; he was truant on several occasions and will probably have to repeat ninth grade.

- Leon was born in Puerto Rico and is the oldest of three children. His family moved to the mainland shortly after his birth, and the primary language at home is Spanish. His father is employed as a janitor and speaks very little English. His mother works as a secretary and has achieved fairly good command of English. He has received no treatment except for consultation with the school social worker.

What Do You Think?

- When conducting a nursing assessment, what would you want to learn about Leon's school performance?
- What information could you provide Leon's parents about pharmacotherapy? About behavior management?

Conduct disorder is characterized by more serious violations of social norms, including aggressive behavior, destruction of property, and cruelty to animals. Children and adolescents with conduct disorder often lie to achieve short-term ends, may be truant from school, may run away from home, and may engage in petty larceny or even mugging.

Epidemiology

Disruptive behavior disorders are more common in boys and are associated with lower socioeconomic status and urban living (Miranda-Mendizabal et al., 2019). These disorders are relatively common in school-aged children and are frequently presenting complaints in child psychiatric treatment settings.

The prevalence of conduct disorder estimates range from 2% up to 10% with a median of 4%. The disorder appears to be fairly consistent across various countries that differ in race and ethnicity. Prevalence rates rise from childhood to adolescence and are higher among males than among females. Males with conduct disorder frequently are involved in fighting, stealing, vandalism, and school disciplinary problems. Females with the diagnosis are more likely to practice lying, truancy, running away, substance use, and prostitution. Whereas males tend to exhibit both physical aggression and relational aggression (i.e., behaviors that harm social relations of others), females tend to exhibit relatively more relational aggression (APA, 2013). Conduct disorder is one of the most frequently diagnosed disorders in children in mental health facilities. Individuals with conduct disorder are at greater risk for experiencing mood or anxiety disorders and substance-related disorders (APA, 2013).

Etiology

The etiologies of oppositional defiant disorder and conduct disorder are complex. More attention has been paid to conduct disorder, probably because it is the more serious of the two. Models used to understand aggressiveness (see Chapter 20) are useful in examining these childhood disorders, which appear to have both genetic and environmental components.

Mental Health Nursing Assessment

The nurse gathers data from multiple sources. Adolescents with these disorders are at high risk for physical injury as a result of fighting and impulsive behavior. Sexual promiscuity is common, resulting in an increased frequency of pregnancy and sexually transmitted diseases.

An important aspect of assessment is to rule out comorbid conditions that may partially explain or complicate the person's lack of behavioral control. These conditions include ADHD, learning disabilities, chemical dependency, depression, bipolar illness, or generalized anxiety disorder. Young people who are chronically depressed may be irritable and easily frustrated. Given the tendency of adolescents to act out their frustration, chronic depression may exacerbate their behavior. Conduct problems can also elevate the risk for depression because young people who regularly elicit negative attention from parents and teachers and are constantly at odds with their environment may become despondent.

Adolescents with conduct problems are usually brought or forced into the mental health system by family, school, or the court system because of fighting, truancy, speeding tickets, car accidents, petty crimes, substance abuse, or suicide attempts. These young people may be hostile, sarcastic, defensive, and provocative. At the same time, they may appear calm, outgoing, and engaging.

Inconsistencies, distortions, and misrepresentations of the truth are common when interviewing these children, so obtaining a clear history may be difficult. Therefore, instead of asking whether an event or behavior occurred, it may be better to ask when it occurred. These adolescents are adept at changing the subject and diverting discussions from sensitive issues. They often use denial, projection, and externalization of anger as defense mechanisms when asked for self-disclosure. The assessment, which may take several sessions, should be conducted in a nonjudgmental fashion. High levels of marital conflict, parental substance abuse, and parental antisocial behavior often mark family history.

Priority of Care

After patient and staff safety are established, improving communication and coping skills should be the patient's priorities. The nurse can help the patient develop insight into the need for enhanced communication and positive coping.

Nursing Interventions

Children with oppositional defiant disorder or conduct disorder who also have specific neurodevelopmental disorders should be placed in appropriate programs for remediation. If a diagnosis of ADHD or depression emerges from the evaluation, appropriate pharmacotherapy should be considered (see previous discussion of ADHD and after the discussion regarding depression). In planning interventions for patients with oppositional defiant disorder or conduct disorder, the focus is on problem behaviors. Therapeutic progress may be slow, at least partly because these patients often lack trust in authority figures.

Social Skills Training

The nurse should communicate behavioral expectations clearly and enforce them consistently. Consequences of appropriate and inappropriate actions also should be clear. Specific approaches for improving social and problem-solving skills are fundamental features for school-aged children and adolescents. Insofar as children and adolescents with conduct problems fail to recognize the adverse effects of their verbal and nonverbal behavior, their deficit can be formulated as an interpersonal problem. Social skills training teaches adolescents with these behavior disorders to recognize the ways in which their actions affect others. Training involves techniques such as role-playing, modeling by the therapist, and giving positive reinforcement to improve interpersonal relationships and enhance social outcomes.

Problem-Solving Therapy

In contrast to social skills training, which proposes that problems of conduct are the result of poor interpersonal skills, problem-solving therapy conceptualizes conduct problems as the result of deficiencies in cognitive processes. These processes include assessment of situations, interpretation of events, and expectations of others that are congruent with behavior. These children often misinterpret the intentions of others and may perceive hostility with little or no cause. Problem-solving skills training teaches these children to generate alternative solutions to social situations, sharpen thinking concerning the consequences of those choices, and evaluate responses after interpersonal conflicts.

Parent Management Training and Education

Parent training begins with educating parents about disruptive behavior disorders, focusing particularly on impulsiveness, impaired judgment, and self-control. Children with long-standing problems in these areas often elicit punitive responses and negative attributions about their behavior from their parents. Ironically, because these parental responses focus on the child's failure, they may contribute to the child's behavior problems. An important second step is to clarify parental expectations and interpretation of the child's behavior. Parent management training may be offered to a group of parents or to individuals.

The aims of education are to provide parents with new ways of understanding their child's behavior and to promote improved interactions between parent and child. The most commonly presented techniques include the importance of positive reinforcement (praise and tangible rewards) for adaptive behavior, clear limits for unacceptable behavior, and use of mild punishment (e.g., a time out) (Box 37.6).

Referral to Family Therapy

Family therapy is directed at assisting the family with altering maladaptive patterns of interaction or improving adjustment to stressors, such as changes or loss in family membership. Multisystem family therapy, which considers the child in the context of multiple family and community systems, has shown promise in the treatment of adolescents with conduct disorder.

Evaluation and Treatment Outcomes

The nurse can review treatment goals and objectives to assess the child's progress with respect to verbal and physical aggression, socially appropriate resolution of conflicts, compliance with rules and expectations, and

---

BOX 37.6

Time-Out Procedure

Labeling behavior: Identify the behavior that the child is expected to perform or cease. The aim of this statement is to make clear what is required of the child. It typically takes the form of a simple declarative sentence: "Threatening is not acceptable."

Warning: In this step, the child is informed that if they do not perform the expected behavior or stop the unacceptable behavior, they will be given a "time out." "This is a warning: if you continue threatening to hit people, you'll have a time out."

Time out: If the child does not heed the warning, they are told to take a time out in simple straightforward terms: "Take a time out."

Duration: The usual duration for a time out is 5 minutes for children 5 years of age or older.

Location: The child sits in a designated time-out chair without toys and without talking. The chair should be located away from general activity but within view. A kitchen timer can be used to mark the time, but the clock does not start until the child sits quietly in the designated spot.

Follow-up: The child is asked to recount why they were given the time out. The explanation need not be detailed, and no further discussion of the matter is required. Indeed, long discourse about the child's behavior is not helpful and should be avoided.

---

better management of frustration. As is true for the initial assessment, evaluation of treatment outcomes relies on input from parents, teachers, and other health care team members.

Continuum of Care

Children and adolescents with conduct disorders may be involved with many different agencies in the community, such as child welfare services, school authorities, and the legal system. Mental health services are requested when a child or adolescent's behavior is out of control or a when comorbid disorder is suspected. Helping the patient and family negotiate their way through this maze of services may be an essential part of the treatment plan.

TIC DISORDERS AND TOURETTE SYNDROME

Tics are a part of several mental health problems. **Motor tics** are usually quick jerky movements of the eyes, face, neck, and shoulders, although they may involve other muscle groups as well. Occasionally, tics involve slower, more purposeful, or dystonic movements. **Phonic tics** typically include repetitive throat clearing, grunting, or other noises but may also include more complex sounds, such as words; parts of words; and in a minority of patients, obscenities. Transient tics by definition do

not endure over time and appear to be fairly common in school-aged children. *Tic disorder* is a general term encompassing several syndromes that are chiefly characterized by motor tics, phonic tics, or both.

> **KEYCONCEPT Tics** are sudden, rapid, repetitive, stereotyped motor movements or vocalizations.

Tourette Syndrome, the most severe tic disorder, is defined by multiple motor and phonic tics for at least 1 year. Because no diagnostic tests are used to confirm this disorder, the diagnosis is based on the type and duration of tics present (Gill & Kompoliti, 2020). Early symptoms of Tourette syndrome typically occur in early childhood, with an average onset between the ages of 3 and 9 years (National Institute of Health, National Institute of Neurologic Disorders and Stroke [NIH NINDS], 2020). The average age when symptoms are most severe is 9 years old. Motor tics generally precede phonic tics, and parents often describe the seeming replacement of one tic with another. In addition to this changing repertoire of motor and phonic tics, Tourette syndrome exhibits a waxing and waning course. The child can suppress the tics for brief periods. Thus, it is not uncommon to hear from parents that their child has more frequent tics at home than at school. Older children and adults may describe an urge or a physical sensation before having a tic. The general trend is for tic symptoms to decline by early adulthood.

Epidemiology and Etiology

Studies estimate that 1 out of every 162 children (0.6%) has Tourette syndrome, of which only half are diagnosed. Among those diagnosed, 37 report moderate to severe symptoms. Symptoms generally occur for around 2 years before receiving a formal diagnosis. Tourette syndrome is more common in boys than girls. Though Tourette syndrome is found in all racial and ethnic groups, non-Hispanic White children are twice as likely to have a diagnosis than Hispanic and non-Hispanic Black children. It is not uncommon for children diagnosed with Tourette syndrome to have a comorbid mental, behavioral, or developmental disorder. More than a third of individuals with Tourette syndrome have OCD. Other comorbid diagnoses include ADHD (63%), anxiety (49%), learning disabilities (47%), ASD (35%), developmental delays (30%), behavioral problems (26%), and depression (25%). In addition, over 40% of children with Tourette syndrome have a co-occurring chronic health condition (CDC, 2020e).

The precise nature of the underlying pathophysiology in this primarily inherited disorder is unclear, but the basal ganglia and functionally related cortical areas are presumed to play a central role. Findings from neuroimaging studies are consistent with the presumption that a dysregulation of the cortico-striatal–thalamic circuitry of the brain underlies Tourette syndrome. Additionally, multiple genes on different chromosomes interacting with environmental factors are involved. Several neurotransmitters (dopamine, serotonin, and norepinephrine) have been implicated in the etiology of Tourette syndrome (Kanaan et al., 2017; NIH NINDS, 2020).

Family Response to Disorder

Before evaluation and diagnosis of Tourette disorder, most families struggle with various explanations for the child's tics. Because tics fluctuate in severity with time and may be more prominent in some settings than in others, family members may have difficulty understanding their involuntary nature. Some parents may be convinced that the tics are deliberate and done to secure attention; others may judge that the tics are "nervous habits" indicative of underlying trouble. Such views require reconciliation with the currently accepted view that tics are involuntary. Some parents may conclude that the child is incapable of controlling any behavior because of Tourette disorder. They may subsequently feel uncertain about setting limits. In these families, delineating the boundaries of Tourette syndrome can be helpful (CDC, 2020e).

On learning that this disorder is probably genetic, some parents may harbor guilt for having passed it on to their child. The nurse can assist such families by listening to these concerns and providing information about the natural history of Tourette disorder—it is not a progressive condition, tics often diminish in adulthood, and it need not restrict what the child can achieve in life.

Evidence-Based Nursing Care for Children with Tourette Syndrome

Mental Health Nursing Assessment

Nursing assessment of a child with tics includes a review of the onset, course, and current level of the symptoms. Goals of the assessment are to identify the frequency, intensity, complexity, and interference of the tics and their effects on functioning; determine the child's level of adaptive functioning; identify the child's areas of strength and weakness in general and in school; and identify social supports for the child and family.

Another important aspect of the assessment is to determine the effects of the tic symptoms on the child and family. Some children and families adjust well; however, others are embarrassed or devastated and tend to withdraw socially. Because of the likelihood of comorbid mental, behavioral, or developmental disorders, in addition to inquiring about tics, the nurse should assess the child's overall development, activity level, and capacity to concentrate and persist with a single task, as well as explore repetitive habits and recurring worries.

Clinical Judgment

Children with Tourette syndrome typically have normal intelligence, but their tics can interfere with their ability to relate to others and perform well in school. The nurse should determine the degree of anxiety experienced by the child, the impact of the tics on the child's ability to cope, and whether the tics contribute to interference with social relationships and interactions.

Nursing Interventions

The approach to planning nursing interventions depends on the primary source of impairment: tics themselves; OCD symptoms; or the triad of hyperactivity, inattention, and poor impulse control. The nurse can provide counseling and education for the patient, education for the parents, and consultation for the school. Most children and their families need some education about Tourette syndrome. Individual psychotherapy with a mental health specialist (e.g., a psychologist or an advanced practice nurse) may be indicated for some children and adolescents with Tourette syndrome to deal with maladaptive responses to the chronic condition. There is evidence that comprehensive behavior therapy is effective in reducing the tics (Pringsheim et al., 2019).

Medications

Two classes of drugs are commonly used in the treatment of tics: antipsychotics and α-adrenergic receptor agonists. Aripiprazole is replacing the use of older antipsychotics, such as haloperidol and pimozide (Yang et al., 2020). These potent dopamine blockers are often effective at low doses. Attempts to eradicate all tics by increasing the dosages of these antipsychotics almost certainly will result in diminishing therapeutic returns and additional side effects. The most frequently encountered side effects include drowsiness, dulled thinking, muscle stiffness, akathisia, increased appetite and weight gain, and acute dystonic reactions. Long-term use carries a small risk for tardive dyskinesia.

Psychoeducation

Teachers, guidance counselors, and school nurses may need current information about Tourette syndrome and its related problems. Discussions with school personnel often include issues such as how to deal with tic behaviors that are disruptive in the classroom, how to manage teasing from other children, and how to handle medication side effects. A careful discussion of the boundaries of Tourette syndrome and tic symptomatology usually can resolve these matters. Teachers who understand the involuntary nature of tics can often generate creative solutions, such as excusing the child to do errands. This strategy allows the child to step out of the classroom briefly to release a bout of tics, thereby reducing stress. In some situations, a brief presentation about Tourette syndrome to the class will reduce teasing and help both teachers and classmates tolerate the tic symptoms (Box 37.7).

Before initiating these interventions with the school personnel, it is essential to identify the child's needs and to pursue these strategies in collaboration with the family and other clinical team members. The Education for the Handicapped Act (Public Law 94–142) ensures that children with conditions such as Tourette Syndrome are eligible for special education services even if they do not meet full criteria for having a learning disability. Thus, if evidence shows that Tourette disorder is hindering academic progress, parents can demand special education services for their child. Nurses can help families negotiate with the school to obtain appropriate services.

Evaluation and Treatment Outcomes

Treatment outcomes will vary over the years and will be influenced by growth and development changes, family interaction and understanding of the disorder, and reduction or elimination of the frequency of the tics. Outcomes should include improvement of the child's quality of life and ability to learn to manage the symptoms of the disorder.

SEPARATION ANXIETY DISORDER

Separation anxiety is normal for very young children, but typically declines between ages 3 and 5 years. When the child's fear and anxiety around separation become developmentally inappropriate, separation anxiety disorder is diagnosed. Separation anxiety disorder is the most common childhood anxiety disorder and occurs at a mean age of 7 years (Vaughan et al., 2017). Although many children experience some discomfort on separation from their attachment figures, children with separation anxiety disorder suffer great worry or fear when faced with ordinary separations or being away from home, such as when going to school. When separation is about to occur, children often resist by crying or hiding from their parents (Phillips et al., 2020). When asked, most children with separation anxiety disorder will express worry about harm to or permanent loss of their major attachment figure. Other children may express worry about their own safety. For a discussion of other anxiety disorders, see Chapter 27.

A common manifestation of anxiety is school phobia, in which the child refuses to attend school, preferring to

---

BOX 37.7 • TICS AND DISRUPTIVE BEHAVIORS

INEFFECTIVE APPROACH

Teacher: I see the tics. He jerks his head, makes faces, and flicks his hands.

Nurse: What do you do about them?

Teacher: What can I do? If he isn't disrupting the class, I leave him alone. Even when he is throwing spitballs.

Nurse: Spitballs! He shouldn't be allowed to throw spitballs.

Teacher: Oh, I thought that was a part of his problem.

Nurse: Well, throwing spitballs has nothing to do with tics.

EFFECTIVE APPROACH

Teacher: I see the tics. He jerks his head, makes faces, and flicks his hands.

Nurse: He cannot help the tics that you are seeing. Tic disorders can exhibit a wide range of severity, from mild to severe and from simple to complex. Some complex tics may be difficult to distinguish from habits or rituals.

Teacher: What about things like throwing spitballs? When he does things like that, I try to ignore that behavior.

Nurse: Sounds like you give him the benefit of the doubt. (Validation) However, throwing a spitball is not a tic behavior.

Teacher: What should I do?

Nurse: How do you usually handle that type of behavior? (A modification of reflection)

Teacher: I'd ask him to stop and sometimes go into the hall.

Nurse: Disruptive behavior that is voluntary in a student with a tic disorder should be handled as you would handle any other child.

CRITICAL THINKING CHALLENGE

• Compare the responses of the nurse in these scenarios. What made the difference in the teacher's responsiveness to the nurse?

stay at home with the primary attachment figure. The term *school phobia* was coined to distinguish it from truancy; whether it is a phobia in the usual sense is a matter of some debate. However, school phobia is common in other disorders such as general anxiety disorder, social phobia, OCD, depression, and conduct disorder. When a comorbid disorder such as depression is identified, it becomes the focus of treatment. In some cases, school phobia may resolve when the primary disorder is successfully treated.

Epidemiology and Etiology

Separation anxiety disorder is estimated at 1% to 4% of school-aged children between ages 5 and 11 years (Vaughan et al., 2017). Insecure attachment, difficult temperaments, and genetic factors contribute to the development of separation anxiety disorder. Anxiety disorders are often familial, so it appears that both environmental and genetic factors affect the risk for separation anxiety disorder. For example, separation anxiety may emerge after a move, change to a new school, or death of a family member or pet.

No single etiologic factor, but instead several risk factors are associated with the onset of the disorder. For example, children of parents with at least one anxiety disorder have an increased risk of also having an anxiety disorder. The risk increases even more when two parents are affected (Lawrence et al., 2019).

Family Response to Disorder

There is no single family response to a child who is experiencing separation anxiety. Parenting style, life events, and environmental factors vary from family to family. The family dynamics related to the child's behavior have to be carefully assessed. In some instances, the family may be undergoing a separation of a significant family member through death, divorce, or military deployment. In other situations, the arrival of a new family member may precede the child's separation anxiety. A family assessment is important in determining the relationship of the child's fears and anxiety and the family dynamics.

Teamwork and Collaboration: Working toward Recovery

An interdisciplinary approach is needed for the treatment of separation anxiety disorder. Effective treatment includes child and parent psychoeducation, school consultation, cognitive behavioral therapy, and selective serotonin reuptake inhibitors (SSRIs) (Vaughan et al., 2017).

Evidence-Based Nursing Care for Children with Separation Anxiety Disorder

School refusal is often what prompts the family to seek consultation for the child. Because school refusal can be a behavioral manifestation of several different child psychiatric disorders, it requires careful assessment. Issues to consider are whether the parents have been aware that the child is avoiding school (separation anxiety vs. truancy); what efforts the family has used to return the child to school; the presence of significant subjective distress in the child with anticipation of going to school; and whether the school refusal occurs in the context of other behavioral, social, or emotional problems. The nurse should also review the purpose and dose of current medications.

The child's developmental history and response to new situations and prior separations provide essential background information for understanding the child's current separation anxiety. The assessment should also include a review of recent life events and the methods the family has used to promote the child's return to school. Finally, the family history with respect to anxiety, panic attacks, or phobias is also informative.

Nursing priorities will depend on the role of the nurse (school nurse, acute care, or community practice) and the relationship with the child and family. In some instances, the nurse will be responsible for education of the child and family. If the child is receiving medication, nursing care related to administration of medications and education should be implemented. Nurses will also be involved in educating teachers and serving as a liaison between treating physicians, family and child, and school.

OBSESSIVE–COMPULSIVE DISORDER

OCD is characterized by intrusive thoughts that are difficult to dislodge (i.e., obsessions) or ritualized behaviors that the child feels driven to perform (i.e., compulsions) (see Chapter 27). Children tend to exhibit both multiple obsessions and compulsions that relate to fear of catastrophic family event, contamination, sexual or somatic obsessions, and overly moralistic thoughts. Washing, checking, repeating, and ordering are the most commonly reported compulsions (Geller, 2016).

Epidemiology and Etiology

The prevalence rate of OCD is estimated at 1% to 2% with two peaks of incidence across the life span, one occurring in preadolescent children and later a peak in early adult life (Geller, 2016). More than half of the cases of OCD in youth involve a comorbid disorder such as a tic, mood, or anxiety disorder. The etiology of OCD in children is thought to be similar to that of adults (see

Chapter 26). However, there is a subset of children whose OCD behavior that may be related to an immune response to group A beta hemolytic streptococcal infections that led to inflammation of the basal ganglia (Geller, 2016).

Family Response to Disorder

Parents' responses to their child's obsessions and compulsions depend on their understanding of the thoughts and behaviors. Because OCD is highly familial, if the parents are recovering from their disorder, they may be able to support their child's ability to begin to deal with the symptoms. Conversely, the parents may find their child's thoughts and behaviors tiring so they become easily irritated with the multiple obsessions and compulsions. Parents need education and support to help their child.

Teamwork and Collaboration: Working toward Recovery

Interdisciplinary treatment including school personnel is important for the child and family with OCD. Cognitive behavior therapy (CBT), including psychoeducation, cognitive training, exposure and response preventions, and relapse prevention, is the treatment of choice.

Evidence-Based Nursing Care for Children with OCD

Recurrent worries and ritualistic behavior can occur normally in children at particular stages of development. The first step in the assessment of OCD in children is to distinguish between normal childhood rituals and worries and pathologic rituals and obsessional thoughts. Obsessional thoughts are recurrent, nagging, and bothersome. Although children may describe obsessions as occurring "out of the blue," external events may trigger obsessions. For example, a child may fear contamination whenever they are in contact with a certain person or object. Likewise, compulsions waste time, cause distress, and interfere with daily life (Box 37.8).

The severity of the child's and family's response to OCD will determine the appropriate interventions. When the obsessions and compulsions emerge, these children or adolescents are in distress because of the disturbing and relentless nature of the symptoms.

Nursing interventions will be guided by the needs of the family and the developmental needs of the child or adolescent. If medication is prescribed, it is important to emphasize safe management of medications. Because the antidepressants have a "black box" warning regarding suicide risk in adolescents, the nurse must discuss with the parents and child the importance of monitoring moods and keeping regularly scheduled mental health appointments.

BOX 37.8 CLINICAL VIGNETTE

Kimberly and Obsessive–Compulsive Disorder

Kim, an 11-year-old fifth grader, comes for evaluation because her mother and teacher have become increasingly concerned about her repetitive behaviors. In retrospect, Kim's mother recalls first noticing repetitive rituals about 2 years before, but she did not become alarmed about these behaviors until recently when they began to interfere with daily living. At the time of referral, Kim exhibits complicated jumping rituals that involve a specific number of jumps and a particular manner of jumping. She also turns light switches off and on and performs complex movements, such as blinking in patterns and thrusting her arms back and forth a certain number of times. Her mother also reports Kim's near-constant request for reassurance about her own safety. In recent months, her incessant demands for reassurance have been more frequent and elaborate. For example, Kim's mother has to answer three times that everything is all right and then say, "I swear to it."

At the evaluation, Kim expresses fears that some ill fate, such as catastrophic illness or injury, will befall her. This fear is triggered by contact with any individual who seems sick, chance exposures to foul smells or dirt, and minor scrapes or bumps. When the fear is triggered, she becomes increasingly anxious and consumed with the fear that she will develop an illness and die. Sometimes her fears are specific, such as cancer or AIDS. Other times her fears are more ambiguous, as evidenced by statements such as, "Something bad will happen" if she doesn't complete the ritual. Kim acknowledges that the ritual is probably not related to the feared event, but she is reluctant to take a chance. If the ritual does not reduce her anxiety, she seeks reassurance from her mother.

Kim's medical history was negative for serious illness or injury. She was born after an uncomplicated pregnancy, labor, and delivery and achieved developmental milestones at appropriate times. Indeed, her mother could recall no unusual problems in the first few years of life except that Kim was typically anxious in unfamiliar situations. Kim's mother reports a prior history of panic attacks, but the family history is otherwise negative for anxiety disorders, including OCD.

What Do You Think?

- What assessment information would you want to elicit from Kim?
- What additional information should be considered from Kim's mother about her history of panic attacks?
- What nursing interventions should be considered if Kim were your patient?

OTHER NEURODEVELOPMENTAL DISORDERS

Other neurodevelopmental disorders are characterized by a narrower range of deficits. These include specific neurodevelopmental disorders generally classified as learning, communication, and motor skills disorders. This section focuses primarily on learning and communication disorders.

Specific Learning Disorders

Generally, a learning disorder (also called learning disability) is defined as a discrepancy between actual achievement and expected achievement based on the person's age and intellectual ability. The definition varies depending on the source and state statute. Learning disorders are typically classified as verbal (e.g., reading, spelling) or nonverbal (e.g., mathematics).

Reading disability, also called **dyslexia**, has been recognized for more than 100 years. It is defined as a significantly lower score for mental age on standardized tests in reading that is not the result of low intelligence or inadequate schooling. This relatively common problem affects about 5% of school-aged children, with some studies reporting higher prevalence. In clinical samples, dyslexia affects boys more often than girls. This discrepancy can be explained by slower and variable processing speed and less inhibitory control in males than females. Verbal reasoning is a strength in males (Arnett et al., 2017).

Although it is clear that no single cause will provide a sufficient explanation for reading disability, the underlying problem appears to be a deficit in **phonologic processing**, which involves the discrimination and interpretation of speech sounds. A disturbance in the development of the left hemisphere is believed to cause this deficit. Both genetic and environmental factors have been implicated in the etiology of reading disability. Data from family studies show that reading disability is familial and that shared environmental factors alone cannot explain the high rate of recurrence in affected families (Becker et al., 2017).

Less is known about the prevalence of specific learning disorder in mathematics (SLDM), with estimates as high as 6% of school-aged children and no apparent difference between boys and girls. In a study of children with SLDM, 20% also had a diagnosis of a language or communication disorder. An association with autism and ADHD was also noted (Morsanyi et al., 2018).

Communication Disorders

Communication disorders involve speech or language impairments. *Speech* refers to the motor aspects of speaking; *language* consists of higher-order aspects of formulating and comprehending verbal communication. Communication disorders are fairly common and are yet more common in children with ASDs, ADHD, anxiety, and conduct disorders (Beitchman et al., 2014). As with reading disability, undoubtedly multiple causes of speech or language deficit may be present.

A delay in speech or language development can adversely affect the child's socialization and education. For example, peers may rebuff or tease a child with an articulation defect or stutter, contributing to withdrawal and a negative self-image. The resulting isolation could limit opportunities to negotiate rules, take turns, and learn cooperation. These same tasks could also be difficult for children with language delay. Moreover, language appears to play a role in the regulation of behavior and impulses (Lyons et al., 2016).

Evidence-Based Nursing Care for Children with Communication Disorders

Nursing assessment of children with a known specific developmental disorder includes (1) evidence of interference in daily life, (2) determination of the child's ability (and limitations) to communicate during the interview, (3) assessment of the child's perception about their disability, (4) observation for impaired learning and communication, and (5) past and current interventions for the learning or communication deficit with data gathered through direct interview of the child and significant others such as parents. Several nursing diagnoses can be generated from these data, such as impaired verbal communication and social isolation.

For the child with learning disabilities, nurses can focus on building self-confidence and helping the family connect with guidance and educational resources that support the child's development into adulthood. For the child with communication disorders, the interventions focus on fostering social and communication skills and making referrals for specific speech or language therapy. Modeling appropriate communication in spontaneous situations with the child can be a useful intervention for some children. The following is an overview of nursing interventions for the child with specific developmental difficulties:

- Introduce strategies for increasing communication skills (e.g., initiating conversation, taking turns in conversation, facing the listener).

- Identify and develop specific intervention strategies for problems secondary to learning communication disorders, such as low self-esteem.

- Provide parental support for coping with the disorder.

- Maintain interdisciplinary medical, dental, and speech therapy, and also educational collaboration.

- Refer to learning or speech specialist for evaluation and assistance.

Continuum of Care

Children with learning disabilities obviously require careful psychoeducational and cognitive testing to identify their strengths and deficits. School or clinical psychologists usually perform this type of specialized testing. When a learning disability has been identified, the U.S. Education for All Handicapped Children Act (Public Law 94–142) mandates that public school systems provide remedial services in the least restrictive educational setting. Families occasionally need help in advocating for these services.

The same is true for children with communication disorders, although the services requested may be different. Speech pathologists conduct the diagnostic assessment of speech and language disorder. Nurses may be involved with formal screening for communication disorders. Services such as speech therapy (directed at the motor aspects of speaking) or social skills groups (directed at the social and interpersonal aspects of language) are often available in school districts and can be obtained if a speech or language disorder has been identified. For some children with communication disorders, the services offered by the school may be insufficient. In such cases, the nurse can help the family locate a facility that can provide these needed services.

OTHER MENTAL DISORDERS

Mood Disorders

Mood disorders in children and adolescents are a major public health concern. The prevalence of depression is estimated to be 13.3% (3.2 million) of the U.S. population. Rates of depressive episodes are higher in females (20%) as compared to males (6.8%). Approximately 60% of adolescents with depression report not receiving treatment for their illness (NIMH, 2019b). Lifetime prevalence of bipolar disorder among adolescents aged 13 to 18 is estimated to be 2.9%, of which 2.6% have severe impairment. Bipolar disorder in adolescents is found to be higher in females (3.3%) than in males (2.6%). (See Chapters 25 and 26 for a complete discussion of these disorders.)

Children with mood disorders may not spontaneously express feelings (e.g., sadness, irritability) and are more likely to show their suffering through their behavior. These children may act out their feelings rather than discuss them. Thus, behavior problems may accompany depression. Reports from parents are important sources of information about changes in sleep patterns, appetite, activity level and interests, and emotional stability.

Priorities of nursing care for children or adolescents who are depressed are similar to those for adults. Treatment goals include improving the mood and restoring sleep, appetite, and self-care. Interventions for responses to mood disorders in children and adolescents are also similar to those for adults. The psychiatric nurse develops a therapeutic relationship with the child and provides parent education and support. Developing sensitivity to the influence of environmental events on the child is important for the nurse, parents, and teachers (Box 37.9).

Children and adolescents may be treated with medication. Antidepressant medications are used for depression and mood antipsychotics for bipolar disorder. The controversy surrounding the use of SSRIs in children reminds us that all treatments involve a risk–benefit

---

BOX 37.9

Questions, Choices, and Outcomes

Mrs. S has just returned with her son Jared to the child psychiatric inpatient services facility after an overnight pass. She reports that the visit did not go well because of Jared's anger and defiance. She remarked that this behavior was distressingly similar to his behavior before the hospitalization. She expressed additional concern because of the upcoming discharge from the hospital. After saying goodbye to Jared, she pulled the nurse aside and stated that she had decided to file for divorce.

Mrs. S indicated that she had not told her husband or the family therapist. When asked whether Jared knew about her decision, Mrs. S suddenly realized that he may have overheard her discussing the matter with her sister on the telephone during this home visit.

How should the nurse approach this situation?

Choice	Possible Outcomes
Discuss her hypothesis about Jared's behavior and his uncertainty	Mother can see relationship between Jared's behavior and her plan for divorce. Mother ignores the nurse. Mother is interested but does not see the connection.
Ignore the statement	Child and family did not learn about the connection between Jared's behavior and the events at home.
Encourage Jared's mother to sort out her problems.	The focus is then on mother's problems.

ANALYSIS

The best response is focusing on the possible relationship between Jared's recent behavioral deterioration and his uncertainty about his family's future. If the nurse ignores the statement or focuses on the mother's interpretation of Jared's behavior, the mother is less likely to appreciate the connection between her pending divorce and Jared's behavior. The nurse should also emphasize the importance of discussing the matter in family therapy.

---

equation. Given the modest benefit of the SSRIs and the potential for side effects, these medications merit careful monitoring in children and adolescents. Patient monitoring should focus on evidence of benefit and side effects, including sleep problems, hyperactivity, sudden changes in mood or behavior, suicidal ideation, or self-injurious behavior.

Childhood Schizophrenia

Childhood (early-onset) schizophrenia is diagnosed by the same criteria as those used in adults (see Chapter 24). Difficulty in diagnosing a psychiatric disorder in children has led to years of debate and controversy regarding whether childhood schizophrenia differs from the adult type or is merely an early manifestation of the same disorder. For many years, it was believed that autism represented the childhood form of schizophrenia. However, today autism and childhood schizophrenia are differentiated. As currently defined, childhood schizophrenia (onset before the age of 13 years) is very rare, but prevalence increases sharply during adolescence, especially in young men (Kodish & McClellan, 2016).

Childhood schizophrenia is usually characterized by poorer premorbid functioning than late-onset schizophrenia. Common premorbid difficulties include social, cognitive, linguistic, attentional, motor, and perceptual delays. Taken together, these findings suggest that early-onset schizophrenia is a more severe form of the disorder.

Nursing care for children with schizophrenia follows an approach similar to that for ASD. Antipsychotic medications are not generally approved for use in children, although the newer atypical antipsychotic medications appear to have a lower risk for neurologic effects; other side effects such as weight gain also warrant careful monitoring.

Development of an individualized care plan for children with schizophrenia begins with a nursing assessment to identify functional problems specific to the child. Similarly, the recognition that childhood schizophrenia is a chronic and severe condition should guide the identification of outcomes. Goals should be realistic; the nurse should pay special attention to the child's support systems. Parent education about the disorder, medications, and long-term management (including use of community resources) is an essential part of the treatment plan. Long-term management also requires monitoring of chronic antipsychotic therapy.

ELIMINATION DISORDERS

Enuresis

Enuresis is the involuntary excretion of urine after the age at which the child should have attained bladder control. It usually involves involuntary bed-wetting at night, but repeated urination on clothing during waking hours can occur (diurnal enuresis). Enuresis is a self-limiting disorder, with most children experiencing a spontaneous remission.

Epidemiology and Etiology

The prevalence of nocturnal enuresis varies with age and gender, being most common in young boys—an estimated 5% to 10% of 5-year-old boys, and 3% to 5% in 10-year-old boys have nocturnal enuresis (Mikkelsen, 2014). The frequency in girls is about half that of boys in each age group. The etiology of enuresis is unknown, with probably no single cause. Most children with nocturnal enuresis are urologically normal. Some evidence has shown that at least some children with nocturnal enuresis secrete decreased amounts of antidiuretic hormone during sleep, which may play a role in enuresis (Mikkelsen, 2014).

Nursing Care

Nursing assessment should include the child's developmental history, the onset and course of enuresis, prior treatment, presence of emotional problems, and medical history. The nurse should also explore the family's home environment, family attitudes about the child's enuresis, and the family's medical history. Routine laboratory tests such as urinalysis and a urine culture are used to identify the presence of infection. The nurse should obtain baseline data regarding toileting habits, including daytime incontinence, urinary frequency, and constipation. They should refer children with persistent daytime enuresis for consultation with a urologist.

In many cases, limiting fluid intake in the evening and treating constipation (if present) is sufficient to decrease the frequency of bed-wetting. One of the most effective methods is the bell and pad. In this approach, the child sleeps on a pad that has wires on it, and when the child voids, a bell sounds, waking up the child. With use, the child either wakes up to urinate or learns to sleep through the night without voiding. A more temporary solution is the use of desmopressin (DDAVP), a synthetic antidiuretic hormone that actually inhibits production of urine. After medication is withdrawn, the enuresis frequently returns (Mikkelsen, 2014).

Encopresis

Encopresis involves soiling clothing with feces or depositing feces in inappropriate places. Additional diagnostic criteria include that the child is older than 4 years; that the soiling occurs at least once per month; and that the soiling is not the result of a medical disorder, such as congenital aganglionic megacolon (Hirschsprung disease). The most common form of encopresis is fecal impaction accompanied by leakage around the hardened mass of stool. Because of the loss of muscle tone in the lower bowel, the child loses the usual urge to defecate and may not feel the leakage. Surprisingly, the child may not detect the smell of the stool because the olfactory apparatus becomes accustomed to the odor. If left untreated, this problem generally resolves independently by middle adolescence. Nonetheless, the social consequences may be substantial (Mikkelsen, 2014).

Epidemiology and Etiology

As with enuresis, encopresis is more common in boys, and the frequency of the condition declines with age. The current estimate of prevalence is 1.5% of school-aged children aged 7 to 8 years old, with boys three times more likely to have encopresis than girls (Mikkelsen, 2014).

The reasons for withholding stool and starting the cycle of fecal impaction are unclear but are not usually the result of physical causes. However, as noted, when fecal impaction occurs, there is an accompanying loss of tone in the bowel and subsequent leakage.

Nursing Care

Assessment includes a detailed interview with the child and parent regarding the pattern of the encopresis. A calm matter-of-fact approach can help to reduce the child's embarrassment. Physical examination is also necessary; thus, collaboration with the child's primary care provider or consulting pediatric specialist is essential. The presence of encopresis does not necessarily signal severe emotional or behavioral disturbances, but the nurse should inquire about other psychiatric disorders. Diagnosis of encopresis is presumed given a history of intermittent constipation and soiling. Collaboration with primary care consultants is often helpful to rule out rare medical conditions, such as Hirschsprung disease.

Effective intervention begins with educating the parents and the child about normal bowel function and the self-perpetuating cycle of fecal impaction and leakage of stool around the hardened mass of feces. The short-term goal of this educational effort is to decrease the anger and recrimination that often complicate the picture in these families. Because encopresis often results in a loss of bowel tone, it may help to motivate children by emphasizing the need to strengthen their anal muscles.

In many cases, cleaning out the bowel is necessary before initiating behavioral treatment. The bowel catharsis is usually followed by administration of mineral oil, which is often continued during the bowel retraining program. A high-fiber diet is often recommended.

The behavioral treatment program involves daily sitting on the toilet after each meal for a predetermined period (e.g., 10 minutes). The child and parents can measure the time with an ordinary kitchen timer. The parents can encourage the child to read or look at picture books while sitting. They can give the child rewards in the form of stars, stickers, or points for complying with the retraining program and add bonuses for successful defecation. The family can tally stickers or points on a calendar, and the child can "cash in" collected points for small prizes.

Caring for children with encopresis on an inpatient unit is a challenge, because very little research provides direction for positive outcomes. Staff can become frustrated with the child's seemingly unwillingness to cooperate. Possible interventions include maintaining discretion, assisting children with the development of age-appropriate social skills and empathy, and providing positive peer pressure (Shepard et al., 2017).

IMPACT OF THE COVID-19 PANDEMIC ON MENTAL HEALTH

The COVID-19 pandemic has had widespread impact on the lives of children and adolescents across the country and around the world. The combination of the public health crisis, social isolation, and economic recession contributes to the development of psychosocial stressors that may result the development of mental health problems or worsen already existing mental health conditions, including an increased risk of post-traumatic stress disorder (PTSD), depression, and anxiety (Golberstein et al., 2020; Guessoum et al., 2020). School closures have affected the lives of an estimated 55 million students across the country, causing significant disruption in students' day-to-day routines. Social isolation and physical distancing resulting in a lack of regular contact with friends is of particular concern in middle childhood and adolescence. Studies have found that when children are out of school, they are more likely to be less physically active, spend more time on electronics/screens, and have inconsistent eating and sleeping patterns (Nearchou et al., 2020). For quite some time, schools have served as a de facto mental health system for children and adolescents. Data from a nationally representative study of adolescents receiving mental health services found that 35% of them received their mental health services exclusively from school settings (Ali et al., 2019). The closure of schools effectively terminates or significantly reduces the availability of some imperative resources. Fortunately, telehealth services have been found to be similarly effective to in-person services, though not all families and schools have the technology to support this. The coordination and partnership of schools and community mental health agencies may allow students to engage in needed mental health treatment (Golberstein et al., 2020). Strategies to help provide stability and support to children and adolescents include establishing and maintaining a normal routine, encouraging expression of thoughts and concerns, providing honest and accurate information, teaching simple steps to maintain health, being attentive to changes in behavior, and reassurance about the child's safety and well-being (Centers for Disease Control and Prevention [CDC], 2020a).

SUMMARY OF KEY POINTS

- An estimated 20% of American youths are affected by a mental disorder that impairs their ability to function.

- In addressing intellectual disabilities, the emphasis is on determining adaptive behaviors (e.g., conceptual skills, concepts, self-direction), social skills, and practical skills. With guidance and education, many children will no longer have a disability as adults.

- Children with ASD benefit from structure and specific behavioral interventions.

- ADHD is defined by the presence of inattention; impulsiveness; and in most cases, hyperactivity. As currently defined, ADHD is the most common disorder of childhood. This heterogeneous disorder affects boys more often than girls. Nursing interventions involve family and child education and support. The family must partner with the school system to help the child receive the best educational experience. Effective treatment of ADHD often involves multiple approaches, including medication and parental education and support.

- Tourette syndrome is a tic disorder characterized by motor and phonic tics. It is a frustrating disorder that requires patience and understanding. About half of the children with this disorder also have ADHD.

- Separation anxiety is relatively common in school-aged children. OCD becomes more common in adolescents. Treatment of separation anxiety and OCD may include medication, behavioral therapy, or a combination of these treatments.

- Elimination disorders include encopresis and enuresis. Behavioral therapy approaches are the most effective treatment for these disorders. Medication may also be used.

- Major depression in children is believed to be similar to major depression in adults.

- Childhood schizophrenia is a rare disorder, so other diagnoses should be carefully considered. Nursing care is similar to care of children with ASDs.

CRITICAL THINKING CHALLENGES

1. Interview parents of a child with an intellectual disability. Determine their approach to providing support in education and socialization.

2. Examine the differences and similarities between ASD with and without intellectual and language impairment. Determine whether differences exist in the nursing care according to the diagnoses. Develop a teaching plan for parents of children who have ASD and are trying to understand the underlying problems related to the disorder.

3. Compare and contrast nursing approaches for a child with ADHD with those used for a child with ASD. How are they different? How are they similar?

4. Learning disabilities and communication disorders are more common in children with psychiatric disorders than in the general population. How might a learning disability or a communication disorder complicate a psychiatric illness in a school-aged child?

5. How would you answer these questions from a parent: "What causes ADHD? Is it my fault"?

6. A child is threatening to kill himself. What information is needed in order to keep this child safe?

 Movie Viewing Guides
Rain Man: (1988). This classic film stars Dustin Hoffman as Raymond Babbitt, a man who has autism (savant). Tom Cruise plays his brother Charlie, a self-centered hustler who believes that he has been cheated out of his inheritance. Discovering Raymond in an institution, Charlie abducts Raymond in a last-ditch effort to get his fair share of the family estate. The story revolves around the relationship that develops as the brothers drive across the country.

Dustin Hoffman brilliantly portrays the behaviors and symptoms of high-functioning autism, such as the monotone speech, insistence on sameness, and repetitive behavior.

VIEWING POINTS: Identify and describe Raymond's ritualistic behaviors. Observe Raymond's language patterns and any distinct abnormalities. What happens when Raymond's rituals are interrupted?

REFERENCES

Ali, M. M., West, K., Teich, J. L., Lynch, S., Mutter, R., & Dubenitz, J. (2019). Utilization of mental health services in educational setting by adolescents in the United States. *Journal of School Health, 89*(5), 393–401.

American Association on Intellectual and Developmental Disabilities. (2021). Definition of intellectual disability. Retrieved January 1, 2021, from https://www.aaidd.org/intellectual-disability/definition

American Psychiatric Association. (2013). *Diagnostic and statistical manual of mental disorders* (5th ed.). Arlington, VA: Author.

Arnett, A. B., Pennington, B. F., Peterson, R. L., Willcutt, E. G., DeFries, J. C., & Olson, R. K. (2017). Explaining the sex difference in dyslexia. *Journal of Child Psychology & Psychiatry.* doi:10.1111/jcpp.12691

Bai, D., Marrus, N., Yip, B. H. K., Reichenberg, A., Constantino, J. N., & Sandin, S. (2020). Inherited risk for autism through maternal and paternal lineage. *Biological Psychiatry, 88*(6), 480–487.

Becker, N., Vasconcelos, M., Oliveira, V., Santos, F. C. D., Bizarro, L., Almeida, R., Salles, J. F. D., & Caralho, M. R. S. (2017). Genetic and environmental risk factors for developmental dyslexia in children: A systematic review of the last decade. *Developmental Neuropsychology, 42*(7/8), 423–445.

Beitchman, J. H., Brownlie, E. B., & Bao, L. (2014). Age 31 mental health outcomes of childhood language and speech disorders. *Journal of the American Academy of Child & Adolescent Psychiatry, 53*(10), 1102–1110.

Bowling, A., Blaine, R. E., Kaur, R., & Davison, K. K. (2019). Shaping healthy habits in children with neurodevelopmental and mental health disorders: Parent perceptions of barriers, facilitators and promising strategies. *The International Journal of Behavioral Nutrition and Physical Activity, 26*(16), 52.

Buckley, N., Glasson, E. J., Chen, W., Epstein, A., Leonard, H., Skoss, R., Jacoby, P., Blackmore, A. M., Srinivasjois, R., Bourke, J., Sanders, R. J., & Downs, J. (2020). Prevalence estimates of mental health problems in children and adolescents with intellectual disability: A systematic review and meta-analysis. *The Australian and New Zealand Journal of Psychiatry, 54*(10), 970–984.

Buitelaar, N. J. L., Posthumus, J. A., & Buitelaar, J. K. (2020). Domestic violence or intimate partner violence: A systematic review. *Journal of Attention Disorders, 24*(9), 1203–1214.

Centers for Disease Control and Prevention. (2020a). COVID-19 parental resources kit- Childhood. Retrieved on January 7, 2021, from https://www.cdc.gov/coronavirus/2019-ncov/daily-life-coping/parental-resource-kit/childhood.html

Centers for Disease Control and Prevention. (2020b). Data and statistics on children's mental health. Retrieved January 1, 2021, from https://www.cdc.gov/childrensmentalhealth/data.html

Centers for Disease Control and Prevention. (2020c). What is ADHD? [Online]. Retrieved on January 2, 2021, from https://www.cdc.gov/ncbddd/adhd/facts.html

Centers for Disease Control and Prevention. (2020d). What is Autism Spectrum Disorder? Retrieved on January 1, 2021, from https://www.cdc.gov/ncbddd/autism/facts.html

Centers of Disease Control and Prevention. (2020e). What is Tourette Syndrome? Retrieved on January 3, 2021, from https://www.cdc.gov/ncbddd/tourette/facts.html

Chang, J. G., Cimino, F. M., & Gossa, W. (2020). ADHD in children: Common questions and answers. *American Family Physician, 102*(10), 592–602.

Chaplin, S. (2018). Diagnosis and management of ADHD in children and adults. *Prescriber, 29*(10), 23–27.

Claudius, I., & Axeen, S. (2020). Differences in comorbidities between children and youth with suicide attempts versus ideation presenting to the emergency department. *Archives of Suicide Research, 6*, 1–10.

Conners, C. K. (1989). *Conners' Rating Scales Manual.* Multi-Health Systems.

Daley, D., Van Der Oord, S., Ferrin, M., Cortese, S., Danckaerts, M., Doepfner, M., Van den Hoofdakker, B. J., Coghill, D., Thompson, M., Asherson, P., Banaschewski, T., Brandeis, D., Buitelaar, J., Dittmann, R. W., Hollis, C., Holtmann, M., Konofal, E., Lecendreux, M., Rothenberger, A., Santosh, P., … Sonuga-Barke, E. J. (2018). Practitioner review: Current best practice in the use of parent training and other behavioural interventions in the treatment of children and adolescents with attention deficit hyperactivity disorder. *Journal of Child Psychology & Psychiatry, 47*(2), 199–212.

Danielson, M. L., Bitsko, R. H., Ghandour, R. M., Holbrook, J. R., Kogan, M. D., & Blumberg, S. J. (2018). Prevalence of parent-reported ADHD diagnosis and associated treatment among U.S. children and adolescents, 2016. *Journal of Clinical Child & Adolescent Psychology, 47*(2), 199–212.

Davico, C., Canavese, C., Vittorini, R., Gandione, M., & Vitiello, B. (2018). Anticonvulsants for psychiatric disorders in children and adolescents: A systematic review of their efficacy. *Frontiers in Psychiatry, 9*, 270.

Deater-Deckard, K. (2017). Parents' and children's ADHD in a family system. *Journal of Abnormal Child Psychology, 45*(3), 519–525.

Del-Ponte, B., Quinte, G. C., Cruz, S., Grellert, M., & Santos, I. S. (2019). Dietary patterns and attention deficit/hyperactivity disorder (ADHD): A systematic review and meta-synthesis. *Journal of Affective Disorders, 252*, 160–173.

Donzelli, G., Carducci, A., Llopis-Gonzalez, A., Verani, M., Llopis-Morales, A., Cioni, L., & Morales-Suarez-Varela, M. (2019). The association between lead and Attention-Deficit/Hyperactivity Disorder: A systematic review. *International Journal of Environmental Research and Public Health, 16*(3), 382.

Feldman, M. E., Charach, A., & Belanger, S. A. (2018). ADHD in children and youth: Part 2-treatment. *Paediatrics Child Health, 23*(7), 462–472.

Feingold, B. M. (1975). Hyperkinesis and learning disabilities linked to artificial food flavors and colors. *American Journal of Nursing, 75*(5), 797–783.

Fuemmeler, B. F., Sheng, Y., Schechter, J. C., Do, E., Zucker, N., Majors, A., Maguire, R., Murphy, S. K., Hoyo, C., & Kollins, S. H. (2020). Associations between attention deficit hyperactivity disorder symptoms and eating behaviors in early childhood. *Pediatric Obesity, 15*(7), 1–10.

Geller, D. (2016). Obsessive-compulsive disorder. In M. K. Dulcan (Ed.), *Dulcan's textbook of child and adolescent psychiatry* (2nd ed.). American Psychiatric Publishing.

Ghandour, R. M., Sherman, L. J., Vladutiu, C. J., Alie, M. M., Lynch, S. E., Bitsko, R. H., & Blumberg, S. J. (2019). Prevalence and treatment of depression, anxiety, and conduct problems in U.S. children. *Journal of Pediatrics, 206*, 256–267.

Gill, C. E., & Kompoliti, K. (2019). Clinical features of Tourette syndrome. *Journal of Child Neurology, 35*(2), 166–174.

Ginsberg, Y., Quintero, J., Anand, E., Casillas, M., & Upadhyaya, H. P. (2014). Underdiagnosis of attention-deficit/hyperactivity disorder in adult patients: A review of the literature. *Primary Care Companion CNS Disorders, 16*(3), PCC.13r01600.

Giupponi, G., Innamorati, M., Rogante, E., Sarubbi, S. Erbuto, D., Maniscalco, I… Pompili, M. (2020). The characteristics of mood polarity, temperament, and suicide risk in adult ADHD. *International Journal of Research and Public Health, 17*, 2871.

Golberstein, E., Wen, H., & Miller, B. F. (2020). Coronavirus disease 2019 (COVID-19) and mental health for children and adolescents. *JAMA Pediatrics, 175*(9), 819–820.

Goyette, C. H., Conners, C. K., & Ulrich, R. F. (1978). Normative data on the Conners parent and teachers rating scales. *Journal of Abnormal Child Psychology, 6*(2), 221–236.

Guessoum, S. B., Lachal, J., Radjack, R., Carretier, E., Minassian, S., Benoit, L., & Moro, M. R. (2020). Adolescent psychiatric disorders during the COVID-19 pandemic and lockdown. *Psychiatry Research, 291*, 1–6.

Hou, Y. W., Xiong, P., Gu, X., Huang, X., Wang, M., & Wu, J. (2018). Association of serotonin receptors with attention deficit hyperactivity disorder: A systematic review and meta-analysis. *Current Medical Science, 38*(3), 538–551.

Huang, Y., Su, H., Au, W., Xu, C., & Wu, K. (2018). Involvement of family environmental, behavioral, and social functional factors in children with attention-deficit/hyperactivity disorder. *Psychology Research and Behavior Management, 9*(11), 447–457.

Kanaan, A. S., Gerasch, S., García-García, I., Lampe, L., Pampel, A., Anwander, A., Near, J., Möller, H. E., & Müller-Vahl, K. (2017). Pathological glutamatergic transmission in Gilles de la Tourette syndrome. *Brain, 140*(Pt 1), 218–234.

Kanner, L. (1943). Autistic disturbances of affective contact. *Nervous Child, 2*, 217–250.

Kim, J. H., Kim, J. Y., Lee, J., Jeong, G. H., Lee, E., Lee, S., Lee, K. H., Kronbichler, A., Stubbs, B., Solmi, M., Koyanagi, A., Hong, S. H., Dragioti, E., Jacob, L., Brunoni, A. R., Carvalho, A. F., Radua, J., Thompson, T., Smith, L., Oh, H., … Fusar-Poli, P. (2020). Environmental risk factors, protective factors, and peripheral biomarkers for ADHD: An umbrella review. *Lancet Psychiatry, 7*(11), 955–970.

Klein, M. O., Battagello, D. S., Cardoso, A. R., Hauser, D. N., Bittencourt, J. C., & Correa, R. G. (2019). Dopamine: Functions, signaling, and association with neurological diseases. *Cellular and Molecular Neurobiology, 39*(1), 31–59.

Kodak, T., & Bergmann, S. (2020). Autism spectrum disorder: Characteristics, associated behaviors, and early intervention. *Pediatric Clinics of North America, 67*(3), 525–535.

Kodish, I., & McClellan, J. M. (2016). Early-onset schizophrenia. In M. K. Dulcan (Ed.), *Dulcan's textbook of child and adolescent psychiatry* (2nd ed.). American Psychiatric Publishing.

Korrel, H., Mueller, K. L., Silk, T., Anderson, V., & Sciberras, E. (2017). Research review: Language problems in children with attention-deficit hyperactivity disorder—a systematic meta-analytic review. *Journal of Child Psychology & Psychiatry, 58*(6), 640–654. doi:10.1111/jcpp.12688

Lawrence, P. J., Murayama, K., & Creswell, C. (2019). Systematic review and meta-analysis: Anxiety and depressive disorders in offspring of parents with anxiety disorders. *Journal of the American Academy of Child & Adolescent Psychiatry, 58*(1), 46–50.

Levy, T., Kronenberg, S., Crosbie, J., & Schachar, R. J. (2020). Attention-deficit/hyperactivity disorder (ADHD) symptoms and suicidality in children: The mediating role of depression, irritability, and anxiety symptoms. *Journal of Affective Disorders, 265*, 200–206.

Li, Y.-J., Xie, X.-N., Lei, X., Li, Y.-M., & Lei, X. (2020). Global prevalence of obesity, overweight, and underweight in children, adolescents and adults with autism spectrum disorder, attention-deficit hyperactivity disorder: A systematic review and meta-analysis. *Obesity Reviews, 21*(12), e13123.

Liu, W.-J., Mao, H.-J., Hu, L.-I., Song, M.-F., Jang, H.-Y., & Zhang, L. (2020). Attention-deficit/hyperactivity disorder medication and risk of suicide attempt: A meta-analysis of observational studies. *Pharmacoepidemiology & Drug Safety, 29*(11), 1364–1372.

Lyons, G. L., Huber, H. B., Carter, E. W., Chen, R., & Asmus, J. M. (2016). Assessing the social skills and problem behaviors of adolescents with severe disabilities enrolled in general education classes. *American Journal of Intellectual Developmental Disability, 121*(4), 327–345.

Maenner, M. J., Shaw, K. A., Baio, J., EdS1, Washington, A., Patrick, M., DiRienzo, M., Christensen, D. L., Wiggins, L. D., Pettygrove, S., Andrews, J. G., Lopez, M., Hudson, A., Baroud, T., Schwenk, Y., White, T., Rosenberg, C. R., Lee, L. C., Harrington, R. A., Huston, M., … Dietz, P. M. (2020). Prevalence of autism spectrum disorder among children aged 8 years—autism and developmental disabilities monitoring network, 11 sites, United States, 2016. *MMWR Surveillance Summaries, 69*(3/4), 1–12.

Matte-Landry, A., Boivin, M., Tanguay-Garneau, L., Mimeau, C., Vitaro, F., Tremblay, R. E., & Dionne, G. (2020). Children with persistent versus transient early language delay: Language, academic, and psychosocial outcomes in elementary school. *Journal of Speech, Language, and Hearing Research, 63*(11), 3760–3774.

Mazza, M. G., Rossetti, A., Crespi, G., & Clerici, M. (2020). Prevalence of co-occurring psychiatric disorders in adults and adolescents with intellectual disability: A systematic review and meta-analysis. *Journal of Applied Research in Intellectual Disabilities, 33*(2), 126–138.

Mikkelsen, E. J. (2014). Elimination disorders. In R. E. Hales, S. C. Yudofsky, & L. W. Roberts (Eds.), *The American Psychiatric Publishing textbook of psychiatry* (6th ed.). American Psychiatric Publishing.

Miranda-Mendizabal, A., Castellví, P., Parés-Badell, O., Alayo, I., Almenara, J., Alonso, I., Blasco, M. J., Cebrià, A., Gabilondo, A., Gili, M., Lagares, C., Piqueras, J. A., Rodríguez-Jiménez, T., Rodríguez-Marín, J., Roca, M., Soto-Sanz, V., Vilagut, G., & Alonso, J. (2019). Gender differences in suicidal behavior in adolescents and young adults: systematic review and meta-analysis of longitudinal studies. *International Journal of Public Health, 64*(2), 265–283. https://doi.org/10.1007/s00038-018-1196-1.

Molina, B., Kipp, H. L., Joseph, H. M., Engster, S. A., Harty, S. C., Dawkins, M., Lindstrom, R. A., Bauer, D. J., & Bangalore, S. S. (2019). Stimulant diversion risk among college students treated for ADHD: Primary care provider prevention training. *Academic Pediatrics, 20*(1), 119–127.

Morsanyi, K., van Bers, B., McCormack, T., & McGourty, J. (2018). The prevalence of specific learning disorder in mathematics and comorbidity with other developmental disorders in primary school-age children. *British Journal of Psychology, 109*, 917–940.

Myers, S. M., Voigt, R. G., Colligan, R. C., Weaver, A. L., Storlie, C. B., Stoeckel, R. E., Port, J. D., & Katusic, S. K. (2019). Autism Spectrum Disorder: Incidence and time trends over two decades in a population-based birth cohort. *Journal of Autism and Developmental Disorders, 49*(4), 1455–1474.

National Alliance on Mental Illness (NAMI). (2021). Mental health conditions. Retrieved on January 1, 2021, from https://nami.org/Learn-More/Mental-Health-Conditions

National Institute of Health, National Institute of Neurologic Disorders and Stroke. (2020). Tourette syndrome fact sheet. Retrieved January 3, 2021, from https://www.ninds.nih.gov/Disorders/Patient-Caregiver-Education/Fact-Sheets/Tourette-Syndrome-Fact-Sheet

National Institute on Drug Abuse (NIDA). (2018). Drug facts: Prescription stimulants. Retrieved on January 3, 2021, from https://www.drugabuse.gov/sites/default/files/drugfacts-prescriptionstimulants.pdf

National Institute of Mental Health (NIMH). (2019a). Attention-deficit/hyperactivity disorder. Retrieved on January 2, 2021, from https://www.nimh.nih.gov/health/topics/attention-deficit-hyperactivity-disorder-adhd/index.shtml#part_145446

National Institute of Mental Health (NIMH). (2019b). Major depression. Retrieved on January 3, 2021, from https://www.nimh.nih.gov/health/statistics/major-depression.shtml#part_155031

Nilsen, F. M., & Tulve, N. S. (2020). A systematic review and meta-analysis examining the interrelationships between chemical and non-chemical stressors and inherent characteristics in children with ADHD. *Environmental Research, 180*, 108884.

Nearchou, F., Flinn, C., Niland, R., Subramaniam, S. S., & Hennessy, E. (2020). Exploring the impact of COVID-19 on mental health outcomes in children and adolescents: A systematic review. *International Journal of Environmental Research and Public Health, 17*, 1–19.

Olusanya, B. O., Wright, S. M., Nair, M., Boo, N. Y., Halpern, R., Kuper, H., Abubakar, A. A., Almasri, N. A., Arabloo, J., Arora, N. K., Backhaus, S., Berman, B. D., Breinbauer, C., Carr, G., de Vries, P. J., Del Castillo-Hegyi, C., Eftekhari, A., Gladstone, M. J., Hoekstra, R. A., Kancherla, V., … Global Research on Developmental Disabilities Collaborators (GRDDC). (2020). Global burden of childhood epilepsy, intellectual disability, and sensory impairments. *Pediatrics, 146*(1), e20192623.

Pelsser, L. M., Frankena, K., Toorman, J., & Pereira, R. R. (2017). Diet and ADHD, reviewing the evidence: A systematic review of meta-analyses of double-blind placebo-controlled trials evaluating the efficacy of diet interventions on the behavior of children with ADHD. *PLoS One, 12*(1), e0169277.

Phillips, K. E., Norris, L. A., & Kendall, P. C. (2020). Separation anxiety symptom profiles and parental accommodation across pediatric anxiety disorders. *Child Psychiatry & Human Development, 51*, 377–389,

Posner, J., Polanzxyk, G. V., & Sonuga-Barke, E. (2020). Attention-deficit hyperactivity disorder. *Lancet, 395*, 450–462.

Pringsheim, T., Holler-Managan, Y., Okun, M. S., Jankovic, J., Piacentini, J., Cavanna, A. E., Martino, D., Müller-Vahl, K., Woods, D. W., Robinson, M., Jarvie, E., Roessner, V., & Oskoui, M. (2019). Comprehensive systematic review summary: Treatment of tics in people with Tourette syndrome and chronic tic disorders. *Neurology, 92*(19), 907–915.

Quiban, D. (2020). Addressing needs of hospitalized patients with Autism: Partnership with parents. *Critical Care Nursing Quarterly, 43*(1), 68–72.

Sciberras, E., Mulraney, M., Silva, D., & Coghill, D. (2017). Prenatal risk factors and the etiology of ADHD-review of existing evidence. *Current Psychiatry Reports, 19*(1), 1.

Shepard, J. A., Poler, J. E., Jr, & Grabman, J. H. (2017). Evidence-based psychosocial treatments for pediatric elimination disorders. *Journal of Clinical Child and Adolescent Psychology, 46*(6), 767–797. https://doi.org/10.1080/15374416.2016.1247356.

Shields, R. H., Kaat, A. J., McKenzie, F. J., Drayton, A., Sansone, S. M., Michalak, C., Riley, K., Berry-Kravis, E., Gershon, R. C., & Widaman, K. F. (2020). Validation of the NIH Toolbox Cognitive Battery in intellectual disability. *Neurology, 94*(12), e1229–e1240.

Sigfusdottir, I. D., Asgeirsdottir, B. B., Hall, H. A., Sigurdsson, J. F., Young, S., & Gudjonsson, G. H. (2017). An epidemiological study of ADHD and conduct disorder: Does family conflict moderate the association? *Social Psychiatry Psychiatric Epidemiology, 52*(4), 457–464.

Strasser, L., Downes, M., Kung, J., Cross, J. H., & DeHaan, M. (2018). Prevalence and risk for autism spectrum disorder in epilepsy. A systematic review and meta-analysis. *Developmental Medicine and Child Neurology, 60*(1), 19–29.

Tamm, L., Loren, R. E. A., Peugh, J., & Ciesielski, H. A. (2020). The association of executive functioning with academic, behavior, and social performance ratings in children with ADHD. *Journal of Learning Disabilities*, 22219420961338.

Torgersen, T., Gjervan, B., Lensing, M. B., & Rasmussen, K. (2016). Optimal management of ADHD in older adults. *Neuropsychiatric Disease and Treatment, 12*, 79–87.

Uchida, M., Driscoll, H., DiSalvo, M., Rahalakshmim, A, Maiellow, M., Spera, V., & Biederman, J. (2020). Assessing the magnitude of risk for ADHD in offspring of parents with ADHD: A systematic literature review and meta analysis. *Journal of Attention Disorders, 00*(0), 1–6.

Uldall, T., & Thomsen, P. H. (2020). The use of diet interventions to treat symptoms of ADHD in children and adolescents: A systematic review of randomized controlled trials. *Nordic Journal of Psychiatry*, 74(8), 558–568.

Um, Y. H., Hong, S. C., & Jeong, J. H. (2017). Sleep problems as predictors in attention-deficit hyperactivity disorder: Causal mechanisms, consequences and treatment. *Clinical Psychopharmacology and Neuroscience*, 15(1), 9–18.

Vaughan, J., Coddington, J. A., Ahmed, A. H., & Ertel, M. (2017). Separation anxiety disorder in school-age children: What health care providers should know. *Journal of Pediatric Health Care*, 31(4), 433–440.

Verdugo, M. A., Aguayo, V., Arias, V. B., & Garcia-Dominguez, L. (2020). A systematic review of the assessment of support needs in people with intellectual and developmental disabilities. *International Journal of Environmental Research and Public Health*, 17(24), 1–26.

Walkley, S. U., Abbeduto, L., Batshaw, M. L., Bhattacharyya, A., Bookheimer, S. Y., Christian, B. T., Constantino, J. N., de Vellis, J., Doherty, D. A., Nelson, D. L., Piven, J., Poduri, A., Pomeroy, S. L., Samaco, R. C.,

Zoghbi, H. Y., Guralnick, M. J., & Intellectual and Developmental Disabilities Research Centers Directors Committee. (2019). Intellectual and developmental disabilities research centers: Fifty years of scientific accomplishments. *Annals of Neurology*, 86(3), 332–343.

Weibel, S., Menard, O., Ionita, A., Boumendjel, M., Cabelguen, C., Kraemer, C., Micoulaud-Franchi, J. A., Bioulac, S., Perroud, N., Sauvaget, A., Carton, L., Gachet, M., & Lopez, R. (2020). Practical considerations for the evaluation and management of Attention Deficit Hyperactivity Disorder (ADHD) in adults. *L'Encphale*, 46(1), 30–40.

Yang, C., Cheng, X., Zhang, Q., Yu, D., Li, J., & Zhang, L. (2020). Interventions for tic disorders: An updated overview of systematic reviews and meta analyses. *Psychiatry Research*, 287, 112905.

Yang, T. X., Allen, R. J., Holmes, J., & Chan, R. C. (2017). Impaired memory for instructions in children with attention-deficit hyperactivity disorder is improved by action at presentation and recall. *Frontiers in Psychology*, 8, 39.

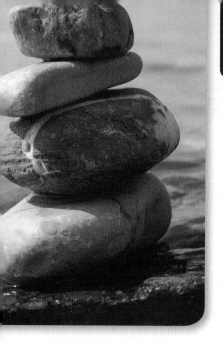

Care of Older Adults

38

Mental Health Assessment of Older Adults

Mary Ann Boyd

KEYCONCEPTS

- Normal aging

- Psychiatric–mental health nursing assessment for the older adult

LEARNING OBJECTIVES

After studying this chapter, you will be able to:

1. Compare changes in normal aging with those associated with mental health problems in older adults.

2. Select various techniques in assessing older adults who have mental health problems.

3. Delineate important areas of assessment in the geropsychiatric nursing assessment.

KEY TERMS

- Dysphagia • Functional activities • Instrumental activities of daily living • Polypharmacy • Xerostomia

INTRODUCTION

The average life span in the United States has increased from 47 years in 1900 to more than 78.7 years in 2018 (National Center for Health Statistics, 2020). Healthcare providers will face new and increased challenges as the Baby Boomers—those born between 1946 and 1964—move into the ranks of the older adult population. Between 2020 and 2060, the number of older adults is projected to increase by 69%, from 56.0 million to 94.7 million. The number of people ages 85 and older is projected to nearly triple from 6.7 million in 2020 to 19.0 million by 2060 (Mather & Kilduff, 2020).

Normal aging is associated with some physical decline, such as decreased sensory abilities and decreased pulmonary and immune function, but many important functions do not change. Intellectual function, capacity for change, and productive engagement with life remain stable. Many myths exist about normal aging. Some people believe that "senility" is normal or that depression or hopelessness is natural for older adults. If family members believe these myths, they will be less likely to seek treatment for their older family members with real problems. For example, although some normal cognitive changes contribute to a slower pace of learning, memory complaints are more likely related to depression than normal aging (Aajami et al., 2020).

The most common mental health problems in older persons are depression, anxiety disorders, and dementia which commonly occur with somatic conditions (Morin et al., 2020). Older adults with mental health problems comprise different population groups. One group consists of those with long-term mental illnesses who have reached the ranks of the older adult population. These individuals usually understand their disorders and treatments. Unfortunately, the changes associated with aging can affect a person's control of their chronic mental illness. Symptoms may reappear, and medications may need to be adjusted. Another group comprises individuals who are relatively free of mental health problems until their elder years. These individuals, who may already have other health problems, develop late-onset mental disorders, such as depression, schizophrenia, or dementia. For these individuals and their family members, the development of a mental disorder can be very traumatic.

Mental health problems in older adults can be especially complex because of coexisting medical problems and treatments. Many symptoms of somatic disorders mimic or mask psychiatric disorders. For example, fatigue may be related to anemia, but it also may be symptomatic of depression. In addition, older individuals are more likely to report somatic symptoms rather than psychological ones, making identification of a mental disorder even more difficult.

The coronavirus disease 2019 (COVID-19) pandemic hit the older adult group especially hard. High morbidity and mortality rates of COVID-19 were observed throughout the world. Those over the age of 65 were impacted disproportionately with serious consequences of severed illness and hospitalizations. Within this age group, members of underrepresented minority were disproportionately affected by COVID-19 (CDC, 2021). This pandemic has had profound psychological and social effects on the older adult leading to social isolation, distress anxiety, fear of contagion, depression, insomnia, and suicidal ideation (Sher, 2020).

The purpose of this chapter is to present a comprehensive geropsychiatric–mental health nursing assessment process that serves as the basis of care for older adults. A mental health assessment is necessary when psychiatric or mental health issues are identified or when patients with mental illnesses reach their later years (usually about age 65 years). The assessment generally follows the same format as described in Chapter 11. However, the overall healthcare issues for older adults can be very complex, so it follows that certain components of the geropsychiatric nursing assessment are unique. Thus, the geriatric assessment emphasizes some areas that are less critical to the standard adult assessment.

| **KEYCONCEPT Normal aging** is associated with some physical decline, such as decreased sensory abilities and decreased pulmonary and immune function, but many important functions do not change.

BOX 38.1

Changes That Affect Mental Status in Older Adults

- Acid–base imbalance
- Dehydration
- Drugs (prescribed and OTC)
- Electrolyte changes
- Hypothyroidism
- Hypothermia and hyperthermia
- Hypoxia
- Infection and sepsis

TECHNIQUES FOR DATA COLLECTION

The nurse assesses the patient using an interview format that may take a few sessions to complete. They also may rely on self-report standardized tests, such as depression and cognitive functioning tools. A wide variety of physiologic disorders may cause changes in mental status for older adults; thus, results of laboratory tests often are significant. For example, urinalysis can detect a urinary tract infection that has affected a patient's cognitive status. Box 38.1 contains a representative listing of common physiologic causes of changes in mental status. In addition, medical records from other healthcare providers are useful in developing a complete picture of the patient's health status.

An important source of patient data is family members, who often notice changes that the patient overlooks or fails to recognize. A patient with memory impairment may be unable to give an accurate history. By interviewing family members, the nurse expands the scope of the patient assessment. Moreover, the nurse has an opportunity to evaluate the caregivers themselves to determine whether they can care for the patient adequately and how they are coping with the situation. For example, a husband may be unable to care for his wife but is unwilling to admit it. If the nurse can establish rapport with the husband, the nurse may use the assessment interview as an opportunity to help the husband to examine his wife's care requirements realistically.

PSYCHIATRIC–MENTAL HEALTH NURSING ASSESSMENT OF THE OLDER ADULT

| **KEYCONCEPT A psychiatric mental health nursing assessment** for the older adult is the comprehensive, deliberate, and systematic collection and interpretation of data based on the special needs and problems of the older adult. The purpose is to determine the current and past health, functional status, and human responses to mental health problems, both actual and potential (Box 38.2).

BOX 38.2

Psychiatric–Mental Health Nursing Assessment for the Older Adult

I. Major reason for seeking help _____

II. Initial information

Name _____

Age _____ Current marital status _____

Gender _____ Caregiver's name _____

Living arrangements _____

III. Level of independence:

High (needs no help) _____

Moderate (lives independently, but needs some help with instrumental activities) _____

Low (relies on others for help in meeting functional and instrumental activities) _____

Physical limitations _____

Level of education completed _____

	Normal	Treated	Untreated
Physical functions: system review	☐	☐	☐
Activity/exercise	☐	☐	☐
Sleep patterns	☐	☐	☐
Appetite and nutrition	☐	☐	☐
Hydration	☐	☐	☐
Sexuality	☐	☐	☐
Existing physical illnesses	☐	☐	☐

List any chronic illnesses _____

Presence of pain (use standardized instrument if pain is present.) No _____ Yes _____

Score _____ Treatment of pain _____

IV. Responses to mental health problems

Major concerns regarding mental health problem

Major loss/change in past year: No _____ Yes _____

Fear of violence: No _____ Yes _____

Strategies for managing problems/disorder _____

V. Mental status examination

General observation (appearance, psychomotor activity, attitude) _____

Orientation (time, place, person) _____

Mood, affect, emotions (GDS should be used if evidence of depression) Speech (verbal ability, speed, use of words correctly) _____

Thought processes (hallucinations, delusions, tangential, logic, repetition, rhyming of words, loose connections, disorganized) *(Describe content of hallucinations, delusions.)*

Cognition and intellectual performance *(Use standardized test scores as well as observations.)*

Attention and concentration _____

Abstract reasoning and concentration _____

Memory (recall, short-term, long-term) _____

Judgment and insight _____

VI. Significant behaviors (psychomotor, agitation, aggression, withdrawn) *(use standardized test if behaviors are problematic.)*

When did problem behavior begin? Has it gotten worse?

VII. Self-concept beliefs about self-body image, self-esteem, personal identity) _____

VIII. Risk assessment

Suicide: High _____ Low _____

Assault/homicide: High _____ Low _____

Suicide thoughts or ideation: No _____ Yes _____

Current thoughts or harming self _____

Plan _____

Means _____

Means available

Assault/homicide thoughts: No _____ Yes _____

What do you do when angry with a stranger? _____

What do you do when angry with family or partner? _____

Have you ever hit or pushed anyone? No ___ Yes ___

Have you ever been arrested for assault? No ___ Yes ___

Current thoughts of harming others _____

IX. Functional status *(use standardized test such as FAQ)* _____

X. Cultural assessment

Cultural group _____

Cultural group's view of health and mental illness _____

By what cultural rules do you try to live? _____

Special, cultural foods that are important to you _____

XI. Stresses and coping behaviors

Social support _____

Family members _____

Which members are important to you? _____

On whom can you rely? _____

Community resources _____

XII. Spiritual assessment _____

XIII. Economic status _____

XIV. Legal status _____

XV. Quality of life _____

XVI. Summary of significant data that can be used in formulating clinical judgment.

SIGNATURE/TITLE _____ Date _____

At the beginning of the assessment, the nurse should determine the patient's ability to participate. A key component in a successful interview with an older adult is the formation of an atmosphere of respect for the person. Use of childlike language with the older adult signifies an ageist attitude and often results in poor communication. For example, if a patient is using a wheelchair, they may have physical limitations that prevent full participation in the assessment. However, physical limitations should not be assumed to indicate decreased mental capacity. The patient must be able to hear the nurse. For a patient with compromised hearing, the nurse must attend to voice projection and volume. Shouting at the older patient is unnecessary. The nurse should remember to lower the pitch of their voice because higher pitched sounds are often lost with presbycusis (loss of hearing sensitivity associated with aging). The nurse should eliminate distracting noises, such as from a television or radio, and ensure that the patient's hearing aid is in place and turned on. Facing the patient and using distinct enunciation will help lip-reading patients understand what is being said. Sometimes deafness is mistaken for cognitive dysfunction. If a patient's hearing is questionable, the nurse should enlist the help of a speech and language specialist. Generally, the pace of the interview should mirror the patient's ability to move through the assessment. Usually, the pace will be slower than the nurse uses with younger populations.

Physical Assessment

Collecting and analyzing data for the physical assessment include areas similar to those discussed in Chapter 11. The assessment components include present and past health status, physical examination results, physical functioning, and pharmacology review. When focusing on physical health, the nurse pays special attention to the patient's general physical appearance as well as any observable manifestations of illness. The nurse should assess how all physical problems affect the patient's mental well-being. For example, pain and immobility are physical problems that can negatively affect mental health. A low-energy level may be immediately apparent. Women with obvious osteoporosis are experiencing pain most of the time. Men undergoing radiation for prostate cancer worry about sexual functioning and urinary incontinence.

Present and Past Health Status

A review of the patient's current health status includes examining health records and collecting information from the patient and family members. The nurse must identify chronic health problems that could affect mental healthcare. For example, the patient's management of diabetes mellitus could provide clues to the likelihood of complications such as retinopathy or neuropathy, which in turn will affect the patient's ability to follow a mental health treatment regimen. The nurse must document a history of psychiatric treatment.

Physical Examination

The psychiatric nurse reviews the physical examination findings, paying special attention to recent laboratory values, such as urinalysis, white and red blood cell counts, thyroid studies, and fasting blood glucose data (see Chapter 8). Results of neurologic tests could indicate compromise of the neuromuscular systems. Many psychiatric medications lower the seizure threshold, making a history of seizures, which can cause behavior changes, an important assessment component. The nurse should note any evidence of movement disorders, such as tremors, abnormal movements, or shuffling. If a patient has been taking antipsychotics, the nurse should consider assessment for symptoms of tardive dyskinesia using one of the appropriate assessment tools (see Chapter 24 for an additional discussion of tardive dyskinesia).

The nurse should take routine vital signs during the assessment. They should note any abnormalities in blood pressure (i.e., hypertension or hypotension) because many psychiatric medications affect blood pressure. Generally, these medications may cause orthostatic hypotension, which can lead to dizziness, an unsteady gait, and falls. A baseline blood pressure is needed for future monitoring of medication side effects. Lying, sitting, and standing blood pressures are especially useful in assessing for orthostatic hypotension.

Physical Functions

The nurse must consider the patient's physical functioning within the context of the normal changes that accompany aging and the presence of any chronic disorders. The nurse should note the patient's use of any personal devices, such as canes, walkers, or wheelchairs; oxygen; or environmental devices, such as grab bars, shower benches, or hospital beds. Specific areas to consider are nutrition and eating, elimination, and sleep patterns.

Nutrition and Eating

Assessment of the type, amount, and frequency of food eaten is standard in any geriatric assessment. Weight loss of more than 10 pounds should be noted. The nurse must consider such nutrition changes in light of mental health problems. For example, is a patient's weight loss related to an underlying physical problem or to the patient's belief that she is being poisoned, which makes her afraid to eat?

Eating is often difficult for older patients, who may experience a lack of appetite. The nurse must assess eating and appetite patterns because many psychiatric medications can affect digestion and may impair an already compromised gastrointestinal tract. A common problem of older adults who live in nursing homes is dysphagia, or difficulty swallowing. **Dysphagia** can lead to dehydration, malnutrition, pneumonia, or asphyxiation. People who have been exposed to conventional antipsychotics (e.g., haloperidol, chlorpromazine) may have symptoms of tardive dyskinesia, which can make swallowing difficult. Thus, the nurse should evaluate any patient who has been exposed to the older psychiatric medications for symptoms of tardive dyskinesia.

Xerostomia, or dry mouth, which is common in older adults, also may impair eating. The nurse should pay particular attention to those who are currently receiving treatment for mental illnesses, particularly with medications that have anticholinergic properties. Dry mouth is also a side effect of many other anticholinergic medications, such as cimetidine, digoxin, and furosemide. Frequent rinsing with a nonalcohol-based mouthwash will help to correct the dry condition. Observe for the frequent use of candy- or sugar-based gum for these clients because dental caries and gum disease provide a portal of entry for sepsis in older adults. Decreased taste or smell is common among older adults and may reduce the pleasure of eating so that the patient may eat less. Making meal times social and relaxing experiences can help the patient compensate for some of the loss of pleasure associated with decreased taste or smell. Preparing favorite foods will also enhance the quality of meals and meal times.

Substance Use

Alcohol use is common in the older adult population and is the substance of choice. Older adults are more vulnerable to the effects of alcohol because of the physiologic changes associated with aging, increases in chronic diseases, and medication use. Alcohol use in older adults has been associated with functional impairments, falls, delirium, and increased mortality. Substance abuse in the older adults is expected to increase as the Baby Boomer generation ages with its higher rates of substances use compared to preceding generation. There is a substantially increased mortality risk for heavy drinkers and a slightly reduced risk for lighter drinkers (Bares & Kennedy, 2020). Indications of alcohol or drug use include observable changes in sleep patterns and unusual fatigue, changes in mood, jerky eye movement, seizures, unexplained complaints about chronic pain or vision problems, poor hygiene and self-neglect, unexplained nausea or vomiting, and slurred speech. Use of an assessment tool such as the CAGE questionnaire (discussed in Chapter 31) may be helpful in this area.

Elimination

The nurse must assess the patient's urinary and bowel functions. Older adults are more likely to experience constipation caused by a change in eating or activity patterns or intentional reduction in fluid intake. Medications with anticholinergic properties can cause constipation, leading to fecal impaction. Abuse of laxatives is common among older adults and requires evaluation. Although the addition of fiber is recommended for constipation, such measures may cause bloating and excessive gas production. Older patients are also more likely to experience urinary frequency because the strength of the sphincter muscles decreases. Because many older adults drink fewer fluids to manage urinary incontinence, fluid intake also becomes an important factor in assessing urinary functioning and constipation. The nurse should remember that urinary incontinence is not a normal age-related finding but a symptom of a disorder that requires follow-up and treatment.

Sleep

During the normal aging process, sleep patterns change, and patients may sleep more or less than they did when younger. The nurse must assess any recent changes in sleep patterns and evaluate whether they are related to normal aging or are symptomatic of an underlying disorder. Insomnia, the inability to fall or remain asleep throughout the night, may be the result of depression or can lead to an increased risk for depression and regular use of sleep medications. Sleep disturbances such as waking after onset of sleep and spending time in bed are associated with apathy, one of the early signs of Alzheimer dementia (Lloret et al., 2020). Disturbed sleep patterns are also associated with interpersonal stress and loneliness (Griffin et al., 2020; Pye et al., 2020). If a patient reports sleep problems, the nurse should ask about the patient's use of alcohol, over-the-counter (OTC) medications, and prescription drugs, which can interfere with sleep (Box 38.3).

Pain

Older adults are more likely to experience persistent pain than younger adults because they are at increased risk for chronic illness and may be experiencing the consequences of a lifetime of injuries. For many older adults, chronic pain is a constant companion and contributes to unexplained behavior and personality changes. Chronic pain assessment is more difficult because of the person's perception of pain or cognitive impairment, which interferes with communication. Older persons are often reluctant to report pain or believe that they have to be stoic about pain and "not make a big deal" about it.

BOX 38.3

Perceptions and Beliefs about Sleep

McPhillips, M. V., Dickson, V. V., Cacchione, P. Z., Li, J., Gooneratne, N., & Riegel, B. (2020). Nursing home eligible, community-dwelling older adults' perceptions and beliefs about sleep: A mixed-methods study. Clinical Nursing Research, 29(3), 177–188. https://doi.org/10.1177/1054773819849348

THE QUESTION: Do nursing home eligible, community dwelling older adults have dysfunctional beliefs about sleep that perpetuate sleep disturbances.

METHODS: Forty Black females over the age of 55 years participated in the study. Qualitative data were obtained by semi-structured interviews and prioritized according to the perceptions and beliefs about sleep. Quantitative measures were obtained by actigraphy (a non-invasive method of monitoring rest/activity cycles.

FINDINGS: The majority of the sample had poor sleep quality and did not get the recommended amount of sleep, regardless of self-perceptions of sleep quality. Despite objective sleep disturbances, qualitative interviews revealed those participants believed their sleep was good.

IMPLICATIONS FOR NURSING: Older adults may not be accurately perceiving their sleep disturbances. Clinicians should proactively assess sleep in this group through qualitative measures. Based on this study, older adults may not recognize a sleep problem making them higher risk for nursing home placement.

While an in-depth discussion of pain assessment is beyond the scope of this text, it is important for the mental health nurse to understand the pain assessment approaches. A common practice of asking a patient if they are experiencing pain on a scale of 1 to 10 is being replaced with a more meaningful assessment of the impact of the pain on the person. The emerging trend in pain assessment is to determine the intensity of the pain and the extent to which the pain interferes with movement (physical activity) and function (performance of daily or overall function). It is important to understand how pain limits their functional ability and mobility. A movement-based pain assessment involves assessing the pain intensity and interference on function during movement or physical activities (Booker et al., 2020).

Pharmacologic Assessment

One of the most important aspects is the pharmacologic assessment. **Polypharmacy**, the use of duplicate medications, interacting medications, or drugs used to treat adverse drug interactions, is common in older adults. The nurse must ask the patient and family to list all medications and times that the patient takes them. Asking family members to bring in all the medications the patient is taking, including OTC medications, vitamins, and herbal

supplements, allows for a careful assessment of polypharmacy. Because older adults are more sensitive than younger people to medications, the possibility of drug-to-drug interactions is greater. When considering potential drug interactions, the nurse should ask the patient about their consumption of grapefruit juice, which contains naringin, a compound that inhibits the CYP3A4 enzyme involved in the metabolism of many medications (e.g., antidepressants, antiarrhythmics, erythromycin, and several statins).

Psychological Assessment

The psychological assessment provides the nurse with the opportunity to identify limitations, behavior symptoms, and reactions to illness. The nurse assesses many of the same areas as in other adult assessments, but again, the emphasis may be different. The following discussion focuses on the responses of older patients to mental health problems, mental status examination, behavior changes, stress and coping patterns, and risk assessments.

Responses to Mental Health Problems

Many older patients are reluctant to admit that they have psychiatric symptoms, particularly if their culture stigmatizes mental illness, and may deny having mental or emotional problems. They may also fear that if they admit to any symptoms, they may be placed outside their home. If patients do not recognize or admit to having psychiatric symptoms, their vulnerability to being taken advantage of or injured increases.

Throughout the assessment, the nurse evaluates the patient's verbal reports, obvious symptoms, and family reports. If a patient flatly denies any psychiatric symptoms (e.g., depression, mood swings, outbursts of anger, memory problems), the nurse should respectfully accept the patient's answer and avoid arguments or confrontation (Box 38.4). If the patient's family members contradict the patient's report or symptoms are obvious during the interview, the nurse can approach the issue while planning care. Nurses may need to use conflict resolution strategies in helping families and patients arrive at mutually agreed on reports.

Mental Status Examination

The areas of special interest in the mental status examination are mood and affect, thought processes, and cognitive functioning. The nurse should interpret the results in light of any accompanying physical problems, such as chronic pain, or life changes, such as loss of a spouse.

Mood and Affect

Depression in older adults is common and associated with the following risk factors: loss of spouse, physical illness, low socioeconomic status, impaired functional

BOX 38.4 • ASSESSMENT INTERVIEW

Tom, 79 years old, is being seen for the first time in a geropsychiatric clinic because of recent changes in his behavior and his accusations that family members are trying to steal his house and car. He locked his wife out of the house, accusing her of being unfaithful. When Susan, the psychiatric nurse assigned to his case, is conducting the assessment interview, Tom cooperates and is very pleasant until the nurse begins the psychological assessment.

INEFFECTIVE APPROACH

Nurse: Have there been times when you have had problems with any members of your family?

Patient: No. (Silence)

Nurse: Have you noticed that lately you have been getting more upset than usual?

Patient: No. Who has been talking to you?

Nurse: Your wife seems to think that you may be getting a little more upset than usual.

Patient: You are just like her. She keeps telling me something is wrong with me. (Getting very agitated)

Nurse: Please, I'm trying to help you. I understand that you locked your wife out of the house last week.

Patient: Leave me alone. (Gets up and leaves)

EFFECTIVE APPROACH

Nurse: How have things been going at home?

Patient: All right.

Nurse: (Silence)

Patient: Well, my wife and I sometimes argue.

Nurse: Oh. Most husband and wives argue. Any special arguments?

Patient: No. Just the usual. I don't pick up after myself enough. I don't dress right to suit her. But, lately, she's gone a lot.

Nurse: She is gone a lot?

Patient: Yeah! A lot.

Nurse: The way you say that, it sounds like you have some feelings about her being gone.

Patient: You're damned right I do—and you would, too.

Nurse: I'm missing something.

Patient: Well, if you must know, I think she's having an affair with the man next door.

Nurse: Really? That must upset you to think your wife is having an affair.

Patient: I am devastated. I feel so bad.

Nurse: Would you say that you are depressed?

Patient: Well, wouldn't you be? Yes, I'm feeling pretty low.

CRITICAL THINKING CHALLENGE

• How do the very first questions differ in the two interviews?

• What therapeutic techniques did the nurse use in the second interview to avoid the pitfalls the nurse encountered in the first scenario?

• How did the nurse in the second scenario elicit the patient's delusion about his wife's affair?

• From the data that the second nurse gathered, how many patient problems can be identified?

status, and heavy alcohol consumption. In older people, other disorders may mask depression. When symptoms are present, they may be attributed to normal aging or atherosclerosis or other age-related problems. Older patients are less likely to report feeling sad or worthless than are younger patients. As a result, family members and primary care providers often overlook depression in older patients.

The term *late-onset depression* refers to the development of depression or depressive symptoms that impair functioning after 60 years of age. In late-onset depression, the risk for recurrence is relatively high. Emerging evidence suggests that late-life depression is associated with changes in the cortical network (Li et al., 2020).

The Geriatric Depression Scale (GDS) is a useful screening tool with demonstrated validity and reliability (Hyer & Blount, 1984). The GDS was designed as a self-administered test, although it also has been used in observer-administered formats. One advantage of the test is its "yes/no" format, which may be easier for older

---

BOX 38.5

Geriatric Depression Scale (Short Form)

1. Are you basically satisfied with your life?	Yes	No
2. Have you dropped many of your activities and interests?	Yes	No
3. Do you feel that your life is empty?	Yes	No
4. Do you often get bored?	Yes	No
5. Are you in good spirits most of the time?	Yes	No
6. Are you afraid that something bad is going to happen to you?	Yes	No
7. Do you feel happy most of the time?	Yes	No
8. Do you often feel helpless?	Yes	No
9. Do you prefer to stay at home rather than go out and do new things?	Yes	No
10. Do you feel you have more problems with memory than most?	Yes	No
11. Do you think it is wonderful to be alive now?	Yes	No
12. Do you feel pretty worthless the way you are now?	Yes	No
13. Do you feel full of energy?	Yes	No
14. Do you feel that your situation is hopeless?	Yes	No
15. Do you think that most people are better off than you are?	Yes	No

Score:——/15. One point for "No" to questions 1, 5, 7, 11, 13; one point for "Yes" to other questions.

Normal	3 ± 2
Mildly depressed	7 ± 3
Very depressed	12 ± 2

From Sheikh, J. I. & Yesavage, J.A. (1986). Geriatric Depression Scale (GDS): recent evidence and development of a shorter version. Clinical Gerontologist, 5(1–2), 165–173. Reprinted by permission of Taylor & Francis Ltd, https://www.tandfonline.com.

---

adults than the Hamilton Rating Scale for Depression (HAM-D), which uses a scale from 0 to 4 (see Chapter 25). This tool is easy to administer and provides valuable information about the possibility of depression (Box 38.5). If results are positive, the nurse should refer the patient to a psychiatrist or advanced practice nurse for further evaluation. Among nursing home residents, the usefulness of the GDS depends on the degree of cognitive impairment. Residents who are mildly impaired may be able to answer the yes/no questions; however, moderate to severely impaired patients will be unable to do the same. The best validated scale for patients with dementia is the Cornell Scale for Depression in Dementia (CSDD) (Alexopoulos et al., 1998). The CSDD is an interview-administered scale that uses information both from the patient and an outside informant.

Anxiety is another important mood for nurses to assess in older adults because it can interfere with normal functioning. In dementia, anxiety is common (Hwang et al., 2020). The Rating Anxiety in Dementia (RAID) scale was developed as a global scale to assess anxiety in patients with dementia (Shankar et al., 1999). The domains that the RAID scale assesses include worry, apprehension and vigilance, motor tension, autonomic hyperactivity, and phobias and panic attacks.

Thought Processes

Thought processes and content are critical in the assessment of older patients. Can the patient express ideas and thoughts logically? Can the patient understand questions and follow the conversation of others? If the patient shows any indication of hallucinations or delusions, the nurse should explore the content of the hallucination or delusion. If the patient has a history of mental illness, such as schizophrenia, these symptoms may be familiar to family members, who can validate whether they are old or new problems. If this is the first time the patient has experienced these abnormal thought processes, the nurse should further evaluate the content. Suspicious and delusional thoughts that characterize dementia often include some of the following beliefs:

- People are stealing my things.
- The house is not my house.
- My relative is an impostor.

Cognition and Intellectual Performance

Cognitive functioning includes parameters such as orientation, attention, short- and long-term memory, consciousness, and executive functioning. Intellectual functioning, also considered a cognitive measure, is rarely formally assessed with a standardized intelligence test in older adults. Considerable variability among individuals depends on lifestyle and psychosocial factors. Some changes in cognitive capacity may accompany aging, but important functions are spared. Normal cognitive changes during aging include a slowing of information processing and memory retrieval. Abnormalities of consciousness, orientation, judgment, speech, or language are not related to age but to underlying neuropathologic changes. Cognitive changes in older adults are associated with delirium or dementia (see Chapter 39) or with schizophrenia (see Chapter 24).

The assessment includes the number of years of education. An inverse relationship between Alzheimer disease and the number of years of education exists. Evidence suggests that severe cognitive deterioration may occur in older adults with schizophrenia. An easy to administer and easily accessible screening tool is the SLUMS (Saint Louis University Mental Status Examination) (see Chapter 39).

Behavior Changes

Behavior changes in older adults can indicate neuropathologic processes and thus require nursing assessment. If such changes occur, it is most likely that family members will notice them before the patient does. Apraxia (an inability to execute a voluntary movement despite normal muscle function) is not attributed to age but indicates an underlying disease process, such as Alzheimer disease, Parkinson disease, or other disorders. Various other behavior problems are associated with psychiatric disorders in older adults, including irritability, agitation, apathy, and euphoria. Other behaviors in older adults who are experiencing psychiatric problems include wandering and aggressive behaviors.

The Neuropsychiatric Inventory (NPI) was developed in 1994 to assess behavior problems associated with dementia. The scale assesses 10 behavior problems: delusions, hallucinations, dysphoria, anxiety, agitation or aggression, euphoria, inhibition, irritability or lability, apathy, and aberrant motor behavior (Cummings et al., 1994). This very popular tool is used in many medication clinical trials. There are two versions. The standard version is used when the patient is still at home; the second version (NPI-NH) is used when the patient is in a nursing home.

Stress and Coping Patterns

Identifying stresses and coping patterns is just as important for older patients as it is for younger adults. Unique stresses for older patients include living on a fixed income, handling declining health, losing partners and friends, and ultimately confronting death. Coping ability varies, depending on patients' unique circumstances. For example, some patients respond to stressful events with amazing adaptability, but others become depressed and suicidal.

Bereavement, a natural response to the death of a loved one, includes crying and sorrow, anxiety and agitation, insomnia, and a loss of appetite. These symptoms, although overlapping with those of major depression, do not constitute a mental disorder. Although bereavement is a normal response, the nurse must identify it and develop interventions to help the individual successfully resolve the loss. Bereavement is an important and well-established risk factor for depression (see Chapter 21).

Risk Assessment

Suicide is a major mental health risk for older adults. An average of one older adult dies by suicide every 57.3 minutes. Older adults make up 16.9% of 2019 population but 19.4% of suicides (AAS, 2020). Depression is the greatest risk factor for suicide and is crucial in maintaining a desire to die. Hopelessness is also a strong factor related to death by suicide. Hopelessness is driven by a low mood,

perceptions of poor physical health, and social isolation (Hernandez et al., 2020). The social isolation associated with COVID-19 contributes to the risk of suicide in the older adult (Sher, 2020). Individuals who are suicidal often believe that they are a burden to their family who would be better off without them (see Chapter 22). In assessing an older patient, the nurse should consider the following characteristics as indications of high risk for committing suicide:

- Depression
- Attempted suicide in the past
- Family history of suicide
- Firearms in the home
- Abuse of alcohol or other substances
- Unusual stress
- Burden to family
- Chronic medical condition (e.g., cancer, neuromuscular disorders)
- Social isolation

NCLEXNOTE Suicide assessment is a priority for the older adult experiencing mental health problems. It is important to carefully assess recent behavior changes and loss of support.

Social Assessment

The social assessment includes determining the patient's interactions with others in their family and community. The nurse targets social support because it is so important to the well-being of the older adult's functional status and because of the potential physical changes that can affect this area and social systems, which encompasses all community resources.

Social Support

Remaining active throughout one's life is one of the best predictors of mental health and wellness in an older patient. People obtain their sense of self-worth through their interactions with others in their environment. A sense of "who one is" is closely tied to the roles that a person play in life. When older adults relinquish such roles because of physical disabilities, become isolated from friends and family, or begin to sense that they are a burden to those around them rather than contributing members of society, a sense of hopelessness and helplessness often follows.

The role of social support is critical to assess in this age group. Social support is a reciprocal concept, meaning that simply receiving assistance increases the person's sense of being a burden. Those older adults who believe that they contribute to the welfare of others are most likely to remain mentally healthy. For this reason, pets are often "life savers" for older adults who live alone. Nothing can be more understanding and accepting of an older adult's behavior or disabilities than a beloved pet.

The nurse should assess the patient's number of formal and informal social contacts. The nurse should ask about the frequency of contacts with others (in person and through telephone calls, letters, and cards). Determining whether these contacts are actually satisfying and supporting to the patient is essential. If family members are important to the patient's well-being, the nurse should complete a more in-depth family assessment (see Chapter 15).

The nurse can use the following questions to focus on social support:

- In the past 2 weeks, how often would you say that family members or friends let you know that they care about you?

- In the past 2 weeks, how often has someone provided you with help, such as giving you a ride somewhere or helping around the house?

- Do you have a family member or a special person you could call or contact if you needed help? Who?

- In general, other than your children, who do you consider a close friend or companion?

For patients who are isolated with few social contacts, the nurse can develop interventions to improve social support.

Functional Status

As part of a complete assessment, the nurse will need to assess the older adult's functional status. **Functional activities** or activities of daily living (ADLs) are the activities necessary for self-care (i.e., bathing, toileting, dressing, and transferring). **Instrumental activities of daily living (IADLs)** include those that facilitate or enhance the performance of ADLs (i.e., shopping, using the telephone, using transportation). These aspects are critical to consider for any older adult living alone. The most common tools used to assess functional status are the Index of Independence in the ADLs and the IADLs (Katz & Akpom, 1976).

Social Systems

Community resources are essential to an older adult's ability to maintain mental health and wellness, as well as to their ability to remain at home throughout the later years. Senior centers are federally funded community resources that provide a wide array of services to the nation's older population. They provide daily balanced meals at a nominal cost. In addition, they provide opportunities for socialization, which is a key to combating loneliness and social isolation. Many senior centers provide annual influenza and pneumonia vaccination clinics and education on such topics as fall prevention and recognition and prevention of elder abuse. Additional community resources that are specific to older adults include geriatric assessment clinics and adult day care centers.

During the assessment, the nurse must determine which community resources are available and if the older patient uses them. Lack of transportation to and from these community resources may be a barrier to use. Most communities have buses available for older or disabled individuals. The nurse may need to assist the older adult in accessing this important resource.

Many older citizens rely on the Social Security Administration for their monthly income. For many, this financial support, although less than adequate in most instances, is their only source of income. In addition to Social Security, the federal government provides basic healthcare coverage in the form of the state-administered Medicare program. Together, these programs contribute to the patient's ability to live independently and receive healthcare. The nurse should assess a patient's sources of financial support. Sometimes nurses are uncomfortable asking for financial information, fearing that they are invading the patient's privacy. However, such data are important for the nurse to determine whether a patient's resources adequately meet their needs. The source of financial support is also important. For example, a patient whose income is adequate and from personal resources is more likely to be independent than the patient who depends on family members for income.

The nurse should ask the patient about accessible clinics, support groups, and pharmaceutical services. Information about available healthcare resources can provide useful data regarding the patient's ability to access services and can also provide potential referral sources. In urban areas that are likely to have adequate healthcare resources, cultural and language barriers may prohibit access. People who live in rural areas where healthcare resources are limited are less likely to enjoy the full range of healthcare resources than are those in urban areas. Overall, the use of mental health services by older adults with mental illnesses is low (Knight & Winterbotham, 2020). If older adults are married and have insurance, they are more likely to seek mental health services.

Spiritual Assessment

Spiritual needs are basic for all age groups and are requirements for establishing meaning and purpose, love and relatedness, and forgiveness. With advanced age, many people begin to reflect on their successes and failures. During such reflection, many seek out God or a higher being to make sense of the past and establish hope for the future.

The process of spiritual assessment involves active listening, thoughtful observing, and sensitive questioning. The nurse may simply ask if the person would find comfort from a visit from a spiritual leader. Many forms of religion use various rituals that are important to the person's daily routine. The nurse should explore and honor these aspects to the extent possible.

Legal Status

A growing trend in the United States is to view older adults as a special population whose rights deserve increased attention. Instances of elder abuse are far too common. Every nurse must consider themselves a patient advocate and be vigilant in recognizing the signs of neglect or abuse, such as unexplained injuries. At times, abuse can take the form of another individual usurping the rights of the older person. Unless the older person is determined to be incompetent, they has the same rights to personal decision-making as any other adult, including the right to refuse treatment.

Quality of Life

A sense of quality of life is closely tied to values and beliefs. For many older adults, quality of life is not reflected in material possessions or physical health. At this stage, quality of life is connected more with contentment over how the person has lived life and the extent to which their life has had meaning and purpose. Keeping close personal contacts with friends and family and having the opportunity to shares stories of lifetime experiences are essential to maintaining mental health and wellness for older adults. For older adults, physical illnesses may affect the quality of life more than psychiatric disorders. The assessment of quality of life becomes especially important when assessing a patient living in a nursing home or isolated in their own home. The assessment of quality of life of older adults is similar to that for younger adults (see Chapter 11).

SUMMARY OF KEY POINTS

- Normal aging is associated with some physical decline, but most functions do not change. Intellectual functioning, capacity for change, and productive engagement with life remain stable.

- Mental health assessments are necessary when older patients face psychiatric or mental health issues. The biopsychosocial geropsychiatric nursing assessment examines many sources of data, including self-reports, laboratory test results, and reports from family members.

- The psychiatric–mental health nursing assessment for the older adult is based on the special needs and problems of the older adult. This assessment examines current and past health, functional status, and human responses to mental health problems.

- The physical assessment involves collecting data about past and present health status, physical examination findings, physical functions (i.e., nutrition and eating, elimination patterns, sleep), pain, and pharmacologic information.

- The psychological assessment includes the patient's responses to mental health problems, mental status examination, behavioral changes, stress and coping patterns, and risk assessment.

- The social assessment includes social systems, spiritual assessment, legal information, and quality of life.

- When conducting an assessment, the nurse may find several tools useful. For patients with possible depression, the GDS may be helpful. For patients with anxiety, nurses can use the RAID scale.

- Coping with the stresses of aging varies among patients. Determining stresses and coping skills for dealing with stresses is important.

- Social support is critical to patients in this age group and requires assessment.

- Determination of the patient's ability to perform functional and instrumental ADLs is critical in the assessment of the older adult.

Unfolding Patient Stories: George Palo

Part 2 (90 years, independent living—when to move to higher level of care)

 Recall from Chapter 21 George Palo, a 90-year-old, is diagnosed with minor neurocognitive disorder, Alzheimer's type, and living independently in a retirement community since his wife died 3 years ago. His daughter has noticed some cognitive decline and social isolation after the recent loss of his dog. What assessments should the nurse perform during a home visit? How can the nurse determine if he is receptive to community resources for supporting his independent living and involvement in activities? Considering his neurocognitive disorder and response to recent loss, how would the nurse approach a discussion on his ability to maintain independence and when he should transfer to a higher level of care?

CRITICAL THINKING CHALLENGES

1. The director of your church's senior center has asked you to be the guest speaker at the monthly meeting of the Retired Active Citizens group. The subject is to be "Maintaining Your Mental Health After Retirement." What key points will you touch on in your presentation? What activities or handouts will you use to highlight your talk?

2. When asking about current illnesses, a patient begins telling you her whole life story. What approach would you take to elicit the most important needed to develop an individualized plan of care for your older patient?

3. A caregiver tells you that her mother has become suspicious of the neighbors and other family members. How would you assess this perceptual experience? What other data should you gather from this patient?

4. A caregiver brings a sack of medications to the patient's assessment interview. What information should you obtain from the caregiver regarding the patient's use of these medications?

5. A woman brings her father, who has a long history of frequent psychiatric hospitalizations for depression, to the clinic. The patient's wife recently died, and the daughter fears that her father is becoming depressed again. What approach would you use in assessing for changes in mood?

6. Obtain a listing of the social services available in your community. Examine the list for areas of duplication and omission of services needed by an older adult living alone in their own home.

Movie Viewing Guides

Dad (1989): Looking like death warmed over, Jack Lemmon plays Jake Tremont, the aging father of John Tremont (Ted Danson). Always proud of being able to fend for himself, Lemmon despises being dependent on others, but his increasingly frequent periods of confusion do not allow him his old independence. For his part, Danson resents having to care for his dad as he would for an infant. To make matters even worse, Lemmon is diagnosed with cancer. As the reality of his imminent death strikes everyone around him, Lemmon retreats into fantasy, recalling the past happy events of his life as though they're happening here and now. The rest of the family humors their dying dad, and in so doing draws closer together than they've been in years.

VIEWING POINTS: Identify the physical impairments that are obvious throughout the movie. Identify specific memory problems that Jake experiences. Are these problems part of normal aging? If you were Jake Tremont's nurse, what key assessment areas would you explore?

REFERENCES

Aajami, Z., Kazazi, L., Toroski, M., Bahrami, M., & Borhaninejad, V. (2020). Relationship between depression and cognitive impairment among elderly: A cross-sectional study. *Journal of Caring Sciences, 9*(3), 148–153. https://doi.org/10.34172/jcs.2020.022

Alexopoulos, G. S., Abrams, R. C., Young, R. C., & Shamoian, C. A. (1998). Cornell scale for depression in dementia. *Biological Psychiatry, 23*(3), 271–284.

American Association of Suicidology. (2020). USA suicide: 2019 official final data. https://suicidology.org/wp-content/uploads/2021/01/2019datapgsv2b.pdf

Bares, C. B., & Kennedy, A. (2020). Alcohol use among older adults and health care utilization. *Aging & Mental Health*, 1–7. Advance online publication. https://doi.org/10.1080/13607863.2020.1793903

Booker, S. Q., Herr, K. A., & Horgas, A. L. (2020). A paradigm shift for movement-based pain assessment in older adults: Practice, policy and regulatory drivers. *Pain Management Nursing: Official Journal of the American Society of Pain Management Nurses*, S1524-9042(20)30171-5. Advance online publication. https://doi.org/10.1016/j.pmn.2020.08.003

Centers for Disease control and Prevention. (2021). COVIDView. *CDC 24/7 Saving lives, Protecting people*. U.S. Department of Health and Human Services. https://www.cdc.gov/coronavirus/2019-ncov/covid-data/covidview/

Cummings, J. L., Mega, M., Gray, K., Rosenberg-Thompson, S., Carusi, D. A., & Gornbein, J. (1994). The neuropsychiatric inventory: Comprehensive assessment of psychopathology in dementia. *Neurology, 44*(12), 2308–2314.

Griffin, S. C., Williams, A. B., Mladen, S. N., Perrin, P. B., Dzierzewski, J. M., & Rybarczyk, B. D. (2020). Reciprocal effects between loneliness and sleep disturbance in older Americans. *Journal of Aging and Health, 32*(9), 1156–1164. https://doi.org/10.1177/0898264319894486

Hernandez, S. C., Overholser, J. C., Philips, K. L., Lavacot, J., & Stockmeier, C. A. (2020). Suicide among older adults: Interactions among key risk factors. *International Journal of Psychiatry in Medicine*, 91217420982387. Advance online publication. https://doi.org/10.1177/0091217420982387

Hwang, Y., Massimo, L., & Hodgson, N. (2020). Modifiable factors associated with anxiety in persons with dementia: An integrative review. *Geriatric Nursing (New York, N.Y.), 41*(6), 852–862. https://doi.org/10.1016/j.gerinurse.2020.06.003

Hyer, L., & Blount, J. (1984). Concurrent and discriminant validities of the geriatric depression scale with older psychiatric inpatients. *Psychological Reports, 54*(2), 611–616.

Katz, S., & Akpom, C. A. (1976). A measure of primary sociobiological functions. *International Journal of Health Science, 6*(3), 493–508.

Knight, B. G., & Winterbotham, S. (2020). Rural and urban older adults' perceptions of mental health services accessibility. *Aging & Mental Health, 24*(6), 978–984. https://doi.org/10.1080/13607863.2019.1576159

Li, J., Gong, H., Xu, H., Ding, Q., He, N., Huang, Y., Jin, Y., Zhang, C., Voon, V., Sun, B., Yan, F., & Zhan, S. (2020). Abnormal voxel-wise degree centrality in patients with late-life depression: A resting-state functional magnetic resonance imaging study. *Frontiers in Psychiatry, 10*, 1024. https://doi.org/10.3389/fpsyt.2019.01024

Lloret, M. A., Cervera-Ferri, A., Nepomuceno, M., Monllor, P., Esteve, D., & Lloret, A. (2020). Is sleep disruption a cause or consequence of Alzheimer's disease? Reviewing its possible role as a biomarker. *International Journal of Molecular Sciences, 21*(3), 1168. https://doi.org/10.3390/ijms21031168

Mather, M., & Kilduff, L. (2020). The U.S. population is growing older, and the gender gap in life expectancy is narrowing. *Population Resource Bureau*. https://www.prb.org/the-u-s-population-is-growing-older-and-the-gender-gap-in-life-expectancy-is-narrowing/

Morin, R. T., Nelson, C., Bickford, D., Insel, P. S., & Mackin, R. S. (2020). Somatic and anxiety symptoms of depression are associated with disability in late life depression. *Aging & Mental Health, 24*(8), 1225–1228. https://doi.org/10.1080/13607863.2019.1597013

National Center for Health Statistics. (2020). Mortality in the United States, 2018. Centers for Disease Control and Prevention. https://www.cdc.gov/nchs/products/databriefs/db355.htm

Pye, J., Phillips, A. J., Cain, S. W., Montazerolghaem, M., Mowszowski, L., Duffy, S., Hickie, I. B., & Naismith, S. L. (2020). Irregular sleep-wake patterns in older adults with current or remitted depression. *Journal of Affective Disorders, 281*, 431–437. Advance online publication. https://doi.org/10.1016/j.jad.2020.12.034

Shankar, K. K., Walker, M., Frost, D., & Orrell, M. W. (1999). The development of a valid and reliable scale for rating anxiety in dementia (RAID). *Aging & Mental Health, 3*(1), 39–49.

Sheikh, J. I., & Yesavage, M. D. (1986). Geriatric depression scale (GDS). *Clinical Gerontologist, 5*(1–2), 165–173.

Sher, L. (2020). The impact of the COVID-19 pandemic on suicide rates. *QJM: Monthly Journal of the Association of Physicians, 113*(10), 707–712. https://doi.org/10.1093/qjmed/hcaa202

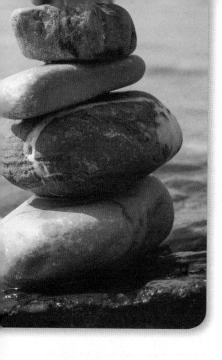

39
Neurocognitive Disorders

Mary Ann Boyd and Rebecca Luebbert

KEYCONCEPTS

- Cognition
- Delirium
- Dementia
- Memory

LEARNING OBJECTIVES

After studying this chapter, you will be able to:

1. Discuss the role of cognition and memory in neurocognitive disorders.

2. Distinguish the clinical symptoms and course of delirium and Alzheimer disease.

3. Analyze the primary theories of delirium and dementia and their relations to cognition and memory.

4. Develop strategies to establish a patient-centered therapeutic relationship with a person with Alzheimer disease.

5. Apply a person-centered nursing process for persons with delirium and Alzheimer disease.

6. Identify medications used to treat people with Alzheimer disease and evaluate their effectiveness.

7. Differentiate types of mental health care provided in inpatient-focused care and community mental health care for persons with Alzheimer disease.

8. Discuss the importance of integration of primary health care for persons with Alzheimer disease.

9. Describe other types of neurocognitive disorders.

KEY TERMS

- Acetylcholine (ACh) • Acetylcholinesterase (AChE) • Acetylcholinesterase inhibitors (AChEIs) • Agnosia
- Amyloid precursor protein (APP) • Aphasia • Apraxia • Beta-amyloid plaques • Catastrophic reactions • Cortical dementia
- Disinhibition • Disturbance of executive functioning • Hypersexuality • Hypervocalization • Illusions
- Impaired consciousness • Neurocognitive disorders • Neurofibrillary tangles • Oxidative stress • Subcortical dementia

INTRODUCTION

Most mental disorders occur in people of all ages and are not unique to the older adult. The first disorder discussed in this chapter, delirium, can occur at any time in a person's life, but it frequently occurs in the older adult. The other disorders discussed in this chapter are unique to the older adult. This chapter focuses on changes in cognitive functioning and **neurocognitive disorders** that are associated with the older adult.

Cognition is an intellectual process of acquiring, using, or manipulating perceptions and information. It involves the perception of reality and an understanding of its representations. Cognitive functions to be noted include the acquisition and use of language, the orientation of time and space, and the ability to learn and solve problems.

Cognition also is the basis of judgment, reasoning, attention, comprehension, concept formation, planning, and the use of symbols (e.g., numbers and letters used in mathematics and writing).

> **KEYCONCEPT Cognition** is based on a system of interrelated abilities, such as perception, reasoning, judgment, intuition, and memory, that allow one to be aware of oneself and one's surroundings. Impairments in these abilities can result in a failure of the afflicted person to recognize that they are ill and in need of treatment.

Memory, a facet of cognition, refers to the ability to recall or reproduce what has been learned or experienced. It is more than simple storage and retrieval; it is a complex cognitive mental function that includes most areas of the brain, especially the hippocampus, which is believed to be essential to the transfer of some memories from short- to long-term storage. Defects of memory are an essential feature of many cognitive disorders, particularly dementia.

> **KEYCONCEPT Memory** is a facet of cognition concerned with retaining and recalling past experiences, whether they occurred in the physical environment or internally as cognitive events.

Neurocognitive disorders are characterized by a decline in cognitive function from a previous level of functioning. These disorders are acquired and have not been present since early life. The diagnosis of a neurocognitive disorder is based on deficits in the following cognitive domains: *attention* (distractibility with multiple stimuli), *executive function* (planning, decision-making, working memory), *learning and memory* (recall and recognition), *language* (expressive including naming, work finding, fluency, grammatical syntax, and receptive language), *perceptual-motor* (visual perception, visuoconstructional, perceptual-motor), and *social cognition deficits* (recognition of emotions, ability to consider another's mental state) (American Psychiatric Association [APA], 2013).

The neurocognitive disorders discussed in this chapter include delirium, a disorder of acute cognitive impairment usually caused by a medical condition (e.g., infection) and dementia, characterized by chronic cognitive impairments. Dementia is differentiated from delirium by underlying cause, not by symptom patterns, which are often similar.

> **KEYCONCEPT Delirium** is a disorder of acute cognitive impairment that is caused by a medical condition (e.g., infection), substance abuse, or multiple etiologies.

> **KEYCONCEPT Dementia** is characterized by chronic cognitive impairments and is differentiated by underlying cause, not by symptom patterns. Dementia can be further classified as cortical or subcortical to denote the location of the underlying pathology.

Cortical dementia results from a disease process that globally afflicts the cortex. **Subcortical dementia** is caused by dysfunction or deterioration of deep gray- or white-matter structures inside the brain and brain stem. Symptoms of subcortical dementia may be more localized and tend to disrupt arousal, attention, and motivation, but they can produce a variety of clinical behavioral manifestations. In this chapter, one type of cortical dementia, Alzheimer disease (AD), is highlighted because it is the most prevalent form of dementia.

DELIRIUM

Clinical Course

Delirium is a disturbance in consciousness and an acute change in cognition and mental status that develops over a short time. It is usually reversible if the underlying cause is identified and treated quickly. It is a serious disorder and should always be treated as a medical emergency.

> **EMERGENCY CARE ALERT** *!* Individuals with delirium are in a state of confusion and disorientation that develops during a period of a few hours or days. If delirium is not treated in a timely manner, irreversible neurologic damage can occur. Delirium is a common complication in patients admitted to intensive care units and inpatient psychiatric units (Jin et al., 2020).

Diagnostic Criteria

Impaired consciousness is the key diagnostic criterion for delirium. The patient becomes less aware of their environment and loses the ability to focus, sustain, and shift attention. Cognitive changes include problems with memory, orientation, and language. The patient may not know where they are, may not recognize familiar objects, or may be unable to carry on a conversation. This problem developed during a short period (compared with dementia, which develops gradually) (APA, 2013). Impaired alertness, apathy, anxiety, disorientation, and hallucinations commonly occur. Delirium can be categorized as *hyperactive* with agitation, increased psychomotor activity, and heightened level of arousal; *hypoactive* with somnolence and psychomotor retardation; or *mixed* with alternating hypoactive and hyperactive states. Hyperactive delirium is easily recognized, but hypoactive delirium is most common (Shenvi et al., 2020). Delirium is different than dementia, although the presenting symptoms are often similar. Table 39.1 highlights the differences between delirium and dementia.

TABLE 39.1	DIFFERENTIATING DELIRIUM FROM DEMENTIA	
Characteristics	Delirium	Dementia
Onset	Sudden	Insidious
24-hr course	Fluctuating	Stable
Consciousness	Reduced	Clear
Attention	Globally disoriented	Usually normal
Cognition	Globally disoriented	Globally impaired
Hallucinations	Visual auditory	Possible
Orientation	Usually impaired	Often impaired
Psychomotor activity	Increased, reduced, or shifting	Often normal
Speech	Often incoherent; slow or rapid	Often normal
Involuntary movement	Often asterixis or coarse tremor	Rare
Physical illness or drug toxicity	One or both	Rare

Source: Lee, L., Weston, W. W., Heckman, G., Gagnon, M., Lee, F. J., & Stoke, S. (2013). Structured approach to patients with memory difficulties in family practice. *Canadian Family Physician, 59*(3), 249–254.

NCLEXNOTE Delirium and dementia have similar presentations. Because delirium can be life threatening, identifying the potential underlying cause for the symptoms is a priority.

Although delirium may occur in any age group, it is most common among older adults. In this age group, delirium is often mistaken for dementia, which in turn leads to inappropriate treatment. Patients with delirium have a reduced ability to focus, difficulty in sustaining or shifting attention, changes in cognition, or perceptual disturbances (Mattison, 2020).

Epidemiology and Risk Factors

Statistics concerning prevalence are based primarily on older adults in acute care settings. Estimated prevalence rates range from 10% to 50% of patients. Delirium is particularly common in older postoperative patients. In some groups, such as those with dementia, the prevalence may be higher. Preexisting cognitive impairment is one of the greatest risk factors for delirium (Mattison, 2020; see Boxes 39.1 and 39.2).

Etiology

Delirium in the older adult is associated with medications, infections, fluid and electrolyte imbalances, metabolic disturbances, hypoxia, or ischemia. The probability

---

BOX 39.1

Risk Factors for Delirium

Advanced age
Preexisting dementia
Functional dependence
Endocrine and metabolic disorders
Bone fracture
Infection (pneumonia, urinary tract)
Medications (anticholinergic side effects)
Changes in vital signs (including hypotension and hyper- or hypothermia)
Electrolyte or metabolic imbalance (dehydration, renal failure, hyponatremia)
Admission to a long-term care institution
Postcardiotomy
AIDS
Pain
Acute or chronic stress
Substance use and alcohol withdrawal

---

of the syndrome developing increases if some predisposing factors, such as advanced age, brain damage, or dementia, are also present. Sensory overload or underload, immobilization, sleep deprivation, COVID-19, and psychosocial stress also contribute to delirium (Duggan et al., 2021).

BOX 39.2

Delirium

Margaret, a widowed 72-year-old woman living in her own home, has been having trouble sleeping. Her daughter visits her and suggests that she try an OTC sleeping medication. Margaret also takes antihistamines for allergies and the antidepressant amitriptyline. Three nights later, a neighbor calls the daughter, concerned because Margaret is wandering the streets, unable to find her home. When the neighbor approached Margaret to help her home, she began to scream and strike out at the neighbor.

The daughter visits immediately and discovers that her mother does not know who she is, does not know what time it is, appears disheveled, and is suspicious that people have been in her home stealing the things she cannot find. Margaret does not recall taking any medication, but when her daughter investigates, she finds that 10 pills of the new sleeping aid have already been used.

WHAT DO YOU THINK?

- Identify risk factors that may have contributed to Margaret's experiencing delirium.
- How could the addition of an OTC sleeping medication interact with the antihistamine and antidepressant to be responsible for Margaret's delirium?

RECOVERY-ORIENTED CARE FOR PERSONS WITH DELIRIUM

Delirium is a medical emergency that is easily misdiagnosed as a dementia. Prompt treatment leads to recovery.

Teamwork and Collaboration: Working Toward Recovery

Although delirium may be recognized and diagnosed in any health care setting, appropriate intervention usually requires that the patient be admitted to an acute care setting for rigorous assessment and rapid treatment. Priority in care is identifying the underlying cause of the delirium. Interdisciplinary management of delirium includes two primary aspects: (1) elimination or correction of the underlying cause and (2) symptomatic and supportive measures (e.g., adequate rest, comfort, maintenance of fluid and electrolyte balance, and protection from injury).

Safety Issues

If possible, the use of all suspected medications should be stopped and vital signs should be monitored at least every 2 hours. Close observation of the patient with particular regard to changes in vital signs, behavior, and mental status is required. Patients are monitored until the delirium subsides or until discharge. If the delirium still exists at discharge, it is critical that referrals for post-discharge follow-up assessment and care be implemented.

EVIDENCE-BASED NURSING CARE FOR PERSONS WITH DELIRIUM

The best management is prevention or early recognition of delirium. Special efforts should be made to include family members in the nursing process.

Mental Health Nursing Assessment

The onset of symptoms is typically signaled by a rapid or acute change in behavior. Delirium is underdiagnosed, and symptoms are easily missed in persons with mental disorders when it is assumed that the cognitive and behavioral changes are related to the mental disorder. An underlying medical cause should always be the first consideration.

Assessing the symptoms requires knowing what is normal for the individual. Caregivers, family members, or significant others should be interviewed because they can often provide valuable information. Family members may be the only resource for accurate information.

Physical Health Assessment

History should include a description of the onset, duration, range, and intensity of associated symptoms. Recent physical illness, dementia, depression, or other psychiatric illnesses should be identified. A physical examination should be conducted. Vital signs are crucial. Changes in activities of daily living (ADLs), use of sensory aids (eyeglasses and hearing aids), pain, and sleep should be documented. Recent laboratory results that might indicate hypoxia, hypoglycemia, and ST-segment elevation myocardial infarction (STEMI) should be considered. Assessment for infections that commonly underlie delirium, such as urinary tract infection, pneumonia, and sepsis from other sources, should be included. An abnormal neurological assessment would suggest a TIA (transient ischemic attack), stroke, intracranial hemorrhage or mass).

Medication Assessment

Many medications are associated with delirium (see Table 39.2). Medications and recent changes in the type and number, including over-the-counter (OTC) medications, should be documented. Combinations of medications can interact and cause delirium. Cold medications, taken in sufficient quantities, may cause confusion, especially in older adults. A substance use history (including alcohol intake and smoking history) should be taken.

Psychosocial Assessment

Mental Status

Rapid onset of global cognitive impairment that affects multiple aspects of intellectual functioning is the hallmark of delirium. Mental status evaluation reveals several changes:

- Fluctuations in level of consciousness with reduced awareness of the environment
- Difficulty focusing and sustaining or shifting attention
- Severely impaired memory, especially immediate and recent memory

Patients may be disoriented to time and place but rarely to person. Environmental perceptions are often disturbed. The patient may believe shadows in the room are really people. Thought content is often illogical, speech may be incoherent or inappropriate to the context. Mental status tends to fluctuate over the course of the day.

Behavior

Persons with delirium exhibit a wide range of behaviors, complicating the process of making a diagnosis and

TABLE 39.2	EXAMPLES OF DRUGS THAT CAN CAUSE DELIRIUM
Class	**Specific Drugs**
Anticholinergic	Antihistamines
	Chlorpheniramine
	Antiparkinsonian drugs (e.g., benztropine [Cogentin], biperiden [Akineton], or trihexyphenidyl)
	Atropine
	Belladonna alkaloids
	Diphenhydramine
	Phenothiazines
	Scopolamine
	Tricyclic antidepressants
Anticonvulsant	Phenobarbital
	Phenytoin (Dilantin)
	Sodium valproate (Depakene, Depakote)
Antiinflammatory	Corticosteroids
	Ibuprofen (Motrin, Advil)
	Indomethacin (Indocin)
	Naproxen (Naprosyn)
Antiparkinsonian	Amantadine
	Carbidopa (Sinemet)
	Levodopa (Larodopa)
Antibiotics	Isoniazid
	Rifampin
Analgesic	Opioids
	Salicylates
	Synthetic narcotics
Cardiac	Beta-blockers
	Propranolol (Inderal)
	Clonidine (Catapres)
	Digitalis (Digoxin, Lanoxin)
	Lidocaine (Xylocaine)
	Methyldopa (Aldomet)
	Quinidine
	Procainamide (Pronestyl)
Sedative—hypnotic	Barbiturates
	Benzodiazepines
Sympathomimetic	Amphetamines
	Phenylephrine
	Phenylpropanolamine
Over-the-counter medications	Compoz
	Excedrin PM
	Sleep-Eze
	Sominex

(Continued)

Class	Specific Drugs
Miscellaneous	Acyclovir (antiviral)
	Aminophylline
	Amphotericin (antifungal)
	Bromides
	Cephalexin (Keflex)
	Chlorpropamide (Diabinese)
	Cimetidine (Tagamet)
	Disulfiram (Antabuse)
	Lithium
	Metronidazole (Flagyl)
	Theophylline
	Timolol ophthalmic

Source: Wynn, G. H., Oesterheid, J. R., Cozza, K. I., Armstrong, S. C. (2009). *Clinical Manual of Drug Interaction: Principles for Medical Practice.* Arlington, VA: American Psychiatric Publishing, Inc.

planning interventions. At times, the individual may be restless or agitated and at other times lethargic and slow to respond.

Family Environment

An assessment of living arrangements may provide information about sensory stimulation or social isolation. Assessing family interactions, support for the patient, and family members' ability to understand delirium is also important. The behaviors exhibited by the person experiencing delirium may be frightening or at least confusing for family members. Some family members may actually contribute to the patient's increased agitation. At the same time, however, the family's presence may help to calm and reassure the patient.

CLINICAL JUDGMENT

If delirium is established as the medical diagnosis, the nurse must address any life-threatening issues related to respiration and cardiovascular impairment. If the patient is combative, de-escalation becomes a priority. Because there are many potential issues that could be underlying delirium, other priorities will be based on the identified causes.

MENTAL HEALTH NURSING INTERVENTIONS

Important interventions include providing a safe and therapeutic environment, maintaining fluid and electrolyte balance and adequate nutrition, and preventing aspiration and decubitus ulcers, which are common complications. Other interventions relate to individual symptoms and underlying causes.

Complementary and Nonpharmacological Interventions

There is strong evidence that complementary and non-pharmacological medicine interventions are effective in reducing agitation and delirium in older adults. Aromatherapy, massage, acupuncture, and therapeutic touch have been used successfully in reducing agitation and aggressive behavior (Leng et al., 2020).

Medications

There is no medication for delirium, but as the underlying medical problem is treated, the person may be given medication to treat the symptoms associated with delirium, such as agitation, inattention, combativeness, insomnia, and psychosis. Dosages are usually kept very low, especially with older adults and the medication is selected in light of the potential side effects (particularly anticholinergic effects, hypotension, and respiratory suppression). Antipyschotics are often used for a targeted group of patients who experience hallucinations or delusions associated with delirium (Ostuzzi et al., 2020). Recent research suggests that supportive measures and treatment of precipitating factors are more effective than antipsychotics (Ali & Cascella, 2020). Benzodiazepines are also used when the delirium is related to alcohol withdrawal. In some patients, benzodiazepines may further impair cognition because of the sedation.

Patients should be monitored for sedation, hypotension, or extrapyramidal symptoms. Although mental status often fluctuates during delirium, it may also be influenced by these medications, so any changes or worsening of mental status after administration of the medication should be reported immediately to the prescriber. Some side effects may also be confused with the symptoms of delirium. For example, akathisia (see Chapter 11), a side effect of antipsychotics, may appear as agitation or restlessness. Medications for treating symptoms related to delirium should be discontinued as soon as possible.

Psychosocial Interventions

Patients with delirium need frequent interaction and support if they are confused or hallucinating. Patients should be encouraged to express their fears and discomforts that result from frightening or disconcerting psychotic experiences. Adequate lighting, easy-to-read calendars and clocks, a reasonable noise level, and frequent verbal orientation may reduce this frightening experience. If the patient wears eyeglasses or uses a hearing aid, these devices should be used. Including familiar personal possessions in the environment may also help. These interventions have been shown to reduce the need for antipsychotic medication and reduced length of hospitalization (Hshieh et al., 2020).

A safe environment is important to protect the patient from injury. A predictable, orienting environment will help to reestablish order to the patient's life. That is, a calendar, clocks, and other items may be provided to help orient the patient to time, place, and person. If the patient is agitated, de-escalation techniques should be used (see Chapter 14). Physical restraint should be avoided.

Families can also be encouraged to work with staff to reorient the patient and provide a supportive environment. Families need to understand that important decisions requiring the patient's input should be delayed if at all possible until the patient has recovered. Although patients may be able to participate in decision-making, they may not remember the decision later.

Psychoeducation

To prevent future occurrences, provide education to the patient and family about the underlying cause of the delirium. If the delirium is not resolved before discharge, family members need to know how to care for the patient at home.

Promoting Safety

Behaviors exhibited by the person with delirium, such as hallucinations, delusions, **illusions**, aggression, or agitation (restlessness or excitability), may pose safety problems. Because individuals with delirium are more likely to fall or injure themselves during a confused state, special precautions and safety measures should be considered. The patient must be protected from physical harm by using low beds, guardrails, and careful supervision. Delirium management and fall prevention may be implemented for any patient at risk for falls.

Therefore, it is important to have several witnesses present.

Evaluation and Treatment Outcomes

The primary treatment goal is prevention or resolution of the delirious episode with return to previous cognitive status. Outcome measures include the following:

- Correction of the underlying physiologic alteration
- Resolution of confusion
- Family member verbalization of understanding of confusion
- Prevention of injury

Resolution of confusion is the primary goal; however, the nursing care provided makes important contributions to

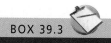

BOX 39.3

Delirium

When caring for the patient with delirium, be sure to include the caregivers, as appropriate, and address the following topic areas in the teaching plan:

- Psychopharmacologic agents, if used, including drug action, dosage, frequency, and possible adverse effects
- Underlying cause of delirium
- Mental status changes
- Safety measures
- Hydration and nutrition
- Avoidance of restraints
- Decision-making guidelines

all four of these outcomes. The end result of delirium may be full recovery, incomplete recovery, incomplete recovery with some residual cognitive impairment, or a downward course leading to death.

Continuum of Care

Patients with delirium may present in a number of treatment settings (e.g., home, nursing home, ambulatory care, day treatment, outpatient setting, hospital). Patients usually are admitted to an acute care setting for rapid evaluation and treatment of the underlying etiology. For more information on caring for patients with delirium, see Box 39.3.

ALZHEIMER DISEASE

Clinical Course

AD is a degenerative, progressive, neuropsychiatric disorder that results in cognitive impairment, emotional and behavioral changes, physical and functional decline, and ultimately death. Gradually, the patient's ability to carry out ADLs declines, although physical status often

remains intact until late in the disease. Although primarily a disorder of older adults, AD has been diagnosed in patients as young as age 35 years.

Two subtypes have been identified: early onset AD (age 65 years and younger) and late onset AD (age older than 65 years). Late-onset AD is much more common than early-onset AD, but early-onset AD has a more rapid progression. AD is also routinely conceptualized in terms of three stages: mild, moderate, and severe. Signs and symptoms of AD change as the patient passes from one phase of the illness to another (Figure 39.1).

Diagnostic Criteria

The diagnosis of AD is made on clinical grounds, but verification is only confirmed during autopsy. The essential feature of AD is cognitive decline from a previous level of functioning in one or more cognitive domains (attention, executive function, learning and memory, language, perceptual-motor or social cognition) (APA, 2013). These deficits interfere with independence in ADLs. Typical deficits include **aphasia** (i.e., alterations in language ability), **apraxia** (i.e., impaired ability to execute motor activities despite intact motor functioning), **agnosia** (i.e., failure to recognize or identify objects despite intact sensory function), or a **disturbance of executive functioning** (i.e., ability to think abstractly, plan, initiate, sequence, monitor, and stop complex behavior).

Mild neurocognitive impairment (MCI) is diagnosed if a modest cognitive decline from a previous level of function is found in one or more of the cognitive domains, but the cognitive deficits do not interfere with independence in daily activities (APA, 2013). MCI is thought to be related to multiple causes and some, but not all, progress to AD. MCI is categorized according to type of memory loss. In *amnestic MCI*, an individual may start to forget important information such as appointments, conversations, or events. In *nonamnestic MCI*, impairment

Dementia/Alzheimer Disease

Stage	Mild	Moderate	Severe
Symptoms	Loss of memory	Inability to retain new info	Gait and motor disturbances
	Language difficulties	Behavioral, personality changes	Bedridden
	Mood swings	Increasing long-term memory loss	Unable to perform ADL
	Personality changes	Wandering, agitation, aggression, confusion	Incontinence
	Diminished judgment	Requires assistance w/ADL	Requires long-term care placement
	Apathy		

FIGURE 39.1 Alzheimer disease progression.

in visual perception, the ability to make sound decisions, or the capacity to judge the time or sequence of steps needed to complete a complex task occurs (Alzheimer's Association, 2021a).

Epidemiology and Risk Factors

In 2020, an estimated 5.8 million Americans had AD, 1 in 10 older than 65 years old. By 2050, the population of America over the age of 65 is projected to grow from 56 million to 88 million. With this increase in population, the number of those with AD will also grow. Almost two thirds of Americans with AD are women. Dementia appears to affect all groups, but studies in the United States reveal a higher incidence in Black or African American individuals and Hispanic or Latinx individuals than in White individuals. Currently, AD is the fifth leading cause of death among older adults in the United States (Alzheimer's Association, 2020).

General Risk Factors

AD can run in families. Compared with the general population, first-degree biologic relatives of individuals with early-onset AD are more likely to experience the disorder. Studies show that those with fewer years of education or those who have had a prior head injury are at higher risk of developing AD (Alzheimer's Association, 2020).

Down Syndrome

People with Down syndrome are at higher risk of developing AD than others, most likely because of the additional copy of chromosome 21. The **amyloid precursor protein (APP)** is a gene found on this chromosome that is involved in the formation of neurons and their survival. This gene is cut into smaller fragments (peptides) by enzymes. The extra copy of chromosome 21 increases the amount of amyloid beta (A-beta) fragments in the brain, which in turn increases the possibility of formation of **beta-amyloid plaques**. By age 40, most people with Down syndrome have increased levels of beta-amyloid plaques and tau tangles in their brain (Alzheimer's Association, 2020).

Metabolic Syndrome

Individuals with metabolic syndrome have a greater risk of developing AD (Alzheimer's Association, 2020). Metabolic syndrome, a cluster of conditions (hypertension, hyperglycemia, abdominal obesity, and hyperlipidemia) that occur together, increases the risk of heart disease, stroke, and diabetes. Metabolic syndrome is associated with microvascular changes in the brain, which in turn appear to cause mitochondrial dysfunction. Insulin resistance is thought to play a key role in the neuroinflammation and loss of synapses (Kellar & Craft, 2020).

Etiology

Researchers have yet to identify a definitive cause of AD, but a combination of genetic, environmental, and lifestyle factors influences a person's risk for developing the disease. There are multiple factors involved in the development and progression of this disorder (National Institute on Aging [NIH], 2019).

Amyloid Precursor Protein

The APP located on the cell membrane appears to have a neuroprotective role in situations of metabolic stress. During an acute stroke, cardiac arrest, or chronic hypoxic–ischemic condition, the APP can promote neuronal survival. Damage to DNA prevents repair of the APP. When APP is cut or cleaved by the beta-site APP Cleaving Enzyme 1, neurotoxic amyloid-beta is released. These peptides can accumulate as amyloid plaques, promoting neurodegeneration (Lin et al., 2020).

Beta-Amyloid Plaques

One piece of the puzzle is partially explained by a leading theory that beta-amyloid plaques, made up of proteins, clump together in the brain and destroy cholinergic neurons. Research suggests that beta-amyloid deposits impair the normal function of pericytes, which are cells important for controlling the removal of protein from the brain. This leads to further accumulation of the protein. Beta-amyloid is hypothesized to interfere with the process of storing memories through interrupting synaptic connection. Symptoms such as aphasia and visuospatial abnormalities are attributable to plaque formation (Sengoku, 2020).

Neurofibrillary Tangles

Neurofibrillary tangles are made of abnormally twisted protein threads found inside the brain cells. The main component of the tangles is *tau*, a protein that stabilizes the microtubules of transport cells. In AD, tau separates from the microtubules. Loose tau proteins tangle with each other, causing the characteristic neurofibrillary tangles. When microtubules disintegrate, the neuron's transport system collapses, resulting in cell death (Sengoku, 2020) (Figure 39.2).

Synaptic Micron RNA and Neurotransmission

In patients with AD, neurotransmission is reduced, neurons are lost, and the hippocampal neurons degenerate. Several major neurotransmitters are affected, such as **acetylcholine (ACh)**, norepinephrine, and

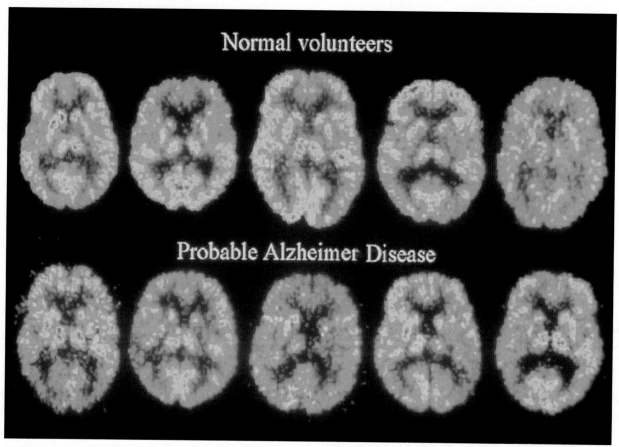

Figure 39.2   Series comparison of older control subjects (*top row*) and patients with Alzheimer disease (AD) (*bottom row*). Although some decreases in metabolism are associated with age, in most patients with AD, marked decreases are seen in the temporal lobe, an area important in memory functions. (Courtesy of Monte S. Buchsbaum, MD, The Mount Sinai Medical Center and School of Medicine, New York.)

serotonin important, in cognitive functioning and memory. Researchers hypothesize that microRNA (molecules involved in gene expression) alterations, occur impacting synaptic transmission (see Chapter 6). See Figure 39.3 are also affected (Kumar & Reddy, 2020).

One of the early hypotheses was that cholinergic dysfunction contributed to cognitive deficits associated with aging and AD. This hypothesis was based on evidence that alterations in the cholinergic systems induced cognitive deficits similar to those in AD and aging. When cholinergic functioning was increased, there were beneficial effects. We now understand that the pathogenesis of AD is much more complicated than a single cause, even though the primary medications for AD target the cholinergic system (Barfejani et al., 2020).

Genetic Factors

Mutations on three genes are identified as causing AD through altering A-beta processing and are transmitted through genetic inheritance—*APP*, *PSEN1*, and *PSEN2*. These mutations explain 5% to 10% of the occurrence of early-onset AD. The majority of early-onset AD cases do not have a clear genetic pattern of inheritance. However, genetic predisposition is estimated to be a factor in 60% to 80% of AD cases, including late-onset AD (Bellenguez et al., 2020).

The *APOE* gene transports cholesterol in the bloodstream. Three forms of the *APOE* gene (e2, e3, and e4) are inherited from each parent. The e3 form is the most common and is believed to neither increase or decrease the risk of AD. e4 is the next most common and is found to increase the risk of developing AD. People with one copy of the e4 form are three times as likely to develop AD compared with those who have the e3 form, and those with two copies of the e4 form have an 8 to 12 times greater risk. The least common *APOE* gene, e2, is relatively rare and may actually decrease one's risk of AD (Alzheimer's Association, 2020).

Oxidative Stress, Free Radicals, and Mitochondrial Dysfunction

It is hypothesized that in AD-affected brains, there is a rapid increase in formation of free radicals (i.e., highly reactive molecules), which can lead to **oxidative stress**

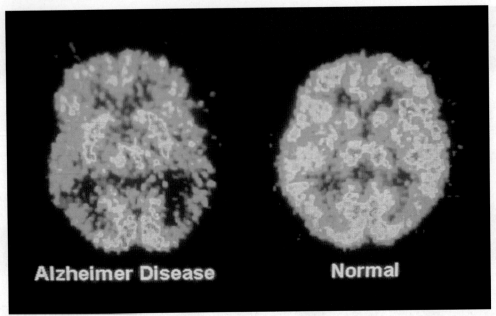

FIGURE 39.3 Metabolic activity in a subject with Alzheimer disease (*left*) and control subject without AD (*right*). (Courtesy of Monte S. Buchsbaum, MD, The Mount Sinai Medical Center and School of Medicine, New York.)

that damages other cellular molecules such as proteins, lipids, and nucleic acid. Recent studies suggest that oxidative stress may result in changes in chromatin (a complex of DNA and proteins), which may lead to dysfunctional gene expression (Tadokoro et al., 2020).

Inflammation

Inflammation is now considered as one of the many factors that contribute to the development of AD. The hypothesis is that inflammation may damage small blood vessels and brain cells, initiating a cascade of pathologic events related to oxidative damage and dysregulated amyloid metabolism (Kacířová et al., 2020).

Gut–Brain Axis Alteration

The gut microbial composition is thought to influence several age-related neurological disorders including AD. It is proposed that alterations in gut microbial composition contributes to the pathogenesis of AD. Normally, the gastrointestinal (GI) tract epithelium and the blood–brain barrier are protective physiological barriers. After aging, these protective barriers become more permeable. If repeated chronic infection occurs, exposure to exotoxins such as lipopolysaccharides (LPS) and bacterial amyloids occurs because they pass more easily through compromised GI tract and blood–brain barrier. Evidence reveals that aging together with repeated chronic infections lead to altered activation of

microglial cells that aggravates inflammatory responses, A-beta fibrillation, and the aggregation of amyloid-beta. in the brain (Kesika et al., 2021).

Family Response to Disorder

Families are the first to be aware of the cognitive problem, often before the patient, who can be unaware of the extent of memory impairment. When finally confirmed, the actual diagnosis can be devastating to the family. Unlike delirium, a diagnosis of AD means long-term care responsibilities while the essence of a family member diminishes day by day. Most families keep their relative at home as long as possible to maintain contact and to avoid costly nursing home placement. The two symptoms that often result in nursing home placement are incontinence that cannot be managed and behavioral problems, such as wandering and aggression.

RECOVERY-ORIENTED CARE FOR A PERSON WITH ALZHEIMER DISEASE

AD has a long clinical course—at least 20 years. AD research is quickly advancing, and it is likely that treatment will provide more options to reduce or reverse the illness trajectory. Hope for the future should be instilled in patients and families. Recovery is an important focus for persons with AD, reminding families that wellness is possible despite the presence of a chronic disease.

Teamwork and Collaboration: Working toward Recovery

The nature and range of services needed by patients and families throughout the illness can vary dramatically at different stages. As with any other patient, the person with AD should be the center of the decision-making process. The plan should include educational and supportive programs individualized for the person's self-identified needs. Ideally, plans should be designed to support self-awareness, self-esteem, maintenance of abilities, and management of behavioral symptoms and health promotion.

Treatment efforts currently focus on managing cognitive symptoms, delaying cognitive decline (e.g., memory loss; confusion; and problems with learning, speech, reasoning), treating the noncognitive symptoms (e.g., psychosis, mood symptoms, agitation), and supporting the caregivers to improve the quality of life for both patients and their caregivers.

Safety Issues

The priority of care changes throughout the course of AD. Initially, the priority is delaying cognitive decline and supporting family members. Later, the priority is protecting the patient from injury because of the patient's lack of judgment. Near the end, the physical needs of the patient are the focus of care.

EVIDENCE-BASED NURSING CARE FOR PERSONS WITH ALZHEIMER DISEASE

Development and implementation of appropriate, effective, and safe nursing services for the care and support of patients with AD and their families is a particular challenge because of the complex nature of the illness. See Nursing Care Plan 39.1.

> **NCLEXNOTE** Needs and problematic behaviors of patients with AD vary throughout the course of the disorder. Early in the disorder, the nurse focuses on support, education, and cognitive interventions for depression. As AD progresses, priority care becomes safety interventions.

Mental Health Nursing Assessment

Physical Health Assessment

A review of body systems must be conducted on each patient suspected of having AD. The neurologic function of the patient with AD is usually preserved through the early and middle stages of the disease, although seizures, gait disturbances, and tremors may occur at any time. In the later stages of the disease, neurologic signs, such as flexion contractures and primitive reflexes, are prominent features.

Physical Functions

Assessment of physical functions includes ADLs, recent changes in functional abilities, use of sensory aids (e.g., eyeglasses, hearing aids), activity level, and assessment of pain. Eyeglasses and hearing aids may need to be in place before other assessments can be made.

At first, limitations may primarily involve instrumental activities of daily living (IADLs) (e.g., shopping, preparing meals, performing other household chores). Later in the disease process, basic physical dysfunctions occur, such as incontinence, ataxia, dysphagia, and contractures. Incontinence can be a major source of stress and a considerable burden to family caregivers. Evaluation of the patient's functional abilities includes bathing, dressing, toileting, feeding, nutritional status, physical mobility, sleep patterns, and pain.

Self-Care

Alterations in the central nervous system (CNS) associated with AD impair the patient's ability to collect information from the environment, retrieve memories, retain new information, and give meaning to current situations. Therefore, patients with AD often neglect self-care activities. Periodically, biologic assessment parameters need to be reevaluated because patients with AD may neglect activities such as bathing, eating, or skin care.

Sleep–Wake Disturbances

Patients with AD have frequent daytime napping and nighttime periods of wakefulness, with little rapid eye movement (REM) sleep. Circadian rhythms are disrupted as the amyloid beta (A-beta) increases. Tau pathology and increases in beta-amyloid plaques are associated with restlessness, irritability, and general sleep impairment (Uddin et al., 2021).

Activity and Exercise

One of the earliest symptoms of AD is withdrawal from normal activities. Motor activity is affected in the mild stages of AD and can lead to early problems in functional performance (Alzheimer's Association, 2020). As the disease progresses, the patient may just sit staring at a blank wall.

Nutrition

Nutritional assessment is very important in light of the recent understanding that changes in gut microbiota

NURSING CARE PLAN 39.1

The Patient with Dementia

Lorine is a 76-year-old widow who lives independently. Recently, her children have noticed that she is becoming more forgetful and seems to have periods of confusion. She has agreed to have someone help her during the day. Her oldest son lives with her and is with her during the evening and night. Lorine refuses to see a health care provider but did agree to go in for a routine checkup. Her daughter helped her get dressed and took her to the primary care office.

Setting: Primary Care Office

Baseline Assessment: A well-groomed woman is accompanied by her daughter. Lorine says there is nothing wrong, but her daughter disagrees. A review of body systems reveals poor hearing and vision but is otherwise unremarkable. Her daughter reports that Lorine has become very suspicious of her neighbors and has changed her locks several times.

Associated Psychiatric Diagnosis	Medications
Probable Alzheimer disease	Galantamine (Razadyne) 4 mg twice a day (BID); titrate to 8 mg BID over 4 weeks.

Priority of Care: Changes in Memory

Important Characteristics	Associated Considerations
Inability to recall information Inability to recall past events Observed instances of forgetfulness Forgets to perform daily activities (e.g., grooming)	Neurocognitive changes associated with dementia

Outcomes

Initial	Long-term
Maintain or improve current memory	Delay cognitive decline associated with dementia

Interventions

Interventions	Rationale	Ongoing Assessment
Develop memory cues in home. Have clocks and calendars clearly displayed. Make lists for the patients.	Maintaining current level of memory involves providing cues that will help the patient recall information.	Contact family members for the patient's ability to use memory cues.
Teach the patient and family about taking an acetylcholinesterase inhibitor. Review expected effects and side effects. Develop a titration schedule with the family to decrease the appearance of side effects.	Confidence and self-esteem improve when a person looks well groomed.	Monitor response to suggestions.
Observe patient for visuospatial impairment. If present, sequence habitual activities such as eating, dressing, and bathing.	Visuospatial impairment is one of the symptoms of dementia.	Observe for appropriate dress, bathing, eating, and so on.

Evaluation

Outcomes	Revised Outcomes	Interventions
Lorine did have some improvement in memory. Suspiciousness and behavioral symptoms improved.	Continue maintaining memory.	Continue with memory cues and galantamine.

could affect the brain's physiological, behavioral, and cognitive functions (Lin et al., 2018). Foods high in fat content and foods highly processed are detrimental to the support of a healthy gut microbiome.

Eating can become a problem for a patient with AD and is associated with rapid cognitive decline. As the disease progresses, patients may lose the ability to feed themselves or recognize that what is being offered is food. Some patients with AD are bulimic or hyperoral (eating or chewing almost everything possible and sometimes with an insatiable appetite). Other patients with AD experience anorexia and have no appetite.

Pain

Although AD is not usually considered a physically painful disorder, patients often have other comorbid physical diseases that may be painful. In the early stages of AD, the patient can usually respond to verbal questions regarding pain. Later, it may be difficult to assess the comfort level objectively, especially if the patient cannot communicate. Some patients in the end stage of AD become hypersensitive to touch.

Subtle behavioral changes, such as lethargy, anxiety, or restlessness, or more obvious physical signs, such as pyrexia, tachypnea, or tachycardia, may be the only indications of actual or impending illness. Observing for changes in patterns of nonverbal communication, such as facial expressions, may help in identifying indicators of pain. **Hypervocalizations** (disturbed vocalizations), restlessness, and agitation are other possible signs of pain.

Psychosocial Assessment

Personality changes almost always accompany AD. Researchers have identified two contrasting patterns. One is marked by apathy, lack of spontaneity, and passivity. The other involves growing irritability, sarcasm, self-preoccupation, and intolerance of and lack of concern for others.

Mental Status and Appearance

The mental status assessment can be difficult for the patient with AD because cognitive disturbance is the clinical hallmark of AD. However, family members should also be a part of any assessment, especially early in the disease process. There are several screening instruments that can be used in detecting symptoms of dementia. The Mini-Cog is used by clinicians in assessing whether an individual has symptoms of AD (Borson et al., 2003). The AD8 Dementia Screening Interview, which is given to a family member, is a brief, sensitive measure that differentiates between those with and without dementia (Galvin

et al., 2005, 2006). The AD8 contains eight questions asking the family member to rate any change ("yes" or "no") in memory, problem-solving abilities, orientation, and ADLs. The higher the number of changes, the more likely dementia is present (Figure 39.4). The nurse should suspect delirium in instances where cognitive deterioration occurs rapidly.

Memory

The most dramatic and consistent cognitive impairment is in memory. Patients with dementia appear mildly forgetful and repetitive in conversation. They misplace objects, miss appointments, and forget what they were just doing. They may lose track of a conversation or television show. Initially, they may complain of memory problems, but rapidly in the course of the illness, insight is lost, and they become unaware of what is lost. Sometimes, they may confabulate, making what appears to be an appropriate explanation of why the information or object is missing. Eventually, all aspects of memory are impaired and even long-term memories are affected. During the interview, short-term memory loss is usually readily evident by the patient's inability to recall three or four words given to them at the beginning of the assessment. Often, the earliest symptom of AD is the inability to retain new information.

Language

Language is also progressively impaired. Individuals with AD may initially have agnosia (difficulty finding a word in a sentence or in naming an object). They may be able to talk around it, but the loss is noticeable. Later, fluent aphasia develops; comprehension diminishes; and, finally, they become mute and unresponsive to directions or information.

Visuospatial Impairment

Deficits in visuospatial tasks that require sensory and motor coordination develop early, drawing is abnormal, and the ability to write may change. An inaccurate clock drawing is diagnostic of impairment in this area (Figure 39.5). Sequencing tasks, such as cooking or other self-care skills, become impaired. The individual becomes unable to complete complex tasks that require calculations, such as balancing a checkbook.

Executive Functioning

Judgment, reasoning, and the ability to problem solve or make decisions are also impaired later in the disorder, closer to the time of nursing home placement. It is

Remember, "Yes, a change" indicates that there has been a change in the last several years caused by cognitive (thinking and memory) problems.	YES, A change	NO, No change	N/A, Don't know
1. Problems with judgment (e.g., problems making decisions, bad financial decisions, problems with thinking)			
2. Less interest in hobbies/activities			
3. Repeats the same things over and over (questions, stories, or statements)			
4. Trouble learning how to use a tool, appliance, or gadget (e.g., VCR, computer, microwave, remote control)			
5. Forgets correct month or year			
6. Trouble handling complicated financial affairs (e.g., balancing checkbook, income taxes, paying bills)			
7. Trouble remembering appointments			
8. Daily problems with thinking and/or memory			
TOTAL AD8 SCORE			

Adapted from Galvin JE et al, The AD8: A Brief Informant Interview to Detect Dementia, Neurology 2005:65:559-564. Copyright ©2005 by Washington University, St. Louis, MO. All Rights Reserved. Please contact otm@wustl.edu for a commercial license, for permission to make modifications, or for any other intended purpose.

The AD8® Administration and Scoring Guidelines

A spontaneous self-correction is allowed for all responses without counting as an error.

The questions are given to the respondent on a clipboard for self–administration or can be read aloud to the respondent either in person or over the phone. It is preferable to administer the AD8 to an informant, if available. If an informant is not available, the AD8 may be administered to the patient.

When administered to an informant, specifically ask the respondent to rate change in the patient.

When administered to the patient, specifically ask the patient to rate changes in his/her ability for each of the items, *without* attributing causality.

FIGURE 39.4 AD8® Dementia Screening Interview.

If read aloud to the respondent, it is important for the clinician to carefully read the phrase as worded and give emphasis to note changes due to cognitive problems (not physical problems). There should be a one second delay between individual items.

No timeframe for change is required.

The final score is a sum of the number items marked "Yes, A change".

Interpretation of the AD8

(Adapted from Galvin JE et al, The AD8, a brief informant interview to detect dementia, Neurology 2005:65:559-564)

A screening test in itself is insufficient to diagnose a dementing disorder. The AD8 is, however, quite sensitive to detecting early cognitive changes associated many common dementing illness including Alzheimer disease, vascular dementia, Lewy body dementia and frontotemporal dementia.

Scores in the impaired range (see below) indicate a need for further assessment. Scores in the "normal" range suggest that a dementing disorder is unlikely, but a very early disease process cannot be ruled out. More advanced assessment may be warranted in cases where other objective evidence of impairment exists.

Based on clinical research findings from 995 individuals included in the development and validation samples, the following cut points are provided:

0 – 1: Normal cognition

2 or greater: Cognitive impairment is likely to be present

Administered to either the informant (preferable) or the patient, the AD8 has the following properties:

Sensitivity > 84%

Specificity > 80%

Positive Predictive Value > 85%

Negative Predictive Value > 70%

Area under the Curve: 0.908; 95%CI: 0.888-0.925

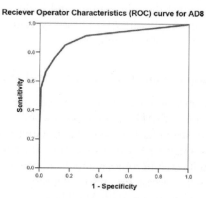

Reciever Operator Characteristics (ROC) curve for AD8

Permission Statement

FIGURE 39.4 *(Continued)*

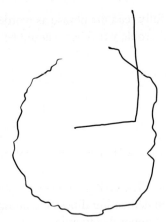

FIGURE 39.5 Clock drawing by a patient with moderate Alzheimer disease. The patient was asked to draw a clock at 3:00 PM.

hypothesized that as the disease progresses, the degeneration of neurons is spread diffusely throughout the neocortex.

Psychotic Symptoms

Delusional thought content and hallucinations are common in people with AD. These psychotic symptoms differ from those of schizophrenia.

Suspiciousness, Delusions, and Illusions

Illusions, or mistaken perceptions, are also common in patients with AD. For example, a woman with AD mistakes her husband for her father. He resembles her father in that he is roughly her father's age when the father was last alive. If an illusion becomes a false fixed belief, it is a delusion.

As the disease progresses, delusions develop in 34% to 50% of the people with AD. These characteristic delusions are different from those discussed in the psychotic disorders. Common delusional beliefs include the following:

- Belief that their partner is engaging in marital infidelity
- Belief that other patients or staff are trying to hurt them
- Belief that staff or family members are impersonators
- Belief that people are stealing their belongings
- Belief that strangers are living in their home
- Belief that people on television are real and not actors

Hallucinations

Visual, rather than auditory, hallucinations are the most common in AD. A frequent complaint is that children, adults, or strange creatures are entering the house or the patient's room. These hallucinations may not seem unusual to the patient. If possible, the content and form of hallucination should be ascertained because this information may suggest a treatable disorder. For example, an auditory hallucination commanding the patient to commit suicide may be caused by a treatable depression, not AD. In some cases, hallucinations may be pleasant, such as children being in the room, or the hallucinations may be frightening and uncomfortable.

Mood Changes

A depressed mood is common, but major depression and AD appear to be separate disorders. Many people with AD experience one or more depressive episodes with symptoms such as psychomotor retardation, anxiety, feelings of guilt and worthlessness, sadness, frequent crying, insomnia, loss of appetite, weight loss, and suicidal rumination. Depressive symptoms are most prevalent in the early stages of AD, which may be attributed to the patient's awareness of cognitive changes, memory loss, and functional decline (Kuo et al., 2020).

Anxiety

Moderate anxiety is a natural reaction to the fear engendered by gradual deterioration of intellectual function and the realization of impending loss of control over one's life. Failure to complete a task formerly regarded as simple creates a source of anxiety in patient with AD. As patients with AD become unsure of their surroundings and the expectations of others, they frequently react with fear and distress. It is thought that anxious behavior occurs when the patient is pressed to perform beyond their ability.

Catastrophic Reactions

Catastrophic reactions are overreactions or extreme anxiety reactions to everyday situations. Catastrophic responses occur when environmental stressors are allowed to continue or increase beyond the patient's threshold of stress tolerance. Behaviors indicative of catastrophic reactions typically include verbal or physical aggression, violence, agitated or anxious behavior, emotional outbursts, noisy behavior, compulsive or repetitive behavior, agitated night awakening, and other behaviors in which the patient is cognitively or socially inaccessible. Factors that contribute to catastrophic responses in patients with progressive cognitive decline include fatigue, a change in routine (e.g., faster pace, caregiver), demands beyond the patient's ability, overwhelming sensory stimuli, and physical stressors (e.g., pain, hunger).

Behavioral Responses

Apathy and Withdrawal

Apathy, the inability or unwillingness to become involved with one's environment, is common in AD, especially in the moderate to late stages. Apathy leads to withdrawal from the environment and a gradual loss of empathy for others. This lack of empathy is very difficult for families and friends to understand.

Restlessness, Agitation, and Aggression

Restlessness, agitation, and aggression are relatively common in the moderate to late stages of AD. Restlessness should be further evaluated to determine its underlying cause. If the restlessness occurs during medication change or adjustment, side effects should be suspected.

Aberrant Motor Behavior

Symptoms such as fidgeting, picking at clothing, wringing hands, loud vocalizations, and wandering may all be signs of such underlying conditions as dehydration, medication reaction, pain, or infection (suggesting delirium). One of the most difficult behaviors for which to determine an underlying cause is *hypervocalization*, a term that refers to the screams, curses, moans, groans, and verbal repetitiveness that are common in the later stages of AD in cognitively impaired older adults, often occurring during a hospitalization or nursing home placement. In the assessment of these hypervocalizations, it is important to identify when the behavior is occurring; antecedents of the behavior; and any related events, such as a family member leaving or a change in stimulation.

Disinhibition

One of the most frustrating symptoms of AD is **disinhibition**, acting on thoughts and feelings without exercising appropriate social judgment. In AD, the patient may decide that they are more comfortable naked than with clothes. Or the patient may not be able to find their clothes and may walk into a room of people without any clothes on. This behavior is extremely disconcerting to family members and can also lead to nursing home placement.

Hypersexuality

A closely related symptom is **hypersexuality**, which is inappropriate and socially unacceptable sexual behavior. The patient begins talking and behaving in ways that are uncharacteristic of premorbid behavior. This behavior is very difficult for family members and nursing home staff.

Stress and Coping Skills

Patients with AD seem extremely sensitive to stressful situations and often do not have the coping abilities to deal with such situations. A careful assessment of the triggers that precede stressful situations will help in understanding a provoking event.

Social Network and Support System

AD interferes with a person's ability to interact socially as much as it disrupts intellectual functioning. The patient's whole social network is affected by AD, and the primary caregiver of a person with AD (usually the partner or offspring in a community setting) is often considered a copatient. It is important to assess the family caregiver's ability to use supportive mechanisms to maintain their own integrity throughout the disease process.

If the patient still resides in the community, a home visit will prove useful because it provides information about the patient in the natural environment. From this assessment, the situational and psychosocial stressors that affect the family and patient can be identified, so interventions to strengthen coping strategies, including the ability to seek help from appropriate community resources, can be developed.

CLINICAL JUDGMENT

The unique and changing needs of these patients present a challenge for nurses in all settings. Priorities of care vary according to the stage of the disease. Early on, memory impairment and confusion may be present. An individual may begin to feel less connected and engaged in usual activities. As the disease progresses, the patient may have difficulty with their ADLs. Safety concerns may be present, especially if the patient is agitated, aggressive, or prone to wondering. In late stages of AD, the patient may be completely reliant on others in meeting basic health care needs.

MENTAL HEALTH NURSING INTERVENTIONS

Self-Care Interventions

Patients should be encouraged to maintain as much self-care as possible. If eyeglasses and hearing aids are needed but not used, patients are more likely to have false perceptual experiences (hallucinations).

Oral hygiene can be a problem and requires excellent basic nursing care. Aging and many medications reduce salivary flow, which can lead to a painfully dry and cracking oral mucosa. Periodontal disease (a persistent low-grade inflammatory condition caused by pathogenic microorganisms) has been linked to increase in the amyloid beta (A-beta) load (Sadrameli et al., 2020). For patients with xerostomia (dry mouth), hard candy or chewing gum may stimulate salivary flow or modification of the drug regimen may be necessary. Glycerol mouthwash can provide as much relief from xerostomia as artificial saliva.

During later stages of AD, bathing can be problematic for the patient and nursing staff. Bath time is a high-risk time for agitation and aggression. The person-centered approach focuses on personalizing care to meet residents' needs, accommodating to residents' preferences, attending to the relationship and interaction with the resident, using effective communication and interpersonal skills, and adapting the physical environment and bathing procedures to decrease stress and discomfort.

Physical Health Interventions

Supporting Bowel and Bladder Function

Urinary or bowel incontinence affects many patients with AD. During the middle phases of the disease, incontinence may be caused by the patient's inability to communicate the need to use the toilet or locate a toilet quickly, undress appropriately to use the toilet, recognize the sensation of fullness signaling the need to urinate or defecate, or apathy with lack of motivation to remain continent.

For the patient who is incontinent because of an inability to locate the toilet, orientation may be helpful. Signs and active training should help to modify disorientation. Displaying pictures or signs on bathroom doors provides visual cues; words should use appropriate terminology.

Sleep Interventions

Sedative–hypnotic agents may be prescribed for a short time for restlessness or insomnia, but they may also cause a paradoxical reaction of agitation and insomnia (especially in older adults). Sleep hygiene interventions are appropriate for patients with AD, although morning and afternoon naps (or rest periods for patients who do not nap) may be the most effective intervention for a patient with altered diurnal rhythms.

Activity and Exercise Interventions

Activity and exercise are important nursing interventions for patients with AD. To promote a feeling of success, any activity or exercise plan must be culturally sensitive and adapted to the patient's functional ability and interests.

The activity or exercise must be designed to prevent excess stress (both physical and psychological), which means that it must be individualized for each patient with AD based on their relative strengths and deficits.

Nutritional Interventions

Maintenance of nutrition and hydration are essential nursing interventions. The patient's weight, oral intake, and hydration status should be monitored carefully. Patients with AD should eat well-balanced meals appropriate to their activity level and eating abilities, with special attention given to electrolyte balance and fluid intake. A Mediterranean diet (vegetables, whole grains and olive oil, fermented dairy products, nuts, seeds and herbs/spices, plant protein and seafood) supports a healthy gut and brain (Flanagan et al., 2020).

Watch for swallowing difficulties that may put the patient at risk for aspiration and asphyxiation. Swallowing difficulties may result from changes in esophageal motility and decreased secretion of saliva.

Pain and Comfort Management

Nursing care of noncommunicative patients who have AD and who also have pain can be challenging. Because of the difficulty in identifying and monitoring the pain, the patients are often undertreated. However, several measures may be used to assess the efficacy of pharmacologic interventions, such as decreased restlessness and agitation. Small doses of oral morphine solution appear to reduce discomfort during routine nursing procedures. The main side effect of morphine is constipation.

Relaxation

Approaching patients in a calm, confident, unhurried manner; maintaining a soothing, quiet environment; avoiding unnecessary noise or chatter around patients and lowering vocal tone and rate when addressing them; maintaining eye contact; and using touch judiciously are likely to promote a sense of security conducive to patient relaxation and comfort. Simple relaxation exercises can be used to reduce stress and should be performed by the patient.

Medication Interventions

Medications have two goals: restoration or maintenance of cognitive function and treatment of related psychiatric and behavioral disturbances that cause discomfort for the patient, interfere with treatment, or worsen the individual's cognitive status. Doses must be kept extremely low, and patients should be monitored closely for any side effects or worsening of cognitive status. "Start low and go slow" is the principle guiding the administration of psychopharmacologic agents in older patients.

Cholinesterase Inhibitors.

Acetylcholinesterase inhibitors (AChEIs) are the mainstay of pharmacologic treatment of AD because they inhibit **acetylcholinesterase (AChE)**, an enzyme necessary for the breakdown of acetylcholine. Inhibition of AChE results in an increase in cholinergic activity. Because these medications have been shown to delay the decline in cognitive functioning but generally do not improve cognitive function after it has declined, it is important that this medication be started as soon as

the diagnosis is made. The primary side effect of these medications is gastrointestinal distress, including nausea, vomiting, and diarrhea.

Cholinesterase inhibitors are indicated for the treatment of AD. These drugs may help to delay or prevent symptoms from becoming worse (see Table 39.3). Cholinesterase inhibitors are oral medications usually taken once or twice a day. The earlier in the disease process these medications are initiated, the more likely they will delay cognitive decline. Although there are no special monitors for the cholinesterase inhibitors, the prolonged concurrent use of nonsteroidal antiinflammatory drugs (NSAIDs) with them can increase the risk of stomach ulcers.

TABLE 39.3   MEDICATIONS TO TREAT ALZHEIMER DISEASE

Drug	Drug Type and Use	Dose	Common Side Effects	Drug–Drug Interactions
Donepezil (Aricept)				
Prevents the breakdown of acetylcholine in the brain	Cholinesterase inhibitor treats symptoms of mild, moderate, and severe Alzheimer	5 mg once a day Increase after 4–6 wk to 10 mg/day	Nausea, diarrhea, vomiting	None observed in laboratory studies. NSAIDs should be used with caution in combination with this medication
Galantamine (Razadyne)				
Prevents breakdown of acetylcholine and modulates nicotinic receptors that release acetylcholine in the brain	Cholinesterase inhibitor treats symptoms of mild and moderate Alzheimer	4 mg BID Titrate to 16–24 mg/day over 8 wk	Nausea, vomiting, diarrhea, weight loss	Some antidepressants, such as paroxetine, amitriptyline, fluoxetine, fluvoxamine, and other drugs with anticholinergic action, may cause retention of excess galantamine in the body. NSAIDs should be used with caution in combination with this medication
Memantine (Nameda)				
Blocks toxic effects of excess glutamate and regulates glutamate activation	NMDA antagonist to treat moderate to severe symptoms of Alzheimer	Initial dose 5 mg once a day; may increase to 10 mg/day, 15 mg/day, 20 mg/day at weekly intervals	Dizziness, headache, diarrhea, constipation, confusion	A total of 174 drugs (1,401 brand and generic names) are known to interact with memantine. Other prescribed medications and substances should be checked for interactions
Memantine Extended Release and Donepezil (Namzaric)				
Blocks the toxic effects associated with excess glutamate and prevents the breakdown of acetylcholine in the brain	NMDA antagonist and cholinesterase inhibitor to treat symptoms of moderate to severe Alzheimer	28-mg memantine extended release mg donepezil once a day	Headache, nausea, vomiting, diarrhea, dizziness	Combined use with NMDA antagonists, anticholinergic medications, succinylcholine, similar neuromuscular blocking agents, or cholinergic agonists
Rivastigmine (Exelon)				
Prevents the breakdown of acetylcholine and butyrylcholine in the brain	Cholinesterase inhibitor treats symptoms of mild to moderate Alzheimer (patch is also for severe)	1.5 mg BID Titrate to 24 mg/day by increasing 3 mg/day every 2 wk	Nausea, vomiting, weight loss, upset stomach, muscle weakness	None observed in laboratory studies; NSAIDs should be used with caution in combination with this medication

Note. BID, twice a day; NMDA, *N*-methyl-D-aspartic acid; NSAIDs, nonsteroidal antiinflammatory drug.

Adapted from USDHHS. (2018). *Treatment of Alzheimer's Disease.* Washington, DC: Alzheimer's Disease Education & Referral (ADEAR) Center, National Institute on Aging, National Institutes of Health, NIH Publication N. 08–3431. Retrieved February 5, 2021, from https://www.nia.nih.gov/alzheimers/publication/alzheimers-disease-medications-fact-sheet#treatment

N-Methyl-ᴅ-Aspartic Acid Antagonists.

In AD, it is hypothesized that the chronic release of glutamate leads to neuronal degeneration. Memantine (Namenda XR) is an *N*-methyl-ᴅ-aspartic acid (NMDA) receptor antagonist that has been shown to improve cognition and ADLs in patients with moderate to severe symptoms of AD (Yiannopoulou & Papageorgiou, 2020).

Memantine and Donepezil Combination

Patients stabilized on daily donepezil may be prescribed Namzaric, a combination of memantine and donepezil in one capsule (Box 39.4). This medication is formulated in various strengths of memantine (7, 14, 21, 28 mg) combined with 10-mg donepezil.

Amyloid Beta-Directed Antibody

In AD, there is a build-up of the amyloid-beta plaque which interferes with neurotransmission. Aducanumab-avwa (ADUHELM®) was approved for the treatment of Alzheimer disease on an accelerated basis by the US Food and Drug Administration in 2021. This medication is a human, immunoglobulin gamma-1 (IgG1) monoclonal antibody that reduces the amyloid-beta plaques. Aduhelm is administered as an intravenous infusion over approximately 1 hour for every 4 weeks and at least 21 days apart. Patients can experience symptoms such as headache, confusion, dizziness, vision changes, or nausea. There can be temporary swelling in areas of the brain that usually resolves over time. Continued approval of this drug will depend on verification of clinical benefits in clinical trials (US FDA, 2021).

Other Medications

Even though antipsychotics are not approved for the use in dementia-related psychosis and have a boxed warning for this population, off-label use of antipsychotics for psychosis is common. There is evidence for the use of antidepressants for treating symptoms of depression and in reducing agitation (Magierski et al., 2020). Benzodiazepines should be used with caution and only on a short-term basis to treat anxiety in older adults. Anticholinergic medications should be avoided in patients with AD if at all possible. See Box 39.5 for examples of medications that are commonly prescribed in older adults that have anticholinergic properties.

Psychosocial Interventions

The therapeutic relationship is the basis for interventions for the patient and family with dementia. Care of the patient entails a long-term relationship needing much support and expert nursing care. Interventions should be delivered within the relationship context.

BOX 39.4
Memantine and Donepezil (Namzaric)

DRUG CLASS: *N*-methyl-ᴅ-aspartate (NMDA) receptor antagonist and cholinesterase inhibitor

RECEPTOR AFFINITY: Low to moderate affinity uncompetitive (open-channel) NMDA receptor antagonist, which binds preferentially to the NMDA receptor, a reversible inhibitor of the enzyme acetylcholinesterase.

INDICATIONS: For treatment of moderate to severe dementia of the Alzheimer type in patients stabilized on 10 mg of donepezil hydrochloride once daily

ROUTES AND DOSAGE: 7-, 14-, 21-, and 28-mg tablets

For patients stabilized on donepezil hydrochloride 10 mg and not currently on memantine hydrochloride, the recommended starting dose of Namzaric is 7/10 mg, taken once a day in the evening. The dose should be increased in 7-mg increments of the memantine hydrochloride component to the recommended maintenance dose of 28/10 mg once daily. The minimum recommended interval between dose increases is 1 week. The dose should only be increased if the previous dose has been well tolerated. The maximum dose is 28/10 mg once daily.

HALF-LIFE (PEAK EFFECT): Terminal half-life, 60–80 hours (peak effect, 3–7 hours). Excreted predominantly in the liver.

SPECIFIC PATIENT AND FAMILY EDUCATION: Caregivers should be instructed in the recommended administration (twice per day for doses above 5 mg) and dose escalation (minimum interval of 1 week between dose increases).

- This drug does not alter the Alzheimer disease process, and the efficacy of the medication may decrease over time.
- Continue using other medications for dementia as prescribed by the health care provider.
- Review the patient information.
- Instruct patients and caregivers to take Namzaric only once daily in the evening, or as prescribed.
- If a patient misses a single dose of Namzaric, the patient should not double up on the next dose. The next dose should be taken as scheduled.
- Instruct patients and caregivers that Namzaric capsules should be swallowed whole. Alternatively, Namzaric capsules may be opened and sprinkled on applesauce and the entire contents consumed. The capsules should not be divided, chewed, or crushed. Warn patients and caregivers not to use any capsules of Namzaric that are damaged or show signs of tampering.
- Advise patients and caregivers that Namzaric may cause headache, diarrhea, dizziness, anorexia, vomiting, nausea, and ecchymosis.
- Do not discontinue the drug or change the dose unless advised by the health care provider.
- Do not increase the dose of memantine if Alzheimer disease symptoms do not appear to be improving or appear to be getting worse; notify the health care provider.
- Namzaric may cause drowsiness or dizziness. Use caution while driving and performing other activities requiring mental alertness and coordination until tolerance is determined.
- Do not use any prescription or over-the-counter medications, dietary supplements, or herbal preparations unless advised by the health care provider.
- Follow-up visits may be required to monitor therapy and to keep appointments.

BOX 39.5

Medications with Anticholinergic Effects

Amitriptyline
Captopril (Capoten)
Codeine
Cimetidine (Tagamet)
Citalopram (Celexa)
Digoxin (Lanoxin)
Diphenhydramine
Dipyridamole (Trental)
Donepezil (Aricept)
Escitalopram (Lexapro)
Furosemide (Lasix)
Fluoxetine (Prozac)
Isosorbide (Ismotic)
Mirtazapine (Remeron)
Nifedipine (Procardia)
Oxybutynin ER
Paroxetine (Paxil)
Phenytoin (Dilantin)
Prednisolone
Ranitidine (Zantac)
Theophylline
Triamterene and hydrochlorothiazide
Tolterodine (Detrol LA)
Warfarin (Coumadin)

Memory Enhancement

The sooner patients begin taking AChEIs, the slower the cognitive decline will be. However, pharmacologic agents are only a small part of the intervention picture. The nursing goal is to maintain memory function as long as possible. When caring for a patient with AD, a concerted effort should be made to reinforce short- and long-term memory. For example, reminding patients what they had for breakfast, which activity was just completed, or who their visitors were a few hours ago will reinforce short-term memory. Encouraging patients to tell the stories of their earlier years will help bring long-term memories into focus. In the earlier stages of AD, there is considerable frustration when the patient realizes that they have short-term memory loss. In a matter-of-fact manner, help "fill in the blanks" and then redirect to another activity. Pictures of familiar people, places, and activities are also important tools in memory retrieval. Using scents (perfume, shaving lotions, spices, different foods) to stimulate memory retrieval and asking patients to relate their memories are also useful. Formalized reminiscence groups also help patients relive their earlier experiences and support maintenance of long-term memories.

Orientation Interventions

To enhance cognitive functioning, attempts should be made to remind patients of the day, time, and location. However, if the patient begins to argue that they are really at home or falsely believes that it is 1992, the patient need not be confronted by facts. Any confrontation could easily escalate into an argument. Instead, either redirect the patient or focus on the topic at hand (Box 39.6).

Maintaining Language

Losing the ability to name an object (i.e., agnosia) is frustrating. For example, the patient may describe a flower in terms of color, size, and fragrance but never be able to name the flower. When this happens while interacting with a patient, immediately say the name of the item. This reinforces cognitive functioning and prevents disruption in the interaction. Referral to speech therapists may also be useful if the language impairment impedes communication.

Supporting Visuospatial Functioning

The patient with visuospatial impairments loses the ability to sequence automatic behaviors, such as getting dressed or eating with silverware. For example, patients often put their clothes on backward, inside out, or with undergarments over outer garments. After they are dressed, they become confused as to how they arrived at their current state. If this happens, it may help to place clothes for dressing in a sequence for the patient so they patient can move from one article to the next in the correct sequence. This same technique can be used in other situations, such as eating, bathing, and toileting.

Interventions for Suspiciousness, Illusions, and Delusions

Delusions often occur when patients are placed in a situation they cannot master cognitively. The principle of nonconfrontation is most important in dealing with formation of suspiciousness and delusion. Efforts should be directed at determining the circumstances that trigger suspicion or delusion formation and creating a means of avoiding these situations.

Frequent causes of suspicion occur when changes in daily routine occur. The common accusations that "someone has entered my room," or "someone has changed my room" can be managed by asking, "Do you want to see if anything is missing?" Such accusations usually arise when a patient cannot remember what the room looked like or when the room was rearranged or cleaned.

Patients with AD often have delusions that a spouse, child, or other significant person is an impostor. If this situation occurs, it is important to assert in a matter-of-fact manner, "This is your wife, Barbara" or "I am your daughter Jenny." More vigorous assertions, such as offering various types of proof, tend to increase puzzlement as to why a person would go so far to impersonate the spouse or child.

BOX 39.6 • THERAPEUTIC DIALOGUE: THE PATIENT WITH DEMENTIA OF THE ALZHEIMER TYPE

Lois's daughter has told the home health agency nurse that on several occasions Lois has been found cowering and fearful under the kitchen table, saying she was hiding from voices. The nurse also knows that Lois denies having any difficulty with her memory or her ability to care for herself.

INEFFECTIVE APPROACH

Nurse: I'm here to see you about your health problems.

Lois: I have no problems. Why are you here?

Nurse: I'm here to help you.

Lois: I do not need any help. I think there is a mistake.

Nurse: Oh, there is no mistake. Your name is Ms. W, isn't it?

Lois: Yes, but I don't know who you are or why you are here. I'm very tired; please excuse me.

Nurse: OK. I will return another day.

EFFECTIVE APPROACH

Nurse: Hello, my name is Susan Miller. I'm the home health nurse, and I will be spending some time with you.

Lois: Oh, alright. Come in. Sit here.

Nurse: Thank you.

Lois: There is nothing wrong with me, you know.

Nurse: Are you wondering why I am here? (Open-ended statement)

Lois: I know why you are here. My children think that I cannot take care of myself.

Nurse: Is that true? Can you take care of yourself? (Restatement)

Lois: Of course I can care for myself. When people get older, they slow down. I'm just a little slower now, and that upsets my children.

Nurse: You are a little slower? (Reflection)

Lois: I sometimes forget things.

Nurse: Such as ... (open-ended statement)

Lois: Sometimes I cannot remember a telephone number or a name of a food.

Nurse: Does that cause problems?

Lois: According to my children, it does!

Nurse: What about you? What causes problems for you?

Lois: Sometimes the radio says terrible things to me.

Nurse: That must be frightening. (Acceptance)

Lois: It's terrifying. Then, my daughter looks at me as if I am crazy. Am I?

Nurse: It sounds like your mind is playing tricks on you. Let's see if we can figure out how to control the radio. (Validation)

Lois: Oh, OK. Will you tell my daughter that I am not crazy?

Nurse: Sure, I would be happy to meet with both you and your daughter if you would like. (Acceptance)

CRITICAL THINKING CHALLENGE

• In the first scenario, how did the nurse's underlying assumption that the patient would welcome the nurse lead to the nurse's rejection by the patient?

• What communication techniques did the nurse use in the second scenario to open communication and set the stage for the development of a sense of trust?

When patients experience illusions, find the source of the illusion and remove it from the environment if possible. For example, if a patient is watching a television program featuring animals and then verbalizes that the animal is in the room, switch the channel and redirect the conversation.

Some patients with AD may no longer recognize the reflections in the mirror as themselves and become agitated, thinking that a stranger is staring at them. Potentially misleading or disturbing stimuli, such as mirrors or art work, can be easily covered or removed from the environment.

Interventions for Hallucinations

Reassurance and distraction may be helpful for the hallucinating patient. For example, an 89-year-old patient with AD in a residential care facility would get up each night, walk to the nursing station, and whisper to the nurses, "There's a man in my bed who won't let me sleep. You should patrol this place better!" If the hallucination is not too disturbing for the patient, it can often be dismissed calmly with diversion or distraction. Because this patient did not seem too concerned by the "man" in her bed, the nurse may gently respond by saying, "I'm sorry you have to put up with so much. Just wait here (or come with me) and I'll make sure your room is ready for you." The nurse should then take the patient back to her room and help her into bed.

Frightening hallucinations and delusions usually require antipsychotic medications to dampen the patient's emotional reactions, but they can also be dealt with by optimizing perceptual cues (e.g., cover mirrors, turn off the television) and by encouraging patients to stay physically close to their caregivers. For example, one patient complained to her visiting nurse that she was being poisoned by deadly bugs that crawled up and down her arms and legs while she tried to sleep at night. Antipsychotic medication may help this patient sleep at night, and she would also likely benefit from reassurance and protection.

Interventions for Mood Changes

Strategies for Depression

Psychotherapeutic nursing interventions for depression that accompanies AD are similar to interventions for any depression. It is important to spend time alone with patients and to personalize their care as a way of communicating the patient's value. Encouraging expression of negative emotions is helpful because patients can talk honestly to a nonjudgmental person about their feelings. Although depressed patients with AD are likely to be too disorganized to attempt suicide, it is wise to remove potentially harmful objects from the environment.

Coping with Stress and Anxiety

Cognitively impaired patients are particularly vulnerable to anxiety. Patients with AD become unsure of their surroundings or of what is expected of them and then tend to react with fear and distress. They may feel lost, insecure, and left out. Failure to complete a task formerly regarded as simple creates anxiety and agitation. Often, they cannot explain the source of their anxiety. In many cases, lowering the demands, simplifying routines, and reducing the number of choices alleviates the anxiety.

Interventions for Catastrophic Reactions

If a patient reacts catastrophically, remain calm, minimize environmental distractions (quiet the environment), get the patient's attention, and softly assure the patient that they are safe. Give information slowly, clearly, and simply, one step at a time. Let the patient know that you understand the fear or other emotional response, such as anger or anxiety.

As nursing skills are developed in identifying antecedents to the patient's catastrophic reactions, it becomes possible to avoid situations that provoke such reactions. Patients with AD respond well to structure but poorly to change. Attempts to argue or reason with them will only escalate their dysfunctional responses.

Interventions for Apathy and Withdrawal

As the patient withdraws and becomes more apathetic, it becomes more challenging to engage the patient in meaningful activities and interactions. Providing this level of care requires knowing the premorbid functioning level of the patient. Close contact with family helps provide ideas about meaningful activities.

Using Behavioral Interventions

Strategies for Restlessness and Wandering

Restlessness and wandering are major concerns for caregivers, especially in the community (home) or long-term care setting. The principal means of dealing with restless patients who wander into other patients' rooms or out the door is to have an adequate number of staff (or caregivers in the home setting) to provide supervision, as well as electronically controlled exits. Wandering behavior may be interrupted in more cognitively intact patients by distracting them verbally or visually. Patients who are beyond verbal distraction can be distracted by physically joining them on their walk and then interrupting their course of action and gently redirecting them back to the house or facility. Many times, wandering is a result of a patient's inability to find their own room or may represent other agenda-seeking behaviors such as trying to find a bathroom.

Interventions for Agitated Behavior

Agitated behavior is likely to occur when patients are pressed to assist in their own care. A calm, unhurried, and undemanding approach is usually most effective. Attempts at reasoning may only aggravate the situation and increase the patient's resistance to care. If unable to determine the source of the patient's anxiety, the patient's restless energy can often be channeled into activities such as walking. Relaxation techniques also can be effective for reducing behavioral problems and anxiety in patients with AD.

TABLE 39.4	MESSAGES, MEANINGS, AND MANAGEMENT STRATEGIES
Possible Underlying Meanings	**Related Management Strategies**
"I'm hurt!" (e.g., from arthritis, fractures, pressure ulcers, degenerative joint disease, cancer)	• Observe for pain behaviors (e.g., posture, facial expressions, and gait in conjunction with vocalizations). • Treat suspected pain judiciously with analgesics and nonpharmacologic measures (e.g., repositioning, careful manipulation of patient during transfers and personal care, warm or cold packs, massage, relaxation).
"I'm tired." (e.g., sleep disturbances possibly related to altered sleep–wake cycle with day–night reversal, difficulty falling asleep, frequent night awakenings)	• Increase daytime activity and exercise to minimize daytime napping and promote nighttime sleep. • Promote normal sleep patterns and biorhythms by strengthening natural environmental cues (e.g., provide light exposure during the day; avoid bright lights at night), provide large calendars and clocks. • Establish a bedtime routine. • Reduce night awakenings: avoid excess fluids, diuretics, caffeine at bedtime, minimize loud noises, consolidate nighttime care activities (e.g., changing, medications, treatments).
"I'm lonely."	• Encourage social interactions between patients and their family, caregivers, and others. • Increase time the patient spends in group settings to minimize time in isolation. • Provide opportunity to interact with pets.
"I need ..." (e.g., food, a drink, a blanket, to use the toilet, to be turned or repositioned)	• Anticipate needs (e.g., assist the patient to toilet soon after breakfast when the gastrocolic reflex is likely). • Keep patient comfort and safety in mind during care (e.g., minimize body exposure to prevent hypothermia).
"I'm stressed." (e.g., Inability to tolerate sensory overload)	• Promote rest and quiet time. • Minimize "white noise" (e.g., vacuum cleaner) and background noise (e.g., televisions and radios). • Avoid harsh lighting and busy, abstract designs. • Limit patient's contacts with other agitated people. • Reduce behavioral expectations of patient, minimize choices, and promote a stable routine.
"I'm bored." (e.g., lack of sensory stimulation)	• Maximize hearing and visual abilities (e.g., keep external auditory canals free from cerumen plugs, ensure that glasses and hearing aids are worn, provide reading material of large print, soften lighting to reduce glare). • Play soft classical music for auditory stimulation. • Offer structured diversions (e.g., outdoor activities).
"What are you doing to me?" (e.g., personal boundaries are invaded)	• Avoid startling patients by approaching them from the front. • Always speak before touching the patient. • Inform patients what you plan to do and why before you do it. • Allow for flexibility in patient care.
"I don't feel well." (e.g., a urinary or upper respiratory tract infection, metabolic abnormality, fecal impaction)	• Identify the etiology through patient history, examination, possible tests (e.g., urinalysis, blood work, chest radiography, neurologic testing). • Treat underlying causes.
"I'm frustrated—I have no control." (e.g., loss of autonomy)	• When possible, allow patient to make their own decisions. • Maximize patient involvement during personal care (e.g., offer the patient a washcloth to assist with bathing). • Treat patients with dignity and respect (e.g., dress or change patients in private).
"I'm lost." (e.g., memory impairment)	• Maintain familiar routines. • Label the patient's room, bathroom, drawers, and possessions with large name signs. • Promote a sense of belonging through displays of familiar personal items, such as old family pictures.
"I feel strange." (e.g., side effects from medications that may include psychotropics, corticosteroids, beta-blockers, NSAIDs)	• Minimize the overall number of medications; consider nondrug interventions when possible. • Begin new medications one at a time; start with low doses and titrate slowly. Suspect a drug reaction if the patient's behavior (e.g., vocal) changes. • Educate caregivers about the patient's medications.
"I need to be loved!"	• Provide human contact and purposeful touch. • Acknowledge or verify the patient's feelings. • Encourage alternative, nonverbal ways to express feelings, such as through music, painting, or drawing. • Confirm a sense of purpose in life, acknowledge achievement, and reaffirm that the patient is still needed.

Note. NSAID, nonsteroidal antiinflammatory drug.

Reprinted from Clavel, D. S. (1999). Vocalizations among cognitively impaired elders: what is your patient trying to tell you? Geriatric Nursing, 20(2), 90–93. Copyright © 1999 Elsevier. With permission.

Interventions for Aberrant Behavior

When patients are picking in the air or wringing hands, simple distraction may work. Hypervocalizations are another story. Direct care staff tend to avoid these patients, which only makes the vocalizations worse. In reality, these vocalizations may have meaning to the patient. Instead, develop strategies to try to reduce the frequency of vocalizations (Table 39.4).

Reducing Disinhibition

Anticipation of disinhibiting behavior is the key to nursing interventions for this problem. Disinhibition can take many forms, from undressing in a public setting to touching someone inappropriately to making cruel but factual statements. This behavior can usually be viewed as normal by itself but abnormal within its social context. Keen behavioral assessment of the patient increases the ability to anticipate the likely socially inappropriate behavior and redirect the patient or change the context of the situation. If the patient starts undressing in the dining room, offering a robe and gently escorting them to another part of the room might be all that is needed. If a patient is trying to fondle a staff member, having the staff member leave the immediate area or redirecting the patient may alleviate the situation.

Psychoeducation for Families

Especially in AD, the needs of family members should also be considered. Caring for a family member with dementia takes its toll. Eighty percent of the home care is provided by family caregivers. Two thirds of the caregivers are women, and 34% are over the age of 65 years. Caregivers' health often declines and directly affects their ability to provide care (Alzheimer's Association, 2020). Caregivers are faced with extreme pressures and often feel isolated, frustrated, and trapped. The potential for patient abuse is significant, especially if agitated and aggressive behaviors are present in the relative.

Caregivers should be encouraged to attend support groups and carve out personal time. Educational and training programs may help in understanding the complex nature of the disorder (Boxes 39.7 and 39.8). Community resources, such as day care centers, home health agencies, and other community services, can be an important aspect of nursing care for the patient with dementia.

Promoting Safety

In the early stages of the illness, safety may not seem to be a prime issue because the individual is cognitively intact. However, early behaviors suggesting AD are often related to safety, such as the patient getting lost while driving or going the wrong way on the highway. Patients may be prevented from driving even though they can continue to live at home. Safety continues to be an issue in the home when patients engage in unsupervised cooking, cleaning, or household tasks. Day care centers provide a structured yet safe environment for these individuals. Family members should be encouraged to assess continually the abilities of members to live at home safely.

During hospitalizations or nursing home care, the safety issues are different. Most geropsychiatric units are kept locked and a dementia unit often has an electronic

BOX 39.7

Tips for Caregivers

When caring for the patient with dementia, be sure to include the caregivers, as appropriate, and address the following topic areas in the teaching plan:

- Psychopharmacologic agents, if used, including drug action, dosage, frequency, and possible adverse effects
- Rest and activity
- Consistency in routines
- Nutrition and hydration
- Sleep and comfort measures
- Protective environment
- Communication and social interaction
- Diversional measures
- Community resources

BOX 39.8

Caregiver Burden and Quality of Life

Zeliha, T., Baykal, D., Erturk, S., Bilgic, B., Hanagasi, H., & Gurvit, I. H. (2020). Caregiver burden, quality of life and related factors in family caregivers of dementia patients in Turkey. Issues in Mental Health Nursing, 41(8), 741–749, DOI:10.1080 /01612840.2019.1705945

THE QUESTION: What are the caregiver burdens and quality of life in dementia caregivers?

METHODS: Family caregivers of persons with dementia (*N* = 102) attending an outpatient dementia clinic were assessed for their caregiver burden and quality of life.

FINDINGS: Caregiver burden was related to quality of life. Compared to the general population with the same age, caregivers of dementia patients had poorer quality of life. Polypharmacy, cognitive function, age of the caregiver, and having limited space at home were predictors of caregiver burden. Having any disease and having limited space at home were predictors for poorer quality of life of the caregivers.

IMPLICATIONS FOR NURSING: Caregivers are at high risk for poorer quality of life than the general population. Nurses should assess caregivers and provide them support as they care for persons with Alzheimer disease.

alarm system to alert staff about patients attempting to leave the secured floor. Staff and visitors need to be vigilant for perilous situations.

Implementing Milieu Therapy

Overstimulating activities (e.g., social outing, family visit) can result in an outburst of delusional accusations or agitation. The nurse should attempt to determine each patient's optimal level of stimulation at various times of the day. It may be that stimulating environments can be tolerated early in the morning but not in the afternoon, when the patient is tired.

Socialization Activities

Overlearned social skills are rarely lost in patients with AD. It is not unusual for patients with dementia to respond appropriately to a handshake or smile well into the disease process. Even patients who are no longer able to communicate coherently will carry on long discussions with people who are willing to listen and respond (to language that does not make sense). The risk for social isolation is strong in patients with AD because of communication difficulties. Reinforcing social remarks and gestures, such as eye contact, smiling, greetings, and farewells, can promote a sense of competency and self-esteem. Pet therapy and "stuffed animal" therapy can also enhance social interaction in cognitively impaired individuals. It is important to remember that patients with AD do not lose their ability to laugh and play, and the psychosocial benefits of humor are well known.

Activities that elicit pleasant memories from an earlier time in the patient's life (reminiscence) may produce a soothing effect. Eliciting pleasant memories may be enhanced by gentle stimulation of the patient's senses, for example, viewing and discussing photo albums, looking at personal memorabilia, providing a favorite food item, playing a musical instrument, or listening to music the person preferred in younger years. It may be useful to incorporate movement or dance along with a singing exercise.

If the patient with AD resists structured exercise, it may be because of a fear of falling or injury or of demonstrating to others that their health is failing. Patients with AD often forget how to move or how to coordinate their movements in relation to objects. Therefore, exercise should be light and enjoyable. Encourage the patient to take rest periods at intervals throughout the activity in an effort to minimize stress.

Evaluation and Treatment Outcomes

The objectives of nursing interventions are to help the patient with AD remain as independent as possible and to function at the highest cognitive, physical, emotional, spiritual, and social levels. The maximum level of functional ability can be promoted when nursing care is related to and based on the remaining abilities of the patient.

Continuum of Care

The goal of in-home and community-based long-term care services is to maintain patients in a self-determining environment that provides the most home-like atmosphere possible, allows maximum personal choice for care recipients and caregiver, and encourages optimal family caregiving involvement without overwhelming the resources of the family network. All services for patients with AD and their families must be provided within a context of continuity of care, a concept that mandates access to various health and supportive services over an unpredictable and changing clinical course.

Nurses working with patients with AD are especially knowledgeable about all aspects of the illness and care. These nurses are often involved in local organizations, such as the Alzheimer's Association. Issues of care and safety and reimbursement for services often require professional expertise and influence.

Inpatient-Focused Care

Comprehensive admission assessment followed by the development of an individualized (and constantly updated) care plan that involves the patient, significant others, and diverse health care professionals is the foundation of an effective and efficient post-discharge plan. Attention to all aspects of this process is necessary to ensure that the goal of continuity of care is achieved. The hospital-based nurse may initiate family education and counseling as part of discharge planning.

Community Care

It is estimated that more than 60% to 70% of older adults with AD live at home, with 86% of home care provided by family and friends. In 2019, unpaid caregivers provided $244 billion of economic worth (Alzheimer's Association, 2020). Use of community-based services (e.g., home health aides, home-delivered meals, adult day care centers, respite care, caregiver support groups) often extends the amount of time an individual with AD or a related disorder can safely remain in the home.

Nursing Home

As the AD progresses, many patients are placed in a nursing home for care. Nursing care in a nursing home is usually delivered by nurses' aides, who need support and direction. Interestingly, people with AD require complex nursing care, but the skill level of people caring for these individuals often is minimal. Education and support of the direct caregiver is the focus of most nursing homes.

Integration with Primary Care

Persons with AD usually have multiple physical health issues and are most likely to be treated by primary care providers. Dementia is often treated in the primary care health care settings until behavioral disturbances emerge. Persons with advancing dementia are then referred to mental health or specialized geriatric providers for treatment of these psychiatric symptoms. The other health care needs continue to be treated by primary care. The mental health specialist integrates care, with the medical health care being provided by the primary care nurse or physicians. If patients are treated with medications, the primary care nurse must be monitoring the patient for changes in target symptoms, side effects and drug–drug interactions.

OTHER DEMENTIAS

Dementia symptoms may occur as a result of a number of disorders and underlying etiologies. The subsequent sections provide a brief description of some of the dementias listed in the *DSM-5*. In each case, the classic symptoms of dementia (e.g., memory impairment with a number of other cognitive deficits) must be present. Nursing interventions for all dementias are similar to those described for individuals with AD.

Vascular Neurocognitive Disorder

Vascular neurocognitive disorder (also known as *vascular dementia*) is a decline in thinking skill caused by conditions that block or reduce blood flow to the brain and the second most common type of dementia. Slightly more men than women are affected. Vascular dementia results when a series of small strokes damage or destroy brain tissue. These are commonly referred to as "ministrokes" or TIAs; several TIAs may occur before the affected individual becomes aware of the symptoms of vascular dementia. Most often, a blood clot or plaques (fatty deposits) block the vessels that supply blood to the brain, causing a stroke. However, a stroke can also occur when a blood vessel bursts in the brain (Alzheimer's Association, 2021b).

Symptoms of vascular neurocognitive disorder usually begin more suddenly rather than in AD. Often, the neurologic symptoms associated with a TIA are minimal and may last only a few days, including slight weakness in a limb, dizziness, or slurred speech. Thus, the clinical progression is often described as intermittent and fluctuating or of step-like deterioration, with the patient's cognitive and functional status improving or plateauing for a period of time followed by a rapid decline in function after another series of TIAs. Treatment aims to reduce the primary risk factors for vascular dementia, including hypertension, diabetes mellitus, and additional strokes.

Dementia Caused by Parkinson Disease

In individuals with Parkinson disease, 75% will develop neurocognitive dementia (APA, 2013). Although investigators do not know why, pathologic overlap is considerable between Parkinson disease and AD. The evidence consistently suggests that low cerebrospinal fluid levels of amyloid-beta predict future cognitive decline and dementia in Parkinson disease. Cognitive-enhancing medications have some effect, but there is no convincing evidence that the progression of dementia can be delayed (Kyle & Bronstein, 2020).

Dementia Caused by Huntington's Disease

Huntington's disease is a progressive, genetically transmitted, autosomal dominant disorder characterized by choreiform movements and mental abnormalities. The onset is usually between the ages of 30 and 50 years, but onset occurs before 5 years of age in the juvenile form or as late as 85 years of age in the late-onset form. The disease affects men and women equally. A person with Huntington's disease usually lives for approximately 15 years after diagnosis (APA, 2013). The dementia syndrome of Huntington's disease is characterized by insidious changes in behavior and personality. Typically, the dementia is frontal, which means that the person demonstrates prominent behavioral problems and disruption of attention.

FRONTOTEMPORAL NEUROCOGNITIVE DISORDER

Progressive development of behavioral and personality change and/or language impairment characterizes frontotemporal neurocognitive disorder, which has distinct patterns of brain atrophy and distinctive neuropathology. Individuals with this disorder have varying degrees of apathy or disinhibition. They may lose interest in socialization, self-care, and personal responsibilities. Family members report socially inappropriate behaviors, but afflicted individuals show little insight. The cognitive deficits are typically in the area of planning, organization, and judgments. They are easily distracted (APA, 2013).

NEUROCOGNITIVE DISORDER WITH LEWY BODIES

Progressive cognitive decline with visual hallucination, REM sleep disorder, and spontaneous parkinsonism characterizes dementia with Lewy bodies, a major neurocognitive disorder. Cognitive symptoms occur several months before motor symptoms. These symptoms fluctuate and may resemble delirium. These individuals are at high risk for falls because of periods of syncope and transient episodes of consciousness. Orthostatic hypotension and urinary incontinence may occur. The cause is unknown, but evidence implies genetic factors and neuroinflammation (Hinkle & Pontone, 2020). The pathology involves Lewy bodies found in the cortical location in the brain, which are thought to be responsible for the disorder.

The estimated prevalence of this dementia ranges from 0.1% to 5% of the general older population, with men slightly more affected (APA, 2013). This onset of disorder is typically in the sixth to ninth decades and is progressive with a 5- to 7-year survival rate. These individuals are more functionally impaired than those with other types of dementia (e.g., AD) and are very sensitive to psychotropic medication, especially antipsychotics.

NEUROCOGNITIVE DISORDER DUE TO PRION DISEASE

Neurocognitive disorder due to prion-related symptoms comprises a group of spongiform encephalopathies including Creutzfeldt–Jakob disease, a rare, rapidly fatal, brain disorder, and mad cow disease, which is a bovine disorder. A prion is a small infectious particle composed of abnormally folded protein that causes progressive neurodegeneration. Many of the symptoms seen in Creutzfeldt–Jakob disease are similar to those found in AD and other dementias. However, changes in the brain tissue are different in Creutzfeldt–Jakob disease and are best differentiated with surgical biopsy or during autopsy (APA, 2013). Common symptoms include fluctuating fever, difficulty swallowing, incontinence, tremors, seizures, and sensitivity to touch and environmental noise.

At present, no effective treatment for the disease exists and nothing has been found to slow progression of the illness, although antiviral drug studies are ongoing. Person-to-person transmission of Creutzfeldt–Jakob disease is rare (but possible), and it can be transmitted from people to animals and between animals. Because of the transmissible nature of Creutzfeldt–Jakob disease and because the virus is not easily destroyed, strict criteria for the handling of infected tissues and other contaminated materials have been developed.

NEUROCOGNITIVE DISORDER DUE TO TRAUMATIC BRAIN INJURY

Traumatic brain injury (TBI) affects about 1.4 to 1.7 million people in the United States each year, resulting in various symptoms including neurological, cognitive, behavioral, and emotional impairments (APA, 2013). Repeated concussions can lead to brain injury with long-term TBI. Evidence suggests that even mild TBI is a significant risk factor of developing dementia (Maigler et al., 2021).

SUBSTANCE- OR MEDICATION-INDUCED NEUROCOGNITIVE DISORDER

If dementia results from the persisting effects of a substance (e.g., drugs of abuse, a medication, exposure to toxins), substance-induced neurocognitive disorder is diagnosed. Other causes of dementia (e.g., dementia caused by a general medical condition) must always be considered even in a person with a dependence on or exposure to a substance. For example, head injuries often result from substance use and may be the underlying cause of the neurocognitive changes (APA, 2013). Prescription drugs are the most common toxins in older adults.

SUMMARY OF KEY POINTS

- Neurocognitive disorders are characterized clinically by significant deficits in cognition or memory that represent a clear-cut change from a previous level of functioning. In some disorders, the loss of cognitive function is progressive, such as in AD. It is important to recognize the differences because the interventions and expected outcomes of the two syndromes are different.

- Delirium is characterized by a disturbance in consciousness and a change in cognition that develops over a short period of time. It requires rapid detection and treatment.

- The primary goal of treatment of individuals with delirium is prevention or resolution of the acute confusion episode with return to previous cognitive status and interventions focusing on (1) elimination or correction of the underlying cause and (2) symptomatic and safety and supportive measures.

- Dementia is characterized by the gradual onset of decline in cognitive function, especially memory, usually accompanied by changes in behavior and personality.

- AD is an example of a progressively degenerative dementia. Treatment efforts currently focus on reduction of cognitive symptoms (e.g., memory loss; confusion; and problems with learning, speech, and reasoning) in attempts to improve the quality of life for both patients and their caregivers.

- Research efforts continue to focus on understanding the relationship among the development of the beta-amyloid plaques, neurofibrillary tangles, and cell death.

- Nursing care of a person with dementia depends on the stage of the disease and the availability of family caregivers.

- Educating and supporting families and caregivers through the progressive cognitive decline and behavior changes is essential to ensuring proper care.

- Several mental health strategies (exercise, education, cognitive stimulation) support and protect a person's cognitive reserve. A healthy cognitive reserve is thought to be protective against neuropathologic insults.

- Other neurocognitive disorders may be related to specific brain changes (Lewy bodies), infections (prion disease), genetic diseases (Huntington's disease), and substances/medications.

CRITICAL THINKING CHALLENGES

1. What factors should be considered in differentiating AD from vascular dementia?

2. Suggest reasons that older adults are particularly vulnerable to the development of neurocognitive disorders.

3. Compare the nursing care of a person with delirium versus one with dementia. What are the similarities and differences in the care?

4. The physical environment is particularly important to the patient with dementia. Visualize your last experience in a health care setting (e.g., hospital, nursing home, day care program, home care setting). Identify environmental factors that could be misleading or stress producing to a person with impaired cognition (dementia) and identify ways to modify this environment to alleviate some of the stressors or misleading stimuli.

5. Mr. J. has been recently diagnosed with mild AD and is asking for advice about deciding on his care in the future. His wife and daughter believe that he does not have the ability to make these decisions and asks for the nurse's advice. How should the nurse respond? Explain the rationale.

 Movie Viewing Guides

Iris (2001): This film tells the story of British novelist Iris Murdoch (played by Kate Winslet and then by Judi Dench when Iris is much older) and her relationship with her husband, John Bayley (played by Hugh Bonneville and Jim Broadbent) during the last 5 years of her life. Based on Bayley's memoir, *Elegy for Iris*, the film depicts Ms. Murdoch's decline into dementia and the stress associated with caregiving. This wonderful movie shows the suffering of a person with AD but also shows the strength of relationships. The film contrasts their relationship at the start, when Iris was an outgoing but dominant individual and John was a timid, shy, scholarly partner, with that between the two older adults who created a loving bond that provided the fabric of the last days of Iris's life.

VIEWING POINTS: Identify the symptoms of the progressive illness throughout the film. Were there any "breaking points" for the caregiver? Were there aspects of Iris's personality that were sustained throughout the course of her life that were evident at the end? What nursing interventions would have been helpful to support her cognitive functioning?

REFERENCES

Ali, M., & Cascella, M. (2020). ICU Delirium. In *StatPearls*. StatPearls Publishing.

Alzheimer's Association. (2021a). Mild cognitive impairment. Retrieved January 30, 2021 from https://www.alz.org/alzheimers-dementia/what-is-dementia/related_conditions/mild-cognitive-impairment

Alzheimer's Association. (2020). 2020 Alzheimer's disease facts and figures. Alzheimer's Association. Retrieved January 30, 2021 from https://www.alz.org/media/Documents/alzheimers-facts-and-figures.pdf

Alzheimer's Association. (2021b). Vascular dementia. Retrieved February 5, 2021 from https://alz.org/alzheimers-dementia/what-is-dementia/types-of-dementia/vascular-dementia

American Psychiatric Association. (2013). *Diagnostic and Statistical Manual of Mental Disorders* (5th ed.). Author.

Barfejani, A. H., Jafarvand, M., Seyedsaadat, S. M., & Rasekhi, R. T. (2020). Donepezil in the treatment of ischemic stroke: Review and future perspective. *Life Sciences*, 263, 118575. https://doi.org/10.1016/j.lfs.2020.118575

Bellenguez, C., Grenier-Boley, B., & Lambert, J. C. (2020). Genetics of Alzheimer's disease: Where we are, and where we are going. *Current Opinion in Neurobiology*, 61, 40–48. https://doi.org/10.1016/j.conb.2019.11.024

Borson, S., Scanlan, J. M., Chen, P., & Ganguli, M. (2003). The Mini-Cog as a screen for dementia: Validation in a population-based sample. *Journal of the American Geriatrics Society*, 51, 1451–1454.

Clavel, D. S. (1999). Vocalizations among cognitively impaired elders: What is your patient trying to tell you? *Geriatric Nursing*, 20, 90–93.

Duggan, M. C., Van, J., & Ely, E. W. (2021). Delirium assessment in critically ill older adults: Considerations during the COVID-19 pandemic. *Critical Care Clinics*, 37(1), 175–190. https://doi.org/10.1016/j.ccc.2020.08.009

Flanagan, E., Lamport, D., Brennan, L., Burnet, P., Calabrese, V., Cunnane, S. C., de Wilde, M. C., Dye, L., Farrimond, J. A., Emerson Lombardo, N., Hartmann, T., Hartung, T., Kalliomäki, M., Kuhnle, G. G., La Fata, G., Sala-Vila, A., Samieri, C., Smith, A. D., Spencer, J., Thuret, S., ... Vauzour, D. (2020). Nutrition and the ageing brain: Moving towards clinical applications. *Ageing Research Reviews*, 62, 101079. https://doi.org/10.1016/j.arr.2020.101079

Galvin, J. E., Roe, C. M., Powlishta, K. K., Coats, M. A., Muich, S. J., Grant, E., Miller, J. P., Storandt, M., & Morris, J. C. (2005). The AD8: A brief informant interview to detect dementia. *Neurology, 65*(4), 559–564.

Galvin, J. E., Roe, C. M., Xiong, C., & Morris, J. C. (2006). Validity and reliability of the AD8 informant interview in dementia. *Neurology, 67*(11), 1942–1948.

Hinkle, J. T., & Pontone, G. M. (2020). Lewy Body degenerations as neuropsychiatric disorders. *The Psychiatric Clinics of North America, 43*(2), 361–381. https://doi.org/10.1016/j.psc.2020.02.003

Hshieh, T. T., Inouye, S. K., & Oh, E. S. (2020). Delirium in the elderly. *Clinics in Geriatric Medicine, 36*(2), 183–199. https://doi.org/10.1016/j.cger.2019.11.001

Jin, Z., Hu, J., & Ma, D. (2020). Postoperative delirium: Perioperative assessment, risk reduction, and management. *British Journal of Anaesthesia, 125*(4), 492–504. https://doi.org/10.1016/j.bja.2020.06.063

Kyle, K., & Bronstein, J. M. (2020). Treatment of psychosis in Parkinson's disease and dementia with Lewy Bodies: A review. *Parkinsonism & Related disorders, 75*, 55–62. https://doi.org/10.1016/j.parkreldis.2020.05.026

Leng, M., Zhao, Y., & Wang, Z. (2020). Comparative efficacy of non-pharmacological interventions on agitation in people with dementia: A systematic review and Bayesian network meta-analysis. *International Journal of Nursing Studies, 102*, 103489. https://doi.org/10.1016/j.ijnurstu.2019.103489

Lin, L., Zheng, L. J., & Zhang, L. J. (2018). Neuroinflammation, gut microbiome, and Alzheimer's disease. *Molecular Neurobiology, 55*(11), 8243–8250. https://doi.org/10.1007/s12035-018-0983-2

Lin, X., Kapoor, A., Gu, Y., Chow, M. J., Peng, J., Zhao, K., & Tang, D. (2020). Contributions of DNA damage to Alzheimer's disease. *International Journal of Molecular Sciences, 21*(5), 1666. https://doi.org/10.3390/ijms21051666

Kacířová, M., Zmeškalová, A., Korínková, L., Železná, B., Kuneš, J., & Maletínská, L. (2020). Inflammation: Major denominator of obesity, Type 2 diabetes and Alzheimer's disease-like pathology?. *Clinical Science (London, England : 1979), 134*(5), 547–570. https://doi.org/10.1042/CS20191313

Kellar, D., & Craft, S. (2020). Brain insulin resistance in Alzheimer's disease and related disorders: Mechanisms and therapeutic approaches. *The Lancet Neurology, 19*(9), 758–766. https://doi.org/10.1016/S1474-4422(20)30231-3

Kesika, P., Suganthy, N., Sivamaruthi, B. S., & Chaiyasut, C. (2021). Role of gut-brain axis, gut microbial composition, and probiotic intervention in Alzheimer's disease. *Life Sciences, 264*, 118627. https://doi.org/10.1016/j.lfs.2020.118627

Kumar, S., & Reddy, P. H. (2020). The role of synaptic microRNAs in Alzheimer's disease. *Biochimica et Biophysica Acta-Molecular Basis of Disease, 1866*(12), 165937. https://doi.org/10.1016/j.bbadis.2020.165937

Kuo, C. Y., Stachiv, I., & Nikolai, T. (2020). Association of late life depression, (non-) modifiable risk and protective factors with dementia and Alzheimer's disease: Literature review on current evidences, preventive interventions and possible future trends in prevention and treatment of dementia. *International Journal of Environmental Research and Public Health, 17*(20), 7475. https://doi.org/10.3390/ijerph17207475

Magierski, R., Sobow, T., Schwertner, E., & Religa, D. (2020). Pharmacotherapy of behavioral and psychological symptoms of dementia: State of the art and future progress. *Frontiers in Pharmacology, 11*, 1168. https://doi.org/10.3389/fphar.2020.01168

Mattison, M. (2020). Delirium. *Annals of Internal Medicine, 173*(7), ITC49–ITC64. https://doi.org/10.7326/AITC202010060

Maigler, K. C., Buhr, T. J., Park, C. S., Miller, S. A., Kozlowski, D. A., & Marr, R. A. (2021). Assessment of the effects of altered amyloid-beta clearance on behavior following repeat closed-head brain injury in amyloid-beta precursor protein humanized mice. *Journal of Neurotrauma.* https://doi.org/10.1089/neu.2020.6989

National Institute on Aging. (2019). Alzheimer's disease fact sheet. Alzheimer's and related Dementias Education and Referral Center. National Institute on Aging. NIH Publication No. 19-AG-6423. Retrieved on January 30, 2021 from https://order.nia.nih.gov/publication/alzheimers-disease-fact-sheet

Ostuzzi, G., Gastaldon, C., Papola, D., Fagiolini, A., Dursun, S., Taylor, D., Correll, C. U., & Barbui, C. (2020). Pharmacological treatment of hyperactive delirium in people with COVID-19: Rethinking conventional approaches. *Therapeutic Advances in Psychopharmacology, 10*, 2045125320942703. https://doi.org/10.1177/2045125320942703

Sadrameli, M., Bathini, P., & Alberi, L. (2020). Linking mechanisms of periodontitis to Alzheimer's disease. *Current Opinion in Neurology, 33*(2), 230–238. https://doi.org/10.1097/WCO.0000000000000797

Sengoku, R. (2020). Aging and Alzheimer's disease pathology. *Neuropathology, 40*(1), 22–29. https://doi.org/10.1111/neup.12626

Shenvi, C., Kennedy, M., Austin, C. A., Wilson, M. P., Gerardi, M., & Schneider, S. (2020). Managing delirium and agitation in the older emergency department patient: The ADEPT tool. *Annals of Emergency Medicine, 75*(2), 136–145. https://doi.org/10.1016/j.annemergmed.2019.07.023

Tadokoro, K., Ohta, Y., Inufusa, H., Loon, A., & Abe, K. (2020). Prevention of cognitive decline in Alzheimer's disease by novel antioxidative supplements. *International Journal of Molecular Sciences, 21*(6), 1974. https://doi.org/10.3390/ijms21061974

Uddin, M. S., Tewari, D., Mamun, A. A., Kabir, M. T., Niaz, K., Wahed, M., Barreto, G. E., & Ashraf, G. M. (2020). Circadian and sleep dysfunction in Alzheimer's disease. *Ageing Research Reviews, 60*, 101046. https://doi.org/10.1016/j.arr.2020.101046

U.S. Food and Drug Administration (FDA). (2021). Aduhelm. Retrieved on June 23, 2021 from https://www.accessdata.fda.gov/drugsatfda_docs/label/2021/761178s000lbl.pdf

Yiannopoulou, K. G., & Papageorgiou, S. G. (2020). Current and future treatments in Alzheimer disease: An update. *Journal of Central Nervous System Disease, 12*, 1179573520907397. https://doi.org/10.1177/1179573520907397

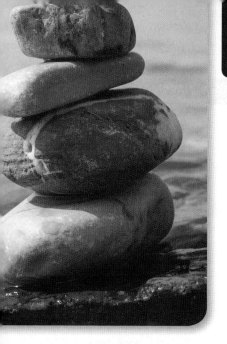

40

Care of Veterans with Mental Health Needs

Mary Ann Boyd

KEYCONCEPTS

- Military Sexual Trauma
- Military Veteran
- Moral Injury
- Veteran Identity

LEARNING OBJECTIVES

After studying this chapter, you will be able to:

1. Describe the military culture.

2. Trace the mental health needs of veterans during various military campaigns.

3. Describe the changing role of women in the military.

4. Discuss the inclusion of underrepresented groups in the military.

5. Analyze mental health needs of veterans.

6. Describe recovery-oriented nursing care for veterans with mental health needs.

7. Describe the mental health services available to veterans.

KEY TERMS

• Active duty • Active duty (regular) service member • Anxious-arousal • Betrayal • Combat-related trauma • Index trauma • Microaggression • Minority stress • Musculoskeletal pain • Non-combat-related trauma • Numbing symptoms • Operation Enduring Freedom (OEF) • Operation Iraqi Freedom (OIF) • Operation New Dawn (OND) • Perpetration • Post-9/11 • Re-experiencing • Reservist • Service-connected disability • Sexual assault • Sexual harassment • Witnessing

INTRODUCTION

The defense and protection of the United States (U.S.) depend upon the U.S. military armed forces. Wars and conflicts not only shape the history of the United States but also affect the long-term health and mental health of military service members and veterans. Throughout this chapter specific health and mental health issues of military members and veterans are associated with the wars in which they served. The aim of this chapter is to discuss the mental health needs and recovery-oriented nursing care for veterans.

U.S. MILITARY ORGANIZATIONS

The U.S. military is a complex institution consisting of three departments (Army, Navy, and Air Force) reporting to the Department of Defense (DOD). The Navy and Marines fall under the Department of the Navy and the Air Force and the Space Force under the Department of Air Force. The Coast Guard, which is a military service and a branch of the Armed Forces, is organizationally housed in the Department of Homeland Security (Council on Foreign Relations, 2020).

There are also seven reserve components that provide trained units and qualified persons available for **active duty** in time or war or national emergency. The Army, Navy, Marine Corps, Air Force, and Coast Guard reserves are under federal control and are activated when they are needed. The Army National and Air National Guards are under the authority of their respective states with the exception of the District of Columbia National Guard, which is exclusively a federal organization. All national guard units can be ordered into federal service if needed (Congressional Research Services, 2021).

The operational names of the conflicts in Iraq and Afghanistan are used frequently to differentiate the time and focus of the military engagement (Box 40.1). The military gives names for different operational phases of a war or conflict. See Table 40.1 for an overview of the military wars and conflicts of the United States (Torreon, 2020).

Active duty (regular) service members are employed full time by the military; the **reservists** and National Guard members are not on full-time active duty but may live on a military base and can be deployed at any time. Enlistment time varies from 2 years to more than 20 years depending on the career goals of the service member. Once service members are discharged from the military, they become veterans and are entitled to varying privileges according to time in service, rank, and situation.

In 1973, the United States ended conscription (compulsory enlistment of males) and transitioned to an

TABLE 40.1	U.S. MILITARY WARS/CONFLICTS
Wars/Conflicts	**Periods of War**
Revolutionary War	1775–1783
War of 1812	1812–1815
Mexican American War	1846–1848
American Civil War	1861–1865
Spanish American War	1898–1902
World War I	1917–1918
World War II	1939–1945
Korean Conflict	1950–1955
Vietnam War	1959–1975
Gulf War	1990–1991
Conflict in Afghanistan	2001–present
Iraq Conflict	2003–2011

Torreon, B. S. (2020). U.S. periods of war and dates of recent conflicts. Congressional Research Service. RS21405 Retrieved on April 28, 2021 from https://crsreports.congress.gov
*Dates may vary depending on proclamations, declarations, laws, or treaties.

all-volunteer force. An estimated 1.3 million currently serve as active-duty personnel, or less than one-half of 1% of the U.S. population. The Army is the largest U.S. military service with 35% of the active duty members (Council on Foreign Relations, 2020).

Military Culture

The military culture is structured to protect and defend the United States. The values, beliefs, and behaviors acquired in the military often last a lifetime. As a hierarchal organization, there is a chain of command with defined authority and responsibility. Leaders protect and maintain the health and well-being of their subordinates. Officers are expected to transmit values of honor, pride, discipline, and loyalty, instill warrior beliefs, and display self-sacrifice behaviors. There is a clear separation of officers and enlisted members with order and discipline being instilled in both groups. Officers and enlisted members are expected to maintain separate social networks. Within the military, there is little room for individuality. Symbols of military order include uniforms and rituals such as saluting officers and military march (Center for Deployment Psychology, 2021).

The Changing Role of Women in the Military Throughout History

Before World War II (WWII), women could only serve in the Women's Army Auxiliary Corps and the Army Nurse Corp., temporary, auxiliary components. They

---

BOX 40.1

Names of Operational Phases of Conflicts in Iraq and Afghanistan

Conflict	Operation Name	Period of Conflict*
Afghanistan (Global War on Terror—GWOT)	Operation Enduring Freedom (OEF)	2001–2014
	Operation Freedom's Sentinel (OFS)	2014–present
Iraq	Operation Iraqi Freedom (OIF)	2003–2011
	Operation New Dawn (OND)	2010–2014
	Islamic State-Operation Inherent Resolve (OIR)	2014–present

Torreon, B. S. (2020). U.S. periods of war and dates of recent conflicts. Congressional Research Service. RS21405 Retrieved on April 28, 2021 from https://crsreports.congress.gov
*Dates may vary depending on proclamations, declarations, laws, or treaties.

were activated only during times of national need such as during a war. These women were released from duty at the end of each war. Their work was often stigmatized and mocked. Sexual harassment was common (Blakemore, 2019).

The *Women's Armed Services Integration Act* signed into law on June 12, 1948 recognized women as full members of the armed forces. This meant that they could claim the same benefits as their male counterparts and it allowed women to make a career in the armed forces. The law limited the number of women who could serve in the military to 2% of total forces in each branch. As a result of a regulation, mothers with dependent children were ineligible to serve in the military.

During the Vietnam War, 7,000 American military women served in Southeast Asia. When the draft ended in 1973, women represented just 2% of enlisted forces and 8% of the officer corps (primarily nurses). Following the elimination of the draft, the need for service members became apparent and women were actively recruited into the military. Women were finally admitted into America's service academies in 1976. Nearly 40,000 women were deployed for Gulf War. In 2020, women represented 16% of the enlisted forces and 19% of the officers. More than 700,000 women have served since post-9/11, including **Operation Enduring Freedom (OEF)** and **Operation Iraqi Freedom (OIF)** (Gorbulja-Maldonado, 2020).

Inclusion of Underrepresented Groups in the Military

Information related to underrepresented groups in the military is very general because of federal racial and ethnic categorization. Federal agencies categorize race according to five groups—**White, Black or African American, American Indian or Alaska Native, Asian, and Native Hawaiian or other Pacific Islander**. Ethnicity is divided into two groups: (a) Hispanic/Latinx and (b) not Hispanic or Latinx. Based upon federal data, we know that a greater proportion of underrepresented groups are found primarily in the lower rather than the higher military ranks. The majority of all service members are White with the overwhelming majority of officers in all military departments also White. In all the services, underrepresentation is higher among female recruits than among male recruits (Council on Foreign Relations, 2020).

For most of the U.S. military history, persons who identified as lesbian, gay, bisexual, transgender, and queer or questioning (LGBTQ) were excluded from military service. In 1993, a DOD *Directive 1304.26*, known as the "Don't Ask, Don't Tell policy," was issued that prohibited military personnel from asking or requiring recruits and service members to reveal their sexuality. Persons were no longer barred from military service based on sexual

orientation. Even though LGBTQ persons could serve in the military service if they concealed their sexual orientation, they could be excluded if they demonstrated "a propensity or intent to engage in homosexual acts, or a homosexual marriage or attempted marriage (DOD Directive, 1993, December 21)." This directive remained in place until 2011 when the policy was repealed following a decision by a federal appeals court that barred further enforcement of the military's ban on openly gay members. In 2016, President Obama allowed transgender individuals to serve openly in the armed forces, but the policy was later reversed by President Trump. In 2021, President Biden lifted the ban and now individuals who identify as LGBTQ can serve openly in the military.

The DOD is strengthening policies and procedures that promote diversity and inclusion and equal opportunity missions. In a 2020 report, the DOD recommended six areas of improvement in recruitment and accessions, retention, barriers, career development, organizational climate, and culture, worldview, and identity (see Box 40.2).

VETERANS OF THE U.S. MILITARY

KEYCONCEPT Military veteran refers to persons who served in the armed services.

Every year, about 200,000 service members transition to civilian life (Inhofe et al., 2019). In 2019, there were more than 18 million veterans in the United States or about 7%

BOX 40.2

Recommendations to Improve Racial and Ethnic Diversity and Inclusion in the U.S. Military

- **Recruitment and Accessions:** Strengthen both community engagement and the narrative about military service opportunities during recruiting to attract more diverse candidates.
- **Retention:** Retain minorities beyond initial commitment and into leadership ranks.
- **Barriers:** Address barriers confronted by minority members in the workplace.
- **Career Development:** Improve advancement opportunities (e.g., promotion boards, command selection, professional military education, assignments).
- **Organizational Climate:** Address command and organizational climate issues that may negatively impact the retention of minority members.
- **Culture, Worldview, and Identity:** Promote inclusion of minority groups in military culture and strengthen aspects of individual and cultural identity.

Department of Defense (2020). Recommendations to improve racial and ethnic diversity and inclusion in the U.S. military. Retrieved May 21, 2020 from https://media.defense.gov/2020/Dec/18/2002554852/-1/-1/0/DOD-DIVERSITY-AND-INCLUSION-FINAL-BOARD-REPORT.PDF of the U.S. population. The veteran population has been declining for years and the decline is expected to continue. By 2040, it is projected that there will be about 12.9 million veterans living in the United States (Vespa, 2020).

The veteran population served in several different departments, wars, and conflicts. The largest cohort of veterans served during the Vietnam Era (6.4 million) which lasted from 1964 to 1975. The second largest cohort served during peacetime only (4.0 million). The median age of veterans today is 65. The **post-9/11 group** (military service after September 2001) is the youngest with a median age of about 37, Vietnam Era veterans have a median age of about 71, and WWII veterans are the oldest with a median age of about 93 (Vespa, 2020).

Veteran Identity

The veteran population consists of men and women of varying ages, ethnicities, races, and military experiences. The common element for all veterans is that their experience in the military helped to shape their adult life and form a veteran identity.

> **KEYCONCEPT A veteran identity** is the degree to which the veteran role is central or important to how they think about themselves and how they want others to view them (Adams et al., 2019).

In order to measure a veteran identity, researchers surveyed the strength of agreement of three questions on a scale of 0–4. The questions are "Being a veteran is an important reflection of who I am." "I have come to think of myself as a veteran." "It is important to me that others know about me as a veteran." (Adams et al., 2019).

The presence of a strong veteran identity is variable among the cohorts. For example, Vietnam veterans tend to have the strongest veteran identity and the Iraq/Afghan veterans show the lowest identity. Veterans with a prominent veteran identity are generally older, non-college graduates, have limited income, and had their first deployment to Vietnam (Adams et al., 2019).

Female Veterans

Women make up a growing share of veterans. In 2021, about 9% of veterans or 1.7 million are women. By 2040, the number of women veterans is projected to increase to 17% (Adams et al., 2021). In 2017, the median age of women veterans was 51 years compared to 65 years for their male counterparts. The middle age group (45–64 years old) represent the largest group of women veteran Veterans Health Administration (VHA) patients (U.S. Department of Veterans Affairs, 2019).

Females tend to be younger and more likely college graduates than their male counterparts (holding similar positions or functions). Females are more likely to serve during the Afghanistan/Iraq War, be deployed in National Guard/Reserve units, and less likely to experience high combat exposure. The female veteran population is more racially diverse than their male counterpart and is less likely to serve multiple tours. Females are more likely to have low resilience and report poor health. Women veterans are more likely to contemplate suicide and experience depression, but less likely to abuse alcohol than their male counterparts (Adams et al., 2021).

HEALTH CARE FOR VETERANS

Health Issues of Veterans

Veterans have distinctive health issues related to the military service. They are more likely to suffer from trauma-related injuries, substance use, and mental health disorders than people who have never served in the armed forces. About one-quarter (24.2% of 18,000.000) of all veterans have a **service-connected disability**, an injury, disease, or disability that active duty either caused or aggravated. The Gulf War and the post-9/11 veterans have the highest number of service-connected disabilities with more than 1/3 of whom had a service-connected disability. The post-9/11 veterans have the highest proportion (17%) of disabilities for all groups (Vespa, 2020).

It is thought that the high rate of post-9/11 veterans service-connected disabilities is related to several factors such as extended tours of duty or difficult service conditions that were not experienced by the other cohorts. Medical advances allow veterans to survive injuries that would have been fatal in past wars. Black, Hispanic, and other underrepresented veterans are more likely than White veterans to have a service-connected disability. While the type and severity of most injuries have remained constant across time, this is not true of posttraumatic stress disorder (PTSD). PTSD is more likely to be reported today than during previous periods (Vespa, 2020).

Transition to Civilian Life

Providing access and care immediately upon separation from the military is critical. The transition from the structured military life to civilian life can be difficult and stressful. The first year after discharge from the military is a high-risk period. Many newly separated veterans report chronic physical or mental health conditions and are less satisfied with their health than their work or social relations. Work satisfaction often deteriorates shortly after beginning a civilian job. Enlisted personnel consistently report poorer health, vocational, and social outcomes compared to their officer counterpart.

War-zoned deployed service members report more health concerns; women have more mental health concerns when compared to their non-deployed female and male peers (Vogt et al., 2020).

The *Transition Assistance Program* supported by the departments of Defense, Veterans Affairs, and Homeland Security provides seamless access to mental health care and suicide prevention resources, particularly during the first year after separation or retirement (Exec. Order No. 13822, 2018). This program provides information on veteran benefits, mental health resources, training, and other resources to service members as they transition from military to civilian life. Psychosocial and peer support are also provided. Registration in the Veterans Administration Health Care System is facilitated to assure access to health care. Veterans can choose to seek health care in the private community systems or the VHA (Figure 40.1).

Veterans Health Administration and U.S. Government Support of Veterans

The U.S. federal government has provided care for veterans since the first Soldier's Home opened after the Civil War in 1866, but it was not until 1946 that the care to the WWII veterans was initiated (U.S. Department of Veterans Affairs, n.d.). In 2021, the VHA is one of the two components of the Department of Veterans Affairs led by the Secretary of Veterans Affairs for Health and operates numerous medical and health care centers. The VA Health Care System has grown from 54 hospitals in 1930 to 1,600 health care facilities including 144 VA Medical Centers and 1,232 outpatient sites of care. The VHA operates one of the largest integrated health care systems in the world (U.S. Department of Veterans Affairs, 2021a).

Nursing attention to the needs of veterans has grown since 2007 when the Department of Veterans Affairs

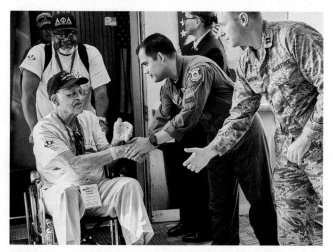

FIGURE 40.1 Active service members thanking veterans for their service.

established the VA Nurse Academy which later became the VA Nursing Academic Partnerships. The goal is to enhance the care of the Veterans through developing relationships with nursing schools and providing educational opportunities for students (U.S. Department of Veterans Affairs, n.d.a.). In 2011, Former First Lady, Michelle Obama and Dr. Jill Biden launched *Joining Forces*, a national initiative to support service members, veterans, and their families. The goal was to bring attention to the needs of service members, veterans, and their families including their wellness needs (Joining Forces, n.d.). In 2021, First Lady, Dr. Jill Biden re-launched this initiative to continue to support service members, veterans, and their families.

MENTAL HEALTH NEEDS OF VETERANS

Mental health needs are pervasive in the veteran population. Post-deployment depression, PTSD, and substance use disorders are disabling to the veterans and their families. Veterans are also at risk for suicide, traumatic brain injury (TBI), and homelessness.

Protective Factors

A strong veteran identity contributes to a positive self-esteem and self-definition and it can be protective of mental health problems such as suicide ideation (Adams et al., 2019). Protective factors also include serving multiple tours, having a rank as an officer, and living in a rural area. In a study comparing mental health factors of rural versus non-rural veterans, the veterans living in the rural areas were more likely to be older, more often White, more often married, and less often college graduates. The rural veterans had few stressful events in the previous year, good overall measure of mental health, and used psychiatric services less often than their urban counterparts (Boscarino, Figley, et al., 2020). Other protective factors include employment, being able to meet basic needs, self-care, living stability, social support, spirituality, resilience, and self-determination (Elbogen et al., 2020).

Risks for Mental Health Issues

Veterans who are exposed to stressors and traumatic events during military deployments are at greater risk for mental disorders than the general population (Meyer et al., 2019). Common risk factors for major depressive disorder and PTSD include having high combat exposure, history of concussion, high stressful life events within the past year, and low social support. Other predictors of PTSD include being female, high lifetime trauma, and low social capital (few connections with neighborhood and neighbors). Female veterans have a greater risk than their male counterpart for lifetime PTSD, depression, suicidal thoughts, and for lifetime use of psychological services (Figure 40.2) (Boscarino, Adams, et al., 2020).

Females veterans living in non-rural areas have an increased risk for PTSD, depression, likelihood of using psychiatric services, and a decreased risk for alcohol problems when compared with the female veterans living in rural locations (Boscarino, Figley, et al., 2020).

National guard and reservists are at risk for post-deployment mental health problems which are more common in the national guard and reserve components than the active duty component. It was initially thought that the national guard and reservists had higher rates of mental disorders because of being less prepared and having less support than the active component. But, research shows that the mental health needs of national guard and reservists were related to combat exposure, lifetime traumatic stress exposures, current life stressors, and current social support (Boscarino, Adams, et al., 2020).

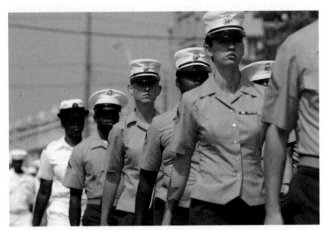

FIGURE 40.2 Female service members are integrated into military formation.

POSTTRAUMATIC STRESS DISORDER

Trauma and stress during military combat are not new. During the 17th to 19th century, the term *nostalgia* described a condition where a longing to return home was experienced by young people in the military. In nostalgia, service members experienced sadness, insomnia, and anorexia which were sometimes linked to psychic trauma. Nostalgia could lead to death (Battesti, 2016). During the American Civil War (1861–1865), a disorder known as *Soldier's Heart* developed after combat and was expressed as fatigue, shortness of breath, sighing respirations, palpitations, rapid heart rate, and sweating, with no observable cardiological abnormality (Bremner, et al., 2020; Da Costa, 1871). During the First World War (1914–1918), a condition known as "shell shock" or "war neurosis" was identified and shared similar, but not all, characteristics of modern day posttraumatic disorder (Pedroso et al., 2017;

Stein & Rothbaum, 2018). In WWII, the terms *Combat Stress Reaction (CSR)* and *battle fatigue* described a psychological condition that soldiers developed. This syndrome was characterized by anxiety, intense autonomic arousal, reliving, and sensitivity to stimuli (Andreasen, 2010). Up to half of the military discharges during WWII were said to be related to combat exhaustion (Friedman, n.d.).

The Korean and Vietnam wars brought attention to the traumatic experiences of service members. When the *Diagnostic and Statistical Manual III* was published in 1980, a stress disorders category was included (APA, 1980). The PTSD diagnostic criteria have evolved into the current diagnosis published in the *DMS-5* (Andreasen, 2010). See Chapter 29. PTSD is now understood to be a complex interplay of biologic and psychological symptoms that are experienced as a result of other traumatic experiences besides the trauma of war.

Epidemiology

The prevalence of PTSD in veterans is difficult to estimate because of the various diagnostic criteria that have been used over several decades. Reliable data on the prevalence of PTSD in veterans from WWII to Vietnam war are not available. Most experts believe the prevalence is much greater than reported. Estimated prevalence data of PTSD from OEF and OIF veterans vary from 11% to 30% (see Box 40.1). Experts agree that veterans who served Iraq and Afghanistan report higher rates of PTSD than non-veteran population. Co-occurring disorders, particularly alcohol use disorder (AUD), are common in veterans with PTSD (Pedersen et al., 2020).

Trauma

To meet the criteria for a PTSD diagnosis, there must be exposure "to actual or threatened death serious injury, or sexual violence (APA, 2013, p. 271)." The trauma can be experienced, witnessed, or learned about such as an accidental or violent event of a family or friend (APA, 2013). An **index trauma** is defined as either the worst single event or closely related multiple events (Priebe et al., 2018; Weathers et al., 2018). When there are multiple traumatic events, it may be difficult to identify one single event that precipitated the PTSD symptoms.

Service members deployed to areas of combat are at high risk for trauma, such as Iraq and Afghanistan. In the recent Iraq/Afghanistan wars battlefield lines were not linear. There was no clearly defined front line or area in the rear where safe operations could be performed. Attacks occurred without warning and battle lines shifted. Witnessing and experiencing combat events in these high-risk locations have provoked traumatic responses and initiated PTSD.

Typical PTSD symptoms related to military trauma include startle reaction with hypervigilance, avoidance of memories with avoidance of external reminders, anhedonia with detachment, being upset when reminded of event (physiological reactivity), and dreams with sleep disturbance (Osório et al., 2018).

Combat Versus Non-Combat-Related Trauma

Military trauma can be categorized as combat- or non-combat-related. **Combat-related trauma** occurs while engaging in warfare activities that involve injuries, loss of comrades on the battlefield, and improvised explosive devices. **Non-combat-related** trauma occurs outside of direct combat and includes trauma such as military sexual trauma (MST), witnessing violence and serious accidents. Both types of traumas can result in PTSD. When combat-related traumas are compared with non-combat-related traumas, differences in PTSD symptom patterns emerge.

In a study of 944 veterans, 63.5% experienced combat-related trauma. They were more likely to be male, White or Hawaiian/Pacific Islander, married or widowed, serve in Vietnam, or OEF/OIF/**Operation New Dawn** (OND). This cohort experienced self-blame, intrusive memories with dreams, detachment, and reckless behavior with lack of positive emotion. The veteran group that experienced non-combat-related trauma were more likely to be female, Black and African American, divorced, separated, or never married and to have either not deployed to a war zone or served in wars other than Vietnam and OEF/OIF/OND. The PTSD symptoms of this group included exaggerated startle, self-blame with distorted beliefs, and concentration problems related to anhedonia (Macia et al., 2020).

Moral Injury

Moral injury is emerging as a significant construct in understanding the consequences of exposure to traumatic events.

> **KEYCONCEPT Moral injury** is "the lasting psychological, biological, spiritual, behavioral, and social impact of perpetrating, failing to prevent, or bearing witness to acts that transgress deeply held moral beliefs and expectations" (Litz et al., 2009, pg. 699).

Moral injurious experiences violate moral beliefs or cause one to question the justness of the world. Three types of moral injury have been identified. **Perpetration** is an act that transgresses or goes beyond personal moral values. **Witnessing** is observing transgression by others. **Betrayal** is being wronged by others' transgressions. For moral injury to occur, there must be an awareness of the discrepancy between personal morals and the injurious experience which results in dissonance and inner conflict. Consequences of moral injury may include self-harming behaviors and demoralization (Litz et al., 2009).

When gender differences in exposure to potentially morally injurious events were examined in post-9/11 veterans (N = 48,965), 27.9% experienced witnessing events, 18.8% reported perpetration by commission or omission, and 41% reported being betrayed by leadership, fellow service members, or others outside the U.S. military. When separating the findings according to gender, women were more likely to experience psychological distress by witnessing and betrayal, whereas men experienced all three–perpetration, witnessing, and betrayal (Maguen et al., 2020).

The consequences of moral injury are apparent in the lives of the veterans. For example, for men who are parents who experienced perpetrating events such as the killing of children in war, they may fear harm to their own children who serve as a reminder of those who were killed. For women, betrayal, such as MST, may be a strong driver of impaired functioning leading to demoralization and self-blame (Maguen et al., 2020).

Violent Combat and Caring for the Wounded

Violent combat is associated with a greater risk of developing **re-experiencing**, a cognitive–sensory experience with an emotional response to current stimuli that resembles the aspects of the index trauma. Violent combat also is associated with **numbing symptoms,** (feeling flat physically and emotionally, unable to fully participate in life) that are likely a result of intrusive memories, nightmares, distress, and physiological reactivity (Osório et al., 2018).

The proximity to wounding and death is associated with re-experiencing and **anxious-arousal** symptoms (cognitive impairment with autonomic symptoms). For example, military personnel who gave aid to the wounded and seriously wounded or handled bodies of killed service members are more likely to re-experience the trauma and exhibit anxious-arousal symptoms (Osório et al., 2018).

Microaggressions and Stress in Underrepresented Groups

Veterans who identify as lesbian, gay, bisexual, transgender, questioning, or queer LGBTQ are under stress because of social attitudes, stigma, and prevailing policies that may include exclusion from the service or reduction of benefits. They have PTSD from experiencing the trauma of war, plus discrimination, **microaggressions** (brief verbal, behavioral, or environmental indignities, whether intentional or unintentional, that communicate hostile, derogatory, or negative slights and insult), and **minority stress** (high levels of stress experience by stigmatized minority groups). These individuals report experiencing paranoia, hypervigilance, drug use, sexual risk taking, and heightened anxiety and depression (Livingston et al., 2020).

Evidence-Based Nursing Care for Veterans with PTSD

As with any patient, a comprehensive, patient-centered, and culturally informed assessment will guide veteran care. Veterans have unique needs which should be considered during the assessment process. Some veterans have a strong veteran identity, but others do not. It is important to determine the significance of the veteran experience and the relationship of the current PTSD symptoms to the military experience. Safety is always a concern. Is the patient having suicide thoughts or behaviors? For combat-related veterans, evidence of detachment, avoidance of people and places and lack of social support are important indications that the veteran is experiencing PTSD symptoms.

The nurse should help the veteran identify the PTSD symptoms and refer patient to PTSD services. Encouragement from friends and family will increase the likelihood of engaging in therapy and the need for interpersonal therapy.

MILITARY SEXUAL TRAUMA

> **KEYCONCEPT Military sexual trauma (MST)** refers to sexual assault and sexual harassment experienced during a veteran's military service (Title 38 U.S. Code 1720D).

MST includes any sexual activity during military service where a veteran is involved against their will. MST can occur on or off the military base (see Box 40.3). Perpetrators can be anyone—mentor or women, military personnel or civilians, commanding officers or subordinates, strangers, friends, or intimate partners.

MST is not a new phenomenon but has become more visible because victims are more likely to report the incident. In earlier wars, such as WWII and Vietnam, MST was underreported. If reported, the prevailing attitudes were that the victim was responsible or "asking for it." **Sexual harassment** (e.g., jokes, images involving sexual innuendos, and comments regarding sexual activity,) is documented by female veterans from before 1973 through 1993. This harassment often occurred in public and work locations. **Sexual assaults** (i.e., intentional sexual touching without the persons consent, groping, rape, and forcing a person to engage in sexual act) occurred

---

BOX 40.3

Military Sexual Trauma (MST)

MST Behaviors

- Pressured into sexual activities—threats of negative consequences for not cooperating
- Unable to consent to sexual activities (i.e., when intoxicated)
- Physically forced into sexual activities
- Unwanted sexual touching or grabbing
- Threatening, offensive remarks about a person's body, or sexual activities
- Threatening and unwelcome sexual advance

Survivor Reactions

- Strong emotions (depressed, intense emotions, angry, and irritable)
- Feelings of numbness
- Trouble sleeping
- Difficulties with attention, concentration, and memory
- Problems with alcohol or other drugs
- Difficulty with reminders of experience
- Difficulties in relationship
- Physical health problems

Adapted from U.S. Department of Veterans Affairs (n.d.b). Military sexual trauma. Mental Health Retrieved April 27, 2021 from https://www.mentalhealth.va.gov/mentalhealth/msthome/index.asp

---

more likely when a woman was alone and on duty. Perpetrators were more likely to be ranked higher than the victim (Wolff & Mills, 2016).

Epidemiology

MST occurs primarily to women, but also to men. One in three women and 1 in 50 men have told their VA health care provider that they experienced sexual trauma in the military (U.S. Department of Veterans Affairs, 2020a). In a study of 60,000 OEF/OIF female and male veterans, approximately 41% of women and 4% of men reported experiencing MST (Barth et al., 2016). LGBTQ individuals are at an increased risk for sexual harassment. There is an increased risk of sexual harassment and assault for those who identify as transgender (Schuyler et al., 2020).

Mental Health Issues Related to MST

MST is a life changing event. MST is highly associated with mental health disorders including PTSD, depression anxiety disorders, eating disorders, suicide, lower satisfaction with interpersonal relationships, and substance use. There is evidence that many victims of MST do not seek mental health care or disclose the trauma. MST represents a morally injurious experience that can profoundly affect their view of the world. There are several barriers that prevent victims from reporting abuse including self-stigma and fear of loss of relationships (Andresen & Blais, 2019). Women victims are often hesitant to seek treatment at the male-dominated VA Medical Centers (Gilmore et al., 2016).

Depression, PTSD, substance use, suicidal ideation, and severe self-directed violence are associated with MST (Forkus et al., 2020; Gross et al., 2020; Livingston, Fargo, et al., 2020). Self-directed violence such as suicide attempt or non-suicidal self-injury following MST occurs in both male and female victims, but female victims have a greater risk of self-directed violence (Gross et al., 2020).

Evidence-Based Nursing Care for Veterans with MST

Screening for MST should be included in any nursing assessment of veterans. If the veteran screens positive for MST, the impact of the MST should be discussed and considered for a referral to an experienced therapist or service for MST. In caring for persons with MST, nurses should follow similar care strategies as anyone who has had been physically or sexually abused (see Chapter 23). The VHA has developed programs to address the needs of women and men who have experienced MST.

DEPRESSION

Depression is common in the U.S. population and is associated with high rates of mortality and morbidity (see Chapter 25). Depression is more common in the veteran population than in the general U.S. population. An increasing number of veterans are reporting depressive symptoms. Depression is highly comorbid with PTSD and suicidal ideation. Trauma exposure is associated with both depression and PTSD, which can ultimately result in suicidal ideation. There is limited research on depression among U.S. veterans (Liu et al., 2019).

Epidemiology

The large study of veterans ($N = 6577$) over the age of 50 in 2006 showed that veteran status was not associated with an increase in anxiety or depression when compared with non-veterans. However, additional analysis showed that Vietnam veterans were twice as likely to have elevated depression and anxiety than WWII or Korean War veterans (Gould et al., 2015). In a study of OEF/OIF/OND service members and veterans, depression, PTSD, and military TBI were associated with a high risk for substantial disability such as getting around, communicating, and getting along with others (Lippa et al., 2015).

When depression data were analyzed in the *National Survey on Drug Use and Health* (NSDUH) from 2005 to 2016, the prevalence of depression (9.6%) in veterans was higher than that of the 6.7% rate of adults in the United States. The rate of depression peaked in 2011–2013 at 12.3% of veterans experiencing depression. Female veterans have a higher prevalence of depression than male veterans. White veterans consistently have a higher prevalence rate of depression than Black and Hispanic veterans (Liu et al., 2019).

Protective Factors

Involvement in community groups and activities, which fosters a sense of belonging and identity, has been shown to be a protective factor for depression and PTSD in veterans. An optimistic disposition appears to be protective of depression. Veterans who are optimistic are more likely to use adaptive and problem-focused coping strategies such as positive reframing of problems and seeking social support (Nichter, Haller, et al., 2020).

Risk Factors

Veterans of racial or ethnic minorities (Black and Hispanic) are at high risk for depression and PTSD. The number of lifetime traumas increases the risk for PTSD and depression. They experience more psychosocial stressors (minority stress and microaggressions) than White veterans that, in turn, interact with PTSD to increase the risk for depression (Nichter, Haller, et al., 2020).

Evidenced-Based Nursing Care for Veterans with Depression

Nursing care for veterans with depression is similar to care of non-veterans. Cognitive therapy, cognitive processing therapy, medications, and transcranial magnetic stimulation are used. The care should be tailored to the needs of the veteran.

Depression in women veterans has been associated with impaired quality of life (QOL), which leads to functional decline and behavioral problems (Devine et al., 2020) (see Box 40.4). Accessing treatment for depression in women veterans can be complicated by discrimination and sexual harassment by male veterans when accessing VHA health care facilities. When inappropriate or unwanted comments or behavior from male veterans occur, the women are more likely to report feeling unwelcome and unsafe. Hence, the treatment is delayed or appointments missed (Klap et al., 2019). Depression and poor QOL improve with treatment that is timely, comprehensive, and gender-specific (Devine et al., 2020).

BOX 40.4

Research for Evidence-Based Practice: Quality of Life Among Women Veterans

Devine, D. T., McMillan, S. C., Kip, K., & Powell-Cope, G. (2020). Quality of life among women veterans. Journal of the American Association of Nurse Practitioners, 32(11), 745–755. https://doi.org/10.1097/JXX.0000000000000445

THE QUESTION: Do women veterans age 40 to 60 years who use VA women's health specialty clinic have a lower quality of life (QOL) compared with normal reference values of women in North America?

METHODS: Records of 51 females veterans age 40 to 60 attending a women's health specialty clinic were retrospectively reviewed. Multiple linear regression models were fit to explore QOL and depression levels with socioeconomic status, parity, years of service, and military sexual trauma.

FINDINGS: Female veterans had significantly lower baseline QOL scores than the comparison group. Following treatment, their QOL and depression improved.

IMPLICATIONS FOR NURSING: Care for female veterans should be individualized with a focus on improving QOL, reducing depressive symptoms, and identifying MST.

SUICIDE

Suicide in the Military

Active-duty military personnel dying by suicide is a relatively new phenomena. For example, WWII (1939–1945) had a reported suicide rate of 5 per 100,000. Between 1945 and 1991, the rate generally stabilized in the low to mid-teens (10–15 per 100,000). Some experts suggest that rates of suicide in earlier wars are likely underreported. They suggest that wars provide other ways to end lives such as rushing from a trench into enemy fire. The military suicide rate began increasing in 2004, peaking 2012 during the Afghanistan and Iraq Wars with 29.7 per 100,000 reported suicides. From 2008 to the present, the annual rate remains within a range of 20.2 to 29.7 per 100,000 (Jones, 2019; Smith et al., 2019). It should be noted that suicide in the general population had increased from 2005 to 2018 (see Chapter 22).

In 2015, almost half of the service members who died by suicide had a history of at least one behavioral health disorder such as substance use disorder, adjustment disorder, or major depression. Stressors associated with suicide included failed/failing intimate-partner relationships and legal proceedings (Pruitt et al., 2019).

Suicide in the Veteran Community

Suicide rates in the veteran community began increasing in 2001 (U.S. Department of Veterans Affairs, 2016). From 2005 to 2018, the veteran suicide rate gradually increased from 18.5 per 100,000 (16.6 per day) to 27.5 per 100,000 (17.6 per day) (U.S. Department of Veterans Affairs, 2020b).

The most common suicide method is firearms with 68.2% of suicide deaths due to a self-inflicted firearm injury (69.4% of males; 41.9% of females). Poisoning and suffocation are the next most frequent methods (U.S. Department of Veterans Affairs, 2020b). Veterans have higher rates of firearm ownership than the general population and are at substantially increased risk of firearm suicide compared to non-veterans. They use firearms mainly for personal protection and generally favor measures to restrict access to firearms among at-risk individuals. Providers are often hesitant to screen and counsel for firearms because of the lack of familiarity with guns, little confidence in intervention effectiveness, or philosophical reasoning related to constitutional rights (Theis et al., 2020).

Epidemiology

The 2018 rates (latest data) of suicide among veterans were higher and rose faster than those among non-veteran U.S. adults. Suicide rate is 1.5 times the rate for non-veteran adults. The suicide rates were highest among White veterans and lowest among Black or African American veterans. Veterans ages 18–34 had the highest rate in 2018 (45.9 per 100,000). Veterans, age 75 and older, had the lowest suicide rate (27.4 per 100,000). The rate of women veteran suicide was 2.1 times that of non-veteran women. Veterans identifying as LGBTQ are more likely to report suicidal ideation and screen positive for PTSD, depression, and alcohol problems than heterosexual veterans (U.S. Department of Veterans Affairs, 2020b).

Protective Factors

The *National Health and Resilience in Veterans Study* (NHRVS), initiated in 2011, is an ongoing study characterizing the longitudinal trajectories of mental and physical health outcomes in U.S. veterans. This study focuses on genetic and environmental risk and protective factors that contribute to these trajectories. Findings from this study show that perceived social support, curiosity, resilience, and acceptance-based coping are protective of suicide. In veterans who had been diagnosed with PTSD and/or major depressive disorder, greater purpose in life, curiosity, and optimism were inversely related to suicide ideation. For veterans who experience moral injury, having a greater global purpose and meaning in life were important in combating suicidal thoughts (Fogle et al., 2020).

Risk Factors for Veteran Suicide

Several risk factors are associated with veteran suicide including economic disparities, race, ethnicities, LGBT disparities, and homelessness. Difficulties translating military-related skills to civilian jobs contribute to lower income and homelessness. Other risks include greater age, loneliness, disability in instrumental daily living (e.g., shopping, cooking), somatic symptoms, and use of denial-based coping (Fogle et al., 2020).

With the COVID-19 pandemic there has been an increase in unemployment among veterans. In April 2020, there were 833,000 more unemployed veterans than in April 2019. As the veteran unemployment rate increased from 2.3% to 11.7%, suicidal ideation was higher for racial and ethnic minority populations (U.S. Department of Veterans Affairs, 2020b).

Suicide rates are higher in veterans with mental health or substance use disorder diagnoses. The risk of suicide is greater in veterans who have been diagnosed with PTSD and/or major depressive disorder (Fogle et al., 2020). In 2018, the suicide rate for VHA patients with a substance use or mental illness was 57.9 per 100,000 veterans; for patients with depression, the rate was 65.6 per 100,000 (U.S. Department of Veterans Affairs, 2020b).

Childhood abuse is associated with suicide behavior in adulthood. Combat-exposed veterans with a history of childhood sexual abuse are nearly three times more likely to contemplate suicide compared to those without a history of abuse. Childhood sexual abuse is a stronger predictor of suicide attempts than either childhood physical abuse or combat exposure. Childhood sexual abuse leads to long-term psychological consequences such as chronic depression, PTSD, and suicide-related outcomes (Nichter, Hill, et al., 2020).

Experiences during deployment contribute to risks for suicide ideation. There is evidence that morally injurious events are associated with suicidal ideation. Many veterans experienced or witnessed transgressive acts that violated their moral code such as killing an enemy or a non-combatant while serving in the military (Cameron et al., 2020).

Evidence-Based Nursing Care for Veterans with Suicide Ideation

The results of the NHRVS studies indicate that a considerable proportion of U.S. veterans experience suicidal ideation, but that ideation may fluctuate over time (Fogle et al., 2020). That is, there may be long periods where suicidal thoughts are absent. Monitoring suicidal ideation by primary care nurses becomes important in identifying veterans' high risk for suicide.

The nursing care of a veteran with suicide ideation begins with engagement in the therapeutic relationship and treatment. The aim of the care is to keep the veteran safe and to help the person develop a safety plan (see Chapter 22). The nurse should recognize that veterans often internalize the stigma that seeking mental health care means weakness and are less likely to engage in care. It is estimated that as many as two-thirds of veterans with suicidal ideation are not engaged in mental health treatment (Nichter, Hill, et al., 2020).

Older male veterans with suicide ideation are less likely to engage in treatment than their younger female counterparts. Concerns about masculinity and gender role expectations are often barriers for male veterans. Veterans are more likely to engage in treatment if they have a diagnosis of depression, a prior suicide attempt, multiple medical problems, or lifetime traumas (Nichter, Hill, et al., 2020).

There are several nursing approaches for the care of veterans. The nurse should always screen for suicide ideation by using a standardized screening tool such as the Columbia Suicide Severity Rating Scale (see Chapter 11). Every veteran should know about the Veterans Crisis Line (Figure 40.3). If the veteran screens positive for suicide ideation, the nurse should refer the patient to a mental health professional. If the veteran is currently thinking about hurting or killing self, looking for ways to kill self, talking about death, dying, or suicide or carrying out self-destructive acts such as drug abuse or using weapons, the nurse should not leave the patient alone and seek available mental health help.

The VHA suicide prevention program is an important resource. Suicide prevention is a VHA clinical priority. Each VA Medical Center has a full-time suicide prevention coordinator who provides active preventive interventions and follows-up with at risk veterans. Suicide prevention teams provide community outreach, coordination of resources, and increases awareness of suicide risks. The VA provides medical screening and assessment of patients at risk for suicide. Patients with

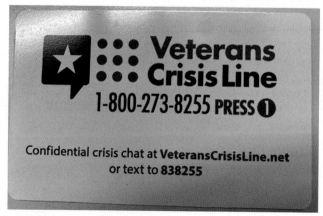

FIGURE 40.3 Veterans Crisis Line

elevated suicide risk receive an enhanced level of care, including missed appointment follow-up, safety planning, follow-up visits, and care plans that directly address their risk factors for suicide (U.S. Department of Veterans Affairs, Office of Suicide Prevention, 2018).

SUBSTANCE USE

Alcohol and Drug Use in the Military

Alcohol and drugs have long been associated with the military and war. Whiskey was used for wounded soldiers, but supplies would disappear and run consistently low. Drinking alcohol was a part of everyday life in the Civil War. Ulysses S. Grant had a well-documented alcohol problem (Chernow, 2017). Morphine was given as an anesthetic and a diarrhea cure, leaving many soldiers with a morphine addiction or *Soldiers Disease*. During World War I, cocaine became the drug of abuse of the frontlines. Amphetamines were the most popular drugs used in WWII. Dextroamphetamine was a popular drug during the Vietnam war. During this war, antipsychotics were also given to soldiers (Tackett, 2019).

The misuse of alcohol and drugs in the military continues to be a problem in 2021. Deployment is associated with smoking initiation, unhealthy drinking, drug use, and risky behaviors. Many service members see drinking as part of the military culture. Military members are at higher risk of developing a drug or alcohol problem than civilians. Substance use is associated with combat, trauma, PTSD, sexual and physical abuse (National Institute on Drug Abuse [NIDA], 2019).

Even though illicit drug use among active duty personnel is relatively low, alcohol and rates of binge drinking are high compared to the general population. Cigarette smoking and misuse of prescription drugs have decreased in recent years (NIDA, 2019).

Use of Substances

Substance use often continues long after military service ends. In the military, service members can face dishonorable discharge or criminal prosecution for a positive drug test. These consequences discourage illicit drug use. Once the service member transitions to civilian life, the protection of the service is gone and substance use becomes more likely. More than 1 in 10 veterans is diagnosed with a substance use disorder. (NIDA, 2019).

Alcohol Use

AUD is one of the most prevalent mental disorders in the United States (see Chapter 31). Veterans are more likely to use alcohol than other substances. They also are more

likely to use alcohol than their non-veteran counterparts. Within 1 year of deployment. 39.2% of OEF/OIF veterans screened positive for AUD. In the U.S. veteran population, 42.2% met criteria for lifetime AUD (Fuehrlein et al., 2018).

Data from the NHRVS identified four veteran trajectories of alcohol consumption over 4 years ($N = 3,157$). *Rare drinkers* (65.3%) were abstinent or rarely drank alcohol; moderate drinkers (30.2%) consistently drank at a moderate level; *excessive drinkers* (2.6%) drank at elevated levels and *recovering drinkers* (1.9%) were excessively drinking and decreased consumption over time. The researchers posited that the low percentage of excessive drinkers was related to the older age of the sample (Fuehrlein et al., 2018).

AUD is highly comorbid with PTSD, major depressive disorder, and suicide (Bohnert et al., 2017; McHugh & Weis, 2019; Straus et al., 2019). Research shows that comorbidity varies among White, Black, and Hispanic veterans. Black and Hispanic veterans with AUD have greater psychiatric comorbidity relative to White veterans. Hispanic veterans with lifetime AUD have worse physical health, cognitive function and QOL. Black and Hispanic veterans with lifetime AUD are more likely to screen positive for depressive disorder (Carr et al., 2021). These results suggest that racial and ethnic minorities with AUD may have higher rates of mental disorders and poorer outcomes. There is a need for race/ethnicity-sensitive approaches to the care and treatment AUD in veterans.

Risks and Protective Factors

Alcohol consumption and use of drugs are risks for the development of lifetime AUD. Other risk factors of AUD include trauma, exposure to military stress and adjustment to civilian life. Due to the stigmatization of mental illness in the military culture, many veterans self-medicate with alcohol rather than access mental health services (Fuehrlein et al., 2018; Straus et al., 2020).

Resilience, purpose in life, dispositional gratitude (believing that there is much in life to be thankful for), and religiosity/spirituality are protective factors for developing AUD. Social support, and secure attachment style (feeling that it is easy to get close to others; feeling comfortable with others) are also protective.

Opioid Use

Opioid addictions are discussed in Chapter 31. The following discussion is specific to the unique challenges the veteran experiences who uses opioids.

Opioid Use in the Military

OUDs often begin with a prescription following an injury. Service members are high risk for trauma and injury requiring the treatment of pain. Injured and sick military personnel are often prescribed pain medication. Because opioids can quickly become addictive, regular use of opioids can lead to addiction. The amount of pain medication prescribed to service members peaked in 2009 but began decreasing in 2011 in response to the prevention and appropriate prescribing initiatives of the DOD (NIDA, 2019).

Opioid Use by Veterans

The lifetime prevalence of OUD in veteran men is an estimated at 418,000 and is not proportionately different than the 2.5 million non-veteran men with OUD. Risk factors for lifetime OUD include a younger age, lower income, and fewer years of education. Racial minority status is associated with a risk of OUD because the general veteran population includes an older generation of adults with OUD who started using heroin when the problem was more prevalent among African American than Caucasians. In recent years, opioid users are more likely to be Caucasians starting with prescription drugs rather than heroin (Rhee & Rosenheck, 2019).

About one-half of veterans using the VHA are diagnosed with chronic pain that is treated with opioids, putting them at higher risk of dependency and overdose (Ahonle et al., 2020). From 2001 to 2009, the percentage of veterans in the VHA system receiving opioid prescription increased from 17% to 24% (Teeters et al., 2017). The VHA launched a system-wide *Opioid Safety Initiative* to address the opioid epidemic. Since 2012, the number of veterans prescribed opioids decreased 56% and co-prescribed opioid/benzodiazepine decreased 83% (Sandbrink et al., 2020).

Polysubstance Use, Comorbidity, and Overdose

The majority of veterans in the VHA diagnosed with OUD appear to have at least one comorbid substance use disorder and many have multiple substance use disorders (Lin et al., 2021). OUD is strongly associated with psychiatric and substance use disorders. In a study comparing veterans with OUD ($N = 61$), veterans without OUD ($N = 2.679$), and non-veterans with OUD ($N = 329$), 63.4% of veterans with OUD and 60.9% of the non-veterans had a comorbid lifetime psychiatric disorder compared with 22% of veterans without OUD ($N = 2.679$) (Rhee & Rosenheck, 2019).

Opioid use is associated with suicide and unintentional overdose (Bohnert & Ilgen, 2019). Some veterans qualify to enroll in both the VA and Medicare Part D where they can receive prescription opioids from both systems. Dual-users are at significantly higher odds of death from opioid overdose than those who receive opioids from the VA only (Moyo et al., 2019). Veterans with an OUD have among the highest rates of suicide when compared to veterans with psychiatric disorders (U.S. Department of Veterans Affairs, Office of Mental Health and Suicide Prevention, 2020b). Comorbid OUD and depression and comorbid OUD and AUD are significantly associated with additive risk of suicide attempts (Ashrafioun et al., 2020).

Tobacco Use

Tobacco use of cigarette and non-cigarette products is prevalent in the U.S. veteran population, especially younger veterans. Nearly half of the veterans who served during September 2001 or later report using tobacco products. These veterans are more likely to have comorbid conditions including poor physical health, poor mental health, other substance use and problematic alcohol use than their non-veteran counterparts. In nearly all age groups, veterans have a higher prevalence of tobacco use than non-veterans (Cooper et al., 2019).

Many veterans were introduced to tobacco use while in the military. Another explanation for such high use of tobacco is that the use is related to the stress associated with re-integrating into civilian life (Cooper et al., 2019).

Evidence-Based Nursing Care for Veterans with Substance Use Disorder

Nursing care for any veteran should include an assessment of substance use. Based on the research, veterans are high risk for multiple substance use which significantly impacts their health and well-being. The U.S. veteran population has complex health needs that that can be complicated by substance use.

The VHA health care system is prepared for treatment of substance use disorders, but not every veteran seeks care in the VHA system. Recognizing the relationship between the substance use and other health and mental health issues will guide the nurse in planning for the appropriate care. The approach to patients should always be non-judgmental and foster a therapeutic partnership and help patient move toward recovery. The nurse should always conduct a medication assessment and determine where the prescriptions are filled. A medication assessment is especially important when the veteran is receiving care at the VA and non-VA facility to prevent over prescribing of medication, particularly opioids.

OTHER ISSUES IMPACTING VETERAN MENTAL HEALTH

The wellness and mental health of veterans are impacted by other conditions. These conditions are related to the mental health needs and recovery and interrelated with other disorders. It is important for nurses to stay informed about the issues and challenges that are unique to military veterans.

Pain

The prevalence of chronic pain (pain lasting longer than 3–6 months) occurs more frequently in veterans than non-veterans (Nahin, 2017). See Chapter 43 for an in-depth a discussion of pain and its treatment. General chronic pain prevalence estimate ranges from 25% to 72% of veterans. Pain type includes most parts of the body from head to neck, chest, and back (Reyes et al., 2020). Individuals with chronic pain experience high rates of disability, decreased QOL, and emotional distress (Brintz et al., 2020).

Chronic back pain in veterans is the most frequently reported type of pain followed by jaw pain, severe headaches or migraine, and neck pain (Nahin, 2017). **Musculoskeletal pain** (MSP) is caused by injuries or disorders of the joints, muscles, tendons, or ligaments to the bones, muscles, nerves, and/or connective tissue. Combat injuries (polytrauma, blast injuries) and non-combat injuries (muscle strain, overuse) lead to which can lead to chronic MSP. In an integrative review of the incidence, prevalence, and risk factors for MSP and headaches in active duty, inflammation and pain from overuse comprised the largest proportion of injury (82% of all non-deployed military personnel). The risk of MSP was highest among active duty, female, Army, enlisted personnel and those with greater time in mother vehicle. For veterans who sustained a TBI, 92% reported headaches (Bader, et al., 2018).

Considering the number of active duty service members who transition each year to veteran status, chronic MSP is a major focus of treatment for this population (Grinberg et al., 2020; O'Neil et al., 2020). Pain is associated with an increased in allostatic load leading to physical manifestations of chronic stress including

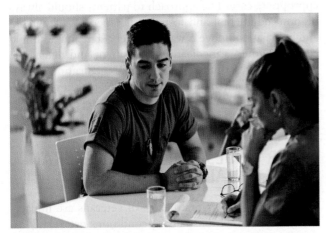

FIGURE 40.4   Veteran being assessed for health problems.

changes in endocrine dysfunction, sleep disturbance, orthopedic problems substance use, depression, and suicide (Figure 40.4) (Frueh et al., 2020). Multifocal pain (i.e., multiple pain sites such as back, knees, hips, knees) is common and leads to poorer outcomes (Bushey et al., 2021). Prolonged opioid use for pain can result in an OUD (Riva et al., 2020).

Traumatic Brain Injury

TBI is often referred to as a "signature injury" of the post-9/11 conflict (OEF/OIF/OND) (Hoge et al., 2008). Pain medication estimates from 49.5 78% of veterans with chronic pain use pain medication. It is estimated that general chronic pain among veterans with a history of TBI is 59% (O'Neil et al., 2020). The estimates of the number of veterans with TBI from 2000 to 2019 was 423,858. Hearing disturbance and headaches are the most frequently reported adverse outcomes of blast-related injuries. Frequent comorbidities associated with the blast-related injuries include PTSD, depression, anxiety, sleep disorders, attention disorders, and cognitive disorders (Phipps et al., 2020).

Homelessness

U.S. veterans who are homeless have served in wars from WWII to the recent war in Afghanistan and Iraq. Nearly half of the veterans who are homeless served during the Vietnam era and two-thirds served the United States for at least 3 years and one-third were stationed in a war zone. It is estimated that there are over 37,000 veterans homeless on any given night (see Chapter 41). The majority are predominantly male with about 9% being female. Roughly 45% are African American or Hispanic, despite only accounting for 10.4% and 3.4% of the U.S. veteran population. About 1.4 million other veterans are at risk of homelessness due to poverty, lack of support networks, and poor living conditions (National Coalition for Homeless Veterans, n.d.).

The VHA has multiple programs to support veterans who are homeless or at risk of being homelessness. The VA conducts coordinated outreach to seek out veterans in need of assistance. Veterans who are homeless or at risk of being homeless are connected with housing, health care, community employment services, and other required supports (U.S. Department of Veterans Affairs, 2021b).

There are multiple factors that contribute to homelessness in the veteran's population. In one study, one-third of the veterans screened positive for lifetime PTSD. Compared with veterans who are not homeless, veterans who were homeless, especially underrepresented groups (Black and Hispanic) were likely to screen positive for

PTSD (Tsai et al., 2020). A higher proportion of veterans who are homeless received high-dose opioid therapy compared with non-veterans associated with increased rates of fatal opioid overdoses (Jasuja et al., 2021).

Veterans who are experiencing homelessness have multiple health and mental health issues. While there are available services for veterans who are homeless, there are multiple barriers as well. Social stigma and perceived lack of support contribute to hesitancy to access services (Bounthavong et al., 2020). Veterans with children make up a considerable component of the female veterans who are homeless. Veterans with families have additional stressors when compared to non-veteran homeless families such as military-related experienced, deployment, reintegration stress, and PTSD or MST (Ijadi-Maghsoodi et al., 2021).

SUMMARY OF KEY POINTS

- The U.S. military consists of three departments (Army, Navy and Air Force). The Department of the Navy is responsible for the Navy and Marines and the Air Force is responsible for the Air Force and Space Force. There are seven reserve components that can be activated in time of war or national emergency. The Army is the largest U.S. military service with 35% of the active duty members.

- The values, beliefs, and behaviors acquired in the military often last a lifetime.

- Historically, women in the military was very limited until the elimination of the draft when the need for service members became apparent. Women were admitted into the service academies in 1976.

- Individuals who openly identified as LGBTQ were excluded from military service until 2016 and reaffirmed in 2021. The majority of all service members are White with the greater proportion of minorities found primarily in lower ranks.

- Every year about 200,000 service members transition to civilian life. The transition year is a high-risk period for physical and mental health issues. The Transition Assistance Program provides support, resources, and training.

- A veteran identity is the degree to which the veteran role is essential or important to how they think about themselves.

- The VHA operates one of the largest integrated health care systems in the world. Nursing plays an important role in the care of the veterans through developing relationships with nursing schools and providing educational opportunities for students.

- Joining Forces is a national initiative to support service members, veterans, and their families.

- Mental health needs are pervasive in the veteran population. Post-deployment depression, PTSD, and substance use disorders are disabling to the veterans and their families.

- Veterans are at risk for suicide, TBI and homelessness. A strong veteran identity can support positive self-esteem and be protective of mental health problems.

- High combat exposure, history of concussions, stressful life events, and low social support are risk factors for depression and PTSD.

- PTSD is associated with both combat and non-combat trauma. PTSD symptoms from combat trauma include self-blame, intrusive memories with dreams detachment, and reckless behavior. PTSD symptoms from non-combat trauma include exaggerated startle, self-blame with distorted beliefs, and concentration problems.

- Moral injury can be a consequence of exposure to traumatic events. Moral injury can be caused by perpetration, witnessing, and betrayal.

- Veterans who identify as LGBTQ experience the trauma of war plus microaggressions and minority stress.

- MST refers to sexual assault and sexual harassment. MST occurs primarily to women, but also to men. MST is a life changing event and is highly associated with mental health disorders.

- Nursing care of veterans should always include a comprehensive assessment that screens for PTSD and MST. Veterans with these disorders should be referred to mental health specialists.

- Depression is more common in the veteran population than in the general U.S. population. Depression is highly comorbid with PTSD and suicidal ideation.

- Suicide is a major mental health problem in the veteran community. The most common method of suicide is firearms followed by poisoning and suffocation. Childhood sexual abuse of veterans is a strong predictor of suicide. Experiences during deployment contribute to risks for suicide ideation especially morally injurious events.

- Veterans are more likely to use alcohol than other substances. Alcohol use often begins in the military service and continues after discharge. AUD is highly comorbid with PTSD, major depressive disorder, and suicide.

- Opioid use by veterans often begins with prescription pain medication putting them at risk of dependency and overdose. Veterans who have opioid use disorder are likely to have at least one comorbid substance use disorder. Opioid use is associated with suicide and unintentional overdose.

■ Tobacco use is more prevalent by veterans than in the general population.

■ Chronic pain, TBI, and homelessness contribute to health and mental health issues of veterans.

CRITICAL THINKING CHALLENGES

1. Describe how the military culture influences the values, beliefs, and behaviors of a veteran.

2. Compare the mental health problems of World War I and II service members with those serving in Iraq and Afghanistan.

3. Trace the role of women in the military from the Revolutionary War through the wars in Iraq and Afghanistan.

4. Discuss the difficulties the LGBTQ community has experienced in the military. Include a discussion about microaggression and minority stress.

5. M.J. was recently discharged from the U.S. Army. M.J. experienced combat in Afghanistan and was treated for PTSD but is reluctant to seek out care in the community. M.J. visits a clinic for an influenza injection and the nurse notices the ARMY insignia on the patient's wallet. What approach should the nurse take in giving the influenza injection? Should the nurse ask about serving in the military?

6. Differentiate combat-related trauma from non-combat-related trauma. Explain the different PTSD symptom patterns.

7. Define the components of a "moral injury" and explain their relationship to PTSD.

8. Discuss the nursing responsibility of screening for MST in veterans.

9. P.S., a Vietnam veteran is attending a health screening at a local community clinic. The veteran is expressing worthlessness and sadness following the death of a life-long partner. Should the nurse conduct a suicide screening on the patient. Explain your answer.

10. During a health assessment, a 32-year-old veteran talks about consuming a six-pack of beer each night before going to bed to sleep. What additional assessment data are needed to determine the likelihood of an alcohol use disorder?

11. Discuss the use of opioids and the treatment of pain in veterans. How should a nurse approach a veteran who is suspected of using excessive opioids for the treatment of pain?

 Movie Viewing Guides
Thank You for Your Service (2017) Adam Schumann (Miles Teller) returns home to Kansas after a 15 month combat tour in Iraq. He returns to his wife, Saskia (Haley Bennett) and two young children, a daughter and an infant son born while Adam was still overseas. Adam suffers from PTSD as manifested by nightmares and frequent flashbacks for which his wife convinces him to seek help from the Department of Veterans Affairs. The movie depicts the struggles of Adam and two service buddies as they transition to civilian life.

VIEWING POINTS: Identify the inherent difficulties in making the transition from military to civilian life. How did the military culture influence Adam willingness to seek help for PTSD? Identify the PTSD symptoms that are characteristic of combat-related trauma. Describe the TBI symptoms that Solo Aeiti (Beulah Koale) manifested. Did you increase your understanding of the difficulties veterans can have when transitioning to civilian life?

Unfolding Patient Stories: Andrew Davis

Part 2 (56 years)

 Recall from Chapter 31 Andrew Davis who admitted himself to an alcohol rehabilitation facility. His alcohol abuse began in early adolescence. What factors can increase the risk for alcohol abuse and addiction as an adolescent? What are the psychosocial influences and consequences of alcohol abuse? What assessments can help the nurse identify the signs of alcohol abuse?

REFERENCES

Adams, R. E., Hu, Y., Figley, C. R., Urosevich, T. G., Hoffman, S. N., Kirchner, H. L., Dugan, R. J., Boscarino, J. J., Withey, C. A., & Boscarino, J. A. (2021). Risk and protective factors associated with mental health among female military veterans: Results from the veterans' health study. *BMC Women's Health*, 21(1), 55. https://doi.org/10.1186/s12905-021-01181-z

Adams, R. E., Urosevich, T. G., Hoffman, S. N., Kirchner, H. L., Figley, C. R., Withey, C. A., Boscarino, J. J., Dugan, R. J., & Boscarino, J. A. (2019). Social and psychological risk and protective factors for veteran well-being: The role of veteran identity and its implications for intervention. *Military Behavioral Health*, 7(3), 304–314. https://doi.org/10.1080/21635781.2019.1580642

Ahonle, Z. J., Jia, H., Mudra, S. A., Romero, S., Castaneda, G., & Levy, C. (2020). Drug overdose and suicide among veteran enrollees in the VHA: Comparison among local, regional, and national data. *Federal Practitioner: For the Health Care Professionals of the VA, DoD, and PHS*, 37(9), 420–425. https://doi.org/10.12788/fp.0025

American Psychiatric Association. (1980). *Diagnostic and Statistical Manual of Mental Disorders-III*. American Psychiatric Association.

American Psychiatric Association (APA). (2013). *Diagnostic and statistical manual of mental disorders* (5th ed.). Author.

Andreasen, N. C. (2010). Posttraumatic stress disorder: A history and a critique. *Annals of the New York Academy of Sciences, 1208*, 67–71. https://doi.org/10.1111/j.1749-6632.2010.05699.x

Andresen, F. J., & Blais, R. K. (2019). Higher self-stigma is related to lower likelihood of disclosing military sexual trauma during screening in female veterans. *Psychological Trauma: Theory, Research, Practice and Policy, 11*(4), 372–378. https://doi.org/10.1037/tra0000406

Ashrafioun, L., Zerbo, K. R. A., Bishop, T. M., & Britton, P. C. (2020). Opioid use disorders, psychiatric comorbidities, and risk for suicide attempts among veterans seeking pain care. *Psychological Medicine, 50*, 2107–2112. https://doi.org/10.1017/S0033291719002307

Barth, S. K., Kimerling, R. E., Pavao, J., McCutcheon, S. J., Batten, S. V., Dursa, E., Peterson, M. R., & Schneiderman, A. I. (2016). Military sexual trauma among recent veterans: Correlates of sexual assault and sexual harassment. *American Journal of Preventive Medicine, 50*(1), 77–86. https://doi.org/10.1016/j.amepre.2015.06.012

Bader, C. E., Giordano, N. A., McDonald, C. C., Meghani, S. H., & Polomano, R. C. (2018). Musculoskeletal pain and headache in the active duty military population: An integrative review. *Worldviews on Evidence-based Nursing, 15*(4), 264–271. https://doi.org/10.1111/wvn.12301

Battesti, M. (2016). Nostalgia in the Army (17th-19th Centuries). *Frontiers of Neurology and Neuroscience, 38*, 132–142. https://doi.org/10.1159/000442652

Blakemore, E. (2019). How women fought their way into the U.S. Armed Forces. History Stories. Retrieved March 2, 2021 from https://www.history.com/news/women-fought-armed-forces-war-service

Bohnert, A., & Ilgen, M. A. (2019). Understanding links among opioid use, overdose, and suicide. *The New England Journal of Medicine, 380*(1), 71–79. https://doi.org/10.1056/NEJMra1802148

Bohnert, K. M., Ilgen, M. A., Louzon, S., McCarthy, J. F., & Katz, I. R. (2017). Substance use disorders and the risk of suicide mortality among men and women in the US Veterans Health Administration. *Addiction (Abingdon, England), 112*(7), 1193–1201. https://doi.org/10.1111/add.13774

Boscarino, J. A., Adams, R. E., Urosevich, T. G., Hoffman, S. N., Kirchner, H. L., Dugan, R. J., Boscarino, J. J., Withey, C. A., & Figley, C. R. (2020). Guard/Reserve service members and mental health outcomes following deployment: Results from the Veterans' Health Study. *General Hospital Psychiatry, 62*, 102–103. https://doi.org/10.1016/j.genhosppsych.2019.03.002

Boscarino, J. J., Figley, C. R., Adams, R. E., Urosevich, T. G., Kirchner, H. L., & Boscarino, J. A. (2020). Mental health status in veterans residing in rural versus non-rural areas: Results from the veterans' health study. *Military Medical Research, 7*(1), 44. https://doi.org/10.1186/s40779-020-00272-6.

Bremner, J. D., Wittbrodt, M. T., Shah, A. J., Pearce, B. D., Gurel, N. Z., Inan, O. T., Raggi, P., Lewis, T. T., Quyyumi, A. A., & Vaccarino, V. (2020). Confederates in the attic: Posttraumatic stress disorder, cardiovascular disease, and the return of soldier's heart. *The Journal of Nervous and Mental Disease, 208*(3), 171–180. https://doi.org/10.1097/NMD.0000000000001100

Brintz, C. E., Miller, S., Olmsted, K. R., Bartoszek, M., Cartwright, J., Kizakevich, P. N., Butler, M., Asefnia, N., Buben, A., & Gaylord, S. A. (2020). Adapting mindfulness training for military service members with chronic pain. *Military Medicine, 185*(3–4), 385–393. https://doi.org/10.1093/milmed/usz312

Bounthavong, M., Suh, K., Christopher, M., Veenstra, D. L., Basu, A., & Devine, E. B. (2020). Providers' perceptions on barriers and facilitators to prescribing naloxone for patients at risk for opioid overdose after implementation of a national academic detailing program: A qualitative assessment. *Research in Social & Administrative Pharmacy: RSAP, 16*(8), 1033–1040. https://doi.org/10.1016/j.sapharm.2019.10.015

Bushey, M. A., Ang, D., Wu, J., Outcalt, S. D., Krebs, E. E., Yu, Z., & Bair, M. J. (2021). Multifocal pain as a predictor of pain outcomes in military veterans with chronic musculoskeletal pain: A secondary data analysis of a randomized controlled trial. *Pain Medicine (Malden, Mass.)*, pnaa409. Advance online publication. https://doi.org/10.1093/pm/pnaa409

Cameron, A. Y., Eaton, E., Brake, C. A., & Capone, C. (2020). Moral injury as a unique predictor of suicidal ideation in a veteran sample with a substance use disorder. *Psychological Trauma: Theory, research, practice and policy*, 10.1037/tra0000988. Advance online publication. https://doi.org/10.1037/tra0000988

Carr, M. M., Potenza, M. N., Serowik, K. L., & Pietrzak, R. H. (2021). Race, ethnicity, and clinical features of alcohol use disorder among US military veterans: Results from the National Health and Resilience in Veterans Study. *The American Journal on Addictions, 30*(1), 26–33. https://doi.org/10.1111/ajad.13067

Center for Deployment Psychology. (2021). Military culture: Enhancing clinical competence. Uniformed Services University. Retrieved on March 7, 2021 from https://deploymentpsych.org/Military-Culture-Enhancing-Competence-Course-Description

Chernow, R. (2017). *Grant*. Penguin Press.

Congressional Research Service. (2021). Defense primer: Reserve forces. Retrieved March 2, 2021 from https://fas.org/sgp/crs/natsec/IF10540.pdf

Cooper, M., Yaqub, M., Hinds, J. T., & Perry, C. L. (2019). A longitudinal analysis of tobacco use in younger and older U.S. veterans. *Preventive Medicine Reports, 16*, 100990. https://doi.org/10.1016/j.pmedr.2019.100990

Council on Foreign Relations. (2020). Demographics of the U. S. military. Retrieved March 2, 2021 from https://www.cfr.org/backgrounder/demographics-us-military#:~:text=Now%2C%20are%20about%201.3,percent%20of%20the%20U.S.%20population._

Da Costa, J. J. (1871). On irritable heart: A clinical study of a form of functional cardiac disorder and its consequences. *American Journal of Psychiatry, 142*, 1341–1343.

Department of Defense Directive (DOD) 1304.26 (1993, December 21). Qualification standards for enlistment, appointment, and induction. Department of Defense. Retrieved March 17, 2021 from https://biotech.law.lsu.edu/blaw/dodd/corres/pdf/d130426wch1_122193/d130426p.pdf

Department of Defense. (2020). Recommendations to improve racial and ethnic diversity and inclusion in the U.S. military. Department of Defense Board on Diversity and Inclusion. Retrieved May 21, 2020 from https://media.defense.gov/2020/Dec/18/2002554852/-1/-1/0/DOD-DIVERSITY-AND-INCLUSION-FINAL-BOARD-REPORT.PDF

Devine, D. T., McMillan, S. C., Kip, K., & Powell-Cope, G. (2020). Quality of life among women veterans. *Journal of the American Association of Nurse Practitioners, 32*(11), 745–755. https://doi.org/10.1097/JXX.0000000000000445

Elbogen, E. B., Molloy, K., Wagner, H. R., Kimbrel, N. A., Beckham, J. C., Van Male, L., Leinbach, J., & Bradford, D. W. (2020). Psychosocial protective factors and suicidal ideation: Results from a national longitudinal study of veterans. *Journal of Affective Disorders, 260*, 703–709. https://doi.org/10.1016/j.jad.2019.09.062

Executive Order No. 13,822. 3CFR, 1513-1514. (January 2, 2018). https://www.federalregister.gov/documents/2018/01/12/2018-00630/supporting-our-veterans-during-their-transition-from-uniformed-service-to-civilian-life

Friedman, M. (n.d.). PTSD History and overview. PTSD: National Center for PTSD. U.S. Department of Veterans Affairs. Retrieved April 2, 2021 from History of PTSD in Veterans: Civil War to DSM-5 - PTSD: National Center for PTSD (va.gov)

Fogle, B. M., Tsai, J., Mota, N., Harpaz-Rotem, I., Krystal, J. H., Southwick, S. M., & Pietrzak, R. H. (2020). The National Health and Resilience in Veterans Study: A narrative review and future directions. *Frontiers in Psychiatry, 11*, 538218. https://doi.org/10.3389/fpsyt.2020.538218

Forkus, S. R., Rosellini, A. J., Monteith, L. L., Contractor, A. A., & Weiss, N. H. (2020). Military sexual trauma and alcohol misuse among military veterans: The roles of negative and positive emotion dysregulation. *Psychological Trauma : Theory, Research, Practice and Policy, 12*(7), 716–724. https://doi.org/10.1037/tra0000604

Frueh, B. C., Madan, A., Fowler, J. C., Stomberg, S., Bradshaw, M., Kelly, K., Weinstein, B., Luttrell, M., Danner, S. G., & Beidel, D. C. (2020). "Operator syndrome": A unique constellation of medical and behavioral health-care needs of military special operation forces. *International Journal of Psychiatry in Medicine, 55*(4), 281–295. https://doi.org/10.1177/0091217420906659

Fuehrlein, B. S., Kachadourian, L. K., DeVylder, E. K., Trevisan, L. A., Potenza, M. N., Krystal, J. H., Southwick, S. M., & Pietrzak, R. H. (2018). Trajectories of alcohol consumption in U.S. military veterans: Results from the National Health and Resilience in Veterans Study. *The American Journal on Addictions*, 10.1111/ajad.12731. Advance online publication. https://doi.org/10.1111/ajad.12731

Gilmore, A. K., Davis, M. T., Grubaugh, A., Resnick, H., Birks, A., Denier, C., Muzzy, W., Tuerk, P., & Acierno, R. (2016). "Do you expect me to receive PTSD care in a setting where most of the other patients remind me of the perpetrator?": Home-based telemedicine to address barriers to care unique to military sexual trauma and veterans affairs hospitals. *Contemporary Clinical Trials, 48*, 59–64. https://doi.org/10.1016/j.cct.2016.03.004

Gorbulja-Maldonado, A. (2020). 'We can do it:' The history of women in military service. The American Legion. Retrieved March 3, 2021 from https://www.legion.org/womenveterans/248582/%E2%80%98we-can-do-it-history-women-military-service#:~:text=President%20Truman's%20determination%20to%20make,members%20of%2-0the%20armed%20forces.

Gould, C. E., Rideaux, T., Spira, A. P., & Beaudreau, S. A. (2015). Depression and anxiety symptoms in male veterans and non-veterans: The Health and Retirement Study. *International Journal of Geriatric Psychiatry, 30*(6), 623–630. https://doi.org/10.1002/gps.4193

Grinberg, K., Sela, Y., & Nissanholtz-Gannot, R. (2020). New insights about chronic pelvic pain syndrome (CPPS). *International Journal of Environmental Research and Public Health*, *17*(9), 3005. https://doi.org/10.3390/ijerph17093005

Gross, G. M., Ronzitti, S., Combellick, J. L., Decker, S. E., Mattocks, K. M., Hoff, R. A., Haskell, S. G., Brandt, C. A., & Goulet, J. L. (2020). Sex differences in military sexual trauma and severe self-directed violence. *American Journal of Preventive Medicine*, *58*(5), 675–682. https://doi.org/10.1016/j.amepre.2019.12.006

Hoge, C. W., McGurk, D., Thomas, J. L., Cox, A. L., Engel, C. C., & Castro, C. A. (2008). Mild traumatic brain injury in U.S. Soldiers returning from Iraq. *The New England Journal of Medicine*, *358*(5), 453–463. https://doi.org/10.1056/NEJMoa072972

Ijadi-Maghsoodi, R., Feller, S., Ryan, G. W., Altman, L., Washington, D. L., Kataoka, S., & Gelberg, L. (2021). A sector wheel approach to understanding the needs and barriers to services among homeless-experienced veteran families. *Journal of the American Board of Family Medicine: JABFM*, *34*(2), 309–319. https://doi.org/10.3122/jabfm.2021.02.200331

Inhofe, J. J., Reed, J., Smith, A., Thornberry, M. (2019). Transitioning servicemembers: Information on military employment assistance centers. U.S. Government Accountability Office (GAO). GAO-19-438R. Retrieved March 17, 2021 from https://www.gao.gov/products/gao-19-438r

Jasuja, G. K., Bettano, A., Smelson, D., Bernson, D., Rose, A. J., Byrne, T., Berlowitz, D. R., McCullough, M. B., & Miller, D. R. (2021). Homelessness and veteran status in relation to nonfatal and fatal opioid overdose in Massachusetts. *Medical Care*, *59*(Suppl 2), S165–S169. https://doi.org/10.1097/MLR.0000000000001437

Joining Forces. (n.d.) Taking action to serve America's military families. Retrieved April 6, 2021 from https://obamawhitehouse.archives.gov/joiningforces/about

Jones, D. S. (2019). In search of historical insight into the problem of military suicide. *JAMA Network Open*, *2*(12), e1917498. https://doi.org/10.1001/jamanetworkopen.2019.17498

Litz, B. T., Stein, N., Delaney, E., Lebowitz, L., Nash, W. P., Silva, C., & Maguen, S. (2009). Moral injury and moral repair in war veterans: A preliminary model and intervention strategy. *Clinical Psychology Review*, *29*(8), 695–706. https://doi.org/10.1016/j.cpr.2009.07.003

Lin, L. A., Bohnert, A., Blow, F. C., Gordon, A. J., Ignacio, R. V., Kim, H. M., & Ilgen, M. A. (2021). Polysubstance use and association with opioid use disorder treatment in the US Veterans Health Administration. *Addiction*, *16*(1), 96–104. https://doi.org/10.1111/add.15116

Lippa, S. M., Fonda, J. R., Fortier, C. B., Amick, M. A., Kenna, A., Milberg, W. P., & McGlinchey, R. E. (2015). Deployment-related psychiatric and behavioral conditions and their association with functional disability in OEF/OIF/OND veterans. *Journal of Traumatic Stress*, *28*(1), 25–33. https://doi.org/10.1002/jts.21979

Liu, Y., Collins, C., Wang, K., Xie, X., & Bie, R. (2019). The prevalence and trend of depression among veterans in the United States. *Journal of Affective Disorders*, *245*, 724–727. https://doi.org/10.1016/j.jad.2018.11.031

Livingston, N. A., Berke, D., Scholl, J., Ruben, M., & Shipherd, J. C. (2020). Addressing diversity in PTSD treatment: Clinical considerations and guidance for the treatment of PTSD in LGBTQ Populations. *Current Treatment Options in Psychiatry*, 1–17. Advance online publication. https://doi.org/10.1007/s40501-020-00204-0

Livingston, W. S., Fargo, J. D., Gundlapalli, A. V., Brignone, E., & Blais, R. K. (2020). Comorbid PTSD and depression diagnoses mediate the association of military sexual trauma and suicide and intentional self-inflicted injury in VHA-enrolled Iraq/Afghanistan veterans, 2004–2014. *Journal of Affective Disorders*, *274*, 1184–1190. https://doi.org/10.1016/j.jad.2020.05.024

Klap, R., Darling, J. E., Hamilton, A. B., Rose, D. E., Dyer, K., Canelo, I., Haskell, S., & Yano, E. M. (2019). Prevalence of stranger harassment of women veterans at Veterans Affairs Medical Centers and impacts on delayed and missed care. *Women's Health Issues: Official Publication of the Jacobs Institute of Women's Health*, *29*(2), 107–115. https://doi.org/10.1016/j.whi.2018.12.002

Macia, K. S., Raines, A. M., Maieritsch, K. P., & Franklin, C. L. (2020). PTSD networks of veterans with combat versus non-combat types of index trauma. *Journal of Affective Disorders*, *277*, 559–567. https://doi.org/10.1016/j.jad.2020.08.027

Maguen, S., Griffin, B. J., Copeland, L. A., Perkins, D. F., Finley, E. P., & Vogt, D. (2020). Gender differences in prevalence and outcomes of exposure to potentially morally injurious events among post-9/11 veterans. *Journal of Psychiatric Research*, *130*, 97–103. https://doi.org/10.1016/j.jpsychires.2020.06.020

McHugh, R. K., & Weiss, R. D. (2019). Alcohol use disorder and depressive disorders. *Alcohol Research: Current Reviews*, *40*(1), arcr.v40.1.01. https://doi.org/10.35946/arcr.v40.1.01

Meyer, E. C., Kotte, A., Kimbrel, N. A., DeBeer, B. B., Elliott, T. R., Gulliver, S. B., & Morissette, S. B. (2019). Predictors of lower-than-expected posttraumatic symptom severity in war veterans: The influence of personality, self-reported trait resilience, and psychological flexibility. *Behaviour Research and Therapy*, *113*, 1–8. https://doi.org/10.1016/j.brat.2018.12.005

Moyo, P., Zhao, X., Thorpe, C. T., Thorpe, J. M., Sileanu, F. E., Cashy, J. P., Hale, J. A., Mor, M. K., Radomski, T. R., Donohue, J. M., Hausmann, L., Hanlon, J. T., Good, C. B., Fine, M. J., & Gellad, W. F. (2019). Dual receipt of prescription opioids from the Department of Veterans Affairs and Medicare Part D and prescription opioid overdose death among veterans: A nested case-control study. *Annals of Internal Medicine*, *170*(7), 433–442. https://doi.org/10.7326/M18-2574

Nahin, R. L. (2017). Severe pain in veterans: The effect of age and sex, and comparisons with the general population. *The Journal of Pain*, *18*(3), 247–254. https://doi.org/10.1016/j.jpain.2016.10.021

National Coalition for Homeless Veterans. (n.d.). Background & statistics. Retrieved April 23, 2021 from https://nchv.org/index.php/news/media/background_and_statistics/

National Institute on Drug Abuse (NIDA). (2019). Substance use and military life drugfacts. National Institutes of Health. Retrieved on April 14, 2021 from https://www.drugabuse.gov/publications/drugfacts/substance-use-military-life

Nichter, B., Haller, M., Norman, S., & Pietrzak, R. H. (2020). Risk and protective factors associated with comorbid PTSD and depression in U.S. military veterans: Results from the National Health and Resilience in Veterans Study. *Journal of Psychiatric Research*, *121*, 56–61. https://doi.org/10.1016/j.jpsychires.2019.11.008

Nichter, B., Hill, M., Norman, S., Haller, M., & Pietrzak, R. H. (2020). Associations of childhood abuse and combat exposure with suicidal ideation and suicide attempt in U.S. military veterans: A nationally representative study. *Journal of Affective Disorders*, *276*, 1102–1108. https://doi.org/10.1016/j.jad.2020.07.120

O'Neil, M. E., Carlson, K. F., Holmer, H. K., Ayers, C. K., Morasco, B. J., Kansagara, D., & Kondo, K. (2020). *Chronic Pain in Veterans and Servicemembers with a History of Mild Traumatic Brain Injury: A Systematic Review*. Department of Veterans Affairs (US).

Osório, C., Jones, N., Jones, E., Robbins, I., Wessely, S., & Greenberg, N. (2018). Combat experiences and their relationship to post-traumatic stress disorder symptom clusters in UK military personnel deployed to Afghanistan. *Behavioral Medicine (Washington, D.C.)*, *44*(2), 131–140. https://doi.org/10.1080/08964289.2017.1288606

Pedersen, E. R., Bouskill, K. E., Holliday, S. B., Cantor, J., Smucker, S., Mizel, M. L., Skrabala, L., Kofner, A., & Tannielian, T. (2020). *Improving substance use care: Addressing barriers to expanding integrated treatment options for Post-9/11 veterans*. Rand Corp.

Pedroso, J. L., Linden, S. C., Barsottini, O. G., Filho, M. P., & Lees, A. J. (2017). The relationship between the First World War and neurology: 100 years of "Shell Shock". *Arquivos de Neuro-psiquiatria*, *75*(5), 317–319. https://doi.org/10.1590/0004-282X20170046

Phipps, H., Mondello, S., Wilson, A., Dittmer, T., Rohde, N. N., Schroeder, P. J., Nichols, J., McGirt, C., Hoffman, J., Tanksley, K., Chohan, M., Heiderman, A., Abou Abbass, H., Kobeissy, F., & Hinds, S. (2020). Characteristics and impact of U.S. military blast-related mild traumatic brain injury: A systematic review. *Frontiers in Neurology*, *11*, 559318. https://doi.org/10.3389/fneur.2020.559318

Priebe, K., Kleindienst, N., Schropp, A., Dyer, A., Krüger-Gottschalk, A., Schmahl, C., Steil, R., & Bohus, M. (2018). Defining the index trauma in post-traumatic stress disorder patients with multiple trauma exposure: Impact on severity scores and treatment effects of using worst single incident versus multiple traumatic events. *European Journal of Psychotraumatology*, *9*(1), 1486124. https://doi.org/10.1080/20008198.2018.1486124

Pruitt, L. D., Smolenski, D. J., Bush, N. E., Tucker, J., Issa, F., Hoyt, T. V., & Reger, M. A. (2019). Suicide in the military: Understanding rates and risk factors across the United States' Armed Forces. *Military Medicine*, *184*(Suppl 1), 432–437. https://doi.org/10.1093/milmed/usy296

Reyes, J., Shaw, L. E., Lund, H., Heber, A., & VanTil, L. (2020). Prevalence of chronic musculoskeletal pain among active and retired military personnel: A systematic review protocol. *JBI Evidence Synthesis*, *19*(2), 426–431. https://doi.org/10.11124/JBISRIR-D-19-00392

Rhee, T. G., & Rosenheck, R. A. (2019). Comparison of opioid use disorder among male veterans and non-veterans: Disorder rates, socio-demographics, co-morbidities, and quality of life. *The American Journal on Addictions*, *28*(2), 92–100. https://doi.org/10.1111/ajad.12861

Riva, J. J., Noor, S. T., Wang, L., Ashoorion, V., Foroutan, F., Sadeghirad, B., Couban, R., & Busse, J. W. (2020). Predictors of prolonged opioid use after initial prescription for acute musculoskeletal injuries in adults: A systematic review and meta-analysis of observational studies.

Annals of Internal Medicine, *173*(9), 721–729. https://doi.org/10.7326/M19-3600

Sandbrink, F., Oliva, E. M., McMullen, T. L., Aylor, A. R., Harvey, M. A., Christopher, M. L., Cunningham, F., Minegishi, T., Emmendorfer, T., & Perry, J. M. (2020). Opioid prescribing and opioid risk mitigation strategies in the Veterans Health Administration. *Journal of general Internal Medicine*, *35*(Suppl 3), 927–934. https://doi.org/10.1007/s11606-020-06258-3

Schuyler, A. C., Klemmer, C., Mamey, M. R., Schrager, S. M., Goldbach, J. T., Holloway, I. W., & Castro, C. A. (2020). Experiences of sexual harassment, stalking, and sexual assault during military service among LGBT and non-LGBT service members. *Journal of Traumatic Stress*, *33*(3), 257–266. https://doi.org/10.1002/jts.22506

Smith, J. A., Doidge, M., Hanoa, R., & Frueh, B. C. (2019). A historical examination of military records of US Army Suicide, 1819 to 2017. *JAMA Network Open*, *2*(12), e1917448. https://doi.org/10.1001/jamanetworkopen.2019.17448

Stein, M. B., & Rothbaum, B. O. (2018). 175 years of progress in PTSD therapeutics: Learning from the past. *The American Journal of Psychiatry*, *175*(6), 508–516. https://doi.org/10.1176/appi.ajp.2017.17080955

Straus, E., Norman, S. B., Haller, M., Southwick, S. M., Hamblen, J. L., & Pietrzak, R. H. (2019). Differences in protective factors among U.S. Veterans with posttraumatic stress disorder, alcohol use disorder, and their comorbidity: Results from the National Health and Resilience in Veterans Study. *Drug and Alcohol Dependence*, *194*, 6–12. https://doi.org/10.1016/j.drugalcdep.2018.09.011

Straus, E., Norman, S. B., & Pietrzak, R. H. (2020). Determinants of new-onset alcohol use disorder in U.S. military veterans: Results from the National Health and Resilience in Veterans Study. *Addictive Behaviors*, *105*, 106313. https://doi.org/10.1016/j.addbeh.2020.106313

Tackett, B. (2019). Drug use in wartime. American Addiction Centers. Retrieved April 14, 2021 from https://www.recovery.org/addiction/wartime/

Teeters, J. B., Lancaster, C. L., Brown, D. G., & Back, S. E. (2017). Substance use disorders in military veterans: Prevalence and treatment challenges. *Substance Abuse and Rehabilitation*, *8*, 69–77. https://doi.org/10.2147/SAR.S116720

Theis, J., Hoops, K., Booty, M., Nestadt, P., & Crifasi, C. (2020). Firearm suicide among veterans of the U.S. military: A systematic review. *Military Medicine*, usaa495. Advance online publication. https://doi.org/10.1093/milmed/usaa495

Title 38 U.S. Code § 1720D–Counseling and Treatment for Sexual Trauma. Retrieved March 30, 2021 from https://www.govinfo.gov/content/pkg/USCODE-2011-title38/pdf/USCODE-2011-title38-partII-chap17-subchapII-sec1720D.pdf

Torreon, B. S. (2020). U.S. periods of war and dates of recent conflicts. Congressional Research Service. RS21405 Retrieved on April 28, 2021 from https://crsreports.congress.gov

Tsai, J., Schick, V., Hernandez, B., & Pietrzak, R. H. (2020). Is homelessness a traumatic event? Results from the 2019–2020 National Health and Resilience in Veterans Study. *Depression and Anxiety*, *37*(11), 1137–1145. https://doi.org/10.1002/da.23098

U.S. Department of Veterans Affairs. (2019). Women veterans health care: Facts and statistics about women veterans. Retrieved April 11, 2021 from https://www.womenshealth.va.gov/womenshealth/latestinformation/facts.asp

U.S. Department of Veterans Affairs. (2020a). Top 10 things all healthcare and service professionals should know about VA services for veterans who experienced military sexual trauma (MST). Retrieved March 31, 2021 from https://www.mentalhealth.va.gov/docs/top_10_public.pdf

U.S. Department of Veterans Affairs, Office of Mental Health and Suicide Prevention. (2020b). National Veteran Suicide Prevention Annual Report. Retrieved April 6, 2021 from https://www.mentalhealth.va.gov/docs/data-sheets/2020/2020-National-Veteran-Suicide-Prevention-Annual-Report-11-2020-508.pdf.

U.S. Department of Veterans Affairs. (2021a). History- VA history. Retrieved March 11, 2021 from https://www.va.gov/about_va/vahistory.asp

U.S. Department of Veterans Affairs. (2021b). Veterans experiencing homeless. Retrieved April 23, 2021 from https://www.va.gov/homeless/

U.S. Department of Veterans Affairs, Office of Suicide Prevention. (2018). VA Office of Mental Health and Suicide Prevention Guidebook. Retrieved on April 11, 2021 from https://www.mentalhealth.va.gov/docs/VA-Office-of-Mental-Health-and-Suicide-Prevention-Guidebook-June-2018-FINAL-508.pdf.

U.S. Department of Veterans Affairs, Office of Suicide Prevention. (2016). Suicide among veterans and other Americans. Retrieved April 8, 2021 from https://www.sprc.org/sites/default/files/resource-program/2016suicidedatareport.pdf

U.S. Department of Veterans Affairs. (n.d.a). VA Nursing Academic Partnerships. Office of Academic Affiliations. Retrieved April 6, 2021 from https://www.va.gov/oaa/vanap/

U.S. Department of Veterans Affairs. (n.d.b). Military sexual trauma. Mental Health Retrieved April 27, 2021 from https://www.mentalhealth.va.gov/mentalhealth/msthome/index.asp

U.S. Department of Veterans Affairs. n.d. VA History In Brief. Retrieved May 24, 2021 from https://www.va.gov/opa/publications/archives/docs/history_in_brief.pdf

Vespa, J. E. (2020). Those who served: America's veterans from World War II to the War on Terror. American Community Survey Report. U.S. Census Bureau. Retrieved March 10, 2021 from https://www.census.gov/content/dam/Census/library/publications/2020/demo/acs-43.pdf

Vogt, D. S., Tyrell, F. A., Bramande, E. A., Nillni, Y. I., Taverna, E. C., Finley, E. P., Perkins, D. F., & Copeland, L. A. (2020). U.S. Military veterans' health and well-being in the first year after service. *American Journal of Preventive Medicine*, *58*(3), 352–360. https://doi.org/10.1016/j.amepre.2019.10.016

Weathers, F. W., Bovin, M. J., Lee, D. J., Sloan, D. M., Schnurr, P. P., Kaloupek, D. G., Keane, T. M., & Marx, B. P. (2018). The Clinician-Administered PTSD Scale for DSM-5 (CAPS-5): Development and initial psychometric evaluation in military veterans. *Psychological Assessment*, *30*(3), 383–395. https://doi.org/10.1037/pas0000486

Wolff, K. B., & Mills, P. D. (2016). Reporting military sexual trauma: A mixed-methods study of women veterans' experiences who served from World War II to the war in Afghanistan. *Military Medicine*, *181*(8), 840–848. https://doi.org/10.7205/MILMED-D-15-00404

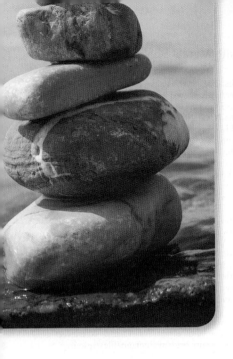

41

Care of Persons Who Are Experiencing Homelessness and Mental Illness

Mary Ann Boyd

KEYCONCEPT

- homelessness

LEARNING OBJECTIVES

After studying this chapter, you will be able to:

1. Define sheltered and unsheltered homelessness.

2. Describe risk factors for becoming homeless.

3. Describe challenges of persons who are experiencing homelessness and have a mental disorder.

4. Discuss personal and societal attitudes and beliefs about homelessness.

5. Describe nursing care of people who are experiencing homelessness and have a mental disorder.

6. Discuss the importance of advocacy for those who are experiencing homelessness with a mental illness.

KEY TERMS

- Assertive Community Treatment (ACT) • Continuum of Care • Day treatment • Housing First • Safe Havens
- Section 8 housing • Sheltered homeless individuals • Shelter Plus Care Program • Supportive housing • Transitional housing • Unsheltered homeless individuals

INTRODUCTION

Homelessness is a word that evokes images and feelings in everyone. Without a stable dwelling place, meeting basic needs is difficult. Homelessness means carrying all of one's possessions in a car, suitcase, bag, or shopping cart or storing necessities in a bus station locker or under the bed of a night shelter. It means no chest for treasured objects, no closet for next season's clothing, no pantry with food to eat, no place to entertain friends or have solitude, and no place for a child to play.

People who are experiencing homelessness tend to be ignored or not seen by the general population, who hurry on their own way. The homeless community is treated poorly by society and often suffers from acts of violence.

Many attacks go unreported. Hate crimes against the homeless community are a vital issue in the United States. Perpetrators of these acts are generally males under age 30 (National Coalition for the Homeless, 2018).

This chapter explores issues relevant to individuals who are experiencing homelessness and who are also experiencing mental health problems. It presents nursing care measures and suggests ways to improve services for the homeless population.

HOMELESSNESS AND MENTAL ILLNESS

Children, adults, and families can become homeless from encountering a natural disaster, home fire, some situational crisis or unexpected overwhelming life situation, or economic hardship. Others find themselves homeless because of problems related to substance use or mental illness. Box 41.1 lists characteristics of people who are experiencing homelessness and are mentally ill.

> **KEYCONCEPT Homelessness** is a lack of a fixed, regular, and adequate nighttime residence, which includes places not designed for or ordinarily used as a regular sleeping accommodation (i.e., car, park, abandoned building, bus/train station), as well as publicly or privately operated shelters or **transitional housing**, including a hotel or motel paid for by government or charitable organization.

The following criteria define homelessness in the United States:

- Individual or family who lacks a fixed, regular, and adequate nighttime residence

- Individual or family who will imminently lose their primary nighttime residence with no subsequent residence identified, and they lack resources or support networks to remain in housing

- Unaccompanied youth under 25 years of age, or families with children and youth who do not have permanent housing

- Any individual who is fleeing or attempting to flee domestic violence, dating violence, sexual assault, stalking, or other dangerous or life-threatening situations related to violence and lack resources or support networks to remain in housing (U.S. Department of Housing and Urban Development, 2021a).

Homelessness can be either sheltered or **Sheltered homeless individuals** obtain temporary or transitional housing operated by public and private agencies for individuals and families who do not have stable housing. **Unsheltered homeless individuals** live in places that are not used for housing, such as cars, parks, abandoned building, tents, or bus/train stations.

As the United States is emerging from the COVID-19 pandemic, homelessness will continue to be a national crisis. Homelessness has been increasing since 2016 as likely consequences of the national recession, economic disparities, and the pandemic (National Alliance to End Homelessness, 2020).

Epidemiology

The homeless population includes people of all ages, economic levels, racial and cultural backgrounds, and geographic areas. In January 2019, more than 560,000 people were homeless on a single night in the United States. Seventy percent of people experiencing homelessness are living on their own or in the company of other adults. The remainder are people in families with children. Sixty percent of all people experiencing homelessness are male. Most underrepresented groups are considerable in the homeless population, with African American individuals making up the largest group. Among individuals experiencing homelessness, one in two are unsheltered (National Alliance to End Homelessness, 2021).

Approximately, one-third of the total homeless population are persons with untreated serious mental illnesses. Many of these individuals suffer from schizophrenia, bipolar disorder, or major depression. Substance use is common, which further impairs these individuals. Many of these individuals were discharged from state and federal facilities with limited opportunities for housing and follow-up treatment. Studies show that persons with psychosis are more likely to be assaulted or threatened while homeless. Stigma and discrimination toward individuals remain pervasive across societies (Mejia-Lancheros et al., 2020).

Homelessness was a major problem for veterans since the early 2000s. Since 2011, the number of veterans experiencing homelessness had dropped by 43.3%, and since 2018, the number dropped another 2.1%. However, in 2019, still more than 37,000 veterans were homeless on a single night (National Alliance to End Homelessness, 2021).

Risk Factors

There are a variety of factors that place individuals and families at risk for homelessness. Adolescents and runaway youths can become homeless because of strained family relationships, family dissolution, foster care struggles, economic instabilities, and instability of residential placements. The consequences of COVID-19-related restrictions, such as remote learning, stay-at-home orders, increase the risk of homelessness for vulnerable youth. Young people experiencing homelessness may resort to drug trafficking and prostitution to support themselves. They are at risk for physical and mental health problems, including substance abuse, HIV infection or AIDS, pregnancy, and suicidal behaviors (Silliman Cohen & Bosk, 2020).

New immigrants and refugees can lose housing when they experience economic problems or conflicts with the sponsoring family or organization. Language barriers and citizenship/documentation status impede Latinx individuals' success in the rental market, increasing the risk of homelessness (Chinchilla & Gabrielian, 2020). Mental health problems arise because of torture experiences, losses suffered in the country of origin, culture shock, and discrimination experienced in the United States. Posttraumatic stress is common in this group; their physical health problems are often complex (Hasanović et al., 2020).

Migrant workers and their families lack residential stability as they move from one geographic region to another for 6 to 9 months of the growing and harvest season. These laborers and their families may be U.S. citizens or foreign born. They are poor and typically lack adequate living quarters and health care. Physical health problems and depression are common in these families. After farm labor is completed, family members may be homeless until they can return to their place of origin or to a relative's home (Blackmore et al., 2020).

Mental illness is significant risk factor for becoming homeless. Symptoms of mental illnesses often interfere with family relationships and impair judgments. Mental illness increases a person's vulnerability to be victimized (see Box 41.2).

The Experience of Being Homeless

The person who is experiencing homelessness spends time hunting for shelter, food, and clothing and lacks consistent ways to meet basic needs. They are at higher risk for disease, infection, and exposure to the coronavirus (Shinn & Viron, 2020). This lifestyle, plus grinding poverty and victimization, especially if the person is mentally ill, leaves little energy for change or reentrance into mainstream society. Panhandling, hustling, doing odd jobs, and selling plasma or aluminum cans are common sources of income, although some people who are homeless receive Social Security or veterans' pension benefits. The longer a person is homeless, the more likely

---

BOX 41.2

Risk Factors for Homelessness among People with Serious Mental Illness

INDIVIDUAL RISK FACTORS

- Symptoms of mental illness, including unpredictable behavior; an inability to manage everyday affairs; and an inability to communicate needs, which results in conflicts with family, employers, landlords, and neighbors
- Youth and adults with a concurrent mental disorder and substance use are at high risk for eviction, arrest, and incarceration in jails or repeated admissions and short stays in mental hospitals
- Coexisting HIV or AIDS with mental illness, chemical use, or both
- Coexisting demographic and societal factors of poverty; single-parent family (usually female headed); dependent child; child in foster home; underrepresented groups; veteran status; single men and women; ex-offender released from jail or prison
- Coexisting physical illness or developmental disability
- Exposure to traumatic events repeatedly, resulting in posttraumatic stress disorder and deficits in independent living skills
- Exposure to victimization (physical and sexual abuse), especially if a family member was the perpetrator
- Inability to cope with or manage the requirements of family, community, or group living home
- Lack of high school education or equivalence
- History of war veteran

ENVIRONMENTAL RISK FACTORS

Mental Health System Factors
- Inadequate discharge planning with a lack of appropriate housing, treatment, and support services
- Lack of funding for community-based services
- Lack of integrated community-based treatment and support services for individual and group therapy, medication monitoring, and case management
- Lack of community-based crisis alternatives for housing, health care, and respite care for families with risk for rehospitalization and loss of residence
- Lack of attention to consumer preferences for autonomy, privacy, and integrated regular housing
- Changing environment, such as loss of home caused by natural or human-made disaster

SOCIETAL AND FAMILY FACTORS
- Lack of affordable housing; affluent economic times have caused housing prices to soar out of reach, to reduce construction of low-cost housing, and to create a tight rental market
- Insufficient disability benefits; Social Security income recipients are below the federal poverty level
- Lack of coordination between mental health and substance abuse systems
- Waiting lists to receive a subsidy that requires the person to pay only 30% of income for rent and utilities
- Lack of job opportunities for disabled people
- Stigma and discrimination; resistance to community housing for people with mental illnesses is widespread
- Poor family relationships; willingness to help the ill person is exhausted as relatives cope with frightening or disturbing behavior and receive insufficient help from the community or medical profession

Substance Abuse and Mental Health Services Administration. (2013). Behavioral health services for people who are homeless. Treatment Improvement Protocol (TIP) Series 55. HHS Publication No. (SMA) 13-4734. Rockville, MD: Substance Abuse and Mental Health Services Administration.

the person is to experience mental illness or engage in substance use (Montgomery et al., 2016).

The healthiest survivors seek support from others, maintain hope for the future, and strive to have valued lives and selves. They believe they are resourceful, can handle uncertainty, and can maintain health. Women with children who are experiencing homelessness have described the need to keep going for the sake of, and to avoid, losing their children. However, women living in temporary or transitional shelters are confronted with insecurity, lack of privacy, isolation, stigma, and disempowerment (Andrade et al., 2020). Some women have preexisting mental health problems that lead to homelessness, while others develop mental illness because of their homelessness. Domestic abuse is often an antecedent to homelessness (Duke & Searby, 2019; see Chapter 23).

Chronic Homelessness

A person is considered to be experiencing chronic homelessness when they spend more than a year in state of homelessness or have experienced a minimum of four episodes of homelessness over a 3-year period (U.S. Department of Housing and Urban Development, 2016). The experience of being homeless for a long time results in a sense of depersonalization and fragmented identity; a loss of self-worth and self-efficacy and a stigma of being "nothing," "a bum," "lazy," and "stupid" (Singh et al., 2019). They may have lived in poverty for years. People who are homeless are often chronically ill, jobless, or have recently lost all financial resources. Educational level varies greatly, from less than an eighth-grade education to doctoral degrees.

Some people wrongly associate all homelessness with mental illness, violence, and alcohol or drug addiction. A person who is homeless for the first time or for a few months is more likely to have a more positive outlook than a person who has been experiencing homelessness for a longer period of time because the chances of recovering economic and social status are greater. Biographies and research describe the tragedy and nightmare of being homeless (Mejia-Lancheros et al., 2020).

Homelessness and Hope

Deprivation of needs, the sense of isolation and stigma, and the lack of accessible resources may be of short- or long-term duration. In turn, self-confidence and sense of competence can be eroded. Persons who have been or are homeless and have mental illnesses have typically endured and coped with constraints or problems with extreme stressors or catastrophes and negative life events. Instilling a sense of hope and possibility of recovery from homelessness and mental illness is important. Many people who experience homelessness maintain hope and a positive attitude, which in turn helps them to reach out to help, take advantage of opportunities, and become part of the housed population (Karadzhov et al., 2020).

Federal Assistance

There are several federal programs that provide assistance to people who are homeless. The McKinney–Vento Homeless Assistance Act (Public Law 100–77, first passed in 1987 as the McKinney Act), signed by President Ronald Reagan and confirmed by President Bill Clinton, provides federal money for homeless shelter programs. This law established the U.S. Interagency Council on the Homeless that provided for the use of funds in a coordinated manner, and for programs to assist the homeless, with special emphasis on older adults, persons with disabilities, families with children, Native American individuals, and veterans. This program is funded through grants to the states.

Substance Abuse and Mental Health Services Administration (SAMHSA) recognizes that housing is critical to recovery from mental and substance abuse disorders and promotes safe, affordable, and permanent support housing in the community with access to benefits and services for individuals, families, and communities. SAMHSA has several initiatives to create safe places for people with mental illness and substance abuse. SAMHSA works closely with the U.S. Interagency Council on Homelessness to support and implement Opening Doors, the federal strategy to prevent and end homelessness. SAMHSA's programs emphasize the importance of employment and education as outcomes and core components of recovery (SAMHSA, 2020).

ETIOLOGY OF HOMELESSNESS

Homelessness has no single cause. People want to have a home and be part of a family or social group. People do not choose or purposefully maintain homelessness and living on the streets. Many factors—unemployment, lack of skills, mental illness, substance abuse, domestic violence—typically combine, with time, to cause the person or family to lose permanent housing. The series of events that results in having no home is the culmination of individual and environmental factors, including factors in the mental health system, society, and family or community (Box 41.3).

The reduction of psychiatric beds has had a huge impact on the increase in the number of persons with mental illness who are homeless. In 1955, there were 337 beds per 100,000 persons. The deinstitutionalization

---

BOX 41.3

Causes of Homelessness

- Poverty; history of childhood family instability
- Lack of affordable housing; doubling up with relatives or friends until the situation is intolerable
- Mental illness or substance abuse and lack of needed services
- Low-paying jobs; unemployment
- Domestic violence; flight from a violent home or abandonment; youth aging out of services
- Eviction for not paying rent; multiple movers
- Limited life coping skills; disturbing behavior
- Changes or reductions in public assistance programs
- Veteran status
- Prison release; having no money, job, or place to go

---

movement decreased the number of state hospital beds to 11.7 per 100,000 by 2016. Even though there has been an increase in community and private hospital expansions to provide mental health services, their beds are primarily occupied by insured patients who have voluntarily sought care (Fuller et al., 2017).

State hospitals that do exist dedicate most of their beds to those who have committed crimes and have court-ordered treatment. Even under these circumstances, there is often a 30-day to 6-month wait for a bed. Many "nonforensic" individuals are detained in emergency departments (EDs) until beds are available (Fuller et al., 2017).

Gentrification, upgrading of inner-city property so that it is affordable only to people who have the resources of upper-middle or upper economic levels, is increasingly a factor in creating homelessness among urban residents. Middle-class and upper-middle-class professionals, mostly White individuals, are relocating to the inner city. Thus, abandoned or substandard buildings are demolished to build modern condominiums or "lofts." People who reside in poverty-stricken urban areas cannot afford the new housing in their regenerated neighborhood. They are often displaced and are at risk of becoming homeless (Tran et al., 2020).

Family Response to Homelessness

Family homelessness, whatever its cause, has an especially adverse effect on children. Underprivileged children move two or three times within 1 year before becoming homeless and moving into a shelter. Children experiencing homelessness are generally school-aged or younger. These children have high rates of both acute and chronic health problems and are more likely than children who are not homeless to be hospitalized, have delayed immunizations, and have elevated lead blood levels. In addition, they are at risk for developmental delays and emotional

and behavioral difficulties. School attendance is disrupted frequently, and they are vulnerable to violence, either as victims or witnesses. Children who experience family homelessness, even for brief periods of time, are significantly more likely to be a victim aggressor or aggressor compared with those who have never experienced homelessness (Andrade et al., 2020).

Living in shelters is stressful for families for several reasons. Many shelters exclude men and adolescent boys older than 12 years; thus, family members are separated. Overcrowding prevents privacy and promotes loss of personal control. Stressors of poverty and reduced social support compound the trauma of these experiences.

A history of abuse and assault is common among homeless. Women have greater mental health concerns, higher rates of diagnosed mental health issues, suicidal thoughts and attempts, and adverse childhood trauma. Mothers who are experiencing homelessness have often left abusive relationships and have difficulty accessing shelter and health care (Milaney et al., 2020).

RECOVERY-ORIENTED CARE FOR PERSONS WITH MENTAL ILLNESS WHO ARE HOMELESS

It is beyond the scope of most mental health services to meet many of the urgent needs for individuals with mental illness who are homeless. The mental health system is often the first contact for the person who is homeless or facing homelessness. The mental health team should have a working knowledge and relationships with community resources that provide housing, physical health care, financial support, and legal support.

Teamwork and Collaboration: Working Toward Recovery

SAMHSA recommends a five-stage process in homeless rehabilitation for persons who are homeless with a mental illness. *Outreach and engagement* is the first step in the process and involves facilitation of the individual into behavior changes. Outreach and engagement involves recognizing the needs of people who are homeless for preventive and basic service and developing a trusting and supportive relationship with these individuals. *Transition to intensive care* occurs when individuals agree to accept health and/or financial benefits, substance abuse/mental health treatment. During this phase, the clinician maintains a relationship with the individual and works with any resistance or concerns the person has. *Intensive care* phase emphasizes the person's participation in defining and managing their own goals. The primary focus of this phase is mental health treatment, accessing benefits, attending to medical problems, accessing housing, and seeking preventive services, such as skills training. *Transition from intensive care to ongoing rehabilitation* is preparation for sustaining the process of recovery. Depending on the individual, some may move quickly into affordable housing and maintain an independent lifestyle. Others may need 1 or 2 more years of supportive recovery and housing. *Ongoing rehabilitation* is an open-ended phase in which people gradually establish an identity as no longer homeless. This stage includes an active and continuing supportive counseling relationship, participation in mental health treatment as needed, and continued participation in prevention programs as appropriate (SAMHSA, 2013).

Safety Issues

Safety needs are always a priority. If an individual is threat to others or self, safety interventions should be implemented. The person may be involuntarily hospitalized for stabilization of symptoms. Overdose of opioids or alcohol intoxication is also a priority care issue. Persons should be referred to emergency services. The nurse may be required to take immediate action to reverse the drug effects by administering naloxone. Other priority issues involve basic needs, including housing and food. Many persons who are homeless are fearful of being incarcerated and resist any attempts to provide shelter.

Screening, Brief Interventions, and Referral to Treatment

Screening, brief interventions, and referral to treatment (SBIRT) integrates initial screening with brief interventions or referral to treatment for people who may have substance use disorders and co-occurring mental disorders (see Chapter 42). SBIRT is particularly useful for individuals who are homeless. The screening requires little time—5 minutes to screen and 10 minutes to provide the interventions (SAMHSA, 2013).

Homelessness and COVID-19

People experiencing homelessness are at high risk for contracting coronavirus. Many people who are homeless live in congregate living settings and might not have access to basic hygiene supplies or shower facilities. Their exposure may negatively affect their ability to find safe housing and the mental health. COVID-19 infection increases the mortality disparity between those who are homeless and those who are not (Tsai & Wilson, 2020).

EVIDENCE-BASED NURSING CARE FOR PERSON WITH A MENTAL ILLNESS WHO IS EXPERIENCING HOMELESSNESS

A holistic perspective is essential for assessing any person or family unit who is experiencing homelessness. Assessing a person who has a mental disorder and does not have a home requires patience and skill. Generally, these individuals have not been following a recommended treatment regimen and are symptomatic.

Mental Health Nursing Assessment

The assessment begins at the point of the person's need; often, it is a physical need or health problem (Box 41.4). The person may be malnourished and most concerned about food and shelter. Because of negative past experiences with the health care system or providers or because of mental illness or substance use, the person may not allow a thorough physical examination or may refuse to answer questions about history at the first visit.

BOX 41.4

Assessment Tips for the Physical Assessment

- Use unobtrusive observation as a part of physical assessment. Some conditions will be immediately obvious. Other conditions may become apparent during the interview.
- Examine—look, touch, palpate, auscultate—the person to the extent that they allow. The person may resist anything more than a superficial conversation and observation. The nurse may need to perform initial palpation of the abdomen or auscultation of the lung through several layers of clothes. If the patient perceives the health care provider as too intrusive, the patient may leave the setting even though they are desperate for care.
- Listen carefully to what the patient does *not* say and pay attention to nonverbal as well as verbal expressions. Avoid unnecessary directness and probing. Give the person time to answer questions. The blood test or urine screen may have to wait; a patient, nonintrusive manner may ensure that the person returns for needed tests or screening.
- Determine whether the person has been prescribed medications in the past. Often, the person who is homeless is not taking medications, even if they are prescribed and essential. The person may have difficulty keeping pills dry and easily retrievable or paying for medications. A daily insulin injection, for example, may not seem practical. Or the person may have been mugged by another homeless person seeking to quiet addictive urges or to sell drugs for cash.

Physical Health Assessment

Provide privacy for any assessment. Be gentle. Avoid hurry. Explain the need for any physical examination. The person may feel very embarrassed about their physical appearance or body odor if there has been no opportunity for physical hygiene or clothing change. Observation of mucous membrane and skin integrity, including the face, torso, limbs, and feet, is essential. Explain your concern about the person's health status and the need to remove clothing, including shoes and socks, and to pull down underwear.

Realize that many people who are experiencing homelessness consider themselves well as long as they can get where they need to go. The individual may believe that refusing to admit illness is adaptive behavior. Be aware of the many health problems that may be present (Box 41.5). Children and adolescents who are experiencing homeless may experience any of those listed, plus diseases that are specific to their age group. If a woman is pregnant and experiencing homelessness, assess indications that she is at high risk for maternal or fetal complications.

BOX 41.5

Common Physical Health Problems Experienced by Homeless People

- Injuries, fractures, epistaxis, or edema from trauma, falls, burns, assault, gunshot wounds
- Influenza, colds, bronchitis, asthma, shortness of breath
- Hypothermia, hyperthermia
- Arthritis, musculoskeletal disorders, headaches, fatigue
- Diabetes mellitus
- Hypertension
- Cardiovascular and peripheral vascular diseases
- Malnutrition
- Pulmonary tuberculosis
- Infestations, such as lice or scabies
- Dermatitis, sunburn or frostbite, bruises
- Foot injury, blisters, calluses
- Sexually transmitted diseases
- Hypothyroidism or hyperthyroidism
- Kidney or liver disease
- Cancer
- Epilepsy
- Impaired vision, glaucoma, cataracts
- Impaired hearing
- Dental caries, periodontal disease

Psychosocial Assessment

Mental Status and Appearance

The mental status examination may have to be done over several sessions (see Box 41.6). Symptoms of schizophrenia may be difficult to differentiate from emotional responses to the stressors of experiencing a homeless

---

BOX 41.6

Assessment Tips for the Psychological Assessment

- Observe for behavior that indicates hallucination and try to validate.
- Listen for delusions or denial over time; try to sense what purpose these serve.
- Observe and listen to what the person defines as a problem and potential solution and what they consider to be a strength or coping strategy; validate and reinforce when applicable.
- View the person and their situation from the individual's perspective; be a patient, nonthreatening listener. Such an approach encourages the person to return regularly; the nurse can then observe the patterns of behavior.
- Determine the extent of stability or integration of the person's sense of self, cognitive appraisals, and overt behavior. Lack of integration or stability indicates the need for continued monitoring and therapy.

---

lifestyle. Required hypervigilance may augment suspicion or paranoid beliefs. The need for constant awareness of possibilities for meeting basic needs can augment self-preoccupation. Blunted affect, lack of communication, loose associations, ambivalence, isolation, and uncertainty may be the result of life on the streets and living in various places. Such symptoms or behaviors may be part of the homelessness experience and reflect healthy coping mechanisms and creative survival techniques rather than pathology.

Substance abuse should be considered because it is common among people who are homeless, including people with mental illnesses. Because people who are experiencing homelessness, especially those with psychiatric disorders, are often victims of crime and violence, the incidence of posttraumatic stress disorder among them may be higher than in the general population. Homeless women are especially in danger of being assaulted, abused, and raped.

When a child or adolescent is homeless, ask about the educational history, if the youth is enrolled in school, and about perceived progress. Homeless children often have difficulty with school; the school district may change every time the parent changes shelters or moves from a temporary residence. Determine whether the child has behavioral or emotional problems and whether they need special education services.

Behavioral Responses

The behavioral assessment should follow the one presented in Chapter 11. The nurse should recognize that the person who is homeless has their own way of being in the world. They may not have insight into their illness and deny that they have a mental health problem. Much of the behavioral assessment will be conducted through observation and listening to the person's explanation of events.

Stress and Coping Skills

Homelessness is stressful. It is important that the nurse understands how the person who is experiencing homelessness copes on a day-to-day basis. The nurse should ask the person how basic needs are met: How the client eats and sleeps? How does the person cope with experiencing homelessness?

Cultural Assessment

Cultural value differences exist between people who are experiencing homelessness and people in the dominant American culture, to which most providers of health care subscribe. Thus, providers and the person who is homeless and needs health care may experience cultural conflict in their norms of health and illness, basic value systems and priorities, and perceptions about health care. Health care providers expect patients, including those who are homeless and mentally ill or chemically dependent, to problem solve, become more independent, and be future oriented. These values affect assessment, treatment, and interactions with the person and can interfere with the nursing process and patient response to the health care system. Consider how the person perceives their everyday life and vary the assessment and therapy approach accordingly.

Support Network and Support System Assessment

Homelessness is an expression of and response to certain family, societal, or environmental conditions, as well as to individual factors. See Box 41.7 for factors included in

the social and family assessment. It is also important to consider that childhood abuse and prior trauma may be continuing to affect the person as a stressor or contribute to interpersonal crises.

Spiritual Assessment

Listen for expressions that convey a spiritual faith, a connection to a transcendent being, or a belief system that helps the person endure. Questions about the spiritual dimension may convey an invitation to talk about an aspect of life that is often ignored but that may be very important to the beliefs, and preferred practices will help determine relevant therapy approaches.

CLINICAL JUDGMENT

A person who is experiencing homelessness has several immediate needs. The first priority is safety from immediate harm to self or others. The next priority will depend upon the current housing situation—do they have safe shelter at night. The nurse should consider whether the gender, mental status, and history of mental disorders. Physical health needs should be a priority before addressing mental health needs.

THERAPEUTIC RELATIONSHIP

Self-awareness on the part of the nurse is important. Often people do not know how to respond to a person who is homeless and who asks for food, money, or interpersonal communication because they hold common stereotypical beliefs about homelessness. Nurses and teachers, for example, who are accustomed to caring for others and giving attention to people who ask for it may find themselves considering various myths when approached by a person who is homeless (Box 41.8). To respond appropriately, one must first examine these myths and one's own feelings about people who are homeless and mentally ill. Relating to people who are homeless requires a gentle and compassionate approach.

MENTAL HEALTH NURSING INTERVENTIONS

Interventions are to be directed at the social system, as well as at the individual or family level. Interventions should take advantage of community resources and the inner resources and support systems of the individual or family. Box 41.9 describes interventions that focus on the individual and social system.

BOX 41.7

Assessment Tips for the Social Assessment

- Ask about support systems, people who could be helpful, and what services have been or could be used.
- Determine whether the person is isolated from the family, and if so, if it is by personal choice rather than by family choice.
- Respect that the person who feels isolated may avoid talking about their biologic family.
- Explore if the patient views a homeless peer, local pastor, counselor, or another health care provider as "family" or as a support system.
- Convey genuine interest in the person and convey that others may also care. Questions may be the catalyst to reestablishing family ties.

BOX 41.8

Myths and Facts about People Experiencing Homelessness with Psychiatric Disorders

Myth #1. People choose to be homeless.
Fact: Most people who are homeless want what most people want: to support themselves, have jobs, have attractive and safe housing, be healthy, and help their children do well in school.
Myth #2. Housing is a reward for abstinence and medication compliance, and society shouldn't house people who have active substance use or mental disorders.
Fact: Housing may be the first step to becoming abstinent and/or entering treatment to address a variety of problems. From a public health perspective, adequate housing reduces victimization, hypothermia or hyperthermia, infectious diseases, and other risks to the population as a whole.
Myth #3. People who are homeless are unemployed.
Fact: Many people who are homeless are employed full or part time.
Myth #4. There are few homeless families.
Fact: Families become homeless for a variety of reasons.
Myth #5. People who are homeless aren't smart enough to make it.
Fact: Keeping things together while homeless takes ingenuity and experience. People who are homeless often have well-developed street skills, resourcefulness, and knowledge of the service system.
Myth #6. Those with substance use or mental disorders need to "bottom out," so homelessness is okay and provides a motivator to make behavioral changes.
Fact: People who have substance use and mental disorders are more responsive to interventions before they become homeless or when placed in housing.
Myth #7. Everyone stands an equal risk of homelessness.
Fact: Although any of us could find ourselves homeless in our lifetime, some people are at higher risk than others. If we can identify people at special risk of homelessness, we may be able to intervene earlier and prevent the devastating effects experienced by people who are homeless and have accompanying mental and/or substance use disorders.
Myth #8. All clients with substance use and mental disorders who are homeless require extensive, long-term care.
Fact: The process of recovery from substance abuse and mental illness is an ongoing and sometimes lifelong process, yet healing often begins with short-term, strategic interventions. Screening, brief intervention, and referral to treatment is a proven method for early intervention with substance use and mental disorders, and it can significantly reduce the impact and progression of illness.

Substance Abuse and Mental Health Services Administration. (2013). Behavioral health services for people who are homeless. Treatment Improvement Protocol (TIP) Series 55. HHS Publication No. (SMA) 13-4734. Rockville, MD: author.

BOX 41.9

Interventions for People Who Are Experiencing Homelessness

- Stabilize physical health status.
- Provide a list with addresses and telephone numbers of shelters and luncheon sites that provide food; discourage rooting through dumpsters and panhandling.
- Provide a list of facilities that are safe, including shelters that provide clothing, a safe place to sleep, and opportunity for basic hygiene and laundry.
- Give information on city ordinances that forbid sleeping on park benches, in building doorways, on sidewalk grates, at bus or train stations, in vacant buildings, or in viaducts.
- Explore sources of income, such as gathering and selling aluminum cans or engaging in temporary day labor. Discourage selling blood or plasma.
- Assist the person directly or by referral to pursue entitlements, such as Social Security, veterans, or other benefits.
- Explore how to stay safe. Even in a night shelter, the person who is homeless may not be safe from assault. It is difficult for the person who is homeless to know who is trustworthy; carrying a bag or case is usually considered a marker for being robbed on the streets.
- Explore how to secure privacy, which is difficult to achieve, and how to cope with loneliness, which can be overwhelming.
- Give a list of names, addresses, and telephone numbers of agencies that offer services and socialization, such as the local mental health agency, the local chapter of NAMI, or the local Emotions Anonymous group.
- Give information about meetings of Alcoholics Anonymous, Narcotics Anonymous, or Cocaine Anonymous if the person is using substances.

---

meaningful goals, but it is important that their primary needs are met. Hospitalization may be needed to treat illness symptoms and providing immediate shelter. The nurse should advocate for finding permanent housing, which is associated with mental health recovery (see Box 41.10).

Overcoming Barriers to Care

Cost and lack of insurance are the biggest barriers to health and hospital care for people who are homeless. Another barrier is the inability of this population to carry out treatment recommendations; survival is their first priority. Compliance with medication and treatment regimens is difficult because successful treatment requires collaboration, monitoring, time for medication and other measures to be effective, and a secure place to keep medication. People with mental disorders who are experiencing homelessness often cannot routinely get prescriptions filled. Medicine may be stolen. It is necessary for the person or family unit to have a place to keep medications that can be reached at the necessary times and to have access to primary care services for regular check-ups, assessment for adverse drug responses, and necessary blood monitoring.

Establishing Recovery and Wellness Goals

Prioritizing the patient's goals will guide the nursing care. The individual may only want to get a warm coat and a bus pass. The nurse should encourage the patient to identify

---

BOX 41.10

Recovery, Homelessness, and Mental Illness

Kerman, N., Sylvestre, J., Aubry, T., Distasio, J., & Schütz, C. G. (2019). Predictors of mental health recovery in homeless adults with mental illness. Community Mental Health Journal, *55(4), 631–640. https://doi-org.libproxy.siue.edu/10.1007/s10597-018-0356-3*

THE QUESTION: What are the strongest predictors of mental health recovery among homeless people with mental illness at baseline?

METHODS: Data from 2,187 participants who had a mental illness, were currently homeless, and 18 years of age were assessed for recovery, mental health symptoms, substance use, community integration, use of social services for 24 months.

FINDINGS: Having fewer chronic medical conditions, fewer mental health symptoms, having a diagnosis of a psychotic disorder, having a close confidante with whom to share personal information, being more involved in community activities, and feeling a greater sense of belonging in the community were most consistently associated with more positive recovery ratings.

IMPLICATIONS FOR NURSING: Many of the predictors for recovery occur within the context of permanent housing. Finding housing facilitates mental health recovery.

NCLEXNOTE The priority for people who are experiencing homelessness is meeting the basic needs—food, shelter, and so on. Care for the response to the mental illness is secondary. Use Maslow hierarchy of needs as the guiding framework when you are planning interventions.

Improving Quality of Life

Interventions that improve quality of life include providing food, clothing, and assistance with housing; addressing physical health problems; promoting safety and self-esteem; and educating the person to decrease the risk of victimization. A trusting relationship with the care provider and ongoing follow-up care is also necessary.

People who have been homeless for several years have greater difficulty readjusting to stability and need more time for healing, depending on illness severity, comorbidity, and available support system. People who are experiencing homelessness, including those with psychiatric disorders, become creative at surviving on the streets. Explore resources with the individual or family (see Box 41.9 for appropriate interventions).

Meeting Spiritual Needs

Depending on the person's beliefs, the nurse may explore ways to meet spiritual needs. In one study, respondents listed the following as ways to meet spiritual needs: pray and put trust in God, hope that things will get better, obtain strength from religious beliefs and say these beliefs to self daily, seek a religious worker and attend religious services, talk about the meaning of the life situation with someone who is understanding and caring, and read devotional material (e.g., the Bible or the Koran).

NCLEXNOTE Providing physical resources, social services, and social and legislative advocacy counter the negative social and emotional effects of homelessness for the person and family.

Evaluation and Treatment Outcomes

There are two outcomes for people who are homeless with a mental illness. Recovery from a mental disorder and living in a housing of choice are primary. In some instances, after the mental disorder is treated and in remission, housing, a job, and positive interpersonal relationships follow. In other instances, finding housing sets the stage for strengthening coping skills to address the mental disorder.

COMMUNITY SERVICES

Diverse services and integrated systems are essential to address all aspects of the life situations of people who are without a home and experiencing psychiatric disorders. Essential components include **Safe Havens** or stable shelters or residences, accessible outreach, integrated case management, accessible and affordable housing options, treatment and rehabilitation services, general health care services, vocational training and assistance with employment, income support, and legal protection. The agencies that provide these services must develop a physical and emotional atmosphere that conveys a sense of caring and community. Often, community agencies are located at one site, much like a shopping mall, so that the person or family does not have to travel to numerous separately located agencies to get their needs met.

Emergency Services

Some agencies provide a street or mobile outreach program. As part of this program, a van travels the streets to areas where homeless people are found outdoors. Food, warm coffee, hygiene kits, and blankets are the first steps in building trust between staff and homeless persons. The person who is homeless may accept an offer to be driven to a local shelter for the night. Following up the next day by van or bicycle provides a way to recontact the individual and invite them to the agency programs or take them to other social service or health care services. Luncheon sites for homeless people are a basic step in emergency services. Some agencies have a health clinic on site for treatment of minor problems.

Integration with Primary Care

Integrating crisis intervention with physical and medical care is essential for individuals with psychosis who are seeking service in a hospital ED. The ED is likely to emphasize triage and rapid disposition while administering essential care. The physical orientation supersedes care for the emotional status of the person. Medication should be supplemented by crisis intervention techniques. The developmental level of the person, regardless of age, should also be considered. Emergency shelters typically provide refuge at night, along with an evening meal and morning coffee. Shelters for homeless women and children usually allow them to remain during daytime hours as well. The child leaves the shelter for school; the mother may attend educational classes, counseling, **day treatment**, rehabilitation, or employment programs.

Housing Resources

Transitional housing may consist of a halfway house, a short-stay residence or group home, or a room at a hotel designated for people who are homeless. Some agencies have a transitional home and stabilization center where the atmosphere and staff are a model for residents, who work on specific goals and a treatment plan. Sharing housekeeping tasks; obtaining psychiatric stabilization; and attending residence group meetings, social skills and budgeting classes, day treatment programs, and vocational training are steps to independent housing and employment. A holistic program reduces readmission to the hospital and reentry to street dwelling.

Housing First is a homeless assistant approach that prioritizes permanent housing to people experiencing homelessness. This approach is adopted by communities in providing services to people who are homeless. It is guided by the belief that people need basic necessities like food and housing before they can attend to other issues such as recovery from a mental illness, secure a job, and develop meaningful relationships. Case management, living skills classes, and other services are provided as "wrap-around" interventions as needed. There is a direct relationship between the safety and security provided by the Housing First program and a decrease in psychiatric symptoms and chronic homelessness, with an increase in a sense of independence, choice, and mastery of living skills.

The HEARTH Act of 2009 consolidated the McKinney–Vento homeless assistance program, **Shelter Plus Care Program**, and Section 8 Moderate Rehabilitation single room occupancy (SRO) Program into one program known as the **Continuum of Care**. Shelter Plus Care provides long-term housing and supportive services for people who are homeless with disabilities, primarily those with serious mental illness, chronic problems with alcohol or drug use, or AIDS or related diseases (USDHUD,

2021b). **Section 8 housing** has been helpful to this population for many years. Section 8 federally subsidized housing units are supervised or operated by the state or city, for which tenants are responsible for paying one-third of the monthly income (e.g., Supplemental Security Income or Social Security Disability Insurance) toward rent. The difference between the tenant payment and the maximum fair market rental price is calculated as the federal Section 8 housing contribution to the housing provider.

Safe Haven programs are found throughout the United States and provide 24-hour residence for an unspecified duration. Safe Havens serve hard to reach people with severe mental illness who are on the streets and have been unwilling or unable to participate in traditional supportive services, meet the following criteria. A Safe Haven provides private or semiprivate accommodations and limits overnight occupancy to 25 persons (USDHUD, 2014).

Supportive housing, permanently subsidized housing with attendant social services, was previously considered too expensive. Today, communities are realizing that such programs for people who are mentally ill and homeless are a good investment. The person who is safely housed is less likely to use other acute care and publicly funded services, such as shelters, although case management services are needed. Use of acute psychiatric and medical services is reduced, and the person is less likely to be arrested or incarcerated (Fuller et al., 2017).

U.S. Military Veterans Services

The Veterans Administration has a national service dedicated to the care of homeless veterans with mental health problems. The Health Care for Homeless Veterans (HCHV) Program provides community-based residential treatment for homeless veterans. The HCHV serves as a hub for housing and other services that provide the Veterans Health Administration with a way to reach and assist homeless Veterans (Veterans Administration, 2021; see Chapter 40).

Case Management

Case management is essential in addressing an individual's needs and preventing the person from becoming lost in the complexity of community services (SAMHSA, 2013). Case management involves systematic assessment, planning, goal setting, counseling and other interventions, coordination of services, referral as necessary, and monitoring of the person's or family's needs and progress. It enhances self-care capability and quality of care, decreases fragmentation, provides for cost containment, and reduces unnecessary duplication of services or hospitalization. The case manager is the gatekeeper and facilitator who may at first network with services on the person's or family's behalf and then encourage them to deal directly with other service providers to obtain bus passes and transportation, children's services and supplies, medical or obstetric care, or housing. The nurse is the ideal team member or case manager because of knowledge about both psychiatric and physical diseases and the ability to develop therapeutic relationships and stay connected with persons or families who are homeless and with the health care system.

Rehabilitation and Education

Day Treatment Programs

Day treatment provides a bridge between institutional and community care for people with mental illness or substance abuse problems. Participation in structured day treatment programs can provide emotional and practical support and strengthen ties to community services and potentially to family and friends. A day treatment program can provide legal assistance, help with finding employment and independent housing, and a mailing address for people who are homeless. It can provide case management, assistance with goal setting and problem-solving, and psychiatric or medical care. The day treatment program may incorporate adult basic education classes to increase literacy and survival skills, and general education development (GED) classes for those who want a high school diploma, and computer skills to improve employment options. A Living Skills Program typically includes content in nutrition, budgeting, parenting, household and family management, tenant responsibilities and rights, and employment readiness. Such classes are especially useful to women who will no longer be receiving welfare benefits. The person can receive assistance applying for government benefits, if qualified, and obtaining identification, such as a birth certificate, if needed. The informal environment of day treatment programs promotes a feeling of camaraderie, self-confidence, trust in staff, and aspirations for independent living.

Alcohol and Substance Use Treatment

The structure of some day treatment programs included alcohol and substance abuse treatment. Sobriety or harm reduction is the goal; the person attends daily meetings, receives necessary psychiatric and medical treatment, and participates in all of the other activities and services available at the day treatment program. No one is terminated for relapse; the person is referred to more intensive services, including hospitalization, if necessary.

Employment Services

Job placement is most likely when an employment program teaches basic job-seeking skills (e.g., resume writing; interview skills; appropriate attire, hygiene, and behavior; and computer skills) and offers job training in settings that prepare the person for the real world and real jobs. Case management during employment training can increase self-confidence, teach budgeting skills and methods of coping with the stresses of regular employment, and link the person with community resources. It can also help to teach various skills for job retention and career development. The employment service should periodically follow up with both the employee and their employer to ensure a successful record and movement to independence.

Integrated Services

Assertive Community Treatment (ACT) programs focus on service delivery to the homeless and mentally ill population by a transdisciplinary team of 10 to 12 specialists with a 1:10 staff–client ratio. A single, integrated, mobile staff team uses outreach, case management, practical assistance and support, and rehabilitation services to maximize the possibility that the most disabled consumers will live independently in the community and have a good quality of life. The team provides counseling and advocacy; monitors the person's management of housing, income, medication use, and leisure activities; and provides opportunities for employment if appropriate. Substance abuse management and physical health care are provided as needed.

Ongoing social support groups; membership in day treatment programs; attendance at meetings of AA, Narcotics Anonymous, or Cocaine Anonymous; or the local National Alliance on Mental Illness (NAMI) or Mental Health Association can help the person remain in the community and live independently or with family. Support groups foster peer socialization and problem-solving, enhance self-esteem, and offer many activities (e.g., art and recreation therapy, legal assistance).

For a number of years, the SAMHSA and the Center for Substance Abuse Treatment have funded treatment programs for women and young children. Long-term stays have been found to predict positive treatment outcomes, including lower rates of drug use, criminal behavior, and unemployment. Improved parenting and mother–child relationships, less child abuse and neglect, improved developmental outcomes in children, and lowered costs for mother and infant health are other benefits.

Advocacy

Nurses can share experiences and research findings with the local chapter or national headquarters of NAMI and with state legislators and members of Congress who are involved in developing legislation and policies related to people who are homeless, mentally ill, and substance abusing. Continued advocacy is essential to convey the perceptions and needs of this population, to influence allocations for needed programs and services, and to end the social injustice of chronic homelessness.

SUMMARY OF KEY POINTS

- People who are experiencing homelessness are a heterogeneous, diverse group, some of whom have a mental disorder and a substance use disorder.

- There are many risks for being homeless.

- People do not want to be homeless.

- Meeting the needs of people who have a mental illness and are experiencing homelessness requires more than mental health services. Housing services are critical.

- The nursing assessment must be holistic; the nurse must listen to the person's perceptions and observe carefully.

- People who have a mental illness or substance use disorder and are without a home may have various physical health problems.

- Intervention must be oriented to the person's or family's perceived needs, culturally sensitive, and compassionate.

- People who have mental disorders and are experiencing homelessness may avoid traditional health care services.

- Nurses must incorporate new trends in providing and improving services for health care and social integration.

CRITICAL THINKING CHALLENGES

1. How do the effects of mental illness, substance use, and homelessness interact with one another?

2. What factors might interfere with the ability of the person who is mentally ill to participate in treatment? What is the impact of exposure to the coronavirus?

3. What barriers to communication might the nurse experience when relating to the person who is homeless and mentally ill?

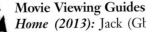
Movie Viewing Guides
Home (2013): Jack (Gbenga Akinnagbe) lives in a group home and is suffering from a mental illness. He wants to have his own home and reconnect with his son. When he moves into an apartment, he finds that living alone is more difficult than expected.

VIEWING POINTS: How does Jack illness limit his ability to maintain his independence? What does having his own place represent to Jack?

West 47th Street (2001, 2003): This documentary describes services offered by Fountain House, the original clubhouse for persons who are homeless and mentally ill, through the eyes of four clubhouse members. Fountain House has celebrated 50 years of providing services and is the model for more than 300 clubhouses nationwide. (This video is available for purchase from Lichtenstein Creative Media, 617-682-3700. Information is also available online.)

VIEWING POINTS: Discuss the range of services needed for people who are homeless and mentally ill. Visit a clubhouse program in your community and compare the services with those of Fountain House.

REFERENCES

Andrade, F., Simões Figueiredo, A., Capelas, M. L., Charepe, Z., & Deodato, S. (2020). Experiences of homeless families in parenthood: A systematic review and synthesis of qualitative evidence. *International Journal of Environmental Research and Public Health*, 17(8), 2712. https://doi.org/10.3390/ijerph17082712

Blackmore, R., Boyle, J. A., Fazel, M., Ranasinha, S., Gray, K. M., Fitzgerald, G., Misso, M., & Gibson-Helm, M. (2020). The prevalence of mental illness in refugees and asylum seekers: A systematic review and meta-analysis. *PLoS Medicine*, 17(9), e1003337. https://doi.org/10.1371/journal.pmed.1003337

Chinchilla, M., & Gabrielian, S. (2020). Stemming the rise of Latinx homelessness: Lessons from Los Angeles County. *Journal of Social Distress & the Homeless*, 29(2), 71–75. https://doi-org.libproxy.siue.edu/10.1080/10530789.2019.1660049

Duke, A., & Searby, A. (2019). Mental ill health in homeless women: A review. *Issues in Mental Health Nursing*, 40(7), 605–612. https://doi.org/10.1080/01612840.2019.1565875

Fuller, D. A., Sinclair, E., Lamb, H. R., Cayce, J. D., & Snook, J. (2017). Emptying the "New Asylums": Beds capacity modeling to reduce mental illness behind bars Treatment Advocacy Center. Arlington, VA. www.treatmentadvocacycenter.org/storage/documents/emptying-new-asylums.pdf

Hasanovié, M., Šmigalović, D., & Fazlović, M. (2020). Migration and acculturation: What we can expect in the future. *Psychiatria Danubina*, 32(Suppl 3), 386–395.

Karadzhov, D., Yuan, Y., & Bond, L. (2020). Coping amidst an assemblage of disadvantage: A qualitative metasynthesis of first-person accounts of managing severe mental illness while homeless. *Journal of Psychiatric and Mental Health Nursing*, 27(1), 4–24. https://doi.org/10.1111/jpm.12524

Mejia-Lancheros, C., Lachaud, J., O'Campo, P., Wiens, K., Nisenbaum, R., Wang, R., Hwang, S. W., & Stergiopoulos, V. (2020). Trajectories and mental health-related predictors of perceived discrimination and stigma among homeless adults with mental illness. *PLoS One*, 15(2), e0229385. https://doi.org/10.1371/journal.pone.0229385

Milaney, K., Williams, N., Lockerbie, S. L., Dutton, D. J., & Hyshka, E. (2020). Recognizing and responding to women experiencing homelessness with gendered and trauma-informed care. *BMC Public Health*, 20(1), 397. https://doi.org/10.1186/s12889-020-8353-1

Montgomery, A. E., Szymkowiak, D., Marcus, J., Howard, P., & Culhane, D. P. (2016). Homelessness, unsheltered status, and risk factors for mortality: Findings from the 100 000 Homes Campaign. *Public Health Reports*, 131(6), 765–772.

National Alliance to End Homelessness. (2020). Homelessness in 2021: Five factors to watch. https://endhomelessness.org/homelessness-in-2021-five-factors-to-watch/

National Alliance to End Homelessness. (2021). State of homelessness: 2020 edition. https://endhomelessness.org/homelessness-in-america/homelessness-statistics/state-of-homelessness-2020/

National Coalition for the Homeless. (2018). *Vulnerable to hate: A survey of bias-motivated violence against people experiencing homelessness in 2016–2017.* Author.

Shinn, A. K., & Viron, M. (2020). Perspectives on the COVID-19 pandemic and individuals with serious mental illness. *The Journal of Clinical Psychiatry*, 81(3), 20com13412. https://doi.org/10.4088/JCP.20com13412

Silliman Cohen, R. I., & Bosk, E. A. (2020). Vulnerable youth and the COVID-19 pandemic. *Pediatrics*, *146*(1), e20201306. https://doi.org/10.1542/peds.2020-1306

Singh, A., Daniel, L., Baker, E., & Bentley, R. (2019). Housing disadvantage and poor mental health: A systematic review. *American Journal of Preventive Medicine*, *57*(2), 262–272. https://doi.org/10.1016/j.amepre.2019.03.018

Substance Abuse and Mental Health Services Administration. (2013). Behavioral health services for people who are homeless. Treatment Improvement Protocol (TIP) Series 55. HHS Publication No. (SMA) 13-4734. Rockville, MD: Author.

Substance Abuse and Mental Health Services Administration. (2020). Recovery integration in homeless service urged. Retrieved February 11, 2021 from https://www.samhsa.gov/homelessness-programs-resources/hpr-resources/recovery-homeless-services

Tran, L. D., Rice, T. H., Ong, P. M., Banerjee, S., Liou, J., & Ponce, N. A. (2020). Impact of gentrification on adult mental health. *Health Services Research*, *55*(3), 432–444. https://doi.org/10.1111/1475-6773.13264

Tsai, J., & Wilson, M. (2020). COVID-19: A potential public health problem for homeless populations. *The Lancet. Public Health*, *5*(4), e186–e187. https://doi.org/10.1016/S2468-2667(20)30053-0

U.S. Department of Housing and Urban Development. (2014). Notice for Housing Inventory Count (HIC) and Point-in-Time (PIT) Data Collection for Continuum of Care (CoC) Program and the Emergency Solutions Grants (ESG) Program. Community Planning and Development. https://www.hud.gov/sites/documents/14-14CPDN.PDF

U.S. Department of Housing and Urban Development. (2016). Notice on prioritizing persons experiencing chronic homelessness and other vulnerable homeless persons in permanent supportive housing. CPD-11. https://www.hud.gov/sites/documents/16-11CPDN.PDF

U.S. Department of Housing and Urban Development. (2021a). Homeless definition. Criteria and recordkeeping requirements for definition of homelessness. https://files.hudexchange.info/resources/documents/HomelessDefinition_RecordkeepingRequirementsandCriteria.pdf

U.S. Department of Housing and Urban Development. (2021b). "Shelter Plus Care Program" [Online]. https://www.hudexchange.info/homelessness-assistance/hearth-act/

Veterans Administration. (2021). Health Care for homeless Veterans (HCHV) program. U.S. Department of Veterans Affairs. https://www.va.gov/homeless/hchv.asp

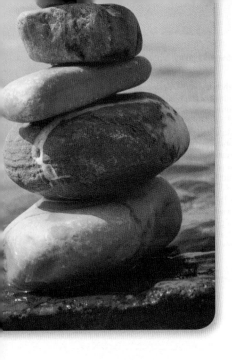

42
Care of Persons with Co-occurring Mental Disorders

Mary Ann Boyd

KEYCONCEPTS

- co-occurring disorders (CODs)
- relapse cycle

LEARNING OBJECTIVES

After studying this chapter, you will be able to:

1. Define the term *co-occurring disorders* (CODs).

2. Describe the cycle of relapse in COD.

3. Discuss patterns of substance use with other mental disorders.

4. Analyze barriers to the treatment of patients with COD.

5. Discuss the significance of integrated health care for persons with COD.

6. Apply a person-centered, recovery-oriented approach for persons with co-occurring disorders.

KEY TERMS

- Assertive Community Treatment (ACT) • Engagement • Integrated treatment • Motivational interventions
- Quadrants of care • Relapse prevention • Recovery • Self-medicate

---

| **KEYCONCEPT The term co-occurring disorders** (COD) refers to coexistence of a mental and a substance use disorder (SUD) in the same person.

INTRODUCTION

Mental disorders and SUDs are each a primary mental disorder even though they do not necessarily appear at the same time. A diagnosis of COD means that at least one disorder of each type can be established independently. However, the person's experience, symptoms, and outcomes are influenced by the interaction of the two disorders, not just the discrete disorders.

The goal of treatment for patients with COD is a comprehensive recovery plan for the complex problems

presented—one that offers the patient a way out of what can be a downward spiral of debilitation. Effective treatment of COD requires an integrated approach based on both an understanding of mental disorder and addiction. **Integrated treatment**, coordinated substance use, and mental health interventions require modifying traditional approaches to both the mental disorder and addiction (Office of Disease Prevention and Health Promotion, 2021).

This chapter presents the epidemiology and etiologic patterns of COD and discusses specific mental disorders and the adverse effects of concurrent substance use. It highlights methods of assessing COD and offers treatment strategies and nursing interventions to address this complex yet common presentation in psychiatric and substance use treatment settings. A complete discussion of related SUDs is provided in Chapter 31.

CO-OCCURRING DISORDERS OVERVIEW

The problem of COD was inadvertently magnified during the community mental health reform movement when there was a rational movement toward deinstitutionalization of people with mental disorders (see Chapter 1). Large numbers of persons with mental disorders were left homeless, lost to local and state mental health systems. Their long-standing mental disorders and protected life in a state hospital increased their vulnerability to exploitation by others, particularly the more astute and streetwise addicts. Along with homelessness came the increased use of drugs and alcohol and discrimination (Mejia-Lancheros et al., 2020; see Chapter 41).

It is impossible to make any meaningful distinction between simple recreational use of a substance and actual substance use with this population because even small amounts of alcohol or other drugs can be damaging to people who have concurrent psychiatric problems. Substances of abuse exert profound effects on mental states, perception, psychomotor function, cognition, and behavior. The specific neurochemical and other biologic mechanisms that evoke these psychological features are discussed in Chapter 31. Table 42.1 lists the psychological effects of substances of abuse.

Clinical Course and Relapse

Although two types of disorders are diagnosed independently, people with COD respond to the interaction of two psychiatric disorders. In many instances, the use of substances serves as a coping strategy for dealing with psychiatric symptoms. Without alternative, effective coping behaviors, the patient will continue to self-medicate (using medication, usually over-the-counter medications, or substances without professional prescription or supervision, to alleviate an illness or condition). Persons with COD have lesser outcomes, such as higher rates of HIV infection, relapse, rehospitalization, depression, and suicide risk (Hides et al., 2019).

A frequent problem of this group is relapse, which leads to repeated hospitalizations or the "revolving-door" phenomenon. When symptoms of the mental disorder are stabilized, the hospitalized patient is discharged. Once in the community, the patient fails to follow the therapeutic regimen and resumes the use of alcohol or drugs. Reappearance of symptoms leads to another episode of hospitalization (Urbanoski et al., 2018). The relapse cycle is characterized by a pattern

TABLE 42.1	PSYCHOLOGICAL EFFECTS OF SUBSTANCES OF ABUSE
Substance	**Psychological Effects**
Alcohol	Alcohol amnestic syndrome, dementia
	Agitation, anxiety disorders, sleep disorders
	Ataxia, slurred speech
	Withdrawal symptoms, which may include hallucinations, confusion, illusions, delusions; protracted withdrawal delirium can occur
	Depression, increased rate of suicide, disinhibition
Cocaine	Anxiety, agitation, hyperactivity, sleep disorders, delusions, paranoia, euphoria, internal sense of interest, and excitement
	Rebound withdrawal symptoms, such as prolonged depression, somnolence, anhedonia
Amphetamines	Similar to cocaine but more prolonged Hyperactivity, agitation, anxiety, increased energy
Hallucinogens (MDMA, or Ecstasy) and phencyclidine	Hallucinations, delusions, paranoia, confusion
	Withdrawal can produce severe depression, somnolence
	Hallucinations, illusions, delusions, perceptual distortions, paranoia, rage, anxiety, agitation, confusion
Marijuana	Acute reactions: panic, anxiety, paranoia, sensory distortions, rare psychotic episodes; patients with schizophrenia use these reactions to distance themselves from painful symptoms and to gain control over symptoms
	Antimotivational syndrome: apathy, diminished interest in activities and goals, poor job or school performance, memory and cognitive deficits
Opiates	Confusion, somnolence
	Withdrawal can produce anxiety, irritability, and depression and can trigger suicidal ideation
Sedative–hypnotics	Confusion, slurred speech, ataxia, stupor, sleep disorders, withdrawal delirium, dementia, amnestic disorder, sleep disorders
Volatile solvents	Hallucinations, delusions, hyperactivity, sensory distortions, dementia

MDMA, 3,4-methylenedioxy-methamphetamine.

of decompensation, hospitalization, stabilization, discharge, and then decompensation (Fig. 42.1).

KEYCONCEPT In the relapse cycle, reemerging psychiatric symptoms lead to ineffective coping strategies, increased anxiety, substance use to avoid painful feelings, adverse consequences, and attempted abstinence until psychiatric symptoms reemerge and the cycle repeats itself.

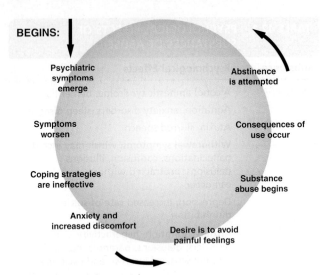

FIGURE 42.1 Relapse cycle.

Epidemiology

The pattern of alcohol and illicit drug use by those with a mental disorder varies, but it is estimated that as many as 9.5 million adults have both disorders (depending on definitions and methodologies). The most commonly used drug substance is alcohol, followed by marijuana and cocaine. Prescription drugs such as opioids and sleeping medicines may also be abused (SAMHSA, 2020a).

The risk for substance use varies among mental disorders. Antisocial personality disorders, bipolar depression, and disorders of childhood, including conduct disorders, oppositional-defiant disorders, and attention-deficit disorders, are strongly associated with SUDs. Having any SUD was associated with at least a threefold increased risk of completed suicide when compared with those having no SUD (Østergaard et al., 2017).

Etiology

There is no one model that explains why mental disorders and substance use occur together so frequently. In one pattern of occurrence, the mental disorder precedes the substance use. As adolescents with emerging mental disorders are exposed to drug use, their disinhibition and impulsivity lead to drug experimentation. Substances are used to self-medicate the underlying mental disorders. In the second pattern, the SUD appears first and leads to the mental disorder. For example, lysergic acid diethylamide (LSD) or cocaine use may change the neurotransmission in the brain that results in panic attacks or psychosis. In the third pattern, there are common causes, either genetic or environmental, that lead to the onset or persistence of both disorders.

Current research is beginning to explain a pattern: The symptoms of the mental disorder generally appear first, followed by the substance use and abuse. Psychiatric symptoms have long been associated with dysregulation of the monoamines and neuropeptides. Drugs of abuse (cocaine, alcohol, marijuana) temporarily potentiate neurotransmission in the brain's reward system, relieving the depression and anxiety for a short period of time. Self-administration of drugs of abuse temporarily masks or suppresses the aversive psychological effects of the dysregulated neuronal systems (see Chapter 31).

BARRIERS TO TREATMENT

High morbidity rates point to the need for effective treatment of individuals with COD. Although it was recognized that integrated treatment should be the standard of care, these patients often face major barriers in obtaining proper treatment. There are many well-documented barriers such as perceived shortcomings of substance use treatment systems, funding barriers, difficulty in communicating with substance use treatment providers, and difficulty reconciling different treatment approaches, and lack of staff (SAMSA). The following discussion highlights some other barriers.

Nature of Co-occurring Disorders

Patients often deny a problem with substances and do not seek treatment because they do not view themselves as needing it. They do not fully understand their mental disorder or the effect of substance use on their mood or behavior. Even those who recognize their disorders are often reluctant to seek mental health treatment. It is confusing to be expected to abstain from alcohol and illicit drugs yet be prescribed medication that also affects their thoughts and feelings. If they take the substance of choice, they experience fleeting moments of joy and escape even though doing so will prompt a decline in overall function and worsen psychiatric symptoms. If they accept prescribed treatments, including medications, they will have higher levels of functioning and better treatment outcomes, but they lose their moments of joy and escape.

Staff Attitudes

Mental health professionals in psychiatric treatment programs are often frustrated in their efforts to assist patients with SUDs. Behavior often associated with addiction, such as denial of substance use, manipulative behavior, and nonadherence with health-related protocols, is often regarded as a sign of treatment failure. This type of behavior can provoke hostility from the staff and can make planning for mental health recovery difficult.

Mental health professionals may have difficulty understanding the compelling nature of drug or alcohol cravings, may not understand differences in drug use patterns and behaviors associated with particular drugs of abuse, and may overdiagnose personality disorders in those who take drugs and commit crimes. In addition, patients or their therapists may excuse substance use because of the patients' psychiatric symptoms.

Stigma

Drug-dependent patients may have the additional stigma of being regarded as criminals because they commit illegal acts every time they purchase, use, or distribute illicit drugs. Strong public feelings about alcohol-related motor vehicle accidents, negative experiences with family members or friends with drinking problems, and cultural biases against public intoxication can prejudice interactions with patients who are alcohol dependent (Miler et al., 2020).

Health Issues

Numerous health hazards are associated with alcohol and drug use (see Chapter 31). The use of alcohol and illicit substances in addition to medications prescribed for mental disorders can lead to drug interactions and may exacerbate side effects of these medications. Homelessness can increase these patients' medical problems with inadequate nutrition, poor hygiene, and the adverse effects of exposure to the elements adding to their difficulties. Health care providers often become frustrated with patients' nonadherence and with what they see as behaviors that are difficult to manage. Their frustration may negatively affect the way they treat patients with COD. Because of the confusion about what is the primary and most immediate problem to treat, these patients are often underserved and only partially treated.

RECOVERY-ORIENTED CARE FOR PERSONS WITH CO-OCCURING DISORDERS

Treatment programs designed for people whose problems are primarily substance use are generally not recommended for people who also have a mental disorder. The **quadrants of care** model is a conceptual framework that classifies patients according to symptom severity, not diagnosis (Fig. 42.2). Developed in 2014, the quadrants of care model continues to be used today. The quadrant can guide an individual's treatment and site of delivery of care. In an integrated treatment model, treatment for both disorders is combined in a single session or interaction or series of interactions.

Patients with COD enter treatment at various stages of recovery. Flexible treatment programs that can meet each patient's needs are the most effective. **Recovery** is sought through commonly recognized stages of treatment, including engagement, persuasion or motivation, active treatment, and relapse prevention. This recovery involves much more than avoiding alcohol and drugs. Individuals must believe that life can be better without drinking, but typically, they test the alternatives before they adopt lengthy remissions (Bradizza et al., 2018). An integrated interdisciplinary team is needed in order to move patients to recovery.

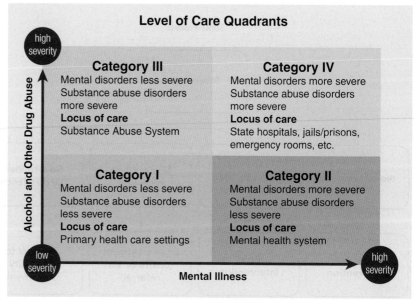

FIGURE 42.2 Level of care quadrants. (From Center for Substance Abuse Treatment. [2013]. Definitions, terms, and classification systems for co-occurring disorders. SAMHSA/CSAT Treatment Improvement Protocols. Rockville, MD: Substance Abuse and Mental Health Services Administration. Retrieved February 16, 2021 from http://www.ncbi.nlm.nih.gov/books/NBK25692.)

Screening, Brief Intervention, and Referral to Treatment

Substance Abuse and Mental Health Services Administration (SAMHSA) initiated and implemented the comprehensive, integrated public health model called screening, brief intervention, and referral to treatment (SBIRT), which provides for services on a full continuum of care, not only the substance use specialty. This intervention model targets people who do not yet meet criteria for SUD and provides strategies for early intervention before the need develops for specialized treatment. This model consists of universal screening, secondary prevention (detecting risky or hazardous substance use or dependence), timely referral, and treatment for people with SUD. This model has been implemented widely in the United States and other countries throughout the world (SAMHSA, 2020b; see Fig. 42.3).

Screening

The screening process identifies individuals who might be misusing or abusing substances but does not identify the exact kind of problem or its seriousness. Screening determines whether a problem exists or whether further screening is needed. Screening should be conducted using a validated instrument to classify the person's pattern of alcohol or drug use. Screening should take 5 to 10 minutes and can be repeated at various intervals over time. The Alcohol Use Disorders Identification Test (AUDIT) (Babor et al., 2001) and the National Institute on Drug Abuse (NIDA) Drug Use Screening Tool (NIDA, 2012) are examples of instruments that can be used. Screening can identify people across the whole spectrum of use—from risky to dependence.

Brief Intervention

A brief intervention is appropriate for persons who are at moderate risk for substance use problems. This is a **motivational intervention** that typically consists of one to several sessions during which the patient becomes interested in seeking treatment. This intervention focuses on increasing a person's insight into and awareness about substance use and behavior change. The primary goal of this stage is to educate the patient and increase their motivation to reduce risky behavior.

Brief Treatment: Brief Intensive Intervention

Brief treatment is a specialty outpatient treatment modality. It is a systematic, focused process that relies on patient engagement and implementation of change strategies. The treatment consists of 6 to 20 sessions of evidence-based, highly focused, and structured clinical sessions (e.g., solution-focused therapy, cognitive–behavior therapy, motivation enhancement). The goals of brief treatment are to change the immediate behaviors or thoughts about a risky behavior, to address long-standing problems with harmful drinking and drug misuse, and to help patients with higher levels of disorder obtain more intensive care. One goal of this intervention is to increase engagement in treatment and help the patient identify their own goals (DiClemente et al., 2017).

Engagement

Engagement entails establishing a treatment relationship and enhancing motivation to make behavior changes and a commitment to treatment. Research has

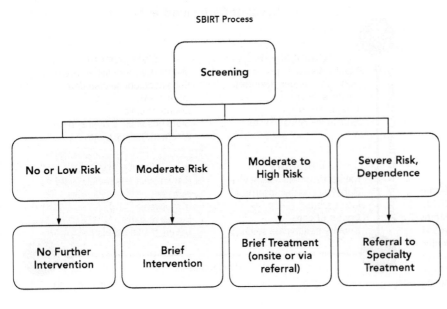

FIGURE 42.3 SBIRT Process. (From Substance Abuse and Mental Health Services Administration. [2013]. Systems-level implementation of screening, brief intervention, and referral to treatment. Technical Assistance Publication [TAP] Series 33. HHS Publication No. [SMA] 13–4741. Rockville, MD: Substance Abuse and Mental Health Services Administration.)

shown that engaged patients are more likely to stay in treatment and have positive outcomes (Thompson et al., 2020). Patients who are abusing substances may experience repeated cycles of detoxification and relapse. They may have prolonged cycles of "revolving-door" admissions and persistent medication nonadherence before acknowledging the need to engage in continuous treatment (Urbanoski et al., 2018). Each admission is a "window of opportunity." Relapse does not mean that a treatment intervention, the health care provider, or the patient has failed. Readmission and clear, realistic goals can further the patient's engagement in the treatment process. Effective programs emphasize a combination of empathic, long-term relationship building, and the use of leverage and possible confrontation by family, other caregivers, or the legal system.

Engagement in treatment is a process that may take many contacts with a patient and requires patience. Patients who struggle with authority and control issues must be convinced that the treatment team members have something to offer and are worth listening to before patients will begin to trust them. The engagement process is enhanced if staff can deal with presenting crises concretely (e.g., provide help in avoiding legal penalties and obtaining food, housing, entitlements, relief from psychiatric symptoms, vocational opportunities, recreation, and socialization). Harm reduction may be a first step toward a goal of abstinence.

The process of engagement is often characterized by approach–avoidance behavior by the patient. Lengthy intake and assessment procedures may discourage the patient from engagement or be intolerable if they are protracted and begin with asking the patient numerous pointed personal questions. These procedures may have to be adjusted to tailor treatment and accommodate the needs or reactions of the patient with COD.

Referral to Treatment

Some individuals will need more intensive treatment than brief treatment. These individuals will be referred to substance use specialty treatment programs.

Assertive Community Treatment

In **Assertive Community Treatment (ACT)**, the delivery of services is in the community (rather than a clinic), with shared caseloads, 24-hour responsibilities for patients, and direct provision of most services. This model was developed for patients with severe mental disorders who do not use outpatient services, are prone to frequent relapses and rehospitalization, and have severe psychosocial impairment (Ponka et al, 2020).

Relapse Prevention

Persons with COD are highly prone to relapse even after they have achieved full remission. Although many relapse factors are the same for those with mental disorders as with the general population, such as interpersonal problems, negative emotions, social stresses, lack of involvement in more satisfying activities, and attempts to escape from painful experiences, there are additional factors that affect this population. Symptoms of the mental disorders recur, and there are inadequate treatment resources in many settings. Many people with mental disorders live in extreme poverty, which forces them into high-crime, drug-infested neighborhoods, which makes them easy targets for crimes. Employment rates are low for this population even though many want to work. Finally, the same neurobiologic dysfunctions may underlie both addiction and mental disorders (Kolodner & Koliatsos, 2020).

Because persons with mental disorders face more challenges, emerging evidence suggests that **relapse prevention** for this population should be different than for the general population. Relapse prevention needs to account for the pervasive cognitive and social dysfunctions that are inherent in many people with COD. Patients usually need assistance in finding and maintaining housing and employment. Learning new skills may be difficult because of cognitive impairments that reduce the effectiveness of learning new skills. Social deficits can lead to isolation and victimization. Relapse prevention for COD involves the following:

- A stable and safe place to live
- A specific, individualized plan for managing stressful times
- Making informed, healthy choices that support physical and emotional well-being
- Purposeful and meaningful daily activities such as a job, school, volunteering, family caretaking, or creative endeavors
- Relationships and social networks that provide support, friendship, love, and hope
- Support for meeting spiritual needs and finding a sense of meaning in life
- Independence, income, and resources to participate in society (SAMHSA, 2021).

EVIDENCED-BASED NURSING CARE FOR PERSONS WITH CO-OCCURRING DISORDERS

It is crucial for patients with COD to be thoroughly assessed for responses to both psychiatric and SUDs. In some cultural groups, recognition of psychiatric and SUDs is difficult because of the lack of access and stigma associated with COD. Nurses in nonpsychiatric, community settings may be the only health care professional contact that some groups have. Assessment should include determination of the patient's willingness to change or level of motivation for treatment.

It is important to delineate the relative contribution of each diagnosis to the severity of the current responses presented and to establish priorities accordingly. Because patients with COD often make unreliable historians or distort the reality of their mental health problems and the severity of their substance use, obtaining objective data is especially important. Ideally, one should obtain an objective history of the patient from family, significant others, board and care operators, other health care providers, or anyone familiar enough with the patient to provide an accurate history. Box 42.1 lists basic assessment tools and methods used for patients with COD. The following concepts are paramount when assessing persons with COD:

BOX 42.1

Assessment of Co-occurring Disorders

Obtain a history and physical examination and laboratory tests (e.g., liver function tests, complete blood count) to confirm medical indicators related to substance use and also to rule out medical disorders with psychiatric presentations.

- Obtain substance use history and severity of consequences and physical symptoms.
- Identify core cultural values; explore meaning of the symptoms.
- Assess mental status examination and severity of symptoms (e.g., suicidal, homicidal, florid psychosis).
- Explore social context—socioeconomic, environment, literacy, and support system.

Interview with and assess family members to verify or determine (1) the accuracy of the patient's self-reported substance use or mental health history; (2) the patient's history of past mental health problems during periods of abstinence; and, if possible, (3) the sequence of the diagnoses (i.e., what symptoms appeared first).

- Conduct interviews with the patient's partner, friends, social worker, and other significant people in the patient's life.
- Review court records, medical records, and previous psychiatric and substance use treatment.
- Perform urine and blood toxicity screens; use a breath analyzer to test the patient's blood-alcohol level.

Revise initial assessment by observation of the patient in the clinical setting; full assessment of the underlying psychiatric problem may not be possible until there is a long (up to 6 months) period of total abstinence.

- Observe the patient for reappearance of psychiatric symptoms after a period of sobriety.
- Assess the patient's motivation to seek treatment, desire to change behavior, and understanding of diagnoses.

- Psychiatric and SUDs can coexist.
- Responses (psychosis, agitation) to both disorders can be similar.
- Substance use can mask other symptoms and syndromes.
- Psychiatric behaviors can mimic alcohol and other drug use problems.

NCLEXNOTE Patients with both mental and SUDs have responses to both disorders. Prioritizing nursing care depends on the immediate issue, but responses to both disorders should be assessed.

Mental Health Nursing Assessment and Clinical Judgment

Psychotic Disorders and Substance Use

Research shows that a high percentage estimated 50% of persons with schizophrenia will have an SUD during their lifetime. There are a number of possible explanations for the high rate of substance use in individuals with this disorder. Individuals with COD (substance use and schizophrenia) score higher on measures of sensation seeking and impulsivity than those without the COD. Stress reduction, symptom reduction, and relaxation are also offered as explanations. A neurobiologic model suggests that a dysregulated dopamine-mediated mesocorticolimbic network in patients with schizophrenia may also underlie substance use. Whereas all people are vulnerable to experiencing psychotic episodes from the use of various drugs, one psychotic episode increases susceptibility to subsequent episodes (Li et al., 2020).

Assessing the needs of people with schizophrenia, who are also chemically dependent, is complicated by the changing interaction among psychotic symptoms, the antipsychotic effects of medications, and the side effects of medications. A patient with a psychotic disorder may have an altered thought process or delusional thinking and may experience auditory hallucinations. They may also be cognitively impaired and have poor memory. These patients can have negative symptoms, such as poor motivation and poor hygiene. They often have low self-esteem and poor social skills and may have a general sense of not belonging to a community. Their sense of self in relation to the world may be altered.

As with all of the CODs, a multifaceted, integrated treatment approach is needed. Atypical antipsychotics continue to be the primary pharmacologic agent for the treatment of patients with comorbid schizophrenia with substance use. Not only do these agents treat the symptoms of schizophrenia, but they also appear to reduce cue-trigger cravings of the substances and prevent relapse

(Li et al., 2020). While monitoring side effects of antipsychotics, the nurse's attention needs to focus on liver functioning because drugs and alcohol are also metabolized by the liver. Relapse is frequently secondary to medication nonadherence, especially if patients experience side effects associated with the use of antipsychotics. Nursing interventions that focus on medication compliance may reduce the chances of relapse.

A confrontational interactive approach does not benefit this population and could even alienate patients. A more supportive approach is appropriate in which relapses are treated as an expected part of the recovery process. Addressing relapse risk is part of treatment planning. Focus on examining behavior, feelings, and the thinking process that led to the relapse. The nurse must avoid blame and guilt-inducing statements.

Social skills training is needed to help the patient learn ways of avoiding peer pressure and social situations that could lead to substance use. The goal is to successfully interact in a sober living situation, develop problem-solving skills, and refine behaviors.

Mood Disorders and Substance Use

Substance use in patients with depression contributes to treatment nonadherence and less positive outcomes (Hunt et al., 2020). Mood disorders may be more prevalent among patients using opiates than among other drug users. Many who use substances self-medicate an underlying mood disorder. Because many of the symptoms of substance use are the same as those of mood disorders, it is difficult to differentiate between them. This is especially true in the case of stimulant use and bipolar disorder. It is often impossible to determine the presence of an underlying mood disorder until there has been a period of abstinence.

Screening for suicide ideation is a priority during the assessment of these individuals. Both mood disorders and substance use are related to suicide (see Chapters 22, 25, and 31). Depression during withdrawal from alcohol, cocaine, opiates, and amphetamines also puts patients at severe risk for suicide. A person's presenting behaviors may not have included depression, but depression may develop as the withdrawal syndrome unfolds. Hyperactivity often appears with stimulant use and at times with alcohol use. Patients may be treated for hypomania or bipolar disorder when they are actually hyperactive. Symptoms usually improve as the person maintains abstinence.

Determining whether mood disorders are the cause or the effect of protracted substance use is difficult. An important nursing assessment is to determine how drug use relates to mood states. Patients may be attempting to alleviate uncomfortable symptoms, such as depression or agitation, or to enhance a mood state (e.g., hypomania).

Symptoms that persist during periods of abstinence are a clue to the degree that the mood disorder contributes to the presenting symptoms.

There is little research regarding pharmacologic interventions for comorbid mood disorders and substance use. Consequently, treatment is similar to that of mood disorders without substance use or abuse. When a pharmacologic agent is selected, attention is paid to its interaction with drugs and alcohol and its potential for dependence. The selective serotonin reuptake inhibitors (SSRIs) are frequently used for co-occurring depression. Higher doses may be required because of the possibility that alcohol use may induce hepatic microsomal activity. In the bipolar disorders, mood stabilizers are used.

Treatment for bipolar disorders and chemical dependency should be individualized to accommodate the specific needs, personal goals, and cultural perspectives of these individuals in different stages of change. Using interventions centered on examining cognitive distortions (e.g., "I'll never get better; no one likes me; alcohol is my only friend") and cognitive therapy techniques can help improve mood. Use of positive self-talk can be helpful for both the depression and the SUDs.

Anxiety Disorders and Substance Use

Research is scant regarding the relationship of anxiety disorders to substance use. Because there are a variety of anxiety disorders with differing clinical symptoms and numerous substances of abuse, it is difficult to develop studies addressing all of the anxiety disorders. Posttraumatic stress disorder (PTSD) is of particular concern because it has been shown to increase the risk of substance use relapse and is associated with poor treatment outcomes (Vujanovic et al., 2020).

The symptoms of anxiety may result from an anxiety disorder, such as panic attack, or may be secondary to drug or alcohol use as part of a withdrawal syndrome. Symptoms are so subjectively disturbing that they can lead to drug or alcohol use as self-medication for the emotional pain; therefore, they require prompt evaluation and treatment. There are many unanswered questions regarding the relationship of the anxiety symptoms, stress, and changes in the hypothalamic–pituitary–adrenal axis response to substance use. More research is sorely needed in this area.

Pharmacologic treatment of patients with anxiety is difficult because the traditional medications used, the benzodiazepines, are themselves addicting. Long-term treatment of the anxiety disorders, particularly PTSD, with the SSRIs maintains and improves quality of life. For PTSD, other medications such as the atypical antipsychotics, non-SSRI antidepressants, and mood stabilizers also appear to result in improvements (see Chapter 29).

Comorbid anxiety disorders and substance use require psychosocial interventions along with pharmacologic treatment. Patients with anxiety disorders should also pay particular attention to their physical health. Regular, balanced meals; exercise; and sleep are ways to decrease and manage stress levels. Patients should avoid excessive consumption of caffeine and sugars. If the patient has a fear of crowds, they may benefit from gradual desensitization techniques.

Personality Disorders and Substance Use

Personality disorders are frequently present in those who use alcohol and other substances. Antisocial personality and borderline disorders carry a high risk of having a comorbid substance use problem (Kaltenegger et al., 2020; Khalifa et al., 2020). The assessment of persons with comorbid personality disorders and substance use focuses on the problems related to the particular personality disorder, as well as the substance use. Individuals with antisocial personality disorder are likely to have a family history of other psychiatric disorders and problems with hostility. Interventions should be individualized according to the disorder and are discussed in the next section.

Substance Use, Mental Disorders, and Coronavirus Disease 2019

The coronavirus disease 2019 (COVID-19) pandemic has profound psychological and social effects, particularly on the most vulnerable populations. Uncertainty, social isolation, and economic problems impact individuals with psychiatric disorders and can exacerbate symptoms and substance use. Most suicide victims have a psychiatric disorder, usually depression. Individuals with CODs are at a greater risk of suicide than before COVID-19. The mental health consequences of the pandemic will be present for a long time. Suicide prevention efforts should be targeted at persons who are at high risk for suicide (Sher, 2020).

Mental Health Nursing Interventions

The nurse who provides care to patients with COD faces numerous challenges. Nurses implement interventions according to their level of practice and knowledge (see Box 42.2). Comprehensive planning within a multidisciplinary team approach is highly successful in the care of such patients. The entire system is organized to care for persons with COD (SAMHSA, 2020b). Community organizations are valuable sources of support as well. Many of the interventions that are indicated for persons with COD are discussed in previous chapters. The following discussion highlights interventions that are modified because of the special needs of this population.

Medication Management

One essential feature of COD treatment is medication management. Medication for a known mental disorder should never be discontinued on the grounds that the patient is using substances. Nonadherence with prescribed medications is associated with increased behavior problems after discharge and is a direct cause of relapse and rehospitalization. Impulsive behavior in response to transient exacerbations of psychotic symptoms, depressed mood, or anxiety symptoms may lead to relapse.

BOX 42.2

Autism Spectrum Disorder and Substance Use

Helverschou, S. B., Brunvold, A. R., & Arnevik, E. A. (2019). Treating patients with co-occurring autism spectrum disorder and substance use disorder: A clinical explorative study. Substance Abuse: Research and Treatment, 13, 1178221819843291. https://doi.org/10.1177/1178221819843291

THE QUESTION: What are explanations for drug and alcohol use by individuals with SUD and autism spectrum disorder?

METHODS: Four men aged 22 to 44 years with autism spectrum disorder whose drug use included amphetamines, cocaine, alcohol, and benzodiazepines engaged in CBT for their substance use. Therapists were provided with autism spectrum disorder education in order to participate in the study. Three of the four participants improved in functioning and symptoms.

FINDINGS: The individuals identified the reasons they use drugs or alcohol, including to reduce anxiety, improve social skills and concentration, and to be able to socialize, find peace, and forget problems and conflicts. They also used drugs and alcohol to feel normal, to stop worrying, and to think clearer. They wanted to stop using drugs and alcohol because they lost their family and job, felt socially excluded, were placed under arrest, and regretted events that happen while intoxicated.

IMPLICATIONS FOR NURSING: Individuals with autism spectrum disorder are susceptible to using drugs and alcohol and may need specially trained therapists to help them stop using.

Treating a patient with COD can be as complex as the presenting symptoms. Errors in treatment can include treating temporary psychiatric symptoms resulting from withdrawal as if they were a permanent feature of the individual, withholding needed medication for a psychiatric disorder, or setting arbitrary limits on medication based on a belief that medication for all psychiatric symptoms should be suspended until the COD is treated. Overall, patients need ongoing help with adhering to a prescribed medication regimen.

Collaboration between the patient's prescriber and other treatment providers is important to minimize the possible misuse or abuse of prescription drugs such as forging prescriptions, acquiring drugs from nonmedical sources, frequent visits to EDs, or seeking multiple prescribers. In addition, caution is essential in prescribing medications that can increase the patient's potential for relapse into abusing the drug of choice. The patient in recovery is often reluctant to use potentially mind-altering drugs, and the nurse should explore any concerns.

Substance Abuse Counseling

With the COD patient, substance abuse counseling is slower and less confrontational than in many traditional substance abuse programs. Content needs to be repeated frequently and motivation for treatment continually assessed.

Cognitive–Behavioral Interventions

Cognitive–behavioral interventions help patients to (1) analyze which situations are most likely to trigger relapses; (2) examine cognitive, emotional, and behavioral components of high-risk situations; and (3) develop cognitive, behavioral, and effective coping strategies and environmental supports. Role-playing ways out of high-risk situations is a technique that these groups often use. Homework assignments help patients create relapse-prevention plans that address new coping strategies for these high-risk situations.

Patient Education

Patient education is an essential element in treating COD. Patients need to learn about their specific mental disorder, substance use and abuse, and their effects. Relapse prevention and recovery should be highlighted. Education can be conducted in individual sessions, but group sessions encourage interaction among patients. Sharing their experiences with their peers, patients can enhance these presentations.

BOX 42.3

Topics for Education Groups for Patients with Co-occurring Disorders

- The effects of alcohol and drugs on the body
- Alcohol, drugs, and medication—what can go wrong?
- What is a healthy lifestyle?
- Triggers for relapse
- What is Alcoholics (or Narcotics) Anonymous?
- What is a sponsor in Alcoholics (or Narcotics) Anonymous?
- What is recovery from mental illness and substance use?
- What are the tools of recovery?
- The disease of addiction
- The relapse cycle
- How to cope with feelings without using alcohol or other drugs?
- Relapse prevention: what works?
- What are cognitive distortions?
- HIV prevention and education
- Leisure time management
- How to manage stress?
- Relaxation training
- Assertiveness and recovery
- Common slogans to live by
- Pitfalls in treatment
- The process of recovery
- Creating a relapse-prevention plan
- What are my goals? How does the use of alcohol and drugs affect them?
- Coping with thoughts about alcohol and drugs
- Problem-solving basics
- Coping with anger
- Negative thinking and how to manage it
- Enhancing social support networks

Topics should be clear; relevant to the group members; and illustrated with charts, handouts, or appropriate films. Each session should be relatively short and not contain too many new or difficult concepts. Reinforcing and reviewing previous discussions can be helpful to remind patients of particularly relevant concepts. Box 42.3 lists some suitable topics for nurse-led discussion groups. Individual patient education can focus on areas of knowledge deficits and reinforce topics discussed in group settings. Group sessions can also assist patients in learning interpersonal skills (e.g., assertiveness) and problem-solving skills and in relapse prevention planning.

Mutual Self-Help Groups

Several mutual self-help groups are appropriate for many patients with COD. Peer-led self-help approaches specifically for persons with COD are being tried with some success. The most common groups are 12-step programs, such as Alcoholics Anonymous (AA) and Narcotics Anonymous (NA) (see Chapter 31). The advisability of a patient enrolling in a 12-step program needs to be evaluated on an individual basis. A health care provider familiar with 12-step concepts can often facilitate patients' attempts to use these programs. The numerous advantages of self-help groups make them a potentially powerful support for continued recovery. Alternative mutual self-help programs similar to 12-step programs are available in some geographic areas. Rational Recovery and Secular Organization for Sobriety are groups that downplay the concept of powerlessness and the spiritual aspects associated with 12-step programs.

Family Support and Education

The families of patients with COD need education and support. Family psychoeducation interventions address mental disorders, substance use, and their interactions. The focus of family support groups, such as those under the auspices of the National Alliance on Mental Illness, has been both to educate and to help the family cope with a mentally ill relative. AA and NA take a similar approach to providing peer support to families of substance users. These self-help groups aid family members in balancing confrontation of the problem, detachment from forcing a solution to it, and support of the treatment process.

Evaluation and Treatment Outcomes

Evaluation of the patient's ability to deal with both the substance use and mental disorder is an ongoing process. Because the goal of recovery is to have quality of life in the community of choice, treatment outcomes should be evaluated for quality of life as well as management of two disorders.

MENTAL HEALTH NURSING INTERVENTIONS CONTINUUM OF CARE

An integrated approach that combines mental health and substance use interventions at the clinical site has been shown to be the most effective. In an integrated system, the same team provides coordinated mental health and substance use interventions and guides the patient toward learning to manage these intertwined disorders. When the mental health and substance use systems are truly integrated, patient outcomes are positive (Carlo et al., 2020).

When Hospitalization Is Necessary

Often, patients with COD can be treated effectively in community mental health settings if their symptoms are stable, they are following their treatment plan, they are compliant with the use of psychiatric medications, and they remain alcohol and drug free. Patients are hospitalized when they have a need for detoxification, exacerbation of comorbid psychiatric or medical disorders, suicide or homicidal ideation, or a disorder that prevents abstinence or outpatient treatment.

Crisis Stabilization

Setting priorities is essential for hospitalized patients with COD. The first priorities are gathering data from a physical examination and nursing assessments, stabilizing psychiatric symptoms, and treating withdrawal symptoms (see Chapter 31). After these issues are addressed, the patient enters the rehabilitation phase of treatment for both diagnoses. Rehabilitative therapy is appropriate if the patient (1) can participate in a group process, (2) can focus attention on groups or reading material, (3) does not engage in behavior that is detrimental to the group process, (4) can listen to and receive feedback from others, and (5) can benefit from the group process.

Early Stages of Recovery from Substance Use

Many patients seeking alcohol or drug use treatment experience transitory cognitive impairment, which usually resolves within the first month of abstinence. Patients often experience difficulties with disorientation, clouding of consciousness, incoherent thoughts, memory loss, and delirium, which may hinder their ability to learn new concepts. These problems are a result of the neurobiologic insult on the brain by these substances and psychosocial factors such as fear of legal or relationship difficulties, depression, grief, and feelings of guilt and shame. However, if Wernicke syndrome, a reversible alcohol-induced amnestic disorder caused by a thiamine-deficient diet, or Korsakoff psychosis, characterized by a loss of recent memory and confabulation (or filling in the blanks in memory by making up facts to cover this deficit) is present, cognitive problems may last longer. Patients with this condition are highly suggestible, have poor judgment, and cannot reason critically. Korsakoff psychosis often follows Wernicke encephalopathy and is also associated with prior peripheral neuropathy (see Chapter 31).

Psychological testing and other methods of assessment determine the patient's level of cognitive functioning in order to select the appropriate treatment. It is also important to determine the extent of the mental disorder and the substance use. The nurse assesses the patient's abilities for self-care, independent living, impulse control, control of assaultive behavior, direction taking, and development of new responses to new situations and ideas. The nurse must also evaluate changes in mental status during the past 6 months and examine previous treatment outcomes.

Clear, direct, simple interventions that avoid extraneous issues and theoretical discussion may be useful for patients with cognitive or memory impairment such as the following:

- Reading material that is relevant to recovery and that can be referred to in short study sessions

- First-person accounts of addiction and recovery found in AA and NA literature

- Basic concepts of recovery, such as those in AA slogans and on patients' need for continuing care after discharge

- Films with scenes illustrating relevant family problems or other problems related to substance use; movies can be more effective than lectures

Social interaction skills and coping skills learned in treatment need to be reinforced in community settings to create or enhance a stable living situation and possible vocational opportunities. Active planning and intervention are needed for housing and employment, or deterioration may occur despite gains made during hospitalization.

Recovery

To move toward recovery, establishing a positive social network is critical. Isolation and alienation from prior sources of support is a problem that most people with comorbid mental disorders and substance use share. Some patients relate poorly to their families, others are overly dependent on their families, and others have difficulty establishing and maintaining social relationships. Some patients' only "families" are peers within the drug subculture who reinforce substance-abusing behavior.

Compliance with an agreed-on treatment plan is integral to recovery. Box 42.4 presents features of a COD outpatient program. Opportunities to socialize, access to positive recreational activities, and a supportive peer group are stabilizing influences on patients who may otherwise drop out of treatment altogether. Part of a comprehensive relapse prevention plan is to establish or reinforce the patient's social support network so that they can obtain (1) opportunities for substance-free socializing, (2) crisis counseling to prevent readmission to a hospital, and (3) support for sobriety.

Supportive housing is also essential for patients with COD. Supportive housing is especially crucial for patients who are being discharged from the hospital because the

---

BOX 42.4

Features of a Co-occurring Disorders Outpatient Program

- *Community meeting and goal setting:* Patients set small, realistic goals for themselves for the day, which aid them in their ultimate goal of better living in recovery.
- *Anger management and social communication:* Patients learn appropriate ways to express anger and how to socialize with others.
- *Group therapy:* Patients discuss interpersonal issues, get feedback from their peers, and learn problem-solving skills.
- *Dual recovery anonymous meetings:* Patient-run meetings (a modified AA meeting) address the specific needs of patients with COD.
- *Leisure planning:* Patients learn skills to enjoy leisure involving clean and sober fun.
- *Gardening, art therapy, music therapy, swimming:* These methods provide alternatives to the use of alcohol and other drugs.
- *Health education:* Patients learn about the effects of drugs and alcohol on the body and about other relevant medical topics.
- *Medication education:* Patients learn about psychiatric medications, their uses, their side effects, and interactions with drugs or alcohol.
- *Relapse-prevention planning:* Patients talk about their last relapse; triggers, feelings, and stresses that contributed to the relapse; and the consequences, and formulate relapse-prevention plans.
- *Individual counseling:* Patients receive individual counseling to develop goals and work on problem-solving techniques.
- *Psychiatric consultation:* Patients are evaluated and followed up for medication and other psychiatric interventions.

Note: Patients are *not* discharged from the program if they are intoxicated. They are asked not to come to the program intoxicated but to return when they are sober to continue work on their recovery.

---

risk for relapse is greatest during the first few months after discharge. Halfway houses for substance users may deemphasize medication compliance, and housing designed for chronically mentally ill individuals may not emphasize abstinence enough. Thus, an important part of the multidisciplinary team approach to discharge planning for patients with COD is to help them find the best possible living situation.

Younger patients with a mental disorder may want and expect to find appropriate employment, but some of these patients may be unrealistic about potential professions. However, this desire can be a significant motivator and a useful tool in a treatment program. Referring patients to halfway houses or residential substance use treatment programs that stress vocational skill training can be beneficial. Use of community vocational rehabilitation services and of educational opportunities can be an important part of a discharge plan.

SUMMARY OF KEY POINTS

- In co-occurring mental disorder and SUD, each disorder is considered a primary disorder. Patients should be treated concurrently with an integrated approach.

- People with COD are at high risk for relapse. The relapse cycle repeats itself without treatment.

- There is not one model that explains why mental disorders and substance use occur together so frequently. The most common pattern is the onset of the mental disorder, followed by the problems with substance use leading to use. It appears that the substance use is an attempt to self-medicate the psychiatric symptoms.

- Barriers for treatment include homelessness, unemployment, and lack of social support. Other barriers include the complexity of the COD, staff attitudes, stigma, and health issues that interfere with treatment.

- Interdisciplinary treatment is through an integrated approach. Patients are moved toward recovery through engagement, motivation, assertive outreach and treatment, and relapse prevention.

- Recovery through commonly recognized stages of treatment—engagement, persuasion or motivation, active treatment, and relapse prevention—involves much more than avoiding alcohol and drugs.

- Nursing assessment of COD often depends on objective data obtained from interviews with family members, reviews of court records, laboratory test results, and physical examination findings. Assessment should include a determination of the willingness to change and motivation for treatment.

- Treatment and nursing care need to be individualized within the context of the specific mental disorder and substances used.

- Interventions that are tailored to the special needs of the patient with a COD are medication management, substance abuse counseling, cognitive–behavioral interventions, patient education, and family support and education. Participation in peer-led self-help groups has had some success.

- An ideal continuum of care is an integrated approach with one team coordinating the mental health and substance use interventions. Patients should not have to negotiate treatment with two separate systems. Hospitalization may be required during periods of crises. Most treatment occurs in the community, where recovery is the goal.

CRITICAL THINKING CHALLENGES

1. An 18-year-old patient, newly diagnosed with schizophrenia, is relatively compliant with their medication and treatment. This patient was recently at a social event where they were experimenting with alcohol and marijuana. Develop a teaching plan for them that includes the risks of developing a SUD.

2. A nurse in an emergency department recommends AA for every patient who is admitted for detoxification. Is that an appropriate referral for a person with comorbid mental disorder and substance use?

3. A community health nurse wants to refer a young person who lives in a poor rural area to an integrated treatment program several miles away. Discuss the likelihood of the patient's actually being able to access services. What barriers would she face, and how could they have access to the care they need?

4. How would you respond to a patient with COD who states, "Once my medication is stable, I will be able to drink again"?

5. Compare traditional substance use approaches to an integrated treatment program.

6. A patient with a COD tells the nurse, "All chemicals are bad for you. I do not want to take my medication." Develop a response to this statement that reflects the use of engagement.

7. Discuss the differences in behavior of a person with schizophrenia who uses cocaine and a person with a mood disorder who uses marijuana.

8. Which COD concepts should be included in patient education?

 Movie Viewing Guides
Love & Mercy (2014): This film is a biographical drama film about Brian Wilson, the musician-songwriter, cofounder of the Beach Boys. There are two periods of time depicted. Paul Dano stars Wilson in the 1960s and John Cusack plays Wilson in the 1980s. Brian's psychiatric symptoms and use of drugs occurred in his early years. He is misdiagnosed and abused by his therapist. This story is about Brian's struggle to regain independence and quality of life.

VIEWING POINTS: How does Brian's mental disorder interact with his substance use? How are you feeling throughout this movie? Do your feelings about the character change? How could a nurse advocate for Brian's recovery?

REFERENCES

Babor, T. F., Higgins-Biddle, J. C., Saunders, J. B., & Monteiro, M. G. (2001). *AUDIT: The alcohol use disorders identification test: Guidelines for use in primary health care* (2nd ed.). World Health Organization. [Online]. https://apps.who.int/iris/handle/10665/67205

Bradizza, C. M., Brown, W. C., Ruszczyk, M. U., Dermen, K. H., Lucke, J. F., & Stasiewicz, P. R. (2018). Difficulties in emotion regulation in treatment-seeking alcoholics with and without co-occurring mood and anxiety disorders. *Addictive Behaviors*, *80*, 6–13. https://doi.org/10.1016/j.addbeh.2017.12.033

Carlo, A. D., Benson, N. M., Chu, F., & Busch, A. B. (2020). Association of alternative payment and delivery models with outcomes for mental health and substance use disorders: A systematic review. *JAMA Network Open*, *3*(7), e207401. https://doi.org/10.1001/jamanetworkopen.2020.7401

DiClemente, C. C., Corno, C. M., Graydon, M. M., Wiprovnick, A. E., & Knoblach, D. J. (2017). Motivational interviewing, enhancement, and brief interventions over the last decade: A review of reviews of efficacy and effectiveness. *Psychology of Addictive Behaviors: Journal of the Society of Psychologists in Addictive Behaviors*, *31*(8), 862–887. https://doi.org/10.1037/adb0000318

Hides, L., Quinn, C., Stoyanov, S., Kavanagh, D., & Baker, A. (2019). Psychological interventions for co-occurring depression and substance use disorders. *The Cochrane Database of Systematic Reviews*, *2019*(11), CD009501. https://doi.org/10.1002/14651858.CD009501.pub2

Hunt, G. E., Malhi, G. S., Lai, H., & Cleary, M. (2020). Prevalence of comorbid substance use in major depressive disorder in community and clinical settings, 1990–2019: Systematic review and meta-analysis. *Journal of Affective Disorders*, *266*, 288–304. https://doi.org/10.1016/j.jad.2020.01.141

Kaltenegger, H. C., Philips, B., & Wennberg, P. (2020). Autistic traits in mentalization-based treatment for concurrent borderline personality disorder and substance use disorder: Secondary analyses of a randomized controlled feasibility study. *Scandinavian Journal of Psychology*, *61*(3), 416–422. https://doi.org/10.1111/sjop.12595

Khalifa, N. R., Gibbon, S., Völlm, B. A., Cheung, N. H., & McCarthy, L. (2020). Pharmacological interventions for antisocial personality disorder. *The Cochrane Database of Systematic Reviews*, *9*, CD007667. https://doi.org/10.1002/14651858.CD007667.pub3

Kolodner, G., & Koliatsos, V. E. (2020). Update on the neuropsychiatry of substance use disorders. *The Psychiatric Clinics of North America*, *43*(2), 291–304. https://doi.org/10.1016/j.psc.2020.02.011.

Li, K. J., Chen, A., & DeLisi, L. E. (2020). Opioid use and schizophrenia. *Current Opinion in Psychiatry*, *33*(3), 219–224. https://doi.org/10.1097/YCO.0000000000000593

Mejia-Lancheros, C., Lachaud, J., O'Campo, P., Wiens, K., Nisenbaum, R., Wang, R., Hwang, S. W., & Stergiopoulos, V. (2020). Trajectories and mental health-related predictors of perceived discrimination and stigma among homeless adults with mental illness. *PLoS One*, *15*(2), e0229385. https://doi.org/10.1371/journal.pone.0229385

Miler, J. A., Carver, H., Foster, R., & Parkes, T. (2020). Provision of peer support at the intersection of homelessness and problem substance use services: a systematic "state of the art" review. *BMC Public Health*, *20*(1), 641. https://doi.org/10.1186/s12889-020-8407-4

National Institute on Drug Abuse [NIDA]. (2012). *Resource guide: Screening for drug use in general medical settings*. https://archives.drugabuse.gov/publications/resource-guide-screening-drug-use-in-general-medical-settings

Office of Disease Prevention and Health Promotion. (2021). Increase the proportion of persons with co-occurring substance use disorders and mental health disorders who receive treatment for both disorders. Health People 2030. Increase the proportion of people with substance use and mental health disorders who get treatment for both — MHMD-07 - Healthy People 2030 | health.gov

Østergaard, M. L., Nordentoft, M., & Hjorthøj, C. (2017). Associations between substance use disorders and suicide or suicide attempts in people with mental illness: A Danish nation-wide, prospective, register-based study of patients diagnosed with schizophrenia, bipolar disorder, unipolar depression or personality disorder. *Addiction*. *12*(7). 1250–1259. https://doi.org/10.1111/add.13788

Ponka, D., Agbata, E., Kendall, C., Stergiopoulos, V., Mendonca, O., Magwood, O., Saad, A., Larson, B., Sun, A. H., Arya, N., Hannigan, T., Thavorn, K., Andermann, A., Tugwell, P., & Pottie, K. (2020). The effectiveness of case management interventions for the homeless, vulnerably housed and persons with lived experience: A systematic review. *PLoS One*, *15*(4), e0230896. https://doi.org/10.1371/journal.pone.0230896

Sher, L. (2020). The impact of the COVID-19 pandemic on suicide rates. *QJM: Monthly Journal of the Association of Physicians*, *113*(10), 707–712. https://doi.org/10.1093/qjmed/hcaa202

Substance Abuse and Mental Health Services Administration [SAMHSA]. (2020a). Key substance use and mental health indicators in the United States: Results from the 2019 National Survey on Drug Use and Health (HHS Publication No. PEP20-07-01-001, NSDUH Series H-55). Rockville, MD: Center for Behavioral Health Statistics and Quality, Substance Abuse and Mental Health Services Administration. https://www.samhsa.gov/data/

Substance Abuse and Mental Health Services Administration [SAMHSA]. (2020b). About screening, brief intervention, and referral to treatment (SBIRT). https://www.samhsa.gov/sbirt/about

Substance Abuse and Mental Health Services Administration [SAMHSA]. (2021). Employee assistance program prescription drug toolkit and fact sheets. Publication No. PEP20-03-02-001. Rockville, MD. https://store.samhsa.gov/sites/default/files/SAMHSA_Digital_Download/pep20-03-002-001.pdf

Thompson, R. G., Aivadyan, C., Stohl, M., Aharonovich, E., & Hasin, D. S. (2020). Smartphone application plus brief motivational intervention reduces substance use and sexual risk behaviors among homeless young adults: Results from a randomized controlled trial. *Psychology of Addictive Behaviors: Journal of the Society of Psychologists in Addictive Behaviors*, *34*(6), 641–649. https://doi.org/10.1037/adb0000570

Urbanoski, K., Cheng, J., Rehm, J., & Kurdyak, P. (2018). Frequent use of emergency departments for mental and substance use disorders. *Emergency Medicine Journal: EMJ*, *35*(4), 220–225. https://doi.org/10.1136/emermed-2015-205554

Vujanovic, A. A., Smith, L. J., Green, C., Lane, S. D., & Schmitz, J. M. (2020). Mindfulness as a predictor of cognitive-behavioral therapy outcomes in inner-city adults with posttraumatic stress and substance dependence. *Addictive Behaviors*, *104*, 106283. https://doi.org/10.1016/j.addbeh.2019.106283

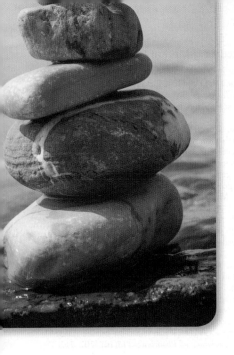

43
Care of Persons Who Are Medically Compromised

Dorothy M. Corrigan

KEYCONCEPT

- chronic pain

LEARNING OBJECTIVES

After studying this chapter, you will be able to:

1. Identify medically ill populations at risk for psychosocial problems.

2. Discuss the impact that both a mental disorder and a medical problem have on patients and their families.

3. Discuss the multimodal approach of treatment of pain, especially for those experiencing chronic pain.

4. Describe assessment and nursing care for patients who are experiencing mental health problems associated with trauma or central nervous system (CNS) disorders.

5. Discuss the importance of integrating the medical aspects of care into psychiatric care for patients with mental health problems.

KEY TERMS

- Allodynia • Beta-endorphins • Bidirectional illnesses • Gate-control theory • Hyperalgia • Hyperesthesia • Ischemic cascade • Nociceptors • Pain mosaic • Pain vulnerability • Plasticity • Postconcussive syndrome • Prostaglandins • Self-efficacy • Substance P • Traumatic brain injury (TBI)

INTRODUCTION

Persons with chronic mental disorders often have one **comorbid condition** which is defined as the presence of a physical illness, injury, or disability that exists simultaneously with another disorder. In some cases, there are several **multimorbid conditions,** the presence of two or more chronic conditions, which overlap each other and influence medical and psychiatric disease complexity. An estimated 68% of adults who have been diagnosed with a mental disorders have at least one medical comorbidity (Avery et al., 2020) and are more likely to describe their own overall health as poor (Walker & Druss, 2017).

Though medical and psychiatric disorders are often intertwined, mental health providers may not recognize medical illness, and medical providers may not screen for mental health problems.

This chapter will discuss some common comorbid and multimorbid medical disorders that are experienced by people who have mental disorders. It will also explore some mental health disorders which are linked to primary medical illnesses. Three special populations will be also be presented: those with comorbid pain, those who have experienced physiologic trauma, and those with mental health issues related to CNS disorders. Psychosocial implications will be explored throughout this chapter.

OVERVIEW OF CONNECTIONS BETWEEN MENTAL AND MEDICAL DISORDERS

The increased presence of comorbid conditions among people with serious mental disorders has long been recognized. As early as 1937, the presence of common comorbidities such as hypertension and diabetes among those with mental disorders had been studied and the connection between comorbid disorders and recurrent hospitalizations within the same population was also observed (Phillips, 1937). We are now aware that mental health problems may diminish the motivation for self-care, impair symptom reporting, and delay treatment. As a result, hospitalization for medical problems may be prolonged, at increased emotional and financial cost to the patient and their family (Šprah et al., 2017).

Although the principal causes of death (cancer and cardiovascular disease [CVD]) among the general population are the same as that of persons with serious mental illness, those with serious mental illness die prematurely of these disorders (Davies, et al., 2021). On average, in the United States, people with chronic mental illness die about 25 years earlier than those in the general population (Olker et al., 2016). For those with psychotic disorders such as schizophrenia, life expectancy is estimated to be about 14.5 years earlier (Hjorthoj et al., 2017). Overall, people with serious mental illness have mortality rates 2 to 3 times higher than the general population and this is likely attributable to cardiovascular risk factors such as obesity, hypertension, and diabetes mellitus (McGinty et al., 2016). However, additional social risk factors such as poverty, lack of safe recreation space for exercise, limited access to full-service grocery stores, unemployment, undereducation, and homelessness also contribute to the presence of medical comorbidities and to the overall experience of decreased health and wellness among those with chronic mental illness. People with mental disorders may be more likely to refuse medical care, may be less likely to maintain their treatment regimen (Swartz, 2018), and may be less able to communicate new health problems or symptoms than those who do not have mental disorders (Carliner et al., 2014; Phan, 2016). Some may simply not have adequate access to health care. To complicate matters further, some health care providers may have the mistaken belief that people with mental disorders are incapable of advocating for and achieving physical health and wellness (Bradford et al., 2016).

The end result of all of this is that care can become fragmented, undermining the possibility of a consistent, holistic, recovery-oriented approach to care. Such fragmentation of care is also expensive. Health care expenditures for individuals with serious mental disorders are approximately 3.3 times higher than for individuals without mental disorders (Lee et al., 2016). Care for persons who are medically compromised requires culturally competent engagement of patients and their families, thorough screening and assessment, systematic monitoring, and comprehensive treatment planning among interdisciplinary team members. This includes lifestyle advice, connection to community services including transportation, and **self-efficacy** (self-care effectiveness) coaching. This is especially critical in the presence of other challenging psychosocial issues, including aging, complex family dynamics, economic hardship, no or inadequate housing, and other issues.

COMMON COMORBID PHYSICAL ILLNESSES AMONG PERSONS WITH MENTAL DISORDERS

It is estimated that at least 68% of those diagnosed with mental disorders have at least one comorbid medical condition (Avery et al., 2020), including obesity (50%), hyperlipidemia (45%), hypertension (44%), asthma (28%), diabetes mellitus (21%), and arthritis (22%) (Razzano et al., 2015). Heart failure, CVD, chronic obstructive pulmonary disease (COPD), kidney disease, cancer, hepatitis B, hepatitis C; and HIV (human immunodeficiency virus) are also diagnosed with frequency and are more prevalent for persons with serious mental disorders than for the rest of the population (Davies, et al., 2021). CVD among persons with mental disorders, for example, is estimated to be 2 to 3 times higher than the general population (Robson & Gray, 2007). This is linked to an increased prevalence of modifiable risk factors, such as obesity, hypertension, and hyperlipidemia among people with mental disorders (Zomer et al., 2017). Subsequently, metabolic syndrome, the clustering of obesity, hypertension, hyperlipidemia, and insulin resistance/glucose dysregulation has been reported at 1.58 times higher among people with mental disorders than among the general population (Vancampfort et al., 2015). With respect to cancers, especially digestive and breast cancer, higher rates of these illnesses have been reported among people with schizophrenia than in the larger population (Bradford et al., 2016). An estimated 88% of the people with schizophrenia have untreated hyperlipidemia and 66% have untreated hypertension (Zomer et al., 2017). Another common comorbidity is poor dental health that can be related to xerostomia from medications as well as limited access to dental care. To complicate this picture, many of these conditions remain untreated. Even more concerning, nurses who care for patients with mental disorders and comorbid or multimorbid health conditions are often unprepared to do so (Avery et al., 2020).

COMMON SECONDARY MENTAL DISORDERS IN PEOPLE WITH CHRONIC MEDICAL ILLNESS

Conversely, persons with chronic physical health issues are at risk for developing comorbid anxiety disorders, substance abuse disorders, depressive episodes, and other mood disorders, and approximately 50% of patients in primary care settings will endorse mental health issues related to their physical health (Hirsch et al., 2016). This is sometimes referred to as "secondary mental disorders" (mental health disorders linked to a medical problem). Chronic illness itself is a stressful event that alters the person's perception of the physical, social, and emotional self (Klein-Gitelman & Curran, 2015). Chronic illness in adults is a risk factor for depression and suicidal ideation (Gurhan et al., 2019). In children with chronic physical illness, the occurrence of secondary mental health disorders is four times that of their peers in the general population (Bennett et al., 2015). Among high school students with asthma, atopic dermatitis, obesity, heart disease, and diabetes, female students were more likely to suffer depression (Kim et al., 2020). For adolescents with chronic physical illness and who are transitioning to adulthood at a critical time of emotional growth, individuation, and unique social pressures, the risks of developing mood disorders, especially depression, are increased (Klein-Gitelman & Curran, 2015). All patients with chronic health conditions should be considered as at risk for developing mental health problems, especially children and adolescents as well as older adults.

Depression has been found to be the most common affective prodrome of many medical disorders (Cosci et al., 2015). Depressive symptoms are often an intrinsic part of the primary pathophysiology of endocrine disorders, metabolic disturbances, malignancies, viral infections, inflammatory disorders, and cardiopulmonary conditions. Table 43.1 lists medical conditions associated with depression. Depression and anxiety often complicate the clinical picture in patients with hyperthyroidism and hypothyroidism, Cushing disease (hyperadrenalism), and Addison disease (hypoadrenalism). Depression has been shown to be an independent risk factor for type 2 diabetes and metabolic syndrome (Kim, et al., 2015). The early onset of vascular disease, multiple infections, and subsequent disability are also associated with increased depressive symptoms. Malignancies have also been associated with anxiety and depression. Depressive syndromes have been associated with cancer in up to 50% of cancer cases and biologic relationships between the two disorders may herald undetected carcinoma. Depression with cancer is associated with poor prognosis and increased morbidity (Wu et al., 2016). Depression can also present as a consequence of antineoplastic therapy and is a risk factor for cancer recurrence (Wen et al., 2018). In people with inflammatory bowel disease (IBS), the odds of developing

TABLE 43.1	MEDICAL ILLNESSES ASSOCIATED WITH SYMPTOMS OF DEPRESSION
Medical Illness	**Symptoms of Depression**
Endocrinopathies	Hypothyroidism and hyperthyroidism Hypoparathyroidism and hyperparathyroidism Cushing syndrome (steroid excess) Adrenal insufficiency (Addison disease) Hyperaldosteronism
Malignancies	Abdominal carcinomas, especially pancreatic Brain tumors (temporal lobe) Breast cancer Gastrointestinal cancer Lung cancer Prostate cancer Metastases
Neurologic disorders	Ischemic stroke Subarachnoid hemorrhage Parkinson disease Normal-pressure hydrocephalus Multiple sclerosis Closed head injury Epilepsy
Metabolic imbalance	Serum sodium and potassium reductions Vitamin B_{12}, niacin, vitamin C deficiencies; iron deficiency (anemias) Metal intoxication (thallium and mercury) Uremia
Viral or bacterial infection	Infectious hepatitis Encephalitis Tuberculosis AIDS
Hormonal imbalance	Premenstrual, premenopausal, postpartum periods
Cardiopulmonary	Acute myocardial infarction Postcardiac arrest Postcoronary artery bypass graft Post-heart transplantation Cardiomyopathy
Inflammatory disorders	Rheumatoid arthritis

generalized anxiety disorder have been shown to be twice the rate of the general population (Fuller-Thomson et al., 2015). IBS is also a risk factor for the development of mood disorders, anxiety, and panic disorder (Simpson, et al., 2020).

CVD deserves special attention because evidence over the years has supported the idea that depression is an independent risk factor in the development and progression of CVD and that this evidence appears to be **bidirectional** (Macchi, et al., 2020). **Bidirectional** refers to a biologic relationship between two separate disease processes, each of which is a risk factor for the other (e.g., heart disease influences the development of depression and depression influences the development of heart disease). Bidirectional markers involving an emerging relationship between depression and CVD include alteration in platelet activity related to thrombus formation, increase in inflammatory cytokines, and heart rate variability. The incidence of CVD is estimated to be around 20% to 50% in patients with depression (Macchi, et al., 2020). In patients who have had a myocardial infarction (MI) risk of cardiac death in the 6 months after an acute MI is approximately four times greater. Despite these risks, depression and anxiety are often underrecognized and undertreated in cardiac patients (Bruyninx, et al., 2020).

Depression is also prominent in neurologic illness. Parkinson disease has a 40% to 50% lifetime prevalence of depression (Lima et al., 2019). Depression commonly co-occurs in both children (Florea et al., 2020) and adults (Silva & Cavalcanti, 2019) with multiple sclerosis. Depression is also a common feature in people who have experienced a cerebral vascular accident (CVA) (Kawasaki & Hoshiyama, 2020).

In addition, some medications used to treat medical disorders are known to be associated with agitation, anxiety, and depressed mood as side effects (Table 43.2). When a drug is suspected of causing mood or mental status changes, it should be withdrawn and an adequate alternative should be tried. When this is not possible, the dosage should be decreased to an effective level at which mood symptoms resolve.

Psychological Aspects of Medical Illness

It is normal for patients to respond to the loss of health with anxiety or depressed mood, particularly when the illness is debilitating, life threatening, and without a clear prognosis. People who have chronic illness are frequently distressed by loss of function and limitations imposed on their daily activities. The person's usual social support systems may also be impacted as the person withdraws from usual activities outside of the home as a consequence of functional loss or pain. Sometimes, relationships are also changed that can further affect healthy coping. Undiagnosed and untreated mental disorders in medically ill people are potentially life threatening because stable moods and cognitive functioning are essential to compliance with the interdisciplinary treatment plan and recovery. In addition, the underuse or overuse of analgesics and reluctance to perform self-care and rehabilitative activities hinder recovery and expose the person to other potential complications. Subsequently, the diagnosis, treatment, and follow-up of a comorbid mental disorders in patients with medical illnesses is crucial.

Clinical Features of Special Significance

Two problems of special significance, psychotic states and suicidal thoughts, are related in that patients with delusions and hallucinations tend to be at greater risk for suicide attempts and are more likely to have compliance issues with respect to their treatment (e.g., to refuse to eat or

TABLE 43.2	MEDICATIONS ASSOCIATED WITH MENTAL DISORDERS SYMPTOMS IN MEDICALLY ILL PATIENTS
Drug Class	**Medication**
Analgesics and NSAIDs	Ibuprofen Indomethacin Opiates Pentazocine Phenacetin Phenylbutazone
Antihypertensives	Clonidine Hydralazine Methyldopa Propranolol Reserpine
Antimicrobials	Ampicillin (gram-negative agents) Clotrimazole Cycloserine Griseofulvin Metronidazole Nitrofurantoin Streptomycin Sulfamethoxazole (sulfonamides)
Neurologic agents	L-Dopa Levodopa
Antiparkinsonism drugs	Amantadine
Anticonvulsants	Carbamazepine Phenytoin
Antispasmodics	Baclofen Bromocriptine
Cardiac drugs	Digitalis Guanethidine Lidocaine Oxprenolol Procainamide
Psychotropic drugs	Benzodiazepines
Stimulants and sedatives	Amphetamines Barbiturates Chloral hydrate Chlorazepate Diethylpropion Ethanol Fenfluramine Haloperidol
Steroids and hormones	Adrenocorticotropic hormone Corticosteroids Estrogen Oral contraceptives Prednisone Progesterone Triamcinolone
Antineoplastic drugs	Bleomycin C-Asparaginase Trimethoprim Vincristine
Other miscellaneous drugs	Anticholinesterases Cimetidine Diuretics Metoclopramide

take medication). It is important to discern the difference between a patient's capacity to exercise the right to refuse lifesaving treatment and a chronically ill and a depressed patient who expresses hopelessness and a desire to die. A clinical evaluation of the effect of depression on the patient's capacity to make competent decisions regarding their care is imperative. Ethics consults are often utilized at this point to clarify the ethical issues at hand and to provide a forum for discussion of possible patient care interventions, including hospice. Patients with primary mental disorders and comorbid chronic medical illness may pose similar problems when their medical condition deteriorates while admitted to a hospital. The use of advance directives helps to address these complex and sensitive issues.

Assessment of Patients with Medical Illness and Secondary Mental Disorders

Mental health assessment should be part of every patient visit regardless of current health status. The Mini-Mental Status examination or a Saint Louis University Mental Status (SLUMS) examination (see Chapter 39) can be helpful to determine baseline cognitive function. Documenting mental health status and cognitive status at each appointment helps establish a baseline and provides for early intervention when there are changes. For patients who have risk factors such as family history of mental health disorders, new psychosocial stressors, current primary mental disorders, or who have chronic medical illnesses, especially CVD, thorough assessment at each visit should always be a priority so that problems can be identified and treated as early as possible. If possible, family and/or caregivers should be engaged as well so that clinical staff can monitor for changes in family dynamics or other new psychosocial issues that could impact the patient's progress and recovery.

The main challenge for clinicians is to determine which signs and symptoms are part of a medical illness and its treatment and which may symptoms signify the presence of a new or worsening mental health disorder. Factors to be considered in assessing mental health problems in medical patients are outlined in Box 43.1. Sometimes, it is difficult to determine whether the presenting symptoms are actually a mix of a psychiatric disorder(s) and chronic medical illness. Some chronic medical illnesses present with decreased appetite, sleep disturbances, and loss of energy as part of the disease process. However, when coupled to feelings of failure, low self-esteem, difficulty concentrating, feelings of hopelessness, and feelings of being punished, a psychiatric liaison referral is needed to determine if depression or anxiety is also present. Side effects of medications for chronic medical illness should also be evaluated. Finally, it is important to recall that changes in mood may signal the beginning of another medical illness for the patient.

BOX 43.1

Factors to Consider in Assessing Mental Health Problems in Medical Patients

- One or more specific medical illnesses
- Past psychiatric history of the patient (before the medical illness)
- Family history of mental health problems
- Current mood, sense of hopelessness, suicidal ideation excessive worry, anxiety
- Current mental health problems, treatment, response to treatment
- Change in sleep or eating (not related to medical illness)
- Sex of the patient

Nursing Interventions for Patients with Medical Illness and Secondary Mental Disorders

Ideally, an interdisciplinary team of care providers that includes a psychiatric liaison nurse should work closely together to deliver optimal treatment of complex medical and mental disorders. Current psychosocial stressors and patient coping mechanisms should be monitored and taken into consideration in developing all plans of care. Most reports suggest that clinicians should be more aggressive in the pharmacologic treatment of mental disorders in medically ill patients. The basic rules for medicating patients include using the minimal dose initially, advancing the dose slowly, and performing frequent blood-level monitoring if appropriate. The person's weight should be carefully monitored at each appointment. Because of pathophysiologic changes associated with the medical illness and likely subsequent changes in pharmacokinetics of medications, doses required to achieve therapeutic blood levels may be less than the usual therapeutic dose and may take longer to titrate. SSRIs (selective serotonin reuptake inhibitors) and SNRIs (serotonin–norepinephrine reuptake inhibitors) are frequently used in the treatment of depression in the medically ill patient population. Both potential interactions and side effects of all medications should be monitored.

Cognitive and behavioral strategies including individual therapy, group therapy, and family therapy are helpful. Assisting the patient and family to understand the nature and relationship of the medical and psychiatric diagnoses may strengthen the support system, alter the perception of caregiver burden, and identify appropriate coping strategies. Mutually agreed-upon goals and therapy actively involve the patient in progress toward recovery and ideally should also include input of caregivers and family members whenever possible. Cognitive intervention should address the areas of the patient's life that can be controlled, despite major lifestyle changes, so that feelings of competence and self-efficacy can be reinforced. At some point, psychodynamic conflicts and maladaptive coping strategies may need to be explored. A referral to clergy or other spiritual support person may also be of value for some patients and their family. In sum, secondary mental disorders can be approached using many of the same strategies that are effective for primary mental health disorders.

MENTAL HEALTH ISSUES RELATED TO PAIN

Pain is one of the most powerful and complex of human experiences and can affect all levels of a person's biopsychosocial and spiritual functioning. It is one of the most common reasons adults seek medical care (Dahlhamer et al., 2018). In the United States, 50 million adults, 15 million of whom are older adults between the ages of 65 and 85, experience chronic pain and an estimated 19.6 million adults experience high-impact pain that interferes with daily life or work activities (Dahlhamer et al., 2018). For children in the United States, chronic pain has been reported to be as high as 15% of the population between 8 and 18 years old (Grout et al., 2018.). Pain is also experienced by neonates who are receiving intensive care. For example, frequently needed eye exams for retinopathy of prematurity (ROP) can produce significant discomfort and distress for premature infants (Corrigan et al., 2020).

Pain can negatively impact the mental health and well-being of anyone and can exacerbate other existing medical conditions. Pain is a frequent comorbidity in persons diagnosed with depressive disorders, anxiety disorders, alcohol use disorder, opioid use disorder, bipolar disorder, and sleep disorders (Borsook et al., 2018). Pain can initiate new or exacerbate existing manic episodes (Stubbs et al., 2015). The presence of pain is considered to be a prominent risk factor for suicide (Kirtley et al., 2020). Pain can stress interpersonal relationships and complicate family systems. In the United States, pain is a serious public health issue that contributes to high health care costs, lower worker productivity, and increased disability (Dowell et al., 2016).

The continuing opioid epidemic in the United States and elsewhere has initiated a long overdue scrutiny of the ways in which we conceptualize, assess, and manage pain. In this new era of pain management, the use of opioids alone, for example, is no longer considered a first-line therapy for pain management (Dowell et al., 2016). Innovative, person-centered approaches to pain have now become clinical necessities. A comprehensive review of pain neuroscience and pain management is beyond the scope of this chapter. However, this section will briefly explore important areas of pain etiology, classification, assessment, and management that are essential for effective nursing of persons with mental health disorders.

Pain Vulnerability and Pain Resilience

Physiological pain is personal. It involves a series of complex, neuro-psychological events that culminate in a highly subjective and deeply individualized experience of discomfort and distress. The experience of pain occurs within each person's biopsychosocial and spiritual ecology where a unique, personal meaning to pain is created by the person who is suffering. **The BioPsychoSocial Spiritual (BPSS) Model for Pain Management and Delivery** (Matteliano, et al., 2014) is one nursing model that takes into consideration the multidimensional complexity of pain and its management. **The Loeser Model of Pain** acknowledges the biopsychosocial experience of pain but importantly identifies **pain behavior** as the end outcome of the pain experience (Loeser & Ford, 1983). Pain behavior may be thought of as the actions and reactions a person has in response to pain. Given the Loeser Model, it is easy to see how comorbid pain complicates care of all patients and especially those with mental health diagnoses. Behaviors such as anger, agitation, isolation, insomnia, change in appetite, lack of focus, and/or depressed mood may represent pain, a change in mental health status, or a combination of both and always require careful nursing assessment.

Recent advances in neuroscience have attempted to partially decode why each person's experience of pain is so individualized. One explanation has suggested that early pain exposure in some neonates may alter and then "prime" pain pathways in the brain. It is theorized that these changes later produce hypersensitivity to nociceptive trauma and greater **pain vulnerability** for some people (Denk et al., 2014). On the other hand, genetics may play a significant role in the mediation of the experience of pain. For example, some people may produce more or different **beta-endorphins**. These are neurotransmitters that exhibit opioid-like behavior. When activated, they diminish pain perception in some people (Choi & Lee, 2019). In doing so they may also improve **pain resilience**, which can be thought of as a diminished susceptibility to suffering from pain over time (Ankawi et al., 2017). There are many other genetic possibilities for pain vulnerability that are being explored.

Age, race, ethnicity, marital status, military veteran status, sex, immune responsivity, socioeconomic status, comorbid medical and mental diagnoses, past psychological or physical trauma, and stress are also factors that contribute to each person's pain vulnerability and pain resilience (Borsook et al., 2018). According to the BPSS pain model, a person's spiritual beliefs and practices are also part of the pain complex. This biopsychosocial complex of risk factors for pain is defined as the "**pain mosaic.**" For example, non-Hispanic White women and non-Hispanic Black women in the United States are more likely to report persistent and bothersome pain than U.S. men of any ethnicity. Military veterans who have been diagnosed with posttraumatic stress disorder (PTSD) and comorbid pain experience worse pain than veterans who have chronic pain but not PTSD (Bair et al., 2020). Older adults who have experienced the biologic changes of aging such as systematic inflammation, altered autonomic function, and changes in neuronal structure suffer increased chronic pain, and they are routinely undertreated for this type of pain (Fillingim, 2017). Among homeless persons with comorbid mental disorders, chronic pain can occur in as much as 64% of that population (Vogel et al., 2017). Finally, chronic pain is also associated with a number of comorbid clinical syndromes. Clearly, many factors must be taken into consideration when caring for people in pain. The presence of mental health issues can certainly complicate pain management. Knowledge of the various biopsychosocial and spiritual risk factors and attentiveness to the unique pain mosaic of each person will ensure adequate pain assessment and appropriate pain interventions.

Classification of Pain

Knowledge of pain types is useful to determine prevention, assessment, treatment, and follow-up care. In the past, pain was usually defined by how long the person had been experiencing it. **Acute pain** has been described as pain that lasts between 3 and 6 months, and **chronic pain** has been described as pain that lasts over 6 months. Given these two limited classifications, identification of pain type has been described in relation to time only. The American Nurses Association (ANA) and the American Society for Pain Management Nursing (ASPMN) have encouraged nursing professionals to reconceptualize pain type along four main classifications of pain: (1) **temporal pattern**—acute, chronic, and episodic; (2) **etiology**—cancer, post-operative, etc.; (3) **tissue injury**—nociceptive and neuropathic; and (4) **mixed**—different pain types and/or the simultaneous presence of both acute and chronic pain (ANA & ASPMN, 2016). See Box 43.2 for more details regarding these classifications

The Nociceptive Pain Pathway and Gate Control Theory

Nociceptive pain is a protective response to noxious stimuli that serves as a warning of tissue injury, inflammation, and pathologic processes that lower the threshold of sensitization. Although current research has further refined the more than half-century-old pain model, gate-control theory continues to offer an adequate general framework for understanding the pain response especially nociceptive pain (Pelaez & Taniguchi, 2016). Gate control theory postulates that there is not a single-pain mechanism but that the processing of pain occurs on at least three levels—peripheral, spinal, and supraspinal. Gate-control theory holds that there are neurologic gates that can either inhibit or allow pain signals to be transmitted to the brain. At the site of the tissue injury, pain receptors (nociceptors) cause the release of prostaglandins (an unsaturated fatty acid that helps control smooth muscle contraction, blood pressure, inflammation,

BOX 43.2
Classification of Pain

Acute Pain: Lasts 3–6 months and has an identifiable cause, e.g., surgery, injury. Described by patients as sharp, throbbing, aching. Resolves when tissues heal and function returns.

Chronic or Persistent Pain: Occurs longer than 6 months or beyond normal healing time and may not have an identifiable cause. Alternation in the dorsal horn of the spinal cord and neuroplastic changes in the brain are thought to be the possible causes. Often associated with mental health comorbidities,

Nociceptive Pain: Pain that elicits the typical response from the nociceptive pathway and is a normal response to noxious stimuli from tissue injury.

Neuropathic Pain: In contrast to nociceptive pain, neuropathic pain originates in a primary lesion of the peripheral or CNS. Described by patients as tingling, burning, numbness, and/or shooting. Allodynia may also be described.

Cancer-related Pain: Can be acute, chronic, or recurrent and is a caused by tumor or metastases, or cancer therapies such as chemotherapy and/or radiation. Often accompanied by malaise, fever, insomnia, and nausea.

Breakthrough Pain: Pain that occurs over baseline pain in a more intense level.

Procedural Pain: Pain associated with any medical intervention.

Adapted from: American Nurses Association (ANA) and American Society for Pain Management Nursing (ASPMN). (2016). *Pain Management Nursing Scope and Standards* (2nd ed.). Silver Spring MD: American Nurses Association.

and body temperature) and substance P (a peptide found in body tissues, especially nervous tissue, that is involved in the transmission of pain and in inflammation), as well as potassium, histamine, leukotrienes (short-range chemical messengers that help regulate the state of blood vessels and airways and influence the activities of some white blood cells), and bradykinin (chemical that dilates blood vessels). These function as transmitters of a relay signal sent to the dorsal horn of the spinal cord that in turn increases the flow of impulses relayed to the brain (Box 43.3). The excitability of this pathway can be altered by inhibitory interneurons at the site of the dorsal horn, closing the gate and lesser or no pain may be experienced. If the cytokines or projection neurons are released, they sensitize and stimulate central pain receptors to spread the pain experience and activate areas of the brain responsible for memory, emotion, and personality (Fig. 43.1). As these ascending pathways signal higher centers, descending noradrenergic and serotonergic pathways are activated and inhibit the release of substance P, which closes the gate and thereby reduces the pain (Fig. 43.2) (Mendell, 2014).

Pain Chronification

For some people who have sustained an injury or trauma, the accompanying acute pain will resolve as the

BOX 43.3
Neurotransmitters Active in Pain Sensation and Induced Plasticity

C-FIBER NEUROPEPTIDES (CYTOKINES) RELEASED BY PERIPHERAL NOXIOUS STIMULATION

Substance P
Bradykinin
Somatostatin
Prostaglandins
Calcitonin gene-related peptide (CGRP)
Histamine
Vasoactive intestinal polypeptide (VIP)
Cholecystokinin

EXCITATORY AMINO ACIDS WITH WIDESPREAD ACTIVITY IN THE CENTRAL NERVOUS SYSTEM (THALAMUS AND SOMATOSENSORY CORTICES)

L-glutamate
N-methyl-D-aspartate (NMDA)

NEUROTRANSMITTERS ACTIVE AS PAIN MODULATORS

Endorphins
Serotonin

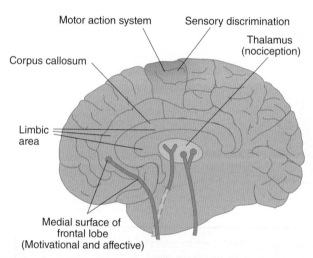

FIGURE 43.1 Pain stimuli activate regions of the brain that influence memory, emotion, and personality.

injury heals. For other people, acute pain does not resolve when the injury heals and instead acute pain transitions into chronic pain. This transition process is known as **pain chronification** and represents potentially permanent changes and modifications throughout the pain pathway and within the brain itself (neuroplasticity). These neurobiological alterations in dendrites, opioidergic and dopaminergic receptors, and cytokine production, to name a few examples, do not occur with acute pain (Borsook, et al., 2018). People suffering from chronic pain report **hyperalgia** (increased sensation of pain), **allodynia** (pain unrelated to noxious stimuli, lowered pain threshold), and/or **hyperesthesia** (increased nociceptor sensitivity). As with pain in general, vulnerability to the transition from acute pain to chronic pain is driven by a variety biopsychosocial and spiritual risk factors that are unique to the person. Environmental factors such as geolocation, atmosphere, and air quality may also play a role (Borsook, et al., 2018). Pain medication itself, including opioids, NSAIDs, and triptans, has also been linked to the transition from acute pain to chronic pain in some people (Borsook, et al., 2018).

Psychosocial Aspects of Chronic Pain

The impact of chronic pain on quality of life can be devastating. When pain persists for an extended period, mood, coping skills, interpersonal relations, and financial and social resources are affected. Pain becomes a preoccupying daily burden. Demoralization, sadness, isolation, loss of interest in life, feelings of worthlessness, self-reproach, excessive guilt, indecisiveness, and suicidal ideation are often associated with chronic pain (Tagliaferri et al., 2020).

Multimodal Pain Management

The treatment of pain, especially chronic pain, is complex and is always interdisciplinary. It requires careful assessment of the patient's pain mosaic and the systematic analysis of the likely mechanisms that are responsible for the experience of pain. In the shadow of the opioid crisis, new models of pain management have been developed. One promising approach is **mechanism-based pain management**, which attempts to target the many unique pain producing mechanisms along the subcellular and molecular pain pathways (Vardeh et al., 2016). Mechanism-based pain management uses simultaneous, **multimodal interventions** to elicit pain mitigation and relief. Once the mechanisms of pain are identified or suspected within the pain pathway, lower-dose traditional analgesia may be used with lower-dose non-traditional analgesia along with non-pharmacological/complementary interventions (Figure 43.3). For example, combinations of traditional analgesics such as local anesthetic agents to block nerve conduction, acetaminophen to inhibit prostaglandin synthesis, NSAIDS to block peripheral and central cyclooxygenase, and/or opioids that can address multiple sites of pain action may be used in combination with choices of nontraditional analgesics including anticonvulsants to inhibit neuronal firing, NMDA-receptor antagonists like ketamine to inhibit glutamate activation, anti-depressants to activate ascending pain pathways, and alpha-2 adrenergic agonists like clonidine to inhibit substance P. Combinations of non-pharmacological interventions such as transcutaneous electrical nerve stimulation, cognitive–behavioral therapies, massage therapy, music therapy, and acupuncture, among many complementary options, complete the multimodal approach (Manworren, 2015). It is important to point out that in the mechanism-based model described earlier, the many types of legitimate complementary treatments are

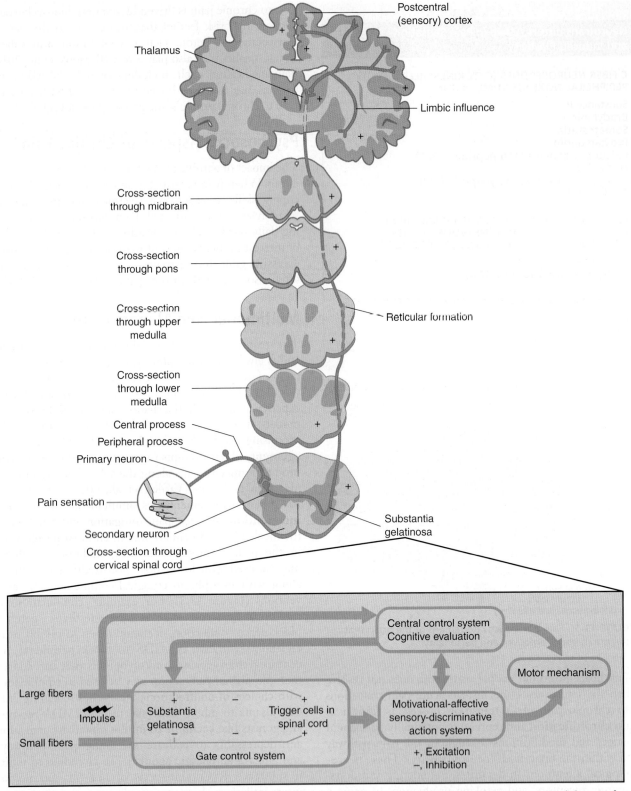

FIGURE 43.2 Ascending sensory pathways: Anterior spinothalamic tract with a schematic diagram of the gate-control theory of pain mechanism.

no longer considered "alternative" or "adjunct." Instead, they are viewed as essential modalities of care to be integrated into the entire pain management plan. There is a growing body of evidence that supports this (Clark et al., 2019). Emerging research has also demonstrated the importance of spiritual interventions for pain relief in patients for whom spirituality can helpful (Siddall et al., 2015). Ritual, prayer, individual and group spiritual

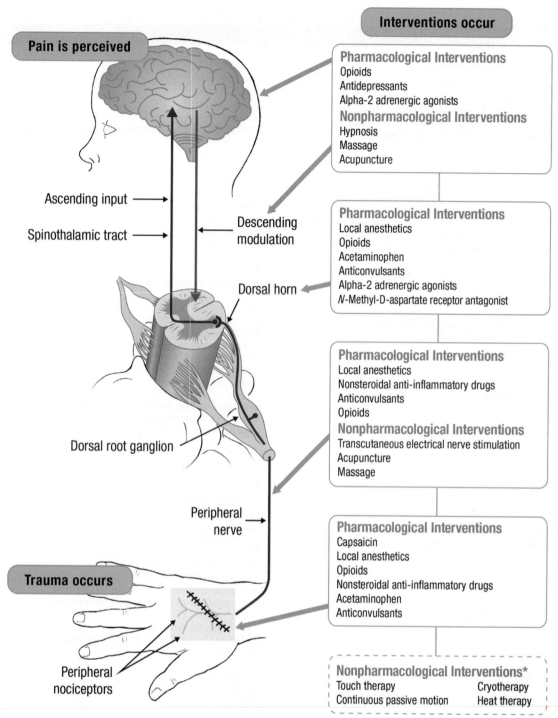

FIGURE 43.3 Mechanism-Based Pain: A multimodal approach Identification of the pain pathway can guide selection of intervention. (Manworren R. C. [2015]. Multimodal pain management and the future of a personalized medicine approach to pain. *AORN Journal, 101*(3), 308–318. https://doi.org/10.1016/j.aorn.2014.12.009)

direction, and other interventions can be included as part of a care plan for some patients (Box 43.4).

Barriers to Care

There are many barriers to effective pain management (Box 43.5). Providers may fail to acknowledge or properly assess pain or may be fearful of providing enough pain relief, especially with pain medications. Patients may experience reluctance to acknowledge the pain and to communicate their distress or discomfort. Maladaptive coping by patients with respect to pain can lead to a fear of pain or a catastrophizing about how intense the pain will become or how long it will last. This can generate

BOX 43.4

Treatment Approaches to Pain

PRINCIPLES OF PAIN TREATMENT

- Establish the correct diagnosis within the context of the person's pain mosaic.
- Recognize that pain reduction, rather than complete pain control, is a reasonable goal.
- Utilize an interdisciplinary, multimodal approach. Opioids are not first-line or routine therapy for chronic pain alone.
- Control other symptoms besides pain. This includes addressing the symptoms that were present before treatment (e.g., depression and anxiety) and any adverse effects associated with the pain therapy. Monitor for signs and symptoms of opioid use disorder.
- Monitor for new mental health issues, including catastrophizing about pain, fear of pain, suicidal ideation, anxiety, depression, mania, psychosis, delirium.
- Treat physical conditions that may initiate or exacerbate the pain.
- Treat the adverse effects of all the agents used.

Examples of Traditional Analgesia Used in Mechanism-Based Pain Management

Nonsteroidal anti-inflammatory drugs (NSAIDs)
Acetaminophen
Acetylsalicylic acid
Oral local anesthetics
Topical agents
Capsaicin
EMLA (lidocaine and prilocaine mixture)
Lidocaine gel
Trigger point injection (TPI)
Epidural steroid injection (ESI)
Facet joint injection (FJI)
Nerve root blocks
Opioids

Examples of Non-Traditional Analgesia Used in Mechanism-Based Pain Management

Baclofen
Neuroleptics
Pimozide
Corticosteroids
Pulsed Glucocorticoids
Calcitonin
Benzodiazepines
Clonazepam
Valium
Drugs for sympathetically maintained pain
Nifedipine
Phenoxybenzamine
Prazosin
Propranolol
Tricyclic and tetracyclic antidepressants
Amitriptyline
Clomipramine
Desipramine

Doxepin
Imipramine
Maprotiline
Nortriptyline
Mirtazapine
Selective and nonselective serotonin reuptake inhibitors
Bupropion
Citalopram
Escitalopram
Fluoxetine
Fluvoxamine
Nefazodone
Olanzapine
Paroxetine
Sertraline
Trazodone
Venlafaxine
Serotonin–norepinephrine or dopamine reuptake inhibitors
Desvenlafaxine
Duloxetine
Ziprasidone
Anticonvulsants
Carbamazepine
Divalproex
Neurontin
Phenytoin

Examples of Non-Medication Treatments: Restorative Therapies, Interventional Procedures, Behavioral Interventions, and Complementary Health Options

TENS (transcutaneous electrical nerve stimulator)
High Frequency Spinal Cord Stimulation (10 kHz)
Cryotherapy
Heat therapy
Massage therapy
Physical therapy
Recreational therapy
Art therapy
Music therapy
Occupational Therapy
Cognitive–Behavioral Therapy
Acceptance and Commitment Therapy
Self-regulatory or Psychophysiological Therapies: Biofeedback
Pain Support Groups
Individual and Group Psychotherapy
Hypnosis
Tai-Chi
Acupuncture
Healing Touch Therapy
Energy Therapies
Meditation/Mindfulness
Yoga
Prayer
Individual and Group Spiritual direction
Ritual

Note: If the patient has failed to experience response to all standard treatments, psychiatric evaluation for underlying problems should be emphasized.

BOX 43.5
Barriers to Pain Management

PROBLEMS OF HEALTH CARE PROFESSIONALS

- Inadequate knowledge and experience with pain management
- Poor assessment of pain
- Concern about regulation of controlled substances
- Fear of patient tolerance and addiction
- Concern about side effects of analgesics

PROBLEMS OF PATIENTS

- Reluctance to report pain
- Concern about primary treatment of underlying disease
- Fear that pain means the disease is worse
- Concern about being a good patient and not a complainer
- Reluctance to take pain medications
- Fear of tolerance and addiction, fear of "addict" label
- Fear of unmanageable side effects

PROBLEMS OF HEALTH CARE SYSTEM

- Cost or inadequate reimbursement
- Restrictive regulation of controlled substances
- Problems with availability of treatment or access to it

hopelessness, despair, and suicidal ideation for some. Improper pain management may also contribute to pain chronification. Nonadherence with sequential prescription changes and combined treatments can be problematic as well. Strategies to assess adherence include awareness of the patient's pain mosaic and monitoring for new changes in it such as recent homelessness, loss of employment, family stress, and new medical diagnoses, to name a few areas. Encouragement of regular self-report by the patient, biochemical assays that check for the presence of medications, and regular outcome assessments can also promote adherence to the treatment plan.

Piecing the Mosaic Together: Assessment of Patients with Chronic Pain

Appropriate diagnosis and treatment of pain begin with a comprehensive biopsychosocial and spiritual history as well as a physical examination. A functional assessment that investigates how the patient's pain affects their daily living should also be completed. Attentiveness to any recent falls due to pain, difficulty completing ADLs (activities of daily living) and IADLs (instrumental activities of daily living), and other diminishments of quality of life is important. When discussing pain, a patient should be asked to describe the pain characteristics, including location and severity, and information about possible factors that may be influencing or producing pain. Patients should also be encouraged to express their feelings, beliefs, and values around pain and suffering. If

the patient is a child, parents should also be included in the discussion.

A direct relationship between the severity or extent of detectable disease and the intensity of the patient's pain may not be evident during the first interaction between nurse and patient. Pain assessment instruments can aid in evaluation. However, using an instrument designed to measure acute pain, such as asking the patient to rate pain on a scale of 1 to 10, is inadequate for assessing chronic pain because the pain may always be a 3 or 4, but the chronic nature of the pain is the problem (Amir et al., 2019). All pain presents over time, so alertness as to whether pain episodically waxes and wanes, is worse at night, or improves with sleep, to name a few factors, is important. Among patients who are critically ill in an inpatient setting, failure to assess pain expeditiously and correctly can result in a variety of complications, including hyperglycemia and increased risk of infection, which among complications may unnecessarily lengthen a hospital stay (Reardon et al., 2015). Attentiveness to the patient's pain mosaic, pain behaviors, levels of pain vulnerability and pain resilience, and acute and chronic medical and psychiatric comorbidities is crucial. Objective data and the patient's own subjective experience of pain must be carefully analyzed so that comprehensive pain management can occur (Box 43.6).

Nursing Response to Chronic Pain

Pain syndromes, especially chronic pain, are very common in the primary care setting (Box 43.7). The nurse–patient relationship is primary for healing and nurses have an important role in helping the patient manage chronic pain. The nurse's therapeutic use of self can help instill hope and improve the patient's self-efficacy and pain resilience. Listening and acknowledging the pain is important because others may ignore or invalidate the impact of the pain. The nurse can help the patient identify circumstances when the pain was diminished and use this information to adjust existing or develop new strategies. Encouraging the patient to engage in all elements of the pain management plan is key. If the patient is taking medications, the nurse should closely monitor therapeutic and untoward effects. Education with the patient and family about approaches to pain mitigation and the patient's particular pain care helps to build compliance.

Pain Management and Nursing Ethics

Patients diagnosed with acute or chronic pain and who have comorbid alcohol or substance abuse or a history of these diseases can present more complex treatment

---

BOX 43.6

Assessing Patients Who Report Pain

QUESTIONS TO ASSESS PAIN

The following questions can guide the nurse in reflecting on the significance of the chronic pain to the individual and family:

- What is the extent of the patient's disease or injury (physical impairment)?
- What is the magnitude of the illness? That is, to what extent is the patient suffering, disabled, and unable to enjoy usual activities?
- Does the person's behavior seem appropriate to the disease or injury, or is there any evidence of amplification of symptoms for any of a variety of psychological or social reasons or purposes?
- How often and for how long does the patient perform specific behaviors, such as reclining, sitting, standing, and walking?
- How often does the patient seek health care and take analgesic medication (frequency and quantity)?

PAIN BEHAVIOR CHECKLIST

Pain behaviors have been characterized as interpersonal communications of pain, distress, or suffering. Pain behavior may be a more accurate indication of intensity and tolerance than verbal reports. Check the box of each behavior you observe or infer from the patient's comments.

- Facial grimacing, clenched teeth
- Holding or supporting of affected body area
- Questions such as, "Why did this happen to me?"
- Distorted gait, limping
- Frequent shifting of posture or position
- Requests to be excused from tasks or activities, avoidance of physical activity
- Taking of medication as often as possible
- Moving extremely slowly
- Sitting with a rigid posture
- Moving in a guarded or protective fashion
- Moaning or sighing
- Using a cane, cervical collar, or other prosthetic device
- Requesting help in ambulation; frequent stopping while walking
- Lying down during the day
- Irritability

BOX 43.7

Pain Syndromes Seen in the Primary Care Setting

- *Migraine headache:* A cerebrovasomotor disorder in which a focal reduction of cerebral blood flow initiates an ischemic headache. It may be preceded by a visual aura and followed by nausea, vomiting, and incapacitating head pain.
- *Low back pain:* Pain arising from the vertebral column or surrounding muscles, tendons, ligaments, or fascia. Causes range from simple muscle strain to arthritis, fracture, or nerve compression from a ruptured disk.
- *Chronic benign orofacial pain:* Temporomandibular joint pain, trigeminal neuralgia
- *Rheumatoid arthritis:* More than 100 different types of joint disease produce inflammation of the joints. Associated with varying degrees of pain and stiffness and eventual loss of use of the affected joints.
- *Reflex sympathetic dystrophy:* A painful burning syndrome that occurs after peripheral nerve injury. Associated with hyperesthesia, vasomotor disturbances, and dystrophic changes caused by sympathetic hyperactivity.
- *Cancer pain:* Pain from malignant tumors that is caused by local infiltration or metastatic spread involving specific organs, bones, peripheral or cranial nerves, or the spinal cord. Pain therapy is aimed at providing sufficient relief to allow maximum possible daily functioning and a relatively pain-free death.
- *Neuropathic pain*
- *Polyneuropathy:* neuropathy involving multiple peripheral nerves
- *Diabetic neuropathy:* neuropathy caused by diabetes mellitus; marked by diminished sensation secondary to vascular changes
- *Inflammatory neuropathy:* neuropathy related to the presence of chemical or micro-organic pathogens
- *Traumatic neuropathy:* neuropathy caused by avulsion or compression
- *Plexopathy:* neuropathy involving a peripheral nerve plexus
- *Peripheral or central neuralgia:* abrupt, intense, paroxysmal pain caused by intrinsic nerve injury or extrinsic nerve compression
- *Herpetic neuralgia:* pain associated with the dermatomal rash of acute herpes zoster
- *Radiculopathy:* pain radiating along a peripheral nerve tract, such as sciatica
- *Vaso-occlusive pain:* Thrombotic crisis of sickle cell anemia in joints and peripheral muscles that is caused by ischemia
- *Myofascial pain:* Pain in palpable bands (trigger points) of muscle; associated with stiffness, limitation of motion, and weakness

---

issues. Social stigma associated with various substance use disorders may prevent such patients from receiving timely and adequate pain management. However, having a current or past substance use disorder does not preclude patients from receiving adequate pain relief including the use of opioids, if necessary, as part of a mechanism-based, multimodal pain management plan. Nurses are morally obligated to advocate for these patients so that adequate pain relief can occur. However, nurses must also be alert to the legitimate concerns of those same patients who may fear an exacerbation or relapse of substance abuse problems. Patient preference regarding pain management options must always be taken into consideration. Multimodal pain management strategies are especially

indispensable for these patients. On the other hand, nurses are also ethically responsible for addressing behaviors with the patient that are not part of the pain management plan. Such behaviors may include lost prescriptions, asking for early refills of pain medications, and/or taking more medications than what was prescribed to name a few such behaviors (ANA & ASPMN, 2016). When this occurs involvement of the interdisciplinary care team by the nurse is crucial to assure proper pain management as well as potential referrals for substance abuse.

MENTAL HEALTH DISORDERS RELATED TO PHYSIOLOGICAL TRAUMA

Physiological trauma can be thought of as sudden onset, severe injury caused by blunt, penetrating, and/ or burn mechanisms. Physiologic trauma activates the overall stress response of the autonomic nervous system. Massive catecholamine release causes certain cardiovascular, muscular, gastrointestinal, and respiratory symptoms that release energy stores and support survival. Tissue destruction, musculoskeletal pain, physical disability, and body image changes all contribute to the physiologic and psychological stress response, which continues long after the traumatic physical insult. Common behavioral responses are hypervigilance, fear, anxiety, and a sense of being overwhelmed. Psychological sequelae may include social isolation, agitation, PTSD, depression, and, in extreme cases, dissociative identity disorders. It may be difficult to distinguish trauma response from existing mental health issues in some people (Lutton & Swank, 2018).

Biologic Basis of the Trauma Response

The neurotransmitters responsible for behavioral responses to fear and anxiety are usually held in balance to maintain a level of arousal appropriate for environmental threat. Information from the sensory processing areas in the thalamus and cortex alerts the amygdala (the lateral and central nucleus). Events that are appraised as threatening activate HPA (hypothalamic-pituitary adrenal axis), which releases adrenal steroids initiating the generalized stress response (see Chapter 19). When the perceived threat is sustained, complex neurochemical processes involving norepinephrine, gamma-aminobutyric acid (GABA), dopamine, and serotonin are overwhelmed, leading to a general dysregulation of the HPA axis. Inappropriate and prolonged secretion of high levels of catecholamines results (Seo et al., 2019).

Adaptation to trauma is related to such factors as the severity of the trauma, the person's maturity and age when the trauma occurs, available social support, and the person's ability to mobilize coping strategies. During adaptation to prolonged stress, the patient's cognitive thought processes and coping behaviors cause dopamine and serotonin to be released in the prefrontal cortex of the brain. These noradrenergic systems are presumed to play a major role in physiologic and emotional coping responses, storage of the trauma experience into memory, and possibly the development of PTSD (Chia-Ying et al., 2015). See Chapters 19 and 29.

Psychological Response to Trauma

An individual's psychological response to trauma depends on the extent of endocrine and autonomic activity that occurs during stress coupled with prior experience, developmental history, physical status, and existing social support. Psychological manifestation of sustained stress and trauma may be manifested as flashbacks, intrusive recurring thoughts, panic or anxiety attacks, paranoia, inappropriate startle reactions, social isolation, and nightmares (see Chapter 29). The patient may become so withdrawn and depressed that they stop participating in activities of daily living. Toward the other extreme, the patient may become agitated and combative, perceiving any treatment as a continued threat.

Assessment of Patients Experiencing Trauma

Complete physical assessment after physical traumatic injury is imperative in life-threatening circumstances. Multiple trauma and head injuries are the major causes of death and disability in young adults in society. Highly trained emergency and intensive care providers look for signs and symptoms of physiologic injury and intervene to stabilize primary and secondary trauma in the general medical setting.

After physical stabilization, the patient should be examined for psychological injury through observation and interview to determine prevalent signs and symptoms of accompanying psychological disorders. This process includes evaluating the patient's adjustment and coping skills, their personal way of dealing with the trauma, as well as current social circumstances, and environmental and life stressors. The majority of people who present for trauma treatment, however, will be older adults who may have significant cognitive and functional deficits (Fisher et al., 2017). Especially with the older adults, assessment must be ongoing to help the patient deal with disfigurement, sudden disability or increased disability, and changes in self-care. The evaluation should include assessment of the patient's perception of experienced stress, feelings related to the stress, dominant mood, cognitive functioning, defense and coping mechanisms, and available support systems. In addition, assessment of the risk for self-inflicted injury or suicide is essential.

Nursing Interventions for Responses to Trauma

Psychiatric clinicians provide an important aspect of emergency care. Interventions that establish trust, reduce anxiety, promote positive adaptive coping, and cultivate a sense of control help the patient to begin recovery and maintain emotional health. Physical trauma involving children has been connected to serious, long-term psychological complications, making early intervention and support critical (Lantz, 2020). Crisis intervention methods, stress management, cognitive–behavioral therapies, psychotherapy, and psychotropic medications, alone or in combination, may be useful in achieving the best possible outcome.

Traumatic death is often sudden and unexpected, and the victim is often young. When trauma causes the patient's death, the family must be informed of the death and allowed to grieve to prevent the development of a pathologic or prolonged grief response. Surviving family members may have a severe emotional reaction to the death. Unhealthy family dynamics, especially maladaptive coping, may become evident during this period. Ideally, the psychiatric–mental health liaison nurse can use family intervention strategies to enhance or improve relationships while the family's motivation to do all that is possible is high.

MENTAL HEALTH ISSUES RELATED TO CENTRAL NERVOUS SYSTEM DISORDERS

Neurologic impairment is most often related to brain cell (neuron) destruction. The primary causes of neuronal damage are traumatic injury, ischemia, infarction (cerebrovascular accident—CVA), abnormal neuron growth (brain tumor), and metabolic poisoning associated with systemic disease. Brain cell loss may also be the result of degenerative processes, such as those that occur in Alzheimer or Parkinson disease. Psychiatric disorders are often complications of these neurologic diseases and may be difficult to distinguish from the neuropathology itself. Therefore, appropriate intervention depends on skilled assessment to discriminate and detect mental status changes related to organic brain injury as well as disorders of mood and thought.

An injury to the brain can destroy brain cells directly or initiate a cascade of cell breakdown from ischemia. This **ischemic cascade** begins with hypoxia and is followed by paralysis of the ion exchange across the cell membrane, edema, calcium influx, free radical production, and lipid peroxidation (oxidative degradation of lipids). The severity of brain injury is related to the degree and duration of ischemia. Complete ischemia results in brain cell death or infarction, commonly known as stroke. The resulting neurologic impairment is related to the size and location of the affected brain area. Some areas of the brain, such as the internal capsule, are extremely sensitive to ischemia. They are typically injured first and contribute to more generalized impairment, such as memory loss, altered judgment, and post-stroke spasticity (Songjin et al., 2020).

Traumatic Brain Injury

Traumatic brain injury (TBI) is an intracranial injury that occurs when an outside force injures the brain. TBI can result in temporary, mild symptoms or symptoms can be permanent and severe, depending on the scope of brain tissue damage. TBI is a major cause of disability for wounded U.S. soldiers and, among those who served in Iraq and Afghanistan, the prevalence of TBI is estimated to be between 9% and 28% (Lindquist et al., 2017). Mild TBI accounts for an estimated 75% to 95% of all TBI cases (Bryson et al., 2017). **Persistent postconcussive symptoms** (PCS), which include fatigue, sleep problems, difficulty concentrating, sensitivity to light and noise, problems with memory, and other mood-related symptoms, can exist a year or longer in those with even mild TBI (Agtarap et al., 2019). PCS, depressive disorders, and PTSD often coexist as distinct, but related, phenomena among military veterans with TBI (Agtarap et al., 2019). Depression is estimated to occur in up to 53% of those with TBI, and PTSD has been found to occur in 44% of veterans with TBI (Agtarap et al., 2019). Patients with TBI are considered to be at risk for suicide (Bryson et al., 2017). The triad of PCS, PTSD, and depressive disorders may become evident in the acute recovery phase or during rehabilitation and often negatively affects survival and recovery. Early evaluation assists in the detection of these and other mental health complications after brain injury.

Ischemic Stroke

Depressive disorder and anxiety are frequent complications of ischemic stroke. Up to one fifth of people who suffer a stroke experience both depression and anxiety within 12 months (Arba et al., 2016). These mood changes are not only a result of the changes in the autonomic and endocrine systems but also a result of the breakdown of biogenic amines after ischemia and brain cell death. Recent studies show that in some parts of the brain (Fig. 43.4), there is actually atrophy and post-stroke high cortisol levels especially at bedtime have been linked to this (Tene et al., 2018). Other symptoms, such as sleep disturbances, cognitive dysfunction, poor concentration, difficulty making decisions, somatic discomfort, poor appetite, social withdrawal, and fatigue or agitation, often accompany the mood disturbance.

Minor and moderate depression may go unrecognized and undiagnosed when patients with stroke describe somatic symptoms and demonstrate lack of motivation in ADLs. There is no one-risk factor for the development of depression and other mood disorders. Among people recovering from strokes, mild depression occurs in about 46%, moderate depression in 38%, and severe depression in 16% (Zhang & Qui, 2020). Men with lower income,

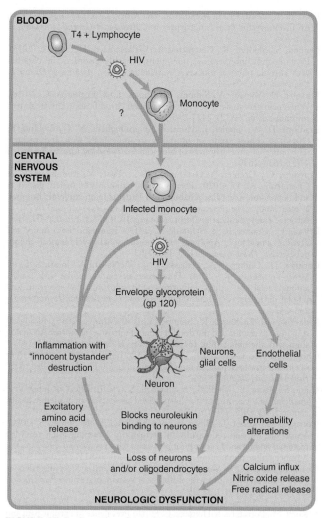

FIGURE 43.4 Functional cerebral anatomy and stroke.

metabolic syndrome, higher neurological deficit, and lower social support are more likely to experience severe depression following a stroke (Zhang & Qui, 2020).

Parkinson Disease

In Parkinson disease and other neuromuscular diseases, there is degeneration in the motor pathways with a loss of dopamine secretion. This dysregulation affects other neurotransmitters. About 35% of patients with Parkinson disease experience depression that contributes to impairment in daily functioning possibly as much as the underlying disease (Yang et al., 2012). However, only about 20% of these patients receive treatment (Frisina et al., 2008). Evidence suggests that altered serotonergic function may be responsible, at least in part, for the depressive symptoms in Parkinson disease and that altered noradrenergic function may underlie some of the associated anxiety symptoms (Kano et al., 2011). Treatment of depression in patients with Parkinson's

is critical because it has been linked to cardiovascular dysautonomia in these patients, which can result in sudden death (Vetrano et al., 2015).

Assessment of Psychological Responses to Central Nervous System Disorders

A thorough neurologic examination is important in determining the location and degree of disability, but is even more critical in establishing the locus of retained function. Cognitive functioning, mood, and functionality are key assessment areas. Many scales exist that accurately assess these areas, are easy to administer, and are generally accepted as reliable tools to detect the degree and limitations of disability. Cognition can be measured using the SLUMS examination (see Chapter 39), and function ability for self-care can be measured using the Barthel index (Mahoney & Barthel, 1965). Evaluation of mood using the Center for Epidemiological Studies Depression Scale (CES-D) or the Beck Depression Inventory (Beck et al., 1961) provides important information for designing intervention strategies for the at-risk neurologic patient. Findings of depressive symptoms indicate the need for a more definitive neuropsychological referral.

Nursing Interventions for Responses to Central Nervous System Disorders

Isolation, lack of companionship, bereavement, and poverty are associated with depressive symptoms in the general population and compound the relative risk of depression developing after brain damage. Prevention strategies should be used as early and include (1) the assessment and provision of social support resources while the patient is hospitalized and as an important component of discharge planning to rehabilitation services; (2) early identification of potential mental health problems with a referral for complete evaluation; (3) education of patient and family about the mental health complications of CNS disorders so they will know when to seek medical attention and treatment to avert major problems; (4) encouragement to seek treatment for mental health problems, including pharmacologic strategies; and (5) enhancement of competence in performing ADLs, with a focus on the use of retained function rather than on adaptation to disabilities only.

SUMMARY OF KEY POINTS

■ Mental disorders are more common in people with systemic or chronic medical illnesses than in the healthy population. Comorbid depression is common in several medical diseases, including endocrine and metabolic disturbances, cancer, viral infections, inflammatory disorders, metabolic syndrome, and cardiopulmonary diseases.

- Mental disorders that accompanies medical illness is often not recognized and treated. Psychiatric symptoms may precede the onset of disease symptoms, and it may be difficult to distinguish between the symptoms of the two conditions.

- Mental disorders in medically ill people is potentially lethal because normal affective–cognitive function may be critical to recovery and compliance with the medical treatment plan. Therefore, it is imperative that mental health is included in the standard health assessment of all medically ill persons and that appropriate referrals be made.

CRITICAL THINKING CHALLENGE

1. You are caring for a patient who is recovering from a stroke who refuses breakfast and a morning bath. Applying what you know about the neurologic damage caused by stroke and the frequency of depression in stroke patients, develop a care plan addressing the patient's biopsychosocial needs.

2. Discuss the pain syndromes you may see in the primary care setting.

3. A patient is being seen for chronic pain. Discuss how you would go about assessing barriers to pain management with this patient.

4. You are a psychiatric–mental health liaison nurse and have been asked to prepare a program for the medical–surgical nursing staff on psychiatric aspects of medical illnesses. What topics would you include, and what would be your rationale for including each?

REFERENCES

Agtarap, S., Campbell-Sills, L., Thomas, M., Kessler, R., Ursasano, R., & Stein, M. (2019). Postconcussive, posttraumatic stress and repressive symptoms in recently deployed U.S. Army soldiers with traumatic brain injury. *Psychological Assessment*, 31(11), 1340–1356.

American Nurses Association (ANA), & American Society for Pain Management Nursing (ASPMN). (2016). *Pain management nursing: Scope and standards of practice* (2nd ed.). American Nurses Association.

Amir, R., Eisenber, E., & Leiba, R. (2019). Anchoring the numeric pain scale changes pain intensity reports in patients with chronic pain but not with acute pain. *Pain Practice*, 19(3), 283–288.

Ankawi, B., Slepian, M., Himawan, L., & France, C. (2017). Validation of the pain resilience scale in a chronic pain sample. *Journal of Pain*, 18, 984–993.

Arba, F., Ali, M., Quinn, T. J., Hankey, G. J., Lees, K. R., & Inzitari, D. (2016). Lacunar infarcts, depression and anxiety symptoms one year after stroke. *Journal of Stroke and Cerebrovascular Diseases*, 25(4), 831–834.

Avery, J., Schreier, An., & Swanson, M. (2020). A complex population: Nurse's professional preparedness to care for medical-surgical patients with mental illness. *Applied Nursing Research*, 52. https://doi.org/10.1016/j.apnr.2020.151232

Bair, M., Outcait, S., Ang, D., Wu, J., & Yu, Z. (2020). Pain and psychological outcomes among Iraq and Afghanistan veterans with chronic pain and PTSD: ESCAPE trial and longitudinal results. *Pain Medicine*, 21(7), 1369–1376.

Beck, A. T., Ward, C. H., Mendelson, M., Mock, J., & Erbaugh, J. (1961). An inventory for measuring depression. *Archives of General Psychiatry*, 4, 561–656.

Bennett, S., Shafran, R., Coughtrey, A., Walker, S., & Heyman, I. (2015). Psychological interventions for mental health disorders in children with chronic physical illness: A systematic review. *Archives of Disease in Childhood*, 100, 308 316.

Borsook, D., Youssef, A., Simons, L., Elman, I., & Eccleston, C. (2018). When pain gets stuck: The evolution of pain chronification and treatment resistance. *Pain*, 59(12), 2421–2436.

Bradford, D. W., Goulet, J., Hunt, M., Cunningham, N. C., & Hoff, R. (2016). A cohort study of mortality in individuals with and without schizophrenia after diagnosis of lung cancer. *Journal of Clinical Psychiatry*, 77(2), 1626–1630.

Bruyninx, G., Grenier, J., Greenman, P. S., Tassé, V., Abdulnour, J., & Chomienne, M. H. (2020). Prevalence of symptoms of anxiety disorders and depression in cardiac rehabilitation Patients in an academic hospital: a case study. *The Psychiatric Quarterly*, 10.1007/s11126-020-09791-w. Advance online publication. https://doi.org/10.1007/s11126-020-09791-w

Bryson, C., Cramer, R., & Schmidt, A. (2017). Traumatic brain injury and lifetime suicidality: Applying the interpersonal-psychological theory perspective. *Death Studies*, 41(7), 399–-405.

Carliner, H., Collins, P. Y., Cabassa, L. J., McNallen, A., Joestl, S. S., & Lewis-Fernández, R. (2014). Prevalence of cardiovascular risk factors among racial and ethnic minorities with schizophrenia spectrum and bipolar disorders: A critical literature review. *Comprehensive Psychiatry*, 55, 233–247.

Chia-Ying, C., La Marca, R., Steptoe, A., & Brewin, C. (2015). Biological responses to trauma and the development of intrusive memories: An analog study with the trauma film paradigm. *Biological Psychology*, 103, 135–143.

Choi, H., & Lee, C-H. (2019). Can beta-endorphin be used as a biomarker of chronic low back pain? A meta-analysis of randomized controlled trials. *Pain Medicine*, 20(10), 28–36.

Clark, S., Bauer, B., Vitek, S., & Cutshall, S. (2019). Effect of integrative medicine services on pain for hospitalized patients at an academic health center. *EXPLORE*, 15(1), 61–64.

Corrigan, M., Keeler, J., Miller, H., Ben Khallouq, B., & Fowler, S. (2020). Music therapy and retinopathy of prematurity screening using recorded maternal singing and heartbeat for post exam recovery. *Journal of Perinatology*. Advance online publication. https://doi.org/10.1038/s41372-020-0719-9

Cosci, F., Fava, G., & Sonino, N. (2015). Mood and anxiety disorders as early manifestations of medical illness: A systematic review. *Psychotherapy & Psychosomatics*, 84(1), 22–29.

Dahlhamer J., Lucas J., Zelaya C., Nahin, R., Mackey, S., DeBar, L., Von Korff, M., Porter, L., & Helmick, C. (2018) Prevalence of chronic pain and high-impact chronic pain among adults - United States, 2016. *Morbidity and Mortality Weekly Report Centers for Disease Control*, 67(36), 1001–1006.

Davies, S., Iwajomo, T., de Oliveira, C., Versloot, J., Reid, R. J., & Kurdyak, P. (2021). The impact of psychiatric and medical comorbidity on the risk of mortality: a population-based analysis. *Psychological Medicine*, 51(2), 320–328. https://doi.org/10.1017/S003329171900326X

Denk, F., McMahon S., & Tracey, I. (2014). Pain vulnerability: A neurobiological perspective. *Nature Neuroscience*, 17(2), 192–200.

Dowell, D., Haegerich, T., & Chou, R. (2016). CDC guideline for prescribing opioids for chronic pain, United States, 2016. *Center for Disease Control and Prevention Recommendations and Reports*, 65(1), 1–49.

Fillingim, R. (2017). Individual differences in pain: Understanding the mosaic that makes pain personal. *Pain*, 158. https://doi.org/10.1097/j.pain.0000000000000775

Fisher, J., Bates C., & Banerlee, J. (2017). The growing challenge of major trauma in older people: A role for comprehensive geriatric assessment? *Age and Aging*, 46(5), 705–712.

Florea, A., Maurey, H., Le Sauter, M., Bellesme, C., Sevin, C., & Deiva, K. (2020). Fatigue, depression, and quality of life in children with multiple sclerosis: A comparative study with other demyelinating diseases. *Developmental Medicine & Child Neurology*, 62(2), 241–244.

Frisina, P., Borod, J., Foldi., N., Tenenbaum, H. (2008). Depression in Parkinson's disease: Health risks, etiology, and treatment options. *Neuropsychiatric Disease Treatment*, 4(1), 81–91.

Fuller-Thomson, E., Lateef, R., & Sulman, J. (2015). Robust association between inflammatory bowel disease and generalized anxiety disorder: Findings from a nationally representative Canadian study. *Inflammatory Bowel Diseases*, 21(10), 2341–2348.

Grout, R., Thompson-Fleming, R., Carroll, A., & Downs, S. (2018). Prevalence of pain reports in pediatric primary care and association with demographics, body mass index, and exam findings: A cross sectional study. *BMC Pediatrics*, 18(1). https://doi.org/10.1186/s12887-018-1335-0

Gurhan, N., Polat, U., Beser, N., & Koc, M. (2019). Suicide risk and depression in individuals with chronic illness. *Community Mental Health Journal 55*(5), 840–848.

Hirsch, J., Sirois, F., Molnar, D., & Chang, E. (2016). Pain and depressive symptoms in primary care: Moderating role of positive and negative effect. *Clinical Journal of Pain 32*(7), 562–567.

Hjorthoj, C., Sturup, A., McGrath, J., & Nordentoft, M. (2017). Life expectancy and years of potential life lost in schizophrenia: A systematic review and meta-analysis. *Lancet Psychiatry, 4*(4), 295–301.

Kano, O., Ikeda, K., Cridebring, D., Takazawa, T., Yoshii, Y., & Iwasaki, Y. (2011). Neurobiology of depression and anxiety in Parkinson's disease. *Parkinson's Disease.* https://doi.org/10.4061/2011/143547

Kawasaki, M., & Hoshiyama, M. (2020). Apathy and depression during the recovery stage after stroke. *International Journal of Therapy & Rehabilitation, 27*(5), 1–12.

Kim, E., Kim, S., Ha, K., Lee, H., Yoon, D., & Ahn, Y. (2015). Depression trajectories and the association with metabolic adversities among the middle-aged adults. *Journal of Affective Disorders, 188*, 14–21.

Kim, E., Lee Y., & Riesche, L. (2020). Factors affecting depression in high school students with chronic illness: Nationwide cross-sectional study in South Korea. *Archives of Psychiatric Nursing, 34*(3), 164–168.

Kirtley, O., Rodham, K., & Crane, C. (2020). Understanding suicidal ideation and behavior in individuals with chronic pain: A review of the role of novel transdiagnostic psychological factors. *Lancet Psychiatry, 7*(3), 282–290.

Klein-Gitelman, M. S., & Curran, M. L. (2015). The challenges of adolescence, mood disorders, and chronic illness. *The Journal of Pediatrics, 167*(6), 1192–1194.

Lantz, A. (2020). Pediatric accidental trauma: Screening and reducing psychological impact. *Pediatric Nursing, 46*(3), 111–114.

Lee, S., Rothbard, A., & Choi, S. (2016). Effects of co-morbid health conditions on healthcare expenditures among people with severe mental illness. *Journal of Mental Health, 25*(4), 291–296.

Lima, T., Ferreira-Moraes, R., Alves, W., Alves, T., Pimentel, C., Sousa, E., Abrahin, O., & Cortinas-Alves, E. (2019). Resistance training reduces depressive symptoms in elderly people with Parkinson disease: A controlled randomized study. *Scandinavian Journal of Medicine & Science in Sports, 29*(1), 1957–1967.

Lindquist, L., Love, H., & Elbogen, E. (2017). Traumatic brain injury in Iraq and Afghanistan veterans: New results from a national random sample study. *The Journal of Neuropsychiatry and Clinical Neurosciences, 29*, 254–259.

Loeser J., & Ford W. (1983). Chronic pain. In Carr, J. E., & Dengerink, H. A. (Eds). *Behavioral Science in the Practice of Medicine* (pp. 331–334). Elsevier Biomedical.

Lutton, S., & Swank, J. (2018). The importance of intentionality in untangling trauma from severe mental illness. *Journal of Mental Health Counseling, 40*(2), 113–128.

Macchi, C., Favero, C., Ceresa, A., Vigna, L., Conti, D. M., Pesatori, A. C., Racagni, G., Corsini, A., Ferri, N., Sirtori, C. R., Buoli, M., Bollati, V., & Ruscica, M. (2020). Depression and cardiovascular risk-association among Beck Depression Inventory, PCSK9 levels and insulin resistance. *Cardiovascular Diabetology, 19*(1), 187. https://doi.org/10.1186/s12933-020-01158-6

Mahoney, F. T., & Barthel, D. W. (1965). Functional evaluation: Barthel index. *Maryland Medical Journal, 14*, 61–65.

Matteliano, F. St. Marie, B.F., Oliver, J., Coggins, C. (2014), Adherence monitoring with chronic opioid T\therapy for persistent pain: A Biopsychosocial-Spiritual Approach to mitigate risk. *Pain Management Nursing, 15*(1), 391–405.

McGinty, E., Baller, J., Azrin, S., Juliano-Bult, D., & Daumit, G. (2016). Interventions to address medical conditions and health-risk behaviors among persons with serious mental illness: A comprehensive review. *Schizophrenia Bulletin, 42*(1), 96–124.

Mendell, L. M. (2014). Constructing and deconstructing the gate theory of pain. *Pain, 155*, 210–216.

Olker, S., Parrott, J., Swarbrick, M., & Spagnolo, A. (2016). Weight management in adult with serious mental illness: A meta analytic review. *Journal of Psychiatric Rehabilitation, 19*(4), 370–393.

Phan, S. (2016). Medication adherence in patients with schizophrenia. *International Journal of Psychiatry in Medicine, 51*(2), 211–219.

Phillips, R. (1937). Physical disorder in 164 admissions to a mental hospital. *British Medical Journal, 2*, 363–366.

Razzano, L., Cook, J., Yost, C., Jonika, J., Swarbrick, M., Carter, T., & Santos, A. (2015). Factors associated with co-occurring medical conditions among adults with serious mental disorders. *Schizophrenia Research, 161*(2–3), 458–464.

Reardon, D., Anger, K., & Szumita, P. (2015). Pathophysiology, assessment, and management of pain in critically ill adults. *American Journal of Health Systems Pharmacy, 72*(18), 1531–1543.

Robson, D., & Gray, R. (2007). Serious mental illness and physical health problems: A discussion paper. *International Journal of Nursing Studies, 44*, 457–466.

Seo, D., Rabinowitz, A., Douglas, R., & Sinha, R. (2019). Limbic response to stress linking life trauma and hypothalamus pituitary-adrenal axis function. *Psychoneuroendocrinology, 99*, 38–46.

Siddall, P., Lovell, M., & MacLeod, R. (2015). Spirituality: What is its role in pain medicine? *Pain Medicine, 16*(1), 51–56.

Silva, M., & Cavalcanti, D. (2019). Evaluation of quality of life in multiple sclerosis patients: Impact of fatigue, anxiety, and depression. *Fistoterapia e Pesquisa, 26*(4), 339–345.

Simpson, C. A., Mu, A., Haslam, N., Schwartz, O. S., & Simmons, J. G. (2020). Feeling down? A systematic review of the gut microbiota in anxiety/depression and irritable bowel syndrome. *Journal of Affective Disorders, 266*, 429–446. https://doi.org/10.1016/j.jad.2020.01.124

Songjin. R., Kivi, A., Urban, P., Wolf, T., & Wissel, J. (2020). Site and size of lesion predict post-stroke spasticity: A retrospective magnetic resonance imaging study. *Journal of Rehabilitation Medicine, 52*(5), 1–4.

Šprah, L., Dernovšek, M. Z., Wahlbeck, K., & Haaramo, P. (2017). Psychiatric readmissions and their association with physical comorbidity: A systematic literature review. *BMC Psychiatry, 17*(2).

Stubbs, B., Eggermont, L., Mitchell, A., De Hert, M., Correll, C., Soundy, A., Rosenbaum, S., & Vancampfort, D. (2015). The prevalence of pain in bipolar disorder: A systematic review and large-scale meta-analysis. *Acta Psychiatrica Scandinavica, 131*, 75–88. https://doi.org/10.1111/acps.12325

Swartz, A. (2018). Smart pills for psychosis: The tricky ethical challenges of digital medicine for serious mental illness. *The American Journal of Bioethics, 18*(9), 65–67.

Tagliaferri, S., Miller, C., Owen, P., Mitchell, U., Brisby, H., Fitzgibbon, B., Huge, M., Van Oosterwijck, J., & Belavy, D. (2020). Domains of chronic low back pain and assessing treatment effectiveness: A clinical perspective. *Pain Practice, 20*(2), 221–224.

Tene, O., Hen, H., Korczyn, A., Shopin, L., Molad, J., Kirschbaum, C., Bornstein, N., Shenhar-Tsarfaty, S., Kliper, E., Auriel, E., Usher, S., Stalder, T., & Assayag, E. (2018). The price of stress: High bedtime salivary cortisol levels are associated with brain atrophy and cognitive decline in stroke survivors. Results from the TABASCO prospective cohort study. *Journal of Alzheimer's Disease, 65*(4), 1365–1375.

Vancampfort, D., Stubbs, B., Mitchell, A., De Hert, M., Wampers, M., Ward, P., Rosenbaum, S., & Correll, C. (2015). Risk of metabolic syndrome and its components in people with schizophrenia and related disorders, bipolar disorder, and major depressive disorder: A systematic review and meta-analysis. *World Psychiatry, 14*(3), 339–347.

Vardeh, D., Mannion, R., & Woolf, C. (2016). Toward a mechanism-based approach to pain diagnosis. *Journal of Pain, 19*(9), 50–69.

Vetrano, D., Pisciotta, M., Lo Monaco, M., Onder, G., Laudisio, A., Brandi, V., La Carpia, D., Guglielmo, M., Nacchia, A., Fusco, D., Ricciardi, D., Bentivoglio, A., Bernabei, R., & Zuccala, G. (2015). Association of depressive symptoms with circadian blood pressure alterations in Parkinson's disease. *Journal of Neurology, 262*, 2564–2571.

Vogel, M., Frank, A., Choi, F., Strehlau, V., Nikoo, N., Nikoo, M., Hwang, S., Somers, J., Krausz, M., & Schutz, C. (2017). Chronic pain among homeless persons with mental illness. *Pain Medicine, 18*(12), 2280–2288.

Walker, E.R., & Druss, B.G. (2017). Cumulative burden of comorbid mental health disorders, substance use disorders, chronic medical conditions and poverty on health among adults in the U.S.A. *Psychology, Health, & Medicine, 22*(6), 727–735.

Wen, S., Xiao, H., & Yang, Y. (2018). The risk factors for depression in cancer patients undergoing chemotherapy: A systemic review. *Supportive Care in Cancer, 27*, 57–67.

Wu, Y., Si, R., Yang, S., Xia, S., He, Z., Wang, L., He, Z., Wang, Q., & Tang, H. (2016). Depression induces poor prognosis associated with the down-regulation brain derived neurotrophic factor of serum in advanced small cell lung cancer. *Oncotarget, 7*(52), 85975–85986.

Yang, S., Sajatovic, M., & Walter, B. (2012). Psychosocial interventions for depression and anxiety in Parkinson's disease. *Journal of Geriatric Psychiatry and Neurology, 25*(2), 113–121.

Zhang, H., & Qiu, L. (2020). Analysis of factors affecting severity of depression in post stroke depression patients at convalescence. *Chinese Nursing Research, 34*(6), 1001–1005.

Zomer, E., Osborn, D., Nazareth, I., Blackburn, R., Burton, A., Hardoon, S., Holt, R., King, M., Marston, L., Morris, S., Omar, R., Petersen, I., Walters, K., & Hunter, R. (2017). Effectiveness and cost-effectiveness of a cardiovascular risk prediction algorithm for people with severe mental illness (PRIMROSE) [Supplement]. *European Psychiatry, 33*. https://doi.org/10.1136/bmjopen-2017-018181

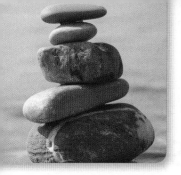

Appendix A
Brief Psychiatric Rating Scale

DIRECTIONS: Place an X in the appropriate box to represent level of severity of each symptom.

	Not Present	Very Mild	Mild	Moderate	Mod. Severe	Severe	Extremely Severe
SOMATIC CONCERN—preoccupation with physical health, fear of physical illness, hypochondriasis.	☐	☐	☐	☐	☐	☐	☐
ANXIETY—worry, fear, overconcern for present or future, uneasiness.	☐	☐	☐	☐	☐	☐	☐
EMOTIONAL WITHDRAWAL—lack of spontaneous interaction, isolation deficiency in relating to others.	☐	☐	☐	☐	☐	☐	☐
CONCEPTUAL DISORGANIZATION—thought processes confused, disconnected, disorganized, disrupted.	☐	☐	☐	☐	☐	☐	☐
GUILT FEELINGS—self-blame, shame, remorse for past behavior.	☐	☐	☐	☐	☐	☐	☐
TENSION—physical and motor manifestations of nervousness, overactivation.	☐	☐	☐	☐	☐	☐	☐
MANNERISMS AND POSTURING—peculiar, bizarre unnatural motor behavior (not including tic).	☐	☐	☐	☐	☐	☐	☐
GRANDIOSITY—exaggerated self-opinion, arrogance, conviction of unusual power or abilities.	☐	☐	☐	☐	☐	☐	☐
DEPRESSIVE MOOD—sorrow, sadness, despondency, pessimism.	☐	☐	☐	☐	☐	☐	☐
HOSTILITY—animosity, contempt, belligerence, disdain for others.	☐	☐	☐	☐	☐	☐	☐
SUSPICIOUSNESS—mistrust, belief others harbor malicious or discriminatory intent.	☐	☐	☐	☐	☐	☐	☐
HALLUCINATORY BEHAVIOR—perceptions without normal external stimulus correspondence.	☐	☐	☐	☐	☐	☐	☐
MOTOR RETARDATION—slowed weakened movements or speech, reduced body tone.	☐	☐	☐	☐	☐	☐	☐
UNCOOPERATIVENESS—resistance, guardedness, rejection of authority.	☐	☐	☐	☐	☐	☐	☐
UNUSUAL THOUGHT CONTENT—unusual, odd, strange, bizarre thought content.	☐	☐	☐	☐	☐	☐	☐
BLUNTED AFFECT—reduced emotional tone, reduction in formal intensity of feelings, flatness.	☐	☐	☐	☐	☐	☐	☐
EXCITEMENT—heightened emotional tone, agitation, increased reactivity.	☐	☐	☐	☐	☐	☐	☐
DISORIENTATION—confusion or lack of proper association for person, place, or time.	☐	☐	☐	☐	☐	☐	☐
Global Assessment Scale (Range 1–100)	☐	☐	☐	☐	☐	☐	☐

From Overall, J. E., & Gorham, D. R. (1962). The brief psychiatric rating scale. *Psychological Reports, 10,* 799–812. Used with permission.

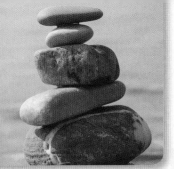

Appendix B

Abnormal Involuntary Movement Scale (AIMS)

		None	Minimal	Mild	Moderate	Severe
Facial and Oral Movements	1: **Muscles of facial expression:** e.g., movements of forehead, eyebrows, periorbital area, cheeks; include frowning, blinking, smiling, grimacing	0	1	2	3	4
	2: **Lips and perioral area:** e.g., puckering, pouting, smacking	0	1	2	3	4
	3: **Jaw:** e.g., biting, clenching, chewing, mouth opening, lateral movement	0	1	2	3	4
	4: **Tongue:** Rate only increase in movement both in and out of mouth, *not* the inability to sustain movement	0	1	2	3	4
Extremity Movements	5: **Upper (arms, wrists, hands, fingers):** Include choreic movements (i.e., rapid, objectively purposeless, irregular, spontaneous), athetoid movements (i.e., slow, irregular, complex, serpentine); *do not* include tremor (i.e., repetitive, regular, rhythmic)	0	1	2	3	4
	6: **Lower (legs, knees, ankles, toes):** e.g., lateral knee movement, foot tapping, heel dropping, foot squirming, inversion and eversion of foot	0	1	2	3	4
Trunk Movements	7: **Neck, shoulders, hips:** e.g., rocking, twisting, squirming, pelvic gyrations	0	1	2	3	4
Global Judgment	8: **Severity of abnormal movements overall**	0	1	2	3	4
	9: **Incapacitation caused by abnormal movements**	0	1	2	3	4
	10: **Patient's awareness of abnormal movements:** Rate only patient's report					

No awareness	0
Aware, no distress	1
Aware, mild distress	2
Aware, moderate distress	3
Aware, severe distress	4

Dental Status			
11: Current problems with teeth or dentures	No	0
	Yes	1
12: Does patient usually wear dentures?	No	0
	Yes	1

Examination Procedure for AIMS

Either before or after completing the examination procedure, observe the patient unobtrusively, at rest (e.g., in the waiting room). The chair to be used in this examination should be a hard, firm one without arms.

1: Ask the patient whether there is anything in his or her mouth (e.g., gum, candy) and if there is, to remove it.

2: Ask the patient about the current condition of his or her teeth. Ask the patient if he or she wears dentures. Do teeth or dentures bother the patient now?

3: Ask the patient whether he or she notices any movements in the mouth, face, hands, or feet. If yes, ask to describe and to what extent they currently bother patient or interfere with his or her activities.

4: Have the patient sit in the chair with his or her hands on knees, legs slightly apart, and feet flat on floor. (Look at the entire body for movements while in this position.)

5: Ask the patient to sit with his or her hands hanging unsupported. If male, between legs, if female and wearing a dress, hanging over knees. (Observe hands and other body areas.)

6: Ask the patient to open his or her mouth. (Observe the tongue at rest within the mouth.) Do this twice.

7: Ask the patient to protrude his or her tongue. (Observe the tongue at rest within the mouth.) Do this twice.

*8: Ask the patient to tap his or her thumb, with each finger, as rapidly as possible for 10–15 seconds; separately with the right hand and then with the left hand. (Observe facial and leg movements.)

9: Flex and extend the patient's left and right arms (one at a time). (Note any rigidity and rate on NOTES.)

10: Ask the patient to stand up. (Observe in profile. Observe all body areas again, hips included.)

*11: Ask the patient to extend both arms outstretched in front with the palms down. (Observe trunk, legs, and mouth.)

*12: Have the patient walk a few paces, turn, and walk back to the chair. (Observe hand and gait.) Do this twice.

*Activated movements.

Reprinted from Guy, W. (1976). *ECDEU: Assessment manual for psychopharmacology* (DHEW Publ No 76–338). Washington, DC: Department of Health, Education, and Welfare, Psychopharmacology Research Branch.

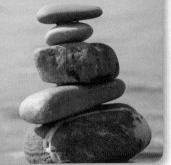

Appendix C

Simplified Diagnosis for Tardive Dyskinesia (SD-TD)

The following instructions accompany the Dyskinesia Identification System: Condensed User Scale (DISCUS). See Box 22.5.

PREREQUISITES. The three prerequisites are as follows. Exceptions may occur.

1. A history of at least 3 months' total cumulative neuroleptic exposure. Include amoxapine and metoclopramide in all categories below as well.
2. **SCORING/INTENSITY LEVEL.** The presence of a **TOTAL SCORE OF FIVE (5) OR ABOVE.** Also be alert for any change from baseline or scores below five which have at least a "moderate" (3) or "severe" (4) movement on any item or at least two "mild" (2) movements on two items located in different body areas.
3. Other conditions are not responsible for the abnormal involuntary movements.

DIAGNOSES. The diagnosis is based upon the current exam and its relation to the last exam. The diagnosis can shift depending upon: (a) whether movements are present or not, (b) whether movements are present for 3 months or more (6 months if on a semiannual assessment schedule), and (c) whether neuroleptic dosage changes occur and effect movements.

- **NO TD.** Movements **are not** present on this exam **or** movements are present, but some other condition is responsible for them. The last diagnosis must be NO TD, PROBABLE TD, or WITHDRAWAL TD.
- **PROBABLE TD.** Movements **are** present on this exam. This is the first time they are present or they have never been present for 3 months or more. The last diagnosis must be NO TD or PROBABLE TD.
- **PERSISTENT TD.** Movements are present on this exam **and** they have been present for 3 months or more with this exam or at some point in the past. The last diagnosis can be any except NO TD.
- **MASKED TD.** Movements **are not** present on this exam **but** this is due to a neuroleptic dosage increase or reinstitution after a prior exam when movements were present. Also use this conclusion if movements are not present due to the addition of a non-neuroleptic medication to treat TD. The last diagnosis must be PROBABLE TD, PERSISTENT TD, WITHDRAWAL TD, or MASKED TD.
- **REMITTED TD.** Movements **are not** present on this exam **but** PERSISTENT TD has been diagnosed and neuroleptic dosage increase or reinstitution has occurred. The last diagnosis must be PERSISTENT TD or REMITTED TD. If movements reemerge, the diagnosis shifts back to PERSISTENT TD.
- **WITHDRAWAL TD.** Movements **are not seen while** receiving neuroleptics or at the last dosage level **but are seen within** 8 weeks following a neuroleptic reduction or discontinuation. The last diagnosis must be NO TD or WITHDRAWAL TD. If movements continue for 3 months or more after the neuroleptic dosage reduction or discontinuation, the diagnosis shifts to PERSISTENT TD. If movements do not continue for 3 months or more after the reduction or discontinuation, the diagnosis shifts to NO TD.

INSTRUCTIONS

1. The rater completes the Assessment according to the standardized exam procedure. If the rater also completes Evaluation items 1 to 4, he/she must also sign the preparer box. The form is given to the physician. Alternatively, the physician may perform the assessment.
2. The physician completes the Evaluation section. The physician is responsible for the entire Evaluation section and its accuracy.
3. IT IS RECOMMENDED THAT THE PHYSICIAN EXAMINE ANY INDIVIDUAL WHO MEETS THE THREE PREREQUISITES OR WHO HAS MOVEMENTS NOT EXPLAINED BY OTHER FACTORS. NEUROLOGIC ASSESSMENTS OR DIFFERENTIAL DIAGNOSTIC TESTS WHICH MAY BE NECESSARY SHOULD BE OBTAINED.
4. File form according to policy or procedure.

OTHER CONDITIONS (partial list)

1. Age
2. Blind
3. Cerebral Palsy
4. Contact Lenses
5. Dentures/No Teeth
6. Down Syndrome
7. Drug Intoxication (specify)
8. Encephalitis
9. Extrapyramidal Side Effects (specify)
10. Fahr Syndrome
11. Heavy Meta Intoxication (specify)
12. Huntington Chorea
13. Hyperthyroidism
14. Hypoglycemia
15. Hypoparathyroidism
16. Idiopathic Torsion Dystonia
17. Meige Syndrome
18. Parkinson Disease
19. Stereotypies
20. Sydenham Chorea
21. Tourette Syndrome
22. Wilson Disease
23. Other (specify)

Sprague, R. L., & Kalachnik, J. E. (1991). Reliability, validity, and a total score cutoff for the Dyskinesia Identification System, Condensed User Scale (DISCUS) with mentally ill and mentally retarded populations. *Psychopharmacology Bulletin, 27*(1), 51–58.

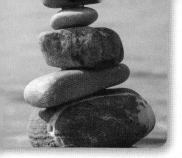

Glossary

ABCDE An acronym for the basic framework of rational emotive behavior therapy.

ABCs of psychological first aid Focusing on A (arousal), B (behavior), and C (cognition).

absorption Movement of drug from the site of administration into plasma.

abuse Use of alcohol or drugs for the purpose of intoxication or, in the case of prescription drugs, for purposes beyond the intended use.

accreditation Process by which a mental health agency is recognized or approved in accordance with established standards to be providing acceptable quality of care.

acculturation Act or process of assuming the beliefs, values, and practices of another, usually dominant culture.

acetylcholine (ACh) The primary cholinergic neurotransmitter. Found in the greatest concentration in the peripheral nervous system, ACh provides the basic synaptic communication for the parasympathetic neurons and part of the sympathetic neurons, which send information to the central nervous system. An important neurotransmitter associated with cognitive functioning; disruption of cholinergic mechanisms damages memory in animals and humans.

acetylcholinesterase (AChE) Key enzyme that inactivates the neurotransmitter acetylcholine. AChE is found in high concentrations in the brain and is one of two cholinesterase enzymes capable of breaking down ACh.

acetylcholinesterase inhibitors (AChEI) Mainstay of pharmacologic treatment of dementia; these drugs inhibit AChE, resulting in an enhancement of cholinergic activity.

activating event The "A" in the ABCDE framework of rational emotive behavior therapy. It represents an external or internal stimulus. Not necessarily an actual event, it may be an emotion, or thought or expectation that is interpreted according to a set of beliefs.

active listening Focusing on what the patient is saying in order to interpret and respond to the message in an objective manner while using techniques such as open-ended statements, reflection, and questions that elicit additional responses from the patient.

acute pain A sudden, severe onset of pain symptoms at the time of injury or illness that generally subsides as the associated condition subsides or the injury heals.

acute stress disorder (ASD) A mental disorder characterized by persistent, distressing stress-related symptoms that last between 2 days and 1 month and that occur within 1 month after a traumatic experience.

adaptation A person's capacity to survive and flourish as it affects health, psychological well-being, and social functioning.

adaptive behavior Behavior that is composed of three skill types: conceptual, social, and practical skills.

addiction A condition of continued use of substances (or reward-seeking behaviors) despite adverse consequences.

adherence An individual's compliance to a therapeutic routine.

advance care directives Treatment directives (living wills) and appointment directives (power of attorney or health proxies) that apply only if the individual is unable to make his or her own decisions because the patient is incapacitated or, in the opinion of two physicians, is otherwise unable to make decisions for himself or herself.

advanced practice psychiatric–mental health nurse A licensed registered nurse who is educationally prepared at the graduate level and is nationally certified as a specialist by the American Nurses Credentialing Center (ANCC).

adverse reactions (adverse effects) Unwanted medication effects that may have serious physiologic consequences.

affect An expression of mood manifest in a person's outward emotional expression; varies considerably both within and among different cultures.

affective instability Rapid and extreme shifts in mood, erratic emotional responses to situations, and intense sensitivity to criticism or perceived slights; one of the core characteristics of borderline personality disorder.

affective lability Abrupt, dramatic, unprovoked changes in the types of emotions expressed.

affinity Degree of attraction or strength of the bond between a drug and its biologic target.

aggression Overt behavior intended to hurt, belittle, take revenge, or achieve domination and control; can be verbal or physical. Behaviors or attitudes that reflect rage, hostility, and the potential for physical or verbal destructiveness; usually occurs if the person believes someone is going to do him or her harm.

agitation Inability to sit still or attend to others accompanied by heightened emotions and tension.

agnosia Failure to recognize or identify objects despite intact sensory function.

agonists Substances that initiate the same response as the chemical normally present in the body.

agoraphobia Fear of open spaces; commonly occurs with panic disorder.

agranulocytosis Dangerously low level of circulating neutrophils.

akathisia An extrapyramidal side effect characterized by the inability to sit still or restlessness; more common in middle-aged patients. Sometimes misdiagnosed as agitation or an increase in psychotic symptoms.

alcohol withdrawal syndrome A syndrome that occurs after the reduction of alcohol consumption or when abstaining from alcohol after prolonged use, causing changes in vital signs, diaphoresis, and other adverse gastrointestinal and central nervous system side effects.

Alcoholics Anonymous The first 12-step, self-help program; a worldwide fellowship of people with alcoholism who provide support, individually and at meetings, to others who seek help.

alexithymia Difficulty identifying and expressing emotion.

allodynia Pain unrelated to noxious stimuli; lowered pain threshold.

allostasis The dynamic regulatory process that maintains homeostasis through a process of adaptation.

allostatic load (AL) An increase in the number of abnormal biologic parameters as a consequence of wear and tear on the body and brain; leads to ill health.

alogia Reduced fluency and productivity of thought and speech. Brief, empty verbal responses; often referred to as *poverty of speech.*

ambivalence Presence and expression of two opposing feelings, leading to inaction.

amino acids Building blocks of proteins that have different roles in intraneuronal metabolism. Amino acids function as neurotransmitters in as many as 60% to 70% of synaptic sites in the brain.

anger An internal affective state, usually temporary rather than an enduring negative attitude, that may or may not be expressed in overt behavior. If expressed, anger behavior can be constructive or destructive.

anger management A psychoeducational intervention for persons whose anger behavior is dysfunctional in some way (i.e., interfering with success in work or relationships) but *not violent.*

anhedonia Inability to experience pleasure.

anorexia nervosa A life-threatening eating disorder characterized by a mixture of biopsychosocial symptoms, including significantly low body weight, intense fear of gaining weight or becoming fat, and a disturbance in experiencing body weight or shape.

anorgasmia The inability to achieve an orgasm.

antagonists Chemicals blocking the biologic response at a given receptor site.

antisocial personality disorder A disorder characterized by a marked pattern of disregard for, and violation of, the rights of others.

anxiety Energy that arises when expectations that are present are not met (Peplau). An uncomfortable feeling of apprehension or dread that occurs in response to internal or external stimuli and can result in physical, emotional, cognitive, and behavioral symptoms.

apathy Reactions to stimuli that are decreased along with a diminished interest and desire.

aphasia Alterations in language ability.

appraisal The process whereby all aspects of a given event or situation are considered—the demands, constraints, and resources are balanced with personal goals and beliefs.

apraxia Impaired ability to execute motor activities despite intact motor functioning.

Asperger syndrome Formerly named Asperger syndrome, it is now diagnosed as autism spectrum disorder with persistent difficulty in social communication and interaction. It appears to be a milder form of autism.

assault The threat of unlawful force to inflict bodily injury on another. The threat must be imminent and cause reasonable apprehension in the individual.

assertive community treatment A model that calls for a multidisciplinary clinical team approach to providing 24-hour, intensive community-based services to help patients meet the requirements of community living during reintegration.

assessment The deliberate and systematic collection and interpretation of biopsychosocial information or data to determine current and past health, functional status, and human responses to mental health problems, both actual and potential.

assortative mating Tendency for individuals to select mates who are similar in genetically linked traits such as intelligence and personality styles.

asylum Safe haven.

attachment Emotional bond formed between children and their parental figures at an early age; attaining and retaining interpersonal connection to a significant person, beginning at birth.

attachment disorganization A consequence of extreme insecurity that results from feared or actual separation from the attached figure. Infants appear to be unable to maintain the strategic adjustments in attachment behavior.

attention A complex mental process that involves concentrating on one activity to the exclusion of others, as well as sustaining interest over time.

attention-deficit hyperactivity disorder (ADHD) A persistent pattern of inattention, hyperactivity, and impulsiveness; typically diagnosed based on teacher and parent reports and direct observation of the behavior patterns described.

atypical antipsychotics Newer antipsychotics that are equally or more effective than conventional antipsychotics but have fewer side effects.

augmentation A strategy of adding another medication to enhance effectiveness.

autism spectrum disorders Disorders characterized by neurodevelopmental delays that are typically diagnosed in childhood. Children with autism spectrum disorders may or may not have an intellectual disability, but they commonly show an uneven pattern of intellectual strengths and weaknesses.

autistic thinking Thinking restricted to the literal and immediate so that the individual has private rules of logic and reasoning that make no sense to others.

autonomic nervous system Part of the nervous system that regulates involuntary vital functions including cardiac muscle, smooth muscles, and glands. It is composed of the sympathetic and parasympathetic systems.

autonomy Concept that each person has the fundamental right of self-determination.

avoidant personality disorder A disorder characterized by avoiding social situations in which there is interpersonal contact with others. Individuals appear timid, shy, and hesitant; fear criticism; and feel inadequate. They are extremely sensitive to negative comments and disapproval and appraise situations more negatively than others do.

avolition Withdrawal and inability to initiate and persist in goal-directed activity.

basal ganglia Subcortical gray matter areas in both the right and the left hemisphere that contain many cell bodies or nuclei.

behaviorism A paradigm shift in understanding human behavior that was initiated by Watson, who theorized that human behavior is developed through a stimulus–response process rather than through unconscious drives or instincts.

behavior modification A specific therapy technique that can be applied to individuals, groups, or systems. The aim of behavior modification is to reinforce desired behaviors and extinguish undesired ones.

behavior therapy Interventions that reinforce or promote desirable behaviors or alter undesirable ones.

belief system The "B" in the ABCDE framework of rational emotive behavior therapy. Beliefs underlying thoughts and emotions are shaped by rationality, which is self-constructive, and irrationality, which is self-defeating.

beneficence The health care provider uses knowledge of science and incorporates the art of caring to develop an environment in which individuals achieve maximum health care potential.

bereavement The process of mourning and coping with the loss of a loved one. It begins immediately after the loss, but it can last months or years.

beta-amyloid plaques Dense, mostly insoluble deposits of protein and cellular material outside and around neurons; pathology of Alzheimer disease.

bibliotherapy The use of provider-assigned books and other reading materials to help individuals gain therapeutic benefit.

binge eating Rapid, episodic, impulsive, and uncontrollable ingestion of a large amount of food during a short period of time, usually 1 to 2 hours, usually followed by feelings of guilt that result in purging.

binge-eating disorder A newly identified eating disorder in its infancy relative to research; individuals binge in the same way as those with bulimia nervosa but do not purge or compensate for binges through other behaviors.

bioavailability Amount of a drug that actually reaches the systemic circulation unchanged.

biogenic amines Small molecules manufactured in the neuron that contain an amine group. These include dopamine, norepinephrine, and epinephrine (all synthesized from the amino acid tyrosine) and serotonin (from tryptophan).

biologic markers Physical indicators of disturbances within the central nervous system that differentiate one disease state from another; found using diagnostic testing.

biopsychosocial model An organizational model consisting of three separate but interdependent domains: biologic, psychological, and social. Each domain has an independent knowledge and treatment focus but can interact and be mutually interdependent with the other dimensions.

biosexual identity   Anatomic and physiologic state of being male or female that results from genetic and hormonal influences.

biotransformation   Metabolism of a drug or substance; the process by which the drug is altered and broken down into smaller substances, known as metabolites.

bipolar disorders   Mood disorders that are characterized by periods of mania or hypomania that alternate with depression. These disorders can be further designated as bipolar I, bipolar II, and cyclothymic disorder depending on the severity of the manic and depressive symptoms.

bipolar I   A type of bipolar disorder that is diagnosed when at least one manic episode or mixed episode is present.

bipolar II   A type of bipolar disorder that has less dramatic symptoms than bipolar I. Hypomania (mild mania) and a major depressive episode are characteristic symptoms.

blood alcohol level   The level of alcohol in the blood; used to determine intoxication.

board-and-care homes   Facilities that provide 24-hour supervision and assistance with medications, meals, and some self-care skills but in which individualized attention to self-care skills and other activities of daily living is generally not available.

body dissatisfaction   A sense of dissatisfaction and low self-esteem when one's own body is perceived to fall short of an ideal.

body dysmorphic disorder   Disorder in which there is a preoccupation with an imagined or slight defect in appearance, such as a large nose, thinning hair, or small genitals.

body image   How each individual perceives his or her own body, including such dimensions as size and attractiveness.

body image distortion   Extreme discrepancy between one's perception of one's own body image and others' perceptions of one.

borderline personality disorder   A disorder characterized by a disruptive pattern of instability related to self-identity, interpersonal relationships, and affects combined with marked impulsivity and destructive behavior.

boundaries   Limits in which a person may act or refrain from acting within a designated time or place. Invisible barriers with varying permeabilities that surround family subsystems.

boxed warning   Serious adverse effects that can occur with the use of a specific medication; noted in issued warning in the package insert.

bradykinesia   An extrapyramidal condition characterized by a slowness of voluntary movement and speech.

brain stem   Area of the brain containing the midbrain, pons, and medulla, which continues beneath the thalamus.

breach of confidentiality   Release of patient information without the patient's consent in the absence of legal compulsion or authorization to release information.

brief intervention   A negotiated conversation between professional and patient designed to reduce alcohol and drug use; any short-term intervention.

bulimia nervosa   An eating disorder in which the individual engages in recurrent episodes of binge eating and compensatory behavior to avoid weight gain through purging methods such as self-induced vomiting or use of laxatives, diuretics, enemas, or emetics or through nonpurging methods such as fasting or excessive exercise.

bullying   Repeated, deliberate attempts to harm someone that are usually unprovoked. An imbalance in strength is a part of the pattern, with most victims having difficulty defending themselves.

carrier protein   A membrane protein that transports a specific molecule across the cell membrane.

case finding   Identifying people who are at risk for suicide to initiate proper treatment. Identification of depression and risk factors associated with suicide.

case management   Service model in which a case manager locates services, links the patient with these services, and then monitors the patient's receipt of these services.

cataplexy   Bilateral loss of muscle tone triggered by a strong emotion such as laughter. This muscle atonia can range from subtle (drooping eyelids) to dramatic (buckling knees). Respiratory muscles are not affected. Cataplexy usually lasts only seconds. Individuals are fully conscious, oriented, and alert during the episode. Prolonged episodes of cataplexy may lead to sleep episodes.

catastrophic reactions   Overreactions or extreme anxiety reactions to everyday situations.

catatonic excitement   Hyperactivity characterized by purposeless activity and abnormal movements like grimacing and posturing.

catharsis   A Freudian concept meaning release of feelings, as in the venting of anger.

cerebellum   Part of the brain that is responsible for controlling movement and postural adjustments; it receives information from all parts of the body.

chemical restraint   Use of medication to control patients or manage behavior.

child abuse   Any action that robs children of rights they should have including the rights to be and behave like a child; to be safe and protected from harm; and to be fed, clothed, and nurtured so the child can grow, develop, and fulfill his or her unique potential.

child neglect   A form of child abuse defined as failure to provide for a child's physical, emotional, health care, or educational needs; failure to adequately supervise a child; or intentionally exposing a child to a dangerous environment.

chronic pain   Pain on a daily basis or pain that is constant for more than 6 months.

chronic syndromes   Symptom patterns that last for long periods of time. Medication-related movement disorders that develop from longer exposure to antipsychotic drugs.

chronobiology   Study and measure of time structures or biologic rhythms.

chronopharmacotherapy   Resetting the biologic clock by using short-acting hypnotics to induce sleep.

circadian cycle   A biologic system that has a 24-hour cycle.

circadian rhythm   Physiologic and psychological functions that fluctuate in a pattern that repeats itself in a 24-hour cycle.

circumstantiality   Extremely detailed and lengthy discourse about a topic.

clang association   Repetition of word phrases that are similar in sound but in no other way, for example, "right, light, sight, might."

classical conditioning   A learning situation in which an unconditioned stimulus initially produces an unconditioned response; over time, a conditioned response is elicited for a specific stimulus (Pavlov).

clearance   Total amount of blood, serum, or plasma from which a drug is completely removed per unit of time.

clinical reasoning   Using critical thinking and reflection to address patient problems and interventions.

closed group   A group in which all the members begin at one time. New members are not admitted after the first meeting.

codependence   An "enabling" method of coping in which an individual in a relationship with a person who abuses alcohol inadvertently reinforces the drinking behavior of the other person.

cognition   A high level of intellectual processing in which perceptions and information are acquired, used, or manipulated; for Beck, verbal or pictorial events in the stream of consciousness. A person's ability to think and know. An internal process of perception, memory, and judgment through which an understanding of self and the world is developed.

cognitive behavioral therapy   A highly structured psychotherapeutic method used to alter distorted beliefs and problem behaviors by identifying and replacing negative inaccurate thoughts and changing the rewards for behaviors.

cognitive distortions   Automatic thoughts generated by organizing distorted information or inaccurate interpretation of a situation.

cognitive interventions or cognitive therapy   Interventions or psychotherapy that aims to change or reframe an individual's automatic thought patterns that develop over time and that interfere with the ability to function optimally.

cognitive reserve   The brain's ability to operate effectively even when there is disruption in functioning.

cognitive schema   Patterns of thoughts that determine how a person interprets events. Each person's cognitive schema screen, code, and evaluate incoming stimuli.

cognitive theory   An outgrowth of different theoretic perspectives, including the behavioral and the psychodynamic, that attempts to link internal thought processes with human behavior.

cognitive triad   Thoughts about oneself, the world, and the future.

cohesion   The ability of a group to stick together.

co-leadership   When two people share responsibility for leading a group.

commitment to treatment statement   Statement in which a patient verbally or in writing agrees to seek treatment or access emergency services if needed.

communication blocks   Interruptions in the content flow of communication, such changes in topic that either the nurse or patient makes.

communication disorders   Disorders that involve speech or language impairments.

communication pathways   An aspect of group interaction based on interaction patterns related to who is most liked in the group, who occupies a position of power, what subgroups have formed, and who is isolated from the group.

communication triad   A technique used to provide a specific syntax and order for patients to identify and express their feelings and seek relief. The "sentence" consists of three parts: (1) an "I" statement to identify the prevailing feeling, (2) a nonjudgmental statement of the emotional trigger, and (3) a statement of what the person would like differently or what would restore comfort to the situation.

comorbidity (comorbid) Presence of a disorder simultaneously with and independently of another disorder.

competence The degree to which the patient is able to understand and appreciate the information given during the consent process; the patient's cognitive ability to process information at a specific time; the patient's ability to gather and interpret information and make reasonable judgments based on that information to participate fully as a partner in treatment.

complicated grief A reaction to the loss of a loved one in which a person is frozen or stuck in a state of chronic mourning.

compliments Affirmations of the patient.

comprehensive family assessment The collection of all relevant data related to family health, psychological well-being, and social functioning to identify problems for which the nurse can generate nursing diagnoses.

compulsions Behaviors that are performed repeatedly, in a ritualistic fashion, with the goal of preventing or relieving anxiety and distress caused by obsessions.

concrete thinking Lack of abstraction in thinking in which people are unable to understand punch lines, metaphors, and analogies.

conditional release Discharge of patients whose psychiatric symptoms have been stabilized and are no longer considered a danger to the community. Patients are monitored on an ongoing basis by the court and must follow established conditions and criteria to maintain their discharged status.

conduct disorder A disorder characterized by more serious violations of social norms, including aggressive behavior, destruction of property, and cruelty to animals.

confabulation Telling a plausible but imagined scenario to compensate for memory gaps.

confidentiality An ethical duty of nondisclosure; the patient has the right to disclose personal information without fear of it being revealed to others.

conflict resolution A specific type of counseling in which the nurse helps the patient resolve a disagreement or dispute.

confrontation Presenting evidence of inconsistencies in a person's thoughts, feelings, and actions.

confused speech and thinking Symptoms of schizophrenia that render the patient unable to respond accurately to the ordinary signs and sounds of daily living.

connections Mutually responsive and enhancing relationships.

constraints Limitations that are both personal (internalized cultural values and beliefs) and environmental (finite resources such as money and time).

containment The process of providing safety and security; involves the patient's access to food and shelter.

content themes Repetition of concerns or feelings that occur within the therapeutic relationship. Themes may emerge as symbolic representations of fears.

continuum of care Providing care in an integrated system of settings, services (physical, psychological, and social), and care levels appropriate to the individual's specific needs in a continuous manner over time, with channels of communication among the service providers.

conventional antipsychotics Also known as typical antipsychotics, "older" medications used to treat psychotic disorders with more side effects than "newer" atypical antipsychotics.

conversion disorder (functional neurologic symptom disorder) When severe emotional distress or unconscious conflict is expressed through physical symptoms.

co-occurring disorders (COD) Refers to the presence of comorbid mental illness and a substance use disorder in the same person.

coordination of care The integration of appropriate services so that individualized care is provided. When several agencies are involved, this allows a person's needs to be met without duplication of services.

coping A deliberate, planned, and psychological effort to manage stressful demands.

cortex Outermost surface of the cerebrum of the mature brain.

cortical dementia A type of dementia that is characterized by amnesia, aphasia, apraxia, and agnosia. Results from a disease process that globally affects the cortex.

counseling (counseling interventions) Specific time-limited interactions between a nurse and a patient, family, or group experiencing intermediate or ongoing difficulties related to their health or well-being.

countertransference The therapist or nurse's reactions to a patient that are based on interpersonal experiences, feelings, and attitudes. It can significantly interfere with the nurse–patient relationship.

court process counseling An approach that educates mentally ill patients about the impending legal procedures and prepares them for courtroom appearances.

craving The urge or desire to engage in a behavior such as drinking.

crisis A time-limited event that triggers adaptive or non-adaptive responses to maturational, situational, or traumatic experiences; results from stressful events for which coping mechanisms fail to provide adequate adaptive skills to address the perceived challenge or threat.

crisis intervention A specialized short-term (usually no longer than 6 hours) goal-directed therapy designed to assist patients in an immediate manner; focuses on stabilization, symptom reduction, and prevention of relapse requiring inpatient services.

Crisis Intervention Teams (CIT) Teams that train police officers to recognize and intervene in crisis situations in the community and determine whether emergency psychiatric services are needed.

Critical Time Intervention (CTI) A "bridge" between inpatient and outpatient treatment by coordinating care between staff in these settings.

cue elimination Emotional and environmental cues are identified and alternative responses are suggested, tried, and reinforced. When a cue or stimulus leads to a dysfunctional or unhealthy response, the response can be eliminated or an alternate, healthier response to the cue can be substituted, tried, and then reinforced.

cultural brokering Act of bridging, linking, or mediating between groups or individuals of different cultural systems for the purpose of reducing conflict or producing change. Cultural competence is a set of academic and interpersonal skills that are respectful of and responsive to the health belief practices and cultural and linguistic needs of diverse patients to bring about positive health care outcomes.

cultural competence A set of academic and interpersonal skills that allows individuals to increase their understanding and appreciation of cultural differences and similarities within, among, and between groups.

cultural identity A set of cultural beliefs with which one looks for standards of behavior; many consider themselves to have multiple cultural identities.

cultural idiom of distress A linguistic term, phrase, or a way of talking about suffering among individuals of a cultural group (*DSM-5*).

cultural syndrome A cluster or group of co-occurring symptoms found in a specific cultural group, community, or context.

culture Any group of people who identify or associate with each other on the basis of some common purpose, need, or similarity of background; the set of learned, socially transmitted beliefs, values, and behaviors that arise from interpersonal transactions among members of the cultural group.

cyberstalking Use of the Internet, e-mail, or other telecommunications technology to harass or stalk another person.

cycle of violence A three-phase pattern of tension, abuse, and kindness in which the abuser engages first in abuse and then in seemingly sincere expressions of love, contrition, and remorse.

cyclothymic disorder Chronic fluctuating mood disturbance. Does not meet criteria for hypomania or depressive disorder.

cytochrome P-450 (CYP450) system A set of microsomal enzymes (usually hepatic) referred to as CYP1, CYP2, and CYP3.

day treatment A bridge between institutional and community care for severely mentally ill and substance-abusing people. Participation in structured day treatment programs provides emotional and practical support and strengthens ties to community services and potentially to family and friends.

debriefing The reconstruction of the traumatic events by the victim as a psychological intervention.

deescalation An interactive process of calming and redirecting a patient who has an immediate potential for violence directed at others or self.

defense mechanisms Coping styles; the automatic psychological process protecting the individual against anxiety and creating awareness of internal or external dangers or stressors.

deinstitutionalization Release of patients with severe and persistent mental illness from state mental hospitals into the community for treatment, support, and rehabilitation as the result of a national movement that began in the 1960s.

delayed ejaculation (DE) Delay or absence of ejaculation.

delirium A disorder of acute cognitive impairment that can be caused by a medical condition (e.g., infection) or substance abuse, or it may have multiple etiologies.

delirium tremens An acute symptom of alcohol withdrawal syndrome that is characterized by autonomic hyperarousal, disorientation, hallucinations, and tremors or grand mal (tonic–clonic) seizures.

delusional disorder A psychotic disorder characterized by delusions that occur in the absence of other psychiatric disorders; includes several subtypes: crotomania, grandiose, jealous, somatic, mixed, and unspecified. Individual can function fairly well and abnormal behavior is not observable.

delusions Erroneous fixed, false beliefs that cannot be changed by reasonable argument. They usually involve a misinterpretation of experience and are unchanged by reasonable arguments.

demands Pulls put on an individual's resources that are generated by physiologic and psychological needs. Includes external pulls (crowding, crime, noise, pollution) imposed by the physical environment and internal pulls (behavior and role expectations) imposed by the social environment.

dementia From the Latin *de* (from or out of) and *mens* (mind); characterized by chronic cognitive impairments. It is differentiated from delirium by underlying cause, not by symptom patterns.

denial The patient's inability to accept loss of control over substance use or the severity of the consequences associated with substance abuse.

dependence The state of being psychologically or physiologically dependent on a drug after a prolonged period of use.

dependent personality Person who clings to others in a desperate attempt to keep them close. Their need to be taken care of is so great that it leads to doing anything to maintain the closeness, including total submission and disregard for self.

depersonalization A nonspecific experience in which the individual loses a sense of personal identity and feels strange or unreal.

depression The primary mood of depressive disorders defined as an overwhelming state of sadness, loss of interest or pleasure, feelings of guilt, disturbed sleep patterns and appetite, low energy, and an inability to concentrate.

depression not otherwise specified A category that includes disorders with depressive features that do not meet strict criteria for major depressive disorder.

depressive disorders Also referred to as unipolar depression, a specific subset of mood disorders consisting of major depression, dysthymia, and depression not otherwise specified (NOS).

derealization Feelings of unreality.

desensitization A rapid decrease in drug effects that may develop within a few minutes of exposure to a drug.

desynchronized Two or more circadian rhythms reaching their peaks at different times.

deteriorating relationship A type of nontherapeutic relationship with several defined phases during which the patient and nurse feel very frustrated and keep varying their approach with each other in an attempt to establish a meaningful relationship.

detoxification Process of safely and effectively withdrawing a person from an addictive substance, usually under medical supervision.

developmental crisis A significant maturational event, such as leaving home for the first time, completing school, or accepting the responsibility of adulthood.

developmental delay An impairment of normal growth and development that may not be reversible. Delays slow a child's progress and can interfere with the development of self-esteem.

dialectical behavior therapy (DBT) An important biosocial approach to treatment that combines numerous cognitive and behavior therapy strategies. It requires patients to understand their disorders by actively participating in formulating treatment goals by collecting data about their own behavior, identifying treatment targets in individual therapy, and working with the therapists in changing these target behaviors.

diathesis A genetic predisposition that increases susceptibility to developing a disorder.

dichotomous thinking Evaluating experiences, people, and objects in terms of mutually exclusive categories (e.g., good or bad, success or failure, trustworthy or deceitful), which informs extreme interpretations of events that would normally be viewed as including both positive and negative aspects.

dietary restraint Instituting severe dieting (e.g., setting rules such as no sweets, no fats) to eliminate out-of-control feelings related to binge eating.

differentiation of self An individual's resolution of attachment to his or her family's emotional chaos. It involves an intrapsychic separation of thinking from feelings and an interpersonal freeing of oneself from the chaos.

difficult temperament Characterized by withdrawal from stimuli, low adaptability, and intense emotional reactions. Four key behaviors are present in a difficult temperament: aggression, inattention, hyperactivity, and impulsivity.

diminished emotional expression One of the core negative symptoms of schizophrenia.

direct leadership The leader controls the interaction of the group by giving directions and information and allowing little discussion.

disaster A sudden overwhelming catastrophic event that causes great damage and destruction that may involve mass casualties and human suffering that require assistance from all available resources.

disconnections Lack of mutually responsive and enhancing relationships.

disinhibition A concept borrowed from physics and biology and based on the idea of a dynamic, self-regulatory model of equilibrium in which equilibrium is defined (Piaget) as compensation for external disturbance; a mechanism for providing the self-regulation by which intelligence adapts to internal and external changes. A symptom of Alzheimer disease in which a patient acts on thoughts and feelings without exercising appropriate social judgment.

disorganized symptoms Symptoms of schizophrenia that make it difficult for the person to understand and respond to the ordinary sights and sounds of daily living. These include confused speech and thinking and disorganized behavior.

dissociation A disruption in the normally occurring linkages among subjective awareness, feelings, thoughts, behavior, and memories (i.e., a person is physically present but mentally in another place).

distraction The purposeful focusing of attention away from undesirable sensations.

distribution The amount of a drug that may be found in various tissues at the site of the drug action for which it is intended.

disturbance of executive functioning Problems in the ability to think abstractly, plan, initiate, sequence, monitor, and stop complex behavior.

dopamine An excitatory neurotransmitter found in distinct regions of the central nervous system involved in cognition, motor, and neuroendocrine function.

dosing Administration of medication over time so that therapeutic levels may be achieved or maintained without reaching toxic levels.

drive for thinness A characteristic of anorexia nervosa in which individuals experience an intense physical and emotional drive to be thinner that overrides all physiologic body cues.

drug–drug interaction Reaction of two or more drugs with each other; may cause unexpected side effects. Can occur if one substance inhibits an enzyme system.

DSM-IV-TR Abbreviation for the *Diagnostic and Statistical Manual of Mental Disorders*, Fourth Edition, Text Revision; contains criteria for the diagnosis of mental disorders.

DSM-5 Abbreviation for the *Diagnostic and Statistical Manual of Mental Disorders*, Fifth Edition, which provides revised diagnostic criteria for mental disorders.

dual process model A model of bereavement where a person adjusts to loss by oscillating between lossorientated coping that includes preoccupation with the deceased and restoration-oriented coping in which the bereaved is preoccupied with stressful events as a result of the death.

dyad A group of only two people who are usually related, such as a married couple, siblings, or parent and child.

dysfunctional The state of a group, such as a family, whose interactions, decisions, or behaviors interfere with the positive development of the group as a whole and its individual members.

dysfunctional consequences Part of the "C" in the ABCDE framework of rational emotive behavior therapy. The result of the interaction between A (an activating event) and B (the person's belief system) that follows from absolute, rigid, irrational beliefs.

dyslexia Significantly lower score for mental age on standardized test in reading that is not caused by low intelligence or inadequate schooling.

dyspareunia Pain during sexual intercourse.

dysphagia Difficulty swallowing.

dysphoric (mood) Depressed, disquieted, or restless.

dysthymic disorder A milder but more chronic form of major depressive disorder that is diagnosed when the depressed mood is present for most days for at least 2 years with two or more of the following symptoms: poor appetite or overeating, insomnia or oversleeping, low energy or fatigue, low self-esteem, poor concentration or difficulty making decisions, and feelings of hopelessness.

dystonia An impairment in muscle tone that is generally the first extrapyramidal symptom to occur, usually within a few days of initiating an antipsychotic. Dystonia is characterized by involuntary muscle spasms, especially of the head and neck muscles.

early intervention programs Community outreach efforts designed to work with infants and preschool-aged children and their caretakers to foster healthy physical, psychological, social, and intellectual development.

early recognition Anticipating aggressive behavior based on the premise that even though behavior is idiosyncratic, it is reconstructable and therefore can provide early signs when violent behavior is likely.

echolalia Repetition of another's words that is parrot like and inappropriate.

echopraxia Involuntary imitation of another person's movements and gestures.

efficacy Ability of a drug to produce a response.

egocentric thinking A type of thinking in which children naturally view themselves as the center of their own universe.

egocentrism Tendency to view the world as revolving around oneself. A preoccupation with one's own appearance, behavior, thoughts, and feelings.

elation Feeling "high," "ecstatic," "on top of the world," or "up in the clouds."

elder abuse Abuse or neglect of adults older than 60 years of age.

elder mistreatment Actions (or inaction) by caregivers or trusted persons that cause harm or the possibility of harm to a vulnerable older adult.

elevated mood A mood that is expressed as euphoria (exaggerated feelings of well-being) or elation (feeling "high," "ecstatic," "on top of the world," or "up in the clouds").

e-mental health The use of electronics and the Internet to provide assessment and interventions.

emotion-focused coping A type of coping in which a person reduces stress by reinterpreting the situation to change its meaning.

emotions Psychophysiologic reaction that defines a person's mood and can be categorized as negative (anger, fright, anxiety guilt, shame, sadness, envy, jealousy, and disgust), positive (happiness, pride, relief, and love), borderline (hope, compassion, empathy, sympathy, and contentment), or nonemotions (confidence, awe, confusion, excitement).

emotional cutoff If a member cannot differentiate from his or her family, that member may flee from the family either by moving away or avoiding personal subjects of conversation. A brief visit from parents can render these individuals helpless.

emotional dysregulation Inability to control emotion in social interactions.

emotional vulnerability Sensitivity and reactivity to environmental stress.

empathic linkage Ability to feel in oneself the feelings being expressed by another person or persons.

empathy The ability to experience, in the present, a situation as another did at some time in the past; the ability to put oneself in another person's circumstances and feelings.

empty nest A home devoid of children and caregiving responsibilities.

encopresis Soiling clothing with feces or depositing feces in inappropriate places.

endorphins Neurotransmitters that have opiate-like behavior and produce an inhibitory effect at opioid receptor sites; probably responsible for pain tolerance.

engagement Establishing a treatment relationship and enhancing motivation to make behavior changes and a commitment to treatment.

enmeshment An extreme form of intensity in family interactions that results in low individual autonomy in a family.

enuresis Involuntary excretion of urine after the age at which a child should have attained bladder control.

enzymes Any of numerous proteins that act as catalysts for physiologic reactions and can be targets for drugs.

epidemiology The study of patterns of disease distribution and determinants of health within populations; contributes to the overall understanding of the mental health status of population groups, or aggregates, and associated factors.

erectile dysfunction Inability of a man to achieve or maintain an erection sufficient for completion of sexual activity.

erotomanic Subtype of delusional disorder characterized by the delusional belief that the person is loved intensely by the "loved object," who is usually married and of a higher socioeconomic status or otherwise unattainable.

ethnopsychopharmacology The study of cultural variations and differences that influence the effectiveness of pharmacotherapies used in mental health; includes genetics and psychosocial factors.

euphoria An exaggerated feeling of well-being.

euphoric (mood) An elated mood.

euthymic (mood) A normal mood.

evidence-based practice The use of current best evidence in making decisions; the search for and appraisal of the most relevant evidence to answer a clinical question.

exception questions Questions used to help the patient identify times when whatever is bothering him or her is not present or is present with less intensity based on the underlying assumption that during these times the patient is usually doing something to make things better.

excitement Phase of the human sexual response cycle marked by erotic feelings that lead to penile erection in men and vaginal lubrication in women. Heart rate and respirations also increase.

excretion The removal of drugs from the body either unchanged or as metabolites.

expansive mood A mood characterized by inappropriate lack of restraint in expressing one's feelings and frequently overvaluing one's own importance. Expansive qualities include an unceasing and indiscriminate enthusiasm for interpersonal, sexual, or occupational interactions.

exposure therapy The treatment of choice for agoraphobia in which the patient is repeatedly exposed to real or simulated anxiety-provoking situations until he or she becomes desensitized and anxiety subsides.

extended family Several nuclear families who may or may not live together and who function as one group.

external advocacy system Organizations that operate independently of mental health agencies and serve as advocates for the treatment and rights of mental health patients.

externalizing disorders Disorders that are characterized by acting-out behavior.

extinction The loss of a learned conditioned emotional response after repeated presentations of the conditioned fear stimulus without a contiguous traumatic event.

extrapyramidal motor system Collection of neuronal pathways that provides significant input in involuntary motor movements; a bundle of nerve fibers connecting the thalamus to the basal ganglia and cerebral cortex.

extrapyramidal side effects See *extrapyramidal syndromes*.

extrapyramidal symptoms (EPS) Acute abnormal movements developing early in the course of treatment with antipsychotic agents. Include dystonia, pseudoparkinsonism, and akathisia.

factitious disorder A type of psychiatric disorder characterized by somatization in which the person intentionally causes an illness for the purpose of becoming a patient.

factitious disorder on another Sometimes called Munchausen's by proxy; involves a person who inflicts injury on another person in order to gain the attention of a health care provider (i.e., a mother who inflicts injury on her child).

fairness In the criminal judicial process, a term meaning that the individual who is charged with a crime should know the legal rules and be able to explain the events surrounding the alleged crime or be "fit to stand trial."

family A group of people connected by birth, adoption, or marriage who have a shared history and future.

family development A broad term that refers to all the processes connected with the growth of a family, including changes associated with work, geographic location, migration, acculturation, and serious illness.

family dynamics The patterned interpersonal and social interactions that occur within the family structure over the life of a family.

family life cycle A process of expansion, contraction, and realignment of relationship systems to support the entry, exit, and development of family members.

family preservation Efforts made by professionals to preserve the family unit by preventing the removal of children from their homes through parental support and education and through work to facilitate a secure attachment between the child and parent.

family projection process In a triangulated family situation, the triangulated member becomes the center of family conflicts.

family structure According to Minuchin, the organized pattern within which family members interact.

fear conditioning A type of classic conditioning that occurs when a neutral stimulus (the conditioned stimulus [CS]) is paired with an aversive unconditioned stimulus (US) that elicits an unconditioned fear response (UR). After repeated pairing, the CS alone will elicit the fear response, which is now the conditioned response (CR).

fetal alcohol syndrome A syndrome that occurs in infants whose mothers abuse alcohol during pregnancy; includes symptoms such as permanent brain damage, often resulting in mental retardation.

fetishism When an object such as women's undergarments or foot apparel is used for sexual arousal.

fidelity Faithfulness to obligations and duties.

first-pass effect Metabolism of part of oral drugs after being absorbed from the gastrointestinal tract and carried through the portal circulation to the liver. Only part of the drug dose reaches systemic circulation.

fitness to stand trial Ability to consult with a lawyer with a reasonable degree of rational understanding of the facts of the alleged crime and of the legal proceedings.

flight of ideas Repeated and rapid changes in the topic of conversation, generally after just one sentence or phrase.

flooding A technique used to desensitize the patient to the fear associated with a particular anxiety-provoking stimulus. Desensitizing is done by presenting feared objects or situations repeatedly without session breaks until the anxiety dissipates.

forensic In mental health, a term that pertains to legal proceedings and mandated treatment of persons with a mental illness.

forensic examiner A mental health specialist, usually a psychiatrist or psychologist, who is certified as a forensic examiner and assigned by the judge to assess and testify to the patient's competency and responsibility for the crime, including the mental state at the time of an offense.

formal group roles The designated leader and members of a group.

formal operations The ability to use abstract reasoning to conceptualize and solve problems.

formal support system Large organizations that provide care to individuals, such as hospitals and nursing homes.

frontal, parietal, temporal, occipital lobes Lobes of the brain located on the lateral surface of each hemisphere.

frotteurism A paraphilia characterized by sexually arousing urges, fantasies, and behaviors resulting from touching or rubbing one's genitals against the breasts, genitals, or thighs of a nonconsenting person.

functional activities Activities of daily living necessary for self-care (i.e., bathing, toileting, dressing, and transferring).

functional consequences Part of the "C" in the ABCDE framework of rational emotive behavior therapy. The results of the interaction between A (an activating event) and B (a person's belief system) that follow from flexible, rational beliefs.

functional imaging The aspect of neuroimaging that visualizes processing of information.

functional neurologic symptoms New name recommended to replace conversion disorder in the *Diagnostic and Statistical Manual of Mental Disorders*, Fifth Edition (*DSM-5*), for which severe emotional distress or unconscious conflict is expressed through physical symptoms.

functional status Extent to which a person has the ability to carry out independent personal care, home management, and social functions in everyday life in a way that has meaning and purpose.

GABA Gamma-aminobutyric acid, the primary inhibitory neurotransmitter for the central nervous system (CNS). The pathways of GABA exist almost exclusively in the CNS, with the largest GABA concentrations in the hypothalamus, hippocampus, basal ganglia, spinal cord, and cerebellum.

gambling disorder (also referred to as pathologic gambling) Persistent and recurrent gambling leading to clinically significant impairment or distress.

gate-control theory The leading explanation of pain; holds that neurologic gates can either inhibit or allow pain signals to be transmitted to the brain. Led to the recognition that there is not a single pain mechanism but that the processing of pain occurs on at least three levels—peripheral, spinal, and supraspinal.

gender, culture, and ethnic differences Factors that must be taken into consideration before planning interventions; for example, when considering interventions for the expression of anger, cultural norms should be understood.

gender dysphoria Incongruence between an individual's experienced/expressed gender and assigned gender.

gender identity A sense of self as being male or female.

gender identity disorders A category of dysfunction in which there is a persistent cross-gender identification with accompanying discomfort about one's assigned sex.

genetic susceptibility A concept that suggests that an individual may be at increased risk for a psychiatric disorder based on genetic transmission.

genogram A multigenerational schematic diagram that lists family members and their relationships.

geropsychiatric nursing assessment The comprehensive, deliberate, and systematic collection and interpretation of biopsychosocial data that is based on the special needs and problems of older adults.

gerotranscendence A concept of Erikson; continued growth in dimensions such as spirituality and inner strength during old age.

glutamate The most widely distributed excitatory neurotransmitter; the main transmitter in the associational areas of the cortex.

grandiosity Elevated self-esteem.

grief An intense, biopsychosocial response that often includes spontaneous expressions of pain, sadness, and desolation, such as with the loss of a loved one.

group Two or more people who develop interactive relationships and share at least one common goal or issue.

group dynamics All of the verbal and nonverbal interactions within groups.

group process The culmination of the session-tosession interactions of the members that move the group toward its goals.

group themes The collective conceptual underpinnings of a group that express the members' underlying concerns or feelings, regardless of the group's purpose.

groupthink The tendency of many groups to avoid conflict and adopt a normative pattern of thinking that is often consistent with the group leader's ideas.

guided imagery The purposeful use of imagination to achieve relaxation or direct attention away from undesirable sensations.

guilty but mentally ill (GBMI) Persons with a mental illness who demonstrate they knew the wrongfulness of their actions and had the ability to act otherwise.

half-life The time required for plasma concentrations of a drug to be reduced by 50%.

hallucinations Perceptual experiences that occur in the absence of actual external sensory stimuli and may be auditory, visual, tactile, gustatory, or olfactory.

hallucinogen A class of drug that produces euphoria or dysphoria, altered body image, distorted or sharpened visual and auditory perception, confusion, uncoordination, and impaired judgment and memory.

harm reduction A community health intervention designed to reduce the harm of substance use to the individual, the family, and society that has replaced a moral or criminal approach to drug use and addiction.

hippocampus Subcortical gray matter embedded within each temporal lobe of the brain that may be involved in determining the best way to store information, especially the emotions attached to a memory.

histamine A neurotransmitter derived from the amino acid histidine that originates predominantly in the hypothalamus and projects to all major structures in the cerebrum, brain stem, and spinal cord. Its functions are not well known, but it appears to have a role in autonomic and neuroendocrine regulation.

histrionic personality Type of person who could be described as "attention seeking," "excitable," and "emotional," with an insatiable need for attention and approval. Also tend to be highly dependent on others, making them overly trusting and gullible. They are moody and experience helplessness when others are disinterested in them. They are also sexually seductive in attempts to gain attention are often uncomfortable within a single relationship.

HIV-associated neurocognitive disorder (HAND) One of the most common CNS manifestations of HIV, it is a chronic neurodegenerative condition characterized by cognitive, central motor, and behavioral changes. HAND can affect any psychologic domain, but the most commonly reported deficits are in attention and concentration, psychomotor speed, memory and learning, information processing, and executive function.

home visits Delivery of nursing care in a patient's living environment.

homelessness State of being without a consistent residence or living in nighttime residences that are temporary shelters or any place not designated as sleeping accommodations.

homeostasis The body's tendency to resist physiologic change and hold bodily functions relatively consistent, well-coordinated, and usually stable. Introduced as a concept by Walter Cannon in the 1930s.

hopelessness A belief that nothing positive will happen or negative events will occur.

hostile aggression Aggression that is intended solely to inflict injury or pain on the victim with no reward or advantage to the aggressor.

Housing First A mental health approach that places people who are homeless, usually also experiencing severe mental illness, substance abuse, or release from prison, into affordable housing.

human sexual response cycle A theory of sexual response described by Masters and Johnson (1966) as consisting of four phases: excitement, plateau, orgasm, and resolution.

hyperactivity Excessive motor activity, movement, or utterances that may be either purposeless or aimless.

hyperalgia Increased sensation of pain.

hyperesthesia Increased nociceptor sensitivity.

hyperkinetic delirium A type of delirium in which the patient demonstrates behaviors most commonly recognized as delirium, including psychomotor hyperactivity, marked excitability, and a tendency toward hallucinations.

hypersexuality Inappropriate and socially unacceptable sexual behavior.

hypervigilance Sustained attention to external stimuli as if expecting something important or frightening to happen.

hypervocalization Screams, curses, moans, groans, and verbal repetitiveness that are common in the later stages of cognitively impaired older adults, often occurring during a hospitalization or nursing home placement.

hypnagogic hallucinations Intense dream-like images that occur when an individual is falling asleep and usually involve the immediate environment.

hypnotic Medication that causes drowsiness and facilitates the onset and maintenance of sleep.

hypochondriasis When individuals are fearful of developing a serious illness based on their misinterpretation of body sensations.

hypofrontality Reduced cerebral blood flow and glucose metabolism in the prefrontal cortex.

hypokinetic delirium A type of delirium in which the patient is lethargic, somnolent, and apathetic and exhibits reduced psychomotor activity.

hypomania A mild form of mania.

hypomanic episode A less intense manic episode in which there is little impairment in social or occupational functioning and normal judgment is mostly intact.

identity diffusion Occurs when parts of a person's identity are absent or poorly developed; a lack of consistent sense of identity.

illness anxiety disorder A preoccupation with having or acquiring a serious, undiagnosed medical illness, but somatic symptoms are not present or, if present, only mild.

illusions Disorganized perceptions that create an oversensitivity to colors, shapes, and background activities, which occur when the person misperceives or exaggerates stimuli in the external environment.

imagery rehearsal therapy A technique in which patients change the endings of the nightmares while awake.

impaired consciousness Less environmental awareness and loss of the ability to focus, sustain, and shift attention. Associated cognitive changes include problems in memory, orientation, and language.

implosive therapy A provocative technique useful in treating agoraphobia in which the therapist identifies individual phobic stimuli for the patient and then presents highly anxiety-provoking imagery in a dramatic, vivid fashion.

impulse-control disorders A disorder that often coexists with other disorders. Characterized by an inability to resist an impulse or temptation to complete an activity that is considered harmful to oneself or others.

impulsiveness The tendency to act on urges, notions, or desires without adequately considering the consequences.

impulsivity Acting without considering the consequences of the act or alternative actions.

incidence A rate that includes only new cases that have occurred within a clearly defined time period.

incompetent A person is legally determined not to be able to understand and appreciate the information given during the consent process.

indirect leadership Leader who primarily reflects the group members' discussion and offers little guidance or information to the group.

individual roles Group roles that either enhance or detract from the group's functioning but have nothing to do with either the group task or maintenance.

inducer Drugs or substances that speed up metabolism, which in turn increases the clearance of the substrate and decreases its plasma level.

informal caregivers Unpaid individuals who provide care.

informal group roles Positions within the group with implicit rights and duties that can either help or hinder the group's process. These positions are not formally sanctioned.

informal support systems Family members, friends, and neighbors who can provide care and support to an individual.

informed consent The right mandated by state laws for a patient to determine what shall be done with one's own body and mind. To provide informed consent, the patient must be given adequate information on which to base decisions about care and actively participate in the decision-making process.

inhalants Organic solvents, also known as volatile substances, that are central nervous system depressants and when inhaled cause euphoria, sedation, emotional lability, and impaired judgment.

inhibited grieving A pattern of repetitive, significant trauma and loss together with an inability to fully experience and personally integrate or resolve these events.

inhibitor Drugs or substances that slow down metabolism, which in turn decreases the clearance of the substrate and elevates its plasma level.

in-home mental health care The provision of skilled mental health nursing care under the direction of a psychiatrist or physician for individuals in their residences. Emphasizes personal autonomy of patient.

insight The ability of the individual to be aware of his or her own thoughts and feelings and to compare them with the thoughts and feelings of others.

insomnia (initial) Difficulty falling asleep.

institutionalization The forced confinement of individuals for long periods of time in large state hospitals. This was the primary treatment for people with mental illness in the period from 1900 to 1955.

instrumental activities of daily living (IADLs) Activities that facilitate or enhance the performance of activities of daily living (e.g., shopping, using the telephone, transportation); these aspects are critical to consider for any older adult living alone.

instrumental aggression Aggression that provides some reward or advantage to the aggressor, is premeditated, and is unrelated to the person's pain.

integrated treatment Treatment for both mental illness and substance use disorders is combined in a single session or interaction or series of interactions.

intellectual disability Limitations in intellectual functioning and adaptive behavior that develop before the age of 18 years. The term is currently used interchangeably with *mental retardation*.

intensive case management An approach targeted for adults with serious mental illnesses or children with serious emotional disturbances. Managers of such cases have fewer caseloads and higher levels of professional training than do traditional case managers.

intensive outpatient program Program focused on continued stabilization and prevention of relapse in vulnerable individuals who have returned to their previous lifestyle (i.e., job or school), usually with sessions running 2 to 3 days per week and lasting 3 to 4 hours per day.

intensive residential services Intensively staffed residential care and mental health services that may include medical, nursing, psychosocial, vocational, recreational, or other support services. May be short or long term.

intergenerational transmission of violence Social learning theory concept that explains the process of violence being transmitted from one generation to the next. Children who witness violence in their homes often perpetuate violent behavior in their families as adults.

intermittent explosive disorder Impulse-control disorder characterized by episodes of uncontrolled aggressiveness that result in assault or destruction of property; the severity of aggressiveness is out of proportion to the provocation.

internal rights protection system Patient protective mechanisms developed by the U.S. mental health care system's organizations to help combat any violation of mental health patients' rights, including investigating any incidents of abuse or neglect.

internalizing disorders Disorders of mood, such as anxiety disorders and depression, in which the symptoms tend to be within the individual.

interoceptive awareness The sensory response to emotional and visceral cues, such as hunger.

interoceptive conditioning Pairing a somatic discomfort, such as dizziness or palpitations, with an impending panic attack.

interpersonal functioning Ability to relate to others with empathy or intimacy.

interpersonal relations Characteristic interaction patterns that occur between human beings that are the basis of human development and behavior and the health or sickness of one's personality.

intervention fit Finding and implementing interventions that are appropriate to a patient's particular needs and circumstances.

intimate partner violence (IPV) Defined by the Centers for Disease Control and Prevention (2009) as psychological, physical, or sexual harm perpetrated by a current or former spouse or partner.

intrinsic activity The ability of a drug to produce a biologic response when it becomes attached to its receptor.

introspective The self-examination of personal beliefs, attitudes, and motivations.

intrusion Thoughts, memories, or dreams of traumatic events occur involuntarily, especially when there are cues that symbolize or resemble the events, causing psychological and sometimes physiological distress.

invalidating environment A highly personal social situation that negates the individual's emotional responses and communication.

invincibility fable An aspect of egocentric thinking in adolescence that causes teens to view themselves as immune to dangerous situations and death.

involuntary commitment The confined hospitalization of a person without his or her consent but with a court order (because the person has been judged to be a danger to him- or herself or others).

inwardly directed anger Anger that is stifled despite strong arousal.

irritable mood Being easily annoyed and provoked to anger, particularly when wishes are challenged or thwarted.

ischemic cascade Cell breakdown resulting from brain cell injury.

judgment The ability to reach a logical decision about a situation and to choose a course after looking at and analyzing various possibilities.

justice Duty to treat all fairly, distributing the risks and benefits equally.

kleptomania A disorder in which the patient is unable to resist the urge to steal and independently steals items that he or she could easily afford. These items are not particularly useful or wanted. The underlying issue is the act of stealing.

Korsakoff amnestic syndrome An amnestic syndrome associated with alcoholism in which there is a problem acquiring new information and retrieving memories involving the heart and vascular and nervous systems; considered to be the chronic stage of Wernicke–Korsakoff syndrome.

label avoidance Type of stigma that occurs when an individual avoids treatment or care in order not to be labeled as being mentally ill.

labile (lability of mood) Changeable mood.

late adulthood The period of life beginning at age 65 years; divided into three chronologic groups: young-old, middle-old, and old-old.

learning disorder A discrepancy between actual achievement and expected achievement that is based on a person's age and intellectual ability.

least restrictive environment The patient has the right to be treated in the least restrictive environment possible for the exercise of free will; an individual cannot be restricted to an institution when he or she can be successfully treated in the community.

lethality The probability that a person will successfully complete suicide, determined by the seriousness of the person's intent and the likelihood that the planned method of death will succeed.

libido The energy or psychic drive associated with the sexual instinct that resides in the id, literally translated from Latin to mean "pleasure" or "lust."

life events Major times or experiences such as marriage, divorce, and bereavement.

limbic system (limbic lobe) A "system" of several small structures within the brain that work in a highly organized way. These structures include the hippocampus, thalamus, hypothalamus, amygdala, and limbic midbrain nuclei.

linguistic competence   The ability to communicate in a way that is easily understood by diverse audiences.

living will   An advanced care directive that states what treatment should be omitted or refused in the event that a person is unable to make those decisions because of incapacitation.

locus coeruleus   A tiny cluster of neurons that fans out and innervates almost every part of the brain, including most of the cortex, the thalamus and hypothalamus, the cerebellum, and the spinal cord.

loose associations   Absence of the normal connectedness of thoughts and ideas; sudden shifts without apparent relationship to preceding topic.

loss-oriented coping   Part of the dual process model of bereavement that includes preoccupation with the deceased.

luminotherapy   Light therapy used to manipulate the circadian system.

maintenance roles   The informal role of group members that encourages the group to stay together.

major depressive episodes   A depressed mood or a loss of interest or pleasure in nearly all activities for at least 2 weeks. Four of seven additional symptoms must be present: disruption in sleep, appetite (or weight), concentration, or energy; psychomotor agitation or retardation; excessive guilt or feelings of worthlessness; and suicidal ideation.

maladaptive anger   Excessive outwardly directed anger or suppressed anger; linked to psychiatric conditions, such as depression, as well as medical conditions.

malingering   To produce illness symptoms intentionally with an obvious self-serving goal such as being classified as disabled or avoiding work.

mania   A symptom of bipolar disorder that is primarily characterized by an abnormally and persistently elevated, expansive, or irritable mood.

manic episode   A distinct period during which there is an abnormally and persistently elevated, expansive, or irritable mood.

maturation   Healthy development of the brain and nervous system during childhood and adolescence.

medical battery   Intentional and unauthorized (without informed consent) treatment that is harmful or offensive.

memory   One aspect of cognitive function; an information storage system composed of short-term memory (retention of information over a brief period of time) and long-term memory (retention of an unlimited amount of information over an indefinite period of time); the ability to recall or reproduce what has been learned or experienced.

mental disorders   Health conditions characterized by alterations in thinking, mood, or behavior. They are associated with distress or impaired functioning.

mental health   The emotional and psychological well-being of an individual who has the capacity to interact with others, deal with ordinary stress, and perceive one's surroundings realistically.

mental health recovery   A journey of healing and transformation enabling a person with a mental health problem to live a meaningful life in a community of his or her choice while striving to achieve his or her full potential.

mental status examination   An organized systematic approach to assessment of an individual's current psychiatric condition.

metabolism   Biotransformation, or the process by which a drug is altered and broken down into smaller substances, known as metabolites.

metabolites   Result when drugs are altered and broken down into smaller substances by metabolism. Substance necessary for or taking part in a particular metabolic process.

methadone maintenance   The treatment of opioid addiction with a daily, stabilized dose of methadone.

metonymic speech   Use of words with similar meanings interchangeably.

middle-age adulthood   A term used to describe adults approximately ages 45 to 65 years.

middle-old   A term used to describe adults ages 75 to 84 years.

mild cognitive impairment (MCI)   A transitional state between normal cognition and Alzheimer disease.

milieu therapy   An approach that provides a stable and coherent social organization to facilitate an individual's treatment; often used interchangeably with *therapeutic environment*. The design of the physical surroundings, structure of patient activities, and promotion of a stable social structure and cultural setting enhance the setting's therapeutic potential.

military sexual trauma (MST)   Sexual assault and sexual Harassment experienced during a veteran's military service.

military veteran   Persons who served in the armed forces.

miracle questions   Patients are asked to use their imagination in crafting their response to very specific questions about a scenario.

mixed episode   When mania and depression occur at the same time, which leads to extreme anxiety, agitation, and irritability.

mixed variant delirium   Behavior that fluctuates between the hyperactive and hypoactive states.

modeling   Pervasive imitation; one person trying to be similar to another person.

mood   The prominent, sustained, overall emotions that a person expresses and exhibits; influences one's perception of the world and how one functions.

mood disorder   Recurrent disturbances or alterations in mood that cause psychological distress and behavioral impairment.

mood episode   A severe mood change that lasts at least 2 weeks that causes clinically significant distress or impairment.

mood lability   The rapid shifts in moods that often occur in patients with bipolar disorder with little or no change in external events.

moral injury   The lasting psychological, biological, spiritual, behavioral, and social impact of perpetrating, failing to prevent, or bearing witness to acts that transgress deeply held moral beliefs and expectations.

moral treatment   An approach to curing mental illness, popular in the 1800s, that was built on the principles of kindness, compassion, and a pleasant environment.

motivation   A goal-oriented attitude that propels action for change and can help sustain the development of new activities and behaviors.

motivational interventions   One to several sessions delivered within a few weeks or less during which a patient is motivated to become involved in treatment.

motivational interviewing   A method of therapeutic intervention often used with those with substance abuse that seeks to elicit self-motivational statements from patients, supports behavioral change, and creates a discrepancy between the patient's goals and his or her continued alcohol and other drug use.

motor tics   Usually quick, jerky movements of the eyes, face, neck, and shoulders, although they may involve other muscle groups as well.

multigenerational transmission process   The transmission of emotional processes from one generation to the next.

multiple sleep latency test (MSLT)   A standardized procedure that measures the amount of time a person takes to fall asleep during a 20-minute period.

Munchausen syndrome   Term (no longer used) used to describe the most severe form of factitious disorder characterized by fabricating a physical illness, having recurrent hospitalizations, and going from one provider to another.

narcissistic personality   Person who could be described as grandiose, with an inexhaustible need for admiration. Beginning in childhood, they believe themselves to be superior, special, and unique, and want recognition for such. They also lack empathy.

negative symptoms   A lessening or loss of normal functions, such as restriction or flattening in the range of intensity of emotion; reduced fluency and productivity of thought and speech; withdrawal and inability to initiate and persist in goal-directed activity; and inability to experience pleasure.

negligence   A breach of duty of reasonable care for a patient for whom the nurse is responsible that results in personal injuries. A clinician who does get consent but does not disclose the nature of the procedure and the risks involved is subject to a negligence claim.

neologisms   Words that are made up that have no common meaning and are not recognized.

neurocircuitry   The complex neural functional networks that link brain structures, including the prefrontal cortex, striatum, hippocampus, and amygdala. Research indicates that a dysfunctional neurocircuitry underlies most psychiatric disorders.

neurocognitive impairment   An impairment in memory, vigilance, verbal fluency, and executive functioning that exists in schizophrenia. May be independent of positive and negative symptoms.

neurodevelopmental delay   When a child's development in attention, cognition, language, affect, and social or moral behavior is outside the norm. It is manifested by delayed socialization, communication, peculiar mannerisms, and idiosyncratic interests.

neurofibrillary tangles   Fibrous proteins, or *tau proteins*, that are chemically altered and twisted together and spread throughout the brain, interfering with nerve functioning in cholinergic neurons. It is hypothesized that formation of these neurofibrillary tangles is related to the apolipoprotein E_4 (apoE_4).

neurohormones   Hormones produced by cells within the nervous system, such as antidiuretic hormone (ADH).

neuroleptic malignant syndrome   A life-threatening condition that can develop in reaction to antipsychotic medications. Patients develop severe muscle rigidity with elevated temperature and a rapidly accelerating cascade of symptoms (occurring during the next 48 to 72 hours), which can include two or more of the following: hypertension, tachycardia, tachypnea, prominent diaphoresis, incontinence, mutism, leukocytosis, changes in level of consciousness, and laboratory evidence of muscle injury.

neuromodulators Chemical messengers that make the target cell membrane or postsynaptic membrane more or less susceptible to the effects of the primary neurotransmitter.

neuron Nerve cells responsible for receiving, organizing, and transmitting information. Each neuron has a cell body, or soma, which holds the nucleus containing most of the cell's genetic information.

neuropeptides Short chains of amino acids that exist in the central nervous system and have a number of important roles, including as neurotransmitters, neuromodulators, or neurohormones.

neuroplasticity The continuous process of modulation of neuronal structure and function in response to the changing environment.

neurosis A category used by Freud and his followers to define those with less severe mental illness but who were often distressed about their problems.

neurotransmitters Small molecules that directly and indirectly control the opening or closing of ion channels.

night terrors Episodes of screaming, fear, and panic while sleeping, causing clinical distress or impairing social, occupational, or other areas of functioning.

nociceptors Pain receptors.

nonbizarre delusions Beliefs that are characterized by adherence to possible situations that could appear in real life and are plausible in the context of the person's ethnic and cultural background.

nonmaleficence The duty to cause no harm, both individually and for all.

non–rapid eye movement (NREM) sleep A sleep cycle state of non–rapid eye movement that occurs about 90 minutes after falling asleep.

nontherapeutic relationship A nontrusting relationship between the nurse and patient. Both feel very frustrated and keep varying their approach with each other in an attempt to establish a meaningful relationship.

nonverbal communication The gestures, expressions, and body language used in communications.

norepinephrine An excitatory neurochemical that plays a major role in generating and maintaining mood states. Heavily concentrated in the terminal sites of sympathetic nerves, it can be released quickly to ready the individual for a fight-or-flight response to threats in the environment.

normal aging Changes that occur with age associated with some physical decline, such as decreased sensory abilities and decreased pulmonary and immune function, but many important functions do not change.

normalization Teaching families what are normal behaviors and expected responses.

not guilty by reason of insanity (NGRI) Persons who demonstrate they had no understanding of their actions and no control over them when they committed the crime.

nuclear family Two or more people related by blood, marriage, or adoption.

nuclear family emotional process Patterns of emotional functioning in a family within single generations.

nurse–patient relationship A dynamic, time-limited interpersonal process that can be viewed in steps or phases with characteristic behaviors during each phase for both the patient and the nurse.

nursing diagnosis A clinical judgment about the individual, family, or community response to actual or potential health problems and life processes. It provides the basis for the selection of interventions and outcomes.

nursing interventions Nursing actions or treatment, selected based on clinical judgment, that are designed to achieve patient, family, community outcomes; can be direct or indirect.

nursing process The basis of clinical decision-making for evidence-based practice.

object relations The psychological attachment to another person or object.

obsessions Excessive, unwanted, intrusive, and persistent thoughts, impulses, or images that cause anxiety and distress and are incongruent with the patient's usual thought patterns.

obsessive-compulsive personality disorder (OCPD) Persons with OCPD do not demonstrate obsessions and compulsions but rather a pervasive pattern of preoccupation with orderliness, perfectionism, and control. They attempt to maintain control by careful attention to rules, trivial details, procedures, and lists.

oculogyric crisis A medication side effect resulting from an imbalance of dopamine and acetylcholine in which the muscles that control eye movements tense and pull the eyeball so that the patient is looking toward the ceiling; may be followed by torticollis or retrocollis.

off-label Use of medication for a condition that is not approved by the Food and Drug Administration.

old-old A term used to describe adults ages 85 years and older.

open communication   Staff and patient willingly share information about relevant topics.

open group   A group in which new members can join at any time, and old members may leave at different sessions.

operant behavior   A type of learning that is a consequence of a particular behavioral response, not a specific stimulus.

opioid   Any substance that binds to an opioid receptor in the brain to produce an agonist action.

oppositional defiant disorder   A disruptive behavior disorder characterized by a persistent pattern of disobedience; argumentativeness; angry outbursts; low tolerance for frustration; and tendency to blame others for misfortunes, large and small.

orgasmic disorder   The inability to reach orgasm or reduced intensity by any means.

orgasmic phase   Phase in the human sexual response cycle that includes ejaculation of semen for men and rhythmic contractions of the vaginal muscles for women.

orientation phase   The first phase of the nurse–patient relationship in which the nurse and the patient get to know each other. During this phase, the patient develops a sense of trust.

oscillation   Part of the dual process model of bereavement that involves a person moving between the process of confronting (loss-oriented coping) and avoiding (restoration-oriented coping) the stresses associated with bereavement.

outcomes   A patient's response to care received; the end result of the process of nursing.

outpatient detoxification   A specialized form of partial hospitalization for patients requiring medical supervision during withdrawal from alcohol or other addictive substances, with or without use of a 23-hour bed during the initial withdrawal phase.

outwardly directed anger   Anger expression particularly the hostile, attacking forms.

oxidative stress   A condition of increased oxidant production in cells characterized by the release of free radicals and resulting in cellular degeneration.

package insert   The approved Food and Drug Administration product labeling that includes approved indications for the medication, side effects, adverse effects, contraindications, and other important information.

panic   A normal but extreme overwhelming form of anxiety often experienced when an individual is placed in a real or perceived life-threatening situation.

panic attacks   Sudden, discrete periods of intense fear or discomfort that are accompanied by significant physical and cognitive symptoms.

panic control treatment   Intentional exposure through exercise to panic-invoking sensations such as dizziness, hyperventilation, tightness in chest, and sweating.

panicogenic   Substances that produce panic attacks.

paranoia   Suspiciousness and guardedness that are unrealistic and often accompanied by grandiosity.

paranoid personality   Marked by traits including long-standing suspiciousness and mistrust of persons in general, a refusal to assume personal responsibility for one's own feelings, and avoidance of relationships in which the person is not in control or loses power.

paraphilias   Problematic sexual behaviors characterized by recurrent, intense sexual urges, fantasies, or behaviors involving unusual objects, activities, or situations. These cause significant distress to the individual or impair social or occupational functioning.

parasuicidal behavior   Deliberate self-injury with intent to harm oneself.

parasuicide   Deliberate, apparent attempt at suicide, commonly called a suicidal gesture, in which the aim is not death (e.g., taking a sublethal drug); also called *parasuicidal behavior*.

partial agonist   A drug that has some intrinsic activity (although weak) to initiate the same response in the body as a chemical that is normally present.

partial hospitalization   A time-limited (usually full or half day), ambulatory, active treatment program that offers therapeutically intensive, coordinated, and structured clinical services for patients with acute psychiatric symptoms who are experiencing a decline in social or occupational functioning, who cannot function autonomously on a daily basis, or who do not pose imminent danger to themselves or others. The aim is patient stabilization without hospitalization or a reduced length of inpatient care.

passive listening   A nontherapeutic mode of interaction that involves sitting quietly and allowing the patient to talk without focusing on guiding the thought process; includes body language that communicates boredom, indifference, or hostility.

paternalism   The belief that knowledge and education authorizes professionals to make decisions for the good of the patient.

patient observation   The ongoing assessment of the patient's mental status to identify and subvert any potential problem.

peak marriage age   An age when the person is most likely to have a successful marriage; currently between the ages of 23 and 27 years.

pedophilia Sexual activity with a child usually 13 years of age or younger by an individual at least 16 years of age or 5 years older than the child.

peer assistance programs Programs developed by state nurses' associations to offer consultation, referral, and monitoring for nurses whose practice is impaired or potentially impaired because of the use of drugs or alcohol or a psychological or physiologic condition.

perfectionism Setting high personal standards for oneself combined with concern over mistakes and their consequences for self-worth and others' opinions.

persecutory delusions Delusions in which the person believes that he or she is being conspired against, cheated, spied on, followed, poisoned, drugged, maliciously maligned, harassed, or obstructed in the pursuit of long-term goals.

personal identity Knowing "who I am" formed through the numerous biologic, psychological, and social challenges and demands faced throughout the stages of life.

personality A complex pattern of psychological characteristics, largely outside a person's awareness, that comprise the individual's distinctive pattern of perceiving, feeling, thinking, coping, and behaving.

personality disorder An enduring pattern of inner experience and behavior that deviates markedly from the expectations of the individual's culture, is pervasive and inflexible, has an onset in adolescence or early adulthood, is stable over time, and leads to distress or impairment.

personality traits Prominent aspects of personality that are exhibited in a wide range of social and personal contexts; intrinsic and pervasive, personality traits emerge from a complicated interaction of biologic dispositions, psychological experiences, and environmental situations that ultimately comprise a distinctive personality.

person–environment relationship The interaction between the individual and the environment that changes throughout the stress experience.

pharmacodynamics The study of the biologic actions of drugs on living tissue and the human body in general.

pharmacogenomics Blends pharmacology with genetic knowledge; understanding and determining an individual's specific CYP450 makeup and then individualizing medications to match the person's CYP450 profile.

pharmacokinetics The process by which a drug is absorbed, distributed, metabolized, and eliminated by the body.

phenotype Observable characteristics or expressions of a specific trait.

phobia Persistent, unrealistic fears of situations, objects, or activities that often lead to avoidance behaviors.

phonic tics Tics that typically include repetitive throat clearing, grunting, or other noises but may also include more complex sounds, such as words; parts of words; and in a minority of patients, obscenities.

phonologic processing Thought to be the cause of reading disability; a process that involves the discrimination and interpretation of speech sounds. Reading disability is believed to be caused by some disturbance in the development of the left hemisphere.

phototherapy Also known as *light therapy*; involves exposing the patient to an artificial light source during winter months to relieve seasonal depression.

pineal body Located in the epithalamus; contains secretory cells that emit the neurohormone melatonin (as well as other substances), which has been associated with sleep and emotional disorders and modulation of immune function.

plasticity Permanent change in central pain interpretation.

plateau Phase of the human sexual response cycle that is represented by sexual pleasure and increased muscle tension, heart rate, and blood flow to the genitals.

polypharmacy Using more than one group from a class of medications at one time.

polysomnography A special procedure that involves the recording of the electroencephalogram throughout the night. This procedure is usually conducted in a sleep laboratory.

polyuria Excessive need to urinate.

population genetics The study of the inheritance of illness or traits from generation to generation.

positive self-talk Countering fearful or negative thoughts by using preplanned and rehearsed positive coping statements.

positive symptoms An excess or distortion of normal functions, including delusions and hallucinations.

posttraumatic stress disorder A mental disorder characterized by persistent, distressing symptoms lasting longer than 1 month after exposure to an extreme traumatic stressor.

potency The dose of drug required to produce a specific effect.

power of attorney As it relates to health care, an advanced care directive through which a proxy, usually a relative or trusted friend, is appointed to make health care decisions on behalf of an individual if that person is incapacitated.

premature ejaculation (PE) The inability to control ejaculation before or shortly after penetration.

pressured speech Speaking as if the words are being forced out.

privacy The part of an individual's personal life that is not governed by society's laws and governmental intrusion.

proband A person who has a genetic disorder or a trait of a mental disorder.

probation A sentence of conditional or revocable release under the supervision of a probation officer for a specified time.

problem-focused coping A type of coping in which a person attacks the source of stress and solves the problem (eliminating it or changing its effects), which changes the person–environment relationship.

process recording A verbatim transcript of a verbal interaction usually organized according to the nurse–patient interaction. It often includes analysis of the interaction.

prodromal An early symptom indicating the development of a disease or syndrome.

prostaglandins An unsaturated fatty acid that helps control smooth muscle contraction, blood pressure, inflammation, and body temperature. One of the most common nociceptive transmitters.

protective factors Characteristics that reduce the probability that a person will develop a mental health disorder or problem or decrease the severity of existing problems.

protective identification A psychoanalytic term used to describe behavior of people with borderline personality disorder when they falsely attribute to others their own unacceptable feelings, impulses, or thoughts.

protein binding The degree to which a drug binds to plasma proteins.

pseudologia fantastica Fascinating but false stories of personal triumph. Stories that are not entirely improbable and often contain a matrix of truth and falsehood.

pseudoparkinsonism Sometimes referred to as *druginduced parkinsonism;* presents identically as Parkinson disease without the same destruction of dopaminergic cells.

psychiatric–mental health nurse A registered nurse who demonstrates specialized competence and knowledge, skills, and abilities in caring for persons with mental health issues and problems and psychiatric disorders.

psychiatric–mental health nursing A specialized area of nursing practice committed to promoting mental health through the assessment, diagnosis, and treatment of human responses to mental health problems and psychiatric disorders.

psychiatric rehabilitation programs Programs that are focused on reintegrating people with psychiatric disabilities back into the community through work, educational, and social avenues while also addressing their medical and residential needs.

psychoanalysis The Freudian treatment of choice; therapy focused on repairing the trauma of the original psychological injury through the process of accessing the unconscious conflicts that originate in childhood and then resolving the issues with a mature adult mind. Includes attempts to reconstruct the personality by examining free associations (spontaneous, uncensored verbalizations of whatever comes to mind) and the interpretation of dreams.

psychoeducation An educational approach used to enhance knowledge and shape behavior by adapting teaching strategies to a patient's disorder-related deficits.

psychoeducational programs A form of mental health intervention in which basic coping skills for dealing with various stressors are taught.

psychological abuse Emotional abuse that includes behaviors such as criticizing, insulting, humiliating, or ridiculing someone in private or in public. It can also involve actions such as destroying another's property, threatening or harming pets, controlling or monitoring spending and activities, or isolating a person from family and friends.

psychoneuroimmunology The study of relationships among the immune system, nervous system, and endocrine system and our behaviors, thoughts, and feelings.

psychopath Also called a sociopath, a person with a tendency toward antisocial and criminal behavior with little regard for others; a term often used by the general public to refer to persons with an antisocial personality disorder.

psychosis A category used by Freud and his followers to define those with severe mental illness that impaired daily functioning. Today, the term is used to describe a state in which the individual is experiencing hallucinations, delusions, or disorganized thoughts, speech, or behavior.

psychosomatic Term traditionally used to describe, explain, and predict the psychological origins of illness and disease.

public stigma Type of stigma that occurs after individuals are publicly "marked" as being mentally ill.

pyromania Irresistible impulses to start fires.

quadrants of care A conceptual framework that classifies patients according to symptom severity, not diagnosis.

rape The most severe form of sexual assault; the penetration of any bodily orifice by the penis, fingers, or an object.

rapid cycling In bipolar disorder, the occurrence of four or more mood episodes that meet criteria for a manic, mixed, hypomanic, or depressive episode during the previous 12 months.

rapid eye movement (REM) sleep A sleep cycle state of rapid eye movement.

rapport Interpersonal harmony characterized by understanding and respect that is established through interpersonal warmth, a nonjudgmental attitude, and a demonstration of understanding.

rational emotive behavior therapy (REBT) A psychotherapeutic approach that proposes that unrealistic and irrational beliefs cause many emotional problems. Its primary emphasis is on changing irrational beliefs into thoughts that are more reasonable and rational.

reappraisal Appraisal after coping that provides feedback about the outcomes and allows for continual adjustment to new information.

receptors Proteins that receive released neurotransmitters. Each neurotransmitter has a specific receptor, or protein, for which it and only it will fit; serves a physiologic regulatory function.

recovery Recovery from mental disorders and/or substance use disorders is a process of change through which individuals improve their health and wellness, live a self-directed life, and strive to reach their full potential.

referential thinking Belief that neutral stimuli have special meaning to the individual, such as a television commentator speaking directly to the individual.

referral Act of sending an individual from one clinician to another or from one service setting to another for care or consultation.

reflection Continual self-evaluation through observing, monitoring, and judging nursing behaviors with the goal of providing ideal interventions.

regressed behavior Behaving in a manner of a less mature life stage; childlike and immature.

reintegration A term used to describe the process of the return and acceptance of a person as a fully participating member of a community through work, educational, and social avenues.

relapse Recurrence or marked increase in severity of the symptoms of the disease, especially after a period of apparent improvement or stability; the recurrence of alcohol- or drug-dependent behavior in an individual who has previously achieved and maintained abstinence for a significant time beyond the period of detoxification.

relapse cycle When reemerging psychiatric symptoms lead to ineffective coping strategies, increased anxiety, substance use to avoid painful feelings, adverse consequences, and attempted abstinence until psychiatric symptoms reemerge and the cycle repeats itself.

relapse prevention An approach that focuses on preventing recurrence of symptoms.

relational aggression A type of bullying, more commonly used by girls, that involves disrupting peer relationships by excluding or manipulating others and spreading rumors.

relationship questions Questions used to amplify and reinforce positive responses to the other questions.

relaxation training A variety of procedures to reduce somatic arousal, such as progressive muscle relaxation, autogenic training, and biofeedback.

religiousness The participation in a community of people who gather around common ways of worshiping.

reminiscence Thinking about or relating past experiences.

repetitive transcranial magnetic stimulation Noninvasive, painless method to stimulate the cerebral cortex, which activates inhibitory and excitatory neurons.

residential services A place for people to reside during a 24-hour period or any portion of the day on an ongoing basis.

resilience Ability to recover readily from illness, depression, adversity, or the like. The ability to recover or adjust to challenges over time. Attaining good mental health despite the presence of risk factors and genetic predisposition.

resolution The termination phase of the nurse–patient relationship that lasts from the time the problems are resolved to the close of the relationship. Also, in regards the human sexual response cycle, the gradual return of the organs and body systems to the unaroused state.

restoration-oriented coping Part of the dual process model of bereavement during which the bereaved person is preoccupied with stressful events as a result of the death (financial issues, new identity as a widow[er]).

restraint The use of any manual, physical, or mechanical device or material that when attached to the patient's body (usually to the arms and legs) restricts the patient's movements.

retrocollis The neck muscles pull back the head.

revictimization A reoccurrence of violence toward the survivor.

rhythm Movement with a cadence. A measured flow that occurs at regular intervals, with a cycle of coming and going, ebbing and rising, to return at the start point and begin again.

risk factors Characteristics, conditions, situations, or events that increase the patient's vulnerability to threats to safety or well-being.

Safe Havens A form of supportive housing that serves hard-to-reach people with severe mental illness.

sandwich generation People with caregiving responsibilities toward the elder generation above and two generations of children below them.

scaling questions Questions that quantify exceptions noted in intensity and in tracking change over time using a scale of 1 to 10.

schema A cognitive structure, or an individual's life rules, that act as a filter that screens, codes, and evaluates the incoming stimuli through which the individual interprets events.

schizoaffective disorder (SAD) A disorder characterized by periods of intense symptom exacerbation alternating with quiescent periods, during which psychosocial functioning is adequate. This disorder is at times marked by symptoms of schizophrenia; at other times, it appears to be a mood disorder. In other cases, both psychosis and pervasive mood changes occur concurrently.

schizoid personality Personality trait characterized as being expressively impassive and interpersonally unengaged.

schizotypal personality disorder A disorder characterized by a pattern of social, interpersonal deficits, and impairments in capacity for close relationships. Perceptual distortions are usually present.

schizotypy Traits that are similar to the symptoms of schizophrenia but less severe. Cognitive perceptual symptoms are a primary characteristic and include magical beliefs (similar to delusions) and perceptual aberrations (similar to hallucinations). Other common symptoms include referential thinking (interpreting insignificant events as personally relevant) and paranoia (suspicious of others).

school phobia Anxiety in which the child refuses to attend school in order to stay at home and with the primary attachment figure. School phobia is a common presenting complaint in child psychiatric clinics and is diagnosed as a separation anxiety disorder.

seclusion Solitary confinement in a full protective environment for the purpose of safety or behavior management.

Section 8 housing Federally subsidized housing units that are supervised or operated by the state or city; tenants are responsible for paying one third of the monthly income toward rent.

sedative–hypnotics Medications that induce sleep and reduce anxiety.

sedatives Medications that reduce activity, nervousness, irritability, and excitability without causing sleep, but if given in large enough doses, they have an hypnotic effect.

selectivity The ability of a drug to be specific for a particular receptor, interacting only with specific receptors in the areas of the body where the receptors occur and therefore not affecting tissues and organs where these receptors do not occur.

self-awareness Being cognizant of one's own beliefs, thoughts, motivations, biases, physical and emotional limitations, and the impact one may have on others.

self-care The ability to perform activities of daily living (ADLs) successfully.

self-concept The sum of beliefs about oneself, which develops over time. Includes three interrelated dimensions: body image, self-esteem, and personal identity.

self-determinism Being empowered or having the free will to make moral judgments. Includes the right to choose one's own health-related behaviors, which at times differ from those recommended by health professionals.

self-disclosure The act of revealing personal information about oneself.

self-efficacy Self-effectiveness; a person's belief in his or her own abilities.

self-esteem Attitude about oneself. Healthy self-esteem includes feelings of self-acceptance, self-worth, self-love, and self-nurturing.

self-harm Deliberate self-injurious behavior with the intent to hurt oneself.

self-identity The development of a separate and distinct personality.

self-medicate Using medication, usually over the counter or substances without professional prescription or supervision, to alleviate an illness or condition.

self-monitoring Observing and recording one's own information, usually behavior, thoughts, or feelings.

self-stigma Type of stigma that occurs when negative stereotypes are internalized by people with mental illness.

self-system An important concept in Peplau model. Drawing from Sullivan, Peplau defined the self as an "antianxiety system" and a product of socialization.

sensate focus   A method of sex therapy in which partners learn what each finds arousing and how to communicate those preferences.

separation anxiety disorder   Developmentally inappropriate fear and anxiety around separation from home or attachment figure.

separation-individuation   A normal developmental process during which the child develops a sense of self, a permanent sense of significant others (object constancy), and an integration of both bad and good as a component of the self-concept.

serotonin   Also called 5-hydroxytryptamine or 5-HT, this is primarily an excitatory neurotransmitter that is diffusely distributed within the cerebral cortex, limbic system, and basal ganglia of the central nervous system. Serotonergic neurons also project into the hypothalamus and cerebellum. Plays a role in emotions, cognition, sensory perceptions, and essential biologic functions (e.g., sleep and appetite).

serotonin syndrome   A potentially life-threatening side effect that occurs as a result of an overactivity of serotonin or an impairment of the serotonin metabolism. Symptoms include mental status changes (hallucinations, agitation, and coma), autonomic instability (tachycardia, hyperthermia, changes in blood pressure), neuromuscular problems (hyperreflexia, incoordination), and gastrointestinal disturbance (nausea, vomiting, diarrhea).

sex role identity   Outward expression of gender.

sex therapist   A therapist who blends education and counseling with psychotherapy and specific sexual exercises.

sexual arousal   A state of mounting sexual tension characterized by vasoconstriction and myotonia.

sexual assault   Any form of nonconsenting sexual activity, ranging from fondling to penetration.

sexual desire   Ability, interest, or willingness to receive or a motivational state to seek sexual stimulation.

sexual disorders   Called sexual dysfunction in the *DSM-5*. A disturbance in sexual desire or sexual response or pain associated with intercourse.

sexual maturation   The aspect of sexual development that encompasses biosexual identity, gender identity, sex role identity, and sexual orientation.

sexual orientation (sexual preference)   An individual's feelings of sexual attraction and erotic potential.

sexual sadism   The real act of experiencing sexual excitement from causing physical or psychological suffering of another individual.

sexuality   Basic dimension of every individual's personality encompassing all that is male or female, undergoing periods of growth and development, and influenced by biologic and psychosocial factors.

Shelter Plus Care Program   A continuum of care program that allows for various housing choices and a range of supportive services.

sibling position   The relative social status of the children in the family based on birth order.

side effects   Unintended effects of medications.

simple relaxation techniques   Interventions that encourage and elicit relaxation to decrease undesirable signs and symptoms.

situational crisis   A crisis that occurs whenever a specific stressful event threatens a person's biopsychosocial integrity and results in some degree of psychological disequilibrium.

skills groups   An integral part of dialectical behavior therapy; skills are taught in group settings in which patients practice emotional regulation, interpersonal effectiveness, distress tolerance, core mindfulness, and self-management skills.

sleep architecture   A predictable pattern during a night's sleep that includes the timing, amount, and distribution of REM and NREM stages.

sleep debt   Interruption of basic restoration after recurrent long-term sleep deprivation.

sleep diary   A written account of the sleep experience.

sleep disorders   Ongoing disruptions of normal waking and sleeping patterns that lead to excessive daytime sleepiness; inappropriate naps; chronic fatigue; and the inability to perform safely or properly at work, school, or home.

sleep efficiency   Expressed as the ratio of total sleep time to time in bed.

sleep latency   Amount of time it takes for an individual to fall asleep. It is the time period measured from "lights out," or bedtime, to initiation of sleep.

sleep paralysis   Being unable to move or speak when falling asleep or waking.

sleep restriction   Deliberately spending less time in bed and avoiding napping.

sleepiness   The urge to fall asleep.

sleep–wake cycle   The biphasic 24-hour cycle that makes up the patterned activity of sleep.

slow-wave sleep   Deepest state of sleep.

social change   The structural and cultural evolution of society.

social distance   Degree to which the values of a formal organization and its primary group members differ.

social functioning Performance of daily activities within the context of interpersonal relations and family and community roles.

social network Linkages among a defined set of people, among whom there are personal contacts.

social skills training A psychoeducational approach that involves instruction, feedback, support, and practice with learning behaviors that help people interact more effectively with peers and children and with adults.

social support Positive and harmonious interpersonal interactions that occur within social relationships.

sociopath Also called a psychopath, a person with a tendency toward antisocial and criminal behavior with little regard for others; a term often used by the general public to refer to persons with an antisocial personality disorder.

solubility Ability of a drug to dissolve.

solution-focused brief therapy A cognitive therapy approach that differs from other cognitive approaches in its deemphasis on the patient's "problems," or symptoms, and an emphasis on what is functional and healthful.

somatic symptom disorder (SSD) Multiple current, somatic symptoms that are distressing and disruptive of daily life. Individuals report all aspects of their health as poor. Physical symptoms may last 6 to 9 months.

somatization Experiencing multiple physical symptoms that are distressing and disruptive of daily life.

somnambulism Sleep walking.

speed–accuracy shift A type of mental processing in which an older adult focuses more on accuracy than speed in responding.

spiritual support Assisting patients to feel balance and connection within their relationships; involves listening to expressions of loneliness, using empathy, and providing patients with desired spiritual articles.

spirituality Beliefs and values related to hope and meaning in life.

splitting Defense mechanism in which the person views the world in absolutes, alternately categorizing people as all good or all bad; also used to describe a person manipulating one group against another.

stabilization Short-term care, usually lasting fewer than 7 days, with a symptom-based indication for hospital admission. Primary focus is on control of precipitating symptoms with medications, behavioral interventions, and coordination with other agencies for appropriate after care.

stalking A pattern of repeated unwanted contact, attention, and harassment that often increases in frequency.

standardized nursing language Language readily understood by all nurses to describe care in order to provide a common means of communication.

standards of practice Standards that guide nursing practice. These are organized around the nursing process and include assessment, diagnosis, outcome identification, planning, implementation, and evaluation.

steady state Absorption equals excretion and the therapeutic level plateaus.

stereotypic behavior Repetitive, driven, nonfunctional, and potentially self-injurious behavior, such as head banging, rocking, and hand flapping, seen in autistic disorder, with an extraordinary insistence on sameness.

stereotypy Repetitive, purposeless movements that are idiosyncratic to the individual and to some degree outside of the individual's control.

stigma A mark of shame, disgrace, or disapproval that results in an individual being shunned or rejected by others.

stilted language Overly and inappropriately artificial formal language.

stimulus control A technique used when the bedroom environment no longer provides cues for sleep but has become the cue for wakefulness. Patients are instructed to avoid behaviors in the bedroom that are incompatible with sleep.

stress A transactional process arising from real or perceived internal or external environmental demands that are appraised as threatening or benign.

stress response Physiologic, behavioral, and cognitive reaction to an appraised threatening person–environment event.

structural imaging The aspect of neuroimaging that visualizes the structure of brain and allows diagnosis of gross intracranial disease and injury.

structured interaction Purposeful interaction that allows patients to interact with others in a useful way.

subcortical dementia Dementia that is caused by dysfunction or deterioration of deep gray or white matter structures inside the brain and brain stem.

substance P A peptide found in body tissues, especially nervous tissue, that is involved in the transmission of pain and in inflammation. It is the most common nociceptive transmitter that is released and transported along the central and peripheral pain synapses in the presence of noxious stimuli.

substrate The drug or compound that is identified as a target of an enzyme.

subsystems A systems term used by family theorists to describe subgroups of family members who join together for various activities.

sudden sniffing death Sudden death for inhalant users when the inhaled fumes take the place of oxygen in the lungs and central nervous system, causing the user to suffocate.

suicidal behavior The occurrence of persistent thought patterns and actions that indicate a person is thinking about, planning, or enacting suicide.

suicidal ideation Thinking about and planning one's own death without actually engaging in self-harm.

suicidality All suicide-related behaviors and thoughts of completing or attempting suicide and suicide ideation.

suicide The act of killing oneself voluntarily.

suicide attempt A nonfatal, self-inflicted destructive act with explicit or implicit intent to die.

suicide contagion Suicide behavior that occurs after the suicide death of a known other (i.e., a friend, acquaintance, or idolized celebrity). Also called *cluster suicide.*

supportive housing Permanently subsidized housing with attendant social services.

symbolism The use of a word or a phrase to represent an object, event, or feeling.

synaptic cleft A junction between one nerve and another; the space where the electrical intracellular signal becomes a chemical extracellular signal.

synchronized Two or more circadian rhythms reaching their peak at the same time.

syndrome A set of symptoms that cluster together that may have multiple causes and may represent several different disease states that have not yet been defined.

systematic desensitization A method used to desensitize patients to anxiety-provoking situations by exposing the patient to a hierarchy of feared situations. Patients are taught to use muscle relaxation as levels of anxiety increase through multisituational exposure.

tangentiality When the topic of conversation changes to an entirely different topic that is within a logical progression but causes a permanent detour from the original focus.

tardive dyskinesia A late-appearing extrapyramidal side effect of antipsychotic medication that involves irregular, repetitive involuntary movements of the mouth, face, and tongue, including chewing, tongue protrusion, lip smacking, puckering of the lips, and rapid eye blinking. Abnormal finger movements are common as well.

target symptoms Specific measurable symptoms expected to improve with treatment for which psychiatric medications are prescribed. Examples include hallucinations, delusions, paranoia, agitation, assaultive behavior, bizarre ideation, social withdrawal, disorientation, catatonia, blunted affect, thought blocking, insomnia, and anorexia.

task roles The group role of an individual that is concerned about the purpose of the group and keeps the focus on the task of the group.

tau A protein that is the main component found in neurofibrillary tangles inside the cells.

temperament A person's characteristic intensity, activity level, rhythmicity, adaptability, energy expenditure, and mood.

therapeutic communication The ongoing process of interaction in which meaning emerges; may be verbal or nonverbal.

therapeutic foster care The placement of patients in residences of families specially trained to handle individuals with mental illnesses. Indicated for patients in need of a family-like environment and a high level of support.

therapeutic index A ratio of the maximum nontoxic dose to the minimum effective dose.

thought stopping A practice in which a person identifies negative feelings and thoughts that exist together, says "stop," and then engages in a distracting activity.

thymoleptic Mood stabilizing.

tics Sudden, rapid, repetitive, stereotyped motor movements or vocalizations.

token economy The application of behavior modification techniques to multiple behaviors. In a token economy, patients are rewarded with tokens for selected desired behaviors that they can then redeem for special privilege or similar.

tolerance A gradual decrease in the action of a drug at a given dose or concentration in the blood. The ability to ingest an increasing amount of alcohol before a "high" and cognitive and motor effects are experienced.

torticollis The neck muscles pull the head to the side.

Tourette disorder The most severe tic disorder. Defined by multiple motor and phonic tics for at least 1 year.

toxicity The point at which concentrations of a drug in the bloodstream become harmful or poisonous to the body.

transaction Transfer of value between two or more individuals.

transfer The formal shifting of responsibility for the care of an individual from one clinician to another or from one care unit to another.

transference The unconscious assignment to a therapist or nurse of a patient's feelings and attitudes that were originally associated with important figures such as parents or siblings.

transition times Times of addition, subtraction, or change in status of family members.

transitional housing Temporary housing such as a halfway house, short-stay residence or group home, or a room at a hotel designated for people who are homeless and looking for permanent housing.

traumatic brain injury (TBI) An intracranial injury that occurs when an outside force traumatically injures the brain.

traumatic crisis A crisis initiated by unexpected, unusual events in which people face overwhelming hazards that entail injury, trauma, destruction, or sacrifice. May affect an individual or a multitude of people at once.

traumatic grief A difficult and prolonged grief.

triad A group consisting of three people.

triangles A three-person system and the smallest stable unit in human relations.

trichotillomania Chronic, self-destructive hair pulling that results in noticeable hair loss, usually in the crown, occipital, or parietal areas, and sometimes of the eyebrows and eyelashes.

23-hour observation A short-term treatment that serves the patient in immediate but short-term crisis. This type of care admits individuals to an inpatient setting for as long as 23 hours during which time services are provided at a less-than-acute care level.

uncomplicated grief Grief that is painful and disruptive within normal expectations after the loss of a loved one.

unconditional positive regard A nonjudgmental caring for a client.

unfit to stand trial (UST) Persons who are determined to be unable to understand the proceedings against them or assist in their own defense because of mental or physical condition.

uptake receptors See *carrier proteins.*

use The drinking of alcohol or the swallowing, smoking, sniffing, or injecting of a mind-altering substance.

vaginismus Condition characterized by a psychologically induced spastic, involuntary constriction of the perineal and outer vaginal muscles fostered by imagined, anticipated, or actual attempts at vaginal penetration.

validation A process that affirms patient individuality and reflects the staff member respect for a patient in any interaction.

veracity The duty to tell the truth.

verbal communication The use of the spoken word, including its underlying emotion, context, and connotation.

veteran identity The degree to which the veteran role is central or important to how they think about themselves and how they want others to view them.

verbigeration Purposeless repetition of words or phrases.

violence (violent behavior) An extreme form of aggression involving the physical act of force intended to cause harm to a person or an object.

voluntary admission (voluntary commitment) The legal status of a patient who has consented to being admitted to the hospital for treatment, during which time he or she maintains all civil rights and is free to leave at any time even if it is against medical advice.

vulnerable child syndrome A phenomenon that occurs when family members view a child as sick despite current good health and as a result are overprotective of the child.

waxy flexibility Posture held in an odd or unusual fixed position for extended periods of time.

Wernicke encephalopathy An alcohol-induced degenerative brain disorder caused by a thiamine deficiency and characterized by vision impairment, ataxia, hypotension, confusion, and coma.

Wernicke–Korsakoff syndrome An alcohol-induced amnestic disorder that includes an acute phase of Wernicke encephalopathy and a chronic phase of Korsakoff amnestic syndrome.

withdrawal The adverse physical and psychological symptoms that occur when a person ceases to use a substance.

word salad A string of words that are not connected in any way.

working memory An important aspect of the brain's frontal lobe function, including the ability to plan and initiate activity with future goals in mind.

working phase The second phase of the nurse–patient relationship in which patients can examine specific problems and learn new ways of approaching them.

xerostomia Dry mouth.

young adulthood A term used to describe adults ages 18 to 44 years.

young-old A term used to describe adults ages 65 to 74 years.

Zeitgebers Specific events that function as time givers or synchronizers and that result in the setting of biologic rhythms.

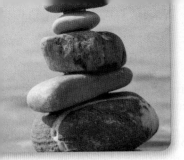

Index

Note: Page numbers followed by *f*, *t*, and *b* indicate figures, tables, and box respectively.